Pre-Feeding Skills
Second Edition

A Comprehensive Resource for Mealtime Development

Suzanne Evans Morris, Ph.D., CCC-SLP

Marsha Dunn Klein, M.Ed., OTR/L

Foreword by
Ellyn Satter, M.S., RD, CICSW, BCD

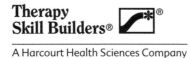

Therapy Skill Builders®

A Harcourt Health Sciences Company

Reproducing Pages From This Book

As described below, some of the pages in this book may be reproduced for instructional or administrative use, not for resale. To protect your book, make a photocopy of each reproducible page. Then use that copy as a master for photocopying.

Library of Congress Cataloging-in-Publication Data

Morris, Suzanne Evans.
   A comprehensive resource for mealtime development / Suzanne Evans
Morris, Marsha Dunn Klein; foreword by Ellyn Satter.— 2nd ed.
      p. cm.
   Includes bibliographical references (p.   ).
   ISBN 0-7616-7407-1
   1. Infants—Nutrition—Study and teaching—Handbooks, manuals, etc.
2. Infants—Care—Handbooks, manuals, etc. 3. Ingestion disorders in
infants—Treatment—Handbooks, manuals, etc. I. Klein, Marsha Dunn. II.
Title.
   RJ216 .M593 2000
   649'.3—dc21
                                    00-009802

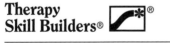
Please visit our Web site at www.PsychCorp.com. Please go to www.tpcweb.com/catg/nf/sub/contact/conforms.htm to comment on this or any of our products. Your feedback is important to us.

To contact Therapy Skill Builders, please call 1-800-228-0752.

About the Authors

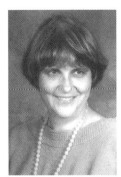
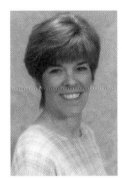

Suzanne Evans Morris, Ph.D., CCC-SLP, a speech-language pathologist in private practice near Charlottesville, Virginia, is recognized for her work in identifying and treating pre-speech and feeding disorders in young children. She is the director of New Visions, an organization that sponsors workshops for teaching feeding-related skills and provides family-oriented clinical services. She has written extensively about assessment and remediation techniques for children who have oral feeding problems. Dr. Morris holds the American Speech-Language-Hearing Association's Certificate of Clinical Competence in Speech. She has completed basic and advanced coursework in pediatrics through the Neuro-Developmental Treatment Association. She and Marsha Dunn Klein co-authored the first edition of *Pre-Feeding Skills: A Comprehensive Resource for Feeding Development,* a best seller in the area for feeding children with special needs, as well as *Mealtime Participation Guide.*

Marsha Dunn Klein, M.Ed., OTR/L, is a registered occupational therapist and a partner in Pueblo Pediatric Therapy, a cross-disciplinary pediatric therapy practice in Tucson, Arizona. She has completed basic and advanced pediatric coursework through the Neuro-Developmental Treatment Association. Her master's degree in special education has contributed to her interest in and skill with a special needs population. Ms. Klein's practice includes direct pediatric treatment, continuing education workshops, consultation and materials development. Previous publications include the first edition of *Pre-Feeding Skills* and *Mealtime Participation Guide,* which she co-authored with Suzanne Morris, and *Feeding and Nutrition for the Child with Special Needs* with Tracy Delaney, Ph.D.

Foreword

In the second edition of *Pre-Feeding Skills,* Suzanne Evans Morris and Marsha Dunn Klein will be telling you over and over in many ways that feeding is far more than getting food into a child. Feeding is a relationship; treating a child's eating behavior and treating the interactions between parent and child around feeding is deeply based on trust. Over the years as I have delivered that message to health professionals, I have found it is not always a welcome one. It is not easy for professionals trained in nutrition, medicine, or another physically oriented field to discover that their endeavor is embedded in social and emotional issues and family dynamics. In this book, you may be asked for the first time to grapple with the impact of a child's social, emotional, and physical milieu as part of helping him or her with eating.

Like Dorothy getting carried up in the tornado, you may have mixed feelings that this topic will so clearly take you out of Kansas! I felt pretty twisted around myself 20 years ago as a nutritionist raising my own children, counseling others on food selection and feeding, and finally writing on the topic. It all seemed so clear before it dawned on me that there is a good bit more to feeding than understanding nutrition. I grappled with those issues, which I came to call the feeding relationship, in my books, *Child of Mine: Feeding with Love and Good Sense, How to Get Your Kid to Eat...But Not Too Much,* and *Secrets of Feeding a Healthy Family.* I continue to grapple with them in articles I have written since that time, many of which are referenced throughout *Pre-Feeding Skills.* Here is a word of encouragement: In time, thinking in the broader context of relationships will become comfortable and automatic to you, too.

Feeding demands a division of responsibility. The parent does the what, when, and where of feeding. The child does the how much and whether of eating. The parent does the feeding; the child does the eating. The division of responsibility assumes that children have considerable capability with eating, but manifesting those capabilities depends on parents effectively executing feeding tasks. Parents are responsible for choosing and preparing food, maintaining the structure of meals and snacks, making eating times pleasant, and providing mastery expectations. Given parents' successful execution of their tasks, children will increasingly gain capability with eating behavior and food acceptance, retain the ability to regulate food intake and grow in a constitutionally appropriate way, and maintain positive eating attitudes and behaviors. The feeding relationship begins and ends with trust: trust that the child wants to eat, knows how much to eat, and wants to grow up with eating. If a child doesn't seem to want to eat, then something is the matter: That child is being forced in some way or insufficiently supported in his or her struggles to grow up.

For children with neuromuscular or cognitive limitations, maintaining that trust and observing a division of responsibility in feeding takes on a special meaning. Let me give you examples of how each of your authors has interpreted that meaning. Suzanne Evans Morris has consistently demonstrated that a child who can't eat enough to maintain nutritional welfare can be trusted in the feeding process. She emphasizes the richness and rewards of the feeding relationship and insists that the child with even severe neuromuscular and or cognitive limitations is entitled to master and enjoy eating to the limits of his or her ability. Tube feedings can be used as an adjunct to feeding but may not replace the feeding for many children. Morris emphasizes that the child does not have to be fully supported nutritionally through his own efforts for feeding to enhance his joy, sense of himself, and the parent-child relationship.

Feeding is about respect and about letting the child be responsible for acting on her own behalf. How can one expect such mastery from a child who is afraid to eat or even to have anything come near her mouth? Many clinicians who do oral desensitization with children resort to control in its various forms: trickery, bribery, cheerleading. Marsha Dunn Klein has the trusting answer to the dilemma. Get the child's permission, she insists. Don't put anything in the child's mouth unless she indicates she is ready to have you do it. Given enough time and a positive and trusting relationship between a child and the feeding therapist (and that child's parents), the child will grapple with his or her own anxiety and determination to grow and eventually do what is feared. Children want to learn and master, but they depend on adults to provide mastery opportunities and to mete out the challenges so they are not overwhelmed. Klein is a perfect wizard at keeping children in control by breaking pre-feeding skills into ever smaller steps to give children manageable opportunities to learn.

In beginning to work with relationships, however, it is important to recognize the limits of your involvement. You are not doing psychotherapy. There is a dividing line between feeding therapy and psychotherapy. I am a psychotherapist in addition to being a nutritionist, and I have been able to define that line. You may certainly work with feelings and, in fact, you must recognize them, encourage their expression, and accept them. People learn better when they are emotionally engaged. However, you are crossing the line into psychotherapy when, in order to achieve feeding goals, you try to change the parent's or the child's feelings or life circumstances. Your task is to satisfy yourself, through the help of *Pre-Feeding Skills* and your own experience, that your behavioral and educational interventions are realistic. If a parent can't apply scrupulously realistic interventions, you can be clear that processes going on within the parents, the child, or in their lives are simply too overwhelming to allow them to change. Before feeding therapy can continue, outside help is needed from a physician, nutritionist, mental health professional, or social caseworker to bring the child and parent to the point where they can be successful with a feeding intervention. In these days of the shrinking health care dollar, you may be asked to do it all. Don't. There is a great deal you can do, but your doing requires reasonably well-functioning parents who are not overwhelmed by unresolved medical or nutritional issues.

Helping a child to be all he or she can be with eating is inspiring and rewarding work that will draw on all of your skills. Through it all, your best guide is your trust in the child and your respect in that child's desire to be all he or she can be. Let me share a story from the toddler chapter in the current edition of *Child of Mine: Feeding with Love and Good Sense*. Thirteen-month-old Tobin had been born with cognitive and neuromuscular limitations and skeletal malformations. He had done just fine with nipple feeding, but at age 4 months when his mother tried to introduce solid foods, it went so poorly that she backed off and didn't offer them for a considerable time. An occupational therapist was working with Tobin to desensitize his mouth, and a physical therapist was helping him with muscle control. He was doing fine. It didn't scare him or turn him off to be offered soft table food. He could mouth and swallow, but he just wasn't interested. His mom complained that it was an all-day job to feed him and during feeding he gagged a lot even on semi-solid food. He seemed to enjoy holding other food, but it was hard for him to get it in his mouth, and when he did, he gagged.

Rather than continuing to work with him on pre-feeding skills, the decision was made to include Tobin in family meals. His parents were game, so they brought him to the table, propped him up in his high chair, and put small pieces of whatever they were having in front of him. The parents were warned not to pressure him in any way to eat and reminded that their cheering and clapping amounted to pressure. Imagine everyone's surprise when Tobin's face brightened up, he focused his attention on the food, and he began to struggle to pick it up. At first he just chased food around the tray, but his mother helped by finding the distance for his arm reach that enabled him to most easily grasp the food. It worked like a charm. Tobin quickly developed the increased muscle control he needed to feed himself, chew, and swallow. Gagging stopped being a problem once he was sitting upright in the chair and feeding himself. You can imagine Tobin's breathless audience and how his parents had to positively sit on their hands and zip their lips to keep from interfering. Awed and astonished and through their tears of joy, the parents could only admire their determined son as he struggled to do it himself.

The feeding therapist made her recommendations based on her understanding of child development and social needs: Tobin was at an age where he was striving for autonomy at the same time as he wanted to be a part of his family. Beyond that, this small miracle could only have happened in the midst of relationship. Tobin's occupational and physical therapist had worked with him so carefully and well that Tobin had retained his positive feelings about eating. The family trusted the feeding therapist, and Tobin trusted both her and the parents. Tobin wanted to be at the family table, he wanted to eat, and he wanted to do it himself. And he did.

—Ellyn Satter, M.S., RD, CICSW, BCD

Acknowledgments

On February 5, 1676, the great British scientist and mathematician Isaac Newton wrote in a letter to his friend, Robert Hooke, "If I have seen further it is by standing on the shoulders of giants." Over the years, this wise comment has become a central part of my perception of my own work and the ideas expressed in this second edition of *Pre-Feeding Skills*. My life has been blessed with giants who have enabled my vision and understanding of feeding and mealtimes to create an even further vision for others—as I, in turn, become their giant. It is with deep gratitude that I extend my thanks and appreciation to the giants, large and small, who have engaged my imagination, challenged my understanding, and extended the depth and breadth of my views. My professional mentors, the thousands of children and families who entered my life, and my family, colleagues, and staff at New Visions have made the writing of this book possible.

—*SEM*

I would like to thank the therapists at Pueblo Pediatric Therapy for their support and feedback during this undertaking. Special thanks to Pam Ellis, Steve Erdman, Debra Houghton, Gigi Larrington, Robyn Lundeen, Penny Ratson, and Elaine Williams for their editorial and therapeutic comments. Heartfelt appreciation to all the children and families who have shared their mealtimes with me and taught me how they needed to be nourished. Thanks to my colleague and friend, Suzanne Evans Morris, who helped inspire my initial interest in feeding years ago! Her love of children and families shows in all she does! And, as always, thank you to Don, Jason, and Brennan, my wonderful family! Without their unending support this would never have been completed.

—*MDK*

We would like to thank Ellyn Satter for her comments in the foreword and for her commitment to children and families and their mealtimes. Special thanks to Miguel, Nakoma and JoLán, Joey and Tina, and Catherine, for decorating our cover with their beautiful faces!

—*SEM and MDK*

Contents

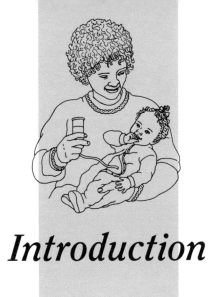

Introduction

When *Pre-Feeding Skills* first was published in 1987, therapists were just beginning to address the challenges presented by children with feeding difficulties. Federal and state legislation had redefined the rights of these children to an appropriate education in the least restrictive environment. Therapists who had never worked with children with sensorimotor difficulties were challenged to provide appropriate services. Early intervention programs for infants and toddlers proliferated, providing the majority of new jobs for clinicians. Clinicians in these new programs needed a book that addressed the philosophical, developmental, and practical aspects of oral feeding. *Pre-Feeding Skills* met that need. Although originally written for professionals involved in feeding programs, it also was adopted by parents who sought a deeper understanding of their children. Its friendly writing style and common-sense approach met the needs of families and professionals.

Following publication of the first edition, we continued to teach continuing education workshops and participate actively in therapy programs with children and their families. We have grown from each encounter and each question we have been asked. We approach the world from the perspective of integration and synthesis. Both of us are constantly asking "how?" and "why?" We are driven by an innate curiosity and desire for a deeper understanding of the issues that are faced by the children, families, and therapists with whom we work. Our quantum growth in linear, intuitive, and emotional understanding is reflected in this edition of the book.

The greatest areas of personal and experiential growth have been in a deepened understanding of the broader concepts of the mealtime and ways in which more specific aspects of feeding can be blended into the life of the child and family.

The Growth of Knowledge and Understanding

The first edition of *Pre-Feeding Skills* emphasized the partnership between the child and the therapist. The second edition focuses on the primary feeding partnership between the parent and the child, and on ways in which the feeding therapist can support that bond.

The professional world also has changed during the past decade. Research has focused more clearly on children and adults with swallowing and feeding disorders. In the 12-year period from 1975–1987 (prior to the first edition), there were 724 journal articles listed by Medline that contained the words *dysphagia* or *swallowing* in the title. The following 12-year period from 1988–2000 (since the first edition), produced 1,719 research papers on this topic—a figure that more than doubled the material and linear knowledge available. There have been comparable increases in information available in each of the areas discussed in this book. It is difficult for the average therapist to keep abreast of this explosion of information. It has been important to do a full literature review and update information that has become available.

Four additional areas of knowledge have profoundly influenced our thinking during this period. These include the perspectives of infant bonding, the influence of children's experiences on their interest in eating, the impact of gastrointestinal dysfunction on feeding, and the role of the ongoing influence of the child's medical issues on the desire to eat and the skill to do so. Therapists are seeing many more infants and children whose lives are changed by the impact of these areas.

The Challenges

The lives of professionals involved with children with feeding problems also have changed during the final decade of the millennium. More therapists have a working knowledge of feeding development as well as a series of strategies and techniques that they can use with children. More children with difficulties have been identified and referred for treatment. The number of therapists with experience and the ability to apply information skillfully remains small compared with the number of children who need the skills of a therapist. Those who become feeding therapists or incorporate feeding into the broader area of their practice do the very best they can with the information they have. Often this information is a series of techniques or a program that has worked for another child or therapist. Even experienced therapists routinely get stuck . . . not because they lack the techniques, but because they are missing the big picture. They have not been taught how to observe children's behavior and learn from it, to know where to begin, and to understand why an approach does or does not work for a given child or family. There is a great deal of discussion and paperwork devoted to family involvement, yet relatively few therapists have made the shift from expert to partner in their work with parents. Therapists still feel pressured to have all the answers, even as they are feeling overwhelmed by the immensity of the challenges presented by the child and family.

In previous decades, therapists were drawn to the area of feeding and mealtimes because they loved the ideas and the work with children with these specific challenges. They worked with youngsters in special schools, hospitals, or programs for children with physical disabilities. At the present time, knowledge and expertise in feeding has become part of the job description for a much larger group of therapists as children with feeding difficulties have been integrated into the majority of schools, clinics, and community programs.

A large number of therapists have grown up in an era of rapid information transfer. The influence of television, computers, and music videos has taught them to process ideas in quick sound bites. They have had less emphasis on and experience with critical thinking. When faced with the challenges of children with complex feeding issues, therapists often want fast answers and quick fixes. They are more oriented toward the end product than the process. They are more involved with destinations than journeys.

This shift in approach has blended with political and economic decisions to move toward more stringent rules and regulations that have influenced payment for rehabilitation services. Managed care has reduced the number of treatment sessions that children receive and has challenged therapists to be more creative and effective with the time they spend with each child. This requires therapists to be able to critically observe and analyze the situation, make appropriate referrals, and work in partnership with parents and children. It requires the ability to select a treatment path or direction and customize the strategies to meet individual needs. This frequently is lacking as therapists often see children through the label of their diagnosis and treat the label, not the child.

The Journey

Pre-Feeding Skills, Second Edition, addresses feeding as part of a total system that is grounded in the personal interactions of the mealtime. The mealtime concept includes the community, culture, family, and child. Eating takes place in an environment of socialization, communication, sharing, and nurturing. Within this context, a child may have difficulties with the sensorimotor aspects of feeding. These problems of physical comfort, sensory processing, and motor coordination must be addressed in therapy to enable the child to become a full participant at mealtime. When therapy takes place as an isolated set of physical exercises to increase the control of parts of the mouth, the main reason for intervening is lost. The purpose of rehabilitation is to help the person participate more fully in the community.

The child and family are at the center of every program. Their values, desires, needs, and personal knowledge combine with the specialized knowledge of the feeding therapist to create an appropriate mealtime program. Together, they envision a destination for the therapy journey or an end product. What will be different for them as a result of therapy? What are the short-term and long-term goals of the program? But they also focus on each step in the journey. What is involved in reaching the next step? The quality of the *journey* is central to the programs that are discussed and supported in this book. You will find a strong emphasis on the process in reaching the feeding goals that are suggested.

A couple of analogies help explain the concept of this journey more clearly.

A weaver creates a beautiful tapestry or rug by taking strands of different colors and textures and weaving them in an interconnected manner that allows each piece to contribute to the final design. The weaver has a pattern, a plan that defines how the strands come together and what the final picture will look like. No strand is more important than any other strand. As more strands are woven into the emerging fabric, the overall design becomes clearer. Weaving is a process of creation that is far more important than the end product of a rug or a piece of cloth. In a similar fashion, the therapist blends the individual pieces or parts of the child's life into the tapestry of therapy. Each piece is valued. Each piece creates the whole.

The spider creates an intricate web with the same artistry as the weaver. The design of the web is internal, programmed into the spider's genetic code. The web is created with a series of connecting pathways that lead into other pathways and connect with still others. Every point on the web is connected with every other point. Movement at any part of the web affects the whole web. It is impossible to jiggle or disturb only one strand. Its impact is felt at every other point. The spider web is a metaphor for therapy. There are many paths to the same end point. Neither the spider nor the child takes the direct route at all times. Therapists can build and understand the interconnections between parts of the child's life and talents, interests and needs. This enables them to begin where the child is at every moment and move in a variety of ways into new areas. It enables them to move from familiar and comfortable areas into those that are newer or unknown. Influences in one area of a child's life have an impact on all other areas. Both the history of gastrointestinal problems and the love of trains are relevant to who the child is at a given moment. Both influence the treatment program to enhance the child's feeding and mealtime skills.

Strategies and Techniques

As professionals, we tend to look for techniques that will make a difference in our therapy program. At one level this is very important. We want to know that what we do has a positive impact on the children and adults with whom we work. Building programs around therapy techniques shifts the focus from an interpersonal relationship with children and families to a relationship with the child's mouth. Feeding therapists often adopt the belief that it is the oral stimulation or the specific blowing exercise that they do that helps the child learn to swallow or eat in a more effective way. The child's key issues often become lost as therapists focus on exercising the tongue or lips rather than looking at the total picture. The key issue may be a gastrointestinal one or a severe sensory-processing disorder or coordination of the body as a whole. When the underlying issues are addressed and understood by the feeding therapist, the child makes more progress than when the focus is placed on the mouth in isolation. When the focus is on the narrow area of oral motor exercises, wedges also may be driven in the mealtime relationship between a child and a parent.

Helping make changes in swallowing and feeding skills goes far beyond the exercises or activities that are provided in therapy. The therapist must find ways of engaging and harnessing the individual's desire and self-directed ability to make positive changes. This ability is present in everyone, and it is not engaged by an exercise approach to treatment. It is engaged by the quality of the time therapists take with the client and with the interpersonal relationship that is established. It is engaged by focusing on mealtimes rather than on feeding and swallowing.

Treatment techniques are important in the overall scheme of the treatment program, but they are not where therapists should focus their main energy. There are many parallels between learning to play a musical instrument well and learning to be an effective therapist. Learning to play an instrument begins with the development of a personal relationship with music and the instrument. There is something within that draws individuals to music and to the particular instruments they have selected. They go to concerts, listen to music recordings, and create the image of themselves as creators of music. As they begin to play, they initially learn the location of the notes on the instrument and ways of producing them. In many ways, this is similar to learning a core number of techniques for addressing a specific problem in therapy. Yet it is not the individual note or the individual technique that is important. A musician can know where all the D notes are on the instrument and play them well, but it is the combining and sequencing of these notes that creates a simple tune. In the same way it is a therapist's knowledge of how to combine and sequence the techniques that creates an initial foundation for therapy. As musicians become more skilled in learning to play their instruments, they learn which notes go together to make chords and harmonies. They learn how to play in different keys with different combinations of notes. They learn a great deal about timing and rhythm. At every phase of learning, they listen carefully to the feedback from the instrument and modify what they are doing according to what they hear and feel as they are playing. As skills improve, musicians begin to play more of the music within them—to improvise on the melody, timing, and rhythm of an existing tune, and to allow new music to flow from within their minds and spirits. Clearly all of these stages and progressions in music have parallels in developing therapy skills. Everyone has heard musicians who are excellent technicians. They play music with exacting accuracy and efficiency. Yet these are not the musicians to whom most people choose to listen because their playing lacks the personal interpretation that results from the interplay of technique and feeling. The techniques of music and the understanding of music theory are very important in learning to play a musical instrument, but they are not the most essential aspects of the music that is played. It is vital for therapists to learn to put techniques in their proper place in the scheme of therapy. It is critical for therapists to take the time and energy needed to really understand the child's most important issues and select treatment strategies that address these issues. The selection of treatment techniques must fit the overall strategy, and the strategy must fit the current needs of the child and family.

Another way of looking at the interplay between treatment strategies and techniques is to consider the difference between a dictionary and a novel. A listing of techniques and the ways in which they are used is similar to having a dictionary. Dictionaries are very helpful aids. They are essential to reading or exploring a new concept or encountering an unfamiliar vocabulary in a novel. The dictionary, however, is not the novel. The novel has specific characters. These characters participate in specific relationships and complex interactions. A narrative or flow creates a plot and a continued story.

In the world of literature, one would never confuse the dictionary and the novel. However, in the world of rehabilitation, the two often are confused. An effective treatment program is similar to writing a novel in that the author consults a dictionary for the precise word to express a portion of the story. In many ways, the feeding therapist's assessment of the child's mealtime and feeding skills is similar to identifying and describing the characters in the novel. The identification of the strengths and needs of the child and family sets the stage for developing specific directions and goals for therapy. In a similar way, an author uses character descriptions and relationships to develop a theme and plot for the novel. Both the author and the therapist work with a sense of flow and progression of a story line. The specific techniques of therapy and the specific events in the novel are selected because they fit the overall strategies developed by the therapist or author.

In *Pre-Feeding Skills,* we have focused primarily on developing strategies for treatment. Many specific treatment examples are provided within the narrative of each chapter. Chapter 17 provides a dictionary of specific treatment techniques that can be incorporated within these strategies.

Keys to Learning

Pre-Feeding Skills evolved from learning ideas and experiences that came predominantly from the fields of accelerated learning, adult continuing education, and direct work with children and their families. It was designed to be an ongoing reference source for the continuous journey of discovery in the realm of oral feeding skills. The ideas within this book are based on the following basic premises:

- Learning is a process of increasing and enriching the connections between what we already know and new ideas and possibilities. It begins with our strengths and interests, gently moving into less familiar areas. Learning enables us to discover how much we already know, even when we initially believe that we are learning for the first time.

- Each person has a preferred style of learning and processing information. Some learn easily through a linear, rational approach to information gathering and reasoning. Others learn best from a global, holistic, intuitive view of the same information. Both groups may reach the same goal, using different pathways for the journey.

- Different sensory modalities take precedence for different learners. Some learn best through hearing. These individuals acquire a great deal of information from listening to audiotapes or lectures. Others learn more easily from visual input, and they thrive in a learning environment that includes pictures, videotapes, and written materials. Still others understand information most clearly when they physically experience what is being taught. For this group, concepts become much clearer when presented through touch and movement.

- A multisensory, multimodal approach to learning offers information in each style and sensory avenue. It enriches the learning process by enabling the learner to experience the same information through a variety of modes and senses. As connections are increased and enriched between our preferred ways and alternate ways, we develop the fullness of our abilities. We experience the ability to look at a situation or problem in a variety of ways, and we allow the questions to emerge that will lead us to a solution.

- Adults communicate their beliefs about learning to the children with whom they work. If adults believe that learning is difficult, children will have difficulty learning. When adults experience learning as an adventure, a way of discovering their world and its richness, children will find the same delight in discovering their emerging abilities.

- In every therapy session with a child, therapists are learners as well as teachers. The child and parents also are simultaneously teachers and learners. Each person learns most fully when each respects the other's expertise. The therapist's role is to trust the child's inner wisdom and to share ideas that will enable development in the direction the individual child wishes to move. It is not the therapist's responsibility to enforce a rigid concept of what that child or family needs in life.

- The questions we ask usually are more important to learning than the answers provided by someone else. When we can look at a situation and find the questions we should be asking, we establish the mechanism for discovering the answers. Many ideas for therapy can be based on our desire to explore a guiding question with a child. For example, suppose we ask, "What role does the auditory environment play for a child who engages in rocking, spinning, and other self-stimulatory behaviors?" To determine the answer, we can observe and record the child's responses when different types and intensities of auditory background are used in therapy. From the question and our observations of one child, patterns may emerge that could be useful with other children. From those observations, formal research may evolve. But without the questions and preliminary observations, research might never begin. Without a desire to explore questions informally, children may be denied valuable treatment approaches that are not yet supported by hard research.

Normal development, assessment, and treatment are the three sides of a learning triangle. Just as the triangle loses its identity if one side is missing, so the learning session with a child becomes incomplete if one of the elements is lacking. Knowledge of normal development gives therapists a baseline and a frame of reference for viewing deviations in movement and feeding behaviors. It enables them, through comparison, to identify movement and sensory patterns that create limitations. This identification of the elements and patterns of a child's feeding behavior is called assessment.

Normal development is composed of a series of connected elements and transitions, not a set of isolated skills. These connections and sequences create the prime elements of normal development. These elements provide ideas that therapists can incorporate into their treatment programs. As concepts of normal development are included in the assessment and treatment program, the child is able to advance along a developmental feeding path.

Assessment and treatment are connected through probes that enable therapists to explore the validity of their diagnostic concepts. During the assessment, they establish working hypotheses and check them out by exploring treatment approaches that are compatible with these hypotheses. Treatment includes assessment observations throughout the session. This enables professionals to evaluate whether their approach with the child is appropriate and effective. Each session with a child becomes a blend of these three elements. The therapist may choose to emphasize one of the components; for example, treatment may be the defined purpose of the session. However, when an awareness and integration of normal development and assessment strategies are present simultaneously, the session is enhanced and changes occur more rapidly.

This book is built on concepts that apply to both the clinician and the child. When therapists and caregivers consider themselves to be learners in each session with a child, they can relinquish the need to be experts and open themselves for further learning. The approaches that are shared in this book are not meant to be a cookbook of treatment recipes but an interweaving of ideas and concepts. By examining different ways of thinking and learning about feeding problems, every therapist and parent will strengthen the skills needed to become an effective observer and problem-solver.

In this book, information is offered in a way that allows for different styles of learning. Information is best learned and retained when an individual participates actively in the learning and discovery process. Many concepts introduced in this book are unproven in the realm of statistical research. Others have a firm research base. Statistical research identifies trends and tendencies. It does not identify whether the findings actually apply to a specific individual. The applicability of each idea or concept presented depends upon the observations and findings of the individual therapist and parent as he or she explores them with specific children. Reproducible charts and checklists are included throughout the book.

We hope that readers will draw from the book what they most need to gain greater depth and breadth of understanding of children with feeding difficulties. *Pre-Feeding Skills* provides a journey from the mouth to the mealtime that can engage each individual's sense of adventure, curiosity, understanding, and empathy. We invite you to take that journey.

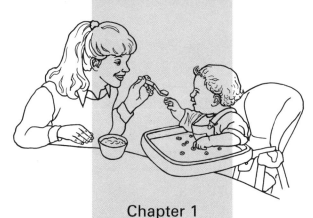

Chapter 1

Foundations for a Mealtime

▪ **What Is a Mealtime?**

As we look beyond the oral motor feeding skills of the mouth and into the mealtime environment, we need a clear understanding of the different meanings of *mealtime*. Meanings shift slightly and reflect the context in which the word is used. Mealtimes may suggest slightly different meanings depending upon where we eat, what we eat, why we are eating, and with whom we are sharing the meal. To understand these meanings, think for a moment about the meals that you have eaten during the past week. Reflect on the environment for those meals.

Reflections on a Mealtime

Where Did You Eat?

Mealtime may have different meanings, a different "feel" in different situations. We adapt our mealtimes to any environment in which we choose to bring food. Meals can take place at home; at the office, school, or hospital cafeteria; or in the car. We may be sitting at a table, standing at the kitchen counter, or lying on a blanket in the park. We may dine in a cafeteria or restaurant, or celebrate with a meal at a birthday party. The physical environment may be quiet and peaceful or noisy and chaotic. Each element of the environment contributes to the type of meal we experience and our enjoyment of that meal.

What Did You Eat?

Our selection of foods for meals varies. Choices correspond with our beliefs about food and nutrition (Brug, Glanz, & Kok, 1997; Dettwyler, 1986; Gibson, Wardle, & Watts, 1998), our economic means, the time available for preparing a meal, the purpose of the meal, personal tastes, gender (Fagerli & Wandel, 1999), age (Birch & Fisher, 1995; Contento, Michela, & Williams, 1995; Cusatis & Shannon, 1996), and family and cultural food traditions (Birch, 1987). Mealtimes bring out a diversity of beliefs, traditions, and lifestyles. Yet within each meal lie the seeds that create a positive mealtime experience. Mealtimes are composed of a series of elements that are woven into the total experience.

Mealtimes may take place when we are alone or with others, sitting down for a hurried breakfast or a relaxed dinner that we have prepared. We engage in many meals by ourselves. We eat with our spouse or friends. We share meals with our children and our extended families and even family pets. The individuals in our mealtime environment add the elements of communication and socialization to the meal. They influence the types of interactions that occur as we eat and our relationship to the food we are eating.

Purposes of a Mealtime

Why do we eat and share meals? This question is at the foundation of our understanding of the richness and diversity of the mealtime experience. Nourishment is central to the mealtime process, but nourishment can be physical as well as emotional and social.

Communication

Mealtimes that are shared with others offer optimum opportunities for interaction and communication. Topics vary from the sharing of the day and the expression of adult beliefs and values to commentary on current events, personal or family plans, and the children's table manners. In some families, mealtime communication focuses on pressuring children to eat what is served. Communication can nourish the mind, emotions, and spirit or it can contribute to psychological distress (Birch, 1998b). Much depends upon the topic of communication and the type of interaction of those sharing the meal.

Socialization

Mealtimes offer children the opportunity to learn social skills connected with family and cultural traditions such as learning to take turns, eating what is served or available, sharing available food and responsibilities, and learning manners and consideration for others at the table (Hammer, 1992). When mealtimes are interactive, children learn to expand conversation skills and develop an interest in and respect for other people.

Adults appreciate the opportunity to get together with family and friends as well as the chance to interact socially with a wider group of acquaintances and make new friends. The sharing and renewing of friendships frequently is associated with getting together for lunch or dinner. Many business agreements are initiated or finalized during a meal away from the office.

Giving and Receiving Love

The preparation and serving of food often becomes a metaphor for expressing love (Kitzinger & Kitzinger, 1991). A mother may spend a great deal of time and energy preparing a nice meal. If the family likes the meal, the mother probably will feel happy that her love was accepted. She may feel rejected or unloved, however, if her husband and children complain about the food, want to watch the ball game on television while they eat, or say they are not hungry.

Children may look at food as the parent's expression of love. If their mother fixes their favorite foods, this could be interpreted that she *really* cares about them. Some parents take great care to serve identical portions of food to each child in the family. If one child receives a slightly larger serving of a favorite food, it could mean that the parent had more love for this child.

Children and adults may highly value foods that are scarce or denied. If children do not get much sugar, for example, they may crave candy bars! Children raised in a family that serves only healthy foods may have access to cookies or candy only when they are away from their parents.

Family dissention may result when grandparents and others offer a child forbidden or discouraged foods such as candy or sweet desserts. Parents may interpret this as trying to buy the child's love. The meaning of sweets is interpreted differently by those who were denied them growing up because of poverty or war and those who grew up with values of highly nutritional foods. On the other hand, when a great deal of pressure is placed on eating certain foods, children are less interested in eating them. For example, when vegetables are pushed, they may be eaten less, contrary to the wishes of health-conscious parents.

Sharing Personal Values Related to Eating

Mealtimes offer opportunities for sharing personal and family values. For example, moral values related to food are communicated through comments such as "You must eat everything on your plate," "We all belong to the Clean-Plate Club in this family," and "Before you throw that food away, think about the starving children in Ethiopia." These comments express values of gratitude for what you have, the importance of not wasting food, and social awareness and empathy for others who are poor or in a state of famine. Adults also share beliefs and messages about self-control, self-discipline, and will power. Parents let children know that there is an appropriate amount to eat and that they should not eat more than this even if they are still hungry. Parents tell children that it is important to develop the self-discipline to eat food that they dislike.

Children may learn to ignore the internal signals from their own bodies to regulate the amount and type of food they eat (Birch & Deysher, 1986; Birch & Fisher, 1997; Fisher & Birch, 1995). They become outer-directed and eat according to the beliefs and expectations of others. Some children respond to the adult onslaught of food-related beliefs with refusals and power contests. They, too, lose sight of their inner relationship to food as they eat or refuse to eat based on the choices of other people. The choices of compliance or resistance often result in inappropriate food intake and difficulties with weight regulation.

The level of appreciation of food and mealtimes is highly individual. Children and adults who have developed a positive physical and emotional relationship to eating look forward to it. Those who have felt physical or emotional pain and discomfort during eating may respond very differently. They may eat when they consciously think about it and look at mealtimes as something you just have to get through.

Sense of Family, Culture, and Community

Sitting at the table for a meal symbolizes the unity of the family or the closeness of friends or partners. Shared mealtimes can reinforce the feeling that the participants belong to a special group; they are not just random individuals living in the same house or working in the same office. When children are disruptive at the table or complain about the food, there is a disruption of family unity.

Personal, family and cultural traditions play the largest role in early feeding practices such as breast-feeding and the age that supplemental foods and liquids are introduced (Bryant, 1982; Kannan, Carruth, & Skinner, 1999; Parraga, Weber, Engel, Reeb, & Lerner, 1988; Skinner, Carruth, Houck, Moran, et al., 1997). They influence the selection of foods we eat at all ages. Some families eat fresh organic vegetables; others eat frozen vegetables; still others rely on canned vegetables. Foods that reflect the ethnic heritage of the family may provide a feeling of family belonging and the sharing of traditions at each meal. A family with a Mexican heritage may include tortillas. A family with roots in Italy may eat more pasta dishes than other families.

Food and mealtimes frequently serve as a link between generations, especially when families have emigrated from their home country. If the grandparents grew up in China, meals may include specialties from the traditional Chinese diet, even if the family is Americanized in other respects. This brings everyone closer to his or her family roots. Food is valued differently in different cultures. For example, a much greater emphasis is placed on the quality of food and its aesthetic presentation in France than in the United States.

Cultural, regional, and class values also are expressed in the foods we eat or don't eat. Grits usually are associated with the South, while a meal of bratwurst and beer reminds one of Wisconsin. A community dinner of chitterlings and greens often becomes a celebration of identity in African American communities in the southern United States.

Children often bring special foods from their family traditions to share with classmates for a holiday party. This provides both security and a sense of identity as the special food is being prepared. A young child who loved peanut butter balls asked his mother to make them for his birthday. As he grew older, he participated in the family ritual of making peanut butter balls in order to share them with classmates as a birthday snack.

Many families in the United States are having difficulty creating meals where the entire family eats together (Jenkins, 1994). Working parents may get home late and have little time or energy to prepare a meal. Children may be involved in after-school organizations, sports, or lessons. It is becoming increasingly difficult to find a time when the whole family is home. Busy families may lean toward convenience foods that can be cooked in a microwave or brought home from a fast-food restaurant. In order to avoid arguments about the likes and dislikes of each individual, the dinner may consist of a different meal for every person.

Celebration

Food is a very important part of any celebration or family gathering. These celebrations call for foods that are traditional to both the culture and the family. Turkey at Thanksgiving and special cake to celebrate a birthday or anniversary are common traditions in the United States. These traditions may be even more specific, declaring that the turkey be prepared in a specific way and accompanied by specific vegetables or desserts. One family may have mashed white potatoes and peas with the turkey. Another may declare that the only vegetables appropriate with a Thanksgiving turkey dinner are candied sweet potatoes and a green bean casserole.

Physical Growth and Health

We eat to take in the nutrients and calories that we need to grow and be healthy. Some people are highly conscious of nutrition. Others are quite informal, serving whatever foods are most convenient or accepted by family members. Still others are limited to foods that are affordable on a very limited income (Margetts et al., 1997). The selection of food to provide physical nutrition often reflects personal and cultural beliefs as well as the ways in which people express love through food. One mother expresses her love through buying and preparing only foods that are high in nutritional value. Another serves only foods that her children enjoy and eat without complaint. These may be lower in nutrition, but are prepared with loving intent.

In their article, *Food as Metaphor,* Kitzinger and Kitzinger (1991) describe nutritional conflicts that evolve between parents and grandparents that are based on their personal experiences and expressions of love. "Many people who give their grandchildren sweets as a treat grew up during the Second World War or immediately after it, when sweets and chocolate were scarce or rationed. Their daughters, on the other hand, ***may be more*** nutrition conscious, and have often read magazine articles and books about healthful eating. Some of these women limit their children's diet to bulky, high-fiber, low-fat foods—which may fill them up before they have had enough calories or protein, and which may inhibit the absorption of minerals such as iron, zinc, and calcium. Such children are at risk for what has been termed 'muesli belt malnutrition', and their grandmothers may be genuinely concerned that the children are not getting enough 'good' food" (p. 46).

Sensory Exploration

Infants and young children delight in the sensory exploration of their world. At mealtimes they pat, poke, smear, taste, and smell the food (Erhardt, 1993). If given the opportunity, their hands, mouths, and eyes become fully involved in the meal. Children's decisions to eat a new food are based primarily on their sensory perceptions of the food. If they don't like the way it looks, smells, or feels when they touch it, they may refuse to taste or have anything to do with it. As the sensations become more familiar, children often accept a food that they rejected before (Birch & Marlin, 1982; Birch, McPhee, Shoba, Pirok, & Steinberg, 1987).

As adults, we appreciate the sensory aspects of our meals, taking pleasure in food and the environment in which we eat. Candles and soft music add a very different ambience and meaning to a meal than bright lights and loud music. We explore the sensory aspects of new foods as we venture into different ethnic restaurants. Our desire to seek new restaurants and eating experiences satisfies an educational curiosity, a desire for discovery, and our need for sensory feasts. We relish the richness provided through the taste and texture of foods such as ice cream and chocolate. If foods that reward us with their sensory input are eliminated from our diet, we grieve their loss and may abandon the diet.

Relaxation

Meals often become a socially acceptable reason to sit down and relax during a busy day. A mother who is nursing her infant simply can't be hurried through the process. Her milk will not flow, and she cannot nurse if she is rushed and divided in her attention to her infant. There are designated meal breaks in the work environment, allowing the employee to leave the work station and renew energy. We digest meals more efficiently when we are relaxed and calm than when we feel hurried and chaotic. Sitting down with others in a social setting usually is more conducive to relaxation than eating on the run. Some people eat in order to reduce stress. Others eat certain foods to make themselves feel better or spoil themselves by eating "comfort food."

Habit

It is easy and comfortable to let patterns guide our day. Many people eat at particular times or in particular places out of habit. There may be an increased sense of comfort and familiarity in having the same foods, eating in the same restaurant, or ordering specific foods in a familiar restaurant. Habits reduce stress and let us use our thinking and creative energies in other areas. A person who has orange juice and toast with orange marmalade for breakfast every morning can prepare breakfast even if not completely awake or while busy getting children ready for school.

Break in Routine

Our days are filled with routines of personal, family, and work events. Meals often are designed to break up the day into more manageable units. The first meal of the day, breakfast, comes from the words *break* and *fast*. Thus, we break the non-eating fast of the night before with an early morning meal. We may eat an early or late lunch as we wait for an appropriate break in what we are doing. At times we even eat out of boredom because we are not happy with the routine in which we are engaged.

Aspects of Nourishment at Mealtimes

Mealtimes provide nourishment that goes beyond physical nutrition for the body. Mental, emotional, and spiritual nourishment supports our lives. The type and extent of nurturing received at mealtimes is highly subjective. Each person brings a history of physical and emotional comfort to the meal. What is nourishing for one person may be neutral or aversive for another. For some, it may be most nourishing to eat with other people. For others, solitary meals are best. The foods most nourishing for one child may be unpleasant for another. For example, a food such as whole grain bread may provide a wealth of healthy nutrients. When eaten, it may satisfy hunger and nutrient needs. If the individual has an allergy to wheat or cannot process the gluten in the bread, the body will not assimilate the food. In addition, the accompanying pain or discomfort may reduce interest in eating.

When emotional conflict accompanies the meal, children can lose interest as well as much of the emotional nourishment provided through eating. Arguments about eating all of the foods served can result in power contests. The child may fight the adult for supremacy or capitulate and eat according to external guidelines. Food loses its psychological ability to nourish, and uninterest in eating can continue into adulthood (Satter, 1986, 1995). The aspects that are most characteristic of nourishing situations cannot be measured or weighed. They are the intangibles that we feel and take into the very core of our being. We need to listen to children at mealtimes. These are some of the thoughts they may want to tell us.

I Feel Nourished at Mealtimes When . . .

- I feel loved unconditionally by another person.
- my value as a person is not determined by what I eat.
- my appetite level and food choices are respected.
- my choice to smother all food with ketchup is respected.
- others listen to my ideas and share in my communication.
- my body receives the calories and nutrients it needs to grow and be healthy.
- nutrients in food are offered in a loving, caring, and respectful way.
- I am served foods that provide comfort through familiarity.
- I am served foods that enable me to make interesting discoveries.
- I can control or guide the meal.
- I feel successful.

I Do Not Feel Nourished When . . .

- I feel an obligation to accept and eat food prepared by another person.
- I must keep eating when I am full.
- I must stop eating when I am hungry.
- others make fun of my food preferences.
- others criticize me for the way I eat or my table manners.
- my diet does not contain the calories and nutrients my body needs to grow and be healthy.
- I am challenged to eat unfamiliar foods too often.
- my meals are boring and offer few opportunities for making discoveries.
- I have no control over the meal and what I eat.
- I feel like a failure.

Creating Nourishing Mealtimes for Children and Families

When children have difficulty with eating and drinking, they and their families may miss out on the most nourishing aspects of the mealtime (Humphry, 1991). It is often difficult to provide a balanced diet and adequate calories. Mealtimes may become stressful because the child takes a long time to eat or eats a very limited repertoire of foods. Parents and therapists often decide what and how much the child will eat at a meal instead of giving the child the autonomy to make these decisions (Babbitt et al., 1994; Johnson & Babbitt, 1993; Sanders, Patel, Le Grice, & Shepherd, 1993; Stark et al., 1996).

Therapists often provide feeding suggestions to parents and other care providers that interfere with the quality of mealtime interactions. The focus shifts from the broad array of mealtime functions to the narrow view of how a tongue works to chew the food. Communication, socialization, a sense of family and belonging, sensory exploration, relaxation, and celebration become lost. Control and frustration often replace love and respect.

Mealtime programs can focus on bringing nourishment of the child and family into every meal. Professionals must discover what is nourishing for the specific child and parent. This will depend upon the beliefs, values, and experiences of each parent as well as those of the therapist. Therapists can model and support a nurturing approach in therapy and in the suggestions they provide for the child's caregivers. Mealtime programs include positive communication and social interaction. They express love for the children and families and are built on a foundation of respect.

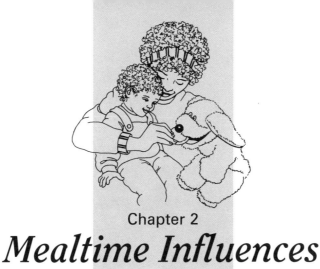

Chapter 2

Mealtime Influences

As we participate in and share mealtimes with friends and family, an assembly of beliefs and experiences guides our decisions, influencing each meal and creating the feedback that tells us whether it was a successful meal. When our experiences at the meal agree with our past experiences and what we believe to be important, we feel satisfied. When the mealtime experience is strikingly different from what we desire or expect, we feel dissatisfied, upset, or angry. Many areas can influence the meal, and these will interact in different ways for different people. For example, a parent who values a strong ethnic identity may be distressed if his child is unable or unwilling to eat specific foods associated with the culture. Another parent may be extremely worried about her child's health and feel she must push the child to eat more fruits and vegetables. The child may be more influenced by a need to declare independence and, understanding his mother's need for a healthy diet, may refuse to eat anything but heavily processed carbohydrates.

Identifying and Understanding Mealtime Influences

Parents and therapists commonly assume that the influences and values surrounding a child's mealtime will be similar to their own. This is not usually the case. The first step in influencing a mealtime is to observe and begin to understand the most important influences for this specific adult and child. Every assessment and treatment program will benefit from a careful review of the following influences on a child's mealtime:

- beliefs
- culture
- parent's history
- child's history
- family dynamics
- socioeconomic factors

- child's health
- child's developmental skills and needs
- child's feeding and oral motor skills
- child's emotional state and temperament
- parent's emotional state and temperament

The mealtime environment that is established will reflect the relative importance of these components.

The Influence of Beliefs

Strong beliefs and attitudes about eating and mealtimes provide expectations and guidance to everyone who participates in the meal. Beliefs are highly subjective and based on the assumption that the truth resides in each individual's specific perception. There is no such thing as a "good belief" or a "bad belief." There are simply beliefs that have specific end results or outcomes. Thus, if I believe that parents are responsible for what and how much their children eat, I will monitor my child's plate until the food I have served has been eaten. If my child protests and refuses to eat green beans or fails to finish a baked potato, I will be uncomfortable unless I push, entice, or coerce him to finish the food.

The beliefs that guide our behavior frequently lie below our conscious awareness (Kaufman, B. N., 1991). We may accept a given belief because others in our family or in our profession have accepted it, even if science has disproven it. For centuries, the world denied the astronomical data of Copernicus, which confirmed that the Earth was not the center of the universe. Despite the data, people continued to believe that the sun and planets circled the Earth. No amount of data could alter their belief! For nearly two decades, physicians have strongly recommended that parents delay introducing solid foods to children until they are 4–6 months old because of the immaturity of the gastrointestinal system (American Academy of Pediatrics, 1980). Despite our objective knowledge that the infant's gut is not mature enough to handle these more complex food molecules prior to 4 months, many parents continue to add cereals and fruits to their babies diets earlier. Skinner, Carruth, Houck, Moran, et al. (1997) found that nearly half of the 98 parents in their study gave their infants smooth solid foods prior to 4 months, with some parents adding cereal to the infant's bottle as early as 1 month.

From the moment we are born, we begin to adopt beliefs from the world in which we live. These come from our parents, teachers, churches, friends, and isolated personal experiences. They create the structure or template through which we view the world and our experiences. Beliefs can even guide or determine our experiences. For example, individuals who hold a positive view of other people are more likely to meet others who are pleasant and cooperative than those who are pessimistic about strangers. This repeated experience, stemming from a positive belief, reinforces the belief and increases the expectation that people basically are happy and willing to cooperate.

We often carry into adulthood beliefs that we've outgrown or don't really accept anymore, yet act as if they still are true. We rarely ask ourselves, "Do I really believe that?" As a child, I may be exposed to the belief that "a parent must be fair to each child." My mother may express this belief by measuring each piece of pie as she divides it among her children and counting the number of gifts under the Christmas tree so that no child receives a larger share. Through observing, I may learn that a good mother is always fair and does not give more to one child than another. When I become the mother of a child with special needs, I may unconsciously carry this belief about parenting into my family and mealtime relationships. I may begin to resent the amount of time spent in therapy or the length of a mealtime because I am spending more time with this child than with my other children.

Mealtime beliefs center on mealtime roles, mealtime responsibilities, personal identity, and food. Think about the following beliefs. Describe the feelings or actions that would result from these beliefs.

- I am responsible for my child's eating enough food.
- It is important to eat everything on your plate.
- Leaving food is wasteful.
- No one can make me eat.
- If I eat that food, it will hurt my tummy.
- Eating is scary. I could choke.
- I've raised children before. I know what you should do about this eating problem.
- That therapist doesn't understand why he doesn't eat. Her ideas are all wrong.
- Sweets are wonderful rewards for good behavior.

- Sweets are bad for my child.
- My child hates broccoli.
- If I serve my children healthy foods, they will be healthy.
- High-fat foods are bad for the body.
- If I'm a good mother, my child eats.
- When someone refuses the food I serve, they reject me and the love I am offering.
- Fathers know how to fix things. When a child has trouble eating, they should be able to fix the problem.
- As a therapist I should have all the answers to this eating problem.
- The mother is responsible for the children. She is the one who feeds the kids.
- Children should have good table manners.
- Children should be neat.
- Mothers cook, fathers take out the garbage, and children do the dishes and clean up after the meal.
- Parents are responsible for their children eating a nutritious meal.
- Parents are responsible for selecting nutritious and appropriate food choices.
- Children are responsible for what they eat and how much they eat.

The Influence of Culture

A culture incorporates the collection of beliefs and traditions associated with a specific group. It can guide the types of food that a family eats, as well as the role of food and mealtimes. Many subcultures have their own values and influence. These include the cultures of gender, ethnicity, and age, as well as the values of the individual family. Different ethnic groups have different beliefs and traditions about specific foods, about the role of food in the family, and the definition of appropriate behavior for children at mealtimes. Many differences in mealtime practices were observed in a study of 45 refugee families from Chile and the Middle East who settled into a city in Sweden (Hjern, Kocturk-Runefors, & Jeppson, 1990). Families from the Middle East introduced infants to solid and semi-solid foods much later than those from Chile. Families from Chile tended to eat their largest meal at noon and serve a very light meal in the evening. Hudson and Distel (1999) found that national groups differed in their judgments of the pleasantness of food odors depending on whether the odor was recognized as representing familiar foods of the culture. They have hypothesized that culture-specific eating experiences may influence an adult's preferences for food-associated odors.

In some ethnic groups, meals are formal, and children are fed separately from their parents. In the United States, there is usually a more informal approach to mealtimes. Even adult-oriented restaurants provide high chairs and booster seats to accommodate families with children. Because of the high value placed on independence rather than interdependence, children are encouraged to feed themselves as soon as they are able and to choose the foods they want to eat. This often results in difficulties with setting limits around mealtimes, and some mothers find themselves creating different meals for each member of the family.

Age and gender also have cultural traditions and proscriptions (Fagerli & Wandel, 1999). In most families, women are the primary caregivers and the ones who feed young children. In some cultural groups this is a fixed responsibility, while in others men increasingly are involved in child rearing. How both parents feel about their roles in feeding children will depend upon the models they learned in their own families and their ethnic background. Behaviors are often age-linked in the culture. Messy eating may be acceptable for the infant or toddler, but not condoned in an older child. Special foods may be offered only to older members of the family when aging implies honor and wisdom.

Each family accumulates a collection of beliefs about the role of children and parents, and expectations about food and mealtimes. A blend of cultural and individual beliefs is passed down from one generation to the next. Grandparents may have a major influence on how young parents manage a child's feeding problems. It is vital for feeding therapists to become familiar with the child-rearing and cultural practices of a family because these family-transmitted beliefs may conflict with suggestions offered by therapists (Lynch & Hanson, 1992). Community or family guidelines may have a stronger impact on family decisions than the unique needs of a single member of the family. In a study of 45 Guatemalan families, researchers examined the unspoken rules by which food was distributed to various family members (Engle & Nieves, 1993). Each family was enrolled in supplementary feeding programs because each had at least one child that was targeted as undernourished. Family members differed in age, sex, earning status, and family role. In most families, individuals considered in the culture to have a higher economic value received a higher percentage of the family's food. Engle and Nieves (1993) wrote, "There was no evidence that mothers were giving the child targeted as undernourished by the health center any more food than any other similar-aged child" (p. 1,605).

The Influence of the Parent's History

Each adult who feeds a child or prepares a meal brings a personal mealtime history to the table. It is important to explore the role played by food in each parent's growing-up and to be aware of the beliefs and family values that were absorbed (McCann, Stein, Fairburn, & Dunger, 1994). One father was astounded when the therapist said she wanted to make mealtimes fun and enjoyable for his son. He stated emphatically that this was not the purpose of a meal. He described being followed around with a spoon all day long by his maternal grandmother who constantly reminded him to eat when he was a child. For him, mealtimes were punitive and unpleasant. As an adult, he saw meals as something he needed to do because his body needed the food. The idea that eating could be enjoyable for him or his son was foreign to him.

Children can have the same set of experiences during mealtimes, yet interpret them differently when they become parents. One mother was raised by parents who took total responsibility for her eating. She was not allowed to leave the table until her plate was clean. As an adult, she realized that she had never learned to respond to internal signals of hunger and satiation. She struggled with unwanted weight gain because she continued to eat what was served, whether or not she was hungry. When she became a mother, she felt strongly about allowing her children to decide what and how much they would eat. She selected and served appropriate foods, but encouraged them to eat only as much as they wished. Another mother had similar experiences as a child. She was never allowed to choose how much food she would eat and was always pushed to eat "just a little bit more." Because she was familiar with this parenting style, she set the same guidelines for her children.

The parent's medical history often plays a large role in mealtimes (Daly & Fritsch, 1995; Drotar, 1991; Duniz et al., 1996). There may be medical issues that influence an adult's energy (Singer et al., 1999; Williams et al., 1999), stamina, emotional state, and ability to make decisions. Physical illness or disability, depression (Field, 1998), mental illness (Weinberg & Tronick, 1998), substance abuse (Burns, Chethik, Burns, & Clark, 1991), cognitive delays, learning disabilities, attention deficit disorders (Daly & Fritsch, 1995), and medication influence how the parent relates to the child at mealtime. Serious problems in these areas may even result in the parent forgetting to feed the child or feeding inadequate amounts for growth (Russell, Treasure, & Eisler, 1998). A mother who is chronically exhausted may approach a meal as something to "get through." She may have very little energy for interaction or for guiding her child into new skills. Opportunities for learning may be delayed because the parent doesn't feel well enough to spend the extra time and deal with the challenges of a child who creates messes while learning a new skill.

It is particularly important to explore the type of relationship that each parent has developed with food. Does the parent find new foods an interesting adventure or consider them risky? Is there a history of food allergies and subsequent dietary restrictions? Is there a history or current problem with an eating disorder such as anorexia or bulimia? Mothers who have experienced anorexia may transfer their beliefs about body size and weight to their young children (Honjo, 1996; Russell et al., 1998). As a result, they may worry that a child is eating too much and will become overweight. They may reduce the amount of food served or engage in verbal battles over food with the child. Research suggests that these features may have an impact on a child's eating patterns.

Mothers who breast-feed their infants provide an extensive range of taste experiences through their breast milk (Mennella, 1995; Mennella & Beauchamp, 1998b). The taste of foods they have eaten transfers to the milk, and the baby has the opportunity to experience many different flavors. When the mother is adventurous and is willing to include novel foods in her diet, the infant's taste experience expands. Moreover, this is correlated with the infant's willingness to try new tastes when supplemental foods are introduced (Mennella & Beauchamp, 1997). Parents continue to influence their children's food habits as they grow older. When they are suspicious of new foods in their personal life, they tend to offer their children primarily familiar foods. Subsequently, their children may limit their own diets because of lack of experience with a wide variety of foods (Koivisto, 1999; Koivisto & Sjoden, 1996).

The Influence of the Child's History

Children also bring their personal histories with them to a mealtime. They expect the current experience to be like past experiences and often will try to avoid situations that have brought them discomfort. A child's history is composed of the factual events that have occurred as well as the child's perception and interpretation of these events. Children respond in unique ways to parental beliefs and practices related to food (Dreikurs & Stoltz, 1964). Some will accept the status quo and cooperate with what is expected. Some will appear to cooperate by giving up and acting helpless as they go along with adult demands. Others will confront adult beliefs and actions and fight them. Still others will find ways of using mealtime situations to enact revenge on parents and others who feed them. It is particularly important to identify children who are engaged in power contests because this becomes a losing battle for everyone. Children can devote 24 hours a day to winning, while most adults cannot. Even when adults overpower children and appear to win the battle by getting them to eat, they have lost. Their children learn that when they are big and strong adults, they can make children do what they want. This is not a lesson most parents and therapists wish to teach children.

If we are to understand a child's responses to food and mealtimes, we must observe whether mealtimes have been both physically and emotionally comfortable. When children experience fear or discomfort with specific foods or types of food, mealtimes can be filled with stress and anxiety. As children try to protect themselves from danger and distress, mealtime battles may emerge. Some children have undiagnosed allergies or sensitivities to the formula or foods that are offered (Rapp, 1991). Others may experience oral or tactile sensory defensiveness (Frick, Frick, Oetter, & Richter, 1996; Wilbarger & Wilbarger, 1991). Still others may have experienced vomiting, gastroesophageal reflux, or retching during oral feedings or tube feedings (Dellert, Hyams, Treem, & Geertsma, 1993; Nelson, Chen, Syniar, & Christoffel, 1998). In each instance, something within the child's system puts up red flags of warning. These guide the child toward behavioral choices that move away from accepting the offending food or eating experience. Unfortunately, some children continue to anticipate trouble even when the initial medical issues have been resolved.

A child's medical history can color his viewpoint about the face, mouth, and the process of eating. Some children have experienced extensive surgery for cranio-facial defects. Some may have had the palate repaired or undergone reconstruction of the head and face. These areas may have been poked and prodded by strange adults in various diagnostic assessments. Some children may have experienced severe pain in the mouth after reconstructive surgery. Others may have been born prematurely and were unable to breathe or eat normally. This may have required ventilation, oral or nasal feeding tubes, and other unpleasant oral experiences. Each of these experiences can evoke memories of pain and discomfort and lead the child toward rejecting any sort of adult-initiated sensory input to the mouth. If there have been periods of hospitalization or a history of doctor visits in a medical setting, the child may generalize the heightened fears and anxieties to any therapist who works in a similar environment.

The Influence of Family Dynamics

Every parent is part of several families. These include the family that each adult grew up in and the new family that has been created with a spouse, partner, or child. Both the nuclear family and extended families play a role in the family dynamics surrounding mealtimes. The family we grow up in is a major source of the beliefs and attitudes that we carry into our adult relationships and immediate family.

Extended families can be very supportive to the new mother and father. For generations, mothers guided their child-rearing practices and their children's feeding development by consulting their own mothers and grandmothers. As families became more geographically mobile and the nature of many families changed, the immediacy of the extended family as a source of knowledge was reduced. Parents have begun to rely more on books, pediatricians, and baby food companies to guide their decisions about eating, nutrition, and mealtimes. Unfortunately, this has resulted in conflicting recommendations, and many parents are more uncertain about their roles at mealtimes.

This conflict is often greater when the child has difficulty eating. The voices of many different physicians and therapists join with the voices of the extended family. When suggestions offered by therapists differ greatly from family traditions, parents have more difficulty being an effective parent. Parents want the best for their children. But which of the many suggestions is really the best? Common sense suggestions of grandparents or other extended family members may be rejected, assuming that the professional knows the best way to feed children. Sometimes the views of the extended family are so strong that parents reject any conflicting recommendations of professionals.

There are many types of family. At one time only the nuclear family consisting of a father, mother, and one or more children was recognized. Now we know that a family may consist of a single mother, a single father, foster parents, stepparents, siblings, and extended families. The two-parent home may consist of the more traditional father and mother or it may be headed by two same-sex parents. The nature of the family will influence the family mealtime. If the child lives in a single-parent family, the parent may have full responsibility for the care of the child with special needs as well as work to provide money to support the family. The parent may feel stressed and chronically exhausted as he or she struggles to meet the many needs of the child and family.

The addition of other siblings in the family can create challenges for the parents to provide a mealtime that meets the needs of the child who has problems. Mealtimes with many young children can be chaotic and noisy. Older siblings may share parenting and mealtime responsibilities with the mother. Often the child with special feeding challenges needs a quieter environment or frequent individual attention from an adult. Parents who experience multiple demands from other children may be unable to create the type of mealtime environment that supports everyone's needs. This can result in frustration and guilt or may be met with the belief that nothing will ever change.

Stepfamilies create a blending of family cultures and traditions. Because the individual parents in the new family have already developed their own parenting styles and a set of mealtime beliefs and practices, there may be conflicts over unspoken assumptions about the way that things are done. Some of the same challenges occur in close extended families. Extended families incorporate grandparents or other adult family members into the home. The effect can be either positive or negative depending on the role played by those outside the nuclear family (Black & Nitz, 1996). In some families, it is the grandmother who makes the major parenting and mealtime decisions for a child. If therapists are unaware of these special family dynamics, the guidelines given to the parents may be inappropriate and actually cause additional mealtime problems. It is vital to discover who makes the decisions in each household and to learn more about the beliefs and guidelines that are part of the family structure. Mealtime responsibilities and roles are influenced by the type of family and by the atmosphere of cooperation or animosity within the family.

Young children do not understand the relationships among the adults in their lives, yet these relationships have a pervasive influence on mealtime. If adults fight or constantly disagree at the meal, mealtime relationships with their children can become strained. The child may respond with increased physical and emotional tension and a reduced ability to eat well.

Often children think it is their fault when parents fight. This can be an easy assumption for a child who needs a lot of physical support or is often out of control because of sensory modulation issues. One parent or siblings may verbally blame the child with disabilities for taking so much of the mother's time. Family members may disagree about the approaches to the child's feeding and mealtime needs that they feel are appropriate. Arguments may break out when one parent feels that the other is interfering with the child's ability to eat.

When a family goes through a divorce, the child's physical, sensory, and mealtime worlds fall apart. The parent who has custody of the children has major child-rearing responsibilities. Feeding may become more difficult for everyone. The stress felt by both the parent and child can contribute to poorer physical and emotional control as each tries to adapt to the new situation. Financial stress increases the overall challenge of being a single parent. Anger at the ex-spouse may be expressed by demands for consistent carryover of the child's feeding program when the child spends time with the non-custodial parent. When parents live in the same city, they may choose to share responsibility for their children. Joint or shared custody often means that the child physically lives with one parent part of the week and with the other parent the rest of the week. Sometimes the child changes homes on alternate months if the parents live far apart or in different school districts. Some children even end up attending two different schools, depending on which parent they are living with at the time. This can create major disruptions for children with physical and sensory issues. It may be very difficult to develop consistency in a feeding or mealtime program.

Raising children can be a challenging adventure that is full of discovery and enjoyment. It also can be a physically and emotionally exhausting roller coaster. When fatigue and frustration enter the picture, it is harder for parents to enjoy their children. This becomes particularly difficult when one parent has the full responsibility for feeding a child every meal (Jones & Heermann, 1992). When no one else can feed the child, the emotional and physical stresses increase. The child may depend totally on the mother and lack confidence that anyone else can feed him. Indeed, when a therapist or baby-sitter tries to feed him, he becomes tense and unable to eat or refuses to open his mouth. This confirms his mother's worst fears—that her child will only be nourished if she is the one who feeds him. This leads to a vicious cycle in which the mother is afraid to let anyone else feed the child, and the child feels secure and comfortable only when the mother offers the food.

The presence or lack of personal support systems plays a large role in how adults respond to their roles as parents (Jones & Heermann, 1992; Mathiesen, Tambs, & Dalgard, 1999). When two adults share the responsibilities of the household, it is easier for one parent to have personal time or get away from the children for short periods. Engaging in personal hobbies, exercise, or a quiet bubble bath can provide the nourishment that is needed to sustain the energy required of all parents. Parents need the option of sharing adult-time with regular evenings away from their children. Some adults set up regular "dates" with their spouses or partners to support their partnership and the relationship that brought them together as a family. This requires the support of child-care providers who are willing and able to care for a child with special needs. This may be difficult to find if the child has a feeding tube, tracheostomy, or other medical condition.

The Influence of Socioeconomic Factors

Socioeconomic factors play a role in the type of mealtime structure that each family creates. These influence the sources of information about feeding and mealtimes that are available to parents (Bryant, 1982), the amount of physical space available for meals, the types of food offered at meals, and the individuals who provide meals for the children.

The type and amount of education that the parents have is related, in part, to their socioeconomic status. Very young parents or those who grew up in poor families may have dropped out of school before high school graduation. A low valuation of education or learning disabilities may have triggered an early departure from school. Parents who are functionally illiterate or undereducated may need additional visual or verbal explanations or teaching geared to their specific learning style to understand how to help their child at mealtime. Parents who are highly educated may hold very high expectations of their child's learning abilities. They may place pressure on the child or become frustrated or angry when the child learns in a different way or takes a longer time to learn.

Families who are poor frequently live in substandard housing or are homeless. They may lodge in crowded apartments with relatives or move from one shelter to another. Migrant families move from one part of the country to another, following the crops. In both urban and rural migrancy, there is little continuity of housing or of therapy services. Children may need special chairs or other pieces of equipment at mealtimes. Many homes and apartments are too small to accommodate equipment suggested by the therapist. Children living in substandard inner-city apartments may not be given the option of playing independently on the floor because of rodents and bugs.

Food budgets are directly related to total family income. When income levels are low, there may not be enough food for children to grow well. To increase the amount of food, parents may purchase less expensive, processed-carbohydrate foods, leaving the diet deficient in protein, vegetables, and fruits that cost more. When there is a bigger budget for food, the diet may consist of a large number of processed convenience foods and restaurant meals, especially if both parents work.

Because of lower incomes and high economic desires, many American families have two wage earners. When both parents work, families often can afford to purchase more services for the child. There may be higher insurance benefits for therapy and more discretionary income for toys and equipment. Parents may experience more work-related stress because of the higher incidence of illness in children with special needs and the large number of professional appointments that the child needs. If the employer is not cooperative about these needs, the parents can become more stressed with conflicting demands of job and family. Sharing job and home responsibilities strongly influences the amount of time that each parent has available to assist the child with feeding difficulties.

When both parents work outside the home, other adults care for the children. In some cases, this is a grandparent or other family member. In many instances, care is provided by a day-care worker, a nanny, or an au pair. Individuals providing child care typically are poorly paid, and the jobs often do not attract highly educated people. Many care providers have poor language and literacy skills (Healy, 1990) and may not speak the parents' language. In addition, each child care provider brings his or her own cultural views of children, mealtimes, and food. These differences may be subtle, but have a strong impact, either positive or negative, on the child and the therapy program.

The Influence of the Child's Health

The child's health plays a major role in feeding and mealtime decisions. When a child is well and does not have extraordinary needs, mealtimes are generally less stressful. If meals are skipped or only small amounts are eaten, most parents are not afraid that this will harm their child. However, if children consistently refuse specific types of food or have specific caloric or nutrient requirements, their parents may become concerned about their health and well being (Singer et al., 1996). Some children lack the energy for new learning. They may be chronically unwell, yet not physically ill. When steps are taken to increase their basic level of health and wellness, they blossom in their ability to learn to eat.

Many children have acute or chronic medical conditions that have a negative impact on their appetite or ability to eat. Acute conditions such as teething, ear infections, colds, or intestinal flu will affect eating for the duration of the health episode. More chronic conditions such as prematurity, cystic fibrosis, cerebral palsy, allergy, and tracheo-esophageal fistula will influence eating for extended periods of time. Eating changes that occur from acute medical conditions often resolve themselves when the condition ends. However, some acute situations, such as a severe choking episode, can have a longer-lasting influence on eating because of the emotional impact of the event. Chronic conditions generally require longer-term support of feeding. Even when positive support is provided, there can be ups and downs in eating skills and appetite depending on the child's current health.

Physical well-being influences children's overall emotions, attitudes, and openness to new experiences. When they are even marginally unwell, children are not as available for learning and may reject new experiences or expectations because they lack the energy or ability to handle anything else.

Children may refuse food or eat very specific foods because of how they feel. Some foods may make a child feel ill or experience reflux. Children eat other foods because they are very easy to handle and don't require much energy.

Gastroesophageal reflux combined with gagging or vomiting creates very unpleasant associations with eating. Mathisen, Worrall, Masel, Wall, and Shepherd (1999) found that infants with gastro-esophageal reflux refused more food, and their mothers had more negative feelings and enjoyed meal-time less. Thus, the reflux reduced the child's interest in eating and the ensuing struggles of the parents interfered with the basic parent-child interaction at mealtime.

Some children require special diets because of allergies or metabolic disorders. This is a "no choice" situation. The child *must* eat (or not eat) specific foods. For example, a child on a ketogenic diet for seizure control must eat a specific number of calories per day with the majority coming from fat (Freeman, Kelly, & Freeman, 1996). The proportion of calories from carbohydrates and protein is sharply reduced. High-fat foods such as cream, butter, cheese, and oils are included in most meals. Some children find it very difficult to eliminate favorite foods that are not on the diet and to adjust to the fatty tastes in everything they eat. Children with cystic fibrosis must maintain a diet that is high in calories and nutrients. Because their bodies overproduce a thick, sticky mucous that blocks the pancreatic ducts, pancreatic enzymes are not available for digestion. To prevent malnutrition and diarrhea, they must take special pills or capsules containing these digestive enzymes with every snack or meal. The regulation of food and external enzymes can be very complex and time sensitive because the right amount of enzymes must be available in the small intestine as the food arrives. In situations where choices are limited because of medical needs, parents are tempted to get into power contests with their children. They know that the child's physical well-being depends upon the amount and type of food eaten. They are reluctant or unable to let the child's hunger and appetite regulate food intake. As a result, they feel that they must push their children to eat what is medically necessary.

Medications also can influence a child's interest in food. Drugs may taste bad or create side effects that reduce a child's interest in eating. This creates a conflict for the parents because they want their child to be well, yet they want him or her to eat. For example, the medication Ritalin (methylphenidate HCl) frequently is given to children who have attention deficit disorder. One of its side effects in children is loss of appetite (Hogan, 1999). Parents may see many positive changes in their child's activity level and ability to pay attention when taking the drug but be very concerned about its effect on eating.

Medications may need to be given on a specific schedule (e.g., 30 minutes before the meal, with a meal at 3-hour intervals). This makes mealtimes much less flexible for both the parent and child. When medications are given at the beginning of the meal or during the meal, the child can associate eating with things that taste bad. If a bad-tasting drug is given by spoon, young children often refuse to eat any food that is offered on the spoon.

Mealtimes also can become a time of major concern and worry when children aren't growing well and are experiencing failure-to-thrive. Physicians often push families to increase the child's caloric intake or the amount of food that the child eats. Often these suggestions are made with little or no understanding of the reasons why the child has poor eating skills. Parents already may be doing everything they can think of to add calories and increase the amount of food that the child will eat. Pressure from professionals to do more can increase their stress and anxiety about meals. This may lead to pushing or forcing the child to eat more. Mealtimes can become a battlefield rather than a playing field. When the child is stressed, the desire to eat is reduced and the child eats less. In addi-tion, when there is stress, digestion may be poorer and the child may assimilate fewer nutrients from the food he eats. The need to increase calories also may result in parents offering empty calories. Fruits and vegetables have fewer calories than foods high in fat or carbohydrate content. Emphasizing calories instead of a balanced nutritional diet can create many nutritional problems later even if the child succeeds in gaining weight. Many children with feeding difficulties limit their intake to a few familiar foods that are easy and comfortable to eat. They may discover the pleasure of sweet-tasting foods that are given to increase weight. Sugar may be added to all foods because the child refuses to eat anything that is not extremely sweet. Gradually, the child's diet becomes more limited nutritionally even though it may contain an appropriate number of calories.

Water makes a very important contribution to children's health (Batmanghelidj, 1995). It is needed to fully hydrate all of the cells of the body, and it contributes to digestion from the stomach to the colon. When there is not enough free water in the system, the child may become constipated. Toxins can build up in the system, making the child feel irritable and unwell. Interest in food may diminish when children do not have easy bowel movements. Many parents, even those of typically developing children, do not offer their children enough water. When children ask for something to drink, they tend to offer juice, milk, or soda pop. These liquid foods also are offered instead of water when the child is having trouble taking in enough calories. Water is viewed as an empty-calorie liquid that can be sacrificed for liquids that contain calories.

The Influence of the Child's Developmental Skills and Needs

Children have different skills and needs at various points in their development. These will strongly influence the mealtime by redefining its roles and relationships. When the role definitions are dysfunctional or do not change as the child changes, feeding and mealtime problems can develop or become exaggerated.

Infants are dependent upon adults to meet their survival needs. Their primary focus is placed on bringing their bodies into a homeostatic balance with the outside world. Sucking and swallowing skills provide a foundation for both physical and emotional nutrition. Infants let their parents know when they are hungry, when they need a pause or a burp, and when they wish to stop eating. As they guide their frequent meals, they are dependent upon parents who can read and respect their communication cues. Parents respond to these cues by providing breast milk or an appropriate formula in a timely and caring way. Child-rearing practices and beliefs will guide the parents into either letting the baby take the lead at mealtimes or into feeling that they are responsible for what and how much the baby eats.

Within reason, parents are more likely to be the "feeding boss" in the first 3 months. Babies are capable of refusing to eat at any age, but they are guided more by hunger signals and automatic sucking and swallowing patterns in the early months. As babies develop more volitional eating skills, their decision to refuse eating for many reasons becomes more of a challenge. For example, premature infants may suck and swallow from the bottle or breast using a very automatic pattern during the early months in the hospital. But as their oral control increases and they are capable of more volitional behavior, they may stop eating if there are respiratory, coordination, sensory, or gastrointestinal issues. At some level they decide that eating causes pain or discomfort or takes too much effort. Their new skills enable them to respond to these internal concerns by stopping the more automatic sucking and swallowing that they used to eat. This tendency becomes even stronger when babies are 8–9 months old and have a real sense of causation. Older infants quickly learn that when they don't eat, their parents become more attentive or upset. Some young children enjoy this feeling of control or power and will begin to use eating or non-eating as a way of meeting their emotional needs.

As infants grow and develop, their feeding capabilities increase. They are interested in new textures in foods and more challenging positions and utensils. They learn to sit in a high chair and accept food from a spoon instead of taking solely the bottle or breast. They gradually expand their experiences with food tastes and textures. They accept new experiences as their physical, sensory, and emotional systems are ready. Problems can arise when parents offer foods that are too challenging or fail to offer new feeding experiences when the child is ready.

Children want to be participants and decision-makers at mealtimes. They begin this process in the early months as they decide what and how much they are going to eat. As their gross and fine motor skills develop, they reach for the spoon, bring toys to the mouth, and want to physically help get the food to the mouth. Toward the end of the first year, they will pick up pieces of food and put them in the mouth, and then learn to use a spoon and cup to feed themselves. This is often a messy process. Some parents discourage self-feeding because they don't want the mess. In response, many busy parents offer their child a sipper cup with a lid so that liquid does not spill when the child tips the cup over or tosses it on the floor. Many 2-year-olds have had no experience drinking from an open cup. They often move directly from the sipper cup to a straw.

As children become 2-year-olds, their developmental agenda shifts toward greater independence. In order for children to learn about themselves and their ability to have an impact on the world, they must feel safe. When limits are set and enforced consistently, children feel safe enough to risk doing more and being independent. Parents set the structure and guidelines for how this independence will be expressed. It may be strongly nurtured, initially discouraged, or redirected depending on the culture and emotional needs of the family. Being more independent early is highly valued in the United States and in busy families with mothers who work outside of the home (Lynch & Hanson, 1992). However, this independence can set the stage for power contests about eating when parents refuse to honor the child's decisions about what to eat and how much. In addition, when limits and guidelines are not defined for children, they attempt to find a structure that is not there and become very demanding and out of control.

The Influence of the Child's Feeding and Oral Motor Skills

Feeding and oral motor difficulties contribute strongly to direct or indirect family stress at mealtimes. Mealtimes are easier for everyone when children can feed themselves easily and well. Even when children are dependent on others for feeding, the ability to suck, swallow, and chew safely makes it easier. Clear interaction and communication skills at mealtime enhance the ability to feed children who have poor feeding skills. When children have many limiting feeding patterns, mealtimes may be stressful and frightening, especially if these patterns increase the risk of choking or aspiration. Feeding is often slow, and parents may worry that the child will get tired and stop eating before taking enough food to meet nutritional needs.

Children with sensory-based feeding issues are among those whose limited feeding patterns and needs are difficult to meet at mealtime. They frequently have a very limited food repertoire and are very erratic in their ability to process sensory information in a way that is comfortable (Quinn, 1995; Sears, 1994). As a result, they often refuse food and need a great deal of sensory preparation in order to sit at the table and participate in the mealtime. The parents of these children also worry about poor weight gain and nutritional status when eating is inconsistent and food variety is limited.

A child's feeding difficulties influence the time and energy that parents have for their own needs and for other family members. Some children take a long time to feed. A parent may spend 60–90 minutes per meal three to five times a day or may give smaller meals to an infant every hour throughout the day. Foods may need to be mixed in a blender or in specific ways that take added time. The child may need an expensive tube-feeding formula that stretches the family's financial resources, creating additional stress.

The Influence of the Child's Emotional State and Temperament

Each child has a unique outlook and approach to the world that begins before birth (Verny & Kelly, 1981). Mothers report that their baby has a distinct style of movement and timing during pregnancy. Some babies are very active and move frequently and vigorously in utero. Others are quieter and move in a more flowing way. Their body rhythms can vary throughout the day with some being more active in the morning and others in the afternoon. Still others awaken the mother in the middle of the night with intra-uterine gymnastic events. These early physiological measures of heart rate and movement frequently are correlated with measures of temperament after the baby is born and into early infancy. Research by DiPietro, Hodgson, Costigan, and Johnson (1996) found that more active fetuses were more difficult, unpredictable, unadaptable, and active infants. Many features of the infant's temperament are evident within a few hours of birth (Medoff-Cooper, 1995). Although a child is born with a variety of temperamental traits, these are not genetically derived (Riese, 1990), and a child's biological predisposition can be altered by the environment (Greenspan, 1995).

A child's temperament is a mix of characteristics that create personality patterns that influence how a child will respond to life events. Many of these traits influence eating and mealtime behaviors. Some children are easygoing and seem to take things in their stride. They handle change well and tend to move through stressful situations such as illness, hospitalization, and family turmoil relatively smoothly. Reflux and intermittent negative feeding events may be distressful while they are happening, but they don't seem to shift the child's belief system toward the perception that "eating is always painful."

Some children are described as difficult for a variety of reasons. Greenspan (1995) refers to them as "challenging children" while Sears (1989, 1996) uses the terms "high-need" or "high-maintenance" children. These often are children who are challenged by their attempts to regulate, modulate, or interpret the complex sensory input of their environment. They may be sensitive to their surroundings and feel overwhelmed or agitated by specific sights, sounds, touches, or smells that they encounter (Wilbarger & Wilbarger, 1991). They may become upset by the faint noise of the clothes dryer that sounds loud and frightening to them. They may pull away from soothing touch because it feels like an attack. As infants and toddlers they may be colicky, finicky, irritable, and demanding (Greenspan, 1995). Some children with vulnerable sensory systems may respond with defiance. They confront adults and refuse to participate if they feel threatened. They try to control the world by attempting to organize their external world and avoid sensory input that feels threatening. Mealtimes may be very upsetting for these children and their parents because of their picky eating patterns and unpredictable emotional upsets.

Some infants and young children show the reduced affect and interaction that suggests clinical depression (Field, 1986; Herzog & Rathbun, 1982; Revol, Rochet, Maillet, Gerard, & de Villard, 1994). These infants and children may sleep excessively and have poor appetites, symptoms of anorexia, and an indifference to the person feeding them (Herzog & Rathbun, 1982; Powell & Bettes, 1992). Many of these children show a primary difficulty with sensory regulation and are underreactive to their environment rather than clinically depressed. They may withdraw to a private internal world and respond to their caregivers passively because it takes a great deal of sensory input to gain their attention. They may show a lack of interest in eating because the food served to infants and toddlers is too bland to hold their attention.

Some children are very cautious observers of the world. They move into new areas and experiences very slowly. They may be shy or have sensory issues that create the need to check things out before making a commitment. They often find change threatening and accept changes more readily if they are introduced slowly as a variation of something familiar. This approach also applies to mealtimes. Cautious children want familiarity and sameness. New foods or mealtime routines are often a major challenge (Pliner & Loewen, 1997). Some children seem to move from being cautious to being quite fearful. This may be related to a strong memory of a negative event such as choking or severe reflux, or of having been forced to eat a food. Occasionally, children will be afraid of anything associated with eating and will cry or become aggressive when they smell food or see a spoon or cup.

In contrast, other children are strong risk-takers. They exhibit a fearlessness that often reflects an impulsive lack of awareness of the consequences of their actions. They are always on the go as they dive headlong into new situations and experiences. This impulsivity may be related to difficulties with sensory modulation (Greenspan, 1995) or may become part of a later personality style that is not necessarily predicted by early emotional traits (Kennedy, 1996; Kennedy & Lipsitt, 1998). They may crave physical input because they underreact to many sensations. At the table they may rapidly grab for food or utensils that are inappropriate for their developmental skills. They impulsively run from the table with a mouthful of unchewed food or with a straw pushed toward the back of the mouth. When they are frustrated at the meal, they may have temper tantrums and aggressively throw food and dishes. Their behavior can be dangerous to themselves and to others.

The Influence of the Parent's Emotional State and Temperament

It is not easy to be the parent of a child with special needs. When these needs include challenges with feeding and mealtimes, many parents may feel overwhelmed, depressed, angry, or afraid that their child will never be able to eat well (Singer et al., 1996). High levels of stress may be related to the parent's belief systems, emotional state, and coping style prior to the birth of the child with a disability (Lambrenos, Weindling, Calam, & Cox, 1996). The parent's emotional state and coping style is a critical component of a child's mealtime. Parents who are relaxed and easygoing in their approach to life participate in mealtimes with less stress than do other adults. They can deal with more mess and handle unexpected events at the meal with less stress. At times, though, they may not see something as a problem that concerns the feeding therapist.

In contrast, parents who are depressed most of the time will have difficulty experiencing and integrating positive experiences. They may become pessimistic and believe that only bad things will happen to them and their child. Several studies have shown that depressed mothers were less sensitively attuned to their infants, and were less affirming and more negating of infant experience (Field, 1998; Murray, Fiori-Cowley, Hooper, & Cooper, 1996). Depression during the mother's pregnancy may even affect her infant's ability to cope with the world after birth. Zuckerman, Bauchner, Parker, and Cabral (1990) found that mothers who experienced high levels of depression during pregnancy were 2.6 times more likely to have infants who were inconsolable or cried excessively as newborns. When parents feel overwhelmed or depressed, mealtimes can become more than they can handle. They may feel less bonded and connected to their infant. They may have difficulty reading and responding to the child's mealtime communication. When children receive a low level of affect and interaction from their primary caregivers, they may withdraw and act depressed. They may give parents fewer cues to their needs and desires at mealtime. Mealtime messages may be confusing or conflicting. Some depressed parents may forget to prepare meals and feed their child or themselves.

Anger is a stage in the grieving process as parents cope with the death of the dream child they imagined during the pregnancy. In most instances, they did not anticipate the birth of a child with exceptional needs. On their journey to acceptance, they pass through the same stages described by Kubler-Ross in patients and families anticipating physical death (Bruce, Schultz, & Smyrnios, 1996). Most parents go through periods where they are angry with the child and with professionals. Therapists must understand that the parents' anger usually is not directed at something they have done. It may be a generalized anger at the loss of the normal child. Some parents may have a more deep-seated anger at themselves or others. They lose patience easily and may strike out at the child when they are frustrated.

Some adults do not feel safe unless they are in control of all situations in their lives. They are particularly vulnerable when parenting a child with special needs. Everything about these children is unpredictable, and this is upsetting to a person who finds reassurance and security in being able to predict and control the world. These parents find it particularly difficult to share mealtime roles and let their children be responsible for what they eat and how much they eat. They may push their children to eat more or to stop eating before they are full.

Parents may be overprotective of children because of their own fears. If a child has been very ill or fragile, the parent may fear that the child will die. If there has been a difficult pregnancy or birth, they are grateful that the child is alive; however, the difficulties that they have experienced may become a shadow that reminds them at every moment that the child could become ill again or die. They often are overly cautious about giving the child new food textures or in encouraging the mastery of new skills. Overprotective parents do not want their children to be unhappy. They recognize the stresses and difficulties that their children have overcome and want to make life easier for them. As a result, they often give in to what the child wants and are slow to set limits. Their children may adopt the parents' cautious approach to experiences and have difficulty moving toward more complex feeding skills. They may become picky eaters who demand that parents prepare special meals that they then refuse to eat!

Perfectionism is a learned approach to life that children adopt from their parents. A study by Vieth and Trull (1999) showed that the degree of perfectionism in college students was positively associated with similar levels in the same-sexed parent. The daughter of a perfectionistic mother is more likely to hold unreasonably high expectations than the son will. When standards of perfection are present, parents of children with feeding difficulties may not recognize small changes because these may not be "good enough." They become discouraged about the child's slow progress and may push the child to work hard. Children of these parents may unwittingly adopt similar beliefs or feel that they personally are unacceptable as they are because they are not "good enough."

Observing and Understanding the Mealtime Environment

We can describe the physical, sensory, communication, and learning characteristics that surround each meal as the mealtime environment. The total mealtime environment incorporates the various influences that have been discussed in this chapter. Each family, consciously or unconsciously, incorporates these elements and influences into its values and coping strategies. Elements of the mealtime environment support or limit a child's ability to participate fully in the meal. Different children and parents will be affected by environmental elements of the meal in various ways, depending upon their physical, sensory, cognitive, and emotional needs. Thus, Jordan, who is very sensitive, may be unable to eat when the television is blaring or when his sisters and parents are arguing. Cathie has no problems with sensory processing and puts all of this noise into the background and ignores it. Maria, whose son is a picky eater and gains weight poorly, feels rejected and overly responsible because she grew up in a family and culture that strongly equated eating with love. She feels that Samuel's rejection of the food she prepares is a rejection of her love and nurturing. She sometimes pushes him to eat more and takes over his role of deciding what and how much to eat. She feels that this communicates her love to him in the same way her mother used food to let her know how much she cared.

The physical environment of the mealtime refers primarily to the physical comfort and support received by the child and the parent. The child's feeding and oral motor skills are strongly influenced by selection of a chair or position on the adult's lap. When children are physically supported appropriately, they have the head and trunk stability that they need to develop the oral motor skills required for eating and drinking. Timmy sits in a high chair with a saddle seat that separates his legs and holds his pelvis against the back of the chair. He is well supported but able to move and interact with the food and those who feed him. An earlier seating solution used straps and a restraining vest to hold him in the chair. He couldn't move and became angry, crying for most meals. His mother became extremely concerned when he seemed to give up and no longer showed any interest in eating.

Many programs look at only the child's physical environment. However, the comfort of the adult who is feeding the child is critical to the success of the meal. When the parent's body is poorly supported, fatigue increases, resulting in physical and emotional stress. Children sense adult stresses but often misinterpret them, assuming that the resulting tension is their fault. Kyle sat on his mother's lap for meals because it was difficult to give him the support he needed in a chair. His head flopped back or pushed strongly when his legs got stiff. His mother sat in a straight chair at the kitchen table and rested Kyle's head on her arm. Her arm became very tired, and her shoulder ached as the meal progressed. She was tense and irritable by the end of the meal. Kyle sensed that something was the matter with his mother and tried to cheer her up by pushing back and spluttering food as he attempted to smile and vocalize. The resulting tension usually resulted in coughing and choking, and a miserable end to the meal.

The sensory environment incorporates all of the sensory areas that are involved in the mealtime. The physical space for the meal may be calm and quiet or noisy and chaotic. A family may eat while watching television or to the beat of loud music. When Mark is fed in a busy school cafeteria or the family kitchen with his five brothers, he often cannot eat. His body becomes more uncoordinated because of the noise, smells, and random visual input of the sensory environment. Jacob experiences extreme sensory discomfort when eating, but he often eats more when he is distracted by an active sensory environment in a restaurant or in front of a favorite video. He seems to use the sensory distraction to refocus his attention, and mentally and emotionally move away from the discomfort created by the food he is eating.

Other aspects of the sensory environment play significant roles for some children. When a child eats slowly, food may become cold and unappetizing. The smell of wet or dirty diapers can reduce everyone's interest in eating and socializing. A child's preference for spicy or bland foods interacts with a parent's personal beliefs about appropriate food choices for a young child. Aaron's parents find it difficult to understand that their toddler wants to begin each meal by chewing on pickles or lemons. Ramon's sensory system rejects hot spicy food, and his parents feel rejected by the rest of the family when they do not serve him the spicy foods associated with their culture's meals and celebrations.

The communication environment predominates at every mealtime. Even when there is very little talking among participants, non-verbal signals are highly expressive. Fatigue, frustration, anger, indifference, and acceptance are expressed in body language and tone of voice. Patience or impatience often are communicated, especially if the child takes a long time to eat or is messy. Some parents offer their children choices at each meal; others do not. Some will include the child in mealtime conversations; others talk about the child, but not to him. Feelings of fear and discouragement intervene when the child doesn't eat enough or vomits everything at the end of the meal. Casey's mother is the only one who can feed him. She has learned how to hold him and put the spoon into his mouth so that he doesn't bite down on it. He is afraid to let anyone else feed him and cries when his father or grandmother tries to give him his dinner. His mother feels overwhelmed by her responsibility. Cameron's parents both feed him. They understand both his needs and their own, and mealtimes communicate a feeling of agreement and harmony. Trisha's parents also take turns feeding her. Each holds different standards for the meal. Her father is comfortable allowing her to decide how much and which foods she will eat. If she eats little or refuses to eat foods that are served, he knows she eventually will become hungry and eat more at the next meal. When her mother feeds her, she goes to the kitchen to prepare other foods when Trisha says she doesn't like something. She fixes macaroni and cheese and Trisha spits it out, saying she wants spaghetti. When she brings the spaghetti back, Trisha has a tantrum and throws the food on the floor, saying she really wants ice cream. Each parent is critical of the other and makes sarcastic remarks in front of Trisha.

Mealtime discussions or non-verbal communication may center on food and what the child is eating or not eating. There may be a general unspoken dialogue of agreement or disagreement that permeates the mealtime. This can create tremendous pressures for the child and elicit counterpressures that result in power contests or learned helplessness. Children can keep their parents very busy at meals with activities that are only peripherally related to eating. All children want to belong and to feel valued and important. Dreikurs and Stoltz (1964) said children are expert observers but they make many errors in interpreting what they observe. They often draw the wrong conclusions as they observe their interactions with others. Unfortunately, they often select mistaken ways of feeling valued that are then misinterpreted by adults.

Children who do not eat well may discover mealtime strategies that help them feel important. Joey felt valued only when he received special attention. He experienced repeated hospitalizations as an infant. Excitement or emotional stress often triggered his severe gastroesophageal reflux. He loved the attention of the nursing staff but received it primarily when he vomited and someone came to change the bedsheets. Each time he went home from the hospital, his parents noticed that his vomiting increased. Carl argued constantly about which foods he would and would not eat. His father said that he must eat all of the food on his plate before leaving the table. Carl admired his father and noticed how powerful he was. He wanted to be just like his dad, but he didn't want to eat many foods. He knew that no one could make him eat vegetables, and he liked the feeling of power he had when he refused to open his mouth for them. Even his father could not make him swallow the carrots! Elena became furious when her parents forced her to eat. On some days she did not feel well, and no one seemed to understand. She tried to tell them, but she couldn't find the right words, and no one seemed to listen anyway. Her mother and aunt held her down and pried her mouth open. They filled it with food and held her nose until she swallowed it. She felt hurt and angry that they would treat her like this. All she wanted to do was hurt them back and get even. She noticed how anxious and upset her family became when she did not eat and decided to stop eating entirely—even on days when she felt well. Mandy was a twin who had been born prematurely. She and her sister both had difficulties learning to suck from the bottle and take food from the spoon. Her sister caught up quickly, and her parents were very excited when Martha finished the whole jar of pears. They encouraged Mandy to eat her serving of pears. Mandy tried to eat them, but her tongue pushed most of the food from her mouth. The more she tried, the less successful she felt. One day, Martha picked up the spoon and fed herself. Mandy watched but decided not to try because she knew that she could never succeed with something that looked so hard. It felt safer to just watch and never try new things. She hated feeling stupid.

These are discouraged children (Dreikurs & Stoltz, 1964). They observe the communication and interaction about their feeding issues, and attempt to feel wanted and accepted by demanding extra attention, seeking power, enacting revenge, or giving up. These attempts to feel valued become mixed with the underlying issues that caused the feeding difficulty.

Mealtimes offer constant opportunities for learning. Foods offer sensory and physical information and challenges. Mastery opportunities can be created that meet the child's current abilities and needs. If children are fearful or resistant, there is no energy or focus for learning. High levels of negative emotion will create strong memories of dislike and resistance for the foods and experiences that accompany the meal. Pressure to eat or to perform at the meal generally is counterproductive and prevents children from learning and doing what adults would like them to.

A physician told Gerald's parents that he was severely retarded and could not learn beyond the level of a 4-month-old. They knew that Gerald tried to feed himself at mealtimes and was very interested in more complicated foods. Nevertheless, they continued to feed him pureed consistencies because they knew that young babies could not be expected to chew or feed themselves. Sharon's family also had been told that her development was delayed. Even though the doctor warned them that they should not expect changes in her skills or behavior, they noticed each small change and celebrated each tiny landmark. Mealtimes were fun and offered many opportunities to explore the food that was served. Sharon was curious about her sensory world and began to make her own discoveries. Each meal became a natural classroom. Soon she was eating the same foods as her brother and sister and knew the names of each food and utensil.

Mealtime environments are like a giant mirror that reflects the most relevant influences that guide a meal. The feeding therapist can begin to understand the most important elements that influence a feeding and mealtime program simply by observing without judging. With understanding comes the possibility of partnership to address changes that are mutually desired by the parent, therapist and child.

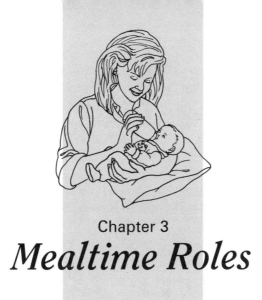

Chapter 3
Mealtime Roles

Humans are born more vulnerable and dependent than most species. In a broad sense, the roles of feeder and baby are clearly defined. The adult must provide nourishment and the baby must eat if the species is to survive. The baby's ability to survive depends on the skills and capabilities of both the adult and child. The adults must understand that the baby needs to be fed and provide that nourishment in a way the baby can use for growth. The baby must be able to take in the food and communicate when more is needed. In the simplest sense, the roles are that of "the one who feeds" and "the one who eats"—the feeder and the eater. However, we really are much more complicated than that. We need emotional nourishment as well as physical nourishment. The mealtime becomes a time where a very vulnerable infant is completely dependent on the adult for nourishment of the body and the spirit.

Our own experiences with physical and emotional nourishment influence our adult style or interpretation of these roles as feeders. The baby's skills at birth, blended with individual personality, temperament, and experiences, influence its interpretation of the role of eater.

Whether we are a parent, grandparent, therapist, nurse, teacher, or other caregiver, we understand feeding from our own history. Some of this history comes from our personal beliefs and culture, while some comes directly from our direct experiences. We all eat. We have all been fed. Some of us can remember our early mealtime interactions. We can imagine ourselves as newborn infants, dependent and looking to "our adults" to provide all of our needs. We can imagine ourselves as toddlers and young children exploring the nourishment of our bodies and emotions.

All societies of the world would agree on the adult responsibility of feeding the child. The interpretation of how that is to be done is personal—personal for the adult and personal for the child. The most important aspect of the feeding, then, becomes the personal communication between the child and the adult. Not all babies need exactly the same nurturing, and not all adults can provide the same type of nurturing. Although the physical need for food will be the same for babies, the style in which it is provided will vary. The core of a successful feeding relationship seems to be in a sensitive communication where the baby lets the feeder know what and how much is needed for physical and emotional nourishment, and the feeder strives to provide those needs.

Mealtimes with a child, therefore, involve a nourishing partnership of two people, usually the parent and the child. Many of us nourish children. Mothers and fathers, grandparents, aunts and uncles, siblings, friends, and day-care providers all share mealtimes with children. Children with special feeding needs expand their mealtime guest list to include lactation specialists, feeding specialists, teachers, nurses, and others. As we continue this discussion of mealtime roles, we will refer to the feeder as the parent in order to describe any adult who assumes the parenting role of giving the child a meal. The parent-child feeding relationship is the closest and, in many ways, the basis of our understanding of mealtime interactions. To refer to the person feeding the baby as the feeder seems too impersonal for this intimate relationship. The roles we describe and the communications we discuss are based on the give-and-take communications seen in the nourishing of children.

◾ The Mealtime Dance

Feeding can be described as a dance in which the child and the parent are partners. As in any well-choreographed dance, each partner's skills influence the timing, smoothness, and overall outcome of the performance. The mealtime dance is influenced by the ability of the mealtime partners to communicate effectively and give and take as the dance routine changes and becomes more complicated. As in any dance, one partner leads and the other follows. This particular dance seems to flow best when the baby is in the lead and the parent in the supporting role. When the mealtime performance is smooth, the child will grow, enjoy the feeding process, and progressively develop more complex mealtime skills. When all is going well, the parent also will enjoy the process and allow the child to develop increasing skills and mastery over the food presented. There are many different dance steps and interpretations of the music in a dance routine just as there are many different communications at the mealtime. Some interpretations make the dance flow more smoothly while others interfere with it.

Babies and parents both bring their own skills and experiences to the mealtime. The babies' needs change with age and maturation of feeding skills. As these needs change, parents must change their ways of support. How well babies communicate their emerging needs and how well parents understand and support these needs will significantly influence the mealtime feeding relationship.

Satter (1983, 1987, 1990, 1999) describes the evolving roles of child and parent in this mealtime dance as a division of responsibility. She writes that parents are responsible for what is presented to eat and the manner in which it is presented. Children are responsible for how much and even whether they eat. Put simply, the parent is responsible for a sensitive preparation and presentation of food. The baby's changing needs dictate the changes in food types and quantities offered, utensils used, where meals are served, and the manner in which the food is presented. Babies are responsible for what they eat of the foods offered and how much. Because this is such a finely choreographed dance, both sides have a responsibility to communicate with the other. Babies do best when they are in the lead role and the parent is the follower, the support role (Satter, 1990). When parents allow the child to accept responsibility for eating or not eating what is offered, they use the natural consequence of hunger and the child's internal body signals to guide a meal (Dreikurs & Stoltz, 1964).

Many authors have described early infant stages of development and attachment as they influence feeding and parent behaviors that support feeding. The following discussion on optimal feeding practices and roles are blended from the early studies of Ainsworth and Bell (1969), feeding scales of Chatoor, Menvielle, and O'Donnell (1989), Price (1983), and Satter (1983, 1987, 1990, 1999) in combination with the experiences of the authors of this book.

Birth to 3 Months—Homeostasis and Mealtimes

The first three months of life have been called the homeostasis stage, or the state of regulation, for the infant (Greenspan, 1985; Satter, 1990). During these first months, infants and parents both have tasks. The infant's job is primarily to stabilize biologic and neurologic functions. The infant has spent the first 9 months of life in utero and needs time to settle into the outside world. While the infant is learning to eat, sleep, and handle all the excitement of this new environment, the parents' job is to learn to understand the infant's needs and to respond in such a way as to support the baby's regulation of state. At this stage, parents are learning to adapt their feeding style to match the baby's needs.

Parents and babies have different roles during this newborn period. Parents are responsible for decisions about what to eat. They make the choice to breast-feed or bottle-feed. If they decide to bottle-feed, then they need to choose formulas, bottles, and nipple styles. If all goes well, babies use their natural skills to root, suck, and swallow. Babies are responsible for taking in what they need. They are learning to relate the hunger feeling in their tummy to feedings followed by hunger satiation as the meal progresses. They eat when they need to and sleep when they need to. Parents learn to listen to the baby and notice what works best. As they mature, babies become more able to let them know when they are hungry, when they are full, what position feels better for feeding, what nipple works best, and when they need to burp.

Positive feeding interactions will depend on the capabilities of both the infant and the parent (Satter, 1990). For feedings to be successful, babies need intact feeding mechanisms. They need to be healthy and medically stable. Babies must become alert enough to engage their parents' attention and let them know what they need. They must be able to respond without becoming overstimulated as their parents try to please them (Morgan, 1987). Parents, on the other hand, need to be sensitive to the cues of the baby and have a desire to please, to work it out during those first few months. Working it out has different meanings in different cultures and in different families. The exact "how" of the feedings (i.e., bottles, nipples, positions, presentations) is not as important as the baby's ability to succeed with the chosen approach or to let the parent know when that approach isn't working. There can be a great deal of flexibility and diversity in the feedings as long as both parent and child are nurtured in the feeding relationship.

Feeding difficulties can arise when infants or parents cannot fulfill their responsibilities in the mealtime process. Babies must be able to achieve physiological stability and be able to minimally communicate. Parents need to be emotionally healthy and sensitively responsive. A baby who has physical limitations, difficulties with sucking and swallowing, or who is medically unstable, may not take in enough food or give appropriate and consistent feeding cues. A parent who is emotionally unavailable or who has other limitations in sensitivity and responsiveness may not be able to read and respond to the baby's cues. When the skills are not there on either side, the relationship can falter and feeding may not go well. During these first 3 months, babies can experience poor growth or colic. Feedings may be stressful to both the parent and the baby. When mealtimes deteriorate in these early months, help with feeding is essential.

4 to 7 Months—Socialization at Mealtime

From about 4 to 7 months, the infant has been described as being in the attachment stage (Satter, 1990; Pridham, 1987). In this stage, the infant's role focuses on learning to engage and interact with the environment. The infant has achieved a more regulated biological and neurophysiological state. By now the infant usually has an eating and sleeping routine. The infant's job is to give clear and specific cues about needs for hunger, sleep, discomfort, and attention. The parents, by now, have learned to read and promptly respond to those cues.

Because the infant is comfortable and secure in these basic biological functions, she has time to play with learning to engage others and interact with the environment. Because the infant trusts she will be fed when hungry, offered sleep when tired, comforted when upset, she can feel secure that her bodily and emotional needs are being met. Movement becomes more purposeful. Infants can physically and socially reach out into the world around them. Social smiles begin and contribute to "falling in love" (Greenspan & Lourie, 1981). Reciprocal communication occurs when infants and parents coo and "make eyes" at each other.

There are a number of ways parents can help infants understand their own biological functions and feel calm enough to reach out and interact with others at feedings. Feedings must be predictable and support the infant's changing needs during the first 7 months.

Feeding disorders during these months complicate the feeding relationship. Feeding difficulties can be related to child issues, parent issues, or both. Some babies have medical problems that cause poor organization and skill development in feeding. Neurological, respiratory, gastrointestinal, and metabolic difficulties will negatively influence the baby's abilities to suck, swallow, and grow. Sometimes the feeding issues are more closely related to unsatisfied feeding interactions. Stresses or problems in the feeding relationship at this age can upset the gastrointestinal system or exacerbate existing medical conditions influencing the gut. These stresses can trigger vomiting or diarrhea and contribute to poor weight gain. We all have experienced feeling upset with a partner at a meal. For some, this may lead to loss of appetite or indigestion. For others, it can result in an upset stomach or vomiting. Young infants often have similar reactions. When there is interplay of medical and interaction issues, mealtimes become very negative for both baby and parent.

Parent and Baby Roles During Infancy

■ **Parents decide the type of feeding for the baby.**

Parents make decisions regarding breast- and bottle-feeding based on experience, cultural expectations, comfort level, work schedules, and a number of personal factors. Once the decision is made, the parent offers the feeding and works to help the baby succeed. It usually takes the mother and baby time to figure out the mechanics of the feedings.

■ **Parents provide an appropriate flow rate of milk or formula.**

The breast-feeding mother needs to understand fully the breast-feeding process so she can ensure the best timing for milk letdown, milk flow, and continuation of milk through the whole feeding. Bottle-fed babies should be provided with nipples with the correct flow. Liquid coming too fast or too slow can be disconcerting for the infant who is trying desperately to understand the entire feeding process and feel safe.

■ **Parents feed promptly when the baby is hungry.**

Babies need to learn that eating can satisfy certain feelings within themselves, such as hunger. They learn that hunger means, "I need to eat," and eating means, "I no longer feel that uncomfortable feeling in my belly." Feeding becomes synonymous with nurturing for babies. A baby who is fed promptly when hungry is comfortable, satisfied, and safe. This helps the baby learn to trust the parents and sets the foundation for love and attachment. Babies who are not fed promptly can become confused about hunger cues and about their relationship with the people feeding them.

■ **Parents provide a physically safe, supported, and comfortable feeding environment.**

Babies should be held firmly but not too firmly. Restrictive holding can be not only uncomfortable for the baby but also discourage adequate food intake. If a baby is held too loosely, it is difficult for the baby to feel secure and stable enough for good control of the sucking-swallowing-breathing process. Proper holding enables the baby to hold the head in a comfortable position with a tucked chin. The head is not way back, and the chin is not cramped too far forward. Arms are comfortably forward and at the side or midline, but not loosely hanging out away from the body. Babies need to be warm and comfortable. They also may appreciate the meal more if they are wearing a dry diaper.

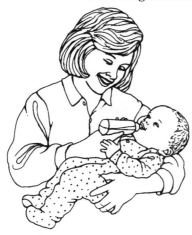

■ **Parents present the breast or the bottle at the appropriate angle.**

When the baby is held securely and positioned as just described for breast- or bottle-feeding, the milk can be presented at a good angle. The angle should allow continuous access to the liquid as the baby compresses and sucks on the bottle or breast. Holding the bottle too low is both uncomfortable when the baby tries to grasp the nipple and allows increased air intake. Holding the bottle too high does not allow the baby to comfortably cup the tongue around the nipple for easy sucking. Jiggling and wiggling the nipple can be disruptive for breast- or bottle-feeding. It can interfere with the rhythm of the suck-swallow-breathe process and can distract the baby from adequate intake.

■ **Parents provide a stable environment that minimizes sensory interruptions.**

Constant face-wiping, unnecessary burping, jiggling, wiggling, and other sensory interruptions can be distracting and unsettling for the baby. Extraneous talking, loud or arrythmical music, and environmental distractions can draw the baby's attention away from the meal. The baby loses control of the pace and the focus. The meal may end before the baby is actually finished with the feeding.

■ **Babies give permission for the nipple to enter the mouth.**

Parents can stimulate the newborn rooting reflex to allow the baby to open the mouth to let them know he is hungry and it is okay to put the bottle or breast in his mouth. Touching the cheek in this way gives the baby some beginning control at mealtime and is important in the trust-building process. Getting permission is a parent's way of giving and trusting the baby's control. As babies get older, they can respond to the sight of the bottle and give or deny permission more quickly rather than waiting for the nipple to touch the lips.

■ **Babies need mealtime socialization.**

Social pauses are those important breaks in feeding (Pridham, 1987) when the baby looks up at the feeder and smiles, reaches for a face or a finger, and "falls in love" (Greenspan, 1985). Babies 3 months and older stop for these social pauses. When they feel secure and know they will be fed as much and as often as they need, they will feel comfortable in mixing social play with the serious work of food intake.

Parents need to encourage and support these social pauses, but not to turn them into a party! Smiling, talking, or cooing softly helps the baby feel loved, safe, and noticed. These gentle interactions create a pleasant social atmosphere for eating. It is important that the interactions do not become overwhelming. This can distract the baby from taking in the appropriate amount of milk.

■ **Babies set the pace of the meal.**

By letting the baby give permission to place the nipple or breast in the mouth, the parent lets the baby start the feeding when ready. The baby needs to set the pace for the rest of the feeding and lead the mealtime dance. The parent should follow. Some babies are serious feeders, and focus well on the feeding and eat quite rapidly. Others need more pauses or playtime and take longer for the feeding.

■ **Babies let parents know when it is time for burping.**

Some babies need frequent burping. Others take a whole feeding without needing to burp. Babies can tell parents when a burp is coming, and may pause or pull away and stop the feeding. New parents may burp their child too often at first but quickly learn to understand the difference between the need to burp and a social pause. Burping too often can be disruptive, and the baby can lose control over the pace of the meal. The baby may become confused or irritated if the feeder interrupts serious feeding attempts with position changes and unwanted burping. Frequent interruptions can distract the baby from taking adequate nutritional intake.

■ **Babies stop the feeding when they have had enough.**

Healthy babies know how much they need to grow. The amount required differs from baby to baby. Studies have shown that babies grow best when they lead and parents follow (Satter, 1999; Morgan, 1987). This includes the when, how much, and pace of meals. Some babies take more food less often. Others eat more frequent smaller meals. Stopping when the baby is done shows the parents' respect and trust in the baby to lead. Pushing the baby to take more when he or she is clearly done can interfere with the baby's trust in the feeder and can lead to an unbalanced mealtime dance. As we look at Satter's division of responsibility, we remember it is the feeder's responsibility to provide developmentally appropriate foods in a supportive manner at appropriate times throughout the day. It is the baby's responsibility to decide what and how much to eat. When babies are in control of their own intake, most of them grow appropriately.

Emerging Independence

Between 8 months and 3 years of age, the baby's needs change, and the parent's role also must change. Mahler, Pine, and Bergman (1975) describe this stage as that of separation and individuation. During this stage, infants actively travel the road to independence. They begin to exert more and more control over their environment and the people around them. The child's job in this stage is one of ever-expanding independence, of exploration, and of trying new ways. The child has more physical skills now and is able to personally explore more aspects of the mealtime routine. In the beginning of this long-emerging stage, the child may be playing with food in the mouth; playing with textures; and picking up, dropping, or throwing food. She will clearly let the feeder know *if* and *when* she will open her mouth for a new food. She'll reach for the spoon and bang a percussion symphony during the previously peaceful mealtime. Part of achieving independence is an active exploration complete with challenging rules and routines. As the child gets older, she will check out the rules about where to eat, about throwing food and utensils, about spitting food, and about finger painting with food. She will stop the meal and then try to get back up in the high chair to see if she can continue it. She will grab the spoons and forks and struggle with her own mastery—even if it does begin with upside-down spoons in the nose or hair! As the child reaches the end of this stage at age 3, she may see if she can demand (and get away with) a potato chip diet!

This can be an exciting and also exasperating time for parents. Their role is to encourage and support the child's independence and exploration while still defining the rules and boundaries of the mealtime. Limits create safe boundaries for children. If parents don't provide them, children will push until they find the parent's limits! Children are much more apt to try something new, be it a food, a spoon or a cup, if their parents are watching, modeling, and supporting. Some parents hold the child on their lap as they introduce new foods. Parents should continue their responsibilities as defined by Satter (1990, 1999), and provide developmentally appropriate food and utensil choices, which demonstrates respect for their maturing child and encouragement for new phases of mealtime development. The child, however, remains responsible for *what* and *how much* he or she eats.

Let's take a more in-depth look at parents' roles and responsibilities as they let the child take the lead while providing support and acceptance of the child's initiative and need for exploration and independence.

Parent and Baby Roles Between 6 and 12 Months

- **Babies indicate when they are hungry. Parents respond by offering food.**

  The feeding schedule followed during the first 6 months of life emerged as the parent began to understand the hunger demands of the baby. This routine will undergo gradual changes as the baby begins smooth pureed foods and finger foods. Parents need to change with the child.

- **Babies mature and indicate readiness for more complex foods. Parents read those cues and present new foods.**

  Babies move from solely breast milk or formula to smooth pureed foods, lumpy foods, solid finger foods, and finally, more textured table foods. Older babies will let their parents know when they are ready to make these transitions. They may look with interest as the parent eats or reach for what the parent is eating or drinking. Perhaps the parent or pediatrician thinks it is time to introduce these foods. Babies will let them know if their hunch was right. Parents need to progress slowly with taste and texture changes as their babies let them know they are ready.

- **Babies gain more skills for sitting upright at mealtimes. Parents understand the need for a change in mealtime position and provide appropriate seating.**

  A baby's developmental motor skills dictates the change from being fed while semireclining in the arms to being fed while sitting on a lap, in an infant seat, or in a high chair. The baby still needs physical support to provide the stable foundation from which to move the fine motor muscles of eating. Parents provide the physical seating support that is best for the child at each change in physical skill development.

■ **Babies and parents create a social atmosphere around the meal.**

Mealtime is a social time, but not *too* social. Parents need to talk in quiet tones, and be there to smile and interact with the baby. As the child becomes older, more social conversation is appropriate. Care must be taken, however, not to overwhelm and distract the child. The attentive social interactions are an important part of the expanding mealtime world. They are the part of mealtime that goes beyond nourishing the body.

■ **Babies give permission for the food to enter their mouths. Parents listen and respect their baby's choice.**

As parents respond to a child's cues of readiness for new food tastes and textures, they must take care to respond sensitively. Parents can offer the food from the spoon, but must wait for the baby to give permission to put it in the mouth. The child may give permission by opening the mouth, grabbing the spoon, or leaning toward the food. Parents learn to recognize these cues and wait for them. Babies usually will look at the parent or open their mouths when they are ready. This helps them feel safe and in control of the meal. Forcing or pushing food at a closed mouth invites a power contest and an unpleasant interaction.

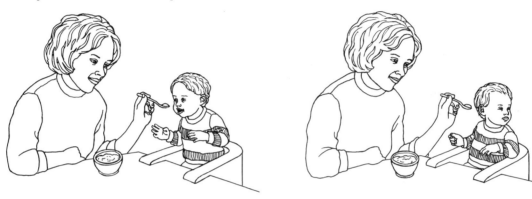

■ **Parents provide encouragement, encouragement, and encouragement!**

Babies learn by the parents' tone of voice and smiles, and by their own positive experiences with food that "this food stuff is okay! It looked different, tasted different, and felt different, but it's not bad!" Babies need supportive adults around when they take the risk to try new foods.

■ **Babies decide the pace of the meal.**

Babies at this age find very creative ways to pace the meal. Some open the mouth widely and cannot get the feeder to shovel it in fast enough. Others carefully take tiny mouthfuls, exploring and contemplating each one. To take breaks in the meal, they may look away, play with the food, drop some food on the floor and watch where it goes, or actually push the feeder away. Parents must be respectful of the child's need to control the pace if all is to go well at the mealtime.

■ **Babies satisfy their need for sensory exploration by playing with food.**

Exploring food is a baby's way of checking it out before it goes into the mouth. Babies become familiar with food by touching it, smearing it on the tray and in the hair, squishing it, and putting it in and taking it out of the mouth. Some of the messiness of this stage comes from unrefined coordination. Squishing a piece of bread en route to the mouth may be a direct result of the baby's inability to grasp it carefully. Experience with foods actually is very helpful in development of emerging finger-coordination skills! The different weights, textures, sizes, and shapes of finger foods provide excellent lessons for finger control. Parents need to remember to support the baby's need for exploration. It is messy, but the sensorimotor learning that occurs will lead

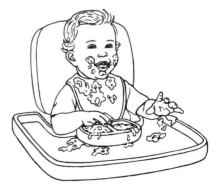

toward neater eating. Early demands for neatness can interfere with the child's willingness to try new foods later.

■ **Parents respect a baby's caution in trying new foods.**

Babies will differ in their enthusiasm for solids, and they let the feeder know how they feel. Sensitive parents will follow their lead and respect differences. Not all babies like green beans. Think about it! Not all adults like green beans! Babies have taste preferences that need to be respected. When parents offer a variety of different flavors, babies are exposed to many different tastes. Many babies thrive on the flavors and variety of commercially available pureed foods. Others reject the more bland flavors and demand more excitement in their diet. Today there is a greater variety of commercially available foods and food combinations, and many parents make their own baby foods.

■ **Babies want to help.**

Babies initially reach for everything, and, of course, bring it to the mouth. This may start out as exploration and quickly move into control. "I want to do it myself!" This is how children master the developmental skills of self-feeding. They should be supported in doing so. Parents must remember, however, that children want this independence in varying degrees. Some are very happy to be fed and make much less effort to do it themselves. Others want to do everything. It is important to honor and respect these differences.

■ **Parents offer choices at mealtimes.**

Parents learn to offer more than one food at a meal. The baby will eat as much as he wants of each food without feeling the pressure of eating one food that he may like only minimally. Serving a familiar food along with a new food gives parents the opportunity to create a safe environment in which to introduce new foods. It gives the child the possibility of making a choice and of being in charge. At one meal, the child may choose to eat lots of cheese. At the next meal, he may eat apples and at the next meal lots of bread. With continued choices and a wide variety of foods, the nutritional balance will even out!

■ **Babies let parents know when the meal is done.**

Parents must listen to the baby. Most babies find obvious ways to let their parents know they are done. Some stop opening their mouths. Others begin playing with the food. Some spit out more than they take in. Others toss the bowl or the spoon, or push them away. It is important to respect the varied cues that the baby is full. It may take a period of trial and error to find out if the baby is really full, tired of a specific food, or just asking for a pause. Most parents can check their initial interpretation in a sensitive way by offering the food again inquisitively and respecting the baby's response.

The Independent Toddler

Mahler et al. (1975) describe the stage of independence as one of separation and individuation that lasts from 8 to 36 months for a reason. It starts early and keeps on going! Most parents actually describe the "independence stage" for many years. Once babies begin to be more mobile, they are capable of moving wherever they like. They can crawl into another room and get into cupboards, climb to new levels to look out of a window, or walk away from any situation. The ability to move farther from the parent often begins to define this stage. These newfound mobility skills and accompanying fine motor skills, paired with an internal desire to "do it myself," can make this Age of the Independent Toddler a challenge.

Brazelton (1993) suggests that "more than any other area of development, feeding is an arena in which parents and baby work out the continuing struggle between dependence (being fed) and independence (feeding oneself). Independence must win. Pushing a child to eat is the surest way to create a problem."

The drive for independence significantly influences mealtimes. Until now the child has been very much dependent on the parent. The baby placed in an infant seat or in parent's arms to be fed usually has stayed there. Now, all of a sudden, the child can climb out of the high chair. Hands, once unskilled, now can reach for and grasp finger foods or the spoon. Cups filled with juice can be tipped over or thrown. The nice control the parent once had over the neatness of the meal disappears. Food exploration that initially happened in the mouth now happens all over the high-chair tray, between the fingers, and in the hair. Toddlers experiment with everything, including "the rules." What does this food feel like? What does this food taste like? Can I crush this food? Does it bounce or splat when it drops on the floor? What does Mommy do when I throw this? What if I only eat the bread? What if I do not want any food at all? These explorers desperately want to be independent, and at the same time, they desperately want to know the rules. They need a routine and a structure from which to seek out new mealtime adventures. Mealtimes seem to work best for these toddlers when the parent provides support for the emerging independence while providing the safe and secure "home base" from which the exploration takes place. Parents must learn to pick their battles carefully. The child needs to learn the mealtime rules, but the rules need not be so restrictive that they don't allow independence and experimentation.

Parents must give toddlers the opportunity to try new foods and utensils. Toddlers need practice with spoons, forks, cups, and straws. They are rapidly learning to enjoy a variety of new tastes and textures of foods. Biting and chewing skills refine with practice until most foods can be eaten safely. These children move from bottle drinking to cup and straw drinking. They move from purees to solids. As Satter (1983) describes so well, "Parents are in charge of what is presented to eat and the manner in which it is presented. They are NOT responsible for how much the child eats, whether he eats and how his body turns out." Each child, therefore, is responsible for eating enough and for choosing which foods he will eat. The old adage applies well here. "You can lead a horse to water, but you cannot make him drink." This is true with children as well as horses! Parents can offer, but they cannot *make* a child eat. Any parent who has tried to force a child to eat knows it does not work. You may win that battle, but you may have started a food war, and children always win in food wars. In addition, when adults win a power contest, they inadvertently teach children that bigger people can use force with smaller people when they want to impose their own way. This is not something that most of us consciously choose to teach children.

Children who have medical issues influencing feeding may become confused about how much to eat. Many times their internal regulation system is not telling them to eat or to eat enough. Parents, worried about their child's growth and development, may be tempted to force, coerce, or bribe their children to eat more. This may only add food battles and mealtime relationship stress to an already existing list of reasons that the child does not want to eat. Throughout this book, we will describe ways to help these children grow, while maintaining a more positive mealtime interaction. Feeders always must remember that the nourishment of meals is emotional as well as physical.

Parent Roles That Encourage Toddlers to Eat

■ **Parents integrate the toddler into a family mealtime routine.**

As babies move past the first year and into the toddler period, their eating needs move from demand feeding toward the participatory routine of family mealtimes. Parents gradually move toward a family structure as the child's eating habits change. Bottle-feeding and breast-feeding tend to decrease as the emphasis on solid foods and other liquids increases. The family's mealtime structure of breakfast, lunch, and dinner is supplemented with nutritious between-meal snacks to keep the growing toddler's hunger satisfied.

■ **Parents are in charge of the menu.**

Parents should offer healthy, developmentally appropriate foods at regular times throughout the day. They remain in charge of the menu, offering foods that expand the child's diet and interest in new foods. Children will let their parents know which food they like—or don't like—on a particular day. Parents need to remember to try these same foods again if they have been rejected. If the toddler says no today, it does not mean no forever. When adults offer food without force or coercion, children's minds remain open to the possibility of eating rejected foods in the near future.

■ **Parents provide mastery opportunities for toddlers.**

Children must have experiences with new foods, different consistencies, and new ways of handling foods (e.g., spoon, fork, cups, straws) to master them. It is the parent's role to provide these opportunities, understanding that mastery takes time and usually includes a *mess!* Children must experiment with the foods and utensils to figure out how best to hold them and to get them to the mouth.

■ **Parents provide structure at mealtimes.**

It is the parent's job to provide a mealtime routine or structure. This includes not only the timing of the meals, but also the mealtime setting. Children seem to eat best when offered foods in a regular schedule of meals and planned nutritious snacks. They eat and grow optimally when they have a defined meal time and place. In one family, lunch could be scheduled at 11:30 with the toddler sitting in a high chair in the kitchen. In another family, the toddler might sit in a booster seat in the dining room at 12:00. We know that children do not develop good eating patterns when they are allowed to walk around with food or drink much of the day and "graze." They are more focused and interested in eating when sitting in a high chair or booster seat at the table during a scheduled meal. It is the child's job to check out the rules! Children may want to nibble all day or to eat in front of the television. They may want to eat a bite, walk away from the table, and then come repeatedly back for more. Parents must set up the structure for eating in a place that helps the child focus on the meal and the mastery opportunities.

■ **Parents offer new foods, but do not force the toddler to eat them.**

Food preferences are highly personal and, with the toddler, quite changeable. What Johnny liked yesterday, he may not touch today! It is the parent's role to offer a variety of new foods so that the child has a chance to taste and experiment with the foods. With the gradual introduction of new textures, the child gains the oral motor skills needed for efficient and safe chewing. It is the child's job to decide if he will eat the food offered. Sometimes the food needs to be offered several times before it is familiar enough to try! Parents should never force the child to eat. Simply offering it in a supportive fashion is enough.

■ **Parents reintroduce rejected foods to expand the child's exposure to new foods.**

In a never-ending effort to be in charge, the toddler may refuse a food for many reasons. Perhaps she does not like it. Perhaps she is full. Perhaps she doesn't feel like eating this specific food today or would rather have the spaghetti that is on the plate. Perhaps she feels pressure to eat the food and is rebelling against parental control. Parents should routinely reintroduce foods that have been rejected. If they believe that their child doesn't like the new food and therefore eliminate it from the list of acceptable foods, they gradually will offer their child fewer and fewer foods and the child will accept choices from a very limited menu.

Parents can learn to keep the options open. If they offered foods again, with repeated exposure, the child would eat many of the new foods. Birch, Johnson, and Fisher (1995) describe neophobia, a rejection of anything new, with children of this age. Research by Birch and Marlin (1982) has shown that children's preference for new foods increases as exposure to the food increases. A new food that was offered on 20 different occasions was chosen more frequently by children than a food that was offered 10 or 15 times. Repeated exposure enhanced acceptance only when children actually tasted a small amount. Simply looking at the food or smelling it was not as effective (Birch et al., 1987). Some children need the visual, tactile, and olfactory exposure first. As they become more familiar with the look, feel, and smell of the food, they can be invited to take a small taste. Hence, parents should offer it again and again. Parents must remember that forcing, bribing, and coercing are not the same as offering. Offering is a neutral act with no expectations that the child will accept or reject it.

- **Parents model mealtime skills.**

  In our busy and changing world, there seems to be less and less structure in the mealtime routine. We eat on the run. Part of the family may be off to soccer practice. One parent may work a later shift and not participate in the family dinner. Children still benefit from the opportunity to watch others eat; to see others using spoons, forks, and napkins; and to participate in the socialization of family mealtime conversation. Children learn a great deal in their attempts to imitate others. They can see how others use forks, and how bagels are eaten. They see others eating broccoli and learn how spaghetti works!

The Older Child

As toddlers turn into preschoolers, their mealtime needs change. Older children are better able to wait for meals and are integrated more easily into mealtime routines and family styles. A schedule of three larger meals divided by two smaller snacks is established securely as the child learns to eat with the rest of the family. As the child gets older, he may challenge the food offered, demand different foods, and ask to eat at different times of the day. Parents are still in charge of the menu, and children still get to decide which foods they will eat. Children continue to expand their food repertoire. Some do this rapidly, enthusiastically eating anything offered, while others are slower and more cautious. We know that pushing this cautious group will not make them more enthusiastic eaters. Parents need to continue to offer and encourage re-tasting of foods periodically, because "tastes change." Parents must remember that forcing food and engaging in power struggles over eating do not help, and actually seem to make children eat less of those foods (Dreikurs & Stoltz, 1964).

Special Feeding Issues

The roles of child and parent can become confused when the child has neurological, developmental, or other medical difficulties that influence feeding. Many times these children are uncomfortable with the feeding process. Their mealtime cues can be difficult to read. It may take awhile for the parents and physicians to figure out what is causing the problem. Sometimes children with disabilities do not have good internal cues. They may stop eating before they actually have had enough nourishment, or they may eat until they are more than full. As we discuss strategies to help them eat, we must make certain we fully understand the impact that the feeding difficulties and our treatment recommendations have had on the feeding relationship. Feeding specialists have the responsibility and opportunity to promote a positive feeding relationship in all therapeutic suggestions.

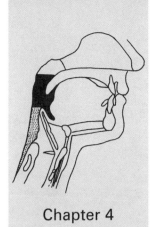

Chapter 4

Anatomy and Physiology of Eating

To fully understand feeding, we need a thorough understanding of the anatomy and physiology of the physical process of eating. We will look at the oral and pharyngeal, esophageal and gastrointestinal structures of eating. Neural control; the processes of swallowing and sucking; and the gastrointestinal, respiratory, cardiac, and oral facial influences on eating and drinking also will be discussed.

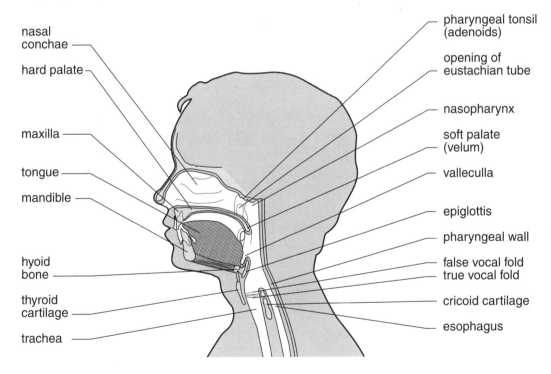

nasal conchae

hard palate

maxilla

tongue

mandible

hyoid bone

thyroid cartilage

trachea

pharyngeal tonsil (adenoids)

opening of eustachian tube

nasopharynx

soft palate (velum)

valleculla

epiglottis

pharyngeal wall

false vocal fold

true vocal fold

cricoid cartilage

esophagus

▓ Oral and Pharyngeal Structures

The oral cavity consists of the maxilla (upper jaw), the mandible (lower jaw), upper and lower lips, cheeks, tongue, teeth, floor of the mouth, hard palate, soft palate, uvula, and anterior and posterior faucial arches. The oral cavity provides the boundaries for the environment of sucking, chewing, and bolus formation. It plays important roles in the preparation of food for swallowing, oral inspiration of air, and sound production.

Both food and air flow through the pharynx. The pharyngeal structures direct air toward the larynx and trachea, and direct the bolus toward the esophagus. In addition to swallowing, the pharyngeal structure allows for maintenance of pharyngeal patency, which allows air to flow properly to the trachea. Proper timing is crucial in the separate movements of air and food thorough the pharynx.

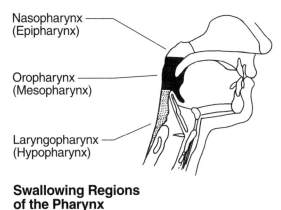

Nasopharynx
(Epipharynx)

Oropharynx
(Mesopharynx)

Laryngopharynx
(Hypopharynx)

**Swallowing Regions
of the Pharynx**

The soft tube of the pharynx is divided into three sections: the nasopharynx, the oropharynx, and the hypopharynx. The **nasopharynx** extends from the nasal choanae to the elevated soft palate. It includes the entrance to the eustachian tube, which equalizes air pressure in the middle ear. The **oropharynx** includes the pharyngeal space between the elevated soft palate and the epiglottis. The faucial arches separate the mouth and oropharynx. The soft palate and the back of the tongue meet during nasal respiration and the oral phase of eating. This connection and the base posterior portion of the tongue form the anterior portion of the oropharynx. The oropharynx includes the valleculae, or bilateral pockets formed by the approximation of the base of the tongue and the epiglottis. The **hypopharynx** includes the pharyngeal structures between the epiglottis and the sphincter at the top of the esophagus. This juncture of the pharynx and the esophagus is sometimes known as the pharyngeal-esophageal juncture (P-E juncture), or the cricopharyngeal sphincter. The mandible, hyoid bone, and thyroid cartilage form the mobile skeleton of the hypopharynx. The hypopharynx includes the pyriform sinuses, which are another set of bilateral pockets within the pharynx formed by the closure of the cricopharyngeal sphincter. These pyriform sinuses, together with the valleculae, form small cavities or recesses into which food can collect before or after the swallow reflex is triggered. Food usually does not remain in these sinuses when the swallow is normal.

The pharyngeal musculature involved in swallowing includes the superior, medial, and inferior pharyngeal constrictors. These give the bolus movement within the pharynx and help shape the pharynx (Donner, Bosma, & Robertson, 1985). The fibers of the inferior pharyngeal constrictors attach anteriorly to the sides of the thyroid cartilage to form the walls of the pyriform sinuses. The lowest fibers of these pharyngeal constrictors function as a valve at the top of the esophagus.

The pharynx also plays an important role in airway protection. Welch, Logemann, Rademaker, and Kahrilas (1993) identified changes in the diameter of the pharynx that were related to head position. Adult subjects held their heads in an upright neutral position and in a chin-tuck position. When the chin was tucked in and down toward the chest, the anterior pharyngeal structures shifted posteriorly, improving protection of the airway.

The larynx, a mostly cartilaginous structure, contains a series of muscular valves that primarily are designed to keep food from entering the airway. These multiple sets of small muscles (the true vocal folds, false vocal cords, and aryepiglottic folds) help to modify the flow of air for phonation, as well as protect the trachea, or airway. The cartilaginous epiglottis is the first structure in the system of airway protection. It is at the top of the system and rests at the base of the tongue. It folds down during swallowing to cover the inlet to the larynx. Stimulation of the edge of the epiglottis also can trigger the swallow reflex (Dua, Ren, Bardan, Xie, & Shaker, 1997). Acting with the epiglottis, the muscles of the true and false vocal folds form three levels of valves at the top of the trachea that can close and protect the airway from the intrusion of food or liquid during swallowing.

There is a great deal of interconnectedness in the anatomy and physiology of sucking, swallowing, breathing, and head and neck control. The skill in one area depends, in part, on the organized functioning in another area. There are numerous structural and muscular connections between these functions. The hyoid bone plays an important role in this interconnectedness. It is a free-floating bone that is held in position by its muscular connections with the scapulae, sternum, cervical vertebrae, temporal bone, mandible, laryngeal cartilage, and tongue. These connections provide the anatomical link between sucking, swallowing, chewing, breathing, and craniocervical posture. When the hyoid bone moves upward and forward during the swallow, some of these muscular connections place a mechanical traction on the upper esophageal sphincter, helping to pull open the upper entryway to the esophagus (Kahrilas, Dodds, Dent, Logemann, & Shaker, 1988; Pouderoux & Kahrilas, 1997; Shaker et al., 1997).

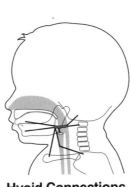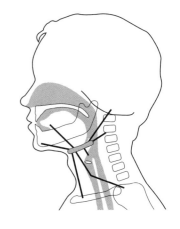

Hyoid Connections

Esophageal and Gastrointestinal Tract Structures

The esophagus is a thin hollow tube 23 to 25 centimeters long that links the pharynx and the stomach (DeNardi & Riddel, 1991). It is a combination of smooth and striated muscles that produces the coordinated, progressive contractions called peristalsis that direct food into the stomach. It is closed by a sphincter at each end. It begins proximally with the cricopharyngeal sphincter or upper esophageal sphincter (UES). When the swallow is triggered and the bolus passes through the pharynx, the UES relaxes to allow the bolus to move into the esophagus. The esophagus distends as the wavelike peristaltic action of the esophageal muscles move the food toward the stomach. The esophagus passes through the diaphragm and ends in the stomach at the lower esophageal sphincter (LES). The gastroesophageal junction is a complex valve composed of a smooth muscle segment (the LES) and a diaphragmatic segment (Kahrilas, 1997). This junction creates a region of high intra-esophageal or intraluminal pressure that relaxes during peristalsis to allow a bolus to enter the stomach.

The LES can be considered a high-pressure zone between the esophagus and the stomach. It is a major factor in providing a barrier against the upward flow (reflux) of gastric contents into the esophagus. It should be closed at rest, relaxing to allow passage of esophageal contents into the stomach. The relaxation occurs within 2 seconds of swallowing and continues for 8 to 10 seconds (Tuchman & Walter, 1994). LES relaxation also occurs during belching, vomiting, and rumination.

The stomach begins proximally at the lower esophageal sphincter and continues to the circular muscle near the duodenal junction called the pyloric sphincter. It consists of the cardia at the base of the LES, the fundus, the corpus, the pyloric antrum, and the pyloric sphincter (Gershon, 1998). The stomach mechanically and chemically digests food. It acidifies ingested foods to help protein digestion, kills microorganisms, secretes an important digestive enzyme (pepsin), and mechanically

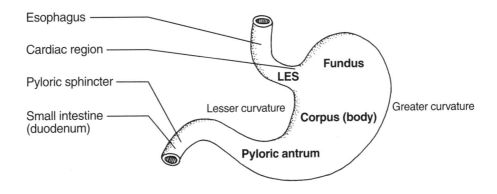

manipulates foods. It ends with the pyloric sphincter, which gates the partially digested food to the duodenum.

The small intestine is the highly coiled organ that provides additional enzymatic and mechanical action to the digestive process. Small molecular nutrients are extracted from the gastric material and absorbed by lining cells, then transferred to the capillaries. It begins with the duodenum, which is the most proximal portion of the small intestine. Bile made in the liver and stored in the gall bladder is discharged into the duodenum through the bile ducts. Pancreatic digestive enzymes also enter the duodenum. The jejunum is the next section of the small intestine. The bulk of the absorption of nutrients takes place through the walls of the jejunum.

The large intestine is used mainly for the absorption of water, vitamins, and minerals. The non-nutritive residue is moved through the rectum and anal sphincter to the outside. Nutrients absorbed through the tract are transported to the liver by way of the hepatic portal system for distribution to the cells of the body.

Form and Function— Cavities, Tubes, and Valves

Consider the anatomy of the feeding system as a system of tubes and valves. The mouth and pharynx share their tubing with both air and food. The initial tube divides in the upper regions to form the nasal and oral cavities. The tube divides into two sections: the trachea leading to the lungs, and the esophagus leading to the stomach. The valves along the tube direct the food rapidly and efficiently toward the stomach, bypassing the pathway to the lungs. Because there are common air and food pathways in the system, timing and coordination are very important.

The lips serve as an initial valve to retain food or liquid in the oral cavity. The posterior portion of the tongue moves upward and backward to keep the food in the front of the mouth and prevent premature swallowing or loss of the bolus. The upward and backward movement of the soft palate and bulging forward of the pharyngeal wall create a separation of the oral and nasal cavities. This prevents the contents of the mouth from moving upward into the nose. During speech, this velopharyngeal valve prevents air and sounds from the larynx from moving through the nose (except when the nasalized consonants /m/, /n/, and /ng/ are desired).

The epiglottis is another valve with major significance in directing food toward the stomach and away from the lungs. It closes the pathway into the trachea during swallowing. The three-fold set of paired muscles within the larynx (i.e., aryepiglottic folds, false vocal folds, and true vocal folds) contract during swallowing to provide additional support to keep food and liquid out of the lungs. If food enters this region, a cough is stimulated to propel the material forcefully away from the trachea.

The cricopharyngeus muscle, which creates the UES at the bottom of the pharynx, acts as a valving mechanism at the top of the esophagus. It contracts at rest and relaxes only when the swallow reflex has been triggered. Because it closes the UES during other activities such as talking and breathing, no food or liquid moves out of the esophagus and into the trachea where it could be inhaled into the lungs. The UES is closed at rest to prevent air from finding its way into the stomach. It quickly relaxes, opening automatically with elevation of the hyoid bone during swallowing and pressure from movement of the bolus of food, allowing food to pass into the esophagus en route to the stomach. This pharyngeal-esophageal junction is an important part of the normal swallowing mechanism. When the swallow reflex is absent, food and liquid that fall into the pharynx can pool at this closed door (i.e., the pyriform sinuses) and eventually spill over into the airway.

The tube continues as the food moves down the esophagus into the stomach. The LES serves as a valve to the entrance of the stomach. Pressure changes allow food into the stomach and prevent food from moving back up into the esophagus. The tube widens in the cardiac region of the stomach, passing food into the fundus and corpus of the stomach, and then into the pylorus for digestion. When the food in the stomach cavity has been sufficiently broken up, sterilized by the acid, and partly digested, it passes into the small intestine through the pyloric sphincter, a valve at the distal end of the stomach. From this point, the long and circuitous tubes of the small and large intestines carry nutrients into the bloodstream and wastes toward the final valve, the anal sphincter. As this valve relaxes, waste materials leave the body.

These valves and sphincters are at work throughout the system to promote the proper flow of food and air by contracting and relaxing mechanically or through changes in pressure gradients.

We've looked at the idea that the system may be conceptualized as a set of larger cavities (e.g., oral cavity, nasal cavity, lungs, stomach) connected by a set of tubes (e.g., pharynx, trachea, esophagus, intestines). We can extend the concept further by imagining a series of smaller cavities or pockets that can contain a small amount of food or liquid as it is en route from the mouth to the stomach. In the areas where food can pool or collect, anatomical pockets are created. These are not functional in assisting the normal swallow, but they can become problem areas when the swallow is uncoordinated.

Anatomically, these pockets are small cavities, recesses, or sulci. Food or liquid may be collected in the mouth in the anterior sulcus and the posterior sulcus. These sulci are cavities or pockets between the lips and teeth or between the teeth and the cheeks. Any food that falls into these sulci is moved into the oral cavity, where it can be projected backward for swallowing. The valleculae and pyriform sinuses also are pockets where food can collect if the swallow is not efficient. Collection of food or liquid in these areas can trigger a delayed swallow reflex or can spill over into the trachea, causing choking, coughing, or aspiration.

▎ Neural Control in Eating

The neural control of eating involves many components. A series of cranial nerves located in the brain stem provide the direct sensory and motor fibers that travel to and from the muscles of the face, mouth, pharynx, larynx, esophagus, and stomach (Dodds, 1989; Dodds, Stewart, & Logemann, 1990). Two sets of specialized nerve tracts in the brain stem have been described as the "swallowing centers." These appear to provide the central pattern or program that selects and guides the movements for swallowing (Miller, 1986, 1993). Other parts of the brain, including the cerebral cortex, cerebellum, and brain stem, contribute sensory fibers and influence the overall coordination of the swallow.

Understanding of the neural control of the gastrointestinal system is in a constant state of change. Although the central nervous system and autonomic nervous system exert a strong influence in digestion and assimilation of nutrients, they are not the only players in the control of the digestive process. Gershon (1998) describes the historical and current understanding of a "second brain" that is located entirely within the gut. This enteric nervous system functions both independently of the central nervous system and in partnership with it. Most of the motility of the gut is handled through the nerves and neurotransmitters of the enteric nervous system. When all connections to the central nervous system are cut, wavelike peristaltic movements of the gut continue. Interestingly, the pyloric sphincter, which must open to release food from the stomach into the upper portion of the small intestine, is totally controlled by the vagus nerve of the central nervous system (Gershon, 1998).

The Cranial Nerves

Although each part of the neural pathway is important in understanding the journey from the lips through the bowel, we have chosen to focus on the role of the cranial nerves. A set of six specialized nerves in the brainstem play a central role in creating the interrelationships among sucking, swallowing, and breathing. There is considerable overlap in neural function for these three important processes. Cranial nerves I, V, VII, IX, X, and XII all have important roles in these processes.

Cranial nerve I, the olfactory nerve, collects the sensory information of smell. Smell strongly influences our perception of taste and our enjoyment of eating.

Cranial nerve V, the trigeminal nerve, innervates muscles that control chewing, movement of the lower jaw, and palatal elevators. These are important for rooting, sucking, and initiation of the swallowing response. The sensory aspects of this nerve provide information from the cheeks, nose, lips, teeth, and the skin over the lower jaw. Sensory information from this nerve provides feedback from the mouth during sucking, from the nose during breathing, and from the soft palate during swallowing. The trigeminal nerve's overlap of function between sucking, swallowing, and breathing supports the interconnectedness of these skills.

Cranial nerve VII, the facial nerve, provides information about taste from the receptors on the anterior two-thirds of the tongue. This part of the tongue provides sweet, salty, and sour taste information. A complete taste experience comes from pairing smell information received from the olfactory nerve with taste input from the facial nerve and the glossopharyngeal nerve.

In addition, the facial nerve has motor fibers to the muscles of facial expression and to the salivary glands. Facial expression is an important aspect of the social interaction and bonding associated with mealtimes. It contributes greatly to the infant-parent bond as the feeding relationship develops. The muscles of facial expression are actively used in giving non-verbal cues. The proper functioning of the salivary glands is important in mixing the bolus with saliva for good bolus production and swallowing. Saliva also mixes the food and moves it so that taste is more efficient.

Cranial nerve IX, the glossopharyngeal nerve, provides sensory information about taste from the posterior one-third of the tongue. This is predominantly for bitter tastes. It also has motor fibers to the muscles used in swallowing and to the salivary glands. This nerve innervates the gag reflex.

Cranial nerve X, the vagus nerve, has motor connections to the pharynx, larynx, and heart. Through its contribution to the autonomic nervous system it is involved in heart rate, smooth muscle activity in the gut, glands that alter gastric motility, respiration, and blood pressure. It innervates the pyloric sphincter, regulating the passage of food from the stomach into the upper portion of the small intestine. The vagus nerve also provides sensory information from the palate, uvula, palatal arch, pharynx, larynx, esophagus, and visceral organs. The sensory and motor fibers of the vagus nerve are critical to the interconnectedness of swallowing, respiration, and visceral control.

Cranial nerve XII, the hypoglossal nerve, is important in the contraction of the muscles of the tongue. This is necessary in bolus preparation, sucking, and swallowing.

The cervical spinal nerves C1–3 innervate muscles between the hyoid, mandible, and shoulder girdle. These influence postural stability as a foundational necessity in sucking, swallowing, and breathing.

There is massive overlap and redundancy in the suck-swallow-breathe pattern. Eating and breathing are so basic to survival that the nervous system has built in multiple backup systems to provide protection. Cervical nerves 1, 2, and 3 are all involved with the motor aspects of sucking, swallowing, and breathing. Cranial nerve IX is involved with the sensory aspects of sucking, swallowing, and breathing.

Table 4.1   Nerve Interrelationships in the Suck-Swallow-Breathe Pattern

Sucking	Motor C 1–3, CN V, CN VII, CN XII
Swallowing	Motor C 1–3, CN V, CN VII, CN IX, CN X, CN XII
Breathing	Motor C 1–3, CN IX, CN X, C 3–7, T 1–12

Suck, swallow, and breathe patterns all have cervical nerves 1–3 in common.

Sucking	Sensory CN IX, CN V, CN VII
Swallowing	Sensory CN IX, CN X
Breathing	Sensory CN IX, CN X, CN V

Suck, swallow, and breathe patterns all have cranial nerve IX in common.

Table 4.2   **Cranial Nerves Associated With Eating**

Cranial Nerve	Type	Function	
I	**Olfactory Nerve**	Sensory	Sense of Smell
V	**Trigeminal**	Mixed	
	Maxillary Branch		**Sensory fibers** from cheek, nose, upper lip and teeth
	Mandibular Branch		**Sensory fibers** from skin over mandible, lower lip and teeth
			Motor fibers to the muscles of mastication
VII	**Facial**	Mixed	**Sensory fibers** from taste receptors on the anterior two thirds of the tongue
			Motor fibers to the muscles of facial expression, salivary glands
IX	**Glossopharyngeal**	Mixed	**Sensory fibers** from taste receptors on the posterior one third of the tongue
			Motor fibers to the muscles used in swallowing and to the salivary glands
X	**Vagus**	Mixed	**Sensory fibers** from the pharynx, larynx, esophagus, and visceral organs
			Somatic motor fibers to the muscles of the pharynx and larynx
			Autonomic fibers to the heart, smooth muscles, and glands to alter gastric motility, heart rate, respiration and blood pressure
XII	**Hypoglossal**	Motor	Contraction of the muscles of the tongue

▉ Swallowing

The Process of Swallowing

Swallowing is the process of moving food from the mouth to the gastrointestinal tract to nourish the body. It has been divided arbitrarily three phases: the oral, the pharyngeal, and the esophageal.

The **oral phase** sometimes is subdivided into an oral preparatory phase and an oral phase. The oral preparatory phase involves biting, chewing, and preparing and organizing the bolus. The oral phase actively propels the prepared bolus to the back of the mouth for swallowing. The process involves breaking the food into small enough particles to be easily swallowed. Food is mixed with saliva to start the digestion process. During this phase, food is collected into a bolus and held in the mouth until it moves toward the pharynx with the trigger of the swallow reflex. The individual's intention to swallow plays a large role in the initiation of the more automatic portion of the swallow. (See Table 4.3 on page 57 for information on the muscles contributing to the oral phase of swallowing.)

The **pharyngeal phase** includes valving the nasal and laryngeal openings to prevent food from entering the airway; the movement of the bolus through the pharynx; and the opening of the cricopharyngeal sphincter to allow bolus movement into the esophagus. As the swallow reflex is triggered, the tongue moves backward, and changes in intraoral pressure gradients propel the food into the pharynx. The soft palate elevates to close the nasal airway. Changing pressure gradients as well as pharyngeal peristaltic action involving more than two dozen muscles transports the bolus from the mouth through the pharynx and into the esophagus. (See Table 4.4 on page 58 for information on the muscles contributing to the pharyngeal phase of swallowing.) To protect the airway, the epiglottis tips downward to cover the opening to the larynx. This directs the bolus toward the esophagus. The hyoid bone and larynx elevate, and the aryepiglottic, false and true vocal folds contract to provide additional airway protection.

The **esophageal phase** involves movement of the bolus through the esophagus and into the stomach. The cricopharyngeal sphincter relaxes and opens through the mechanical pull of the elevated hyoid bone during the swallow combined with pressure from the base of the tongue and the volume of the bolus in the pharynx. The upper esophageal sphincter closes immediately after a bolus enters the esophagus to prevent upward movement of the bolus back into the pharynx. A combination of gravity and esophageal peristaltic action moves the food into the stomach. The esophageal phase involves a coordinated effort of opening and closing with the UES and LES. After the bolus has entered the stomach, the LES should close to prevent upward movement of the gastric contents.

Sequence of Adult Swallowing

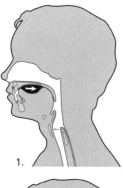

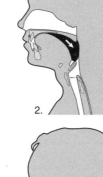

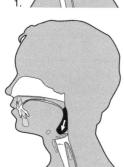

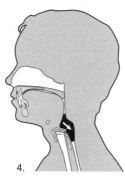

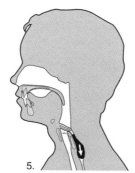

1. Voluntary initiation of the swallow occurs with backward movement of the tongue. The tongue and palate prevent the bolus of liquid from entering the pharynx before the swallow reflex is triggered.

2. The swallow reflex is triggered. As the tongue moves backward, it propels the bolus into the pharynx. The soft palate elevates to close the nasal airway.

3. The bolus passes through the pharynx through peristaltic contraction of the pharyngeal constrictors. The epiglottis moves backward to cover the opening to the airway. The larynx elevates and the true and false vocal folds contract, providing additional airway protection.

4. The bolus bypasses the airway and moves through the cricopharyngeal sphincter into the esophagus. The sphincter closes immediately, preventing reflux into the pharynx.

5. Peristaltic movement of the esophagus carries the bolus into the stomach. The LES at the base of the esophagus relaxes to allow food to pass into the stomach. It then closes to prevent reflux of stomach contents.

Comparison of Infant and Adult Anatomy for Swallowing

There are significant differences between the oral-pharyngeal anatomy of newborns and that of adults (Bosma, 1963a, 1963b, 1967). These differences will predominate and support an infant's functional abilities until the age of 3 to 4 months. A newborn's lower jaw is small and retracted. The small size of the oral space that results gives the impression of an oversized tongue. The tongue fills the entire oral cavity and touches the floor and roof of the mouth simultaneously. Laterally, the tongue contacts the gum ridges and, often, the inside of the cheeks. A full-term newborn has a set of sucking pads that consist of fatty tissue depositions encased in more fatty tissue within the muscles of the infant's cheeks. This gives the baby a "pudgy-cheeked" look. The sucking pads are important for the baby's development because they create a firmness of the cheeks that provides the infant with some stability in the oral system to support early sucking patterns. This is important because the newborn does not have any stability in the region of the temporomandibular joint. When this stability of the cheeks is combined with the small size of the oral cavity and the relatively large size of the tongue, the mouth is able to achieve better compression and suction in extracting liquid from a nipple.

The amount and direction of tongue movement is limited in newborns and young infants because of the small oral space. Because the tongue at rest is in direct contact with the palate, there is no additional space to support up-down tongue movements. This is one of the reasons why the early direction of tongue movement in the suckle is backward and forward. Young infants do not chew, partly because there is insufficient neurological and digestive maturity for handling chewable foods, but also because there is no room in the mouth for lateral tongue movements. Thus, both neurological maturity and the anatomical form and relationships determine function in the system.

Newborns tend to be nose breathers, though they are no longer considered *obligate* nose breathers as was previously believed. More recent studies have shown that oral breathing is possible for short periods of time in neonates, but is done at the expense of respiratory efficiency (Miller et al., 1985; Miller, Martin, Carlo, & Fanaroff, 1987). Infants must work against a complicated anatomical predisposition for nasal breathing. This pattern of preference toward nasal breathing is created because the mouth is filled with the tongue, and the soft palate and epiglottis are touching. The flow of air is directed efficiently through the nose, bypassing the more cluttered oral passageway. To breathe orally, the baby must open the lips, create enough muscle tone to separate the touching of the soft palate and the tongue, and maintain separation of these parts during breathing. It is, therefore, much easier to breathe nasally.

The infant's epiglottis and soft palate are in direct approximation until the child is 3 or 4 months old. This structural difference from the adult anatomy provides additional protection against food randomly falling over the back of the tongue and into the airway. The larynx rides very high in the infant neck and is in much closer proximity to the base of the tongue than in the adult. Because it is directly under the tongue and epiglottis, the larynx is fully protected when it elevates during the swallow. There is less need for coordinated closure of the vocal folds to protect the airway at this stage of development. In the adult, elongation of the neck and pharynx changes the relationship of the larynx, tongue, and epiglottis. The increased vertical space causes the larynx to ride lower in the neck and receive less anatomical protection from the epiglottis during the swallow. Therefore, there is a greater need for coordinated valving at the epiglottis to protect the airway during the swallow. Many infants whose vocal folds are paralyzed in an open position will have no difficulties with swallowing during the early months. As the larynx receives less anatomical protection, they become more vulnerable for choking and aspirating, especially if they also have other difficulties with muscle tone and coordination. The airway protection needed for survival during eating is, thus, supported anatomically in the early months at a time when neurological coordination and timing are immature.

The structural differences in cavity size and relationships also contribute to the nasality of infant sounds. The infant has relatively few options for producing oral sounds. The tongue fills the mouth, and there is little room for the airflow to come out the mouth. In addition, the approximation of the epiglottis and soft palate forms a barrier to airflow through the mouth, directing all air and sound through the nasal cavity. The young infant's typical sound play is a series of nasal vowels. Vowels that are produced orally and consonants that require specific valving activity will develop as the cavity size enlarges, giving the tongue and lips greater opportunities for movement, exploration, and valving.

The infant's eustachian tubes run horizontally from the middle ear on each side into the nasopharynx. The horizontal course of the tubes contributes to the high incidence of middle ear infections in infants and young children. The sucking, swallowing, and breathing mechanisms of infants and young children are less sophisticated than those of older children and adults. There is greater opportunity for food and liquid to reflux into the nasal cavity and transport bacteria-laden food and mucus to the entrance of the eustachian tubes. The horizontal pathway of the tubes provides a direct track to the middle ear that can contribute to middle ear infections in children who are prone to this type of illness. As the infant grows toward adult proportions, the tube runs in a more vertical direction, reducing the incidence of middle ear infection.

Anatomical Differences Between the Newborn and the Adult Mouth and Pharynx

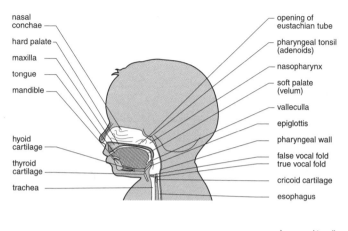

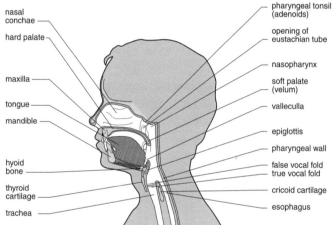

1. The intraoral space of the newborn is small.
2. The lower jaw of the newborn is small and slightly retracted.
3. Sucking pads are present in infants but not in adults.
4. The tongue takes up more relative space in mouth of the newborn due to the diminished size of the lower jaw and the presence of sucking pads in the cheeks.
5. The tongue shows restrictions in movement partially because of the restricted intraoral cavity in which it resides.
6. Newborns prefer nasal breathing.
7. The epiglottis and soft palate are in approximation in the newborn as a protective mechanism.
8. The larynx is higher in the neck of the newborn than in the older infant or adult. This reduces the need for sophisticated laryngeal closure to protect the airway during swallowing.
9. The hyoid is formed of cartilage, not bone in the infant.
10. An infant's eustachian tube lies in a horizontal position. It assumes a more vertical angle in the older child and adult.

Infant Anatomical Maturation and Function

Anatomical changes begin by 4 to 6 months of age and continue throughout the first year. Additional changes will continue into adolescence with changes in dentition and the growth of the skull toward its adult size and shape. In infancy, the intraoral space increases as the lower jaw grows downward and forward. The sucking pads begin to be absorbed, and the oral cavity elongates vertically. Thus, the oral space grows as the infant's head begins to mature toward the adult size and shape. The tongue gradually has more space in which to move. Sucking patterns that were mechanically reflexive now begin to acquire a voluntary overlay. The early stage of continuous tongue-oral cavity contact was essential to the acquisition of sensorimotor information. This provides a base of information and experience upon which the system can build. As the tongue gains more space in which to maneuver, it simultaneously gains greater neurological control with which to move and explore its new home. Through play and exploration, the tongue discovers its possibilities and creates new possibilities for itself. The tongue begins to move in an up-down direction, varying this with a return to the familiar backward-forward direction it has known for the past 6 months. With this new movement, the familiar sensory contact with the hard palate is re-established.

The up-down movement of the tongue joins forces with a greater capacity for control of the valving of the lips. This combination improves negative intraoral pressure for expressing milk from the nipple or drawing food from a spoon. Improvements in tongue and lip valving as well as the increased intraoral space establish the foundation for an increase in oral motor play and exploration. When these movements are combined with vocalization, the baby discovers and produces a wide variety of sounds.

Initial changes in the intraoral space are a function of growth of the mandible and absorption of the sucking pads in the cheeks. The baby's initial need for the stability provided by the sucking pads diminishes as neurological control develops. Greater control of jaw opening and closing possibilities at the temporomandibular (jaw) joint leads toward an internal postural stability that does not depend upon the support provided initially by the sucking pads. With less stiffness, the cheeks and lips acquire greater mobility and exploratory movement. Greater precision of movement control in the jaw, lips, cheeks, and tongue reduces the need for the deep vertical grooving of the tongue used by the young infant to propel the bolus to the back of the tongue for swallowing. A shallower cupping remains and is combined with greater skillfulness of the cheeks and tongue in organizing and propelling the bolus. This prepares the infant for pureed foods that require greater skill in forming the bolus. Further changes in the vertical dimensions of the mouth are provided as the teeth erupt, creating new possibilities for movement and the exploration of sensory receptors that lead toward biting and chewing.

As the hyoid and larynx grow downward, there is a greater separation between the epiglottis and larynx. The exquisite timing of events in normal development supports more mature protection of the airway. With neurological maturation and the improved timing, rhythm, and coordination of sucking, swallowing, and breathing, the infant no longer needs the additional anatomical support provided by the extra protective covering of the larynx by the epiglottis.

These structural changes in infant anatomy make possible the more mature patterns of sucking, swallowing, biting, and chewing. They also can complicate the development of oral motor skill and efficiency for the neurologically impaired infant whose system does not participate in the coordinated dance between neurological and anatomical maturation. Many older infants and children who retain a less mature neurological system have lost the anatomical backup systems that were designed to offer increased protection from incoordination.

Sucking

The Process of Sucking

Sucking is the intake phase of eating liquids and soft solids. Some would consider it a portion of the oral phase of the swallow. It involves taking the liquid into the mouth and moving it to the back of the oral cavity for swallowing. It is a rhythmic pattern of the infant's mouth at the breast, bottle, fingers, or a toy. It has nutritive value and provides nonnutritive support for calming and organizing the body.

Sucking can be seen in utero as early as the second trimester. Premature infants as young as 32 weeks gestation have begun demonstrating the ability to coordinate sucking and swallowing during breast-feeding. Bottle-fed babies seem to develop the coordination somewhat later. Between 34 and 37 weeks, infants continue to refine their sucking skills. Bu'Lock, Woolridge, and Baum (1990) have reported that sucking, swallowing, and breathing are skills that mature with age. Their data showed that these skills do not seem to be consistently achieved until 37 weeks post-conception age. The 37-week mark may well be when most infants are neurologically ready to fully support their nutritional requirements orally.

The Mechanics of Sucking

The infant sucks liquid into the mouth with a combination of actions that cause pressure changes. Positive and negative pressure combine to promote strong and efficient sucking (Colley & Creamer, 1958; Wolf & Glass, 1992). **Positive pressure** or compression extracts the fluid from the breast or bottle. The baby compresses the nipple with the gums against the base of the nipple or with the tongue against the palate. This positive pressure on the nipple makes the liquid push out into the mouth. **Negative pressure** is described as a suction that draws fluid into the nipple and then out of the breast or bottle into the mouth. Suction is created as the oral cavity is sealed around the nipple and the jaw moves downward. The back of the tongue depresses, enlarging the oral cavity and changing the intraoral pressure. This combination acts to refill the nipple and draw in fluid from the breast or bottle (Woolridge, 1986). To create this suction, the oral cavity must be sealed or there will be no change in intraoral pressure. Both positive and negative pressure seem to be used in the sucking process of infants (Ardran, Kemp, & Lind, 1958a, 1958b; Colley & Creamer, 1958). Compression alone with the bottle does not seem to work efficiently. Bottle-fed babies seem to need more negative pressure suction to attain enough milk for growth. Breast-fed babies seem to need a combination of both pressures to nurse most efficiently.

Hunger levels and liquid flow influence the pace of sucking for most infants. At the beginning of the meal when the infant is hungry, sucking generally is more rapid than it is toward the end when satiation sets in. The breast-fed infant will begin the meal with the more rapid nonnutritive suck of approximately a rate of two sucks per second. Once the letdown reflex has occurred and the mother's milk begins to flow, the infant slows to the nutritive sucking rate of one suck per second. Swallowing typically occurs with each suck toward the beginning of the meal, but may move toward more sucks per swallow as the infant finishes the meal. Infants use a pattern of sucking bursts separated by brief pauses during the meal. Both the strength of the suck and the relationship of sucking bursts and pauses are influenced by the amount and timing of the milk flow through the nipple (Mathew, 1988; Mathew & Bhatia, 1989).

■ Digestion

Into the Stomach

The health of the gastrointestinal system strongly influences eating and appetite (Gershon, 1998; Phillips & Wingate, 1998). Digestion begins as food enters the mouth, is chewed or formed into a bolus, and is mixed with saliva. The digestive enzyme, amylase, is present in saliva as well as in breast milk (Hegardt, Lindberg, Borjesson, & Skude, 1984; Hodge, Lebenthal, Lee, & Topper, 1983; Valdez & Fox, 1991). Some authors (Gershon, 1998; Mandel, 1987) have suggested that food does not remain long enough in the mouth for any digestion to take place and that the salivary digestive enzymes are inactivated by stomach acid. Although the amylase that is released into the small intestine by the pancreas is the primary player in fat and starch digestion, salivary amylase also plays a small role. It may be particularly significant for neonates and patients with cystic fibrosis who have pancreatic insufficiency.

Saliva plays another role in early digestive transport. Because saliva is alkaline, it covers the tissues of the pharynx and esophagus with a protective coating that decreases the duration of acid contact with the mucus of the esophagus. This can protect against esophagitis and other damage to the esophageal tissues during episodes of acid reflux.

The mixture of food and saliva moves through the esophagus and into the stomach with efficient motility and appropriate opening and closing of the relevant upper and lower esophageal sphincters. The stomach produces a digestive enzyme, pepsin, which breaks down proteins in food into the small particles called peptides that can be used by the body. Because pepsin requires a very acidic environment in which to work, the stomach produces hydrochloric acid, the main stomach juice that mixes with the food whenever it needs it. In order to protect its own surface cells from

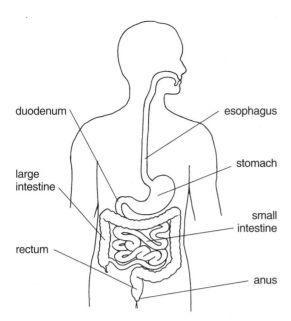

duodenum

large intestine

rectum

esophagus

stomach

small intestine

anus

being eaten up, the stomach produces a protective mucous gel that coats its walls and neutralizes both pepsin and hydrochloric acid (Gershon, 1998). Batmanghelidj (1995) points out that stomach mucus consists of 98% water along with an inner scaffolding that traps the water. Sodium bicarbonate, an alkaline solution, is trapped in this layer of watery mucus and neutralizes any acid that tries to pass through to the cells of the stomach lining. He states that within a half hour of drinking a glass of water, the water is absorbed in the intestine and an almost identical amount is then secreted into the stomach through the mucosal layer. This provides the additional liquid that the stomach needs for efficient food breakdown.

The stomach has an incredible ability to expand in order to store large amounts of food without increasing its internal pressure. Stimulation of sensors in the wall of the stomach provides information on how much the stomach wall is expanding to contain the food. Our perception of the relative amount of stomach expansion is interpreted as fullness or satiation. The muscles of the stomach knead and churn the food, breaking larger pieces of food into tiny particles that can be handled by the small intestine. The enteric nervous system acts as a food monitor that regulates and synchronizes the overall secretion of digestive materials and the movements that are needed. Most of the active digestion of the food occurs in the pyloric region of the stomach after the food has been ground and broken up. This area of the stomach contains a complex feedback system that monitors the level of acidity, increasing it as necessary to complete the gastric digestion of the food. Specialized cells in the stomach also contain receptors for the neurotransmitter, histamine. These receptors are different from the histamine receptors involved in colds and allergies. In the stomach, histamine arouses the special cells that produce acid and keeps them more alert to produce the correct amount of acid.

Into the Intestinal Tract

When the partially digested food is ready to leave the stomach, it passes through the pyloric sphincter into the upper portion of the small intestine known as the duodenum. This occurs in tiny amounts that can be handled easily by the upper intestine. The pyloric sphincter remains closed until the stomach has prepared the food. Like the esophagus at the upper end of the stomach, the small intestine doesn't have cells that secrete a protective mucous coating. However, pancreatic ducts secrete a watery bicarbonate fluid that is alkaline. This helps neutralize the stomach acid that accompanies the food coming through the pyloric sphincter and prevents cell damage. In most circumstances, cranial nerve X, the vagus nerve, regulates the opening and closing of the pyloric sphincter. If the vagus nerve is cut, the pyloric sphincter is paralyzed in a closed position. If this is remedied by a surgical procedure (pyloroplasty) that destroys the sphincter, the enteric nervous system takes over the regulation of the rate of gastric emptying (Gershon, 1998). Once again, we see the existence of anatomical and neurological backup systems that support the vital act of eating.

Once food enters the small intestine, additional digestion occurs through the pancreatic secretion of digestive enzymes (protease, lipase, and amylase) that further reduce protein, fat, and carbohydrate into a form that can be assimilated by the body. Additional substances secreted by the liver and gallbladder contribute to both digestion and the cleansing of body waste materials. Once again, the specialized enteric nervous system orchestrates the secretions and the peristaltic movement through the system.

When digestion is completed, absorption occurs through the intestinal lining, moving the nutrients into the bloodstream. This is done efficiently because the wall of the small intestine is comprised of a complex series of folds that contain more folds, which contain even more folds.

Gershon (1998) states that 1 centimeter of intestinal lining contains enough surface membrane to cover a doubles tennis court! In order for nutrient absorption to happen efficiently, the mixture in the small intestine must be very wet. The body has mixed a large amount of watery fluid with the food at every point in the transport process. It now needs a way of conserving this water and moving waste materials through the remainder of the digestive tract. This is accomplished in the colon, part of the large intestine.

The main function of the colon is to minimize water loss from the body through a system that reabsorbs water from the feces. This is done by pumping salt out of the large intestine, a process that pulls most of the water through the intestinal walls and back into the body's cells. This creates a more solid mass of stools that are propelled downward through the remainder of the colon. Bacteria and dead cells also become concentrated in the stool that is ultimately passed from the body through the anus.

The proper functioning of the whole system is influenced by the structural integrity of the gastrointestinal (GI) tract, proper physiological functioning, general health, medications, and emotions. Difficulties in any part of this process can affect appetite, growth, and the feeding relationship.

The Respiratory and Cardiac Systems

The respiratory system has a powerful influence on eating. A well-functioning respiratory system provides a balance of oxygen and carbon dioxide in the blood throughout the day as we move from one activity to the next. Different activities such as feeding, sleeping, and playing place different respiratory requirements on the body. The common tubing of the feeding and respiratory systems means these systems must work in a highly sophisticated and coordinated fashion. Proper timing is essential. Good feeding and growth will depend on the coordination of the sucking, swallowing, and breathing processes.

Difficulties with respiration decrease interest in eating. Given a choice of eating or breathing, the child must choose breathing. The child must be able to make the respiratory adjustments necessary to move into the activity of eating. Eating is work for infants, and work requires respiratory changes. The infant must have the respiratory systems in place to make the necessary changes to modify oxygen and carbon dioxide levels. This can be done with changes in respiratory rate, depth of respiration, heart rate, and the work of breathing. When the respiratory rate is too rapid or breathing is too shallow, the infant is unable to coordinate the breathing phase of the suck-swallow-breathe synergy efficiently.

The heart rate and the efficiency of its stroke influence the amount of oxygen and carbon dioxide in the blood. Some cardiac conditions will influence the rate and efficiency of the heart and may lead to increased heart rate during feedings. Other conditions can cause low oxygen levels in the blood or poor circulation, making increased demands on the respiratory system during feeding. Feeding endurance is directly affected, and suck-swallow-breathe coordination may be indirectly influenced by the interplay of cardiac and respiratory systems.

Table 4.3	**Muscles Contributing to the Oral Phase of Swallowing**

Muscle	Primary Action
Levator labii superioris	Elevate upper lip
Levator labii superioris alaque nasi	Elevate upper lip
Levator anguli oris	Elevate corner of the mouth
Zygomaticus major	Elevate corner of the mouth
Zygomaticus minor	Elevate upper lip
Risorius	Laterally displace corner of mouth
Depressor labii inferioris	Depress lower lip
Depressor anguli oris	Depress corner of the mouth
Mentalis	Protrude lower lip; depress jaw
Obicularis oris	Close and purse lips
Buccinator	Flatten cheeks
Platysma	Depress mandible and lower lips
Temporalis	Elevate and retract jaw
Masseter	Elevate jaw
Medial pterygoid	Elevate jaw
Lateral pterygoid	Depress and medially displace jaw
Intrinsic muscles of tongue	Shape tongue
Genioglossus	Protrude and depress tongue
Styloglossus	Retract and elevate tongue
Hypoglossus	Depress tongue

Anatomical and Physiological Overview. (1991). In B. Jones & M. W. Donner (Eds.), *Normal and abnormal swallowing: Imaging in diagnosis and therapy* (p 9). New York: Springer-Verlag. Reprinted with permission.

Table 4.4   **Muscles Contributing to the Pharyngeal Phase of Swallowing**

Muscle	Primary Action
Mylohyoid	Propel bolus; elevate and anteriorly displace hyoid and larynx
Anterior digastric	Propel bolus; elevate and anteriorly displace hyoid and larynx
Tensor veli palatini	Elevate soft palate to seal nasopharynx
Geniohyoid	Propel bolus; elevate and anteriorly displace hyoid and larynx
Hyoglossus	Propel bolus; elevate and anteriorly displace hyoid and larynx
Styloglossus	Seal pharyngeal outlet
Pterygopharyngeus	Seal pharyngeal outlet
Palatoglossus	Seal pharyngeal outlet
Palatopharyngeus	Seal pharyngeal outlet
Stylopharyngeus	Seal pharyngeal outlet
Salpingopharyngeus	Seal pharyngeal outlet
Levator veli palatini	Elevate soft palate to seal nasopharynx
Musculus uvulae	Elevate soft palate to seal nasopharynx
Stylohyoid	Seal pharyngeal outlet
Posterior digastric	Seal pharyngeal outlet
Superior constrictor	Seal pharyngeal outlet
Thyrohyoid	Depress and posteriorly displace hyoid and larynx
Sternohyoid	Depress and posteriorly displace hyoid and larynx
Sternothyoid	Depress and posteriorly displace hyoid and larynx
Omohyoid	Depress and posteriorly displace hyoid and larynx
Hypopharyngeus (mid. constrictor)	Clear bolus
Thyropharyngeus (inf. constrictor)	Clear bolus
Cricopharyngeus (inf. constrictor)	Clear bolus
Aryepiglottic	Protect airway; adduct vocal cords
Lateral circoarytenoid	Protect airway; adduct vocal cords
Transverse arytenoid	Protect airway; adduct vocal cords
Oblique arytenoid	Protect airway; adduct vocal cords
Thyroarytenoid	Protect airway; adduct vocal cords
Cricothyroid	Protect airway; adduct vocal cords

Anatomical and Physiological Overview. (1991). In B. Jones & M. W. Donner (Eds.), *Normal and abnormal swallowing: Imaging in diagnosis and therapy* (p 13). New York: Springer-Verlag. Reprinted with permission.

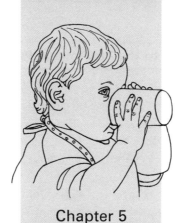

Chapter 5

Normal Development of Feeding Skills

As feeding therapists accept the challenge of designing and implementing appropriate and effective programs for children, they must be able to address three important questions:

1. What pre-feeding and feeding skills does this child already have?
2. What sensorimotor difficulties are interfering with a continued progression toward competent and efficient feeding skills?
3. What specific feeding areas is this child ready to work on, and what is the best progression or sequence for teaching these skills?

The guidelines or answers for these questions may be found in an in-depth familiarity and understanding of pre-feeding and feeding skills. A working knowledge of the normal developmental sequences of feeding provides a solid foundation for understanding when feeding development varies or deviates. It creates a frame of reference that we can use to determine whether a child's current feeding movements will lead to higher skills or create a roadblock that precludes additional growth. Developmental sequences also provide the building blocks for creating treatment programs.

As you explore the richness of normal development, discover how looking at the process in different ways creates a new understanding that enables you to say, "I really know how children develop feeding skills." Many therapists were introduced to normal development as a series of facts along with a checklist to memorize. In a sense, development was taught as a series of small destinations or developmental landmarks. Unfortunately, most people review material taught in this style, pass an examination, and promptly forget most of the information. We conceive of development as a journey, rather than a destination. We are fascinated with the information and skills that infants and young children bring to their feeding journey at each step along the route to competence and efficiency. We are more interested in the interrelationships and interconnections than in any single developmental landmark. How do infants arrive at the ability to remove food from the spoon with the top lip? What skills have they developed in other areas that enable the lip to move freely? What does this new mouth skill prepare the baby for in other areas (such as cup drinking or chewing)? We see the relatedness of everything we observe. We know that this gives us a series of working models for understanding a child's skills and needs during an assessment. From a participatory understanding of the journey, we can identify skill components that indicate where to begin in therapy. Out of an awareness of the progressions selected by most typically developing infants, we can design treatment strategies and specific techniques that support easy and successful learning.

This chapter includes a broad overview focusing on a set of familiar concepts in the developmental process. When we realize that the underlying concepts of feeding development are identical to the concepts found in all sensorimotor development, we are able to link the newer feeding observations with familiar ideas. Learning involves the establishment of associations and interconnections between the familiar and the new; it is not defined by the amount of isolated new facts that can be acquired.

Individuals vary greatly in their learning styles. To meet their differing needs, we have incorporated two ways of looking at the same developmental information. We have organized our discussion of feeding development both sequentially and globally. The sequential approach takes the view of developmental feeding skills through a detailed look at specific skill areas, the component parts of feeding maturation. For example, we can look at the development of sucking skills from birth to 2 years as they emerge with the bottle and breast, the cup, and the spoon. Developmental sequences are examined again, this time using a global approach to the learning and organization of information. The global approach presents an overview of the child's acquisition of feeding skills at a specific developmental period. The interaction and interconnection of specific feeding skills are emphasized. Each component that previously was viewed and analyzed sequentially is placed in the context of total feeding development. The Appendix contains two developmental checklists that summarize this information, the Developmental Pre-Feeding Checklist: A Sequential Approach and the Developmental Pre-Feeding Checklist: A Global Approach. Both may be reproduced and used in recording your observations.

Although it is extremely valuable to read about infant feeding development or to observe videotapes of infants eating and drinking, nothing replaces self-discovery as a tool for learning. The original edition of *Pre-Feeding Skills* included a large number of Participatory Experiences that invited readers to use their own bodies to discover the sensations and movements experienced when drinking and eating different types of liquids and food. Because of the popularity of these experiences and the enthusiasm shown by readers for this type of learning, these experiences were expanded and placed in a companion volume, *Mealtime Participation Guide* (Klein & Morris, 1999). We have included four examples (Physical Limitations No. 5: Retraction Patterns, Spoon No. 1: Smooth Food From a Spoon, Spoon No. 15: Lip Variations in Spoon Feeding, and Imaginings: Sensory No. 12: Sensory Defensiveness to Touch in the Mouth) on pages 743–753 of the Appendix.

Normal development of feeding is both intriguing and exciting. It is not a one-dimensional topic. Like the hologram that enables us to view a photograph from every angle and perspective, the developmental picture is enriched each time we shift our perspective. We invite you to enjoy this chapter and to make it truly your own as specific areas remind you of your own initial feeding experiences or those of children whom you already know. Normal development has roots and connections in every aspect of our work with children with special feeding needs. We suggest that you return to this chapter after you complete the assessment and treatment chapters.

We have incorporated information from a wide selection of researchers who have documented various aspects of the developmental process. Many of the studies cited are historical studies whose early observations have been confirmed through more current research. Others add new perspectives to specific areas of feeding and oral motor skill development. Because the sources are numerous and the results often are repeated in additional studies, we have not attempted to attribute each developmental landmark to specific authors and studies. Some are included where newer research studies or concepts are pertinent to the conclusions about development that are presented. A collection of major sources is included in the reference section.

A substantial amount of developmental information was drawn from two unpublished studies by Suzanne Evans Morris. Between 1974 and 1977, Morris completed a longitudinal study of six typically developing Caucasian infants (Morris, 1978). Gross motor, feeding, respiratory-phonatory, and phonological abilities were filmed between birth and 3 years. The infants were filmed monthly from birth to 12 months and at 3-month intervals during the second year. A final filming occurred at 36 months. The subjects were three female and three male full-term infants who were products of uneventful pregnancy, birth, and neonatal periods. Two infants were breast-fed for the first 3–5 months while four infants were bottle-fed.

Specific developmental trends in sucking, swallowing, biting, and chewing were identified in the research study. Morris clinically observed the action of the jaw, tongue, and lips/cheeks in these areas as each child used an appropriate variety of foods and utensils (e.g., liquids; soft, smooth solids; lumpy solids; chewable solids; bottle; cup; spoon; straw). An extensive list of components was created for each skill area (e.g., jaw in sucking, unstabilized jaw movement with the cup, external jaw stabilization through biting on the edge of the cup, internal jaw stabilization through muscle co-activation at the temporomandibular joint, jaw separates from the tongue in sucking).

All film segments were analyzed to determine the age at which the infants first showed each developmental component. Data for the six infants were combined to identify the age range during which these babies first showed the developmental component, the age at which the component was present in two-thirds of the group, and the age range during which earlier or more primitive components disappeared. These skill components and ages were incorporated into the development of the *Pre-Speech Assessment Scale: A Rating Scale for the Measurement of Pre-Speech Behaviors from Birth Through Two Years* (Morris, 1982).

Formal reliability studies were not done for all feeding behaviors and age levels. However, informal measures showed that the primary examiner identified the same oral motor behaviors (e.g., upper lip removing food from the spoon, tongue elevation when swallowing liquids) 96% of the time when a random sample of 50 filmed segments was viewed on three occasions at 1-month intervals. Interexaminer reliability also was addressed with 75 therapists who had been trained to recognize and score these normal oral motor behaviors in typically developing infants and in young children with cerebral palsy. Forty-eight random samples were drawn from each of the 16 feeding areas on the *Pre-Speech Assessment Scale*. The level of behavior recognition and scoring agreement was identified for each of the 16 areas. The percentage of agreement ranged from 82% to 87%.

A second study was completed between 1992 and 1994 (Morris, 1994). This was carried out as part of a longitudinal study of 98 infants and mothers that looked at specific physical, sensory, and communication cues that could be used as feeding "readiness cues" (Carruth et al., 1994; Skinner et al., 1998). Because very broad guidelines exist for introducing infants to new feeding areas such as pureed foods, lumpy foods, and cup drinking, many parents are uncertain when their baby is ready. It was hypothesized that specific clusters of physical, sensory, communication, and mouth skills could identify when an individual baby was prepared to advance to a new level of feeding skill (Morris, 1992).

As part of the two-year project, a cross-sectional study was conducted, involving 28 typically developing infants and toddlers (white, African American, and Asian). A group of six infants age 4 to 5 months was videotaped. A year later, 22 additional infants age 6 to 28 months were videotaped. Two-month intervals were selected, and two infants were taped at each age level (i.e., 6, 8, 10, 12, 14, 16, 18, 22, 24, and 28 months). The videotapes were reviewed in relationship to the feeding patterns and component skills identified in the initial feeding development study in 1974–77. Morris also noted changes related to cultural differences in children's opportunity to master new experiences. For example, in 1974, very few children were introduced to straw drinking until they were 18 to 24 months old. In the 1990s, it has become common to give infants straws when they are 8 to 12 months old. Today's children are drinking from spout cups for extended periods. Unlike toddlers 20 years ago, many of today's children have no experience drinking from an open cup until they enter preschool. These variations in experience can influence developmental landmarks for skill mastery.

The Influence of Normal Movement Development

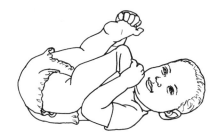

It is important to look at feeding and oral motor skills within the context of the whole body. Issues and patterns that affect normal motor development certainly influence the mouth; everything is connected (Alexander, Boehme, & Cupps, 1993).

We will explore and discover the connections between the mouth and the body, and the characteristics of normal gross motor and oral motor development that are common to both.

Stability and Mobility

The development of a progressive and changing interaction between the components of stability and mobility seems to be characteristic of all areas of sensorimotor development. We must have a stable base from which to develop movement and functional skills. Without that stability, our function or mobility is less controlled or even impossible.

An infant initially shows random disorganized, undirected, and uncontrolled movements. Those movements gradually become more organized, directed, and controlled as the infant begins to establish a means of stabilizing portions of the body. Generally, the central or proximal parts of the body are the first to develop stability or become controlled. From a controlled, proximal base of stability, the infant can have the possibility of greater mobility and more refined distal control.

In all areas of sensorimotor development, we can observe the influence of two types of stability. Initially, stability tends to be external or positional. This type of stability is achieved by supporting one part of the body against another part or against an external source, or by gaining support through a specific anatomical relationship of body parts. This external support provides an initial basis for controlled movement. By stabilizing a proximal part, a dynamic and discrete balance of control of the muscles on both sides of a joint can occur. The external environment initially provides the support or stability necessary for the child to gradually achieve more internal control or stability. Internal or postural stability is a more advanced, dynamic, and changing type of control. It is achieved without reliance on an external aid or support. Postural stability relies on the balance of contraction between agonist and antagonist muscles around a joint, and it can be achieved while the child moves through space.

Let's look at how this stability occurs in normal development. Before a child can reach and grasp efficiently for a toy, he or she must develop some control and stability at the shoulder. Refined grasp with reach is difficult without it. Initially, however, reaching is random and undirected. The child achieves initial external stability positionally by lying supine with the floor or bed supporting or stabilizing the scapulae and shoulder girdle. A child experiences initial success in more controlled reach from this position or from a supported sitting position on a parent's lap while leaning into the support of the adult's body. Moving from this position of support, the child begins to balance the cocontraction of shoulder agonist and antagonist muscles around the joint to develop internal control. As the child spends more time in prone on elbows, the positional stability of the elbow on the floor and the child's movement over the elbow, with weight shifting from side to side and forward and back, provide the external stability that leads to the development of internal stability. Therefore, another point in the development of stability is that weight bearing and then weight shift into the joint help provide the option for dynamically balancing agonists and antagonists.

The concept of mobility developing from a proximal base of stability affects the refined development of distal oral motor skills. Oral stability is dependent upon the development of neck and shoulder girdle stability, which are dependent upon trunk and pelvic stability. The head is distal, and the neck and shoulders are proximal to it. You could imagine that the head and neck sit on the proximal "floor" of the shoulders. If that floor is unstable, then all distal functions are influenced. The concept of proximal-to-distal control is highly relevant when discussing functions of the oral area. The terms are relative and dependent upon the relationship between the two areas or structures being compared. The head and neck are distal to the body. The jaw, however, can be viewed as proximal to the distal lips, cheeks, and tongue. The ability to stabilize the jaw creates the needed prerequisite for the development of skilled and refined tongue and lip movements. Clearly, there is a precise interchange between stability and mobility that influences skills in the oral area.

Separation of Movement

Precision of movement progresses from the presence of total body movement toward the refinement of specific skills. Children's movement patterns proceed from gross motor to fine motor development as proximal stability creates the possibility for more distal mobility. For example, children need head control, trunk control, rolling skills, and sitting balance before they can learn refined hand skills, purposive transfers, precise grasp, and specific toy manipulation. Oral skills also are considered a fine motor progression. They require the gross motor base of stability for the development of skilled movement to unfold.

A gross-to-fine progression also is present within skill areas. In the development of hand skills, the first grasps are palmar or whole-hand. These are considered gross hand skills. Through weight shifts and emerging stability, children gradually develop isolation of the index finger and refined two-finger pincer grasp. These skills are at the more precise end of the gross-to-fine motor continuum.

The same gross-to-fine motor progression occurs in the mouth area. As with the entire body, the progression is influenced by the ability to dissociate one part from another. At first, jaw and tongue movements are gross and unrefined. Jaw movements are wide in excursion, with limited control in the midranges of movement. This reflects the lack of internal jaw stability. The tongue moves with the jaw and is unable to move separately from it. There is not yet a dissociation of the jaw and tongue. As children gain more internal stability of the jaw and use this new control to explore biting and chewing of more difficult foods, they can separate tongue from jaw movements. With jaw stability, they can move the tongue independently to lick their lips or retrieve food that has fallen into the cheek cavity.

The ability to dissociate one movement from another and separate the movement of different parts of the body is necessary in the developmental progression toward refinement of gross and fine motor skills. Eating skills are fine motor sequences. The development of stability and the dissociation of parts are key factors in the maturation of oral skills.

Straight Planes of Movement to Rotation

Infants tend to develop in straight planes of movement before they develop lateral, diagonal, or rotary skills. Infants' initial movements are random and undirected, and tend to be a combination of alternate pulls from extensor or flexor muscle systems. As they discover that they can gain stability by leaning against an external support or against another part of their own body, children begin to develop some internal stability by balancing these straight plane extensor and flexor movements. Using extensor and flexor systems together with graded function, children can accomplish lateral righting reactions and, later, the more mature diagonal and rotational patterns of the equilibrium reactions.

Normally developing infants initially show a tendency toward active movement of the extensor muscles of the neck and, later, the back. They use these muscles while lifting the head in prone. Because the extensor system tends to develop before the flexor system in normal development, it is not unusual to see these extensor patterns predominate in infant movement up to 3 or 4 months of age. As children gradually develop better control of the counterbalancing flexor muscles, we begin to see more graded or smooth function. By playing with the balance of neck extension in prone and flexion in supine, for example, children demonstrate more stability in head control, which gives them the possibility of laterally flexing or righting the head while rolling over. As rolling and weight shifting combine with pivoting, children demonstrate more diagonal and rotary movements.

Oral motor skills also develop from straight planes toward lateral and rotary movements. We first see the jaw open and close to achieve extension and flexion for chewing. As children are introduced to soft cookies, the munching that emerges first is basically an alternating straight plane of extensor (opening) and flexor (closing) patterns. As the skill level and food textures change, we begin to see lateral movements of the jaw as food moves from side to side in the mouth. Eventually, a circular-rotational movement emerges as food is ground between the molars and transferred smoothly to the opposite side of the mouth.

Midline Development

Development of the body midline has assumed an important role in our studies of normal maturational sequences. We usually think of the midline as a vertical line separating two sides of the body. However, in our understanding of normal developmental sequences, it is important to look at the concept of four midlines of the body: vertical, horizontal, and two diagonals.

We gain an internal sense of our midline by becoming fully aware of our edges. Let us consider the edges or corners of the trunk to be the shoulders and hips, or the proximal joints. When children are prone on their forearms, they are putting weight from the flexed elbows and forearms into the shoulders, and they are weight shifting from side to side. This enables them to develop a part of their sense of vertical midline. They continually shift weight from one set of hips and shoulders to the other.

As children are in prone, lifting up the head and pushing up on the elbows, they develop an early sense of a horizontal midline. This continues to develop as they are in supine, playing with knees or feet. Rolling, pivoting, crawling, and creeping can help children feel the internal sense of a diagonal midline.

These are only a few examples of important influences on midline development. Any weight shift to or from a proximal joint can influence midline development. The use of the term midline does not automatically imply that the body is divided into two equal parts by the imaginary line. The horizontal midline, for example, creates a smaller upper portion of the body than the lower, because the legs and lower torso are longer in proportion than the arms and upper torso. As we move from an examination of gross motor skills toward fine motor skills, we see the influence of the midline concept on the development of the hand, foot, and oral control.

To be able to use separate parts of the hand as needed in a refined grasp, we need an internal awareness of the midpoint. This is achieved through a variety of weight-bearing and weight-shifting activities that provide stability to the weight-bearing side. This enables the other side to learn to separate or dissociate from the hand as a unit. When the baby lies on the tummy and reaches up or out for a toy, his or her body weight is shifted to the outer border of the non-reaching hand. The inner portion of the hand with the thumb and index finger separates from the whole hand and becomes more capable of developing the precise skills that will be available for self-feeding. Likewise, the weight shifting that occurs vertically, horizontally, and diagonally over the foot provides the sense of midline or the center of the foot necessary for refined balance reactions in the foot.

The midline awareness in the mouth is important in helping children find the center, the "home base," the resting place for the tongue. In newborns, the oral cavity is very small and is filled entirely by the tongue. The richness of sensory contact of every inch of the tongue's surface with the boundaries of the cavity allows the tongue to experience the totality of its own boundaries. A deeply cupped or grooved tongue configuration is part of the normal suckling pattern that is present at birth in full-term infants. This sharp delineation of a vertical midline creates a channel through which milk can pass from the nipple to the back of the tongue for swallowing. The tongue initially moves up and down with the jaw. As it does so, the tongue's lower and lateral boundaries become clearer. A point is reached when the elevated jaw moves downward and away from the tongue, leaving the front third of the tongue stuck briefly in its familiar point of contact on the roof of the mouth. This sense of a horizontal dividing line, or midline, is expanded as children develop tongue-tip elevation. As small lumpy foods are introduced, the tongue begins to drift or move laterally toward the stimulus of the food. It also develops a clearer sense of the sides of the mouth as the teeth erupt. The diagonal and rotational sense of a midline emerges through the experiences of biting and rotary chewing of more fibrous foods that require some grinding action. When children have experienced and defined horizontal, vertical, and diagonal oral midlines, they have a clearer sense of the center of the mouth.

The sense of center, whether it is developed in the trunk, hand, foot, or mouth is important for helping children focus attention. If a child's energies move away from the center or if there is no sense of midline, it becomes extremely difficult to obtain and maintain focused attention to tasks. Eating is an activity that requires attention and concentration, and the developed sense of midline can help both.

Reversion to Earlier Patterns of Movement

There is a tendency to revert to an earlier pattern of movement as a more difficult component of movement is perfected. When children concentrate on acquiring a new skill, some of the previously learned postural control and stability may be forfeited temporarily. When children first learn to walk, they do so with arms held high and with movements in straight planes. This gives them the look of a new walker. As they practice walking, they gain more hip and shoulder stability, and then begin to incorporate more lateral flexion and rotation into their movements. They bring their arms down to their sides, and their walking becomes smoother, less awkward, and more mature. When the same children begin to run, they revert to the straight plane of movement. Running initially lacks rotation and resembles the early stages of walking. Even though they have the necessary proximal stability for walking, children need to integrate it into their new running patterns.

We often see this reversion to earlier, more primitive patterns of movement in the development of oral motor skills. Children whose chewing experience is predominantly with softer foods use a munching pattern with some tongue lateralization. As their experience broadens to include more precise bits of food, tongue lateralization increases to meet the demands of the food. Eventually, they lateralize the tongue whenever needed and use it to transfer food across the vertical midline and support a rotary chewing pattern. If food becomes stuck in the mouth, however, they immediately revert to an extension-retraction tongue pattern that is more characteristic of an immature suckle-swallow. In the same way, children who demonstrate a good suck-swallow-breathe rhythm with a bottle may regress to a more primitive coping method when a cup is presented. They may cough, spit, and choke in ways that have not occurred with the bottle for months.

Sensory Input in the Direction and Selection of Movement

Sensory input from the environment can influence the direction and selection of movement. The touch of the floor on a child's back provides the positional stability that enables and encourages the child to move from it. The visual sighting of a toy can provide a reason to move toward the toy. The size and shape of a toy can determine the angle of reach and the type of grasp needed to pick it up.

Sensory input also affects the types of oral motor response that children select and use. The sensory aspects of food (including the size of the mouthful, texture, temperature, taste, and acidity) can make a difference in the type of movement they choose. Younger infants have fewer options available to them in choosing an appropriate movement pattern. As children mature and their developmental skills increase, a larger pool of options enables them to select the most efficient way of handling a particular food. A child may select one option with one type of food and another option with a different food type. When chewing a graham cracker, a vertical munching pattern meets the needs for mashing and dissolving the food, but when chewing a chunk of dried apricot, a more mature rotary chew is required to break down the food.

Different sensory properties of food can bias the volitional selection toward particular types of movement responses. For example, even though we assume that children gain lip control as they mature, we cannot assume that when chewing occurs it will be with lip closure. There seems to be no consistent lip pattern during chewing that is totally based on age or skill level. Lip closure appears to be strongly influenced by the sensory input offered by the type of food that is being handled. The child is more likely to close the lips during chewing if the mouthful is large and if food is apt to fall out. If the mouthful is small, the child may not need lip closure to keep the food in and may choose the easier pattern.

Sensory input also can affect spoon feeding. If the feeder puts the spoon into the child's mouth and removes it quickly, the child does not have time to use the top lip to clean the spoon. When the spoon is presented more slowly so there is time to respond, the child will stabilize the jaw in an open position and use a discrete downward movement of the top lip to remove food from the spoon. If the food is too hot, oral reactions will be rapid, and limited chewing will be used in an attempt to swallow the uncomfortable food as quickly as possible. Depending on the circumstances, the child also might respond by spitting, crying, or choking. Presenting food at a proper temperature enables children to select a more mature motor response.

Awareness that the sensory properties of food can influence the child's system toward different oral movements helps us select the type of food that is more likely to elicit advanced or mature movements. This is particularly helpful when we are evaluating a child's oral-feeding skills. Sensory variables such as size, shape, speed, temperature, taste, acidity, and texture can affect oral motor responses. In Chapters 13 and 17, we will discuss food selection in detail.

Economy and Efficiency of Movement

Young children will select the movement option that is the most efficient and economical. When two or more possibilities exist, they will choose the movement that requires the least effort. For example, most infants tend to reach for a toy placed on the left side with the left hand rather than crossing over the midline, rotating, and reaching with the right, even when both options are possible.

When eating, babies also use the most economical and efficient movements when making choices. For example, if children have the option of keeping the lips open or closed during chewing, they select the more complex act of closing the lips only if they need to keep the food from falling out (e.g., if the mouthful is particularly large or juicy, if tongue movements are immature). However, if the tongue, jaw, and cheeks can keep the food in without lip support, open mouth chewing will predominate. This point of view is supported by Gisel's study on the influence of food texture on oral-feeding movements in children 6 months to 2 years old (Gisel, 1991). She observed that up to 10 months of age, children suckled in response to applesauce but shifted to a munching strategy for Cheerios®. She concluded, " … the transitional infant uses the feeding method that requires the least effort. If food can be ingested by suckling, the child will not munch." (p. 76)

Ease and efficiency of movement often are compromised as children get older and move toward adulthood. Certain patterns are repeated more frequently and are perceived as more comfortable or familiar. Others are selected or rejected based on periods of physical discomfort. For example, a child may develop a preference for chewing predominantly on one side of the mouth. This asymmetrical pattern may become stronger if there is pain from a dental cavity or canker sore on the other side. Eventually it may feel very strange if food moves toward the unfamiliar side, and the child will move it quickly into the comfort zone.

Rhythmicity

Rhythmicity is a concept that surrounds and nourishes each of the preceding components. It is perhaps the most basic and encompassing issue of normal development. All living organisms are oscillators that change and pulse rhythmically. The human body consists of a series of electromagnetic impulses, pulsing in different but complementary time relationships. When two or more oscillators in the same general field pulse at nearly the same time, they lock together so that eventually they pulse at exactly the same time. This is called entrainment. Nature appears to seek the most efficient energy state. Entrainment is a feature of this efficiency because it requires less energy to pulse in cooperation than in opposition.

The idea of entrainment is important in the development of feeding and early communication skills. We know, for example, that a speaker makes tiny movements of the body that are precisely synchronized with changes in the syllables, words, phrases, and sentences of speech. These movements follow a definite rhythm, and the speaker's body functions as an oscillator with an entrainment between speech and body movements. Listeners also move in a special shared rhythm with the speaker. As the speaker's words and body movements change, the listener's body produces a similar set of movement shifts. The listener is in physical harmony with the speaker, blending and reflecting the special rhythms and nuances of the speaker's speech-body relationship. These pre-speech rhythms of relationship also are present in newborns listening to adult speech (Condon & Sander, 1974). This implies that the infant has acquired the rhythmical structure of language and relationship in utero.

In some children, these inner rhythms are impaired or different (Condon, 1975). These youngsters experience difficulties in bonding and communication, and often retreat into rhythmical patterns of rocking and spinning to organize a world that confuses and overwhelms them. We can speculate that entrainment or shared rhythms underlie the most basic aspect of our humanity. Our close feelings for another person may be related to our ability to share rhythms.

When a child moves stiffly or with movements that are random and uncontrolled, it may be more difficult for the parent or therapist to feel close and loving. A special link in the development of empathy and understanding of the other person is missing or distorted. This is very important when we consider the highly communicative and interactive nature of the mealtime and the feeding movements that accompany it.

Rhythm is the most consistent characteristic of feeding patterns during the first 3 months of life. Long before feeding reflects the influence of jaw stability or separation of movement, there is rhythm. The newborn begins sucking with a rapid, efficient, and regular movement. The pattern of bursts and pauses is unique to each infant and is as personal as a signature or voice print. Irregularities in the sucking rhythm have been identified as one indicator of brain dysfunction or damage in newborns.

We have rhythm generators for all body systems. Rhythms in the circulatory, respiratory, digestive, and sleep systems are familiar to everyone. The feeding system also has a set of rhythm generators (Dick, Oku, Romaniuk, & Cherniack, 1993). Patterned interrelationships exist between swallowing and breathing. Sucking and chewing rhythms and tempos are similar in everyone; simultaneously they carry with them the subtle variation in tempo that reflects each person's uniqueness. A regular rhythm with a speed of 1 act or cycle per second is common in sucking and chewing patterns. The tempo and rhythm of these feeding patterns is similar to the heel-to-toe gait in walking and the resting tempo of the heartbeat. The tempo of 60 cycles per minute (or 1 cycle per second) is an important reflection of a significant body rhythm-tempo.

When a baby moves from the bottle to the cup or spoon, he or she must develop new coordination patterns. In the beginning stages, the rhythm pattern is irregular, and the timing and coordination of the new skill is immature. The development of a smoother rhythm pattern gives a more mature appearance to the evolving sucking, swallowing, and chewing patterns. The timing with which each part of the total pattern (that is, the individual contributions of the jaw, tongue, lips, cheeks, and palate) interacts with the others to create the whole determines the level of skill and function.

Cultural Influences

Cultural values and beliefs influence the opportunities that children are given to master physical and social skills (Lynch & Hanson, 1992). As a result, children from different cultural groups may reach some developmental milestones at different ages. Children who grow up in cultures that value interdependence over independence may develop self-care skills at a somewhat later period. In 1992, the American Academy of Pediatrics responded to international research that showed a relationship between sudden infant death syndrome and the prone-lying position for sleep (Lockridge, 1997). They recommended that parents place infants only in supine or sidelying for sleep. Since then, studies have shown a delay in reaching motor milestones that are influenced by movement experiences on the tummy such as rolling from prone to supine, sitting, creeping, crawling, and pulling to stand (Davis, Moon, Sachs, & Ottolini, 1998; Jantz, Blosser, & Fruechting, 1997). Because the age of walking was not affected, it is assumed that infants catch up and develop the necessary motor components in other ways.

In the United States, most infants are introduced to cup drinking through use of a cup with a special sipper or spout. In the past, these spouted cups were phased out by the end of the first year and babies had experience drinking from an open cup held by an adult. This is not the case today. The wide variety of spouted cups on the market reflects a cultural desire for children to be independent in their cup drinking, yet not messy. Most 2-year-olds and many 3-year-olds continue to use this type of cup. They typically move from the spouted cup to a straw or sports bottle rather than to an open cup for drinking.

Morris (1978) found that all six infants in her longitudinal study used a pattern of external jaw stability in drinking by biting the edge of the cup for stabilization by the time they were 24 months. This movement pattern was noted as early as 11 months in one infant and was seen in two-thirds of the children by the time they were 18 months old. A cross-sectional study noted that in a group of 16 children between 12 and 28 months old, all continued to use a spouted cup and none had much experience with an open cup (Morris, 1994). All of the children used a wide unstabilized jaw excursion with both the familiar spouted cup and an open cup used during the evaluation. Jaw stabilization during drinking was not seen in any of these children.

As societal and cultural patterns are added, children and adults may not select the most economical movement alternatives. They will select the one that enables them to fit in at the mealtime. For example, in most western countries, it is considered impolite to chew with the mouth open. Despite the fact that it requires more muscle movements and oral coordination to hold the lips closed while moving the jaw up and down, mouth closure during eating is used by most older children and adults. In Korea and many North African countries, this is considered extremely rude. Eating with an open mouth, smacking the lips, and even belching tells the host that the meal is being enjoyed.

Theme and Variations

Normal sensorimotor development is based on a series of themes that fit most babies and an abundance of variations that fit each individual baby. Variations in movement experiences and opportunities are provided by the way a baby is held and positioned, by the sensory input that is available, and by the baby's prior experiences. Variations in feeding skills are based on a complex intermixture of movement coordination, sensory input from food and utensils, and parent and cultural preferences. It is critically important for children to develop the flexibility within their sensorimotor system that enables them to adjust to small variations in the environment.

For example, infants acquire the ability to sit steadily through developing movement patterns of flexion and extension. The majority of infants will begin to develop the extensor component by lying on their tummies, supporting themselves on their forearms, and lifting their shoulders and heads from the floor. Some infants whose parents never place them on their tummies (even for play) develop different sorts of extensor movement experience and control through other activities such as pushing back when sitting in a supported position on the lap or held upright over the shoulder. These may lead toward the same end point or destination through a different route.

The Influence of Oral Sensory Development

Sensory Windows

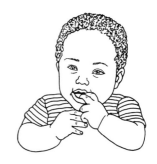

The normal development of the infant's sensory systems also has a major impact on oral sensorimotor skills. Sensation is involved at every point in movement. Most movements are initiated through intention and sensory stimuli that prepare or set the muscles for movement to implement the intention. Thus, if I wish to reach for a glass of water, I am guided initially through my sense of thirst, the visual stimulus of the glass, or an inner thought that I want to take a drink from the glass. My prior experiences with the type of glass and my knowledge of its location and weight enable me to get the muscles of my trunk, shoulder girdle, arms, hands, and fingers ready to reach for the glass, lift it from the table, and bring it to my mouth. If the glass is full, the muscles will prepare themselves to lift a heavier load than if I know the glass is almost empty. As I reach, lift, and bring the glass to my mouth, the sensory receptors in the muscles give constant feedback on the correctness or effectiveness of the physical movement. Based on this sensory feedback, the muscles constantly correct and adjust any errors in the movement plan.

The mouth and hand have the highest number of sensory receptors per square inch of any other part of the human body. Moreover, the sensory receptors of the mouth are the earliest to emerge in fetal development. After birth, the infant seems to explore and learn predominantly by bringing everything to the mouth.

The intraoral mouth space of the newborn is small. It is completely filled by the tongue, which is in constant sensory contact with the palate and dental arches. This provides the infant with a highly evolved sensory feedback of the shape and movement of the mouth at all times (Bosma, 1967). As the lower jaw grows downward and forward between 4 and 6 months, this sensory contact is more variable. With greater inner mouth space and neurological maturation, the tongue engages in a wider variety of movements with corresponding sensory contacts.

Early mouthing activities provide the infant with abundant oral sensory input. This may stimulate rhythmical non-nutritive sucking for self-calming or provide interesting sensory experiences through feeling the fingers or environmental objects. Infants seem to prefer the sensory input of their own body during early mouthing activities. When they are well supported, they can bring their own hands to the mouth. When adults hold a toy to their mouths for sucking and mouthing, they may be satisfied and continue to seek its input. However, if their own hand contacts the mouth, they often lose interest in the toy, preferring the feeling of their own body. The input of the hand may be more interesting because the baby is receiving simultaneous sensory input from both the hand and the mouth rather than from the mouth alone. Sensory responses are difficult to measure directly during infancy. Our perceptions of the baby's response to shifts in sensory information are made on the basis of motor responses. When the infant changes facial expression or increases, decreases, or changes physical or oral movements, we presume that the movement response was in direct response to sensory awareness, perception, and preference.

Taste

Researchers now know that even newborns have strong taste preferences. A variety of research studies have shown that the taste of foods eaten by mothers is transmitted through breast milk, making it a rich source of flavor information for the baby (Mennella, 1995; Mennella & Beauchamp, 1998a). For example, the smell and taste of garlic is known to permeate the breast milk of a mother who has consumed it, and infants show a preference for milk flavored with garlic (Mennella & Beauchamp, 1991; Mennella & Beauchamp, 1993b). The tastes and odors from the mother's diet also are transferred to amniotic fluid, and bottle-fed infants show a preference for the odor of their mother's amniotic fluid over the smell of their formula (Marlier, Schaal, & Soussignan, 1998; Mennella, Johnson,

& Beauchamp, 1995). Nursing babies from different cultures may actually become familiar with the flavors of their culture long before solids are presented (Mennella 1996; Mennella & Beauchamp, 1993a; Weber, Woolridge, & Baum, 1986).

Studies suggest that young animals are more likely to accept unfamiliar foods if they experienced a wide range of flavors during suckling (Bassette, Fung, & Mantha, 1986; Nolte, Provenza, & Balph, 1990). Likewise, during weaning, breast-fed infants strongly preferred cereal that had been mixed with their mother's milk over cereal mixed with water (Mennella & Beauchamp, 1997). Breast-fed infants who had been exposed to vanilla and ethanol flavors in their mother's milk showed a clear preferential response for a vanilla-scented toy, a neutral response to an unscented toy, and a negative response to the ethanol-scented toy (Mennella & Beauchamp, 1998b). This indicated that infants could detect and retain information about their chemical sensory experiences in breast milk and were able to generalize their responses in an unfamiliar context.

In comparison with breast-fed babies, one wonders how predominantly bottle-fed babies experience early flavors. Perhaps their reduced experience with flavors during formula feeding influences generalized acceptance of new foods later on in life. This information can have a strong influence on how we introduce new flavors to children developmentally and therapeutically.

Infants and young children also are predisposed to prefer tastes that are sweet and to reject those that are bitter or sour (Birch, 1998a). This presumably has survival value because most sweet foods in nature are safe to eat, while many poisonous foods are bitter. Positive response to salty tastes increase during early infancy but are based on other features of the food as well as the child's prior experiences with different tastes (Beauchamp & Cowart, 1985; Beauchamp & Moran, 1984). For example, in one study, 3-year-olds enjoyed a salty soup broth, but immediately rejected even small amounts of salt in water (Cowart & Beauchamp, 1986).

The work of Birch and her colleagues shows that 2-year-old children who actually are ready to increase their dietary variety become extremely neophobic (Birch, 1998a; Birch, Johnson, et al., 1995; Birch & Marlin, 1982). They refuse a new food, but gradually increase their acceptance as they repeatedly are exposed to the taste. Birch hypothesizes that this built-in caution also is an adaptive response of the species. In a broad sense, children are suspicious of new food because it could be dangerous. Through repeated exposure without becoming ill, they learn that it is safe and can be eaten without harm.

The Influence of Non-Feeding Oral Motor Development

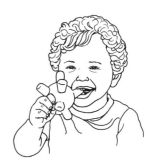

When we think of normal feeding development and the transitions to more complex feeding skills, we usually focus on the infant's changing response to different foods, liquids, and utensils. However, we also can look at the non-feeding skills that the baby is developing and examine their relationship to emerging changes in eating and drinking.

Mouthing

Because sensations in the mouth are more highly developed than in any other part of the body, the mouth is truly the baby's "window to the world" (Gibson, 1967). Many babies use the mouth before they are born to suck their fingers and make discoveries about their intrauterine world. After birth, babies continue to put their own hands in the mouth, and suck or mouth the fingers of a parent, the edge of a blanket, clothing, pacifiers, and other objects that come in contact with the mouth. We call this period *generalized mouthing*, which predominates during the first 4 to 5 months of life. Through this type of mouthing, babies become familiar with general sensations of softness, firmness, and hardness. These sensations familiarize children with the sensations they will encounter as they move from the nipple to the spoon or cup.

An active gag reflex protects the infant who lacks the coordination to chew and swallow food. The gag occurs when an object or food touches the back three-quarters of the tongue. As sensorimotor skills increase and the child is ready to handle solid foods, the strong gag is no longer critical to survival. Between 4 and 6 months, most typically developing babies reduce the strength of the gag through placing their fingers and toys further back in the mouth. Eventually the gag is only triggered when food is stuck on the back one-quarter of the tongue. This is a gradual process that usually begins before the child is ready for more complex foods.

By 6 months, infants typically can sit without support, push up on their arms when lying on the abdomen, and reach for toys. They have developed greater stability in the trunk and shoulder girdle, which creates a foundation for more skillful movements of both the hand and mouth. Children now can hold toys without dropping them, and turn and move them around in the mouth to explore all surfaces. The jaw makes more skillful adjustments in opening and closing, the tongue moves with greater freedom in the mouth, and the lips come forward like a pair of small hands to feel the surface of anything entering the mouth. With this new stage of *discriminative mouthing*, children use the mouth to extract all types of sensory information from whatever enters it. By exploring the toy with the tongue, lips, and jaw, they find out about size, shape, surface texture, taste, and weight. When children are introduced to solid foods, they encounter the same sensory features that they have explored with toys. They are free to expand their sensory awareness and discrimination, learn how to move smaller pieces around, and swallow safely and comfortably.

During this same period, sensations from the gums draw children's awareness to the mouth during teething. This increases the desire to put things in the mouth. Children discover sensations that increase comfort, and increase their biting, chewing, and oral exploration of toys.

Mouthing skills appear to provide a variety of experiences and opportunities that may prepare the mouth for the next step in oral-feeding development. Babies encounter a wide variety of random sensory input in the form of differing amounts of pressure on the lips, cheeks, and tongue. The location of the sensory information changes, and the timing with which it is introduced varies. This expands awareness of the temporal and spatial cues that can be used to help organize a more complex bolus of food. As the tongue and lips develop the ability to move and surround the finger or toy in different ways, babies have the opportunity to learn about shape, surface texture, and size.

Mouthing provides opportunities both for sensory awareness and discrimination and for movement experience related to specific sensory input. Babies who are ready for the challenge of pureed foods from a spoon already are familiar with long spoon-like objects that enter the mouth as a finger or toy and random sensory contact with different parts of the mouth. They learn quickly that they can organize the new food and move it backward for swallowing by beginning a rhythmical suck. Older infants who have explored their world with discriminative mouthing are well prepared for the adventure of lumpy foods. They already recognize texture, size, shape, and location in the mouth. They have learned to move the tongue to explore toys, and enjoy the feeling of biting down with the gums and making small chewing motions on toys or fingers. Most babies learn to adapt these familiar experiences to the new challenge of textured and chewy foods.

Non-Nutritive Sucking

Babies engage in two different types of sucking. Nutritive sucking is used to obtain nourishment and is observed when the infant is breast-feeding or bottle-feeding. Non-nutritive sucking is used for state regulation, calming, and organization; to satisfy the desire to suck; and in exploration. This type of suck is organized in patterns of bursts and pauses that are unique to a specific infant. Approximately two up-down cycles of the jaw occur per second during non-nutritive sucking.

Non-nutritive sucking supports early infant development in a variety of ways. Most infants use sucking on their hands or a pacifier as a major means of self-calming and organization when they are upset or overstimulated. When infants have difficulty bringing their hands to the mouth for self-initiated sucking, they often show more irritability and difficulty with self-regulation. Breast-feeding infants often use a non-nutritive suck at the breast with little or no secretion of milk when they are distressed or need to be calmed. Infants and toddlers who have difficulty with sensory-processing skills frequently increase the amount of non-nutritive sucking they do throughout the day. From infancy through adulthood, sucking and mouthing activities may help organize the sensory system, and assist with sensory regulation and the focus of attention (Oetter, Richter, Frick, 1988).

Research has shown that sucking on a pacifier reduced fussing, crying, and overall behavioral distress during painful procedures (DiPietro, Cusson, Caughy, & Fox, 1994; Field & Goldson, 1984), improved oxygen saturation (Treloar, 1994), and reduced heart rate (Shiao, Chang, Lannon, & Yarandi, 1997). These changes may explain how growth may be enhanced in preterm infants who engage in non-nutritive sucking on a pacifier (Woodson & Hamilton, 1988).

Numerous research studies have shown that sucking on a pacifier during gavage feedings or prior to sucking from a nipple helped the premature infant's transition from tube to oral feedings. Field et al. (1982) replicated an original study by Measel and Anderson (1979). The preterm infants who were given pacifiers during tube feedings averaged 27 fewer tube feedings, started bottle feeding 3 days earlier, averaged a greater weight gain per day, and were discharged 8 days earlier than babies in the control group who were not given a pacifier. These and other studies have shown that during oral feedings, babies who were given pacifiers showed fewer state changes, were more calmly alert, showed less oxygen desaturation, and had a stronger initiation and duration of the first nutritive suck burst (Pickler, Frankel, Walsh, & Thompson, 1996; Pickler, Higgins, & Crummette, 1993).

Non-nutritive sucking also influences gastrointestinal function during tube feeding. Widstrom et al. (1988) studied seven preterm infants during two tube feedings. The infants sucked on a pacifier during one of these meals. Feeding time was significantly decreased and gastric emptying time was shortened for five infants when sucking the pacifier. This was attributed to the release of gastrin and somatostatin, two peptide hormones that stimulate gastric motor function and facilitate digestion.

Although the majority of studies support the view that non-nutritive sucking improves the nutritional outcome and gastrointestinal well being of premature infants, two studies did not. Ernst et al. (1989) fed a group of infants a carefully controlled formula and assessed weight gain, linear growth, and gastric emptying time weekly. They found no effect of non-nutritive sucking on any of these measures. Orenstein (1988) evaluated the non-nutritive sucking of a pacifier on infants younger than 6 months of age with severe gastroesophageal reflux. She found that pacifier use increased the frequency of reflux episodes in infants who were placed in a prone position after a meal, but decreased it in infants who were placed in a sitting position. Non-nutritive sucking did not affect the clearing of reflux episodes or the total reflux time.

A Sequential Look at Feeding Skills

The normal development of oral feeding skills follows a sequential pattern that is similar in most babies. Yet each infant is unique, with a unique nervous system, a unique set of experiences, and a unique inner agenda. This will result in a timetable of development that is a range of months and a slightly variable sequence of steps. Some infants seem determined to spend their waking hours moving and learning to conquer the world through physical interaction. Others are more interested in understanding the environment by carefully watching, listening, and considering. They engage themselves physically, but to a lesser extent. Some children are determined to master cup drinking as soon as they see a parent drinking from a glass. Others seem very happy with the bottle or breast and have less early interest learning to use the strange object their parents call a cup.

We know that there is a readiness period when the central nervous system has reached a stage of development that supports each new skill (McGraw, 1966). Providing more practice and experience before a child is developmentally ready to learn a skill does not result in earlier acquisition of the skill or a higher level of ability. Four of the six subjects in a study by Morris (1978) were bottle-fed infants who were spoon fed pureed foods by 1 month of age, a frequent practice in the mid-'70s. The two children who were breast-fed began spoon-feeding at 3½ months and 5½ months. The ability to bring the upper lip down and forward to help clean food off the spoon emerged between 5 and 8 months with two thirds of the infants developing this skill at 7 months. Morris found no relationship between the infant's amount of experience with spoon feeding and the age at which this skill was observed.

The ages and stages listed in this sequential discussion of feeding development are approximate. Individual parents will offer their infants the opportunity to learn a new skill at different times. Individual children will differ in their personal timing and readiness to learn.

Feeding Positions

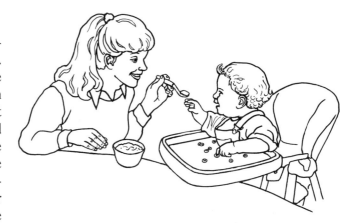

Infants are fed in a variety of positions during their first 3 months. Positions are varied to provide the greatest physical comfort for both the mother and the child. The infant may be fed supine with the head slightly elevated, prone on the mother's chest, reclining at an angle of less than 45 degrees, in a supported semi-sitting position greater than 45 degrees, or in sidelying. The choice of position often is guided by the type of feeding the mother has selected. Infants who are breast-fed are held consistently in a position that provides some elongation of the neck combined with a tipping downward of the chin so that it appears to be tucked neatly into the front of the body. This slightly upright, chin-tucked position increases sucking efficiency and reduces the amount of air swallowed during nursing. It improves digestion and reduces colic. There is greater variability when infants are fed by bottle. A straight bottle often requires the infant to be reclined with the head tipped slightly backward in order to suck the final ounces. When a bottle with an angled neck is used, a position similar to that used by the breast-fed baby is possible, thus reducing colic.

At 3 months, infants are larger and have increased muscle tone, giving them more strength and control. It is common for babies of this age to be held or positioned in an infant seat in a supported semi-sitting posture, reclining at an angle that varies between 45 and 90 degrees. Again, this will vary with the feeding method used by the feeder. In ensuing months, the position will move more and more toward the upright, tracking the infant's overall physical progression toward sitting and standing.

By 7 months, babies are sitting independently. Although independent sitting may support the infant's needs for simple play and gross motor skills, it does not provide sufficient stability for oral feeding and other fine motor skills. They need extra support because the addition of feeding activities places stress on the newly learned sitting pattern. Children of this age typically are fed while sitting in a high chair, infant chair, or special chair with the seat back at a 90-degree angle. Rolled towels, pillows, or a tray provide external support. Alternately, the feeder may provide the necessary external support by holding the child.

With maturation and practice, the child improves sitting skills. By 9 months, infants have developed more trunk and pelvic stability, leading to greater security in sitting. The parents may continue the same high chair or seating arrangement used at 7 months, but the baby no longer needs the pillows or towels that provided extra support and security.

Most parents continue to use high chairs or other type of restrained, supportive seating arrangement for infants until the children are 18 to 24 months old. The high chair and seat belt provide physical security for babies who are curious, adventurous, and fearless of falling out. They also provide peace of mind for the parent, who can focus on the feeding interaction rather than the child's physical insecurity and risk of falling or climbing out of the chair. By the time a child is 18 months, parents usually have other physical positioning options. Sitting balance has been well established, and the child can sit securely and engage in many new fine motor skills without risk of tumbling over. If they choose, they can use a small child's chair and table, a junior chair at the family table, or a booster seat placed on an adult chair at the table. The child is able to sit well without the external support of the high chair back. Parents may continue to use the high chair at home or when eating out because of its convenience and ability to provide a physical restraint during mealtime.

Food Quantity

The amount of food and liquid consumed by a full-term infant varies according to size and weight, appetite, and cultural feeding patterns. As children get older, their caloric intake and meal size typically increase (Pearcey & De Castro, 1997). Infants generally extract from the breast the amount of milk needed to maintain an appropriate level of growth and nutrition. The amount of food taken at each feeding depends on how frequently the infant is fed and on the caloric density or richness of the food (Matheny, Birch, & Picciano, 1990). More frequent feedings usually imply less food and liquid per meal. Even premature infants seem able to regulate the volume of intake according to caloric density when placed on demand feedings (Pridham et al., 1999). When meals contain many high calorie foods, the child may eat less food or reduce the amount of food eaten at the next meal (Birch & Deysher, 1986).

During the first month after birth, the infant usually takes from 2 to 6 ounces of liquid per feeding. This gradually increases so that up to 7 or 8 ounces are consumed by 3 months and up to 9 or 10 ounces are taken at 5 months. By 7 months, the baby is taking 11 or more ounces of food and liquid. This amount will continue to vary during the first 2 years, according to the child's needs and desires.

Sometimes it is difficult for parents to trust that their baby's intake is directed by an inner knowledge or wisdom. Power contests around eating and the progression toward obesity frequently begin when the parent decides that the child has not eaten enough (Birch & Fisher, 1995; Johnson & Birch, 1994; Skinner et al., 1998). Eating is an area where the infant can take full responsibility for the amount ingested. The child is the expert who knows how much is enough.

Food Types and the Transition From Liquids to Table Foods

Full-term infants are born with the reflex mechanism necessary to suck and swallow liquids. Their oral motor skills and digestive system are designed to support the intake of nourishing liquids from their mother's breast. These basic abilities become slightly modified if the mother prefers to use a prepared formula and a latex or silicone nipple. The earliest suckle and swallow movements are highly automatic. They function in a more reflexive fashion that increases their predictability and reduces the amount of movement choice available for handling other types of food. Normal movements become less automatic and more voluntary as the nervous system matures. The oral reflexes gradually become integrated and incorporated in similar movements that the infant can control and direct at will.

By the time babies are between 4 and 6 months old, digestive and motor skills have reached a level where new types of food can be introduced (American Academy of Pediatrics, 1980). Many infants receive only breast milk until they reach 6 months. The increasing need for iron and lack of an adequate amount of this mineral in the mother's milk makes it necessary to add supplemental smooth solids or a mineral supplement by 6 months. Parents usually introduce smooth solids, such as strained or pureed foods, during this period. In a longitudinal study of 98 infants (Skinner, Carruth, Houck, Moran, et al., 1997) found that the mean age for adding cereal to the diet was 3.8 months while juice, fruit, and vegetables were added at an average of 5 months. She and her colleagues found a wide variation in the specific ages at which different foods were introduced. For example, 18 infants were given cereal by 2 months while 14 were older than 5 months.

As head control and stability in sitting improve, a more secure foundation emerges for skilled mouth movements to develop. By 8 to 9 months, babies eat smooth solids well and begin to participate in the feeding process by feeding themselves baby cookies and other simple finger foods. They begin to handle lumps and textures in food, and their diet gradually shifts toward lumpy solids such as ground, Third Stage foods, or mashed table foods.

By the first birthday, babies can handle coarsely chopped table foods, including moistly cooked ground meats, bologna, and other lunchmeats, baby meat sticks, and soft cooked chicken and fish. Skinner, Carruth, Houck, Moran, et al. (1997) found, however, that baby food was still a major component in the diet at 12 months. Babies are now active participants in the feeding process.

At 18 months, toddlers can handle and enjoy coarsely chopped table foods, most meats, and many raw vegetables. They have many food preferences. Some toddlers pass through stages of wanting only one food that they love, and they may fall in love with a food today and hate it tomorrow. This is a period of learning and discovery. Mealtimes become an adventure as these children gain practice in independence and refine their feeding skills.

Although the child's coordination for handling more complex foods increases through the preschool years, certain foods may be dangerous if the child swallows them whole and chokes (Byard et al., 1996; Harris, Baker, Smith, & Harris, 1984). Firm, round foods that are similar in size and shape to the child's airway should not be given or should be cut into smaller pieces until the child is 3 or 4 years old. These include round candy, nuts, popcorn, grapes, raw carrots, pieces of apple, corn chips, and circular pieces of hot dog and sausage that have not had the skin cut off.

Culture and family preferences strongly guide the type of foods offered to infants and young children and the timing of their presentation. Infants usually are offered smooth pureed semi-solids before they are given lumpy or chewy solids. This, however, is not true of all infants. In some families and cultural groups, the baby is breast fed exclusively through 6 months of age. As weaning begins, some infants receive pureed foods for a brief period, but others are offered lumpy foods or soft, chewable foods right away. Some typically developing infants do not like pureed foods and are very unenthusiastic when they are given. They may become very eager eaters when offered foods with more texture and flavor. This pattern also is true of many toddlers and preschool children who have difficulty processing oral sensory information. These youngsters typically have a very difficult time accepting pureed foods and may begin their eating experience with foods that are firm and crunchy. Thus, the ability to take pureed foods during the transitional period between breast milk (or formula) and solid foods may be based on cultural and individual infant preferences rather than the infant's developmental needs. By the time babies are 6 months old, they have developed the physical and oral sensorimotor skills that support learning to chew and handle lumpy foods. Perhaps it is only in societies that introduce supplemental foods earlier than 6 months that a smoother transition food is necessary.

Newborn Oral Motor Reflexes

Infants are born ready to suck and ready to survive. Their ability to feed well at birth can be attributed to a combination of reflexive responses that enables them to locate the source of nourishment, to suckle, and to swallow the liquid. Infants use the rooting reaction to locate the source of food. Touching or stroking infants' cheeks or lips causes them to turn toward the touching object. This is how they initially find the breast. This food-seeking response appears to prepare the infants for feeding. The suck-swallow reflex appears at or soon after birth. The mouth opens and sucking movements begin when light touch is applied to the corners or center parts of the lips. Normally developing infants experience sucking movements before birth. As early as the fifth month of pregnancy, the fetus is able to make suckling movements when the lips are touched. Many newborns have red, swollen thumbs from sucking vigorously in utero. Sucking is elicited in full-term infants shortly after birth by many types of stimuli, including taste, touch, and temperature. Touch to the cheeks or forehead may elicit reflexive sucking in the newborn. After several days, the response becomes more specific, and sucking is elicited only when stimuli are applied to the immediate area of the mouth—to the lips, cheeks, and inside of the mouth.

Most oral and pharyngeal reflexes have one purpose—the survival of the baby. Through the suck-swallow reflex, the infant is nourished. Through a cough reflex, the airway is protected from foreign objects. The gag reflex is present and is quite sensitive at birth. It, too, is a protective pattern, designed for survival.

A transverse tongue reflex is elicited by touch or taste stimulation applied to the lateral or side of the tongue. When the tongue is stimulated, it moves toward the stimulus. This response is an example of an automatic reflexive pattern that has little functional significance for the newborn. However, it provides the pattern of movement for tongue lateralization in chewing that will emerge at a volitional level when the infant is 6 to 8 months old.

Infants are born with several reflexes that remind us of the neurological and functional connections that exist between the hand and mouth. The palmomental reflex is activated by touch to the palm of the hand. This stimulus elicits a wrinkling of the mentalis muscle in the chin. Babkin's reflex is another hand-mouth reflex. When the base of the palm is pressed, the mouth opens, the eyes close, and the head moves forward. Newborns also have an active grasp reflex. The pressure of a finger placed in the palm and providing slight traction against the finger flexors causes the baby's hand to grasp and hold tightly. Babies can suspend their full weight from their hands, holding an adult's fingers or a rod. The grasp reflex is closely connected with the sucking reflex. When the baby sucks, the grasp tightens without the stimulus of traction against the finger flexors.

These three hand-mouth reflexes have little relevance for human infants who are well cared for by their mothers. For other animal newborns, a reflex pattern such as the increase of the grasp with sucking can play a major role in survival. Ape mothers are not as careful while holding their babies for feeding. An ape infant uses the grasp reflex to hold the mother. The tightening of the grasp when sucking is initiated is very handy if the mother decides to move around. The grasping, kneading reactions of a newborn kitten while nursing are similar in the functional interaction between the mouth and hand. This basic interconnection in the human is useful to remember. Although the patterns have little significance for infant survival, their impact can be felt as the baby learns to become a self-feeder. In the normal child, they support the coordination between hand and mouth. If the reflexes do not become integrated, they can trigger limiting oral-feeding patterns when the child tries to use the hands to bring food or a spoon to the mouth.

Automatic reflex patterns support the baby's survival. They assure that the infant can find and take in the milk that will provide nourishment for future growth and development. The reflex patterns provide one model for learning as integration takes place through slow change. New patterns evolve from old ones. Portions of a familiar pattern become the core elements for learning a new pattern. Earlier, we observed that learning occurs through the interconnections made between familiar and new information. In a similar fashion, infants do not learn to move through the simple additive fashion of isolated bits of new movement. Learning is an evolution and a creation of new variations on old patterns. Components of movement are combined in new and unique patterns and combinations to create the landmarks of normal development. This blending of the new and old can be seen in all aspects of feeding development. The automatic reflexes that are programmed into the human system provide the building blocks from which similar responses will emerge at a voluntary level. This movement from automatic to voluntary is a slow dance gradually moving toward volitional control. It is never a case of an automatic pattern one day and a fully volitional one the next day or even the next week. Although age ranges have been described for the duration of the reflex, it is difficult to define in a clearly age-related manner. Most of the early reflex patterns begin to lose their obligatory aspects and become modified between 4 and 6 months, when cortical development begins. Babkin's reflex, the palmomental reflex, the increased grasp with sucking reflex, and the transverse tongue reflex have been described at birth and in the infant of 1 or 2 months. No normative studies have been reported that indicate the age period in which one would no longer see these responses.

Sucking Liquids From the Bottle or Breast

Newborn oral reflexes provide the foundation for the nutritive sucking and swallowing that forms the basis for all growth and development. Sucking can be described as the intake phase of eating liquids and soft foods. It is sometimes referred to as the oral stage of the swallow. It involves taking the food or liquid into the mouth, and moving it to the back of the oral cavity for swallowing. Sucking movements need to be easily initiated, rhythmical, strong, sustained, and efficient. The newborn begins to suck as soon as the stimulation of breast or bottle touches the face. The movement is rhythmical and creates a pattern of sucks, pauses, and swallows that is characteristic of the individual baby. Just as our handwriting or a voiceprint can identify us, the newborn can be identified by variations of the rhythmical pattern in the timing, strength, and relationship between sucking bursts and pauses. This has sometimes been called the infant's "sucking signature."

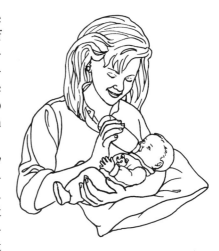

The suck is strong and sustained. When the mother gently pulls the nipple from the baby's mouth, she will feel a tightening of the suck and a resistance to taking away the food source. This strength also allows the baby to suck an adequate amount before tiring. The infant continues to suck, sustaining the pattern for 5 to 10 minutes or until needing to be burped. Most infants obtain whatever amount of milk they need in 20 to 30 minutes. When the infant is breast fed, there is no measure of the volume of milk taken at the meal. The mother simply knows that if she nurses about 10 minutes on each breast, her baby will get everything he needs. We can describe this combination of adequate amount within a reasonable time as a reflection of the baby's sucking efficiency. The infant uses only those movements of the tongue, lips, and jaw that are needed to draw the liquid into the mouth and swallow it.

Two distinct phases of sucking development occur in infant development.

Suckling is the earliest intake pattern observed in infants. The lower jaw and front of the tongue elevate together, placing pressure on the base of the nipple. This provides a positive pressure that helps to extract the milk. The tongue begins a distinctive, rhythmical, backward-forward stripping movement that helps draw liquid into the mouth and propels it toward the pharynx for swallowing. As the jaw moves slightly downward and the back of the tongue depresses, a slight negative pressure is created within the mouth. This creates a suction that allows the nipple to refill. This down-back tongue movement is followed by the up-forward tongue movement that draws the milk out of the nipple and into the mouth. Although the tongue moves in a forward direction for half of the suckle pattern, the backward phase is the most pronounced, and tongue protrusion does not extend beyond the border of the lips. The movements are similar for breast-feeding and bottle-feeding with the exception of a more forward movement of the tongue position during breast-feeding. The early suckle-swallow pattern in newborns and in very young infants has been extensively studied using radiographic and ultrasound technology. The characteristic backward-forward tongue movements are clearly observable in most infants as the nipple is removed from the mouth and during spoon feeding of smooth solids.

Sucking appears to emerge gradually from the negative pressure component of the initial suckle. The tongue eventually loses the backward-forward stripping motion that predominates in suckling and shifts to an up-down movement. The baby seems to use firmer closure of the lips, and there is less liquid loss during nursing, bottle feeding, and spoon feeding. The better closure of the oral cavity appears to allow the older infant to use more negative pressure to draw soft food and liquid into the mouth more efficiently. The baby does not rely on the movement of the jaw for drawing the milk into the nipple and expressing it into the mouth. Therefore, the extent of jaw movement usually is less during sucking. Greater closing activity of the lips appears clinically to be a major factor in the shift of tongue patterns from an in-out to an up-down direction. Although elements of the sucking pattern are present at birth and in the early months, it does not predominate until the baby shows a greater coordination of tongue and lip/cheek movements. At this point, the earlier backward-forward suckling movements of the tongue begin to phase out. Instrumental research studies documenting and describing the movement from suckling to sucking are difficult to find. Data for this shift comes primarily from studies that have used longitudinal clinical observations of infants.

Throughout this book, the term **sucking** will be used as a generic word to refer to the organized intake of a liquid or soft solid as well as to the more mature pattern of intake just described. The term *suckle* will be used when it is important to document this action of the mouth in a specific developmental sequence. In discussion of infants younger than 6 to 9 months, the words *sucking* or *suck* may indicate the suckle or mixture of suckle and suck that is characteristic of many infants in this age range.

Newborns have a strong suckle with major reflexive components. The crowded space in the uterus during the final months of pregnancy places the infant in a very rounded, flexed position. Much of this physiological flexion is present at birth and for the initial month of life. Both suckling and sucking are considered flexor patterns. Babies often have more active closure of the lips and less up-down jaw movement during the first weeks or month of life because of the increased flexor activity in the entire body. As a result, many newborns do not lose liquid from the borders of the lips, a pattern seen in most infants between 1 and 6 months. As the baby develops more extension in the body and loses the early physiological flexion, more liquid is lost during suckling. The earlier control will appear at a more integrated level when the infant begins the shift from suckling to sucking movements of the tongue between 6 and 9 months.

There are similarities as well as differences between the suckle and suck patterns. Both involve a raising and lowering of the jaw and tongue together to create the pressure needed to express the liquid and draw it into the mouth. In both cases, the sides of the tongue move upward to create a central groove or gutter that helps form the liquid bolus and direct its movement to the back of the mouth for the swallow (Bosma, Hepburn, Josell, & Baker, 1990). The differences lie primarily in the direction of tongue movement and the degree of valving or closure of the lips.

Nutritive sucking patterns often are related to internal changes in the infant's hunger level throughout the meal. There seems to be an initial, continuous burst of sucking, with the bursts becoming shorter as the meal progresses. At the end of the meal, there are longer and longer pauses. Swallowing occurs with each suck at the beginning of a meal, but may move to more sucks per swallow as the infant finishes the meal.

It is important to remember that there are two distinct components of sucking pressure that support movement of liquid from the breast or bottle into the mouth. Both positive and negative pressure are essential to the process. Positive pressure consists of tongue squeezing or compression of the nipple (Ardran et al., 1958a). Colley and Creamer (1958) described the importance of depression of the tongue in creating negative-pressure sucking. It appears as though newborns use compression, or positive pressure, immediately after birth and improve the negative pressure suction component within approximately an hour (Ellison, Vidyasagar, & Anderson, 1979). Both types of sucking pressure seem to be necessary for breast-feeding. Bottle-feeding seems to require more negative-pressure suction. This is seen clearly with babies who have a cleft palate and are unable to achieve the intraoral vacuum needed for efficient negative-pressure suction. They tend to use the positive-pressure, tongue-squeezing compression, making efficient sucking difficult in a standard presentation.

At 3 months, infants show variations in the suckle that indicate the pattern is becoming less automatic and more voluntary. With the increased development of extensor tone, liquid often dribbles from the center and corners of the lips.

The anatomical relationships of the jaw and face begin to change between 4 and 6 months. As the lower jaw moves downward, the space within the mouth increases. Now there is greater opportunity for the tongue to move in an up-down direction. The tiny mouth space of the newborn seems more conducive to the in-out pattern. Neurological maturation has included the beginnings of cortical control of many movement patterns. The anatomical and neurological changes support a gradual shift from the primitive suckling pattern to the more mature suck. Form and function in the mouth change gradually, and for many months, babies alternate between the two patterns.

By 6 months, infants rarely lose liquid from the mouth during continuous sucking movements. Jaw excursions are smaller and more refined because, in part, of improvements in head and shoulder girdle control. The baby is beginning to sit independently, with good head control providing a better foundation for jaw stability. The development of proximal stability creates the opportunity for distal control and movement. The jaw depends upon head and trunk stability to develop controlled mobility and a balance of flexor and extensor movements that lead to jaw stability. Between 3 and 6 months, movement control of the jaw is refined. At 6 months, when the nipple is inserted or removed, the mouth is less stable. With reduced stability, the more immature pattern of liquid loss may be seen. Between 6 and 24 months, the jaw has enough stability to support skilled and precise movements of the tongue and lips.

The gradual transition from the suckle to a sucking pattern continues between 6 and 9 months. At 9 months, babies primarily use a sucking pattern with a mixture of suckling. Liquid loss when the nipple is inserted and removed is rare. By 12 months, most babies have made the transition to the cup, although a child may continue to take the bottle or breast before naps or at bedtimes until 2 years old.

Sucking Liquids From a Cup

As the infant makes the transition from bottle or breast to a cup, we begin to apply the word *drinking* to the sucking and swallowing action that is used. Variations of the drinking process occur with cups of different sizes and shapes, with a soda bottle, and with straw drinking. The developmental descriptions in this section are based on Morris' longitudinal study of infants drinking from an open cup (Morris, 1978). Later informal observations suggest that older infants and toddlers today may remain on a spouted cup for longer periods and have fewer opportunities to master the open cup. This would suggest that the guidelines described here represent an infant's underlying ability to coordinate the mouth for drinking at different ages.

The spouted cup can provide advantages and create limits in the development of drinking skills. The lid and spout of different cups influence the drinking process in different ways. For example, a wide, thick spout gives the lips a broad resting area. The spout fills the corners of the mouth and reduces the amount of liquid lost in drinking. This can be advantageous for younger infants who are just learning to drink from the cup. However, the thick spout may encourage a wider opening of the jaw during drinking and reduce the baby's ability to develop gradations in jaw movement control. This type of cup offers no room for the baby to develop the active control at the corners of the lips that reduces spillage. The mouth and lips remain passively supported by the cup's spout and lid as the cup now reduces opportunities for the baby to master this small step in active control of drinking. The positioning of the spout on the child's tongue usually encourages the continuation of an early suckle pattern and delays the transition to the more mature suck that is used for drinking from an open cup. A more detailed discussion of the interplay between feeding movements and equipment is found in Chapters 17 and 18.

Most infants are introduced to the cup by 6 months. Before that time, they receive all nutrition from the bottle or breast. When the cup is presented initially, the baby approaches it with the same movement patterns and sequences that were familiar with the bottle. The suckling pattern predominates even if the infant has begun to incorporate more efficient up-down suck movements with the bottle or breast. In normal development, there is a tendency to revert to an earlier pattern of movement as a more difficult component of movement is perfected. When a baby concentrates on cup drinking, the previously learned up-down movement of the tongue and lip closure are replaced by the earlier in-out suckle of the tongue and minimal lip closure. Often the infant is able to develop a coordinated sucking rhythm as long as the feeder holds the cup tightly against the mouth. This provides a type of positional or external stability that supports a more coordinated action of the tongue and lips. Whenever the feeder offers or removes the cup, the child is required to reorganize the movement pattern.

At 6 months, infants use a wide excursion of the jaw, causing a substantial amount of liquid loss. Although stability has developed for head and trunk control in sitting, the stability does not yet carry over to the jaw. Jaw movements at this age are wide and ungraded. Babies begin to hold the jaw in a stable, open position as the cup approaches. This sets the stage for the emergence of jaw stability during the next year.

Changes in the drinking pattern occur gradually over the next 6 months. By the time a child is 1, the cup-drinking pattern has shifted toward the more mature sucking pattern. The extension-retraction movements of the suckle are rarely seen even as the cup is offered and removed. Most children keep the tongue in the mouth while drinking, but a few will rest the tongue beneath the cup as if seeking the same tactile contact they experienced with the nipple. This strategy also may contribute to greater overall stability of the mouth for drinking.

In general, the increased positional stability provided by the coordinated movements of the tongue and jaw enables the child to lose less liquid during drinking. Jaw excursions still are wide. These may alternate between up-down and backward-forward directions. Twelve-month-old infants have developed the precursors of controlled jaw movement in drinking. The jaw stabilizes in an open posture when the cup is presented for drinking and in a closed position while holding a cookie or other firm solid in the mouth for biting. The ability to stabilize the jaw in both open and closed positions is a prerequisite skill for developing graded movement and control during drinking.

Between 15 and 18 months, children develop a new strategy for drinking. Progress in the development of skilled tongue and lip movements depends upon stability of the jaw. As in other aspects of development, the child discovers that stability can be attained and regulated by using a holding bite on the edge of the cup. This increase in stability enables the child to bring the upper lip down to close on the edge of the cup. The tongue no longer protrudes beneath the cup (if this option had been selected initially). Some liquid still may be lost as the cup is offered and removed.

By 24 months, children use a mature sucking pattern and create the necessary jaw stabilization internally. It is no longer necessary to hold the edge of the cup to stabilize. The jaw opening and closing muscles work in a coordinated fashion to provide internal jaw stabilization at the temporomandibular joint. Because of its greater efficiency for long drinking sequences, this stabilized pattern tends to occur most often when a child combines three or more sucks and swallows. The presence of internal jaw stabilization does not assure that it will always be the pattern selected for drinking. Some of the earlier strategies, such as biting on the edge of the cup or using a slight up-down movement, may be selected into adulthood. New movement patterns offer the child a choice. They do not demand selection.

Sucking Liquids From a Straw

No known studies have described the child's progression in learning to suck from a straw. Researchers observed differences in the type and amount of fluid contact with the teeth following a swallow in a study of adults using an open cup and straws with two different internal diameters (Edwards, Ashwood, Littlewood, Brocklebank, & Fung, 1998). They suggest that oral movements and placement of the straw direct the liquid to different areas of the mouth during straw drinking.

The age at which the straw is introduced appears to vary extensively. Infants as young as 7 months have been observed drinking from a straw. Two infants were observed during their first experience with the straw from a juice box at 8 months (Morris, 1994). Both learned to draw liquid up the short straw and maintain a rhythmical drinking sequence within 5 minutes. These infants rested the straw on the tongue and used a forward-backward motion combined with lip closure to draw in the liquid.

Morris (1978) did not introduce straws in her longitudinal study until the children were 15 months old. Informal observations showed that most children used a stronger, more rounded lip position while drinking. Tongue movement was not visible. Some children indented the straw slightly with their teeth as they drank, but none bit down firmly enough to stop the flow of liquid.

Sucking Soft Solid Foods From the Spoon

The sucking of soft, solid or pureed foods from the spoon provides a different experience and requires different skills from those used to suck liquid from the bottle, breast, or cup.

The mature, adult manner of sucking or drawing soft, solid foods into the mouth can be summarized in this way: As the spoon approaches, the body inclines forward to meet it. The tongue may cup and move slightly forward as well if some of the food is likely to fall off the spoon. Through a combination of visual cues and previous experience with the food, the mouth opens just enough for the spoon and food to enter. The jaw stabilizes in this partially open position, and the tongue rests quietly until the spoon has entered the mouth. There is no wasted energy from an extra-wide opening or unstabilized up-down movement. As the spoon enters, there is simultaneous activity of the jaw and lips to draw the food off the spoon and bring it into the mouth. The jaw closes slowly with a controlled and graded movement. The upper lip moves forward and downward to scrape the food from the spoon, while the lower lip draws inward to bring in any bits of food that cling to the bottom of the spoon or were dropped onto the lips. As the jaw and lips draw in the food, the tongue begins to move. Independent up-down sucking motion draws the food further into the mouth and prepares it for swallowing. A food such as applesauce or yogurt is a mixture of sweet, sour, bitter, or salty tastes. The tongue and cheeks often swish the food around so that all of the taste buds are stimulated and the blending of the food with saliva allows its full taste to be appreciated.

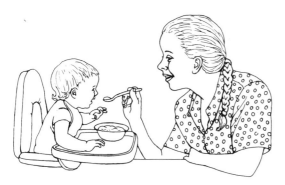

The normal infant will move along a path of development toward this end point. Pureed food usually is not presented to infants younger than 4 months because of their digestive immaturity. When it is introduced earlier, suckling movements of the tongue can be observed as soon as the spoon approaches the mouth or touches the lower lip. The baby has begun to recognize the spoon visually and anticipate the food that is approaching. The upper lip moves slightly forward in anticipation but does not move downward toward the bowl of the spoon. At this age, the infant does not have the maturity to use the top lip to help remove the food from the spoon. The baby quickly trains the feeder to scrape the food off the upper gums or lip. Food that enters the mouth often is spit out, scraped off the chin, and recycled back into the mouth. This scenario continues until the feeder has gotten enough food down the baby for the meal. The "put it in and spit it out" routine occurs because of the in-out suckle pattern of the tongue and the relative inactivity of the lips.

By 6 months, infants consistently recognize the spoon visually as it approaches. Neurologically and digestively, they are ready for smooth, solid foods. As they see the spoon approach, they open the mouth in anticipation of the next bite. If they are involved in another activity, such as playing with spilled food on the high chair tray or watching something interesting across the room, they may wait until they feel the touch of the spoon on the lower lip before opening the mouth. If they are fed with a regular rhythm for presenting the spoon, this rhythm may become the cue for getting ready for the next bite. Six-month-old babies are able to hold the mouth open in a stable, quiet position while waiting for the spoon to enter. The tongue no longer moves in and out in the suckle, but is quiet in the open mouth. This ability to quiet the tongue and jaw in readiness for the food to enter the mouth provides the stable foundation for developing precise movements of the upper lip in clearing food from the spoon.

At 6 months, many infants begin the initial stages of cleaning the spoon with the upper lip, but the inward motion that works most efficiently to remove the food from the spoon usually does not follow the downward movement.

Between 6 and 9 months, infants perfect the ability to use the upper lip to remove food from the spoon. The upper lip moves forward and downward, and postures on the spoon as it enters the mouth. The lower lip also begins to turn inward as the spoon is removed, in preparation for the cleaning by the teeth. This ability to coordinate the inward movement of the lip and a scraping motion of the upper teeth will be present by the time the child is 12 to 15 months old.

By 15 months, children use the upper front incisors to actively clean any food from the lower lip as it draws inward. The up-down tongue motion of the suck has emerged between 9 and 12 months, and by 15 months, it is the predominant pattern used. The earlier suckle becomes mixed with the suck intermittently. Fifteen-month-old babies are explorers and experimenters. They play with the new movements they have experienced in a wide variety of contexts. They may playfully bite the spoon or put it in the mouth straight or sideways, right side up or upside-down.

By age 2, children demonstrate a mature basis for the lifelong pattern of removing soft, solid foods from a spoon. The tongue moves freely in and out of the mouth to clean foods that have gotten onto the lips. Tongue elevation and depression are precise, and they occur independently of jaw movement. Tongue-tip action is skillful. The sucking pattern predominates, but isolated instances of the suckle will occur through adulthood. Although 2-year-olds have all of the components of the adult pattern, tongue precision and skill will continue to develop for another year.

Swallowing Liquids

During the first 2 years of life, children gradually develop the mature swallowing pattern of adulthood. For the first few months, the swallow is actually a suckle-swallow pattern. As the baby initiates a rhythmical suckle pattern, the swallow follows systematically during the retraction portion of the extension-retraction motion of the tongue. Most infants will swallow once for every suckle motion that brings liquid into the mouth.

As the up-down tongue motions of the suck emerge between 6 and 8 months, a new type of swallow begins. Babies can initiate the swallow without a preliminary suckle to move the tongue in a backward direction. Although the in-out suckle-swallow pattern continues, the baby also can use a simple forward protrusion at the point of swallow. Many speech pathologists and dentists often call this a tongue thrust swallow (Fletcher, Casteel, & Bradley, 1961; Lewis & Counihan, 1965). (Note: This is not the same tongue thrust that is classified as an interfering movement pattern and that limits further development in some children with neurological problems.) Liquid is still lost from the mouth during the swallow because of lax closure of the lips.

The free elevator ride upward is no longer available to the tongue when the jaw stabilizes for drinking. However, increased neurological maturity and the sensory awareness of contact points for the tip of the tongue and hard palate make it possible for the tongue tip to elevate independently during sucking and swallowing.

Two-year-olds show more consistent elevation of the tongue tip during swallowing. No loss of liquids occurs while drinking from the cup. The lips remain closed after the cup is removed from the mouth, resulting in only minimal loss of liquids at the end of the drinking sequence. The earlier pattern of extension-retraction of the tongue generally is not seen. A few children will continue a pattern of simple tongue protrusion between the lips, but usually this alternates with the more mature pattern of elevation. Drinking is done smoothly, with easy lip closure and a relaxed swallow.

The development of jaw stabilization and independent upward movement of the tongue tip depend on the type of cup that the child uses for drinking. When a cup with a spout is used, the child may not learn to stabilize externally through biting and may continue to use only the unstabilized up-down jaw movements. The presence of the spout in the mouth usually prevents tongue-tip elevation and separation of tongue movement from jaw movement.

There is very poor agreement in the literature on the labeling of different tongue movements used by young children when they swallow, the developmental periods when these movements are present, and the significance of different tongue movements for speech development. The pattern of gentle protrusion between the teeth during swallowing has been called a tongue thrust by many speech-language pathologists and orthodontists. Bell and Hale (1963) observed that a forward protrusion of the tongue against the teeth during swallowing was present in 82% of 353 5-year-old and 6-year-old children. Hanson and Cohen (1973) found that this tongue-thrust swallow pattern

Table 5.1	**Movement Characteristics of the Tongue**	
Tongue Movement and Configuration	**Suckling**	**Sucking**
Configuration	Flat, thin, cupped or bowl-shaped.	Flat, thin, cupped or bowl-shaped.
Direction of movement	Extension-retraction; an in-out movement on a horizontal plane. Up-down movement with the jaw provides positive pressure components during nursing.	Up-and-down movement on a vertical plane. Gradual separation of the up-down tongue movement from the up-down jaw movement.
Range of movement	Extension or protrusion no further out than the middle of the lips.	From the mandible to the anterior hard palate.
Strength or force of movement	Nonforceful; easy, normal strength of protrusive movement.	Nonforceful; easy upward movement.
Speed or velocity of movement	Normal speed of movement: approximately one extension-retraction cycle per second.	Normal speed of movement: approximately one up-down cycle per second.
Timing or rhythm of movement	Movement is rhythmical. There appears to be equal time for the extension and retraction portions of the cycle or a slightly greater time duration on the retraction or "in" phase.	Movement is rhythmical. There appears to be equal time for the up and down portions of the cycle, or a slightly greater time duration or stress on the downward phase that draws the liquid into the mouth.
Normal stage of movement	Normal movement pattern of early infancy.	Normal movement pattern of later infancy and adulthood.

gradually diminished with age. Their study showed that 57.9% of their subjects had a tongue thrust at 4 years 9 months while 35.4% showed this pattern at 8 years 2 months. Hanson (1976) points out that some of these children will continue to use this pattern in a way that negatively influences their speech and dental patterns.

Swallowing Semisolids

The pattern of swallowing soft, smooth, semi-solid foods follows the developmental pattern of swallowing liquids; however, the maturity of the pattern often lags behind that seen with liquids. In general, infants gain swallowing skills with liquids first. If pureed foods are presented as early as 4 months, the primitive suckle-swallow pattern is used to move food toward the pharynx. The baby pushes a great deal of food out of the mouth, requiring the feeder to scoop it from the chin and replace it in the mouth.

The outward push of the food comes not only from the easy in-out tongue movement of the suckle, but also from the forward push or protrusion of the tongue as the infant swallows. Gagging or choking may occur when the infant is not yet able to collect the bolus and move it backward with efficiency. Occasionally, food sticks to the back of the tongue or falls over the back before the swallow is triggered, resulting in the protective action of a gag or cough.

Six-month-old babies are more motorically ready for pureed foods. Only minor losses of food occur with the suckle. By 9 months, the suck pattern has emerged, and the suckle-swallow diminishes and alternates with the more mature, simple tongue-protrusion pattern at the point of the swallow. At 1 year, children are able to swallow with easy lip closure. Some periodic tongue protrusion continues, but this decreases as the tongue tip becomes elevated for the swallow. This is the same progression we observed as the infant takes liquids. By 2 years, the extension-retraction movements of the tongue have disappeared and the predominant pattern is one of tongue-tip elevation. Simple protrusion of the tongue between the teeth may occur during an occasional swallow. Tongue-tip elevation during the swallow gradually becomes the sole pattern as the child moves into the third year.

Swallowing Solids

Swallowing solid foods requires a slightly different type of control than is used for liquids or semisolids.

By 6 to 8 months, babies generally are introduced to solid foods such as graham crackers or baby cookies. Although the baby chews and sucks these first foods, they usually dissolve or are reduced to soft tiny lumps by the time they are swallowed. This is similar to the ground or lumpy solids that are added to the diet during this period. Swallowing occurs with the same general strategies used for nonchewy foods. Simple protrusion mixed with the suckle-swallow predominates.

By 12 months, babies are swallowing ground, mashed, or chopped table foods with noticeable lumps. As with swallowing semi-solids, an intermittently elevated movement of the tongue is used. Simple tongue protrusion alternates with the elevated pattern. The more primitive extension-retraction movement usually is not present.

Eighteen-month-old children swallow solid foods with easy lip closure and lose little food or saliva during the swallow. Tongue-tip elevation predominates for the swallow, although simple tongue protrusion may occur periodically.

By the time children are 2 years old, they can swallow most solid foods with easy lip closure. As solids that require more prolonged chewing are given, children must add another strategy. The mixture of chewed food and saliva must be swallowed while any remaining pieces that require further chewing are retained. This ability to swallow only part of a mouthful of food without losing the remaining portion requires a great deal of skill. Combination foods such as vegetable soup, dry cereal with milk, gelatin with fruit pieces, and unpeeled fruits such as apples or pears are among the most difficult that children learn to handle. Choking or drooling of liquid occurs for a few months as children learn to swallow these complex foods.

Coordination of Sucking, Swallowing, and Breathing

When taking the bottle or breast, most infants use a pattern of one suck, one swallow, and one breath. They stop the breath briefly during the swallow so that the liquid can bypass the airway and move directly into the esophagus. This 1:1:1 feeding ratio may be altered at some points in the feeding for some infants who take two or three short sucks before they swallow (Fletcher et al., 1961; Bu'Lock et al., 1990). At one time, infant specialists thought that the higher position of the larynx in the neck between birth and 4 months allowed liquid to slide over the sides of the epiglottis, enabling very young infants to breathe and swallow at the same time. More recent work has shown that this is not true, and even newborn infants inhibit their breathing when they swallow (Weber, Woolridge, & Baum, 1986).

By 3 months, the baby sequences 20 or more sucks and coordinates these smoothly with swallowing, with no discernible pauses in the sequence. When the baby is hungry, pauses for breathing are not frequent. The infant may occasionally choke or cough, indicating poor coordination of the suck-swallow-breathe sequence.

By 6 months, infants continue to use the long sequences with the bottle or breast, pausing only for burping or resting. As cup drinking is introduced, incoordination occurs as they try to transfer the familiar longer sequences to the cup. When liquids come rapidly with the cup, the infant is unprepared for the volume of liquid that reaches the back of the mouth. The baby may respond to this in a variety of ways. Long continuous sucks may bring liquid into the mouth, but swallowing does not occur and the unswallowed liquid flows or spurts from the mouth. Large mouthfuls may result in coughing, choking, and gasping for breath with much of the liquid lost.

Infants soon learn that the long sequential sucks that are appropriate for the bottle are not efficient for the cup. By 9 months, they use a sequence of one to three sucks, and they pull away from the cup to stop the inflow of liquid and allow a pause for breathing. They continue to use the longer sequences with the bottle. Coughing and choking occur infrequently.

Coordination gradually improves. Longer sequences begin to emerge by 12 months. The overall balance and stability provided by the neck and shoulder girdle at 15 months contribute to the development of jaw stability during drinking. These abilities provide greater skill and efficiency of tongue and lip movement, and enable the child to drink long drafts of liquid with good coordination. When the child is thirsty, it is possible to drink at least 1 ounce of liquid with a series of coordinated suck-swallow-breathe movements.

Control of Drooling

Control of drooling occurs gradually in a child's development. It is related primarily to position, activity, oral motor control, and the level of motoric integration that has been achieved. Drooling often occurs when the child is learning a new motor skill, and it may continue until the skill has become automatic. Drooling is common during, before, and just after the child cuts a new tooth.

Despite immature physical and oral development, infants produce very little saliva before 3 months of age. Saliva mixes with food, helps bind it together, and begins the digestive process with the salivary enzyme amylase. Little mixture is needed when the infant's sole diet is breast milk or formula. Thus, the body produces the minimum amount needed to keep the mouth moist. As the time approaches to introduce cereals and other semisolid foods, more saliva is produced and the infant must learn to handle amounts that fill the mouth during nonfeeding times.

As greater amounts of saliva are produced, control may be seen in a supine or reclining position, where gravity assists the swallow. When gravity does not assist and babies initiate early motor skills of head lifting and turning, drooling may occur.

By 6 months, infants can control drooling in supine, prone, and supported sitting unless they are teething or using their hands for reaching or manipulating objects. When they progress to tasks that require concentration or fine motor control, the level of oral control is reduced, causing the child to drool. Feeding also may contribute to drooling as the baby begins to salivate before, during, or after the meal.

Nine-month-old babies can move through early-acquired gross motor skills such as rolling, sitting, and belly crawling without drooling unless they are cutting teeth. They may drool at mealtime when eating certain foods, but generally drooling is absent before or after eating.

By 15 months, children no longer drool while moving in and out of newly acquired advanced gross motor skills such as walking. Drooling still may occur when they are teething or concentrating on early fine motor tasks such as self-feeding, undressing, or random play.

By the time children are 24 months old, they have developed the motoric organization to engage in advanced fine motor tasks such as drawing, fine finger movements, manipulation of small objects, and two-word speech combinations without drooling.

Jaw Movements in Biting

Biting can occur independently as a means of breaking off a piece of a larger chunk of food and drawing it into the mouth. It also is a part of the chewing pattern. Infants under 5 months of age will suck any food that comes into the mouth. Some chewing practice is occurring at this age during the mouthing of fingers and toys.

By 5 or 6 months, the normal phasic bite-and-release pattern occurs reflexively as a cookie touches the teeth or gums. This is not a functional bite. It is a rhythmic stereotyped bite followed by a release when the gums or teeth are stimulated. The repetitive biting rhythm that occurs at this age on the cookie, toy, or finger provides an initial experience with a stronger jaw force and the release that follows. Although a controlled bite does not occur when a softer cookie is given, small pieces may break off during this phasic bite. It is important to watch the infant carefully when soft cookies are given at this age. Some babies may not have the skill to control the little pieces that break off.

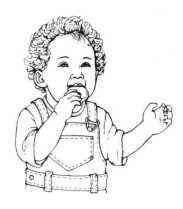

By 9 months, infants can hold the cookie between the gums or teeth. The jaw is stabilized in a closed position as the feeder breaks the cookie, allowing the child to chew and swallow the portion that is in the mouth. The phasic bite has been integrated during activities such as biting and releasing toys, socks, fingers, teething ring, and harder cookies. It still may be seen occasionally as the infant perfects biting skills with food.

At 12 months, children use a controlled, sustained bite through a soft cookie. If the child has both upper and lower incisors, the controlled bite also may occur with harder cookies. An unsustained bite may occur because of lack of teeth or an inadequate biting power. At these times, the child may revert to the phasic bite.

By 18 months, children bite through hard cookies or other solid foods such as apples with a controlled, sustained bite. However, overflow or associated movements of the arms, legs, or head may be present. The head may pull back, the hands or toes may tense, or the child may drool. These associated movements may help the child add more power to the bite.

By 21 months, children can bite through a hard cookie with a controlled and sustained bite while the rest of the body remains quiet. Overflow movements in the arms and legs no longer occur. The head does not need to extend to assist with biting. Regardless of the thickness of the food, children still tend to open the mouth wider than necessary in anticipation.

By 24 months, children can bite most foods with a controlled and sustained bite while beginning to grade the jaw opening to the appropriate size for foods of different thickness. The head may turn toward the side to increase the strength of the bite if food is placed on the side of the mouth. By age 3, children can bite firm solids while keeping the head in midline.

Jaw Movements in Chewing

If chewable food is offered to 5-month-old babies, they usually chew with a phasic bite-and-release pattern. Remember that the 5-month-old has had few controlled biting experiences with food.

During the 6th month, the vertical jaw movement seen during the phasic bite becomes less reflexive. When combined with the up-down motion of the tongue, the vertical bite pattern of the jaw is described as "munching." Munching is actually the earliest form of chewing. The tongue flattens and spreads as the jaw moves up and down. This munch is not efficient for all forms of food. Although the munching pattern continues to be the basis for adult chewing, its later combination with lateral tongue and jaw movements provides the possibility for skilled chewing. As the 6th and 7th month progress, jaw movement continues to be in a vertical up-down direction, but it loses the stereotypic quality seen in the phasic bite. If food is placed on the side of the baby's mouth, both the tongue and jaw will move toward that side. This pattern has a diagonal component, as the jaw movement is simultaneously moving downward and to the side. This is the beginning of the "diagonal rotary" movement of the jaw that will continue through adulthood.

Chewing at 9 months combines a nonstereotypic vertical movement with diagonal rotary jaw movements. This new pattern occurs when the child transfers food from the center of the tongue to the side, or when food is specifically placed between the gums on the side of the mouth. The phasic bite-and-release patterns may continue to form the basis of biting through foods such as cookies or raisins with the front upper and lower incisors. Many children play with food, using this more stereotyped bite-and-release chewing pattern. Although the phasic bite provides the basic pattern that is used, it is more voluntary and less automatic at this age.

Table 5.2   Jaw Movement in Biting and Chewing

Jaw Movement	Direction of Movement	Type of Movement
Phasic Bite	Up-down movement.	A rhythmical bite-release pattern of jaw opening and closing stimulated by touch to the teeth or gums.
Unsustained Bite	Upward movement followed by rapid or irregular opening.	A closing of the teeth on the food, followed by a hesitation and a new attempt to bite through the food. Biting through the food in a smoothly graded fashion does not occur.
Graded Bite	Upward, controlled movement followed by easy opening for chewing.	The teeth close on the food and bite through it gradually. This is followed by an easy release for chewing.
Munching With Stereotyped Vertical Chew	Up-and-down movements of the jaw.	Rhythmical opening and closing based on the primitive phasic bite. This is a stereotypic, automatic pattern that is elicited by stimulation of the teeth and gums.
Munching With Non-Stereotyped Vertical Chew	Up-and-down movements of the jaw.	A chewing pattern characterized by up-and-down movements of the jaw that vary in both opening width and timing.
Diagonal Rotary Chew	From the medial position jaw movement is downward-and-lateral. From the lateral position jaw movement is downward-and-medial.	A chewing pattern characterized by movement of the jaw that gives the impression that the jaw is moving diagonally. These jaw movements are observed as the tongue moves food to the side or from the side to the middle of the mouth.
Circular Rotary Chew	From the lateral position, the jaw swings downward, central, and to the opposite side.	A chewing pattern characterized by circular or semicircular jaw patterns. These jaw movements occur as the tongue moves food from one side of the mouth across the midline to the opposite side. This pattern is used primarily with firmer or tougher foods as the child uses the molars to grind food.

By 15 months, children are using smooth, well-coordinated diagonal movements of the jaw. This mixture of vertical and diagonal rotary jaw movements continues into adulthood.

When children are able to transfer food from one side of the mouth to the other without pausing in the middle (sometime between age 2 and 3), they add a third pattern to the vertical and diagonal rotary movements. The jaw appears to swing from the center to the side where the food is initially located. Without pause, it swings smoothly toward the other side of the face, helping the tongue carry the food to the opposite side. Because of the circular swing, the pattern has been called a "circular rotary" movement.

Tongue Movements in Chewing

Infants spontaneously begin to move the tongue to the side of the mouth to assist with chewing between the ages of 6 and 7 months. This lateral movement is present at birth during the transverse tongue reflex (Weiffenbach & Thach, 1973). Then it had little functional significance, yet it appears to have created the underlying pattern for the volitional use of lateral tongue movements in chewing. As cookies and other bits of solid foods are given to the baby, the tongue makes a gross rolling movement when the food is placed between the gums on the lateral biting surface. The tongue can be said to bias toward the touch of the food. When food is held in place on the molar area, the child's tongue may drift laterally in the direction of the food. Once the food has broken off inside the mouth, the more primitive pattern of suckling the food usually occurs. Babies cannot move the food from the center to the side or transfer it from side to side at 6 months.

As rotation develops throughout the body, we begin to see aspects of rotation emerge in the mouth. Between 7 and 9 months, children use rotary movements to move in and out of sitting and to roll from the tummy to the back and from the back to the tummy. They pivot and rotate during play, moving through lateral and diagonal movements. The foundation is set for rotation and lateralization in the mouth. Tongue lateralization occurs consistently when food is placed between the biting surface of the gums on the side of the mouth, and as babies begin to transfer food from the center of the tongue to the side of the mouth. This transfer occurs intermittently, and often it is seen only to one side. In-out tongue movements may continue to occur with difficult transfers.

By age 1, most children spontaneously transfer food to either side if it is placed in the center of the tongue. In-out movements may continue to occur during difficult transfers. These children may appear to be moving food from one side of the mouth to the other, but the movement is not a single cross-midline transfer. In reality, they are moving food from one side to the center, pausing briefly, and continuing the transfer from the center to the other side.

Two-year-olds often can move food placed between the molar biting surfaces to the other side in a smooth and spontaneous movement across the middle of the mouth. The success of this transfer usually depends upon the size and consistency of the food. Children make these transfers automatically, and they may have difficulty if asked specifically to move food to a particular location in the mouth (Gisel, Schwaab, Lange-Stemmler, Niman, & Schwartz, 1986). Some in-out movements occur if food gets stuck or is out of control.

By age 3, children have learned to transfer food comfortably across midline or to any location within the mouth as needed. Consistency and refinement continue. Motor-planning skills develop, and children are able to transfer food across midline on command by the time they are 3 (Gisel et al., 1986). In-out movements no longer occur with difficult transfers. Side-to-side transfers that are requested by an adult continue to increase in speed and skillfulness until the child is at least 8 years old (Gisel, 1988b).

Lip Movements in Chewing

For chewing, 6-month-olds use a munching pattern based on the phasic bite. They draw in either the upper or lower lip as food is presented. They also may tighten the corner of the mouth slightly when food is placed on the lips. If food is placed in the side of the mouth, the lip and cheek on that side will tighten to help keep the food in the mouth and prevent it from falling into the cheek pocket.

By 9 months, an infant's lips and jaws are active together during chewing. The lips make contact at the sides or in the center as the jaw moves up and down. The upper or lower lip may draw inward when food is on the lip. The upper lip comes down and moves slightly forward during chewing.

Twelve-month-old children can use the incisors or gums to clean food off the lower lip as it is pulled inward. Although greater activity is seen in the lips than was possible at 9 months, food and saliva still are lost during chewing. The cheeks continue to play a major role in controlling placement and movement of the food, and the tongue, lips, and cheeks work together to keep food over the grinding surface of the teeth for efficient chewing.

By 18 months, children can chew with their lips closed—and they do so now and then. The lips are closed primarily when the mouth is stuffed with food and the child does not want any to fall out. When less food is in the mouth, tongue movements alone can prevent its loss. Often, it is more efficient for the child to chew with the lips open. Food and saliva still can be lost during chewing. This occurs primarily when the food is juicy or when several food textures are in the mouth.

By 2 years, children lose little food or saliva while chewing. They are capable of chewing with the lips closed, but do not need to do so to keep food in the mouth. During their preschool years, they can be taught the table manners of Western culture that include chewing with the mouth closed. Gisel attempted to observe tongue movements during swallowing in 2- to 8-year-old Canadian children (Gisel, 1988c). She found that the jaw and lips were open for swallowing in only a small percentage of 2- to 4-year-olds. By age 5, all of the children used lip closure during swallowing.

Chewing Efficiency

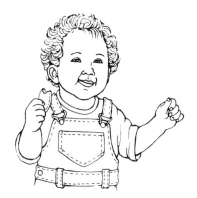

The studies of Erica Gisel and her colleagues (Gisel, 1988a, 1991; Schwaab, Niman, & Gisel, 1984, 1986) have examined the organization of oral movements that results in more skilled and efficient chewing patterns. Although one can break down the process and look at the separate functions of the jaw, tongue, lips, and cheeks, this does not reflect the growing skill and coordination that is seen as children develop higher-level eating skills. In her research, Gisel made careful measurements of changes in chewing duration and the number of chewing cycles in normally developing children from 6 months to 8 years. She defined the chewing duration as the number of seconds between placement of food in the mouth and the completion of the swallow. A chewing cycle was defined as one down-and-up movement of the jaw. She determined a time/cycle ratio by dividing the chewing duration by the number of cycles. These studies showed that the texture of the food determined the duration of chewing. Between 6 months and 2 years, solid foods remained in the mouth for longer periods than viscous or pureed foods. As children got older, the chewing time decreased for each texture. The number of cycles that a child chewed on the same bite of food also decreased. Thus, they became more efficient at chewing a comparable bite of food. These studies showed that a reduction in the length of time for each bite was more significant between ages 2 and 3 years than between 3 and 4 years. However, small increases in chewing efficiency were measured between 5 and 8 years (Gisel, 1988a).

■ A Global Look at Feeding Skills

Newborns

Newborns are ready to suck at birth. During the final trimester of the pregnancy, as space in the uterus becomes cramped, physiological flexion gradually increases as the fetus continues to grow. Thus, full-term babies show many flexor patterns at birth. Sucking can be described as a flexion skill. In addition to the oral reflexes of sucking and swallowing, the rooting reaction aids in the search for liquid. Newborns are motorically dependent, receiving all stability from external support. Generally, they are held in a reclining position with the head and upper body elevated to less than a 45-degree angle. Feedings are given every 3 to 4 hours. Two to four ounces of liquid are taken per feeding. Most of the oral stability for sucking is provided by the sucking pads. The jaw and front of the tongue provide positive pressure on the nipple that is followed by a lowering of the jaw and back of the tongue to add a negative pressure component. This early in-and-out suckle movement of the tongue provides a stripping action that extracts the liquid from the bottle or breast. Swallowing then usually follows sucking by a brief pause to breathe. Because of the amount of flexor tone, the lips may provide an efficient seal with no liquid loss and the tongue may show more frequent up-and-down movements. These more mature patterns gradually will diminish as the physiological flexion is lost and the baby begins to develop control of extension.

3-Month-Old Infants

By 3 months, an infant's motor capabilities have matured substantially. Head and neck control improve, allowing these infants to lift and turn the head while lying on the tummy if they have been given this opportunity during periods of wakefulness. The asymmetric tonic neck response influences neck and shoulder muscle tone in that position by influencing weightshifting on the face and providing a pattern for dissociating the neck from the trunk, and the jaw from the neck. Three- to 4 month-old babies frequently put fingers, fists, clothing, and anything else that is placed in the hand to the mouth for mouthing and sucking.

Because of greater control of the head, 3- to 4-month-old babies usually are held in a more upright position for feeding (that is, at an angle of 45 to 90 degrees). Four to six feedings are provided daily. Seven or eight ounces of liquid are taken per feeding as the nutritional and caloric requirements increase with age. The suckle pattern continues to be used to draw the liquid into the mouth, supported by the stability of the sucking pads. Although the movement patterns are still considered reflexive, they have begun the process of integration that will shift them from more stereotyped automatic patterns to the more varied volitional patterns. Because these infants have lost their early physiological flexion and have not replaced it with the postural control of flexor movements, there may be some loss of liquid during a sucking pattern that is less tight than it was at birth.

6-Month-Old Infants

By 6 months, babies are motorically and cognitively prepared to be more active participants in the feeding process. In the process of learning to move in prone and supine, they have moved on, over, and around the shoulder joints. Head righting reactions are now present in all planes of movement, so that when children are tipped off balance, the head will right itself to a face-vertical, mouth-horizontal position to the pull of gravity. These infants can roll to and reach for desired toys or objects. They begin to sit without support. The shoulders and neck, which provide the proximal foundation for the more distal oral motor skills of feeding, have become more organized and stable. Their hands easily reach for and grasp toys and other objects, and they bring them to the mouth for exploration. The world is discovered through the mouth as they begin to learn about shape, texture, weight, and taste.

At 6 months, babies eat and drink in an upright posture with some support from the high chair or feeder. They recognize and eagerly await the approach of the bottle or spoon. They can hold the bottle independently or throw it on the floor when they have finished or decide to play.

The oral reflexes that once dominated feeding skills now are more integrated as new voluntary skills are perfected. The early suckle pattern still predominates, but is mixed with more frequent up-and-down tongue movements that mark the gradual shift to the more mature suck pattern. As with all new skills, there is an overlapping period when one skill is fading and a new one is emerging. Both the suckle and sucking patterns will be present between 6 and 12 months until sucking becomes dominant. With the beginning refinement of jaw and lip control, liquid is no longer lost regularly during sucking, although it may occur occasionally as the nipple is inserted or removed from the mouth.

Soft, smooth solids are usually introduced by spoon between 4 and 6 months. By that time, these babies recognize the sight or touch of the spoon. Between 6 and 7 months, they learn to open the mouth and hold it in a quiet, stable position as the spoon approaches. Before then, the suckling movements of the jaw and tongue begin as soon as children see the spoon and continue throughout the meal. The new ability to quiet the tongue and jaw in readiness for the food to enter the mouth creates the possibility for precise movements of the upper lip in clearing food from the spoon. The upper lip begins to move forward and downward, and postures on the spoon as it enters the mouth. At this age, the inward motion that works most efficiently to remove the food from the spoon usually does not follow the downward movement. The mixture of suckling and sucking movements of the tongue also is seen during spoon-feeding. Swallowing is accomplished either by the suckle-swallow or by a simple protrusion of the tongue at the point of swallow. Because of these outward motions of the tongue during swallowing, pureed foods may be pushed out of the mouth when they are first introduced.

Soft baby cookies may be introduced during this period. The infant may suck the cookie or attempt to bite it using the stereotyped up-down movement of the phasic bite-and-release pattern. The lower central incisors help this if the tongue is not in the forward sucking position. If a small piece of cookie breaks off in the mouth, a munching pattern may be used alternately with a suck or suckle. Lateral movements of the tongue are seen only if the feeder places the piece of food on the side between the biting surfaces of the gums. When a child uses a munching pattern to chew the food, the jaw moves in a nonstereotypic vertical direction. Diagonal rotary patterns of the jaw are seen when the tongue moves laterally to find food placed on the side.

Cup drinking is introduced between 4 and 6 months. When infants begin to learn about the cup, they may be surprised at the rapid flow of liquid. The larger amount of liquid and irregular flow may result in choking or coughing rather than a coordinated swallow. Parents usually deal with this problem by offering liquid first in a cup with a spout that controls some of the liquid flow. The suckle-swallow or a simple tongue protrusion between open lips as the cup is withdrawn occurs during the swallow. A substantial amount of liquid may be lost as the baby moves toward the new coordination that is required. Some infants do not experience liquid loss if they are drinking from a cup with a wide or thick spout that helps with lip closure by providing greater stability.

9-Month-Old-Infants

By 9 months, babies are mobile and active explorers in the environment. They roll, crawl, or creep to desired toys or people. Their sitting balance has improved, enabling them to use their hands for play and object exploration rather than for stability. They explore everything by mouthing, banging, shaking, grasping, and releasing. Nine-month-old babies have improved their reach so that it is quite functional. Refinement of grasping and finer manipulative skills has begun. The mouth continues to play the primary role in sensory discovery. Although eye and hand skills have improved, these babies prefer to learn about sensory properties through the mouth. New objects are usually taken to the mouth for sensory identification before they are explored with the hands and eyes.

These children can sit in a high chair without the need for side cushions, rolled towels, or other physical restraints. Tray support is optional, being required primarily to encourage the infant to remain in the chair. Liquids are fed by bottle or breast and by cup, and smooth and lumpy solids are fed by spoon. Foods for biting and chewy solids also are included more frequently at 9 months. The sensory experiences provided by discriminative mouthing between 6 and 9 months have set the stage for a successful transition to lumpy solids. Because of increased awareness of cues for texture, size, shape, weight, and temperature, these children have developed an initial sensorimotor strategy for dealing with similar characteristics in food. The protective gag reflex becomes less vigilant as they prepare to expand their diet. They are invited to participate in the meal by holding the bottle and feeding themselves simple finger foods. An awareness of the differences between edible and nonedible foods has not yet emerged, and parents are learning to clean up interesting pieces of dirt and other small objects from the floor when the mobile 9-month-old is exploring!

The sucking of liquids and soft, pureed solids is characterized primarily by the up-down movement of the tongue and increased lip activity of the suck. Suckle movements still occur intermittently, especially if the baby continues to take liquids from a spouted cup. When drinking, the baby has developed better control over the flow by pulling back from the cup after taking one to three sucks. It is extremely difficult to describe developmental skills with the cup at this age because so much depends upon the characteristics of the cup that the child is using. Many babies also are drinking from a straw at 9 months.

The lips are more active during eating. During spoon-feeding, the upper lip comes forward and moves downward and inward to remove the food from the spoon. When handling foods that require some chewing, the upper lip is active and there is more contact between the upper and lower lips as the jaw moves up and down.

Nine-month-old children bite by holding a soft cookie between the gums or teeth and maintaining this stabilized hold while the feeder breaks off the piece of cookie that is in the mouth. Once the food is in the mouth, the baby can move it from the center to either side for chewing. A sustained lateral pressure from the tongue and inward pressure from the cheek keeps the food aligned between the biting surface of the gums until it is sufficiently chewed for swallowing. Jaw movement during chewing follows the transfer action of the tongue, moving in the diagonal rotary pattern during movement of the food to the side and in a nonstereotyped vertical direction during the munching that occurs between transfers.

This 9-month period is an important one in the development of feeding skills. The baby has begun to separate and refine movements of the separate parts of the feeding system. The tongue begins to separate from the jaw in lateralization and swallowing. The lips close as the jaw moves up and down during chewing, and they move with a forward and downward motion to clean the spoon. The sides, center, and tip of the tongue begin to differentiate in the process of collecting and swallowing a bolus of lumpy foods.

12-Month-Old Children

Activity, independence, and interaction are words that can be used to describe children at age 1. They are very mobile as they creep, pull to stand, move along, climb up on furniture, and take their first independent steps. They have refined their reach, grasp, and release. The ability to isolate the movement of the index finger allows many poking and pointing actions in play and communication. They can pick the tiniest piece of cereal from the high chair tray. In a growing desire for independence, they reach for the cup, spoon, or any food presented, and try to pull it into the mouth. With enthusiasm and partial self-feeding, they get as much food on themselves or on the floor as they get in themselves!

The foods they can handle tend to be coarsely chopped table foods and some easily chewed meats. They have no difficulty with lumps, and they can separate the lumps that are ready to be swallowed from those that require more chewing. Food is easily transferred from the center to the side of the mouth and back to the center for swallowing. The lips are active during chewing, and the upper teeth are used to clean food from the lower lip when it is drawn inward. A controlled bite is used through a soft cookie. Success of biting through hard cookies will depend upon the presence of teeth and the ability to control the force of the bite. Because of the greater difficulty and variability with hard foods, a year-old child may revert to a phasic bite with firm foods.

These children take liquids by bottle, breast, cup, or straw. They usually are given the bottle or breast before sleep times and offered cup drinking at snacks or meals. They may use straws when eating out with the rest of the family. Movement control with the cup varies at this age, depending upon the type of cup used. Liquid is lost from the mouth whenever the cup is removed. Control is assisted during the drinking sequence by the stabilizing pressure of the cup on the lower lip or into the corners of the mouth. The up-and-down tongue action of the suck occurs consistently during drinking if the child has had extended experience drinking from an open cup. With this type of cup, intermittent tongue tip elevation also occurs during the swallow. Some coughing or choking may occur if the flow of liquids is too fast. A thirsty child may sequence three or more suck-swallow movements while drinking an ounce or less of liquid.

15-Month-Old Children

Fifteen-month-old children continue to refine eating and oral motor skills. Chewing improves as the timing and coordination of food transfers matures. More frequent diagonal rotary movements occur as these children are given more challenging foods that require breaking up by chewing. The cheeks help the teeth keep the food over the grinding surfaces with greater skill. The corners of the lips and the cheeks draw inward to assist the control of placement and movement of food in the mouth.

Drinking skills also are more refined. Less spilling occurs during drinking and as the cup is removed. Jaw stabilization through biting on the edge of the cup begins by 15 months, freeing the tongue and lips to develop independent control. As this occurs, the tongue is no longer able to move into the elevated position passively as the jaw moves up and down. There is now sufficient neurological maturation to enable the tip of the tongue to elevate independently as it seeks the familiar sensory contact with the front of the palate. This pattern may not develop while the child is on a spouted cup because the spout lies on top of the tongue, preventing tongue-tip elevation. Choking and coughing rarely occur as long sucking sequences are used while drinking an ounce or more of liquid.

18-Month-Old Children

By 18 months, toddlers are quite ambulatory, walking and running with exuberance as they explore the world. They no longer need the external support or security provided by the high chair, and they may be fed at the family table while sitting in a tall child's chair or a booster seat. They can feed themselves with their fingers or a spoon, and they can handle the cup independently. They are capable of chewing with the lips closed, and they do so when the mouth is stuffed and they need to prevent food from falling out. At other times, the mouth usually is open for chewing with no loss of food or saliva. They can bite through a hard cookie using a sustained bite, but they show overflow or associated movements in the arms or legs. The head may move backward into slight extension to assist with the biting.

When drinking from an open cup, they achieve external jaw stabilization by biting on the edge if they have had prior experience with this type of cup. The upper lip moves downward, contacting the edge of the cup for improved skill in drinking. Swallowing occurs with easy lip closure and with an elevated tongue-tip position. There is better overall control of food and liquid and minimal loss during eating.

2-Year-Old Children

By 24 months, the foundation has been set for a lifetime of skilled eating patterns. Although refinements in movement, skill, and social manners will continue for several years, the basic set of patterns is complete. Two-year-olds eat independently and tackle every kind of food and liquid that appeals to them. At this age, the types of food eaten vary because of personal tastes and preferences—not usually because of a lack of coordination and skill.

Chewing is accomplished with nonstereotypic vertical, diagonal rotary, or circular rotary jaw movements as needed. The type of movement depends upon the consistency and texture of the mouthful of food. The tongue transfers food easily across the midline of the mouth with skill, speed, and precise tongue-tip elevation. The tongue also is used to help clean food from the upper and lower lips. Tongue elevation and depression now are accomplished independently of jaw movement. Biting is sustained and carefully graded through a variety of textures without the presence of associated movements in the rest of the body.

Children continue to drink using the up-down movement of the suck if they have had experience with an open cup. Greater control, precision, and speed are possible as these children begin to shift from biting on the cup for external stabilization to an internal means of jaw stabilization. This occurs through balanced contraction of the jaw opening and closing muscles around the temporomandibular joint. Long drinking sequences are common when children are thirsty, often enabling them to finish an entire glass in one long drink. If a child continues with a spouted cup or straw, the amount of unstabilized vertical movement of the jaw decreases, moving gradually toward more stable control as the child gets older.

Tongue protrusion during swallowing has been replaced by tongue-tip elevation in many children. The lips close easily to minimize food and saliva loss during eating.

Older Children

The refinement of oral motor control during feeding continues well beyond the first two years. Although most studies have not looked at older children, those of Gisel and her colleagues (Gisel, 1988a, 1988c; Gisel & Schwob, 1998) have looked at aspects of chewing in children through their 8th year. The mouth continues to change in shape and size as children lose and then gain new teeth. New foods provide a wider array of experience with different tastes and textures that provide different oral sensorimotor experiences. Each of these areas contributes to the number of movement choices from which a child can select for different food and liquid experiences.

Developmental Perspectives

Recognition of developmental landmarks and knowledge of when to expect them is essential in assessing feeding skills. The feeding therapist who knows that the baby's upper lip does not come down and forward to help clean food off the spoon until age 6 to 8 months will consider this in an evaluation. She will not state in the assessment report, "Sarah is missing the ability to use her top lip to clean food from the spoon" when Sarah is 4 months old. Nor would she write "Sam does not lateralize his tongue and transfer food from one side of his mouth to the other" because Sam is only 6 months old and no one would expect him to have this skill. When statements like these appear in a clinical report as deficit statements, it implies that there is something wrong with the child.

Most of our knowledge of normal feeding development comes from careful observation of infants and not from carefully controlled research. Although basic research is important, it is usually defined by its ability to look at a single area by reducing the number of variables involved. Real-life observations of normally developing infants and children with feeding difficulties are not unidimensional. They are the interplay of many interconnected features of the child's meal. Physical position, food placement, food texture, taste, smell, temperature, interaction with the feeder, and prior experiences are involved. These and other variables interact to create a mixture of potential responses from the child.

Children must have the developmental readiness to move to a more complex level of eating and drinking. However, they must also have the experiences that enable them to learn to apply the underlying readiness skills to the new eating challenge. Once they have developed a new set of eating movements, they depend on the sensory input of the overall environment, food, and utensils to select the specific movements they will use.

Carol is 15 months old. Her diet consists of commercially prepared pureed baby foods. When she was a year old, her mother offered her finely mashed table food. She gagged and refused to open her mouth for more. Based on this initial response, her mother continued to give her only smooth, soft foods. During an evaluation of her feeding skills, the therapist placed a small piece of graham cracker in the center of Carol's tongue and observed that the tongue did not move the food to the side for chewing. Carol held her mouth closed and let the graham cracker dissolve before she sucked on it. Based on her age, history, and lack of other developmental problems, we may assume that Carol has developed the underlying neurological readiness to chew a soft cookie—a skill seen in most infants between 6 and 9 months. However, Carol has had no experience with anything that would stimulate her latent chewing abilities. When given the sensory stimulus of a more solid piece of food, she uses the more familiar sucking strategy that she knows. When the therapist asked her mother to put the graham cracker on the side of the mouth, Carol began to mash it between her gums. Soon her tongue had moved to the side to begin some early chewing.

Martin's parents were concerned about his messy eating. During the feeding evaluation the therapist observed the 3-year-old chewing graham crackers. He noted that Martin moved the food from the center of his tongue to both sides. However, he stated that Martin had not yet developed the ability to transfer food from one side of his mouth to the other. Because he did not observe Martin with any firmer food, he did not know whether Martin actually had this ability. Graham crackers and other soft cookies dissolve readily in the mouth and usually are not moved for chewing on both sides of the mouth.

The most important key to understanding the normal development of feeding skills lies in our understanding of the sensory variables, timing and sequencing of a series of interrelated skills. In the same way the secret to effective therapy lies in selecting appropriate goal-directions and a set of strategies that help move toward the goals. Unless we understand how children develop these skills we cannot identify goals and strategies that are appropriate for a specific child.

When we understand the strategies, progressions and variations used by the typically developing child, we have a built-in set of strategies that lead toward very specific therapy techniques. Therapists can find many guidelines in this area from the normally developing infant.

Allison has been fed through a gastrostomy tube for 10 months. She sucked on a pacifier, swallowed her own saliva, and seemed interested in taking tastes of food. Her therapist felt she was ready to move toward some oral feeding. However, when he began to give her small amounts of soft food from the spoon, Allison made disorganized movements with her tongue and then began to choke. The therapist remembered the importance of rhythmical movements in early infant feeding and began to use rhythm to stimulate a more organized movement of Allison's mouth. He initially stimulated a strong, rhythmical sucking pattern with her pacifier. He encouraged her to suck on her finger after playing with her hand in water. He gradually added small tastes to the water. When the tasty finger or pacifier went in her mouth, Allison continued to use a strong suckle movement. Gradually she began to swallow the small amounts of liquid without difficulty. Over time he increased the amount of taste and moved toward a smooth, pureed consistency. Allison gradually learned to take smooth food from the spoon.

John began a strong suckle movement of his tongue as soon as the spoon came toward his mouth. His jaw moved up and down, and he became very excited. His mother scraped food off the spoon with his upper teeth, and John did not use his lips to help clean it. His therapist was working to help John use his top lip. For 6 months, she had done stretching activities with the lip and cheek before the meal and used her finger to help bring the lip down on the spoon as it entered the mouth. However, John did not have the underlying component of jaw stability and tongue quieting that would make it easier to develop precise mobility of the upper lip. When the therapist worked first on developing a quiet, stable opening of the lower jaw with a quiet tongue, John's top lip began to move more. It took much less stimulation to help him develop the downward and forward movement to help clear the spoon. Within 2 weeks, he was using his top lip on the spoon.

The application of our study of normal feeding development does not end with this chapter. We will include examples throughout this book that demonstrate how treatment approaches, strategies, and techniques can come from a developmental model.

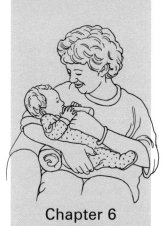

Chapter 6

Factors That Limit Feeding Skill Development

Typically developing infants progress smoothly from one stage in the developmental process to the next. Their internal computer program is clear and direct as they coordinate movements of the jaw, tongue, palate, lips, and cheeks, and advance toward a skillful, mature feeding pattern. Their direct feeding movements are supported by their overall physical and sensory functioning, and the gastrointestinal, respiratory and cardiac systems. When they encounter obstacles on the normal path, the progression for eating and drinking may be stressful, uncomfortable, awkward, or limited to the earliest patterns of coordination.

In referring to movement, sensory, and oral motor patterns, these obstacles traditionally have been called "abnormal" patterns. There is often a fine line between the patterns used by normally developing infants and those used by a child who has a neuromotor problem. The major functional issue is not whether the pattern is objectively normal, but whether it limits the child's further acquisition or refinement of the overall skills required for successful participation in the mealtime. Throughout this text, we will use the more descriptive phrase, "factors that limit feeding skills," to describe patterns that differ from the normal in a restrictive sense.

In earlier chapters, we developed a deep appreciation for the range and complexity of systems and skills that affect a child's ability to participate successfully in a meal. Critical systems include the family, communication, gastrointestinal, respiratory, cardiac, motor, sensory, and oral-sensorimotor systems. Impairment in any of these systems generally has an impact on some aspect of the child's relationship to food and mealtimes. Eating may be uncomfortable. Enjoyment may be limited. Meals may be fatiguing. Eating or drinking may be dangerous or awkward.

The concept of limiting factors reflects a belief in dynamic change. Although we will describe many of the factors that get in the way as children move toward efficient eating, we are not describing fixed, unchanging conditions. **A limit simply describes how and why development is "stuck."**

The following four children show very describable limits in the physical, oral-sensorimotor, oral-structural, gastrointestinal, and sensory areas. Yet each of these limits is changeable. **The limit is a *now* behavior—not a *forever* label.** Limiting factors are influenced by all aspects of the environment in which they occur. They may change rapidly from moment to moment or over time as different aspects of the environment change.

At 7 years old, Zach pushes back in his wheelchair and thrusts his tongue strongly forward when the spoon enters his mouth. He then shifts to a rhythmical suckle movement of the tongue until he has swallowed all of the food. Zach does not chew. It appears that his initial roadblock to chewing occurs when he pushes his body and head backward and thrusts his tongue forward. The strong thrusting pattern also serves as an initial limit to the early suckle pattern. Because Zach strongly suckles everything that comes into his mouth, this pattern has become a roadblock or limit to his ability to develop controlled biting and chewing skills.

Zach's tongue thrust disappeared when his mother put her arm around his shoulders and brought him slightly forward toward the spoon. This stopped the backward push of his pelvis and shoulder girdle. Because his body was not pushing stiffly, the tongue thrust was not elicited. Gradually, Zach learned to quiet his jaw and tongue so that his therapist could place food between the biting surfaces of his teeth. He began to learn some chewing movements, which he used when his mother fed him at home. With these environmental changes, Zach had fewer oral-sensorimotor limits for eating. When Zach became excited or upset, it was difficult for him to control his body. He pushed back to communicate his feelings. At these times, his tongue thrust became very strong, and the roadblocks for successful eating became stronger and more limiting.

José was born with a bilateral cleft of his lips and clefts of both the hard and soft palate. After birth he had difficulty sucking from the breast and bottle. The structural difficulties with his mouth created limits that became roadblocks to eating. Because of the open clefts, he was unable to generate negative pressure in his mouth to assist with sucking.

José was a strong, healthy baby. His cleft lip was repaired a week after birth. A feeding therapist helped his mother find a comfortable position for holding him that supported early communication interaction. She provided a special bottle and nipple that did not require a negative-pressure suckle to extract milk successfully. Within a week, José was taking the bottle well, and mealtimes were enjoyable for him and his parents. The changes through lip surgery, body positioning, communication interaction, and the type of nipple greatly reduced the initial limitations that José experienced when he tried to eat. When he was a year old, he had surgery to repair his palate. When his mother offered the bottle or spoon, José seemed to struggle with eating. He initially cried when his mother first put the nipple in his mouth. It was as if he had forgotten how to eat. Initially the palatal surgery increased his roadblocks or limitations to eating. José essentially had a new mouth. The mouth was sensitive and somewhat painful after surgery. It also worked differently from the mouth he had known for 12 months.

Two-year-old Tamika ate very little. She picked at her food and ate only two or three bites. She often acted as if she didn't feel well and sometimes threw up what she had eaten. She was losing weight, and everyone was worried about her. When her mother pushed her to eat "just one more bite," Tamika clamped her mouth closed and refused to eat. As her mother became more worried, she tried other ways to get her daughter to eat. Tamika became very upset and ended most meals with screaming and crying. Through diagnostic testing her family learned that Tamika had severe gastro-esophageal reflux with painful esophagitis. Her original limitation was the pain and discomfort caused by the reflux. She ate small amounts because she was hungry, but when the initial hunger signals diminished, she was uninterested in eating. A second roadblock to eating developed as her mother pressured her to eat. Tamika began to exert a counterpressure against her mother's actions and grew to hate the very idea of eating.

After gastroesophageal reflux was diagnosed, the doctor gave Tamika medication to reduce the amount of acid her stomach produced and increase the speed with which it emptied the food. She initially showed slightly greater interest in eating and stopped vomiting; however, she quickly returned to the original mealtime battles with her mother. She did not eat larger amounts of food and did not gain weight. Gradually, her eating became worse. The doctor talked to her mother about putting in a feeding tube. He ordered diagnostic tests to find out if she still had reflux and delayed stomach emptying. Both tests showed that these problems were no longer present. Tamika's initial limitation came from the pain and discomfort of reflux. Diagnostic testing supported the suggestion that the medication increased her interest in eating and reduced vomiting, thus increasing her physical comfort.

However, her mother anticipated that Tamika would approach meals with enthusiasm when the reflux was reduced. She was disappointed when change did not happen rapidly. Tamika was already in a power contest with her mother over how much she ate. When her mother's disappointment and anger increased, Tamika's refusal to eat became stronger. The limits and roadblocks increased. With guidance, her mother began to understand that it always takes two people to keep a power contest going. She realized that she could not change Tamika's choices, but she could change her own beliefs and actions at mealtime. She began to serve Tamika small portions of food and returned the responsibility for eating to her daughter. Within a week, Tamika was eating an appropriate amount and variety of food for her age. Her mother's actions reduced the major roadblock that was limiting Tamika's ability to participate comfortably at mealtime.

Elizabeth had just started school. She was in a regular kindergarten classroom. As an infant she experienced many difficulties with internal self-regulation. She had trouble settling down for sleep. During breast-feeding she would nurse for brief periods and then stop and look around. She was easily distracted. She often had temper tantrums when her parents took her to the grocery store or restaurants. When she joined her classmates for lunch in the school cafeteria, Elizabeth's behavior flew out of control. She refused to eat and annoyed the other children by snatching food from their plates and throwing it. Elizabeth experiences many sensory limitations. Her nervous system does not regulate or modulate sensory input well. The cafeteria is a busy, noisy place. Her sensory system is bombarded with high levels of sound and visual distractions as well as accidental physical contact with other children. She becomes totally overwhelmed and internally disorganized. This becomes a major roadblock or limitation to her ability to eat.

Elizabeth experienced total sensory overload when she was in the school cafeteria. She was unable to eat because of her internal chaos. She didn't know how to use words to describe what she was feeling. Her disruptive behavior, however, reflected her ambivalence and her total state of upset. At one level, she wanted to participate in the meal with her friends. At another level, she wanted to escape from the noise and confusion. She chose a food-related behavior to tell others that she was a part of the mealtime. When she grabbed food from other children and threw it, her teacher usually removed her from the cafeteria and had her sit in a time-out chair in the classroom. Elizabeth was not disruptive when the other children came back to the classroom. Her teacher knew she was hungry and brought her lunch into the room. Elizabeth ate happily and promised that she would never be a "bad girl" in the cafeteria. However, this scene was repeated day after day. Elizabeth's removal from the cafeteria immediately reduced the sensory overload that was driving her choice of behavior. As she sat quietly in the time-out chair she began to feel better. When her lunch and the other children arrived, she was able to eat and was no longer disruptive. However, she was developing the belief that she was a bad girl because she had to go to time-out every day. She did not like this self-image, yet recognized that this was the only way she could get the relief that she needed. The school occupational therapist suggested that the teacher form a small lunch club that could meet daily in a corner of the classroom. Elizabeth was invited to participate in this special group of four children instead of going to the cafeteria. In addition to reducing the limitation of the sensory environment of the cafeteria, this choice provided a positive way in which Elizabeth could be part of the mealtime with her peers.

In this chapter, we will examine many of the specific factors that influence eating. Although we will look at each area separately, limiting factors rarely are seen in isolation. Difficulties in the cardiac system usually affect the respiratory system. Gastrointestinal problems can create respiratory complications. Pain from surgery or gastroesophageal reflux may reduce the child's interest in eating. Sensory and movement difficulties may cause problems with eating and drinking coordination. These factors can contribute to weight loss and increase parental worry. Pressure to eat can distort the entire mealtime interaction and place additional limitations on the child's ability to participate easily. Normal functioning of each of these areas is discussed in Chapters 2 to 5. It may help to review this information for a point of reference as atypical or limiting aspects are introduced. Chapter 8 includes information on tests and procedures that help diagnose many of these problems.

Structural Limits

We begin with the structure or scaffolding of the feeding system, because without structure there is no physiology. Structure gives form to each system and provides a master, interconnected set of physical relationships to the total system that supports the development of feeding skills. The feeding system is an interconnection of cavities, tubes, and valves suspended on a bony skeletal frame. The movement, timing, and coordination that give life and action to these structures are guided by neurological programming that appears to have a set of central patterns or templates. It is important to remember that this central programming is designed for a specific structural system. We may think of it in the same way that computer hardware is designed for specific operating systems and software programs. Thus, when structure is changed or limited in some aspect, the physiology will be affected. A change in one system will influence the function or require change in another system.

Types of Structural Limitations and Their Influence on Feeding

Structural limits that affect feeding influence the system by:
- creating connections or openings between two or more cavities or tubes that are usually separated
- failing to create separations, divisions, or openings in a tube or cavity
- altering the size or shape of a bony structure or muscle
- altering the stiffness or mobility of a muscle, joint, or valve

These structural limits affect eating and drinking by:
- interfering with the ability to take food into the mouth
- interfering with the buildup of negative oral pressure during sucking
- leaking food from the nose during sucking and swallowing
- interfering with breathing
- interfering with efficient handling of food in the mouth
- reducing the effectiveness of swallowing
- reducing the coordination and timing of the suck-swallow-breathe sequence
- contributing to aspiration
- contributing to gastrointestinal reflux and discomfort
- leaking food from the esophagus into the airway
- blocking the flow or preventing food from passing into the stomach
- preventing food from passing into or out of the intestinal tract

Structural Limitations Through the Feeding System

Oral-Facial

Let's look at some of the major structural limitations that affect eating skills throughout the system. Eating begins with the structure of the face and mouth. A wide variety of craniofacial disorders influence the initial intake of food. During embryonic development the choanae, or bony channels within the nasal cavity, are closed or occluded. When this early condition continues after birth, there is no passageway from the nasal cavity through the nostrils, a condition known as ***choanal atresia***. Because infants are strongly programmed to breathe through the nose, there generally are severe feeding difficulties when the choanae on both sides are affected (Cozzi, Steiner, Rosati, Madonna, & Colarossi, 1988). There is a high risk for aspiration when the baby attempts to breathe through the mouth while sucking and swallowing. Although infants can breathe through the mouth, it takes a great deal of energy because of the relationship between the mouth size and the tongue in the newborn. These babies have a lot of breathing failure and restrictions even when they are not eating.

The initial expression of milk into the mouth will be affected by a cleft or lack of anatomical closure of the upper lip, making it more difficult for the lips to conform to the shape of the breast or nipple and interfering in some cases with negative pressure for sucking. The hard and soft palates form the anatomical divider between the oral and nasal cavities. Structural difficulties with the hard or soft palate can cause difficulty with feeding. When an infant has a hole because of a cleft or hole in the palate, he will have difficulty building up sufficient negative pressure within the mouth to obtain an efficient feeding pattern. Food or liquid may be lost through the cleft and dribble from the nose. The tongue may rest in the open hole. Because the widest portion of the cleft is in the back of the mouth, the resting position of the tongue often is retracted. A more detailed discussion of the limitations created by a **cleft lip** or **cleft palate** is found in Chapter 25.

We have seen that the relative size and shape of the face, mouth, and pharynx are different in the newborn and young child than those in the adult. These differences seem to be specifically designed to support more efficient sucking and swallowing in an infant whose neurological control is immature. When tongue, mouth, and jaw size are changed by a structural limitation, the efficiency and safety of eating can be affected. One of the more common structural deviations is a small, recessed lower jaw known as **micrognathia**. Because of the small size of the mandible, the tongue is usually pulled toward the back of the mouth. Many children with micrognathia also have accompanying neurological problems with the regulation of muscle tone and movement. This may cause the base of the tongue to flop back into the pharyngeal airway, severely interfering with the infant's ability to breathe.

When micrognathia is paired with upper airway obstruction and a cleft palate, it is referred to as Pierre-Robin malformation sequence. Feeding these children first requires careful consideration of airway opening. If breathing is obstructed during feeding, these infants will be unable to suck and swallow. Supine and typical feeding positions can cause increased airway obstruction from the gravitational influence on the tongue position. Prone positioning may be needed for feeding in order to use gravity to bring the tongue into a more forward placement. Sucking often is impaired in these infants. Compression of the nipple with the tongue is difficult because of the posteriorly positioned tongue. Suction is impaired because of the airway and respiratory compromise. Coordination of sucking, swallowing, and breathing is impaired because each component is influenced. With slow growth, mandibular size increases, decreasing the negative effects of the micrognathia (Vegter, Hage, & Mulder, 1999). The infant, must, however, be well nourished to grow. Oral feedings are preferred if they can be done safely to maintain or develop good sucking and swallowing skills.

Methods of nutritional intake must be carefully considered because the degree of feeding difficulty usually is proportional to the degree of respiratory obstruction (Tomaski, Zalzal, & Saal, 1995). Simple prone positional changes paired with careful consideration of correct nipples will work for some infants. Some situations, however, require supplemental or complete nasogastric tube feedings. Sometimes a surgical tongue-lip adhesion procedure is performed to maintain the tongue in a more forward position until mandibular growth improves the oral dynamics. Surgeons also may contemplate more complex procedures to help the baby develop a more functional nasopharyngeal airway.

The tongue is designed to fit comfortably into the small newborn mouth. In some genetic syndromes, the infant's tongue is too large. Usually this is because of too much muscle tissue, a condition called **macroglossia**. A tongue also can appear to be too large, relative to the amount of space inside the mouth, if the muscle tone is very low. The low tone in the tongue allows it to spread out too much and move either out of the mouth or into the pharyngeal airway. In either case, the disproportionate size of the tongue can cause problems with breathing and the handling of food in the mouth.

Shape, size, and freedom of movement within the mouth also are influenced by dental structures. This appears to be a reciprocal relationship in which the shape of dental structures is influenced by oral tone and movement. The shape and height of the hard palate and the relationship of the dental arches and teeth play a significant role for some children. **Dental malocclusions** can be related to the way in which bony tissue came together before birth or they may be secondary features related to the relative pressures of the tongue and lips. We know, for example, that minimal pressures that are sustained will move bone and teeth. This is evident in the field of orthodontia where braces that are adjusted at intervals have a significant long-term effect on the shape of the mouth and placement of teeth.

The same principle is at work in the early formation of the dental arches and the angle of the teeth. The normal resting tone and placement of the infant's tongue exerts an even pressure on the full hard palate as well as a gentle outward pressure on the lateral dental arches. This results in the typical low palatal vault and nicely spread dental arches. If tone is low in the tongue or the tongue is in a position that does not provide the pressure for lateral movement, the palate can become very highly arched and the mouth may be narrower than usual because the dental arches have not spread. As the teeth come in, an imbalance of pressure among the tongue, lips, and cheeks can cause them to be out of alignment. Retraction of the tongue, especially if combined with increased muscle tone in the lips, will cause the teeth to tip backward. Forward pressure of the tongue, combined with low tone in the lips and cheeks, can contribute to teeth that jut forward in an overbite. If the tongue rests in a forward position between the teeth, the teeth may grow only until they contact the tongue, resulting in a hole or open-bite malocclusion when the child's teeth are brought together. These dental patterns can make it more difficult for a child to bite and chew efficiently. Food may become stuck in a highly arched palate if a child's tongue movement is unskilled. An open bite makes it more difficult for a child to learn to swallow with the tongue inside the mouth.

Oral structural problems negatively influence eating and drinking predominantly when difficulties in other areas make it hard for the child to compensate for the structural difference. This interplay of form and function can be observed clearly when children have a **short lingual frenulum**. At one time, every child whose tongue movement was restricted by a short band of tissue from the front of the tongue to the floor of the mouth had this frenulum clipped. This was supposed to prevent the negative effects of the tongue-tie on the development of feeding and speech. However, dental surgeons now are more cautious and conservative about doing this frenuloplasty on every child (Velanovich, 1994). The tongue restriction from a short frenulum may play a very major role in the feeding difficulties of some children. For example, the breast-feeding infant may have more difficulties than the bottle-fed infant simply because the tongue must come farther forward during breast-feeding to latch on to the nipple and draw it into the mouth (Notestine, 1990). Children who have mild problems with oral coordination may have major problems compensating for this type of tongue restriction, especially during chewing. However, if the child has low tone in the mouth, this structural restriction may actually provide better stability and improve oral functioning.

Gastrointestinal

Structural disorders of the gastrointestinal system play a major role in passage of food through the digestive system. Because they affect tissues that are not subject to volitional control or modification, they usually have a stronger impact on the development of feeding skills than structural problems of the face and mouth. These disorders can vary from a narrowing or stricture in the esophagus that causes food to slow down or get stuck to an atresia, or blind pouch, at any point in the system that totally prevents the passage of food.

Children can be born with an **esophageal stricture** or they may develop it later as the result of acid damage from gastroesophageal reflux. Often the stricture is not discovered until the child developmentally transitions to more solid foods. Clinically, the feeding therapist may see a child who refuses to eat solid foods or gags or vomits on foods that have more texture than liquids or purees. The gagging or vomiting usually is not at the lips, tongue, or swallowing level, but occurs after the food appears to be swallowed and moved down the esophagus some. Often the child only vomits the particular mouthful that was restricted or blocked in its passage through the esophagus. Children with this type of problem rarely vomit a whole meal. Strictures usually are diagnosed by upper GI or esophageal endoscopy procedures. Esophageal dilitation may be successful in stretching the stricture to improve the passage of solids.

Although an esophageal stricture limits the passage of food into the stomach by creating a narrowing of the opening, **pyloric stenosis** impedes movement of food from the stomach to the intestines. The working diameter of the pyloric valve is narrowed by either an increase in size or number of cells of the pyloric muscle (Oue & Puri, 1999). This results in discomfort during feeding and projectile vomiting.

More serious dysfunction occurs when a tube ends in a blind pouch called an atresia. This occurs primarily in the esophagus or the anus. Both conditions usually are identified at birth and must be dealt with by surgical reconstruction before the child can eat orally. When the esophagus does not connect with the stomach, it is called an *esophageal atresia* (EA). Reconstructive reconnection with the stomach is performed when there is enough esophageal tissue. When there is not enough tissue, the physicians may place a tube into the proximal blind pouch to remove secretions until the reconnective surgery is performed. Sometimes, doctors may perform an esophagostomy to bring the upper portion of the esophagus out through an opening in the neck where an ostomy bag collects secretions. In this case, sham feedings often can be done. The child can learn to eat and drink; however, the foods or liquids taken orally drain through the esophagostomy site. From a feeding perspective, this gives the child the advantage of more normal oral motor experiences from an earlier age so that these skills are not forgotten or adversely influenced by long-term tube placement. The child will need a feeding tube for nourishment during this period. When there is an *anal atresia*, the child will use a colostomy bag to collect waste materials until the physician can do reconstructive surgery.

Children with an esophageal atresia often have a related structural problem known as a *tracheoesophageal fistula* (TEF) in which there is a fistula or hole that improperly connects the trachea and the esophagus (Ein & Friedberg, 1981). This clearly interferes with the normal separation of the tubes for breathing and eating.

There are a number of variations of EA and TEF, though the lesions are commonly grouped into five categories by presence or absence of the TEF and by the configuration of the esophagus.

Therapists and parents frequently deal with complications that can occur in feeding after surgical intervention for esophageal atresia and tracheoesophageal fistula (Cavallaro, Pineschi, Freni, Cortese, & Bardini, 1992; Dowling, 1977; Kramer, 1989). Tracheomalacia, esophageal dysmotility, chronic pulmonary disease, gastroesophageal reflux, and eating sensitivities all can influence eating, appetite, and growth. These physiological difficulties are discussed later in this chapter.

On its final path to the stomach, the esophagus passes through a hole in the diaphragm. Ordinarily this is a smooth passage with secure muscle and ligament connections. Structural problems can occur in this area when the diaphragm does not provide a clear separation because of a weakness or herniation of its wall. The most limiting of these conditions is called a *congenital diaphragmatic hernia*. In the same way that a TEF can cause an opening between the esophagus and trachea, an opening between the thoracic and abdominal cavities causes the diaphragmatic hernia. Stomach contents move upward into the chest. Corrective surgery is required; however, surgery doesn't solve all of the problems. Many children with this condition have associated respiratory, cardiac, and gastrointestinal problems. A less serious type of herniation occurs with a *hiatal hernia* in which the lower esophagus, often with a portion of the stomach, shifts upward through the normal hole in the diaphragm. This is one of many conditions that can increase esophageal reflux.

Structural differences or deviations also are seen in the size and shape of the child's stomach. Some of these may be congenital anomalies, but the majority that affect feeding function are created as a side effect of surgery for gastroesophageal reflux. This can affect both the size and motility of the stomach. When conservative treatments for reflux are ineffective, a surgical procedure called a fundoplication frequently is done. A portion of the stomach (i.e., the fundus) is surgically wrapped around the lower esophageal sphincter, eliminating or reducing the upward refluxing of stomach contents. Because the tissue to create this wrap must come from the stomach itself, a fundoplication automatically reduces the size of the child's stomach. Depending on the child and the surgeon, this can reduce the storage area minimally or by a very large percentage. Some children who have had a fundoplication get full very easily and need to eat more frequently because they don't have a normal amount of storage space for a full-sized meal.

A similar acquired limitation of the gastrointestinal tract is seen in *short bowel syndrome.* The most common cause of this condition is necrotizing enterocolitis, a serious illness of premature

Table 6.1 Categories of Lesions

	Type A	Type A is esophageal atresia without a fistula. Both ends of the esophagus are blind pouches and are not connected to each other or to the trachea. This occurs in 8% of the lesions.
	Type B	Type B has a fistula in the proximal portion of the esophagus and a blind pouch in the lower portion.
	Type C	The most common lesion is Type C (85%). The upper end of the esophagus ends in a blind pouch and the lower portion has a fistula to the trachea.
	Type D	In type D, both upper and lower portions of the esophagus have a fistula into the trachea.
	Type E/H	Type E is also called the H type. There is no atresia present. The esophagus connects to the stomach, but also has a fistula connecting directly to the trachea. This type of fistula may be hardest to detect because both the esophagus and trachea are still intact. The baby may demonstrate coughing or choking during feedings, and may have recurrent bouts of pneumonia.

infants. A portion of the intestines may be removed to save the baby's life. Recall the amazing functional surface of the small intestine with its multiple layering of folds. When a length of this tract is removed, often there is insufficient surface to support the proper absorption of nutrients. Depending upon the active length of the gut and the healing of the portion that has been resected, the child usually goes through a period of parenteral feeding in which a nutrient solution is given directly into the bloodstream, bypassing the gastrointestinal system. Many children eventually develop the structure and function for gastrointestinal absorption. However, the reintroduction of enteral feedings may take quite a while, and progress is usually slow as the gut gradually adapts to tiny presentations of food. The infant's appetite is negatively influenced, normal sucking and swallowing experiences are disrupted, and long-term tube feedings often are required—all of which can have a serious impact on oral feeding skills.

Respiratory and Cardiac

Structural disorders of the respiratory and cardiac systems also play a role in children's feeding abilities. These interfere predominantly by placing a heavy physiological stress on breathing, which in turn negatively influences either the suck-swallow-breathe coordination or the energy that is required for eating. The disorders *tracheomalacia* and *laryngomalacia* create this stress by obstructing the respiratory passageway so that the child is unable to take in an adequate amount of oxygen with each breath (Baxter, 1994; Cogbill, Moore, Accurso, & Lilly, 1983). As these infants and children breathe in and out, they make a harsh, noisy sound called stridor, which is produced as air passes through the restricted area. When the cartilaginous rings in the trachea lack adequate tone or are weak, as in tracheomalacia, they may collapse when the child exhales. In laryngomalacia, the flaccid or weak structures are in the walls of the larynx, which tend to collapse inward when the child breathes in. A large number of these infants have difficulty with neuromuscular tone and control of the larynx and trachea (Belmont & Grundfast, 1984). Some infants will experience this type of respiratory obstruction as part of a more generalized hypotonia in the body.

In most instances, tracheomalacia and laryngomalacia are mild, self-limiting disorders, and the child gradually grows out of these conditions during the first 2–5 years without formal intervention. In approximately 10% of infants, the situation is more severe and a tracheostomy must be provided to support breathing until the tracheal or laryngeal structures can work independently.

When there are structural defects in the cardiac system, the basic situation is similar to the types of structural limitations we have discussed in the other systems. Areas that should be separate at birth remain connected (e.g., **pulmonary atresia**) or narrowed (e.g., **pulmonary stenosis, aortic stenosis, coartation of the aorta**) so that blood cannot pass through. Other areas that should function independently at birth are connected because of holes in the heart (e.g., **ventricular septal defect, atrial septal defect, Tetrology of Fallot**) or the failure of fetal blood vessels to separate properly (e.g., **patent ductus arteriosis**). In still others, a critical area of the heart may be underdeveloped (e.g., **hypoplastic left heart**) or vessels may be connected to the wrong parts of the heart (e.g. **transposition of the great arteries**), placing massive stress on the total functioning of the cardiac system.

These and other cardiac defects interfere with efficient blood flow to the heart and lungs. In many cases they are life threatening. In other instances, milder difficulties with heart valves may not be diagnosed until a child is older and receives a physical examination for school or summer camp.

Structural disorders of the respiratory and cardiac systems primarily affect the physiological interplay of these systems with the swallowing and gastrointestinal systems.

Physiological Limits

Just as the physiology of eating is influenced by the system's structural components, it is also influenced by the neural, hormonal, and neurotransmitter systems. These systems control and monitor the movement of food from the mouth to the anus and the timing and coordination of valves that support or stop the transition of food from one part of the system to another. Third, it is influenced by the structure and physiology of the respiratory and cardiac systems that contribute to the overall comfort and safety involved in eating. Physiological function related to eating usually is due to the interplay among two or more systems. Although this section will discuss limits of the swallowing, gastrointestinal, respiratory, and cardiac systems, its primary emphasis will be on the interaction of systems.

We briefly will mention and discuss some of the physiological limits of the motor, sensory, and oral motor systems. However, we have devoted Chapter 7 to a more in-depth look at these issues and their direct effect on sucking, swallowing, biting, and chewing.

Types of Physiological Limitations and Their Influence on Feeding

Physiological limits that affect feeding influence the system by:
- reducing the timing and coordination of the movement of food through the valves of the system
- reducing the amount or efficiency of movement of food through the digestive tract
- causing pain, discomfort, and structural damage due to gastroesophageal reflux
- negatively affecting the respiratory system

These physiological limits affect eating and drinking by:

- interfering with the safe and efficient movement of food from the mouth into the stomach
- reducing the ability of food and acid to remain in the stomach, leading to the pain and discomfort of gastroesophageal reflux
- causing aspiration and contributing to the development of pneumonia
- reducing the efficiency of breathing and interfering with the coordination of breathing with sucking and swallowing
- reducing the efficiency of movement of food through the stomach and intestinal tract
- reducing the efficiency of movement of waste products through the colon and out of the body
- reducing energy and endurance for feeding

Physiological Limitations Through the Feeding System

Oral-Pharyngeal

When the series of upper channels and valves carrying food from the mouth to the stomach does not work well, *aspiration* becomes a high risk for oral feeding. Some children have no swallow reflex, and the system remains in the configuration designed for breathing. The nasal airway remains open, the laryngeal airway remains open, and the top of the esophagus remains closed. Any food that falls or is propelled over the back of the tongue eventually will move into the open airway and the lungs. In most instances a swallow is present and possible. However, it may be delayed, and timing and coordination prevent the protection of the airway, which causes intermittent aspiration. When pharyngeal movement is not active enough to clear all food from its walls after a swallow, the remaining residue eventually may end up in the airway. An open airway due to the paralysis of a vocal cord also contributes to complications. Although the lungs certainly are not designed to hold swallowed food and liquid, they can accept some without causing long-term damage. The greatest damage to the lungs, however, comes from the refluxing of acidic gastrointestinal contents into the lungs. The mechanism of swallowing dysfunction and its impact on eating will be discussed in Chapter 7.

Gastrointestinal

The most frequent and pervasive physiological limit is *gastroesophageal reflux* (GER), which accompanies a high number of other feeding difficulties. When the lower esophageal sphincter does not work competently, stomach contents can backwash into the esophagus. Food and acid can move up the esophagus and even into the pharynx itself. If there is enough force behind the reflux, the child will vomit. This situation leads to a wide variety of primary feeding problems as well as a long list of related complications in other systems. Most people reflux occasionally. Many babies spit up as a normal part of the maturation of their gastrointestinal (GI) system. Although inconvenient for parents, it usually has minimal effects on feeding and will be outgrown with maturity of the GI system and increased postural control. However, when the chronic reflux symptoms cause changes in the child's health, appetite, and growth, then gastroesophageal reflux disease (GERD), or pathological gastroesophageal reflux, is diagnosed.

Some of the symptoms of reflux are overt, such as vomiting, while others are much more subtle, making the accurate diagnosis more complicated. Unlike the stomach, which has a protective coating of mucus, the esophagus is extremely vulnerable to repeated floods of acid. The discomfort leads to the painful and subjective symptoms adults call heartburn. Usually some refluxed material is cleared by peristalsis of the esophagus paired with increased salivation and swallowing, which can neutralize the acidity of the refluxed material. Acid allowed to stay in the esophagus can cause inflammation of the delicate esophageal tissues. This *esophagitis* can cause symptoms from mild nauseousness, gagging, irritability, and heartburn to severe pain or the development of strictures. Many children who have experienced frequent or painful reflux simply don't want to eat, particularly if the situation is complicated by problems in other areas. Others may choose to eat a small amount until their basic hunger is satisfied but then stop before they become too uncomfortable.

Gastroesophageal reflux influences and is influenced by many other parts of the body. For example, when there are motility problems of the stomach or difficulties with opening of the pyloric sphincter, large amounts of food remain in the stomach for a long time. This places pressure on the lower esophageal sphincter and contributes to gastroesophageal reflux.

Respiratory disease can cause gastroesophageal reflux, which then can cause respiratory disease (Halstead, 1999). Pressure changes in the chest that are associated with labored breathing in asthma and bronchopulmonary dysplasia also contribute to upward movement of stomach contents and reflux. The lungs of children with conditions such as bronchopulmonary dysplasia, cystic fibrosis, and asthma may overinflate, altering the shape and configuration of the diaphragm. This can reduce the resting pressure of the lower esophageal sphincter. The increased abdominal pressure associated with coughing also can promote GER. Additionally, some of the medications used to manage the respiratory stress, such as theophylline, also can promote GER by decreasing LES pressure.

Refluxed material can move into the airway, irritating the larynx and causing a cough or hoarseness (Irwin, French, Curley, Zawacki, & Bennett, 1993; Putnam & Orenstein, 1992). It can cause or exacerbate problems with an unstable airway due to laryngomalacia (Matthews, Little, McGuirt, & Koufman, 1999). Chronic microaspiration of refluxed stomach contents can lead to chronic bronchitis, pneumonias, and symptoms that mimic reactive airway disease and asthma. It can cause an asthma-like syndrome with cyanosis, tachycardia, wheezes, and rales (Goodall, Earis, Cooper, Bernstein, & Temple, 1981; Matthews et al., 1999). Children who become noisier during a feeding accompanied by increased wheezing often are suspected of having microaspiration from the feeding. Although aspiration of acidic stomach contents has been shown to cause the most acute and profound pulmonary damage (Orenstein, 1992), chronic aspiration of more neutralized feedings and even antacid neutralized liquids have been shown to cause pulmonary inflammation and damage as well as aspiration pneumonias (Orenstein, 1992). Aspiration of saliva and a food or liquid bolus during, just before, or just after swallowing also can lead to microaspiration. Because lung tissues have already been weakened by respiratory complications, children with lung disease may be more prone to developing pneumonia if food is aspirated during swallowing or as a result of gastroesophageal reflux.

Both nasopharyngeal reflux and gastroesophageal reflux have been associated with apnea episodes in some children (Gomes & Lallemand, 1992; Plaxico & Loughlin, 1981; Thach, 1997) Apnea is the stopping of airflow longer than 20 seconds and is associated with cyanosis, abrupt color change, hypotonia, and bradycardia. It has been suggested that reflux of acid into the distal esophagus or nasopharynx may stimulate the mucosal receptors that change the respiratory mechanics by way of the vagal nerve reflexes. Apnea can be brief and not damaging or can be life threatening. These episodes can be very frightening to the observer because they generally are characterized by some combination of color changes, changes in muscle tone, choking, or gagging. In some situations, the observer fears the child is dying. Damage to the child's brain can occur if the frightened adult tries to alert the child through shaking (Lancon, Haines, & Parent, 1998). It is important to note that in studies of infants with life-threatening events, most of them did *not* have a history of vomiting that otherwise might have led to an earlier diagnosis of the GER that precipitated the severe apnea (Kahn, Montauk, & Blum, 1987).

All of these issues can make eating less pleasant and less safe for children. To protect themselves, children can become very picky about what they will eat. Appetite may be suppressed. Growth can be affected. Greater detail on gastroesophageal reflux and its impact on eating safety and desire will be provided in Chapter 22.

Other motility problems of the gastrointestinal tract play a role when children have difficulty with feeding. ***Esophageal dysmotility*** can be caused by neurological difficulties, by structural problems associated with strictures, or as a result of the surgical repair of an esophageal atresia or tracheoesophageal fistula. The motility difficulties can be within the body of the esophagus itself or can be due to ***achalasia***. During achalasia, the resting pressure of the lower esophageal sphincter is increased so that the LES fails to relax following swallowing (Kahrilas & Ergun, 1994). The esophagus itself becomes stretched as it expands to contain the bolus of food while the opening of the LES is narrowed, blocking movement of the bolus into the stomach. Achalasia often is accompanied by an incomplete or absent peristalsis in the body of the esophagus. Occasionally, achalasia is the result of failure of the LES to open at the site of a Nissen fundoplication procedure that is too tight. Dysmotility of the proximal portion of the small intestine also has been identified in many individuals with achalasia (Schmidt et al., 1999).

Children with esophageal achalasia can have vomiting, difficulty swallowing solids or liquids, weight loss, painful swallowing, recurrent pneumonias, and a feeling of foods getting stuck. These symptoms also are common in children whose esophagus does not move well because of surgical reconstruction of esophageal tissue (e.g., esophageal atresia, tracheoesophageal fistula). These motility issues must be taken into account during feeding.

Clinically, the timing of swallows may need to be slowed. Some foods will be more difficult than others. Even adults with a normally functioning esophagus have more difficulty clearing the esophagus with a single swallow when eating bread (Pouderoux, Shi, Tatum, & Kahrilas, 1999). Liquids may need to be alternated with solids to pass food more easily through the esophagus when there are difficulties with peristalsis.

We know that functioning of the stomach depends on well-timed and controlled muscular and digestive activity. Disorders of **stomach motility** disrupt the system in many ways. The distal portions of the stomach, the corpus and antrum, act as a muscular pump to break up food into small particles as it becomes mixed with hydrochloric acid. Gastric contractions coordinate with duodenal contractions to allow gastric contents to move through the pylorus into duodenum, the beginning of the small intestine. Movement of food through the stomach, therefore, requires appropriate muscular activity paired with properly working proximal and distal stomach openings. We have already seen the difficulties that develop when the LES at the proximal end of the stomach is not properly functioning. Obstruction at the lower end of the stomach will prevent or delay the emptying of the stomach contents at that end.

Abnormal or inconsistent muscular activity in the stomach can lead to **delayed gastric emptying**. These delays can contribute to gastroesophageal reflux and projectile vomiting (Cannon & Stadalnik, 1993; Papaila et al., 1989). Persistent vomiting with delayed emptying also can be caused by an ulcer, irritation, or growth in the stomach near the pylorus. Food sensitivities and allergies also can cause delayed gastric emptying and contribute to GER.

In addition, stomach emptying that is too rapid can cause major problems. This condition, known as **dumping syndrome**, often is a side-effect of a Nissen fundoplication or a pyloroplasty (Samuk et al., 1996; Pittschieler, 1991). Children are extremely uncomfortable during a dumping episode because food enters the duodenum at the top of the small intestine too suddenly, causing severe difficulties with the regulation of insulin and sugar. Typical biochemical changes include hyperglycemia shortly after meals, followed by hyperinsulinemia and reactive hypoglycemia (Rivkees & Crawford, 1987). This frequently results in total autonomic nervous system symptoms such as increased salivation, nausea, sweating, lethargy, and pallor (Veit, Heine, & Catto-Smith, 1994). Delayed gastric emptying and dumping syndrome can increase the risk of developing retching after a Nissen fundoplication (Jolley, Tunell, Leonard, Hoelzer, & Smith, 1987).

In addition to the uncomfortable symptoms of reflux or dumping, infants and children with delayed gastric emptying may feel full all the time. Because the stomach doesn't empty properly, they may still have a large portion of a prior meal in the stomach when it is time to eat again. They may eat very small amounts and cause adults to worry because they are not getting enough calories to grow well. Gastric emptying time can be increased with improved positioning and with medications. Often babies are positioned in prone or right sidelying after or during meals to optimize stomach emptying. Medications used to treat gastroesophageal reflux often improve stomach emptying. Sometimes, when more conservative measures have failed to achieve good stomach emptying, a pyloroplasty is performed to open up the distal stomach and accelerate movement of the food into the intestines.

The major motility difficulties of the intestines affect all aspects of later digestion and absorption of nutrients as well as the movement of waste products from the body. **Chronic intestinal pseudo-obstruction** (CIP) is the most severe form of abnormal gastrointestinal motility. Children with CIP have many of the same symptoms as those with actual physical blockages in the bowel. This condition, however, is the result of poor strength or coordination of the muscle contractions of the intestines. Children complain of poor appetite, nausea, vomiting, heartburn, abdominal pain, and constipation. They may not grow or develop at the expected rate. This is a rare condition that is often difficult to diagnose. Many children with CIP will receive their nutrition through a feeding tube for most of their lives; others seem to outgrow the condition and can eat comfortably by mouth. Children with **Hirschsprung's disease** also experience problems with intestinal motility. However, their condition is related to the lack of nerve cells in the wall of the bowel that enable the intestinal muscles to move the stool through the large intestine. Stool becomes trapped in the colon and cannot be released. Because the colon expands as it fills, the condition sometimes is called a megacolon. Like many conditions, there can be many gradations of difficulty with colonic motility. Some children are severely affected because a large area of the colon is affected. Others do not become chronically ill, but develop discomfort from chronic constipation and abdominal distention. Children initially receive a colostomy so that stools can pass from the body. This is followed by surgery to remove the affected bowel and rejoin the healthy segments. Most children do not have long-term complications after surgery, but some continue to have some difficulties with releasing or holding the stool.

Two relatively common intestinal motility issues are familiar to most parents and therapists. You will recall that the function of the large intestine is to conserve the correct amount of water and remove it from the liquid fecal wastes, allowing a solid yet pliable stool to pass out of the body. When not enough water is removed, the child has **diarrhea**. When too much water is removed, there is a problem with **constipation**. Both of these conditions can be related to internal or external causes. For example, diarrhea is most commonly the result of the body's response to an acute gastrointestinal illness such as influenza or a bacterial insult or a chronic condition such as sensitivity to a food or medication. It also can be precipitated by the body's response to emotional stress. Constipation commonly occurs when the body has an inadequate amount of water in the system. Stools may be too dry or too poorly lubricated to pass easily through the colon. Diets of children with oral motor feeding difficulties may contain insufficient fiber. When children are on a liquid diet, such as a tube-feeding formula, the diet also may not contain enough fiber to create and move a solid stool. Abnormal muscle tone in the gastrointestinal tract and poor physical activity also can contribute to constipation. Constipation can be a side effect of medication or an allergy to cow's milk (Iacono et al., 1995). Constipation becomes a problem when children experience pain as they try to pass a stool. Just as children who experience gastroesophageal reflux often don't want to eat because it hurts, children who experience constipation may resist having a bowel movement because it hurts. The holding of stools causes additional problems that may lead to a chronic cycle of withholding, increased constipation, attempts to pass a large painful stool and more withholding and constipation (Seth & Heyman, 1994).

Many children with feeding disorders and growth problems are prone to constipation. Their oral motor limitation may make it a challenge to take in enough fiber and fluid. Their muscle-tone limitations may decrease their physical activity and limit the movement of the abdomen. Families must find creative ways to present fiber and fluids, and provide as much physical movement as possible for the child. Abdominal massage may need to be incorporated into the daily routine. A regular or adapted toileting routine may need to be established.

Respiratory-Cardiac

The physiological function of the respiratory system has a powerful influence on eating. A well-functioning respiratory system provides a balance of oxygen and carbon dioxide in the blood throughout the day as the child moves from one activity to the next. There are different respiratory requirements on the body with differing activities of feeding, sleeping, and playing. The common tubing of the feeding and respiratory systems creates the necessity for these systems to work in a highly sophisticated and coordinated fashion. Proper timing is essential. Good feeding and growth will depend on the coordination of the sucking, swallowing, and breathing processes.

Physiological difficulties with the respiratory system already have been discussed in terms of structural limitations of the system and in relationship to the pervasive effects of motility issues such as gastroesophageal reflux on other systems. Most difficulties with respiration decrease a child's interest in eating. Given a choice of eating or breathing, the child must choose breathing. The child must be able to make the respiratory adjustments necessary to move into the activity of eating. Eating is work for infants, and work requires respiratory changes. The infant must have the respiratory systems in place to make the necessary changes to modify oxygen and carbon dioxide levels. This can be done with changes in respiratory rate, depth of respiration, heart rate, and the work of breathing.

Respiratory rate is the number of breaths needed for proper oxygen exchange. It changes with the work being done as well as with the health of the alveolar and lung tissue. Conditions such as **bronchopulmonary dysplasia**, which reduce the number and effectiveness of the alveoli, can affect the respiratory rate by causing the need for increased frequency of breaths. The damaged alveoli create fewer gas exchange sites, leading to an increased number of inspirations as compensation for the reduced oxygen exchange in each breath.

The depth of breathing is the amount of oxygen taken in during each breath. This is influenced by the strength of the child's respiratory musculature, the freedom of movement of the muscles between the ribs, strength of the diaphragm, health of the organs of respiration, and thoracic support.

For many children, disruptions of respiration are based on postural tone and movement and on spinal structure. Severe **scoliosis** or **kyphosis** creates postural changes, which decrease the depth of respiratory volume. Others have **hypotonia** and overall decreased physical strength and control, which provide a poor basis of respiratory control. Still others have difficulties with increased tone or **hypertonia**. They may have a resultant decrease in the freedom of movement of the muscles that expand the chest for breathing. Children whose muscle tone and neurological status reduce the normal maturational experiences may develop compensatory methods of respiration that provide less respiratory support to the work of feeding. These children may not fully develop the use of the muscles of the abdominal-pelvic girdle, which supports efficient breathing by stabilizing the lower rib cage so that the upper chest can move for deeper breathing.

The heart rate and the efficiency of the heart's stroke influence the amount of oxygen and carbon dioxide in the blood. Some cardiac conditions will influence the rate and efficiency of the heart and may lead to increased heart rate during feeding. Cardiac conditions such as **congestive heart failure** can cause low oxygen levels in the blood or poor circulation, making increased demands on the respiratory system during feeding.

There are a number of feeding problems commonly associated with significant respiratory and cardiac conditions. Most commonly, there is a decrease in feeding endurance. These children fatigue easily and often will tire out before taking in enough food. They may be weak overall and not have the oxygenation to support the work demands of feeding, becoming cyanotic or short of breath as they eat. They might be quite hungry, starting a feeding rapidly, and then tire easily, becoming short of breath and irritable and then falling asleep exhausted before the end of the meal.

Children with respiratory and cardiac issues often have poor growth and malnutrition if they depend solely on oral feedings. They don't consume enough calories for proper growth, healing of lung tissue, and development. Their nutritional issues are influenced by fatigue and weakness, but also may be affected by delayed gastric emptying and poor gastrointestinal motility. Fluid overload is an issue in congestive heart failure. This may influence the ability to take in enough fluids. Many of these infants need supplemental tube feedings to provide the nutrition necessary for growth or to prepare them nutritionally for surgery. Children who have corrective heart surgeries frequently gain weight and improve their overall health after the surgery.

Breathing takes more work when either the respiratory or cardiac system is compromised. Many infants with chronic respiratory disease come home from the hospital on supplemental oxygen. The oxygen level is reduced as the baby demonstrates the ability to maintain appropriate levels of oxygen saturation during respiration. Feeding generally requires more oxygen than other activities because it takes a lot of energy for some infants. For this reason it is very important to routinely check oxygen saturation levels during feeding and even increase these levels at mealtimes to make it easier for these children, even after oxygen support has been reduced for maintenance breathing.

Children with tracheomalacia, laryngomalacia subglottic stenosis, or other chronic respiratory disease may require a tracheostomy tube for prolonged ventilatory support. Oral feeding can be done while the child has a tracheostomy, but this must be done very carefully. The tracheostomy provides oxygenation but does not improve the underlying structural problems and function that created the need for additional respiratory support. The infant may continue to fatigue easily and have the increased respiratory rates and poor coordination of sucking, swallowing, and breathing associated with them.

The tracheostomy apparatus and placement can mechanically restrict upward movement of the larynx, which is important for efficient swallowing and protection of the airway. In some cases, the placement of the tracheostomy can lead to a desensitization of the larynx that may further reduce protective reflexes and lead to uncoordinated laryngeal closure. Some children who have tracheostomies have pharyngeal scarring or damage from the prolonged use of an endotracheal tube prior to placement of the tracheostomy. These situations can increase the risk of aspiration during swallowing.

Wellness Limits

Wellness is not simply the absence of illness. Many children and adults are not sick, yet they are not well either. They lack the inner strength and balance that allow them to live without limitations in physical, emotional, and spiritual health. There may be subtle imbalances in these systems that reduce the inner vigor and hardiness that enable these people to be healthy and participate fully in life.

For example, let's look at two children who were born with the same heart defect. Each has had the condition corrected surgically. Both parents say that they are glad that their daughter is no longer sick and that she is well. Yet the two children are quite different in their ability to participate in their lives. Lindsey smiles a lot and seems curious about everything around her, including food. She seems to have a strong resistance to getting colds, flus, and ear infections that are common among the other children in her preschool. Although she is often tired at the end of the day, her energy picks up after a short nap. She sleeps well and eats the wide variety of foods that are characteristic of a balanced diet. Julie often has chronic nasal congestion and low energy. She has trouble falling asleep and is often quite restless during the night. Her mother says that she usually is not sick; however, she is more prone to picking up colds from other children. She gives Julie many non-prescription medications to help her breathe and sleep better at night. Each winter, Julie gets three or four ear infections that are treated with antibiotics. Although she used to be more interested in eating, she now picks at her food and says she isn't hungry. She doesn't like many foods, so her parents serve her only foods they think she might accept. Her diet consists primarily of white bread, hot dogs, and french fries. Since her surgery, she has become more fussy and irritable, especially at times of change or stress.

Types of Wellness Limitations and Their Influence on Feeding

Limitations in wellness that affect feeding influence the system by:
- reducing the strength of the immune system
- increasing the number of medications that the child is given
- reducing the strength of taste and smell senses in the enjoyment of food

- reducing the nutritional adequacy of the child's diet
- reducing the child's overall feeling of well being
- reducing the child's endurance at mealtime

These limitations to wellness affect eating and drinking by:
- lowering resistance to illness and increasing the number of upper respiratory infections
- reducing the child's appetite and desire to eat
- causing the child to stop eating before consuming enough calories or nutrients because of fatigue
- increasing allergies and food sensitivities
- causing side effects such as nausea, constipation, gastroesophageal reflux, and appetite reduction

Wellness Limitations Through the Feeding System

Doctors frequently prescribe antibiotics for children with developmental disabilities. This is a reflection of the high use of antibiotics in general medical practice. However, many articles in medical textbooks and peer review journals support the view that antibiotics are over-prescribed (Schmidt, Smith, & Sehnert, 1994). One study indicated that 40–60% of all antibiotics in this country are misprescribed. For example, 51% of patients seeing doctors for the common cold (a viral infection) were given an antibiotic. Antibiotics can save lives when given for a severe bacterial infection. However, their overuse has resulted in the development of strains of bacteria that are highly resistant to all or most antibiotics, and the massive destruction of the friendly bacteria in the intestines.

Antibiotics act in a non-discriminative fashion when they attack bacteria. Yet the gastrointestinal system is colonized by billions of bacteria that live in a cooperative relationship with the body (Chaitow & Trenev, 1990). These friendly bacteria manufacture B-vitamins, provide the enzyme lactase that helps digest milk-based foods, enhance protein digestion and absorption, increase intestinal peristalsis, and control potentially harmful yeasts such as ***candida albicans***. Although antibiotics kill bacteria that contribute to illness, most of them also kill friendly bacteria. The balance of friendly bacteria in the gut also is altered by stress and low levels of hydrochloric acid in the stomach (Schmidt et al., 1994; Chaitow & Trenev, 1990).

Antibiotics, reduced hydrochloric acid, and stress often are chronic companions of the child with a feeding disorder. Medications and antacids that alter the pH by reducing stomach acidity are commonly given if a child has gastroesophageal reflux. Anything that changes the degree of acidity in the gut changes the habitat for all bacteria. A reduction in the acidity kills friendly bacteria and allows an overgrowth of unfriendly bacteria and yeasts.

The most serious gastrointestinal consequence from the use of antibiotics is the uncontrolled growth of the ***candida albicans*** yeast (Schmidt et al., 1994; Trowbridge & Walker, 1986). Candida is present in every gastrointestinal tract, to some degree. It is kept in balance and prevented from colonizing in the wall of the intestine by the friendly bacteria. When antibiotics wipe out these bacteria, rampant candida growth occurs. During this period of overgrowth, the yeast shifts to a more invasive form that causes increased permeability of the intestinal tract. This condition, sometimes called "leaky gut," allows substances into the bloodstream that stimulate the immune system to defend itself. These antigenic substances may contribute to food allergies or sensitivities in some children.

Children with food and environmental allergies and sensitivities typically do not feel well. Symptoms can occur in any system of the body, including the neurological, respiratory, and gastrointestinal areas (Rapp, 1991). In addition to feeling ill or unwell, many children with food allergies begin to associate these feelings with eating. They may become picky or unenthusiastic eaters.

Limitations in the development of high-level wellness create limitations in children's desire to eat, in their physical comfort with eating, and with their coordination of eating skills. Parents and feeding therapists must be aware of health and wellness issues and address them in feeding and mealtime programs.

Experiential Limits

All children and adults have a diverse series of experiences that relate to food, eating, drinking, and mealtimes. Most of our food-related experiences are appreciated or disliked at the moment and then pass from our memory as new experiences take their place. Some experiences, however, make a bigger impression and are remembered longer because they strongly arouse our emotions or have a special meaning to us. For example, if delicious mashed potatoes are always served when I visit my favorite grandmother's home, they may become associated in my memory with the visits themselves. Some of my preference for mashed potatoes is connected to these memories and to an inner sense that I am moving toward something that will bring me pleasure. If eating strawberries made me feel ill, I may get strong inner warnings that I should stay away from strawberries anytime they are served. These warnings may occur whether or not I actually would become ill if I ate them.

Types of Experiential Limitations and Their Influence on Feeding and Mealtime

Experiential limits that affect feeding influence the system by:

- protecting a child from experiences that are perceived as uncomfortable, painful, or dangerous
- increasing the child's and family's stress levels at mealtime
- allowing a child to feel important or valued in the family
- allowing a child to feel in control
- shifting the locus of responsibility for eating from the child to the adult

These limitations in the child's experience affect eating and drinking by:

- removing the child from the situation that is feared
- reducing the child's trust in adults
- reducing the child's opportunities for and openness to learning feeding-related skills
- limiting the amount and variety of food the child will eat
- promoting power contests around eating
- increasing coercive or forced-feeding patterns at mealtime
- contributing to obesity

Experiential Limitations Through the Feeding and Mealtime System

Let's look at some of the experiences that children with feeding difficulties have had and consider how they may limit their growth toward efficient and competent mealtime and feeding skills.

Physical and Sensory Experiences

As discussed previously, many children have experienced medical difficulties that required extensive intervention. Many of these interventions have assaulted their physical and sensory systems. These children repeatedly have encountered the invasion of intubation tubes down their throats as well as orogastric and nasogastric tubes passed through the mouth, nose, and throat. They have felt themselves unable to breathe and have felt the relief and the invasion from suctioning tubes. They have been in pain in all parts of their bodies and have felt the numbing of experience provided by medications. They particularly have felt pain during and after eating. Most of them have been young an[d] non-verbal and unable to tell others how they felt except through crying. If they have been on a v[enti]lator or tracheostomy, even their crying voice has not been heard.

They have been cared for by parents and professionals who love them and care abou[t] [feel]ings and their needs. They also have been cared for by some adults who perceive them [as-a-]need, not as a child-in-need. These are adults who forget the importance of the infa[nt] part of the stomach or lung that is being treated. They are children who have had little control over their lives because others have assumed control so that they might live.

Whether these experiences create limitations on feeding depends, in part, on the meaning the child attaches to the experience. Children are resilient and frequently bounce back from even the most negative situations without long-term harm. However, when experiences are repeated in a consistent pattern, are associated with strong fear or threat, or occur without the loving support of others, the child understandably may choose to avoid similar experiences in the future. If the child has a sensory system that is easily overwhelmed or experiences the intense discomfort of sensory defensiveness, even less intense experiences may be perceived as dangerous or painful.

Many children who have experienced *respiratory distress* related to prematurity, bronchopulmonary dysplasia, or other reasons appear to have an almost innate fear of situations that place stress on respiration. Eating is one of the major stressors because sucking and swallowing demand a fine-tuned coordination with breathing. For many, it is almost as if there is a cellular memory of the moments after birth when they could not breathe and may have felt close to death. When they begin to take small amounts from the bottle or breast, they must stop breathing for a moment while they swallow. Many older infants and toddlers who are ready to begin to eat strongly resist the process. Although there might be other reasons for their refusal to eat, some have referred directly or indirectly to the scary feelings. One 5-year-old who took tiny single sips of liquid said she could not drink big drinks because she could not breathe.

Some children have a disability that affects their ability to process and integrate sensory information. Children may experience aspects of the sensory world in a very different way from others. Problems with *sensory modulation* and *sensory defensiveness* can contribute to intensely negative feeding experiences. Some children seem to be overly sensitive to certain types of input. Others are undersensitive. Still others will perceive and interpret some types of sensation as highly noxious. Some smells may be overpowering. Certain sounds will be painfully loud. Lumpy food may feel like a mouthful of small stones. The sensation may alert their system to fight or run away.

Many children with feeding issues have experienced substantial *gastrointestinal discomfort* associated with eating. They may vomit during or after meals. They may feel severe pain and discomfort from gastroesophageal reflux. Many children whose reflux has been controlled through a Nissen fundoplication experience side effects from the fundoplication. They begin to gag and retch. They have gas cramps and bloating because gas and air becomes trapped within the stomach. These symptoms increase the discomfort they feel during tube-feeding meals. They often learn to associate eating with this discomfort. They perceive that they have no control over the food that is coming into their stomachs. However, when adults suggest that they can eat food by mouth, they recognize this as an area that they can control. They anticipate being uncomfortable and refuse to eat. If they gradually learn to accept small amounts by mouth, they often stop before they have eaten enough. The feeling of a full or filling stomach causes anticipation of gastrointestinal discomfort, and they stop while they still feel safe.

Children with *allergies* and food sensitivities also may associate eating with discomfort. It is especially a problem when a food sensitivity or allergy is unidentified and children are given foods that make them uncomfortable. As a small child, Susan repeatedly told her parents that she hated milk and often refused to drink it. She insisted that milk made her tummy feel sick. Because she did not act sick or throw up or get diarrhea, the pediatrician did not see a need for testing. He told Susan's mother that her body needed milk and she had to drink it. Battles over milk products continued until Susan left for college. Because of severe hay fever, she had been tested for allergies and had severe reactions to many pollens as a child. When Susan's allergic reactions grew worse as a young adult, her allergist began to test for food allergies. The most severe positive reactions were for milk and other dairy products—those foods that she had tried to tell her parents about throughout childhood. Although she frequently was disciplined for not eating many foods containing dairy products, Susan did not develop long-term feeding problems.

Many life-supporting medical interventions include invasive procedures to the face and mouth. The most negative of these for many children is the use of **orogastric** and **nasogastric tubes** for tube-feedings. These are inserted through the oral cavity or nasal cavity and threaded down the pharynx and esophagus to the stomach. This is invasive and uncomfortable for many children. They often fight the insertion and try to pull off the tape securing the tube to their face. Because of this experience, many young children conclude that anything coming toward their nose or into the mouth is dangerous or uncomfortable. During the time when a nasogastric tube is in place, mouthing activities and swallowing dislodge the tube and move it around in the pharynx. This may be uncomfortable and lead the child to conclude that swallowing also is uncomfortable.

Emotional Experiences

Some children experience high levels of emotional stress that have a strong impact on their eating patterns. Children who have experienced **physical** or **sexual abuse** involving the mouth may be extremely cautious or fearful of any adult who approaches this area. If the child already has feeding or oral motor issues for other reasons, oral abuse may increase the problem to the point where the child will not eat or will refuse to be fed by an adult. Christina was a non-verbal 2-year-old who had difficulties lateralizing her tongue for chewing. Her therapist had been placing long strips of food on the side of her mouth for repeated biting. Although she initially had been extremely cautious, she now enjoyed the activity and her oral motor skills were improving. One day, Christina suddenly clamped her hand over her mouth as soon as the therapist entered the room. When the therapist got out the food strips for chewing, Christina began to scream. Although there were changes in many areas of her behavior, the greatest regression occurred in feeding skills. She gradually refused to take any food other than her bottle. These problems were eventually linked to sexual abuse from her father that had escalated into the oral area.

Dislike or discomfort may escalate into actual **fear** for some children. This may be related to the intensity or repetition of the original event. The key is that the child responded with intense fear. The memory of the event persists for a wide variety of reasons, and the child's fear often escalates. Mark, who was fearful of eating because of a choking episode, became very upset and refused to enter a room where food was present. If he was forced to enter the room, he began to vomit. If he saw pictures of food in a book, he cried and began to gag.

All young children go through periods when they want to do things their way and be in control. Some children learn that they feel safe only when they have **control**. They learn that eating is one area where they can be in control. Children learn early that others cannot make them eat and swallow. These discoveries often set the stage for later power contests at mealtime if parents feel that they must be in control of what and how much their child eats. Many children who demand control at mealtimes are frightened and extremely cautious about certain eating situations or foods. Others simply have discovered that if they demand or protest during the meal, adults often do what they want or engage them in delightful battles.

Mealtime Experiences

Some physical and emotional experiences become strongly focused around mealtime beliefs and the mealtime relationship. These can be the major limits to developing positive feeding and mealtime behaviors for many children. Many children who do not have physical, sensory, or gastrointestinal limitations for eating can develop dysfunctional eating patterns because of a stressful mealtime environment.

In Chapter 3 we discussed the development of a mealtime feeding relationship that reflects the partnership between children and those who feed them. At each stage in development, the relationship changes slightly as the baby's developmental skills and agendas change. Although mealtime changes evolve as children and relationships change, the roles assigned to parents and children remain consistent. Parents are responsible for preparing an appropriate diet and offering it to the child in a developmentally appropriate way. Children are responsible for what and how much they eat.

When children say "You can't make me eat that," they actually may be reflecting their intuitive recognition that deciding what to eat is their role, not the adult's.

In Chapter 2 we explored many influences on mealtime. Although each of the components listed plays a role, certain areas have a stronger influence on mealtime roles and relationships. These include beliefs, family dynamics, and parent's history. Limiting mealtime experiences evolve when **_disagreements about the nature of the mealtime partnership and responsibilities_** occur. When a mother strongly believes that her child should eat everything on the plate, problems may begin to erupt when the child does not hold the same belief. If the mother has other beliefs about what and how much the child must eat, the child may actively contest her position.

Marsha was not very hungry at dinnertime. She ate a little, but quickly lost interest in the food. Her mother noticed that there was still a great deal of food on her plate. She tried to keep feeding her. Marsha clamped her mouth closed and turned her head away. Her mother told her she had to eat more. Marsha grabbed the spoon and bowl and threw them on the floor. Her mother became angry and scooped food back into the bowl and continued to try to feed her. Marsha screamed and spit food in her mother's face until her mother angrily let her get down from the table. Gradually, Marsha learned how much her refusals upset her mother. She realized that her mother wanted the food to disappear and also was worried if she did not eat enough. If her mother served a new food or something she did not like, she refused the first bite and then whined until her mother went to the kitchen to get one of her favorite foods. Her mother had taken over her role of deciding how much to eat. Now she has taken over her mother's role of deciding which foods to serve!

Some children will not contest the parent's position. They may continue to eat although they are experiencing internal signals of satiation. This pattern began in early infancy for Chrissy. During her early months, Chrissy had had difficulty with sucking coordination. It took her a long time to take a bottle, and her mother was often worried that she was not getting enough to eat. As Chrissy's eating coordination improved, her mother was delighted with the amount she was able to eat. With assistance, Chrissy made the transition to pureed foods and a spoon. As Chrissy began to get full, she let her mother know by looking away, closing her mouth, and pushing the spoon away. Her mother always insisted that she take two or three more bites. Chrissy wanted to please her mother, so she did not protest. Her mother was pleased that she could usually get her to take 5 or 6 more bites. She felt like a good mother because her daughter was eating so well and ate everything that she gave her. Over time, Chrissy lost touch with her inner signals of hunger and satiation, and developed many problems with obesity.

Parents often believe that they know how much food the child needs to thrive. Their beliefs or past experiences become the reference point for monitoring the child's intake. This often leads to a **_mismatch between the child's hunger and appetite and the adult's expectation_**. Many parents expect that their child will eat the same amount at each meal or each day. However, this rarely happens. Appetites vary from meal to meal, depending on the caloric content of the food and the amount of food eaten at previous meals. A child who has eaten a high-calorie, high-fat snack (e.g., candy bar, ice cream) before dinner will be less hungry for the meal than a child who has not had a snack or has had a low-calorie snack (e.g., raw carrots, apple slices). The amount eaten at snack time may be similar, but because the nutritional content was different, the child's hunger at the next meal will vary.

Tomaso received his meals through tube feedings for his first 2 years. Each meal was the same size and the same number of calories. The dietitian emphasized that he needed the same amount at each meal in order to grow. When Tomaso began to eat more by mouth, his parents were quite worried that at some meals he ate a lot and at other meals he seemed uninterested and ate very little. As his tube feedings were reduced, Tomaso's parents continued to be worried about their son's eating patterns, which actually were very typical of other 2-year-olds. Their experience with tube-feedings had taught them that children must eat the same amount at every meal. When Tomaso did not eat in this way, they were worried. They began to push him to eat more food. They offered him special high-calorie desserts to increase his intake. Gradually, he lost interest in eating fruits and vegetables and waited until dessert arrived.

As infants approach the age of 8 months, they begin to move into a stage of emerging independence, which culminates by age 3. This is a period of exploration, trying new ways of doing things, and becoming more independent. If parents and therapists are not responsive to this developmental agenda, major mealtime feeding limitations will develop. The most common is the birth of the power contest. The child's actions say, "I will do it this way." The parent's counter-actions say, "No you won't. You will do it this way." The child's response is, "That's what you think. Just make me do it!" The most important aspect of the ***power contest*** is that it always requires two players. Many young children enjoy the "game aspects" of a power contest. Often for the first time they witness an important adult becoming upset or angry because of their actions. They now have a strong sense of cause and effect, recognizing their power in causing adults to act in a particular way. They feel powerful when they provoke adults when they behave contrary to what the adult wants. Adults must realize that children can devote 24 hours a day to winning the power contest. Most adults don't have that kind of time or stamina. The best approach for adults is to stay out of power contests. The challenge of the power contest overrides the child's internal signals of hunger and satiation. When power contests limit mealtime skills, they must be dealt with from the beginning. Otherwise, the child is not free to expand his or her feeding and mealtime abilities.

Power contests may escalate into ***force-feeding*** for some adults and children. This may take many forms and even be guided by professionals who believe that a child must not be allowed to get away with a specific behavior. Often, force-feeding is rooted in fear and discouragement. Because the child refuses to eat, parents may become terrified that she will become ill or even die of starvation. Because they have established a routine where they take responsibility for what and how much the child eats, they continue to believe that it is their duty to get food into their child. Other children end up being force-fed because they are making very slow progress in accepting oral-feedings. Bryan had been on tube feedings for 3 years. After 2 years of therapy, he showed very little interest in food and took only a few tastes of familiar foods. Both his parents and therapist were discouraged. They initiated a program to make him eat 3 spoonfuls of food at every meal. At first they tried to talk him into eating by bribing him with toys if he would take a bite. Bryan clamped his mouth closed and said, "No." Then they made him sit at the table until he ate his 3 spoonfuls. Bryan said, "No," and sat at the table until his parents gave up. The power contest was clearly in place. His feeding therapist suggested that they force him to eat, with the hopes that he would give in and decide that he could actually like the food. She suggested that one parent hold his arms and legs so that he couldn't struggle while the other parent held his nose until he opened his mouth. When the mouth was open, they inserted the spoonful of food and held his mouth closed until he swallowed. If he didn't swallow immediately, they were told to hold both his nose and mouth until a more automatic swallow began. Many force-feeding programs are implemented in a less drastic way; however, all include an adult physically or emotionally overpowering the child. In some instances, the child gives in and becomes a passive eater. In others, the child continues to find ways to reject eating. One little girl began to vomit strongly after every tube feeding, effectively getting rid of all food that entered her body. When the gastroenterologist placed her on continuous drip feedings, she began to produce a stronger stomach acid that caused her feeding tube to disintegrate. She effectively had decided that she no longer wished to live when treated in this way.

Lost Experiences

Experiential limitations are not always negative experiences. They may take the form of lost opportunities in which the child misses experiences that provide the building blocks for other skills. Lost opportunities can occur at many points on the feeding development continuum. A child may miss stages such as mouthing, the transition to solid foods, and play and exploration with food. Most children learn to adapt to these missing pieces. Others, however, do not. Sometimes the lost opportunities are related to a child's illness or to sensorimotor difficulties that interfere at particular developmental periods. Other opportunities are lost because of parenting beliefs and styles.

Brandon had been a fussy baby who calmed down only when his mother breast-fed him. He sucked small amounts, spending long periods grazing at the breast and cuddling. His mother kept him with her constantly and was very responsive to his needs. Brandon was not interested in sucking on his own fists and had not learned this strategy for self-calming. His mother was always there to give him the breast for calming. Brandon gagged when his mother offered him the spoon and pureed food at 6 months. He struggled and did not like this new experience. During the next 4 months, he reluctantly took the spoon several times a day and gradually adapted to the sensation of the spoon and smooth food. When he was a year old, his mother introduced small finger foods and lumpier baby foods. Brandon gagged and threw up. He screamed and clamped his mouth closed. He seemed to be very uncomfortable every time the new food entered his mouth. A feeding therapist described Brandon as having "oral defensiveness." Brandon's early history included many lost opportunities to prepare his mouth for feeding-related sensory experiences. He did not seek out mouthing activities spontaneously. When he showed little interest in this, his mother provided the substitute of non-nutritive sucking on the breast, but did not recognize the importance of other kinds of mouthing experiences. His strong rejection of textured foods may have reflected a state of early oral-sensory defensiveness. However, they may also have reflected a child with a nervous system that was more sensitive to change and a total lack of experience with textures in the mouth.

Babies learn to feed themselves by reaching for a parent's spoon and banging on the table, by getting their hands in the food, and smearing food on the tray or in their hair! They discover that they can put a food-covered hand in the mouth and pick up a piece of food on the tray. Eventually they figure out how to hold a spoon and bring it to the mouth without spilling the food. It is a messy and adventuresome process. Some babies are born to parents who have a very low tolerance for mess. Some babies have a very high need to explore the sensory world with their hands. When these parents and babies share the same household, you can call this a "messiness mismatch." Jason was raised by a father who cared for the children and managed the household while his wife worked as an executive manager of the local bank. The father took great pride in his home and family and valued the time he was able to spend with his two young sons. At 6 months, Jason loved to get his hands into everything. When he began to sit in the high chair for meals, he started to pat and bang and smear food. His father was appalled. He hated the mess, and the feeling of food on the back of his hands made him feel very upset. He found a way to keep Jason's hands under the tray and kept bowls and food off the tray. Although Jason was not happy about this, he was hungry and kept eating. As his baby son got older, the father told him "no" every time he reached for the spoon or tried to get his hands in the bowl. Jason got upset, but kept eating as his father put the food into his mouth. Eventually Jason showed no interest in feeding himself. When his parents tried to teach him how to bring the spoon to his mouth independently, Jason pulled his hands away and opened his mouth for the adult.

Environmental Limits

At times, the environment places limits on the child that are related to socioeconomic factors or personal limitations in parents or caregivers. These may have a profound impact on the child's development of feeding skills.

Types of Environmental Limitations and Their Influence on the Family at Mealtime

Environmental limits that affect the family influence the system by:
- causing malnutrition
- limiting housing options
- interfering with bonding, attachment, and separation
- contributing to high levels of stress and anxiety in parents
- contributing to depression and other mental health problems

These limitations in the environment affect the child's mealtime, eating, and drinking by:

■ reducing the amount and variety of food available for a nutritional diet
■ providing multiple caregivers with multiple approaches to mealtimes
■ reducing the financial resources available to deal with a child's feeding difficulties
■ reducing the parents' emotional and physical energy to deal with a child's feeding difficulties

Environmental Limitations Through the Feeding and Mealtime System

We have discussed limitations for feeding that are directly related to the child's physical, sensory, or emotional status or to the family's relationship to the many aspects of feeding. There are, however, many circumstances that impact indirectly on a child's feeding and mealtime skills that are related to issues within the socioeconomic or mental-health issues of the family.

When a family is dealing with poverty, there may be few personal or financial resources to address a child's feeding issues. Although some financial resources are available to provide basic food, housing, and medical care, families must know how to access these resources. Many require a great deal of persistence and paperwork to obtain what is needed. Rules and regulations are often arbitrary and overwhelming and do not fit the needs of a specific child or family. Feelings of personal self-worth often are reduced by an impersonal system, especially when a family has recently experienced poverty because of unemployment. Food may be in limited supply, and children may not get enough to eat or enough of the nutritious foods that support growth. Many parents do not know how to buy or prepare a nutritious diet on a limited income. When income is limited, families may live in crowded conditions or move from one home or shelter to another. Children may move from one school district to another, resulting in frequent changes in therapists and teachers as well as a lack of consistency in the feeding program.

Inconsistent mealtimes and caregiving don't support a child's ability to learn feeding skills through a regular, daily routine. When children spend most of their waking hours in a day-care setting, many different people may feed them. Staff turnover in less expensive day-care programs often is high, and mealtime consistency may be low. In comparison, many infants and young children adopted from orphanages in other countries often have experienced severe environmental deprivation and malnutrition. They have not been able to bond well with a single adult care provider, and they show mental, emotional, and physical delays when they reach their new home and family. Children in both these situations have feeding delays and problems that stem from their early environmental limitation and lack of bonding with a caregiver. Mothers, on the other hand, may feel overwhelmed after an infant's birth and go through severe postpartum depression because of hormonal changes. This makes it more difficult to bond with the infant and begin successful breast-feeding. When depression is a chronic problem, the mother may miss her baby's mealtime communication cues and have a great deal of difficulty developing a satisfying mealtime relationship. Matters can be further exacerbated when parents have their own complicated relationship with food. Anorexia and bulimia may influence their interactions with food, and this all too often has an impact on their beliefs and approach to feeding their children.

Relating to Factors That Limit Feeding Skill Development

The first step toward change is the recognition and understanding of factors that prevent change. This chapter has begun that journey. It offers a broad overview of the many components that may come together in a child's feeding and mealtime history. We must begin by understanding the roles played by structural, physiological, wellness, experiential, and environmental limits. This understanding gives us the foundation to understand how specific physical, sensory, and oral motor skills limitations have an impact on eating and drinking.

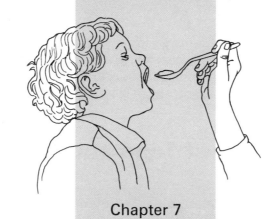

Chapter 7
Factors That Limit Oral Motor Skills

In Chapter 6 we explored the concept that feeding is influenced by a diverse interplay of structure, function, and experience. Specific structural and physiological features of the oral-facial, gastrointestinal, respiratory, and cardiac areas define the medical issues and experiences that create a foundation for eating. These areas interact with the child's level of health and wellness and with the unique meaningful experiences that the child brings to feeding and mealtime. These areas, in turn, influence the child's comfort and endurance during eating, as well as the desire to eat. As we have seen in Chapter 4, eating and drinking require highly specific, well-coordinated movements of the jaw, tongue, lips, cheeks, palate, and pharynx. Movement and coordination problems in these areas have very specific effects on a child's ability to suck, swallow, bite, and chew. In this chapter, we will look at the limiting movement patterns of these individual oral structures and then examine how these limitations may come together to impair a child's ability to eat and drink. Finally, we will discuss limits in body movement and sensory processing that have an impact on the feeding process.

We have incorporated information from a wide selection of physicians and clinicians who have documented various aspects of the developmental process. Because it frequently is difficult to identify the initial source of terms that have been used in the clinical realm for decades, we have not attempted to attribute each description to specific authors and publications. Most of the implications of these limiting patterns on feeding come from our many years of clinical experience.

It may be helpful for you to simulate the body and oral motor patterns discussed. By experiencing them, you can better understand through your inner senses how each oral structure works, both independently and in connection with the rest of the body. Through this experience, you will know how tone and movement support efficient eating when it is working well and how significantly it limits efficient eating patterns when it is not working well. By experiencing the movement patterns, you also can better understand the interconnectedness of all the oral structures. The *Mealtime Participation Guide* (Klein & Morris, 1999) is built around an extensive series of participation experiences that guide therapists and parents through simulation of normal and limiting patterns of eating. We have included several of these experiences in the Appendix to give you a model for this type of learning experience.

Limiting factors are roadblocks that get in the way of a more functional or typical movement pattern. It is important to remember that they may be present at one moment and absent at others. They are influenced by movement and position, sensory input, communication, and emotional stimulation. In the mouth, they are changeable and will increase or decrease depending upon what else is going on in the environment.

The Terminology of Tone and Movement

When we discuss movements that limit the development of the mouth, we must begin with a common frame of reference. Descriptive terms such as retraction or thrust have a similar essence whether they are applied to a tongue or a jaw or a shoulder.

We can think of any movement as having five basic components:
- a degree of tension or tonicity
- a direction of movement
- a speed or timing
- an intensity or force
- a pattern of distribution

Muscle Tension

Normal movement has a degree of tension to give us stability or steadiness around our joints yet it has enough relaxation to allow us to simultaneously move. There is an extensive range of normal muscle tone, depending upon the individual nervous system and the overall degree of activation from environmental stimulation.

Low Tone

Muscle tone that is low is sometimes referred to as floppy tone or hypotonia. Low tone is on a continuum from a muscle or joint that feels very relaxed to one that has so little tone that it cannot move. Low tone results when the muscle cells are not working (e.g., mitochondrial myopathy, muscular dystrophy), when a muscle is not innervated by a peripheral nerve cell (e.g., spinal cord paralysis, Erbs palsy), when a cranial nerve or nucleus is damaged (e.g., vocal fold paralysis, Moebius syndrome), or when there are specific types of dysfunction in the central nervous system (e.g., central hypotonia, hypotonic cerebral palsy, ataxia). Low tone may be seen in a single body part or may be generalized throughout the body.

High Tone

Muscle tone that is high is sometimes referred to as tense tone or hypertonia. High tone is on a continuum from a muscle or joint that feels slightly stiff to one that is so tense that it does not move. Primary high tone typically results from damage to the brain or spinal cord. It may be due to a specific neurological dysfunction such as spasticity or rigidity. A secondary increase in muscle tension results when an individual attempts to compensate for the low tone and reduced postural stability of low tone. If tone provides inadequate stability for movement, the child or adult volitionally tenses the muscles to create more stability. This pattern is sometimes called "fixing." As this pattern is repeated, it often becomes a more permanent part of the child's frame of reference for movement and occurs automatically. High tone may be seen in localized areas or may be generalized throughout the body.

Fluctuating Tone

Muscle tone that moves back and forth between low and high is called fluctuating tone. This type of movement is most typical in children with athetosis or athetoid cerebral palsy. Resting tone may be low, high, or normal. As thoughts, intentions, or actual movements begin, tone may shift toward greater tension, then alternate back and forth among many gradations in tone. This gives the impression of limbs that often are in constant involuntary motion.

Direction of Movement

The direction of movement is limited by the physical structure of the body and the relationships among bones, joints, and muscles.

Extension

Extension is a movement of straightening or opening. Straightening the body or stretching it out is a movement of extension. Straightening the arm, opening the jaw, and sticking out the tongue are all extensor movements.

Flexion

Flexion is a movement of bending or closing. Bending the body forward and curling up is a movement of flexion. Bending the arm, closing the jaw, and pulling the tongue back in the mouth are all flexor movements.

Retraction

Retraction describes a pulling-back movement that is part of the extensor family. When we retract the shoulder girdle, we pull the shoulders back so that the shoulder blades move closer together. We also can retract the elbow, jaw, lips, and tongue.

Protraction and Protrusion

Protraction describes a pulling-forward movement that is part of the flexor family. When we protract the shoulder girdle, we round the shoulders forward so that the shoulder blades move farther apart and the tips of the shoulders move closer together. The term frequently is used to describe movements of the shoulders but is not typically applied to arm or mouth movements. Protrusion usually is used to describe the forward and outward movement of the tongue or lips.

Exaggerated

The adjective exaggerated is often used to describe a movement that goes slightly too far in a normal range of movement. For example, normal jaw movement during sucking is in an up-down direction. When the movement goes slightly too far without disrupting other aspects of the movement, we may say that there is an exaggerated jaw opening. Exaggerated movements are usually combined with low muscle tone.

Timing and Intensity of Movement

The speed or timing of a movement refers to how rapidly it occurs, especially in relationship to other movements that are part of the total pattern.

Thrust

The term thrust usually refers to a sudden and rapid movement. We think of a boxer thrusting the arm forward in a quick jab during a fight. Thrusting movements generally are motions directed away from the center of the body. An arm thrusts forward. A jaw or tongue thrusts forward. A jaw also may thrust downward, but not backward. Most thrusting movements also have a strength or high intensity of muscle power. Although thrusts that are weak or slow are possible, they are not as common as those that are stronger, more sudden, and fast.

Distribution of Movement

Many terms have been used to describe the location or distribution of tone or movement limitations in the body. These may include terms such as quadriplegia (four limbs), hemiplegia (one side of the body), monoplegia (one limb), diplegia (lower half of the body). In reference to the mouth and eating, the terms symmetrical and asymmetrical are of particular relevance.

Symmetrical

This term refers to a distribution of muscle tone and freedom of movement that is equal on both sides of the body. If we draw an imaginary central line from the center of the forehead, through the nose, mouth, chin, trunk, and crotch, we would divide the body into two equal parts. When tone and movement potential are the same in both parts, we say that there is symmetry.

Asymmetrical

This term refers to a distribution of muscle tone and freedom of movement that is unequal on the two sides of the body. The imaginary line may be crooked for many reasons. Muscle tone may be higher or lower on one side of the body. Movement may be more skilled on one side than the other.

Problems With Function of Individual Oral Structures

We can look at some of these obstacles on the normal feeding path by initially examining difficulties with each part of the mouth involved in oral-feeding skill development. Limiting movement patterns in the mouth have been given a wide variety of names. It is confusing to sort out the different labels because often there is inconsistency. Different people and different professional groups use many of the terms in different ways. The term tongue thrust has been used to describe the forceful forward protrusion of the tongue seen in many children who have cerebral palsy. It also has been applied to the early normal pattern of gentle forward movement and protrusion of the tongue during swallowing. It also is used by some therapists to describe a backward-forward movement of the tongue that interferes with the production of certain speech sounds. Terms such as reverse swallow, tongue-thrust swallow, and suckle-swallow have been used to describe the same movement pattern. To avoid misunderstandings in communication, it is important that we define any specialized words used to describe a particular child's movements.

As these patterns are described, bear in mind that each can show different degrees of limitation or severity. A limiting pattern may be present in a strong, total way or it may be weaker or less frequent. The more a movement pattern interferes with the development of normal progressions for feeding, the more severe and the more limiting that pattern is for the child.

Jaw

Jaw limits affect eating and drinking by:
- reducing the ability to open the mouth
- reducing the ability to close the mouth
- reducing endurance during eating
- causing accidental biting of hands, toys, and utensils
- interfering with the development of controlled movements for biting and chewing
- contributing to dislocation or contractures of the temporomandibular joint (TMJ)
- reducing coordinated movement of the tongue
- reducing coordinated movement of the lips and cheeks
- grinding down the surfaces of the teeth and contributing to pain and/or misalignment of the teeth, or both

The jaw is the most important partner on the inner feeding team. It is the foundation upon which all other oral skills are built. Skillful distal movement is dependent upon adequate proximal stability. The lips, cheeks, and tongue require the proximal stability of the jaw for their distal functioning. The ability to stabilize the jaw and to vary the type and amount of stability enables the lips and tongue to operate from a stable, secure base. Rapid, skillful food transfers in chewing and precise lip movements cannot occur when abnormal or very delayed control of the jaw is present.

Infants with neurological involvement tend initially to have low postural tone and very poor central stability of the neck and trunk. If the head is tipped back in extension, there may be greater difficulty keeping the jaw closed. The mouth may hang open or show excessive up-down movement when the baby tries to suck the bottle or breast. This **exaggerated jaw movement** slows down the baby's sucking. It often results in an inefficient sucking pattern with an increased feeding time and reduced feeding intake. This pattern often is related to a more generalized picture of **jaw instability** in which the jaw slips and shifts forward or to the side. This usually is related to the combination of low tone and poor control of the TMJ. It also may be caused directly by problems of the TMJ.

Postural tone usually increases as babies get older; it is most common for this to occur first in the extensor muscles of the body. Babies and young children with neurological impairment may show more neck extension and shoulder retraction. Some pushing back may be observed in the hips and pelvis. As this occurs, the stage is being set for greater difficulties in controlling the jaw. When strong extension patterns are seen in the jaw, it is described as a **jaw thrust**. This is defined as a strong downward extension of the lower jaw that occurs when the bottle, breast, cup, or spoon is presented. It also may occur when food is already in the mouth, or as a social or communicative response. The strength, tension, and frequent loss of the food or the feeding utensil assist in identifying a jaw thrust. Sometimes the jaw thrust will include sudden shifts forward or to the side. If the thrusting is strong or sudden, it can cause a dislocation of the jaw at the TMJ. This can be extremely painful for a child.

A jaw thrust is distinctly different from the young infant's normal full mouth opening. Normal infants open widely to accept the spoon or cup because they have not learned how to adjust the jaw opening to the appropriate size for the utensil. This knowledge of size and the ability to kinesthetically match movement of the jaw with visual information about size and shape develops slowly during the first year. The normal lack of jaw grading is an easy downward movement. It lacks the force and suddenness that characterizes a jaw thrust. It also occurs only as the food is being taken into the mouth. The jaw thrust can occur at any point in the food handling process. The jaw may even become stuck in the open position, making it difficult for the child to close the mouth to begin eating.

Two types of bite reflexes influence control of the jaw. Normal infants pass through a stage on the way to chewing in which stimulation of the gums elicits a rhythmical opening and closing of the jaw and a gentle nibbling on an adult's finger if it is in the baby's mouth. This is known as the ***phasic bite reflex***. The word *phasic* means a repetition or alternation of movement. All bite reflexes are not the same! When the baby or child does not release the bite easily or when there is tension associated with the bite, we call it a ***tonic bite reflex***. The word ***tonic*** means tone or tense. This is a limiting pattern that interferes with all aspects of feeding. It can be elicited from the biting surfaces of the gums or teeth. Sometimes children bite their own fingers or hands accidentally when bringing them into the mouth in play. This can be very frightening, and it quickly discourages self-exploration of the mouth.

It is important to distinguish between the biting down of the tonic bite reflex and biting as a way of achieving stability. Children who demonstrate excessive jaw instability with frustratingly wide jaw excursions may compensate by biting down on the cup or spoon just to gain some stability and stop the excess movement. This ***stability biting*** is seen in normal stages of feeding development as the child bites the cup or straw initially to achieve the external stability necessary for success. As internal stability is achieved, this stability biting no longer becomes necessary. When internal stability is delayed, stability biting is seen more frequently.

If the baby attempts to close the mouth, it may be done with effort. As tension develops, the jaw develops a tight preference for remaining closed. This pattern of ***jaw clenching*** is particularly common in children who show strong flexor patterns in the neck, shoulder girdle, and arms. (Remember that jaw opening is part of the extensor pattern, and jaw closing belongs to flexion.) It is seen also when the infant experiences discomfort in the mouth from oral hypersensitivity, or from constant suctioning or oral hygiene. The child decides to actively prevent others from invading the mouth. The result may be a very clenched jaw. If a reflexive bite occurs as the teeth are stimulated, jaw clenching can be the result of self-stimulating the tonic bite as the upper and lower teeth come into contact. The more constant the closure, the greater the risk of shortening of the muscles and connective tissue that would enable jaw opening. A limitation of movement at the TMJ (jaw joint) may be the long-term result.

Jaw clenching implies that the tight closure of the jaw has reached an involuntary stage. Tightness has developed that is beyond the child's voluntary ability to regulate. It is important to distinguish this type of tight jaw closure at mealtime from the child's behavioral way of refusing food or keeping adults from invading the mouth.

Jaw retraction occurs in some children. This pulling backward of the jaw sometimes makes it difficult to open the mouth fully.

Tongue

Tongue limits affect eating and drinking by:

■ reducing the size of the pharyngeal airway and interfering with breathing

■ making it difficult to insert the bottle or spoon into the mouth

■ stopping the rhythmical flow of movement during sucking

■ interfering with organizing a bolus for efficient movement to the back of the mouth

■ increasing swallowing difficulty

■ causing food or liquid to be pushed out of the mouth

■ interfering with the full range of movement and coordination needed for chewing

The low postural tone and accompanying instability seen in young infants with developing neuro-motor disability can influence tone and mobility in the tongue. Because of the anatomical connections between the tongue and the neck, variations in movement of the head, neck, and shoulder girdle can influence the range and type of movement in the tongue. When there are limits in postural tone, a baby or child frequently will retract or pull back the shoulder girdle. The neck may be hyper-extended, with the chin tipped upward. This contributes to a condition known as ***tongue retraction***. The base of the tongue forms the front wall of the pharynx. When the tongue is pulled backward, the airway becomes smaller. A total falling back or retraction of the tongue can make breathing difficult or impossible. The tip of the tongue is not even with the gums or in approximation with the lower lip as it would be in a normal infant. Many infants compensate for this difficulty by pressing the tongue against the middle of the hard palate. This stops it from being pulled or drawn further into the airway. This is an advantage for the infant because strong tongue retraction can make breathing very difficult. Although this compensation meets the goal of better breathing, it creates additional problems with feeding and the development of sounds. It is difficult for the feeder to insert the nipple or the spoon when the tongue is stuck against the palate, and it is harder for the infant to begin the suck and to sustain an easy sucking pattern. If the tongue is fixed against the palate to provide stability, it is not free to move and participate in sound play simultaneously. Even a mild amount of tongue retraction will cause the baby to use more effort or develop other ways of compensating for the difficulty.

As postural tone increases and infants develop more extension throughout the body, new ways of dealing with tongue retraction emerge. Older infants or children may discover that the airway can open more if they push the tongue forward. This forward movement can occur in two ways. It may take the form of full extension and retraction movements in which the emphasis is on the outward or extensor phase. This **exaggerated tongue protrusion** maintains the easy flow of movement seen in the normal suckle pattern; however, the protrusive movement is exaggerated. Exaggerated tongue protrusion is commonly seen in infants whose low postural tone predominates. It is the most typical tongue movement used by children who have Down syndrome. An infant with a primary respiratory disorder, such as respiratory distress syndrome or bronchopulmonary dysplasia, may hold the tongue in a protruded position between the gums as a way of enlarging the airway.

Some children use a very different type of protrusion as they bring the tongue forward. A **tongue thrust** is a very forceful protrusion of the tongue from the mouth. It is a stronger movement than the extension-retraction movements seen in either the infantile suckling pattern or the mildly limiting exaggerated tongue protrusion. Movement frequently is arrhythmical. Its intermittent occurrence can break a previously sustained rhythm. The thrusting of the tongue makes inserting the nipple or spoon difficult and may cause food and liquid to be pushed out of the mouth.

The limiting movement patterns described as tongue retraction, exaggerated tongue protrusion, and tongue thrust refer to difficulties in controlling the muscles that attach the tongue to other structures of the body and move it in different directions. Differences that limit skill also can occur within the muscles that control the shape and configuration of the tongue. Through these muscles, the tongue can become thin, thick, flat, bunched, pointed, cupped, or humped. The ability of the tongue to change shape contributes to the efficiency and skill with which food can be organized and controlled in the mouth cavity. Low or high tone in the tongue can interfere with these abilities. The most common **difficulty with tongue configuration** in infants is a low-toned tongue that lacks the ability to flatten, thin, and cup. The low-toned tongue is usually thick and bunched, and lacks the central groove that helps move the food or liquid bolus from the front of the mouth to the back for swallowing. The increased rounding or humping of the tongue also may be the result of increased muscle tone. This thick, bunchy tongue shape may or may not also push in a forward protrusion. This bunchiness makes presentation of the spoon and bottle difficult by interfering with comfortable placement.

A partial paralysis of cranial nerves VII (facial) or IX (glossopharyngeal) also can contribute to unusual configurations of the tongue. The tongue may be weak, bunched in areas of muscle contraction and flaccid in areas of paralysis.

Lips and Cheeks

Lip and cheek limits affect eating and drinking by:

- reducing the seal at the front of the mouth that creates a negative intraoral pressure
- interfering with bolus formation for swallowing
- creating food and saliva loss from the front of the mouth or into the buccal cavities

- reducing the ability to remove food from the spoon
- reducing the efficiency of chewing

The lips and cheeks work together. Differences and limitations of tone and function in one will affect the efficiency of the other. When muscle tone is low, the cheeks do not create an efficient barrier to food that is moved against the gums or teeth. It is very easy for food to fall into the cheek cavity. *Low tone in the lips* reduces the ability to keep food and saliva from falling out of the mouth.

If muscle tone is too high, there is a tendency for the lips and cheeks to be pulled into a tight, retracted position. *Lip retraction* occurs when the lips are drawn back so that they form a tight horizontal line over the mouth. In this position, it becomes difficult for the lips and cheeks to assist in sucking from the bottle or breast, removing food or liquid from the spoon or cup, transferring food, and retaining food that has been placed in the mouth. Lip retraction also is influenced by extension and retraction patterns in the neck and shoulder girdle.

Lip pursing is seen in some children when they attempt to counteract the effects of lip retraction. When the lips are pulled forward from a tightly retracted position, it appears as if the lip muscles are being drawn closed in the puckered way that we see when a cloth laundry bag is closed by a drawstring.

The lips work in partnership with the tongue during chewing. Inward pressure from the cheeks is balanced by sideward pressure of the tongue to keep the food centered over the lateral surfaces of the teeth for chewing. The inner surface of the cheeks also provides the movement that helps direct chewed food from the teeth to the center of the tongue to form a bolus for swallowing. Any limiting pattern of cheek movement will negatively influence the precise coordination needed for chewing.

A partial paralysis or underdevelopment of the cranial nerve VII (facial) can result in a facial paralysis. This is seen in Moebius syndrome where the child has difficulty with smiling and frowning. Because of lip and cheek paralysis, infants with this condition have problems with sucking and later with drooling.

To deepen your personal understanding of this aspect of limiting oral motor patterns, see the Physical Mealtime Participation Experience from *Mealtime Participation Guide* (Spoon No. 15: Lip Variations in Spoon Feeding) in Appendix C on page 748.

Palate

Palatal limits affect eating and drinking by:

- creating a loss of liquid and food through the nose
- contributing to apnea spells in young infants when there is nasal reflux
- reducing or limiting the seal of the oral cavity required for the negative pressure component of sucking

The palate forms the anatomical divider between the oral and nasal cavities. Structural or coordination difficulties with the hard or soft palate can cause difficulty with feeding. Chapter 25 provides information on problems with a *cleft palate*. When a hole occurs because of a cleft palate condition, the infant has difficulty building sufficient negative pressure within the mouth to obtain an efficient feeding pattern. Food or liquid may be lost through the cleft and dribble from the nose. The tongue may rest in the open hole. Because the widest portion of the cleft is in the back of the mouth, the resting position of the tongue often is retracted. Young infants may experience apnea spells with bradycardia when liquid refluxes upward into the nasopharynx.

Difficulty in coordinating movements of the soft palate may occur even among children who do not have a cleft palate. *Velopharyngeal insufficiency* results in a soft palate that is too short due to a birth defect or as the result of insufficient tissue to repair a cleft palate. If the palate is short or if the timing of elevation of the palate during swallowing is inaccurate, the child can have problems with nasal loss of food and liquid. Overall difficulties with postural tone and movement also can contribute to *timing and coordination difficulties* with resulting inefficiencies of palatal movement.

Most children who have a ***high, narrow, hard palate*** do not experience feeding problems. However, if the child also has other oral coordination difficulties, the tongue may push food into the palate rather than gathering it into an efficient bolus for chewing and swallowing.

Problems With Motor Processes

We have discussed difficulties that are related to the motor coordination of the mouth. However, it is important to recognize that the mouth is directly or indirectly connected to every other part of the body. Problems with postural tone and movement in the feet, legs, pelvis, trunk, shoulder girdle, arms, hands, and neck can affect oral movement and function.

Motor limits affect eating and drinking by:

- increasing tension and limiting movement patterns in the mouth
- stimulating total patterns of automatic or reflexive movements that include the mouth
- reducing the head and trunk control that provides the postural stability supporting oral movement

Many movement patterns in the mouth can be related directly to similar movement patterns in the body. A movement of extension in the pelvis or neck may trigger or activate a movement of extension in the jaw or tongue such as a jaw or tongue thrust or lip retraction. A movement of forward flexion in the neck and shoulder girdle may include a stronger flexor pattern of jaw closure, making it more difficult for the child to open the mouth. These interconnections are guided by neural pathways as well as muscle kinesiology. Some children may show an extremely strong reflexive connection between the body and mouth. As the head turns to the side and the arms and legs assume an asymmetrical movement pattern called the asymmetrical tonic neck reflex (ATNR), the jaw and tongue may also pull to the side. Other children may show a more delayed response or a very weak connection. If the child has fewer automatic or reflexive patterns and more volitional control, there may be minimal connection between specific patterns of the body and those of the mouth. However, during periods of effort or stress, a more visible connection may emerge. The degree of overall tension or muscle tone in the body often is reflected in the oral-pharyngeal system. Children who have patterns of low tone throughout the body are more likely to have low tone in the mouth. Children whose bodies are in a frequent state of increased tension are more likely to experience greater hypertonicity in the mouth.

Movement patterns of the body and mouth are of two distinct types: primary movement patterns and compensatory movement patterns.

Primary patterns are those that reflect the child's underlying muscle tone and the automatic movement patterns that are programmed into the central nervous system. For example, children with primary low tone may be quite unsteady or unstable when upright against gravity. The mouth may fall open because there isn't enough muscle tone in the muscles that close the jaw. The tongue may be thick and rounded rather than thin and slightly cupped at rest. When these low-toned children want to move and be actively involved, they may figure out ways of increasing their steadiness by tensing some of their muscles to increase stability. They may pull their shoulders up toward the ears or retract the shoulder girdle. They may clench the jaw and tighten the lips. These movement patterns compensate for the underlying issue of low tone and instability. This is why they are called ***compensatory patterns***.

Let's consider some other common examples. It is important to look at the movement dynamics before deciding whether a specific pattern is primary or compensatory. For example, head and neck extension may be part of a primary pattern of total extension. It also may be part of a compensatory pattern if the child is sitting so that the shoulders are protracted and pulling downward. If the rounding of the upper spine were complete, the child's head would be down and visual attention would be on the lap. Most children are more interested in looking around at other things in the room than at their lap. If the downward pull isn't too strong and they have enough control in the neck, they probably will lift the head and rest it in extension on the shoulders. The neck extension in this instance becomes a compensatory pattern. With the neck in extension and the head back, the child's mouth is in a position that favors extension. If the child has a strong jaw thrust or lip retraction (both extension patterns), we might see one of these primary patterns during feeding.

Many therapists and parents have been taught to bring the child's head into a chin-tuck position and do not encourage feeding with the neck in extension. Moving toward this goal is extremely important for most children. However, we first must identify why the child holds the head back in a hyperextended position. At least six different possibilities will be appropriate depending on the nature of the limiting pattern. Each possibility implies a different solution.

1. The head-neck extension may be part of a total primary pattern of extension. This would be confirmed if we see or feel the pushback or extensor tone in other parts of the body (e.g., pushing back with the feet or pelvis). Treatment would address the primary extensor patterns.

2. The head-neck extension may be a compensation for the primary pattern of pulling into flexion. This would be confirmed by feeling for a pull-down and forward pattern in the shoulder girdle and a rounding of the back. Treatment would address the primary flexor patterns.

3. The head-neck extension may be a compensation for the primary pattern of low tone and poor physical endurance. This would be confirmed if the child felt very floppy yet was able to bring the head up to look around. This pattern is often seen in children who are strapped into wheelchairs and held with a vest or supports to keep them from falling forward. Treatment would address the low tone and would work toward developing greater postural stability.

4. The head-neck extension may be a compensation for the primary pattern of poor lip control. Children who have low tone in the lips or lip retraction often lose food from the mouth when they eat or drink. Many of them discover that they don't lose so much if they rest their head back in hyperextension. Treatment would focus on developing more competent lip and cheek activity and mouth closure.

5. The head-neck extension may be a compensation for the primary pattern of reduced respiratory support and poor control of the pharyngeal airway. Neck extension slightly enlarges the diameter of the pharyngeal airway, making it easier to breathe. Treatment would seek ways of increasing respiratory and pharyngeal airway control.

6. The head-neck extension may be a compensation for the underlying problem of bumping into a ventilator or trach tube if the head is kept in a more tucked position. The pattern can persist as a habit or to assist breathing even after the child is no longer on oxygen. Treatment may not address the head-neck extension while respiratory equipment is needed.

Because each of these possibilities requires a different treatment strategy, it is important to understand and identify movement patterns that are primary and those that are compensatory. If you suspect that the pattern is compensatory, figure out the underlying primary pattern or issue. This is the issue that must be addressed in treatment. Children will not let you take away compensations that are working for them unless you can help them discover why they no longer need the compensation.

To deepen your personal understanding of how limiting movement patterns influence oral motor patterns, see the Physical Mealtime Participation Experience from *Mealtime Participation Guide* (Physical Limitations No. 5: Retraction Patterns) in Appendix C on page 743.

■ Problems With Sensory Processes

We have considered difficulties that are related to the motor coordination aspects of feeding. The sensory side plays a big role in determining the type of coordination that will be used or even whether the child will explore and experience learning new movement patterns for feeding. Difficulties can occur when the central nervous system does not control and process an appropriate amount of sensory information at a comfortable level. We can describe normal sensory capacities as a combination of:

1. appropriate acuity or the ability of the sensory organs to receive sensory input,
2. appropriate gating or control of the total amount of information that is being processed by the brain, and
3. the ability of the brain to interpret or perceive the sensory message.

Difficulties in any of these areas can seriously affect the feeding process. The ability to interpret the sensory information, and then integrate and modulate the motoric response is mandatory for efficient functioning of the oral mechanism for feeding.

Sensory limits affect eating and drinking by:

- increasing the level of intensity of sensations surrounding eating to an uncomfortable level
- reducing the level of intensity of sensations surrounding eating so that there is not enough information to alert the system
- triggering sudden changes in muscle tone or movement during mealtimes
- causing sensations associated with eating to be perceived as extremely unpleasant and dangerous or threatening to the system
- making it difficult to eat in noisy or chaotic places such as restaurants, shopping malls, or school cafeterias
- contributing to distractibility and hyperactivity at mealtimes
- reducing the variety and quantity of foods that a child is willing to eat
- contributing to a refusal to eat

Deviations can fall within two broad categories. When the sensory threshold is lowered, the system must cope with too much sensory information; often this is referred to as hypersensitivity. When the sensory threshold is elevated, the system is processing too little sensory information; this is called hyposensitivity.

A problem arises in using these generic terms to describe a specific child. We do not observe sensations; we observe reactions. Therefore, it would be more accurate to use terms that refer to the specific nature of the child's reactions. Moreover, based on these reactions, one may hypothesize that what we call hypersensitivity or hyposensitivity is not a homogeneous disorder. For some children, the response seems to be an overreaction (hyperreaction or hyporeaction) to the sensory stimulation. For others, the response has a defensive or guarded quality; this can be called sensory defensiveness. For still others, the response varies according to the complexity and amount of the sensory input; this can be called sensory overload.

Alterations in the sensory threshold can influence a child's response to feeding. In the case of hypersensitivity, lowering of the sensory threshold can make feeding uncomfortable and unpleasant for the child and the feeder. When the deviation occurs in the touch, smell, or taste areas, these children can become very picky about the foods they eat. Their diet may become limited to those foods that are perceived to be safe and comfortable. In the case of hyposensitivity, elevation of the sensory threshold results in a smaller amount of information reaching the child's awareness. Children may be unresponsive to food because either it lacks taste or they are unaware of remaining food particles in the mouth.

Let's look specifically at categories of response that can occur when the child has difficulty receiving, processing, and interpreting sensory information.

Hyperreaction

Some children appear to have stronger reactions to a specific sensation than would be expected. We might call their response a *hyperreaction*. The sound of the refrigerator opening can cause the mouth to fly open in full anticipation of being fed. Increases in postural tone and automatic reflex patterns appear to reduce the sensory threshold to touch and movement for many children. A child who has been on tube feedings for several months may shudder and make faces when foods are reintroduced.

The taste of food can be strong and unpleasant after a period of oral food deprivation. Each of us has experienced the lowered sensory threshold that results in hyperreaction. Smells can contribute to nausea, lights can make the eyes hurt, and noise can be intolerable when we are coming down with the flu. When we are physically tense, we may startle or respond with a full body movement to a sudden noise. Most people can recall specific instances when they were suddenly surprised by a strong food taste, smell, or temperature. We can only imagine what it would be like to have that type of response on an ongoing basis. Reductions in the sensory threshold can make living in the world a very intense experience.

Hyporeaction

Some children show a more reduced reaction to specific sensations than would be expected. We might call their response a *hyporeaction*. Technically, we can consider problems with acuity as being an organ hyposensitivity. Reduction in the acuity of taste, smell, and touch-pressure receptors in the mouth can cause severe motor-feeding disorders or indifference toward eating. Severe visual impairment reduces the child's ability to anticipate and prepare the mouth for the next bite when the feeder gives only visual cues that the food is coming.

Some children with normal sensory acuity show weaker or lessened reactions to specific sensation than would be expected. Low postural tone often is accompanied by elevations of the sensory threshold, so that the child's ability to perceive small amounts of sensory information is reduced. High levels of anticonvulsant medication also can elevate a child's sensory threshold and reduce overall responsiveness. Most people can recall the low level of sensation and sensory awareness in the mouth after receiving a shot of novocain at the dentist's office. The memory of that experience can help us imagine the reduced awareness of the sensations in the mouth as we eat and drink. It is harder to control the lips, cheeks, and tongue, and it is much more difficult to feel and find the food in the mouth. Some food may be clearer and easier to handle than other food. It is harder to collect food and liquid into a bolus for swallowing, and eating is very messy.

Sensory Defensiveness

For some children, the shift in sensory threshold is not simply a question of being too much or too little input. The ability to discriminate the real nature of the sensory input is altered. Our primary response to sensory information involves using sensory discrimination skills to check out very specific aspects of the input. We examine sensory input by asking, "What is it?" "How intense is it?" "Where is it in my mouth?" We also have an older, survival-based sensory processing system whose function is to keep us safe and alive. It asks "Is it safe?" or "Is it dangerous?" This is the system that is activated in sensory defensiveness. When the system perceives a sensation as dangerous, it immediately prepares for survival and moves into the primitive fight-or-flight mode. At the most basic level, these children know they are being threatened by what they perceive. The response is highly emotional. Often anger and fear are involved. Because of the defensive nature of the child's reaction, this type of hypersensitivity is called *sensory defensiveness*.

One or several sensory systems may be involved. Children may totally refuse to eat the food that looks, feels, tastes, or smells dangerous to the system. Some become very fearful of all foods, and they may limit their food intake to a very few familiar foods. Others carefully check out foods before trying them; they look them over, smell them, or perhaps touch them cautiously to the lips or tongue before putting them in the mouth. Their emotional responses to the situation and duration of the effects of the emotional responses can include screaming, hitting, gagging, vomiting, and throwing the food.

If these children are unable to get rid of the sensation physically, they may block out all awareness of it by shutting it out of their consciousness. A child who has selected this means of survival may appear to be deaf, blind, or profoundly retarded.

To deepen your personal understanding of how limiting sensory patterns influence oral motor patterns, see the Sensory Imagination Experience from *Mealtime Participation Guide* (Imaginings: Sensory No. 12: Sensory Defensiveness to Touch in the Mouth) in Appendix C on page 751.

Sensory Overload

Children who have a lowered threshold to sensory information are at a distinct disadvantage in this busy, chaotic world. Our physical and emotional survival is based on our ability to regulate sensory information and select the amount and type of input that is most important to focus on at the moment. The focus of attention and overall receptivity to input is constantly shifting. The neurological gates that control the amount and type of input give us only what we need at each moment. Certain sensations are given foreground importance while everything else is perceived as background or remains unnoticed. We experience this gated effect every night when we are asleep. Familiar sounds that are unimportant for us to be aware of do not reach our conscious awareness. If we are city dwellers, this might include the noise of traffic and police sirens. Although we can sleep through fairly intense noise that is meaningless to us, we will awaken at the first cry of our infant or the noise of a stranger on the stairway.

Many infants and children are bombarded with sensory input and cannot modulate or regulate the amount and type of information that is consciously processed. They may feel overwhelmed and unable to function. Some children will become hyperactive and distractible at mealtime. Attention may flit from one thing to another during a meal. A noise in the next room may draw attention away from the feeder and the food in the mouth. The feeling of an itch on the foot may shift into the foreground, leaving the more important awareness of unchewed food particles in the mouth ignored. This can be an intermittent experience for many tired adults who are eating in a noisy restaurant after a busy day and find it hard to focus on a conversation. For many children with *sensory overload*, this happens much of the time.

If the sensory overload becomes too great for mental, physical, and emotional well being, the child may cope by shutting out the world or trying to organize it through rhythmical behaviors such as rocking, thumb-sucking, flapping the hands, or spinning objects. Avoidance of eye contact and inconsistencies in response to sound are common coping mechanisms.

■ Problems With Feeding Processes

Individual structures used for eating and the overall response to sensation are important. However, the combination of difficulties with coordinating the jaw, tongue, lips, cheeks, and palate determine what a child's feeding will be like. Again, we can look at things in another way. We have looked at each part; now it is time to shift our perspective and perceive the whole.

Limits with feeding processes affect eating and drinking by:
- restricting the types of utensils the child can use
- limiting the types of food and liquid the child can eat or drink
- reducing the safety of eating and drinking
- reducing the enjoyment of eating and drinking

Sucking

Sucking requires the ability to hold, grasp, or retain a utensil as well as the ability to draw food or liquid into the mouth. It requires the ability to organize the liquid or food into a central mass or bolus, and propel it efficiently to the back of the tongue for swallowing. The movements need to be easily initiated, rhythmical, strong, sustained, and efficient.

Difficulties with the jaw, tongue, lips, cheeks, or palate contribute heavily to problems with these features of feeding movement. Problems with sensory organization, jaw extension or thrust, tongue retraction, and lip retraction interfere with the easy initiation of bottle- or breast-feeding. This poses a major problem for breast-feeding, which requires that the infant's tongue draw the nipple and part of the surrounding areola into the mouth, elongating it. The nipple must be held securely in the mouth. Sucking movements must be strong and sustained enough to trigger a letdown reflex that allows milk to flow from the mother to the baby. Even if the infant eventually is able to latch onto the breast and initiate sucking, an excessively wide jaw excursion, lip retraction, or jaw thrusting can interfere with the ability to sustain a strong enough suck to begin the flow of milk. The infant may tire and give up before the milk starts or before getting enough to eat. If the tongue cannot grasp the nipple and remain in a forward position, a rapid, nonnutritive suck may occur instead of a slower, nutritive suck. Because a swallow doesn't follow a nonnutritive suck, the baby doesn't get very much, even if there is some milk in the mouth. A child's problems with oral hypersensitivity and the tonic bite reflex can lead to great discomfort for the mother. Body and head positioning, combined with attempts to create a more normal reaction to sensory stimulation, become critical to assisting the mother who wishes to breast-feed her baby.

The bottle-fed infant usually has similar problems with sucking. However, the length and shape of the nipple can be varied somewhat by using products from different manufacturers. Although this may reduce one problem, it might create new problems. Temptations to poke larger holes in the nipple may flood the baby and reduce the need to develop a stronger suck. Softer nipples can collapse and eliminate milk flow when the infant uses a clenching of the jaw or fixes the tongue against the palate for stability.

When tongue configuration is humped or bunched rather than grooved, it is difficult for the liquid to flow in an uninterrupted stream to the pharynx. It is like the difference between rain rushing down the gutter of a street into a sewer and rain that falls on top of a ridge and flows over the sides in many directions.

Similar difficulties can occur with the cup or spoon. Variations are seen as the child shows different combinations and severity of limiting movement patterns.

Table 7.1   **Sucking Characteristics Summary**

Normal	Limited
Easily initiated	Poorly initiated
Rhythmical	Arrhythmical
Strong	Weak
Sustained	Unsustained
Efficient	Inefficient

Swallowing

When children have difficulty organizing the food or liquid bolus and moving it toward the back of the mouth, swallowing becomes stressed. The slower and more inefficient the food movement, the greater the risk of accidental choking. The movements used to create this bolus organization in drinking, spoon feeding, and chewing are classified as part of the oral phase of the swallow. Organizational problems will be created any time there are limitations in the muscle tone of the oral and facial structures, or when difficulties with reflexive movements pull the tongue, lips, or jaw in one direction.

It is important to recall that during swallowing, the system must shift rapidly and smoothly from a system designed to support breathing to one that is designed to support eating and digestion. It does this through opening and closing strategic valves along a system of shared passageways. When backward movement of the bolus, intention, or both fail to trigger the pharyngeal swallow reflex, the airway remains open and unprotected. The upper esophageal sphincter remains closed, preventing food entrance into the esophagus and indirectly biasing its movement into the open airway.

Difficulties with sensory awareness, inefficient organization of the oral bolus, and problems with strength, timing, and coordination of movement may cause portions of the bolus to enter or remain in the pharynx during periods of airway opening. This creates a risk of aspiration before, during, or after the swallow has been triggered.

Pooling of the bolus in the sulci or cavities formed by the valleculae and pyriform sinuses can delay penetration of the airway by the bolus. Because of this delay, it can appear clinically as if the bolus has been swallowed. Coughing or choking may signal entrance of the food into the laryngeal vestibule or penetration of the airway that occurs during the third or fourth small bolus.

Infants and children with primary respiratory difficulties (e.g., respiratory distress syndrome, bronchopulmonary dysplasia) often protect their vulnerable respiratory systems through a central inhibition of the swallowing reflex or a voluntary refusal to swallow. This may be observed even when the child is receiving respiratory assistance through a ventilator or additional oxygen.

Swallowing disorders that are centered in the pharyngeal and esophageal phases of the swallow are difficult to identify without special imaging procedures described in Chapter 8.

Biting

The ability to control the bite through a piece of food requires normal jaw control and normal sensory perception of thickness, hardness, and size. With a tonic bite reflex, the bite through the food is sudden, tense, and completed with poor release. The phasic bite lacks the sustained contraction of muscles needed to bite through thicker or harder foods. Although this is a movement pattern that is seen in early normal development, a child can become stuck at this level and never develop a controlled bite. Stability biting can interfere with the normal flow of food removal from the spoon, bottle, cup, and straw when a child has jaw instability and excessively wide excursions of the jaw.

Chewing

The early munching-chewing pattern is a combination of the up-down sucking movements of the tongue and the repetitive gum contact seen in the phasic bite. More mature chewing requires a balance and coordination of jaw movements and lateral tongue movements. Any patterns that interfere with these normal movements will prevent a child from developing chewing. The greatest contributors to limited chewing movements are jaw thrust, jaw clenching, tonic bite, tongue retraction, and tongue thrust. Children who have poor tone and movement of the lips and cheeks will have difficulty keeping food in the mouth and making efficient transfers of food from the side to the center of the mouth. Chewing also requires a special timing that organizes the separate movements of the jaw, tongue, and lips into a smoothly flowing coordination. Some children show normal movements of each separate part but are unable to coordinate the total movement of chewing.

Children who have difficulties with sensory acuity or perception frequently refuse foods that have texture, and they do not develop mature chewing skills. If solids are accepted, they may learn to swallow the food whole, without chewing. (Chewing requires a longer, more sustained contact with the food.) If oral perception is poor, the child may be unaware of food that remains in the mouth after a meal. This accounts for some of the squirreling of food in the cheek cavity that is seen in children with milder feeding problems.

Oral Motor Limitations Glossary

Limiting Oral Motor Patterns

These are oral motor patterns of movement that differ from the normal in a restrictive sense.

Limiting Jaw Patterns

- **Exaggerated jaw movement:** An exaggerated opening of the jaw. The jaw opens wider than is necessary for the mouthful and with decreased control of grading.
- **Jaw instability:** Jaw movements that are poorly graded and unstable, providing a poor base of support for lip and cheek and tongue skills.
- **Jaw thrust:** A strong, sudden downward movement of the lower jaw that occurs with presentation of the bottle or spoon, when food is in the mouth, or when communication is attempted. It sometimes includes sudden shifts of jaw movement forward or side to side.
- **Phasic bite:** A rhythmical, repetitive opening and closing of the jaw that occurs with gum or teeth stimulation. It appears as a gentle nibbling on the object. It is seen in normal development. Some children can become stuck here.
- **Stability bite:** The voluntary biting of a surface to achieve the jaw stability necessary for a particular oral motor activity.
- **Jaw clenching:** A tight closure of the jaw that has reached an involuntary stage. This clenched jaw pattern is particularly common in children who show strong flexor patterns in the neck, shoulder girdle, and arms. (It is important to distinguish this type of tight jaw closure at mealtime from the child's behavioral way of refusing food.) It is seen also when the infant experiences discomfort in the mouth from oral hypersensitivity or from constant suctioning or oral hygiene.
- **Tonic bite:** A forceful or tense biting pattern that interferes with all aspects of feeding. It is elicited from the biting surfaces of gums or teeth. It often is difficult for the child to release the bite and can be frightening for the child.
- **Jaw retraction:** A pulling backward of the jaw, making it difficult to open the mouth fully.

Limiting Tongue Patterns

- **Bunched or bunchy tongue:** The tongue configuration is humped or bunched rather than grooved.
- **Tongue retraction:** A pulling or falling back of the tongue, making breathing and sucking difficult. The tip of the tongue is not even with the gums or in approximation with the lower lip as it would be in a normal infant.
- **Exaggerated tongue protrusion:** Extension and retraction movements of the tongue in which the emphasis is on the extensor portion of the movement. The tongue retains its rhythmical movement but moves forward beyond the gum ridge or teeth.
- **Tongue thrust:** A very forceful protrusion of the tongue from the mouth. It is a stronger movement than the extension-retraction movements seen in either the infantile suckling pattern or the mildly limiting, exaggerated tongue protrusion. Movement frequently is arrhythmical. Its intermittent occurrence can break a previously sustained rhythm.

Limiting Lip Patterns

- ***Low-tone lips:*** Reduced muscle tone in the lips, diminishing the ability to keep food and saliva from falling out of the mouth.
- ***Lip retraction:*** The pulling back of the lips so tightly that they form a horizontal line over the mouth.
- ***Lip pursing:*** A reaction to lip retraction. When the child tries to close the lips from a retracted position, it appears as if the lip muscles are being drawn closed in a puckered way, as when a laundry bag is pulled closed by a drawstring.

Limiting Sensory Factors

- ***Hyperreaction:*** Stronger reactions to a specific sensation than would be expected.
- ***Hyporeaction:*** Reduced or delayed reactions to a specific sensation than would be expected.
- ***Sensory defensiveness:*** A defensive, guarded, or emotional quality to a sensory response. The ability to discriminate the real nature of the sensory input is altered. The unpleasantness that is immediately perceived when the sensation is present is related to the defensive need to survive through the fight-or-flight mechanism.
- ***Sensory overload:*** A sensory response that varies according to the complexity and amount of the sensory input. Many infants and children are bombarded with sensory input and cannot use the type of filtering system that allows a small portion of the input to be attended to.

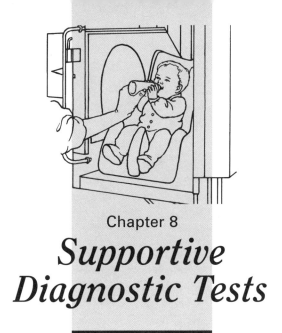

Chapter 8
Supportive Diagnostic Tests

Health-care professionals use a number of tests to aid in the diagnoses of medical problems that influence the eating process. These tests are used most appropriately after the completion of a good feeding history and clinical observations. However, it is important to be familiar with the options these tests provide before doing a clinical evaluation. Feeding therapists can provide invaluable clinical information to the team that is trying to better understand these feeding processes. Their input into the timing, nature, and interpretation of the studies and resultant feeding recommendations makes them pivotal members of the feeding therapy team.

Although a number of studies provide information related to feeding, it is important to note that the studies should not be used in isolation. No single study gives all the answers that help to understand the exact nature of a feeding problem and how it influences a particular child's growth, appetite, and feeding skills. There are so many influences, and the studies provide only a small part of the big picture. Parent feedback and feeding clinician observations are a critical part of the picture.

The videofluoroscopic swallowing study often has been considered the gold standard in the assessment of dysphagia. Although this study can provide important information, it may not be the best procedure for all children who are referred with feeding disorders. It is important for the team to understand the variety of diagnostic tests available and to determine which are appropriate for each child. This chapter will look at commonly available diagnostic test procedures and the information they can provide to the feeding management team.

▨ Evaluation of Swallowing Function

Videofluoroscopic Swallow Study

The videofluoroscopic swallow study (VFSS) is commonly used to further the clinical understanding of the swallowing process. A VFSS, often referred to as a modified barium swallow study or a cookie swallow study (Logemann, 1993), is used to analyze the swallow mechanism. It is used to determine what works and does not work in the process of swallowing. It can help define the nature and pathophysiology of the swallowing impairment, provoke the system to recreate swallowing difficulties experienced during regular feedings, and identify adaptations that can be made to facilitate improved performance in swallowing.

When to Refer?

Generally, a VFSS is used when the team wants to analyze the anatomical and physiological function of swallowing and look for complications of swallowing disorders such as aspiration. If aspiration does occur, the VFSS then can be used to determine when it occurs, why, with what size bolus, and on what consistency of food or liquid. This can give the clinician better ideas for feeding-management options for the child. Some clinics use the VFSS liberally and others are considerably more conservative. Although some believe the VFSS should be a part of each feeding evaluation, others believe it should be used only if the information received would change the treatment plan in some way.

Procedure

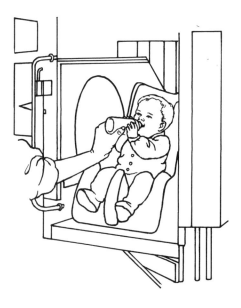

Many authors have described, in detail, the VFSS procedures and interpretations (Arvedson & Lefton-Greif, 1998; Fox, 1990; Logemann, 1993, 1997). In most clinics, the radiologist and speech-language pathologist work together to perform and interpret this study. Every attempt should be made to duplicate the usual feeding scenario. The child is semi-upright in a supportive chair or seating system. The parent or primary feeder usually accompanies the child to keep him as calm as possible. Barium is presented in a bottle, cup, or spoon to make the study as close to a regular feeding situation as possible. Different textures of barium can be used— from the thinnest liquid to puree to textured or solid foods. The child is fed the barium while the entire procedure is videotaped for later review. The focus of the procedure is the oral, pharyngeal, and esophageal aspects of swallowing. Some clinicians routinely follow a bolus through the esophagus and into the stomach while others do not. Lateral and anterior-posterior views are taken, as appropriate for particular swallowing difficulties.

An important component of the VFSS is simulating a typical swallowing situation as much as possible. This is difficult because the study suite is nothing like having a meal at home! Clinicians may ask the parents to bring the child into the fluoroscopy suite before the study to familiarize him with the situation. They may ask that the child bring his favorite stuffed toy to accompany him into the study. It works best when the parents are with the child during the whole procedure and are asked to do the feeding as they normally would. Favorite bottles, cups, or spoons may be brought from home. A favorite flavor of formula or strained food may be used to mix with the liquid or paste barium. In optimum studies, the clinician and the radiologist stop the study if the child becomes upset, spending time to reassure him so that the best swallowing can be viewed.

Limitations in Performing a VFSS

The study looks at swallowing on that particular day, under those particular circumstances, for those particular swallows. Sometimes the situation is such that the child who regularly aspirates does not demonstrate aspiration during the study. In other circumstances, aspiration is seen during the study but is not usually seen, or it may occur in greater quantities than usual because of the stress of the study. The physiological and emotional tension that can result just from the study process can cause some children to become less coordinated in their ability to swallow. Aspiration may result that is atypical for the child who may swallow appropriately when fed during a period of wellness, at home, or in a supportive therapy setting. The stress of a study generally does not affect the swallowing safety of a child who has good swallowing abilities. It may, however, bias the results toward aspiration of the child who has a more vulnerable and fragile swallowing system.

Let us look at some of the stresses of the VFSS for children. Although every attempt can be made to simulate a typical feeding situation, a VFSS can never be the same as a natural feeding in the calm surroundings of the home. The radiology suite of a hospital can be a very frightening place for an infant or young child. The unfriendly or scary looking equipment, adults with lead aprons and gloves, and expectations that the child *will* eat or drink at that moment can contribute to major upsets for some children. When children are asked to suck and swallow liquid or food that tastes unusual because of the barium, they may become confused or resistant. Children who are usually fed in the parent's arms may find the required positioning unusual. The head position may be different from usual despite attempts to make it as similar to the daily routine as possible.

To complicate the testing, sometimes the seating options available actually improve the child's position for swallowing rather than duplicate the feeding situation at home. At times the barium provided is actually a heavier, more viscous liquid in contrast to the thin water or juice that may cause the child trouble at home. In some of these situations, a child may swallow *more* safely during the study than at home. The child may actually be an aspirator but not demonstrate the aspiration during the study.

Stopping the study to adjust and reassure a child takes time. Sometimes the radiologist is not able to spend the time necessary for the optimum swallowing situation. Some children unfortunately and inappropriately end up being tested when they are crying and actively protesting. Others are evaluated when they are tipping or pushing their heads back into extension, making it more difficult to swallow safely.

Although every attempt is made to narrow the fluoroscopic viewing area and keep the timing of the study as short as possible, there is still X-ray exposure.

Invaluable Information the VFSS Can Tell Us

Despite the limitations of just doing the study, the VFSS can provide invaluable information. The information obtained, however, must be paired with a good understanding of the child's feeding history and issues as well as a serious look at circumstances surrounding the swallow study. Sometimes a repeat swallow study is needed to ensure the accuracy of the results.

Following are benefits of doing a VFSS.

- The clinician can use VFSS to document some eating and **swallowing characteristics**. It can be used to identify timing and oral control in the initiation of the swallow. The clinician can observe the duration of the pharyngeal swallow and the ability to clear the bolus from the pharynx safely.

- A VFSS can help the clinician **identify aspiration** that occurs during the study. When a child aspirates during the swallowing study, the clinician can observe it through the fluoroscopy and review it with the videotape after the study. The exact timing of the aspiration before, during, and after the swallow can be noted. The clinician can document factors that indicate high-risk vulnerability for aspiration even if actual aspiration does not occur. The vulnerability of the swallow is an important consideration because it suggests that the child may aspirate at other times when there is physical and emotional stress.

- A VFSS can be used to identify children who have **silent aspiration**. When food or liquid enters the airway, a protective reflex typically triggers a cough to propel the food upward and prevent it from entering the lungs. Children who cough and choke during feeding are at high risk for aspiration because part of the meal may have entered the airway while initiating a cough reflex. Coughing is a good sign but it does not tell us that the child always protects the airway and does not aspirate. A swallowing study can tell us whether the child coughs out everything that goes astray or whether some food enters the lungs in spite of the cough. Many children do not cough when they aspirate. Low sensory awareness or difficulty controlling the movement of the vocal folds can allow food or liquid to pass through the airway and penetrate the lungs. The silent aspirator does not receive immediate feedback that the liquid has been misdirected. The VFSS can be used to help verify this clinically silent aspiration.

■ The VFSS can help the therapist **identify consistencies of food** or liquid that the child can swallow safely. A great advantage of the VFSS is that different liquid and food consistencies can be used and compared during the study. Some children do well with one or more consistencies yet aspirate others. Although a swallow study often is conducted to rule out aspiration, its primary clinical value is to identify situations in which swallowing is more or less safe for the child. When aspiration is documented, the clinician can try different textures or temperatures of foods and liquids to determine the optimum diet consistency for that child. Many children who aspirate thin liquid can handle thickened liquids. These children may be able to remain oral feeders if the thin liquids are eliminated from their diet.

■ A VFSS enables the clinician to identify **risk factors for aspiration**. Children who do not aspirate during the brief period of the swallowing study may still be at high risk for aspiration in other circumstances. The child who collects liquid in the valleculae may experience overflow of liquid into the open airway when he moves or when the valleculae are too full. Food residue may cling to the walls of the pharynx when the pharyngeal movement is inadequate. When a child changes position or in other ways loosens the residue, it can fall directly into the airway and result in aspiration.

■ The anterior-posterior view of the VFSS can be very helpful when used selectively to rule out **asymmetries** in movement of the soft palate, larynx, and pharynx. Strokes, brain tumors, vocal-fold paralysis, and other neurological or cardiac conditions, such as vascular rings that increase the likelihood of asymmetries, would suggest this view be taken. This view can be somewhat difficult to obtain in infants because of the need to hyperextend the neck to move the mandible out of the way. The barium-filled bottle tends to get in the way for bottle-fed babies. Babies and young children with poor head control further complicate this procedure.

■ The clinician can use the VFSS to demonstrate **changes in swallowing patterns** over time. A child who once frequently aspirated may now be able to swallow safely. A child who used to aspirate all liquids and foods may now only aspirate thin liquids. Conversely, children who used to swallow safely may develop swallowing problems because of postural and physiological changes.

■ Swallowing studies can be **combined with other monitoring devices or specialized studies** to give more information to the team.

Sometimes, pulse oximetry is set up to monitor baseline oxygen levels and subsequent changes in oxygen saturation during the swallowing process. This can document oxygen saturation during the study and pinpoint the timing of any desaturation during the swallowing process. The clinician can document conditions such as central apnea, gastroesophageal reflux, vascular rings, or tracheoesophageal fistula, as well as poor suck-swallow-breathe coordination.

The VFSS can be done in combination with a cardiorespiratory monitor to document drops in heart rate or bradycardias during the sucking and swallowing process.

The VFSS can be done in combination with an upper GI (UGI) study. In this situation, the VFSS is usually performed first with the focus on the swallowing mechanism. The UGI then follows with an in-depth view of the esophagus, stomach, and intestines as per the standard UGI protocol. This combination can be very helpful if gastroesophageal reflux is suspected either because of the clinical history presented or because of findings of the VFSS. In some VFSS procedures, refluxed material moves up the esophagus and into the pharynx. Actual vomiting may be documented, or cricopharyngeal spasms may be observed. This combination VFSS and UGI also can be useful in looking at structural abnormalities that influence efficiency and timing of swallowing such as esophageal strictures or tracheoesophageal atresia or fistulas, as well as motility disorders of the esophagus.

Chest X-rays are routinely taken before and after a VFSS of children considered at high risk for aspiration. They are likely to be performed after a child demonstrates aspiration during the VFSS, although they do not tend to be highly sensitive to microaspiration because it usually takes 12–24 hours after an aspiration event for small amounts of material in the lungs to show up on X-rays.

What a VFSS Cannot Tell Us

■ A VFSS cannot tell us that a child does not ever aspirate. It gives us information about swallows performed on that day and time. In order to limit the child's exposure to radiation, a VFSS observes a small set of swallows. If a child's swallowing ability varies under different conditions, aspiration may not occur during the swallows that are filmed. Some children, for example, swallow well at the beginning of the meal but tire 10–15 minutes into the meal. When they are fatigued, their swallowing may deteriorate and cause aspiration. Other children have a great deal of difficulty getting themselves organized to eat. They may do poorly at the beginning of the meal but do well once they have established the comfortable suck-swallow rhythm. Although efforts may be made to "catch" the time when the child has the most trouble swallowing, it is not always achieved. It is critically important to integrate clinical observations of the child eating a full meal with the information from the swallowing study.

■ The VFSS cannot tell us how often or in what circumstances the child will aspirate. It tells us only that the child did aspirate during the study. This is a very small sample of the child's abilities.

■ A VFSS alone cannot tell us whether oral feeding should be discontinued. The information from the swallowing study should be integrated with the other knowledge about the child and family. It is only one part of the objective and subjective data that is taken into consideration in making a decision about oral feeding. It is important to talk with parents about what they want and what their child wants.

■ A VFSS cannot predict whether the child will be able to eat orally safely in the future. A swallowing study tells us about the present moment. With maturation and therapy, many children who once aspirated are able to eat and drink safely. Other children who did not show aspiration when they were younger may begin to aspirate during periods of illness or if their overall coordination deteriorates.

Questions to Consider Before a VFSS

There are a number of questions that should be considered when referring and preparing a child for a swallowing study.

■ **Has an in-depth feeding evaluation been performed on the child before the study?** Sometimes the feeding evaluation is performed by the same therapist who does the study, and sometimes by a different clinician. It is important that the VFSS clinician receive the feeding evaluation information before the study to help determine the parameters of the study. Perhaps the feeding evaluation showed the child to have more difficulty at the end of the meal when fatigued. Perhaps liquid was the biggest problem. Perhaps the feeding therapist is wondering about the gurgling sound the child has in the throat after the meal. Perhaps the child becomes cyanotic during or after a meal. There are a great many possibilities that must be considered. The VFSS clinician should be made aware of the clinical issues being addressed so that the proper positioning, timing, and liquid or food consistencies can be chosen. Having this information in advance can help the study run smoothly with the most accurate and efficient results. Often the feeding therapist attends the study as an observer to understand the client's feeding needs more fully.

■ **What are the specific questions needing to be answered during the study?** The VFSS should be able to address a specific list of questions to be asked during the study. These questions can come from the referring physician, feeding therapist, and parents. These questions come from the feeding evaluation and from the medical history. A swallowing study can tell us so much more than whether the child is aspirating. Each study should be centered on a set of questions that have been prioritized. In order to reduce a child's exposure to radiation, the clinician may choose to not take the time to address all the questions.

- ■ **What are the most important questions for this child at this time?**
  — Is there a delay in the swallow with any consistency of food or liquid? A delayed swallow indicates that the child may be at risk for aspiration even when aspiration does not occur during the swallowing study.
  — Is swallowing ability influenced by the consistency of the food or liquid? Are there differences between thin versus thicker liquids? Are there differences between thick liquids and pureed consistencies? This information can help identify the consistency that promotes the coordinated and safe swallow.
  — Is swallowing ability influenced by the amount of food or liquid? Is there a difference in swallowing when a single swallow of food or liquid is compared with two to three consecutive swallows? Some children are very safe when they take a few swallows and then have a short pause. A child might do very well with small sips but may aspirate when drinking multiple consecutive suck-swallows.
  — Does the timing of the meal influence swallowing ability? Is there a difference between the beginning of a feeding and the end? Some children do very well at the beginning of a meal, but the swallow deteriorates as they get tired. If the child typically does better at the beginning of the meal and begins to have more trouble after 20 minutes, ask the VFSS clinician and radiologist to set up the swallowing study in two parts. They would evaluate the swallow at the beginning of a meal and then stop filming as the parent continues to feed the child a regular meal for another 20 minutes. When the child begins to fatigue with eating, they again would videotape the swallows. Other children are poorly coordinated at the beginning of a meal but improve their eating abilities as the rhythm of the meal continues. These children also benefit from testing at two different points in the meal.

- ■ **Is a speech-language pathologist with a background in swallowing part of the evaluation?** Physicians often ask only whether the child is aspirating. When a therapist is involved in the evaluation, a stronger focus is placed on therapeutic questions related to the child's positioning, food amount and consistency. This provides more information that can help in the development of an appropriate therapy program for the child.

- ■ **Does the radiaographic suite have a special chair or seating system so that the baby or young child can be carefully positioned?** Is the position available in the radiographic suite similar to the feeding position used at home? Some positions during the studies provide better support than the position used at home, making the results less accurate compared with the home-feeding situation. Some feeding positions are difficult to duplicate during the study. Having the information ahead of time enables the VFSS clinician time to creatively tackle this issue.

- ■ **Can the consistency that challenges the child be duplicated in the study?** Barium is thicker than water. Can it be watered down sufficiently to provide accurate results? Does this information change how the results will be interpreted?

- ■ **Are the radiologist and VFSS clinician sensitive if the child becomes upset during the study?** Are time allowances made during the studies for such situations? Some radiologists are better at this than others. We hope that children will cooperate with the test, but sometimes the equipment and the strange situation are frightening. Children may cry or protest about eating under these conditions. It is important to look for a radiologist who is willing to take time with children and stop the study if the child continues to cry. Some physicians seem to believe that the study is more important than the child. They might use an open mouth as an opportunity to pour liquid into the mouth of a screaming child. The child may struggle and be forcibly held down as the mouth is pried open to take a sip of liquid. Any information collected in this manner is meaningless. There must be cooperation from the child in order to have a meaningful study.

- ■ **Is the child ready for the study?** The child needs prior experience with swallowing and must be able to swallow enough material (⅓ teaspoon) to provide information during the study. The child may need special oral motor therapy ahead of time that enables him or her to explore tastes and touches in the mouth and learn basic swallowing rhythms. The child may need to have had oral taste experiences with foods the same color as barium. Some therapists have prepared the child ahead of time with actual tastes of tiny amounts of barium to simulate the study, if the team has determined this option acceptable. During the study, the therapist may need to provide a calming or favorite music tape or other interesting distractions to help the child be as still as possible. Care must be taken to provide a positive experience so that the study does not set back the child in his or her oral and feeding progress.

What to Do With the Results of a VFSS?

The team of physicians, therapists, and parents should consider the results of the VFSS. The information obtained at the time of the study is part of a greater picture of health and mealtime experiences. We hope the study provides information that helps the physician better understand the underlying influences that feeding has on the child's health and can act accordingly in treatment. The study can provide the feeding therapist with information regarding the situations that allow for safety and pleasure in swallowing. If it is found that a child aspirates, the study can give information that helps the team determine the best circumstances for nutritional intake. Can the child eat by mouth under certain circumstances, in certain positions, at a certain pace, and with certain foods? Does the child need to be fed completely by tube? Saying the child needs a tube merely because he aspirated is unfair to the child and family. Some children may need a tube for some or all of their nutrition, but some may not. Modifications in food or liquid consistency may make enough of a difference to forego tube feedings.

The feeding therapist can use the information from the VFSS to enhance treatment and home recommendations for the child. The therapist can glean valuable information about food and liquid consistencies, swallowing timing, and optimum circumstances for food intake.

Ultrasound

Ultrasound imaging is a safe and non-invasive way to evaluate the oral preparatory and oral phases of the swallow. Although its primary use has been with adults (Shawker, Sonies, Hall, & Baum, 1984; Sonies, Wang, & Sapper, 1996), it is being used more frequently with infants and children at centers whose professionals are trained in its use (Bosma, Hepburn, et al., 1990; Casas, Kenny, & McPherson, 1994; Casas, McPherson, & Kenny, 1995; Smith, Erenberg, Nowak, & Franken, 1985).

Procedure

Ultrasound uses high-frequency sound waves that pass through soft tissues and are reflected back to a special transducer (Shawker, Sonies, Hall, et al., 1984). The information is assembled into a video image that shows the real-time movement of the tongue, floor of the mouth, and oropharynx. You also can observe the timing relationships between movements of the mouth and the pharynx.

Advantages of Ultrasound

The procedure uses a small wandlike transducer coated with a special gel that is placed under the chin or on the cheeks. Because it is easy to distinguish the food in the mouth from the tissues of the mouth, no contrast materials such as barium are added to the food. Ultrasound is safe and relatively non-invasive for infants and children (Bosma, Hepburn, et al., 1990; Weber, Woolridge, & Baum, 1986), especially in comparison to videofluoroscopy. The equipment is portable so it can be used in a familiar therapy room. The child can sit on a parent's lap or in the chair and position typically used for eating. Because there is no exposure to radiation, there are no inherent limitations to how much time is spent viewing different aspects of the child's swallow. The procedure can be repeated frequently to observe changes with different foods, different size boluses, and at different points in the meal. It can be used to assess the effectiveness of different treatment strategies.

Limitations of Ultrasound

Ultrasound has its limitations. Because the sound waves do not pass through bone, many parts of the system cannot be observed. Some bony tissues such as the hyoid cast a shadow whose movement can be tracked. The swallow beyond the point of its pharyngeal initiation cannot be tracked with ultrasound because the larynx casts a shadow that obscures the view of the airway. Thus, ultrasound cannot tell us anything about the presence or absence of aspiration. It provides minimal information about the presence of residue in the valleculae or pyriform sinuses. Although ultrasound equipment is available at most major medical centers, it often is hard to find qualified staff trained in its use as a diagnostic tool for swallowing.

Fiberoptic Endoscopic Evaluation of Swallowing (FEES)

A fiberoptic endoscopic evaluation of swallowing (FEES) can help the clinician evaluate the laryngopharynx or upper aerodigestive tract in a dynamic fashion in a child who is awake and in a static fashion in a child who has been anesthetized. The otolaryngologist usually conducts the test, often in partnership with a speech-language pathologist (SLP). In some settings, the SLP is the primary clinician. The flexible fiberoptic endoscope enables the examiner to evaluate the airway and the pharynx from the nasal vestibule to the glottis with full assessment of laryngopharyngeal movements and anatomy of respiration even during swallowing (Tunkel & Zalzal, 1992).

Procedure

The FEES usually is done with a child who is awake and in an upright position. The fiberoptic scope is passed through each nostril after topical anesthesia has been applied and is moved gradually to the region just above the valleculae. Nasal and choanal patencies are assessed. The nasopharynx is checked for lesions and adenoid size. For older children who can speak during the examination, velopharyngeal closure is assessed. Difficulties with palate or pharyngeal wall motion that influence hypernasal speech or regurgitation can be documented. The supraglottic larynx, the base of the tongue, and the hypopharynx then are viewed from this nasopharyngeal vantage point. The FEES can be used to identify pooling of secretions or food in the pyriform sinuses and valleculae.

Supraglottic structures involved during breathing and the specific dynamics of the epiglottis can be observed. Laryngomalacia can be diagnosed from this position. Lesions of the true vocal cords and vocal cord mobility can be viewed during speech, crying, or respiration to determine vocal cord paralysis and symmetry. If laryngeal inflammation is found, this can be suggestive of gastroesophageal reflux. FEES can be used to identify the presence of aspiration before or after a swallow (Leder, Sasaki, & Burrell, 1998). Assessment of the subglottic larynx and the trachea cannot be done safely on a child who is awake because of the risk of respiratory compromise and laryngospasm. These areas usually are evaluated under general or local anesthesia with sedation (Tunkel & Zalzal, 1992).

Langmore and colleagues compared the results of the FEES with videofluoroscopy, finding 90% agreement in identifying aspiration. This indicates that FEES is a valid tool for evaluating oropharyngeal swallowing problems (Langmore, Schatz, & Olson, 1991). Wu and colleagues found similar results but believed that the FEES was a more sensitive tool than videofluoroscopy for detecting aspiration and risk features that could lead to aspiration (Wu, Hsiao, Chen, Chang, & Lee, 1997).

Advantages of FEES

FEES has many of the same advantages of ultrasound. It is relatively safe because there is no radiation exposure. Swallowing studies can be repeated frequently and under a variety of clinical conditions (Leder, 1998). Real food and liquid are used, and there is no need for a contrast material such as barium. Like ultrasound, the equipment is portable and the study can be conducted in an environment that is familiar and non-threatening to the child.

Limitations of FEES

Although FEES now is being used with children, its most frequent use is with adults. It requires cooperation from the child, and the presence of the endoscope in the nasopharynx and oropharynx is invasive and uncomfortable for many children. It is extremely difficult to use this procedure with children who have severe movement disorders. FEES offers a specialized view that provides information about nasal, pharyngeal, and laryngeal structures before or after swallowing. It does not allow a view during the actual swallow, making it impossible to view the interactions of the different parts of the system. It may tell us that food has entered the airway, but it does not tell us why this has occurred.

Cervical Auscultation

Procedure

Cervical auscultation is a procedure used to amplify the sounds made during swallowing and breathing. The examiner places a stethoscope or special microphone over the thyroid cartilage. Special sounds indicate the presence or absence of a swallow and the number of sucks prior to a swallow.

Advantages of Cervical Auscultation

Because the sounds heard during cervical auscultation are usually inaudible to an unassisted ear, their amplification can augment information from clinical observations (Bosma, Vice, Heinz, Giuriati, & Hood, 1990). This study can pick up the noises made as the child breathes before, during, and after a swallow. The sounds of the swallow and their timing with those of breathing also are audible. A gross estimation can be made of size of bolus and timing between oral presentation and swallow elicitation (Tuchman & Walter, 1994).

Limitations of Cervical Auscultation

When used clinically, cervical auscultation is a highly subjective test. Because the examiner cannot simultaneously see the movements of the swallowing system while listening to swallow sounds, the sounds cannot be correlated with specific events except by clinical inference. Sounds of breathing and swallowing made by infants are not the same as those made by adults, so the examiner must be specifically trained to use cervical auscultation with a pediatric group. Nonetheless, in the hands of an experienced listener, the procedure is less invasive and less expensive than any of the other tools that have been discussed.

Evaluation of Gastrointestinal Function

Upper GI Series

An upper GI series (UGI), also called a barium swallow or esophagram, is a radiographic study that is used to evaluate the anatomy and function of the GI tract, specifically the esophagus and the stomach. A UGI often is used to diagnose structural abnormalities, such as tracheoesophageal fistulas, esophageal atresias, esophageal strictures, hiatal hernias, pyloric stenosis, tumors, obstructions, or malrotations. It can provide some information about the functioning and motility of the GI tract by looking at esophageal motility, stomach emptying, and spontaneous gastroesophageal reflux (GER) as the barium flows through the esophagus and into the stomach. Sometimes the radiologist will attempt to elicit GER by providing pressure to the abdomen. It is used to rule out anatomic etiology for persistent vomiting. Swallowing is sometimes briefly scanned at the beginning of the study, but the main focus of the study is the esophagus, stomach and duodenum. Although some radiologists continue to use this procedure as a tool for observing swallowing, the UGI is extremely limited in this area.

Procedure

Barium is taken into the esophagus. This is done orally with the child drinking the liquid by bottle, syringe, or cup. If the child is unable to swallow large amounts of barium orally, a nasogastric tube will be inserted into the esophagus to administer the barium. The child is restrained in supine on a board or on the fluoroscopy or X-ray table during the presentation of the barium. The child is immobilized through swaddling and is restrained by the technicians. The child's arms are extended above the head and restrained at the ears. The head is positioned at the midline. If a board is used, it can be rotated so the barium can flow into all parts of the esophageal and stomach anatomy. The radiologist then can observe these structures from all angles. When a board is not used, the technicians tilt the child to the side to coat the anatomy and review the structures. Parents often are out of the room. Real-time events are viewed, though usually only still photographic X-rays are taken for later study.

Advantages of the UGI Series

This study is very appropriate for evaluating structural abnormalities in the esophagus, stomach, and duodenum. It can demonstrate esophageal motility. If gastroesophageal reflux is seen, the duration and height of the refluxed material can be documented.

Limitations of the UGI Series

This is usually a radiographic study with both fluoroscopic and X-ray exposure. There is increased area of X-ray exposure. There are a number of limitations with using the UGI series for the diagnosis of gastroesophageal reflux. There have been high false positives and negatives noted. The study is short in duration and, therefore, episodes of gastroesophageal reflux are apt to be missed if the child is not cooperating. The amount of barium taken may be inadequate when compared with a full feeding size. GER may not be elicited in this testing situation. When GER is seen, the radiologist can document that GER episodes were observed; however, it is then difficult to extrapolate the frequency of these episodes. This study is done in the supine position and the parent is usually not present. The infant is restrained and often unhappy. Thus, the situation is not at all like a typical feeding situation in terms of position and comfort. Information relating to swallowing function can be suspect because of the conditions. Nipple holes often are enlarged to allow for easy flow of the barium. When fluoroscopy is not used, no videotape is made, so it is impossible to review the results of the study at a later time.

There appears to be considerable variability in procedure techniques and interpretations. Radiologists vary in the amount of barium delivered, hence the impact on the stomach and potential for GER are varied. Different amounts can have an impact on stomach emptying. More volume will stress the stomach capacity more and may promote more GER. There are inconsistencies regarding whether the radiologist determines usual bolus feeding size before the study is done. The barium itself is an inert liquid that moves more rapidly through the stomach than nutrient-dense formulas. Whether the barium is given pure or mixed with a percentage of formula may have a significant impact on stomach-emptying interpretations. When it is mixed with formula, it must be noted what formula was mixed, the caloric density of the formula, and by what percentage the barium was diluted. Until these procedures are more standardized, the interpretation of the results related to feeding may be extremely variable and unreliable. The physician and feeding therapist should share specific questions that they want addressed with the radiologist at the time of the referral rather than after completion of the study.

Implications for the Feeding Therapist

It is important to rule out any structural abnormalities of the esophagus and the stomach. Abnormalities such as strictures, hernias, fistulas, atresias, and pyloric stenosis greatly influence feeding behaviors. Tracheoesophageal fistulas often are complicated and difficult to discover. They sometimes require repeat studies, turning the child, and viewing from several different angles in order to fully assess this condition. Any anatomical issues discovered must be taken care of medically before positive changes in feeding can take place.

It is important for the feeding therapist to understand the whole picture regarding GER and related diagnostic testing. Knowing the limitations of the tests can provide perspective in interpreting the results. If GER is documented during the study, the frequency, intensity and effect on the esophageal tissue cannot be determined. The UGI cannot quantify the intensity of the effect of the GER for that particular child and his or her particular feeding and growth issues. For a child who is clinically assumed to have GER, the UGI results can be confusing if no GER is observed. It may well be that on that day, during that particular study, no GER episodes occurred. It is not appropriate to completely rule out GER as an influence on feeding for children who have demonstrated no episodes of GER during an upper GI.

Table 8.1   **Comparison of Videofluoroscopy and Upper GI Series**

Videofluoroscopic Swallow Study	**Barium Swallow UGI**
Focuses on physiology of mouth, pharynx, and upper esophagus with swallowing	Focuses on esophagus, stomach, and duodenum
Feeding therapist or speech-language pathologist is present with radiologist	Radiologist present
Primary feeder present	Primary feeder often not present
Fluoroscopy videotaped for later review of process and timing; X-rays taken	Real-time view with fluoroscopy
Attempts to duplicate the feeding position	Supine position
Attempts to duplicate the feeding utensils, bottle, etc.	Uses syringe or bottle
Uses variable food consistencies (thin or thick liquid or solids)	Uses liquid barium
Lateral and anterior/posterior (AP) views can be viewed	AP view with some rotation done to view anatomy of stomach and intestines
Management options are tried	No treatment options are explored

Table 8.2   What an Upper GI Can and Cannot Tell the Feeding Therapist

Can tell	Cannot tell
Whether there are anatomical abnormalities – tracheoesophageal fistula – esophageal atresia – hiatal hernia – pyloric stenosis – tumors/blockages – other structural GI conditions	
General information about esophageal motility	Esophageal motility changes with different food textures
General information about esophageal emptying	
Functioning of a Nissen fundoplication	
General information about stomach emptying	
Number of episodes of GE reflux	How the GE reflux affects the child
Duration of GE reflux episodes	The child's frequency of reflux
Amount of barium the child can take before GE reflux occurs	How the reflux affects esophageal tissue
	If the child has no reflux during the study, the clinician cannot say the child will not have reflux at another time
	If the child has GE reflux before or after the study
Information regarding why – GE reflux occurs – there is stomach blockage – there is slow stomach emptying – the lower esophageal sphincter is lax – there is intermittent relaxation of the LES	

Understanding the variability in radiographic procedure techniques, the feeding therapist can work with the physician to ask specific questions before the study. May the parent be present to relax the child and make the procedure more comfortable? How much barium will be given? How much barium was given when the GER was documented? Did the study allow the child to have the amount of barium he usually receives in a bolus? If stomach emptying is considered, could the barium be mixed with the formula that the child usually receives? Asking these and other specific questions will help make the information received more meaningful as it is interpreted within the mealtime setting for that child.

pH Probe

The pH probe, also called the intraesophageal pH probe or intraluminal pH monitoring, is a study used to quantify the frequency and duration of gastroesophageal reflux into the esophagus over a specified time. It can be used to document episodes of GE reflux, duration of reflux episodes, body position, meals, and the sleep and awake states.

Procedure

A special microelectrode sensor is inserted through the nose and into the distal esophagus, just above the lower esophageal sphincter. It continually monitors acidity. Most pH probes are kept in place for 24 hours. A constant bedside graph is kept of all acid occurrences at the sensor level of the esophagus. Meals, movement changes, and other circumstances that can influence esophageal reflux can be documented for later correlation with the pH results. Apple juice is given initially to test the probe placement.

Data is collected regarding the number and duration of acid episodes. Special attention is paid to episodes lasting longer than 5 minutes. A reflux score is determined and compared to established norms.

When gastroesophageal reflux is suspected as a factor in upper airway symptoms (e.g., chronic cough, asthma), a double pH probe may be used. In addition to the standard distal probe that is placed in the esophagus, a second probe is placed in the nasopharynx or hypopharynx near the laryngeal opening of the airway. This second probe picks up acid that directly affects the respiratory system (Conley, Werlin, & Beste, 1995; Little et al., 1997).

pH probe studies can be performed in combination with pulse oximetry, a pneumogram, or both so that heart and respiratory rates or oxygen levels can be correlated with the findings. Many centers now use probes in different settings with the data fed into a central location to be read later. This provides more flexibility in usage.

Advantages of the pH Probe

The pH probe offers an extended (24-hour) look at the acidity of the esophagus correlated with the infant's activities of eating, sleeping, and moving. This may be preferable and more reflective of the actual physiology of the esophagus than the short documentation received in an upper GI. The correlation with activity can be important for management. The length and frequency of the acid episodes can be documented precisely. The time needed for each of these acid episodes to clear can be discovered, giving a hint about how long the acid may be influencing the esophagus. We know, for example, that it takes a typical child swallowing basic saliva less time to clear or neutralize the esophageal acid than it takes a neurologically involved child with poorer swallowing skills. The pH probe can be used in combination with other studies to determine the influence of esophageal acidity on respiratory rate, oxygen saturation, and heart rate.

Limitations of the pH Probe

The pH probe is a procedure that requires close prolonged observation. It is often done in a hospital, although outpatient procedures can be done. It is an invasive procedure in that it requires the placement of an indwelling naso-esophageal probe. pH probes are restricted to only documenting episodes that cause changes in pH and only chart acid events. They, therefore, are unable to detect acid reflux during the postprandial period (i.e., after mealtimes) because many foods buffer the gastric acidity for varying periods of time and interfere with the ability of the probe to detect the reflux episodes. Feeding specialists are well aware that many episodes of reflux occur after a meal when the stomach is most distended or still has food contents. Most of these reflux episodes are missed with current pH studies. Some researchers have suggested that presenting at least one feeding of an acid material such as apple juice during the study would provide more helpful information although this is not yet common practice. Others recommend that all feedings be given with apple juice during the study. This also is not a common practice and has come under question because of the likelihood that such feedings are handled differently in the GI tract than infant milk.

Once a pH probe documents GER, the therapist still doesn't have information about why it exists. Is it slow stomach emptying? Is it a lax lower esophageal sphincter? Is it a part of a disease process? What else is going on? The management decisions must take into consideration why the GER is there.

Keeping it in Perspective

It is important to keep a grounded perspective on referral for this and other tests looking for gastro-esophageal reflux. Most gastroenterologists and feeding therapists who take a good history can determine many children who have GER without this or other invasive procedures. Children who are refluxing often show clear clinical signs. They may spit up or vomit food regularly, be irritable, arch backwards during or after eating, sleep poorly, and demonstrate frequent facial grimaces that often accompany acid reflux in the pharynx. Many of these children simultaneously have poor appetite or growth patterns. Treatment for presumed reflux can be initiated based on clinical symptoms alone. Further efforts may be needed to determine the cause of the GER. A pH probe may only provide further confirmation that the GER is there, but it offers no clues about the cause. In this case, it probably is a redundant procedure. On the other hand, there are children with GER who never vomit or show clear behavioral signs of reflux. Their symptoms, which can include weight loss or uninterest in eating, can be confusing. Those children may need the pH probe to document the GER. Sometimes this study is done before placement of a gastrostomy tube to determine the extent of GER and help in the decision about whether a fundoplication procedure is necessary.

It is important to note that all the data in the world about the frequency and duration of a child's GER still does not tell us how it affects that particular child. Some children can throw up 20 or 30 times a day and still grow and thrive and eventually outgrow the GER. Others spit up once or twice a day but arch and fuss and refuse to eat because of the discomfort. As with all diagnostic tests, the data collected *must* be kept in perspective and interpreted as a part of the whole picture, which includes the child's history, the family reports, the child's growth, and his or her overall health.

Upper Gastrointestinal Endoscopy

In this procedure, the gastroenterologist uses an endoscope to directly view the upper gastrointestinal tract. The pediatric upper gastrointestinal endoscopy uses small video optic or fiberoptic endoscopes for direct visualization of the esophageal mucosa and stomach lining (Godfrey, Avital, Maayan, Rotschild, & Springer, 1997). Tissue biopsies can be performed. This visual examination plus biopsies provides increased understanding of the GI issues that can influence feeding. The physician can look for histologic changes in the esophagus that might be consistent with chronic GER-induced esophagitis. Esophageal narrowing and strictures can be observed. Lower esophageal sphincter functioning can be viewed. Endoscopies can be used in foreign body removal. The endoscope also is used for the placement of a percutaneous endoscopic gastrostomy (PEG) tube. Endoscopy allows for observation of the health of the esophageal tissue as the PEG-tube is being placed.

Procedure

The procedure is done as an outpatient procedure in the GI lab of a hospital or clinic. The procedure should be explained to the child and family in advance. The child is sedated and the sedation level monitored throughout the procedure. Conscious sedation or general anesthesia is used. The child is given enough pain medication to be comfortable and a tranquilizer to alter anxiety, memory, and awareness state. Some at-risk patients need to be given deep sedation or general anesthesia for the procedure. Parents are encouraged to bring transition objects, such as a favorite stuffed toy or blanket, for before and after the sedation. Parents should remain with the child for as long as possible. This is usually until the child is sedated completely. Sometimes, however, parents are asked to leave earlier if their presence is too stimulating for the child.

Fiberoptic endoscopes, which transmit light through tiny fiber bundles, electronic endoscopes, or videoendoscopes, which transmit images to a video screen, are used for this procedure. A flexible fiberoptic tube is used to directly observe the structures within the body. The physician inserts the endoscope through the mouth and pharynx and into the entire distance of the esophagus. The physician advances it as she notes normal and abnormal features of the esophagus, as well as esophageal tissues or tissue changes. The stomach and duodenum can be entered for visual inspection. Tissue biopsies can be taken along the way as indicated by questionable findings, such as esophagitis, ulcers, or tissue changes caused by the chronic GER.

Gastroesophageal Scintigraphy

Gastroesophageal scintigraphy or nuclear scintigraphy also may be referred to as a technetium scan, milk scan, or gastroesophageal scintiscan. The purpose of the study is to evaluate esophageal function and provide information on stomach emptying. Information on the extent and severity of gastroesophageal reflux also can be obtained.

Procedure

A small amount of a radionuclide-labeled formula (radionuclide isotope, 200u Ci technetium-labeled sulfur colloid or Technetium-99) is added to a liquid or solid feeding. This radioactive material marks the food for counting of specific gamma information later. This is not absorbed after oral administration and does not become attached to the GI mucosa. The baby is fed in the usual fashion (i.e., by bottle, cup, or adapted breast-feeding) and then positioned in supine under the camera. A special gamma-counter camera takes images of the esophagus and portions of the oropharynx and stomach every 30 to 60 seconds for more than an hour after the feeding. Using computer processing, specific areas of interest can be focused on as food transit time and intraluminal (esophageal) volumes are determined. Episodes of refluxed material are recorded, as is the height of the refluxed material in the esophagus. These numbers are compared with norms for the child's age. Gastric emptying is determined by calculating the percentage of food remaining in the stomach at certain intervals. In their study of 49 infants and children, Seibert, Byrne, and Euler (1983) found that infants had emptied 48% of the meal while children had emptied 51% during the hour's period. Tolia, Kuhns, and Kaufman's study (1993a) of 27 infants under 1 year of age showed a gastric emptying of 36% during the first hour. Scintigraphy has been shown to have poor sensitivity in detecting aspiration in known aspirators.

Advantages of Scintigraphy

The gastroesophageal scintiscan is readily available and has a number of advantages over some other GI tests. It is noninvasive and exposes the patient to minimum doses of radiation—much less than fluoroscopy. It measures gastric emptying rates over at least an hour, which is an advantage over the upper GI procedure. It can pick up images of refluxed material any time it is present in the esophagus, whether it is acid or postprandial (after the meal) food-buffered alkaline material. The pH probe only documents acid episodes. When children were simultaneously observed with scintigraphy and a pH probe, scintigraphy identified substantially more reflux episodes than the probe. Most of these occurred during the first half hour after the child was fed when nonacid reflux would be most visible (Vandenplas, Derde, & Piepsz, 1992). The height of the refluxed material can be documented, whereas the pH probe only documents the occurrence but not the intensity or height of the reflux.

This procedure helps determine how rapidly a child's stomach empties after a meal. When food remains in the stomach for long periods after a meal, the risk of GER is increased (Hillemeier, Lange, McCallum, Seashore, & Gryboski, 1981). Thus, it can help a physician know whether a drug that helps the stomach empty more rapidly may control reflux episodes. It is also an essential procedure if the physician is considering doing a fundoplication procedure to help control reflux. Because complications of retching and gagging appear to be higher in children with problems of gastric emptying, it is important for the physician to know whether there are problems of gastric motility before the surgery is done. A delay in gastric emptying time may suggest that a pyloroplasty or gastric antroplasty procedure might be done at the time of the fundoplication to assist stomach emptying.

Limitations of Scintigraphy

Gastroesophageal reflux is monitored for only an hour. In contrast, the pH probe monitors GER for a 24-hour period. Episodes that occur after the first hour are missed. The study has been described as having a high false-positive rate of GER. Thus, it may indicate that some children are refluxing who actually are not in everyday life. This may be because the position of choice for the gamma counter is supine. This back-lying position has been correlated with increased episodes of GER. Measurements are taken every 30–60 seconds so that there is not a continuous record of activity. The procedure also is complicated by a poor resolution of the image, along with poor sensitivity for detecting small amounts of aspiration, even in known aspirators. Scintigraphy does not provide either the image sensitivity or clarity of the upper GI procedure in ruling out obstructions. As physicians consider this test, they find that there may be little value in documenting and quantifying GER through scintigraphy. Its value lies predominantly in gaining a clearer picture of the child's gastric emptying time.

Esophageal Manometry

Esophageal manometry is used to determine competence of the upper and lower esophageal sphincters by measuring the pressure within them. This procedure quantifies the force of the contraction of the muscular wall of these sphincters and the esophageal body. It measures motor activity, strength, speed, direction, and duration of the muscle contraction. It can be used to evaluate the LES pressure after a Nissen fundoplication is performed.

The indications for the use of this study include diagnosis of esophageal motility disorders such as achalasia (failure of the LES to relax following swallowing) and the absence of peristalsis in the esophagus (Gilger, Boyle, Sondheimer, & Colletti, 1997). Subtle differences in timing between the pharynx and the UES and the esophageal body and the LES can be documented.

This test involves the placement of a water-filled sleeve with strategically placed sensors into the esophagus. As the esophagus contracts in a peristaltic wave, the muscles move against the sleeve, and the pattern and force of muscle contraction can be measured (Kaul & Rudolph, 1998). The test tends to be expensive and usually is saved for confusing esophageal difficulties that require more information. The upper GI or the VFSS done in combination with the upper GI also can describe peristaltic problems with the esophagus.

Evaluation of Respiratory Function

Bronchoscopy With Bronchoalveolar Lavage

The endoscopic evaluation of the upper airway is called a laryngoscopy, and the endoscopic evaluation of the lower airways is called a bronchoscopy. Pulmonologists usually use these procedures to identify abnormalities in the airway structures. When it is suspected that food is being aspirated into the lungs, a bronchoalveolar lavage (BAL) is performed to look for lipid-laden macrophages (Godfrey et al., 1997). These fat-containing cells are associated with the aspiration of food into the lungs. A positive determination of lipid-laden macrophages documents that food aspiration is occurring. It does not, however, provide the information about whether the food is being aspirated during swallowing or if it is coming from refluxed material. Further studies—including a VFSS, upper GI, pH probe, or all three—may be necessary to understand this finding and determine the next step in treatment of the child.

Table 8.3   Comparison of the Most Commonly Used Diagnostic Tests

Test	Videofluoroscopic Swallow Study
Indications	Analyze the swallow mechanism Rule out aspiration Determine point of aspiration
Advantages	Fluoroscopy, not static X-ray Videotaped Position simulates feeding Primary feeder presents the food Familiar feeding utensils, bottle, cup, and spoon Use of liquid, puree, and solid Lateral and anterior/posterior view Can determine when aspiration occurs Investigation of treatment options Can be paired with other diagnostic studies
Disadvantages	Difficulty in completely simulating a normal feeding Child must be able to swallow an appropriate amount of barium Results reflect that particular date and time Aspirator may not aspirate that day Study environment may increase aspiration Some radiation exposure from fluoroscopy
Test	**Upper GI Series**
Indications	Analyze anatomy and motility of esophagus, stomach, and duodenum
Advantages	Clear contrast image of upper GI anatomy Documents GER if it occurs during study Documents height of GER that occurs during study Observes esophageal motility Observes mechanism for stomach emptying
Disadvantages	X-ray exposure Not routinely videotaped Supine position Barium flow rate may not simulate bottle-feeding Primary feeder often not present High rate of false positives and negatives for GER May miss GER altogether Variability in procedure standards

(continued)

Table 8.3	**Comparison of the Most Commonly Used Diagnostic Tests (continued)**
Test	**pH Probe**
Indications	Quantifies the frequency and duration of GER
Advantages	24-hour study
	Documents effect of movement, sleep, and meals on GER
	Documents frequency and duration of GER
	Documents time necessary for clearance of acid
	Can be combined with other monitoring instruments
Disadvantages	Invasive procedure
	Unable to document GER in postprandial period
Test	**Pediatric Gastrointestinal Endoscopy**
Indications	Provides a direct view of the upper gastrointestinal tract
Advantages	Direct observation of esophageal and stomach tissues for changes that may have occurred with chronic GER
	Biopsies can be taken to further study tissue
Disadvantages	Invasive procedure
	Visualization does not tell the extent that tissue changes impact on that child's feeding
	Study cannot tell frequency of GER
Test	**Gastroesophageal Scintigraphy**
Indications	Evaluate esophageal function and provide information on stomach emptying
Advantages	Documents stomach-emptying rate
	Noninvasive procedure
	Less radiation exposure than fluoroscopy
	Reviews GER and stomach emptying for at least an hour
	Documents height of GER
	Documents postprandial GER
Disadvantages	Does not document frequency of GER
	GER is documented only an hour
	Supine position may cause high false positives
	30–60 second views do not allow for continuous documentation of GER
	Poor resolution of image as compared with UGI
	Poor sensitivity in detecting microaspiration

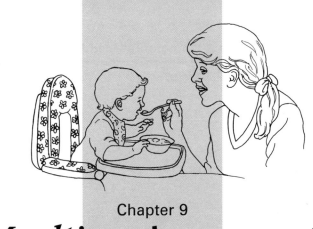

Chapter 9

Mealtime Assessment

■ Foundations

A mealtime assessment is often like an extended mystery novel. The story begins by setting the overall scene. Gradually, the reader gets to know the setting, the individual characters and their relationships, and the problems that bring the detective onto the scene. As the detective explores each element, the essence of the plot begins to emerge. Additional pieces of information are added, and the reader begins to wonder how the various elements of the story will come together. In some cases, the crime or problem area is handled by the legal system through a process of discovery and trial. Various aspects are presented, considered, and debated. The reader may suspect one character or situation and then another of committing the crime. Often he is surprised when the most evident aspects are not the most important and may be shocked in the final pages to discover someone or something that he did not initially suspect. Yet, if the reader reviews the story, he can always trace the clues and elements that led to the final solution.

The Elements of the Story

This scenario is similar to what happens in a mealtime assessment. The clinician is presented with a problem or challenge to solve. In most instances, the challenge is to discover more about a child's eating, drinking, and mealtime patterns. The therapist is asked if there are problems, to identify the problems, to find the reasons for the problems, and to identify some solutions to the problems. She interviews the family, observes the child, and collects data and evidence. The therapist looks at how the different pieces of evidence come together, identifies patterns that lead in specific directions, and collects additional data. She may send some of the data to specialists for additional tests or confirmation of a theory. Finally, the therapist organizes the many pieces of information and identifies the situations that can explain the most important elements of the child's mealtime problem.

The mind-set of the person conducting the feeding assessment requires the same elements as those of the detective. An effective detective is open to all possibilities. He does not enter the case with a fixed point of view and then proceed to collect data that supports only that point of view. The detective looks at the connections among suspects and pieces of data because these connections generally hold the key to a solution.

The clinician explores the ***history of the problem***. What situations or components have led to the referral for an assessment? What past concerns have brought the different individuals in this mealtime story to the feeding or mealtime assessment?

During an evaluation, the clinician wants to know ***the present situation***. What is the current feeding and mealtime like, and what aspects create concern for each person? What is the mealtime situation like for the child? What is each parent's perspective and concern about the child's eating and drinking? What is the feeding therapist's perspective as mealtimes are observed and discussed?

The analogy to the detective novel breaks down at this point. In most fictional stories, the final resolution includes a punitive solution. The perpetrator of the crime is caught and sent to jail or punished in some way. In contrast, the effective mealtime assessment looks for peaceful and equitable resolutions to the problem. There are no good or bad guys who must be punished—only strengths and abilities that can be expanded and limiting factors that can be changed. When the clinician sees something as good or bad in an assessment, she brings in judgments that often cloud a view of the bigger picture. When the therapist thinks of something as interfering, there is more freedom to release it without anger and with the ability to see all of the pros and cons of a situation.

During and following the evaluation, the clinician wants to gain insight toward ***solutions to the problem*** that will be effective. Many potential resolutions to portions of the problem may be explored within the context of the evaluation. Others will be scheduled for discovery and trial at a later time.

The therapist may return to the situation to get feedback on the initial solution. At this point, she reviews what has happened in the interim and focuses on ***future directions***. These may include a more in-depth exploration of the situation, the addition of information from consultants, and the assignment or confirmation of the individuals who will be involved in implementing a long-range plan.

Seeking the Answers

Unfortunately, many feeding assessments continue to examine a very limited portion of the data. They use a deficit model of assessment that includes information primarily on what the child is unable to do. Many feeding professionals who are responsible for the assessment begin with a bias or theory and seek data that supports that theory. Others collect a great deal of unorganized data and present this as the assessment, with no hint of how the pieces relate to each other. Many proposed solutions blame and convict the child or parent. These are not helpful in gaining a true picture of what is happening and in proposing what changes might lead to a resolution of the problem.

The main function of a mealtime assessment is neither the collection of data nor the identification of a diagnosis. An assessment is a descriptive and interpretive process that leads to a resolution of the problems that initiated the assessment. Its primary focus is on the process that leads to a solution, not on the solution itself. It gives equal weight to supporting aspects of the process and those that create limits or roadblocks.

Professionals involved in the mealtime assessment are interested in discovering what is preventing the child or family from moving through the process and arriving at a specified level of feeding or mealtime skill. They also are interested in what strengths, skills, and interests are available to support the journey. They are aware of areas that are unclear and the questions they must ask to begin to understand the unknown aspects of the child's mealtime difficulties.

Professionals and parents constantly seek answers to the problems that distress and puzzle them. Yet, many years ago a wise professor of education (J. Powell, personal communication, 1958) told his students that the greatest myth in education lies in the search for answers. Paraphrased, he said that the purpose of education is not to provide answers but to identify the questions that every student should be asking. If students understand and ask the right questions, the answers will find them.

Assessment is the constant search for the right questions and the internal review of the possible answers or solutions that can make a difference in the life of a child and family. As therapists seek to define the questions, they also remain open to many different answers that reflect aspects of the whole. You may recall the familiar Hindu story of the six blind men and the elephant. Each felt separate parts of the elephant and was asked to describe the elephant. The one who felt the trunk thought it much like a snake, the one who felt the leg argued that indeed an elephant was like a tree, and the one who held the tusk insisted that it was like a sword. Each argued for a limited set of perceptions and point of view. To fully understand what the elephant was like, they needed the whole picture. Each person needed to ask a complete set of questions that would lead to the broader picture of the elephant. The data in isolation was misleading.

The Process

Assessment can be approached in a number of ways. Because an assessment involves the processing and interpreting of information, it is helpful to review the different ways in which the human brain and mind are structured for information processing. What the therapist can learn about a child and family during an assessment is directly dependent upon how she develops the information-gathering process and how she deals with what is learned.

The brain is a highly versatile organ that can process information in many ways. The discussion of learning and the brain can be simplified by saying that the brain is a unitary organ that is divided along preferential lines for information processing. The cortex of the brain is divided into right and left hemispheres that work together while simultaneously specializing in different ways of looking at the information (Ornstein, 1998; Springer & Deutsch, 1997). The left hemisphere interprets information in a very linear, sequential, rational, language-based fashion. The right hemisphere processes the same information globally, holistically, spatially, and visually. The left hemisphere works from the individual parts or data; the right hemisphere works from the whole. The left hemisphere examines information rationally; the right hemisphere perceives the same information intuitively. The left hemisphere analyzes information; the right hemisphere synthesizes it.

The subcortical areas of the brain also contribute to learning and knowledge (Herrmann, 1988). The limbic system is a subcortical group of centers that contribute heavily to emotion, movement, and memory. Creativity and intuition appear to be handled primarily by the limbic system and the right hemisphere of the cortex. Strong interconnections between the limbic system and the cortex allow for an enrichment of learning and understanding.

Learning depends upon the connections that are made between different parts of the brain. The richer the connections between sensations, different ways of looking at information, and experience, the more complete the learning. Thus, the goal in an assessment is to look at the information provided by the child and family in as many ways as possible.

Rational and Intuitive Approaches

Most clinicians, in their academic and professional education, have had extensive experience with the rational model for gathering and interpreting information. This is the scientific model that reaches its conclusions in a linear fashion after each piece of data has been considered. In a rational approach to a mealtime assessment, the examiner observes each aspect of the child's abilities and disabilities, and then moves in a step-by-step fashion toward the conclusion. Only information that makes sense and can be verified objectively is included.

In contrast, an intuitive approach to the assessment is based on hunches. A global impression is obtained from the child and family. The impression also is created (at least in part) from factual data, but questions may be more open-ended, and observations begin from the global perspective. The global data may be refined and specific points checked out by more specific questions and observations. The examiner responds strongly to subtle nonverbal messages and an intuitive knowledge or hunch that either promotes further investigation or leads directly to a conclusion. Information does not have to make sense to be considered in the conclusion because making sense out of something implies that it has been subjected to a rational analysis. Much of the information used within the intuitive approach cannot be validated objectively at the time it is perceived to be accurate. The intuitive approach leads to quantum leaps in understanding. It is an essential component of creativity.

Bear in mind that the objective is to process information in a total way; then the assessment will include both approaches in gathering and interpreting information and in arriving at goals for treatment. Following are more specific styles that incorporate elements of both rational and intuitive approaches to assessment.

Global Overview

The therapist obtains a general concept of feeding and mealtime strengths and needs by discussing the questions brought by the parents, observing the child's interaction with the family, and briefly observing feeding skills. From this, the therapist can gain a general sense of the physical, sensory, and communication issues related to feeding as well as define the most important issues and questions. Part of this global perspective will include the clinician's hunches and impressions as well as those of the parents. Follow-up of these hunches will be incorporated into a more in-depth sequential analysis of the child's abilities.

Sequential Analysis

Once the basic questions have been defined through the global overview, the therapist can begin a sequential analysis and observe each specific area for its details. The details are linked together into a pattern that makes sense in relation to the whole. Then the therapist can check the details against the initial impressions or hunches and make further observations. She may use formal assessment forms or tests to gather objective information that can be compared with other children's scores.

Although both types of information processing are important in the evaluation, most people have a preferential way of gathering and interpreting information. Because of prior experience or brain dominance, some people always approach a learning or problem-solving situation with a detailed, analytical strategy. All information may be gathered in a linear, analytical style. When intuitive information and general hunches play a minimal role in arriving at a conclusion, full information processing has not occurred. Others may find that impressions or answers occur suddenly in intuitive flashes. Although many of these may be accurate, it is impossible to move to a deeper level of understanding and check out the impressions without a more linear, sequential approach.

Most individuals who incorporate both styles will have a preferred way of beginning to observe. Some will begin with the parts, build them into a whole picture, and allow the answers to incubate until they intuitively feel right. Others will observe globally, filling in the sequential details with guidance from their intuition. Answers will be checked out through analysis, and their accuracy will be evaluated intuitively.

Specific Applications to the Feeding Assessment: Jason

Jason, a 1-year-old infant with cerebral palsy, tended to cough and choke when his mother fed him by mouth. His breathing was noisy, and he would make gasping sounds as he moved food in his mouth and prepared for swallowing. He was held in an upright sitting position on his mother's lap. From time to time, his head and body would arch backward and he would become stiff from head to toe. Because of his severe feeding difficulties and poor weight gain, he received most of his nourishment through a gastrostomy tube. Jason often appeared to be unhappy. He fussed and squirmed, and frequently he fell asleep during the meal. His mother had been told that the extensor spasms that caused him to arch backward should be stopped and that he should be repositioned whenever they occurred. She had been shown how to stimulate his lips with her finger and the spoon to help him get a stronger sucking pattern. Jason was able to eat about 1 ounce of pureed food at each meal. This usually took 30 to 45 minutes.

The first impression of Jason was one of discomfort and general unhappiness. Why did he seem so upset and agitated? Were the strong extensor movements simply random, involuntary spasms of the central nervous system? Intuitively, these patterns seemed more important than the specific movements of the mouth (a global observation). Therefore, they were examined initially in greater detail (a sequential observation). When did they occur? Were they associated with any other events or activities? His agitation and upset increased as his breathing became louder and more stressed. The extension occurred primarily when food was placed in his mouth during times when the breathing was stressed.

A number of reasons for this relationship of events were possible. Inner agitation for an unidentified reason could cause incoordination of breathing, resulting in noisy sounds. Poor swallowing of the food also could stress the breathing patterns and cause physiological timing problems with respiration or anxiety related to fear of choking. The upright position on the lap could cause tension throughout the body. The constant effort to work against gravity could stress the muscles that control breathing and swallowing. Jason's desire to communicate his unhappiness with the entire feeding situation could account for the breathing incoordination and the strong extension of the body.

It would be possible to systematically check out each of the possible relationships. However, this is time-consuming. The process can be simplified through shortcuts, enabling time to be spent on the most important aspects. This is where global impressions and hunches based on information, experience, and intuition come into the evaluation. The basic impression of Jason was that the tension of his body increased as he was positioned upright against gravity. This contributed to poor coordination of breathing with swallowing and made oral feeding more difficult. As his mouth filled with unswallowed food, Jason tried to tell his mother that he wasn't ready for more food. He did this by the only movement he had consistently available to him—moving away from the spoon with extension and fussing. The basic problem appeared to be one of bodily tension, an inconsistent delay in the swallowing pattern, and a communication pattern that accentuated the extensor pattern of movement.

This hypothesis was checked out through a set of systematic changes in the mealtime and careful sequential observations. Jason was observed without food. During general movement and handling, there was an increase in tension in Jason's trunk and shoulder girdle whenever he was brought into a sitting position. Breathing became noisy, and the therapist could hear gurgling sounds in Jason's throat. A reclining position reduced the noisy breathing but increased his tendency to arch into extension. When Jason was moved into sidelying on his left side, he immediately appeared to be more comfortable. Tension diminished in his body, and Jason's facial expression appeared happier. From time to time, the strong extension returned. This seemed to occur when his face was touched or when he was touched or moved without warning. Each time a spasm began, it continued into a full extensor arch, and Jason cried and appeared to be quite unhappy. Each time the initial increase in tension began, the therapist stopped whatever she was doing and asked Jason, "Do you want me to stop?" or she said, "You're telling me you are uncomfortable. Let's try it another way." Gradually, the frequency of the extensor spasms diminished; and when they began, he was able to stop them before they reached the point of no return. He seemed interested in what was being said to him, and he smiled. This supported the original hunch that Jason was using some of the extensor movement to say "No!"

The therapist introduced food on her finger rather than by spoon. This resulted in a smaller amount to deal with in the mouth. Jason did very well with the first bite. His breathing remained quiet, and his body was without tension. As the therapist presented the second fingerful, he began to squirm. When the therapist returned the food to the bowl, Jason became calm and quiet. The therapist observed Jason swallow and then stare at the bowl. The therapist again offered food on a finger. This time, Jason accepted the food with ease.

During the remainder of the evaluation, the therapist observed:

> Jason's breathing became stressed when tension in his body increased, when he had not cleared food out of the mouth and was expected to accept another bite, and when the adult did not understand what he was trying to communicate.

Jason used strong extension in his body to indicate that he was unhappy, to tell the feeder hat he was in trouble with his swallowing, and to indicate that he wanted to stop an activity.

Jason's sucking and swallowing were more coordinated when he was positioned on his left side, when a quiet body and quiet breathing were used to signal his readiness for more food, and when he was able to indicate his readiness to the feeder.

By the end of the assessment, Jason was able to choose food or water by looking at the bowl he wanted, and he was able to use his hand to help the therapist guide her finger to his mouth whenever he was ready for more food. His breathing was quiet, and the strong extensor spasms no longer occurred.

This series of events, leading to a successful identification of the child's problems and assets, was possible in a relatively short time because the therapist shifted rapidly among different ways of observing, processing, and interpreting information. A global view of Jason's unhappiness and physical struggle was important to explore before specific aspects of sucking and swallowing could be made. Intuitive hunches became the basis for sequential observation and exploration.

As the variables of position, stimulation, and communication were changed, the therapist was able to observe behavior changes and form further hunches about the meaning of those behaviors for Jason.

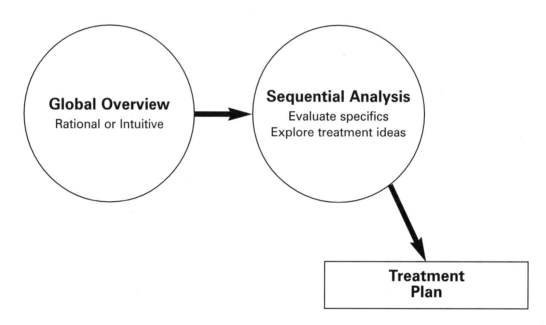

The components of an assessment constitute only the elements from which the whole is created. The flow or movement between components and the underlying philosophy of the assessment are the unifying force. A powerful assessment is one that:

- identifies the child's strengths and needs,
- identifies actions or movements that the child enjoys and wants to do,
- integrates observations from those who know the child best,
- explores differences in the child's behaviors in a series of environments, and
- leads logically and intuitively to changes that will enable the child to move toward the highest potential.

Observations that lead to an effective treatment program can be obtained through the following process.

■ Approaches to Gathering Information

There are a number of ways to gather information about the child's specific feeding and mealtime issues. The child and family are central to any assessment. Information must be obtained from the parent and child, from interview and observation. The type of information gathering depends on the specific situation. Is the child in the home or a hospital environment? Can a home visit be made or will the child be going to a clinic? Will the parent be available for interview? What will be the best way to observe the child's eating skills? Is there an imposed limit on the number of assessment sessions available? How difficult is it to access other team members? The following is a look at some information-gathering options.

Interview and Parent Questionnaire

It is helpful to interview a parent as the first step in the assessment. The parents know the child best. Usually, a parent is the primary feeder. The parent knows the child's best position for mealtime, particular likes and dislikes, typical utensils used, mealtime routine, and the areas of feeding that are working comfortably, as well as those that are not. Sometimes it works best to discuss the mealtime issues with both parents, as they may have different perspectives and concerns about the feedings. The parents are the individuals who will play the major role in implementing changes in the child's feeding environment and eating behaviors. Parental concerns need to be addressed in order for long-range changes to be made.

A formal questionnaire can be given to the parent to be filled out before the feeding observations. It can serve as the basis for a series of interview questions asked directly of the parent at the initial meeting, or it can be discussed by phone before the face-to-face assessment.

Sample Parent Mealtimes Questionnaires are found at the end of this chapter. They include a Parent Questionnaire for eating and drinking skills (pages 175–178) and one for tube-feeding and beginning oral-feeding skills (pages 179–183). Additionally, see the Gastroesophageal Reflux Parent Questionnaire on pages 581–583. The Appendix contains a Spanish translation of this material.

Observation of the Child

Observation Settings

Observations of the child eating can be done in many different settings. Ideally, the therapist would observe the child eating in the home. This can provide the clearest perception of a typical meal. Home observation allows the child to eat in a familiar environment with familiar utensils and foods. Often, more than one observation session is needed to understand the mealtime environment and dynamics. Home observations are not always possible. Some children may need to be seen in a clinic situation. When this is necessary, it helps to have the parents bring familiar utensils and foods, and even special seating, when possible. Parents might be asked to bring foods that show the child's best and most challenged eating skills. This may not be as ideal as a home observation, but the foods, utensils, and seating may add some familiarity for the child. Many times, families are asked to bring a videotape of the family meal. This is a helpful way to see how the child eats within the family mealtime environment. Whether the observation is done in the home or at the clinic, frequently a series of observations is needed to provide the most accurate mealtime assessment.

Parent-Child Feeding Interaction

By watching a parent feed a child, the therapist has an opportunity to observe the aspects of feeding that are familiar to child and parent. What position is used for feeding? How fast is food given? What type of interaction occurs between parent and child? How has the parent learned to deal with challenges presented by the child's feeding problems? What is working in the mealtime interaction and what is not?

When the therapist feeds the child first, it is difficult to discover whether the child's feeding behaviors and movements reflect typical patterns or are a way of saying that the situation is new, the feeding presentation is foreign, and the food is not wanted.

Therapist's Observations From Feeding the Child

Once the therapist has observed the child eating with the parent, she needs to take a turn at feeding. By feeding the child, the therapist can obtain another perspective of the child's needs and abilities. It is possible to feel changes in postural tone in the child's body and obtain a closer view of the child's feeding movements. The therapist can try different foods, utensils, speed of food presentation, and positions, as well as observe the child's responses to these changes. Observations of what the child likes, wants in various situations, and in which activities he wishes to participate provide important knowledge of what works best for the child and what changes could be made to improve mealtime.

Recording Mealtime Assessment Data

After completing the parent interview and reviewing information from the Parent Mealtimes Questionnaire, the therapist should observe the parent feeding the child. She then should become more directly involved in the child's mealtime. During this period, it is important to record rough notes that serve as reminders when it is time to write a more formal evaluation report. The therapist forms an impression of the child's prerequisite and developmental pre-feeding and feeding skills. Attention shifts from the minute details and task analysis of the individual components of feeding to a focused view of the whole picture. This supports an overview of the broader influences that are involved in the child's eating skills, and enable the therapist to blend them with previous observations.

A sample Mealtime Assessment Guide is provided on pages 184–186. It may be photocopied or used directly, or it may serve as a catalyst to the therapist's imagination as she creates an assessment form.

Following are the kinds of information that might be included on the form, divided into sections of History and Concerns, Feeding History, Mealtime Observations, and Summary Planning. The therapist should record the information in a way that feels most organized to her.

Parent Concerns

It is very important that parent concerns and priorities are well understood in the beginning of the assessment. This provides a starting point for looking at specific feeding and mealtime issues. It helps the therapist understand what is most important to the parent and family. Any assessment that does not address parent concerns will fail to have meaning to the people who are most apt to have influence over changes in the feeding and mealtime situations.

Other Concerns

It is important to consider concerns from other team members, too. Perhaps the physician is worried about the child's weight and is coordinating a workup for cardiac difficulties. Maybe there is concern from the pulmonologist that there is aspiration with feedings. The dietitian may have concerns that the child's growth is falling off the growth curve. The psychologist or social worker may have serious concerns about attachment issues for a foster child. The teacher may be wondering how best to feed the child in the school situation. The physical therapist may be designing a new wheelchair for the child. Whenever there are other professionals involved with the child, their concerns should be considered in the assessment. Sometimes these concerns are made known before the initial interview and observation. Sometimes the input may be requested as a part of the information-gathering process.

Diagnoses and Medical History

A specific discussion about medical history and diagnoses to date is an important part of the assessment process. This can include birth history with gestational age and birth weight. It includes surgeries the child has had and possible future surgeries. It is helpful to know what physicians are treating the child. Past and recent health histories are important, especially as they relate to systems that influence feeding.

Previous Therapies and Assessments

Many children who have feeding difficulties have had a multitude of tests and assessments done before a feeding assessment. Some have had no feeding-related testing and part of the therapist's assessment process may be to initiate requests for specific testing procedures. The therapist should document any specific feeding-related procedures such as UGI, pH probes, endoscopy, and stomach-emptying procedures. She should find out when these were done and by whom, and what the results were.

Many children may have received various direct and consultative therapies before this referral for a feeding evaluation. Other children, on the other hand, are coming for an initial evaluation. The therapist should discover what has worked and not worked in previous therapies.

Current Therapies and School

Anytime a feeding assessment is done, it is important to know what direct or consultative therapies the child is receiving. If there is feeding or oral motor therapy, what is the approach and focus of the therapist?

The school that the child attends can be listed along with pertinent information and concerns. Staff from the child's school may need to be interviewed as a part of the assessment process. The parents may want the therapist to share recommendations with these individuals.

Feeding History

A specific feeding chronology provides the clinician with a historical view of when feeding difficulties began and how the infant responded to those problems. When did the parent first notice difficulties with feeding? The therapist should discuss early feeding skills. Was the child breast-fed or bottle-fed and how did he do? What formulas was the child on? Were there any formula intolerances? When were pureed baby foods and solids introduced? How did the child do in the transitions from liquids to purees and purees to solids? Were there any tube feeding experiences? Were there pleasant or unpleasant associations with mealtimes? These early experiences should be documented as they can influence the sensory, emotional, and experiential aspects of current eating patterns. Often, the feeding history helps the clinician understand how a child's progression from primarily medical, sensory, or neurological issues may begin to overlap with an emotional overlay attached to mealtimes.

Current Medications

The therapist should document what medications the child is taking and the reason for each. It is very helpful for the therapist to understand the appetite-related gastrointestinal side effects of each medication as she looks at the whole feeding picture.

Growth Parameters

Whenever possible, the therapist should document the child's current height, weight, head circumference, and height-to-weight ratio. Obtaining a growth chart also will help document the child's growth trends over time. The therapist should be sure the growth charts used have been appropriately adjusted for prematurity, and that specialty growth charts have been used, where appropriate (i.e., Down Syndrome charts).

Mealtime Routine

It is helpful for the therapist to ask the parent to describe a typical day to better understand the current mealtime routine for the child. When does the child first take nourishment in the morning? About what time is that meal given? What and when does the child eat or drink during the remainder of the day? Where does the child eat and in what position? What textures does the child eat? What utensils does she use? It is important for the therapist to have a picture of the whole day and the family mealtime patterns as she reviews mealtime interactions and appetite.

Child's Developmental Skills

The child's overall developmental skills provide an understanding of the foundational skills that are available to support feeding, mealtime skills, and mealtime behaviors. The therapist should document head control, trunk control, rolling, sitting, crawling, walking, and climbing skills.

Mealtime Relationship and Interactions

The therapist should describe the specifics of mealtime interactions. Is the feeding interaction positive for the child and the parent? Does the child provide consistent and clear cues? Does the parent respond appropriately to those cues? Does the parent support the developmental feeding stages of the child?

Mealtime Communication Skills (Strengths and Challenges)

It is important to document the child's individual style(s) of communication. Does the child have the opportunity to communicate with the feeder? How does the child communicate? What primary areas express the child's communication signals (e.g., eye gaze, vocalization, facial expression, body movement, mouth movements, words)? Does the child point or use sign language, picture boards, or other augmentative communication system? Are the child's cues consistent and easy to interpret, or are they inconsistent and difficult to read? Does the child's intent to communicate have an impact on body skills or interfere with feeding skills?

Mealtime Physical Skills (Strengths and Challenges)

Positioning and Seating

This section includes observations on physical challenges for the child and the feeder. It includes information on the usual setting for mealtime (e.g., alone, with the entire family, next to the feeder, across from the feeder). The therapist should note the specifics of the actual feeding position of the child. Is a specific seating system used? The therapist then should observe the feeder's position. Is the feeder physically comfortable? Does the feeder's position support the child's needs? What aspects of positioning are working or not working for the child and the feeder?

Tone and Posture

The therapist should describe the child's muscle tone at rest and during feeding, noting specific difficulties with body control that influence feeding abilities as the child is fed or attempts independent feeding.

Mealtime Sensory Skills (Strengths and Challenges)

It is important to document the sensory strengths and challenges of the child that are related to the food as well as to the mealtime environment. The clinician should note the child's abilities to register, modulate, and integrate sensory information. She should document the texture, taste, and temperature of foods and liquids that the child enjoys as well as those that give the child trouble. In general, the therapist needs to know the child's reaction to many aspects of sensation during feeding as well as at non-feeding times. Does the child experience hyper- or hyposensitivities to specific types of sensory input?

Mealtime Oral Motor Skills (Strengths and Challenges)

Active components of normal feeding skills tell the therapist what is already working for the child. These become the building blocks for the feeding plan. The therapist should record the normal components of each separate part of the mouth, jaw, lips, cheeks, and tongue, and then describe how they are coordinated during sucking, swallowing, biting, and chewing.

Areas of oral motor development that limit acquisition and refinement of oral-feeding skills create the roadblocks to progress. The information that is recorded in this area depends on the nature of the physical and sensory patterns that are observed (e.g., problems with rhythmicity, grading of movement, tongue thrust, lip retraction).

Treatment Explorations

During the evaluation, the therapist will refine diagnostic assumptions by exploring a variety of changes in the areas listed previously. Each of these explorations can provide a learning opportunity to clarify the child's abilities and needs as well as to develop the initial approach to a treatment plan. The therapist should list the ideas explored and how successfully they met the criteria of obtaining a desirable change without also producing an undesirable change.

Ongoing Questions

What are the questions that remain unanswered? What information is still needed? Does the therapist need to see birth or growth records? Why does the child receive a specific medication that may interfere with growth or appetite levels? Does a neurological evaluation or vision evaluation seem appropriate? This section serves as a reminder for the ongoing gathering of information.

Challenges

This section offers an initial opportunity to list the challenges facing the child and family. The therapist should summarize ideas related to goals and objectives for the child and a general direction for the future.

It is important to create an interim plan or set of recommendations. The nature of this plan depends on the type of setting in which the assessment takes place. Some programs allow for a single diagnostic session with a child and family. Others support the option of follow-up evaluations at short intervals. Some are completed by a single therapist. Others involve the input from a full team of professionals. Some of the following questions must be addressed: Who is going to take responsibility for different recommendations? What is the time line for these recommendations? What is the plan for following up with other team members? Are more assessment sessions necessary? What degree of treatment is recommended? What beginning strategies are suggested? Did the feeding therapist make specific requests of the parents (i.e., to present food in a specific way, get a growth chart, record certain behaviors, try to change the position of the child or feeder)?

Developing a Feeding Plan With the Parent

Every assessment should address the most immediate parental concerns with a Feeding Plan. This is created jointly at the time of the assessment and addresses the most important and most easily changeable areas that the therapist observed during the assessment. The clinician may develop a more detailed treatment plan if she has additional opportunities to work with the child and parents in a diagnostic-therapy setting or short-term treatment program. It may be very risky and discouraging to the family if the therapist chooses to create a long and detailed treatment plan based on a short, one-time assessment. Children may show very different physical, sensory, and eating patterns and behaviors at different times. Very specific suggestions and treatment protocols based on a single session may be inaccurate and inappropriate for the specific child and family, although they may fit the larger overview of a child with the specific cluster of feeding issues. Following are some general strategies that are important in helping families develop an initial direction for addressing and changing the mealtime and feeding issues. Chapter 10 provides a more detailed approach to moving from the assessment into setting priorities for a treatment program.

At the end of the period of observation and exploration, the clinician should summarize for the parent her perceptions of the child's strengths and needs. The therapist may discuss and explore these observations at the time that the parent is feeding the child or at a slightly later point in the evaluation. Ideally, the therapist has had the opportunity to record observations and review notes before offering specific suggestions. What changes that were explored have made positive changes in the child's feeding behaviors? What changes does the child willingly accept? What issues or behaviors are creating the greatest blocks to the child's spontaneous development of more advanced feeding skills? These observations must be related to the specific concerns or questions of the family. The clinician and the parents can discuss and explore a few changes that may make mealtime more pleasant and easier for both the parent and child. The therapist should remember that change occurs in small steps. No one can or should try to change everything at once. Changing mealtime skills is an ongoing process that occurs in many stages. Follow-up of the initial suggestions will be essential in the creation of long-range changes. This period toward the end of the assessment becomes a dialogue in which the therapist offers perceptions and suggestions, and the parents respond and modify ideas to blend with the reality of their home and resources.

Throughout the assessment process and collection of information, the focus has been on issues of the child, parent-child interactions, and the mealtime process. The child's learning strengths and weaknesses have been analyzed in an effort to determine the best approach to treatment. As the mealtime and feeding plan is developed, the parents' learning styles also must be considered. Each parent comes to the mealtime assessment with his or her own experiences and attitudes, as well as a foundation for learning. As the therapist shares information with the parents, it is very important that she looks at the specific parent learning styles (M. D. Klein, 1999). How the information is shared will depend on how best that parent learns.

Some parents want to watch the therapist feed the child, and they can easily imitate the components of the presentation that work. Others can observe the same demonstration and have a harder time imitating it. The clinician's familiarity with the techniques may make it look so easy to the parent who then may become frustrated during initial trials to repeat it. Some parents, too, have their own motor-planning issues that make motor imitation more of a challenge.

Other visual learners want to read all about the recommendations. They like to read a very detailed report and recommendations, and see pictures, drawings, instant photographs, or videotapes to reinforce the visual learning. Some of these parents want all of these visual supports; others need one or two.

Some parents are auditory learners who process best by hearing all about the theory and the feeding techniques or strategies. They may want the therapist to describe each part of the presentation technique. They may ask in great detail about the rationale for the approach.

For many parents, feeling the experience is the only way to learn it. The therapist may demonstrate the feeding technique on the parent, providing the same support for jaw control or spoon holding recommended for the child. This way, the parent can feel the precise pressure, timing, and subtleties of the presentation. For these parents, mealtime participation experiences are very helpful. They may want to try the participation experiences in *Mealtime Participation Guide* (Klein & Morris, 1999). Parents are guided through simulated physical and sensory feeding difficulties, developmental feeding challenges, and imagined feeding interactions. Participation can be a powerful tool in parent understanding of the challenges their child faces in feeding.

Many parents learn best from a combination of these teaching strategies. Therapists can use discussion, demonstration, participation experiences, handouts, notes, pictures, drawings, videotapes, and instant camera pictures creatively in combination to provide a rich sharing of information. Just as the child may learn best from a multisensory approach, so might the parent benefit from a combination of visual, verbal, and physical guidance.

Exploring the Initial Feeding Plan

Demonstrate the Feeding Plan

The therapist should demonstrate the new procedures, then allow the parent to experience feeding the child in the new way. A parent can become overwhelmed by the first feeding evaluation. There is so much to remember, and the emotional aspects of new reactions to the therapist's perceptions can block long-term memory. Parents often tell clinicians, "It looked so easy when you did it." When they get home, they may not be able to remember all the new procedures and achieve the desired results.

Children learn what to expect from each feeder. When an unfamiliar person explores new ways of feeding, the child has no preconceived notions of how the meal should progress. Changes often become possible because of the therapist's adventurous approach to the meal and the implication that change is possible. This is quite different from the expectations held by the parent-child partnership. Each knows what is familiar and expected. These expectations often form a set of unspoken suggestions that maintain the status quo. Furthermore, if the parent is persistent in implementing a change that the child is resisting, the child may temporarily increase the undesirable behaviors as a way of telling the parent that the old ways are more acceptable.

The therapist's success in making the desired feeding changes may be frustrating to some parents. They may have tried very hard to make the same changes, and they may perceive the ease with which the clinician makes them as evidence of their incompetence. The contrast between what is and what might be can be very frustrating. The situation demands a great deal of tact and sensitivity to their feelings. The clinician needs to make suggestions as a set of open-ended possibilities and explore them with the parent and child. The therapist also should encourage the parent to feed the child in the new way while guiding her verbally or physically. "What would happen if you lowered the spoon as you presented it?" or " See if slowing down the meal helps." or "Do you think it might be easier for Johnny if he were sitting up a bit taller?" As the parent tries these ideas, the therapist can give immediate, relevant feedback. The therapist can support the parent's nervousness and awkwardness at the newness of the approach. If a specific technique is involved, she may try to demonstrate it by actually feeding the parent. This participation experience enables the parent to understand the new methods through feeling. If the parent prefers to learn by observation, the therapist needs to respect the personal preference, especially if the therapist tends to be a strong kinesthetic learner who needs a hands-on approach to understand. Each parent's individual style of learning must be respected. When a relaxed, stress-free learning environment can be created for the parent, understanding will evolve. The therapist should ensure that the parent experiences some success with the process before ending the session. A therapist's haste to teach the parent everything at the end of the evaluation can create a stressful, hurried environment that compromises what might be possible.

Establishing a Follow-Up Plan

The therapist must establish a follow-up date, which could be scheduled a day, a few days, or perhaps a week later, for receiving and providing feedback. If a parent knows that support by phone or a follow-up visit is available, the initial steps in applying the information will be easier and less stressful.

Creating the Report

Who and What?

The report that follows the assessment is designed to communicate the findings and recommendations to others. The first decision that the feeding professional must make is determining who will be the primary consumer of the report. Is this a report that is written predominantly or exclusively for other professionals? Does it serve primarily as a supportive reminder for the parents? Is it a report that will be used equally by professionals and nonprofessionals who have contact with the child?

The target audience will guide the selection of language and recommendations that are made at the end of the descriptive portion of the report. For example, if the gastroenterologist has requested an assessment to determine the nature of the child's swallowing ability, the report will focus more heavily on the supporting and limiting aspects of the oral-pharyngeal mechanism that relate to swallowing. Other aspects of the full evaluation will be mentioned, but greater emphasis will be placed on the results of the clinical observations and diagnostic tests that identify the child's swallowing function. Most gastroenterologists would not be interested in recommendations describing how to improve the child's ability to form a bolus during chewing. They might, however, welcome suggestions that relate the most effective ways of positioning the child for future diagnostic testing. For example, if a child lies more quietly on a table with the knees slightly bent and a pillow under the head, this would become an important recommendation for conducting a reliable test of gastric emptying.

If the assessment were requested by the child's regular feeding therapist who is seeking appropriate directions for the therapy program, a very different type of report would be written. This report would address the questions of the most important areas for intervention and ways of relating to the child and family that would make progress in an ongoing treatment program more effective. It would offer treatment directions and strategies as a way of creating a more structured path for the therapist.

In many instances the report is written primarily for parents or other nonprofessionals. This is often the case when the therapist who conducts the evaluation is the same individual who is seeing the child for therapy. This type of report may contain specific goal-directions or recommendations for changes or updates in the child's mealtime program. If the therapist knows the child and family well, the report may contain very specific suggestions that serve as reminders of ways that the family can include therapeutic ideas at home. When there is not an ongoing relationship with the child and family, it is risky and even harmful to provide a list of specific things others should be doing for the child. Often, these suggestions turn out to be very inappropriate, or they are misunderstood when parents or other therapists do not have an in-depth understanding of the mealtime, oral motor, and feeding interrelationships.

How?

After completing the assessment, a narrative report may be written following the same general sequence as the assessment notes form. For example, the general report structure for someone using the Mealtime Assessment Guide (see pages 184–186) would include the following areas:

History and Concerns

Medical and Therapy History
Mealtime Concerns

Mealtime Observations

Developmental Skills
Mealtime Relationship and Interactions
Mealtime Communication Skills
Mealtime Physical Skills
Mealtime Sensory Skills
Mealtime Oral Motor Skills

Summary and Conclusions
Recommendations
Future Plans

If it is appropriate to make more specific recommendations of treatment strategies or specific techniques or equipment, the recommendations section becomes a more detailed *Feeding Plan*. The organization of the observations in the body of the report can lead naturally into the creation of the initial feeding plan. It is designed to help the child and family make changes in the mealtime patterns. This plan should follow the same sequence as the assessment. In each section of the feeding plan, the therapist should list the changes and goals that she has decided upon in these areas:

Learning Environment. What learning approaches and tools will be explored or included to allow the child and family to know that positive changes can be made? What changes would help the child focus attention during the meal?

Communication Environment. How should the environment be set up to maximize the feeder-child interaction? Should seating positions be changed to increase opportunities for eye contact? Should different language, pictures, signs, or gestures be used? Can the child be given more choices?

Physical Environment. What environmental seating and positioning changes should be made? Are the feeding utensils appropriate? Should the time for meals be changed?

Sensory Environment. What foods can be added to the child's meals? Are there any foods that are not currently appropriate? What changes can be made in taste, temperature, texture, or touch? Should there be more, less, or different background sounds during the meal?

Expansion of Oral Motor Skills. The therapist should describe the specific methods of feeding that she recommends. How should the food be presented? How long should the therapist wait for a specific response? Where does the child need physical support?

Follow-Up. What plans have been made to help the family carry out the therapist's suggestions? When will the therapist see the child again? Will she maintain interim telephone or written contact with the family? What support will she provide to the school program? When will a formal reevaluation be scheduled?

■ Links Between Assessment and Treatment

The Feeding Team

Feeding is a complex process. It involves a mouth, a jaw, teeth, a neck, shoulders, a trunk, hips, sitting skills, a digestive system, a mealtime environment, communication, a relationship to the feeder... the list is infinite. Feeding strategies that are appropriate for the child require input from a great many people. It involves team problem-solving and team creativity. A look at the team players and their roles in the feeding assessment is helpful.

The Child

The child is the most important team player. The clinician must listen and watch for the child's guiding clues about needs and approaches that will be successful.

The Parents

The parents usually are the child's primary feeders. They have the day-to-day insights into the feeding needs of their child. They have a sense of their child's abilities, and they know what improves or diminishes these abilities. Parents come with feeding concerns. They are the individuals to whom the therapist gears her recommendations.

When the clinician makes suggestions, the inner responses of the parents serve as reflectors of their knowledge of the child. Some ideas ring true, while others are rejected. This inner filter is constructed from their knowledge of their child's needs. Parents sometimes are told that the professional is the one who knows the child. A gap of discomfort may develop when what they are told does not coincide with their knowledge. Parents create the feeding environment at home and have the most direct impact on the mealtime process for the child. The therapist should listen and watch for their cues. She should teach them with words, demonstrations, photographs, written descriptions, and direct experience of the techniques. The therapist should learn from what they tell her about their child, home, beliefs, and priorities. She should enable them to continue their primary role as the child's parents by incorporating suggestions for therapeutic approaches that enhance their parental interaction and relationship with their child.

The Feeding Therapist

The therapist who plays the role of detective in the discovery of oral motor strengths and needs for eating can be called the feeding therapist. This person could have many different professional labels. Special training in the area of feeding is the primary prerequisite. A feeding therapist could be a speech-language pathologist, an occupational therapist, a physical therapist, a nurse, a dietitian, or a special educator. When many specialists become involved with the child and family, the individual with the strongest interest and background in the assessment and treatment of feeding problems can assume the role of the feeding therapist.

The Speech-Language Pathologist

The speech-language pathologist can play a vital role in helping other team players listen to or read the child's communicative signals at a meal. Additional ways of enhancing or augmenting the communicative process can be explored. The SLP has a strong understanding of the anatomy and physiology of the oral structures for speech. If specific training in the use of these structures in feeding has not been included in the professional education program, the SLP who is interested in developing these skills already has a basic knowledge of the systems that are involved.

The Occupational Therapist

The occupational therapist can determine the child's sensory and motor readiness for self-feeding. With a professional emphasis on movement and sensory abilities, the occupational therapist can help with questions related to seating and the child's active physical participation in the meal. Many occupational therapists have an interest or background in the areas of perception and sensory integration. They can provide valuable input for the child with feeding problems related to these areas.

The Physical Therapist

The physical therapist also has a strong background and orientation to postural tone and movement. Work that the feeding therapist includes to develop head and trunk control will be done in coordination with the child's physical therapy program. Many children are able to eat with better physical control when a feeding therapy session or a meal follows the physical therapy session. The physical therapist frequently has received training in the selection or construction of special seating systems and can help the feeding therapist develop a seating system that will provide an appropriate degree of support and control.

The Physician

The physician determines the overall level of health and wellness of the child. Specialty physicians can determine the specific health of the gastrointestinal tract, growth rate, allergic reactions, and neurologic status. In many settings, the physician assumes the role of team leader and coordinates the specific services received by the child.

The Dietitian

The dietitian understands the areas of nutrition, caloric intake, and caloric expenditure. Recommendations can be made to the team for the quantity and types of food needed by the child. Many dietitians are now taking special courses on the development of oral-feeding skills and ways of working with children who have feeding difficulties to increase their ability to take in a higher quality diet. Their recommendations can be made with a clearer understanding of the child's physical and sensory needs and abilities.

The Teacher

The classroom teacher is an important feeder at school. Because they are involved with feeding snacks and lunches each day, teachers can assess the effectiveness of feeding recommendations and suggest alternative proposals. In programs where children receive very few direct therapy services for feeding, a specially trained teacher will assume the role of the feeding therapist.

The Dentist

The pediatric dentist can provide important information on the status of a child's oral health. Many feeding problems become exaggerated because of disease of the teeth and gums and structural malformations of the mouth. The dentist is a primary team member when a child has a craniofacial malformation such as Pierre Robin sequence or cleft palate.

Other Medical Specialists

Gastroenterologists, pulmonologists, allergists, neurologists, radiologists, endocrinologists, and other medical specialists can be involved in the detective work needed to fully understand the child's growth and feeding issues.

The Social Worker and Case Manager

Social workers or case managers often are involved in supporting the social and community services available to the family. These team members can be very supportive in finding funding for needed supplies and services and in coordination of some of the multitude of services often offered these children.

The Psychologist

Psychologists may become involved with the feeding team when parents or children are having emotional and relational difficulties that interfere with the child's development of mealtime and feeding skills.

The feeding team functions best when an integrated, sharing model is used. Each member learns from other members of the team and applies total concepts across discipline boundaries. A family and child may see each member of the team individually, but each team member incorporates the broader needs and perspectives into recommendations that are given. Thus, a physical therapist becomes skilled at understanding the child's nonverbal communication signals, and the dietitian provides food recommendations in textures and quantities that the child can handle in a reasonable time period. The feeding therapist understands the possible medical issues and complications that can arise with the child and is able to make educated guesses that call for direct medical consultation. A phone call to discuss concerns and a request for further consultation can increase the efficiency with which medical care is provided for the child.

A feeding team needs to work together. Effective teamwork is characterized by common goals and a willingness to cooperate. Teamwork has the potential to create the best possible feeding program for a child. Individual team members are challenged to create for themselves an openness to learning, a desire to improve individual skills, and the willingness to develop their abilities to interact positively with others. When each person makes such a commitment, programs can improve and grow to meet the ever-changing needs of each child.

The Process

Assessment and treatment are sides of the same coin. Each assessment contains treatment probes to discover the most effective approaches to remediating the difficulties that have brought the child and family for the evaluation. Each treatment session contains short assessments during every session. The feeding therapist briefly evaluates the situation at the beginning of the session and assesses the child's response to different strategies and techniques used during therapy.

The most effective treatment programs are those that are built on an in-depth understanding of the feeding and mealtime dynamics and the interrelationships that are identified in the more formal assessment. Chapter 10 will explore ways of organizing information from the assessment that lead logically and intuitively into appropriate goal-directions for treatment.

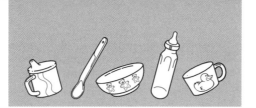

Parent Mealtimes Questionnaire
Eating and Drinking Skills

Child's Name _____ Today's Date _____

Date of Birth _____ Child's Age _____

Parent Name(s) _____

Primary Care Doctor _____

Name of Parent Completing This Questionnaire _____

History and Concerns About Eating and Drinking

What are the feeding concerns you have for your child?

What illness or surgical procedures has your child had?

Is your child on medications? If yes, what are they?

What previous feeding assessments or studies has your child had?

Is a dietitian working with your child? If yes, who and how often?

Is your child receiving therapy? If yes, what kind and with whom?

Does your child attend a preschool or school program? If yes, where?

(continued)

Parent Mealtimes Questionnaire (continued)

Describe your child's early feeding history:

☐ Breast-fed? How long? Problems?

☐ Bottle-fed? Problems?

What formula(s) was/is your baby on?

How did your baby tolerate formula?

When did you introduce pureed foods (e.g., First Foods or homemade)?

How did your child do with pureed foods?

How did your child do with the transition to lumpy and solid foods?

When did the feeding problems begin?

Current Feeding Routine

How often does your child eat and drink? What are his or her usual meal and snack times?

What foods/liquids does your child usually eat for:

Breakfast

Lunch

Dinner

Snack(s)

(continued)

How is the food prepared? (Check all that apply.)

☐ Regular liquid

☐ Thick liquid

☐ Commercial pureed baby First or Second Foods

☐ Prepared in the blender

☐ Ground or commercial Third Foods

☐ Mashed soft table foods

☐ Regular table food (easy)

☐ Regular table food (hard)

☐ Other (Please specify.)

Which of these types of food are easiest for your child?

Which of these types of food are hardest for your child?

What do you usually use when feeding your child? (Check all that apply.)

☐ Breast	☐ Fork	☐ Bottle
☐ Fingers	☐ Cup	☐ Straw
☐ Spoon		

Which of the following can your child use independently?

| ☐ Fork | ☐ Spoon | ☐ Bottle |
| ☐ Fingers | ☐ Cup | ☐ Straw |

Does your child have favorite food tastes? What are they?

Does your child have favorite food textures? What are they?

Does your child prefer food at a certain temperature (e.g., cold, warm, hot, room temperature)?

(continued)

Who usually feeds your child?

Who else can feed your child?

Where is your child fed (e.g., in a chair, on your lap)?

How long does it take to feed your child?

What is the average amount of food and liquid your child takes during that time?

Does your child have any food allergies that you are aware of?

Do any other family members have allergies (e.g., food, chemicals, pollens, molds)?

Does your child have problems with:
  Gagging? (Please describe.)

  Gastroesophageal Reflux? (Please describe.)

  Vomiting? (Please describe.)

  Constipation? (Please describe.)

Other comments:

_____

Parent Signature

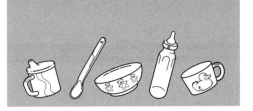

Parent Mealtimes Questionnaire

Tube Feedings and Beginning Oral Feedings

Child's Name _____ Today's Date _____

Date of Birth _____ Child's Age _____

Parent Name(s) _____

Primary Care Doctor _____

Name of Parent Completing This Questionnaire _____

History and Concerns About Tube Feedings

What are the feeding concerns you have for your child?

What illness or surgical procedures has your child had?

Is your child on medications? If yes, what are they?

What previous feeding assessments or studies has your child had?

Is a dietitian working with your child? If yes, who and how often?

Is your child receiving therapy? If yes, what kind and with whom?

Does your child attend a preschool or school program? If yes, where?

Describe your child's early feeding history:
    ☐ Breast-fed?   How long?   Problems?

    ☐ Bottle-fed?   How long?   Problems??

What formula(s) was/is your baby on?

(continued)

How did your baby tolerate formula?

When did you introduce pureed foods (e.g., commercial or homemade)?

How did your child do with pureed foods?

How did your child do with the transition to lumpy and solid foods?

When did the feeding problems begin?

Describe your child's history with a feeding tube

What diagnostic tests have been done? When?

What type of tube does your child have?
- ☐ Nasogastric?
- ☐ Gastrostomy?   If so, which kind: ☐ Button?   ☐ Jejeunostomy?
- ☐ Catheter?
- ☐ Other?

Why was your child given a feeding tube?

When did your child have the tube placed?

Who placed the tube? Where?

(continued)

Did your child have a fundoplication? If yes, when?

What was your child's response to the fundoplication?

What physician monitors your child's tube-feedings?

How has your child adjusted to the tube placement?

Current Feeding Routine

What formula do you put in the tube?

Who usually feeds your child?

Who else can feed your child?

Where is your child tube-fed (e.g., in a chair, on your lap, in bed)?

What is your child's current tube-feeding schedule?
   Daytime?
   Nighttime?

If bolus tube feedings are given, how long does each feeding take?

Do you or your child have difficulties with tube feedings? If there are problems (e.g., amount, timing, retching, gagging, vomiting), please describe them. When do they happen and how do you handle them?

(continued)

Fill out the following if your child takes any food or liquid by mouth.

Who usually feeds your child?

Where do you usually feed your child (e.g., in a chair, on your lap, in bed)?

What foods or liquids do you offer your child?

Does your child have favorite food tastes? What are they?

Does your child have favorite food textures? What are they?

Does your child prefer food at a certain temperature (e.g., cold, warm, hot, room temperature)?

How long does each oral feeding last?

Do you or your child have difficulties with the beginning oral feedings? If there are problems (e.g., interest, coughing, mouth movements), please describe them. When do they happen and how do you handle them?

Does your child have food or other allergies that you are aware of?

Do any other family members have allergies (e.g., food, chemicals, pollens, molds)?

(continued)

Parent Mealtimes Questionnaire (continued)

Does your child have problems with:

Gagging? (Please describe.)

Gastroesophageal Reflux? (Please describe.)

Vomiting? (Please describe.)

Constipation? (Please describe.)

Other comments:

Parent Signature

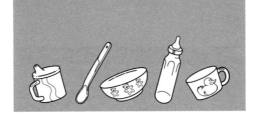

Mealtime Assessment Guide

Child's Name	Assessment Date(s)
Date of Birth	Chronological Age Adjusted Age
Parent Name(s)	
Primary Care Doctor	Today's Date

History and Concerns

Parent Concerns

Other Concerns

Diagnoses/Medical History

Previous Therapies/Assessments

Current Therapies/School

Feeding History

Current Medications   Side effects?

Growth Parameters   Growth Chart Available?   ☐ Yes   ☐ No
     Height   _____ %
     Weight   _____ %
     Head Circumference   _____ %
     Height-to-Weight Ratio   _____ %

Mealtime Routine

(continued)

Mealtime Observations

Child's Developmental Skills (e.g., overall head and trunk control, rolling, sitting, walking)

Mealtime Relationship and Interactions (e.g., emotions, type of relationship, type of interaction)

Mealtime Communication Skills (e.g., facial expression, gestures, ACC system, speech)
    Strengths

    Challenges

Mealtime Physical Skills (e.g., muscle tone, seating, utensils)
    Strengths

    Challenges

Mealtime Sensory Skills (e.g., registration, modulation, integration, taste, smell, texture)
    Strengths

    Challenges

(continued)

Mealtime Oral Motor Skills (e.g., suck, swallow, bite, chew, spoon, cup, straw, jaw, tongue, lips/cheeks)

Strengths

Challenges

Summary Planning

Treatment Explorations

Ongoing Questions

Challenges

Plan

Send Report To:

Feeding Clinician

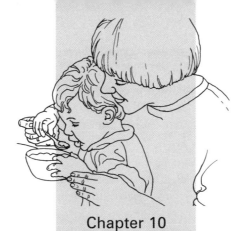

Chapter 10
The Bridge to Treatment: Setting Priorities and Problem Solving

Organizing Information

Treatment planning based on a careful assessment of the child's strengths, needs, and desires is the most critical aspect of building an effective therapy program. The treatment plan begins at the time of the evaluation, as information from the evaluation becomes organized into its basic elements. Isolated bits of information are sorted out and observed in relationship to each other. Memory and understanding are easier when information fits into a pattern. If a person is asked to remember a list of 25 foods to purchase at the grocery store, he may have some difficulty if they are placed in random order. If, however, the list is organized by departments in the grocery store (e.g., dairy, produce, paper goods, bread), it will become easier. It may be easier still if the person knows that these are all items for a picnic and the list is formed of food clusters (i.e., hot dogs, buns, ketchup, mustard, lettuce, tomato, cucumber, salad dressing). Meaningful associations are helpful to remembering and seeing the patterns that lead to other helpful observations.

As therapists begin to organize their observations and notes about a child, their first job is to be able to clearly describe what they have observed and learned about the child. The language that they choose also allows them to be clear about the differences between an objective description and an interpretation.

Their second job is to identify ways of organizing the information so that patterns become clear, and they can sort out and prioritize the most important elements for their attention. Many therapists create treatment recommendations and programs that work on individual splinter skills. Often these splinter skills are inappropriate for the child because the child needs prerequisite skills. For example, one therapist developed a program around the treatment goal to teach 5-year-old Chandler to chew. She worked diligently with recommendations and techniques to obtain tongue lateralization. She placed food between the lateral biting surfaces of the teeth as Chandler's tongue moved in and out of his mouth, and he grimaced and complained. She tried holding his mouth closed to keep the tongue inside. Another therapist showed her how to stimulate the sides of the tongue with a Nuk Massage brush, and Chandler began to cry. She developed a program to reinforce his positive attempts to move his tongue and to punish his complaining and crying. Chandler hated coming to therapy, but still the therapist persisted in her goals to help him develop chewing skills. The therapist was correct in identifying Chandler's lack of chewing skills. However, she did not associate his strong suckle pattern of the tongue and his oral sensory defensiveness with his lack of chewing. Chandler hated any stimulation in his mouth. He had never put his fingers in his mouth and had never mouthed or explored toys. He barely accepted the feeling of pureed food on the spoon. If she had spent their time helping him develop a comfortable relationship with non-food sensory input in the mouth, he would have developed many of the separate skills that depend on this foundational skill. She also would have avoided developing the stressful adversarial relationship that evolved. The most important thing that Chandler learned was to hate therapy and be extremely cautious and suspicious about anyone who approached his mouth.

Therapists can organize information in a wide variety of ways, looking at an overall picture or pattern as well as at very specific functional skills. They can build from the more specific view to the larger view or they can get a sense of the major patterns involved and then explore the detailed organization.

This chapter will introduce a number of alternative ways of organizing and prioritizing information as a bridge to an appropriate and effective therapy program. The Mealtime Assessment Guide (pages 184–186) provides a structure for initially organizing mealtime observations into the broad categories of Developmental Skills, Mealtime Relationships and Interactions, Mealtime Communication Skills, Mealtime Physical Skills, Mealtime Sensory Skills, and Mealtime Oral Motor Skills. Information within each section is organized according to the child's strengths and challenges.

Typically, therapists begin with a global look at the child's assessment and a broader gestalt for organizing information. It is initially very helpful to think in terms of Major Feeding Clusters (pages 188–189), What Works?/What Doesn't Work? (page 193), or Big Picture (pages 205–208) models for organization and problem solving. More linear ways of organizing, such as the Pattern Clusters (pages 196–197) or Component Skills models (pages 208–211), are very helpful in breaking down specific areas in a more linear manner and arriving systematically at problem resolutions.

Major Feeding Clusters

As therapists gather information on children, overall impressions will emerge. It is helpful to initially select four major clusters or categories and gain a sense of a child's overall issues. As therapists view children, their assessment results, and their treatment needs, four distinct groupings or clusters of feeding problems emerge. Although most children do not fall neatly and exclusively into one group or another, most show predominant issues and needs in one of the following groups. Other children will show such a complex mixture of these four areas that the therapist must identify the basic category along with additional groups or clusters that have developed as compensations or from lack of experience.

Motor-Based Feeding Problems

Children with motor-based feeding problems show primary difficulties with postural tone and movement. Their muscle tone is high, low, or fluctuating. Their movement patterns often reflect automatic or total reflexive movement synergies that interfere with more precise and volitional movements. Most of these youngsters have difficulty with the coordination and timing of movement. In the feeding area this is reflected in the incoordination of mouth and body movements. It also affects the coordination and timing of sucking, swallowing, and breathing. Highly specific problems with oral motor control during feeding are common in motor-based feeding problems.

Sensory systems frequently are involved in children with motor-based difficulties. Because of tense muscles and total patterns of movement, input that is unexpected or accompanied by high levels of anticipation or emotion becomes exaggerated and further reduces movement control. Sensory guidance and feedback of movement is affected, making it difficult for children to monitor, correct, or repeat specific movement patterns.

Many of these youngsters have an emotional response to lack of control. They may repeatedly, but unsuccessfully, try to do something. They become discouraged and give up. There is often a high level of learned helplessness in this group of children who may feel that they are victims of their bodies (Seligman, 1991). Other children in this group experience intermittent success with movement and temperamentally become determined to do what they want to do.

Maxwell is a child with cerebral palsy. His overall coordination difficulties contribute to major feeding difficulties. When food initially enters his mouth, he retracts his tongue slightly into the pharyngeal airway, which contributes to a noisy, stressed breathing pattern. Oral movements are disorganized, and he frequently loses control of the food and coughs. Maxwell is a child with a motor-based feeding problem.

Kelsey has mild low tone and postural instability. She enjoys eating, and sucks and swallows soft food relatively easily. She has difficulty with chewing because of her low tone. Biting is weak and poorly sustained. Although she can move her tongue to the side when food is placed between her teeth, she has difficulty keeping it in place while she chews. Food falls into her cheek cavity or onto the back of her tongue before she has finished chewing. She sometimes gags and chokes because she cannot physically control the movement of solid food. Kelsey is a child with a motor-based feeding problem.

Treatment strategies for this group of children center on the overriding issues of physical movement coordination and its influence on feeding. Preparation for the meal through positioning and handling becomes particularly critical for the successful use of any oral motor strategy or technique. These children may benefit from specific techniques to increase or guide movements in the mouth. Specific ideas for this group of children are introduced in Chapter 15. Overt or silent aspiration may be a particular risk when motor-control issues dominate. Children with motor-based feeding issues may receive tube feedings because they cannot swallow safely or eat enough food to grow and thrive.

Sensory-Based Feeding Problems

Children with sensory-based feeding problems have difficulty eating because their sensory systems do not support the complex process of eating and drinking. In some instances the actual sensory intake system is affected. Paralysis or dysfunction of cranial nerves I, V, VII, IX, and X result in a lack of sensory input to various areas of the nose, mouth, and pharynx that are involved in eating and drinking. Smell or taste may be affected, or the child may lack the sensory guidance in specific muscle groups that is critical to coordinated movement. Children who are blind must learn to compensate for the impact that their visual loss has on eating, especially in the area of self-feeding.

The majority of children in this group have difficulty modulating and integrating the sensory input that they receive. They overreact or underreact to their environment and to specific oral sensory information. They may experience sensory overload at mealtimes or deal with sensory defensiveness through one or more sensory channels. Some children with sensory-based feeding problems receive their meals by feeding tube and do not eat orally because they cannot stand the sensory feelings involved in eating. Diagnostic testing of swallowing coordination is usually normal. Others eat orally but are very picky eaters, limiting their intake to foods that feel or look safe and comfortable to them. They may be highly distractible at mealtimes or have strong emotional reactions when something threatening or uncomfortable occurs. Because of their discomfort with sensory input to the mouth or hands, many of these children have a history of limited mouthing and oral exploration.

Many children with sensory-based feeding difficulties also have difficulties with muscle tone and motor coordination. Problems with mild low tone and postural instability are common. Although the overall treatment program should address these issues, they have a much lower priority than the sensory issues.

Sensory experiences have a profound influence on this group of children who seem to remember painful, uncomfortable, or stressful respiratory, gastrointestinal, emotional, or medical experiences for a long time. They become linked with children's basic drive to survive and protect themselves from danger. The fight-or-flight system is chronically activated during sensory defensiveness (Wilbarger & Wilbarger, 1991). Because many of the original experiences become linked with this system, the system becomes reactivated when the child is reminded of the past events. A past or current history of gastroesophageal reflux or other form of gastrointestinal discomfort is highly significant in this group of children.

Many of these sensory responses at mealtime trigger strong negative emotions. Some children have major temper tantrums or act aggressively against others at mealtime. Others will fall apart and retreat as far as possible from engaging with others at the meal. Ritualistic behaviors often give them the external sense of control that they lack internally.

Noah, age 3, has recently been diagnosed with pervasive developmental disorder (PDD). He is extremely sensitive to many sounds and dislikes being touched. He was an irritable, colicky infant who had difficulty with sleep. He was able to breast-feed well in short spurts but had a great deal of difficulty remaining on the breast for extended periods. His feeding problems began when his mother introduced pureed foods. He hated the spoon, cried, and spit out the food. He now takes rice cereal and creamed corn but still receives his primary nutrition through breast-feeding. He becomes extremely upset at the sight or smell of any other foods. Noah has a sensory-based feeding problem.

Erica, age 4, has been tube-fed since birth. She had severe gastroesophageal reflux with vomiting as an infant and was placed on a feeding pump for 20 hours a day. Bolus tube feedings are difficult to introduce because she continues to experience discomfort when given more than 1 ounce at a time. She often will panic and begin to cry and push the syringe away after a 1/2 ounce. Erica intensely dislikes wet or dirty feelings on her face or hands. She hates the sensation of walking or sitting in the grass, and she cries when her family takes her to the beach. Erica never puts toys in her mouth and screeches whenever her mother tries to brush her teeth. She began to eat small amounts of food when her therapist introduced her to pickles and lemons. She seems to enjoy strong bitter and sour tastes. She rejects all other foods. Erica is a child with a sensory-based feeding problem.

Treatment strategies for this group of children center on the predominant issues of sensory processing and their influence on feeding. Getting ready for the meal by preparing the entire sensory system becomes particularly critical in helping the child accept and integrate the specific sensory input of the meal. The specific techniques used are totally different for these children than those used when children have a motor-based feeding problem. They may benefit from specific techniques to shift sensory awareness, increase sensory comfort and organization, or increase sensory discrimination in the mouth. Specific ideas for this group of children are introduced in Chapter 14.

Structurally Based Feeding Problems

Children with structurally based feeding problems may be a very distinct group characterized only by their structural limitations. They may also be a very mixed group with structural limitations combined with motor or sensory problems. The initial feeding issues center around issues such as cleft lip and palate, contractures at the temporomandibular joint, tracheoesophageal fistula, esophageal atresia, or short bowel syndrome. The original structures that were designed to support efficient feeding are altered in a way that is incompatible with safe eating or that require the child to use compensatory movements to succeed.

Children whose structural problems involve the face and mouth are usually fed with modifications of the feeding position, nipple, and bottle. When sensory and motor systems are intact, these children generally acquire functional feeding skills. When the structural problems affect the esophagus or gastrointestinal system, tube feedings may be the initial or long-term option.

Most of these children experience multiple surgeries that involve invasion, pain, or discomfort in the mouth and throat. Surgery that reconstructs a mouth or an esophagus changes the physical and sensory organization that the child has been using for swallowing. In a sense, the child has a new mouth that works differently from the old mouth. New sets of movements and sensations are involved. Old compensations are no longer necessary. In addition, scar tissue may limit or restrict some movements. When an esophagus has been reconnected or reconstructed, its motility often is reduced.

Many of these children are extremely protective of their mouths. They guard themselves from oral examinations and feeding techniques that invade the mouth because of their prior experiences. A great deal seems to depend on their sensory status and temperament; however, many children in this group respond as if they have experienced trauma to the face and mouth and will do anything to protect themselves.

Motility problems of the esophagus and gastrointestinal system often are technically physiological rather than structural. Children whose feeding limitations are strictly because of reflux or the physiological response to surgical procedures such as a fundoplication also may fall into this group. Their underlying physical and sensory processing is in the normal range. Medical or surgical correction of their motility issues usually results in a functional ability to eat. However, complications from surgery or side effects of medications can contribute additional problems that affect the child's ability and desire to eat.

Rosa, age 18 months, was born with massive craniofacial anomalies. She was missing several bones in her skull and had a full cleft of the hard and soft palates. She spent long periods in the hospital undergoing reconstructive surgery. She will require more surgery to add to the bone of the hard palate when she is older. Although she has a warm smile and loves people, Rosa immediately becomes guarded if anyone approaches her mouth. This has become a problem for her mother, who must insert a small plastic obturator in the front of her hard palate each morning. Rosa screams and becomes extremely upset. She takes formula from a Haberman Feeder but has difficulty coordinating her mouth for more solid foods. Rosa is a child with a structurally based feeding problem.

Many children with structurally based feeding problems do well when therapy is geared toward providing position, food, and equipment modifications for eating and helping them learn compensatory movements to support eating. However, major difficulties arise when children with structural challenges also have mild coordination or sensory limitations. These children often lack the ability to use compensatory movements to adjust to their underlying structural difficulty. They may have exceptional difficulties adjusting to the changes in sensory feedback after surgery, or they strongly reject adult intervention that could help them reorganize their oral-sensorimotor coordination. They may develop survival and protective behaviors around eating because of their original surgical experiences or lack of positive oral experiences (Di Scipio & Kaslon, 1982; Dowling, 1977; Geertsma, Hyams, Pelletier, & Reiter, 1985). Specific ideas for children in this group with gastrointestinal discomfort or cleft lip and palate are introduced in Chapters 22 and 25.

Experientially Based Feeding Problems

Children with experientially based feeding problems are characterized by the behavioral choices they have made to feel safe, comfortable, or accepted. These choices may represent a more general approach to life or be very specific to eating and mealtimes. Some of these children have underlying physical, sensory, or structural feeding problems. However, the initial issues surrounding eating have become buried under the child's defensive or offensive strategies to win food wars. Most of these children are engaged in a battle that distorts mealtime roles and relationships. Their battles are typically waged against the adults who feed them. Children may attempt to usurp adult roles by demanding specific foods and feeding routines. Adults may insist on regulating what and how much the child eats. Each recognizes that the other is imposing in an area that is not theirs and fights for their rights. Power contests emerge. Initial belief systems about roles and relationships become more entrenched and force-feeding often results. Children refuse to eat, eat a very limited diet, or insist that parents prepare specific foods before they will eat.

In some instances, the adult or child finds it easier to give in and give the other person what he is demanding. Consequently, children eat to the point of obesity, and adults prepare and offer only foods that they know the child will eat. Neither side feels happy or fulfilled.

Often these battles are extremely subtle. Parents who are concerned about a child's poor weight gain will insist on "just one more bite." Children may learn to eat through a system of bribes or rewards that shifts their attention from an internal to an external guidance system for eating. Children may choose not to eat because they are uncomfortable, remember a painful eating experience, or remember abuse to the face or mouth. As a group, these children feel out of control unless they demand control at mealtimes. They learn very quickly that no one can make them eat.

Gerry is 2. He is growing well but has mild delays in fine motor and speech development. His diet is limited to hot dogs, bologna, chicken, hash brown potatoes, bananas, crackers, and cookies. He chews well, uses a spoon and fork, and drinks from a wide variety of cups. His appetite for food is limited because he demands milk and soda all day. He typically drinks 3 quarts of milk throughout the day and will drink only sodas at mealtime. Gerry is a very powerful, demanding child whose mother gives him whatever food or drink he requests. He cries if he doesn't get his own way and tantrums if someone tells him "no." His mother doesn't like him to make a fuss at meals and will avoid his tantrums by giving in to all of his demands. Gerry is a child with an experientially based feeding problem.

Marissa, at 21 months, has cystic fibrosis. She has many dietary restrictions because of her lung and pancreatic problems. Her body has high caloric needs, but Marissa has a low appetite level. If she eats when she feels too full, her stomach hurts. Her mother knows that her health needs require her to eat more food, and she pushes Marissa to eat more at each meal. Marissa refuses, and her mother pushes more food. Marissa pushes back and each meal ends in unhappiness. As Marissa feels more upset, she is less hungry and eats less. Her mother becomes frantic and forces the spoon into her mouth. Marissa is a child with an experientially based feeding problem.

Treatment strategies for this group of children center around helping the parent and child find a different mealtime relationship. In most cases this involves moving toward a division of responsibility in which the parent decides on the menu, time, and place for the meal. The child decides what and how much to eat. This is often a gradual process that must address belief systems about eating and parental fears that the child will not eat or eat enough to thrive. It involves helping parents reorganize the structure of the child's day and mealtimes, offer a variety of foods, and reintroduce foods that the child has rejected in the past.

Combination Feeding Problems

Many children have a primary basis for their feeding problem that is in one area. The problem can easily be just a motor problem, a sensory problem, a structural problem, or an experiential problem. However, many feeding problems are more complicated than that. As can be seen from the previous examples, many children who have motor-, sensory-, structural-, or experiential-based feeding difficulties develop complicated combination feeding problems. Although the basis for the difficulty usually starts out as one of these four factors, the emotional and interactional nature of feeding can quickly complicate the reactions of the child and the parent. As the therapist looks at the basis for a feeding problem, it is important to prioritize and understand the initial feeding problem and then look at the resultant compensations that combine to complicate that original reason for the feeding difficulty.

A child may have a motor-based feeding problem that causes a severe choking episode because of poor bolus control. This may lead to fear and refusal of new foods, which then adds an experiential component. The primary motor-based feeding problem is then combined with an experiential problem. Sensory-based feeding difficulties can end up looking like motor-based feeding problems because of the exaggerated or unusual movements the child uses in responding to sensations of the food presented or the poor ability to organize the mouth in response to the sensation of food. Thus, a sensory-based feeding problem can become a combination problem with sensory and motor components. Children with early repeated negative oral experiences, such as long-term ventilation or orogastric or nasogastric tube placement and replacement, can develop sensory-based feeding difficulties related to increased oral sensitivities and motor-based feeding problems because of a lack of normal oral sucking and swallowing experiences. Here, the experientially based feeding problem may develop into a combination feeding problem with sensory and motor components.

Donald is 11 months old. He has a history that includes prematurity with repaired tracheoesophageal fistula and esophageal atresia. A gastrostomy tube was placed in him shortly after birth. He had an oral replogle tube in place to suction the blind esophageal pouch until enough growth had taken place to allow surgery. At 5 months of age, he had surgery to reconnect the esophagus and then had weekly dilatations to stretch the narrowed esophageal repair site. Donald now is very upset as his mother tries to present foods by mouth. He clamps his mouth shut, turns away, or cries whenever she presents the spoon or bottle. His oral protectiveness comes from his oral experiences that he found unpleasant or negative. His refusal to eat is, for him, imperative for survival. Donald is a child with a structurally based feeding problem. Although structural repairs have been undertaken, he is still dealing with the post-surgical need to keep the esophagus open and the effects of scar tissue. External pressures from the surgeon and his mother have increased the intensity of the frightening and unpleasant experiences associated with management of these structural problems.

At the moment, his primary feeding issues are related to the acquired or compensatory experiential component. In addition, there are strong motor and sensory components from lack of practice with the oral skills necessary for sucking and swallowing. Feeding treatment for Donald must begin by addressing the experientially based components of this combined problem. It must include pleasant oral experiences and exploration to begin to rebuild the trust necessary as a foundation for feeding. Starting with the sensory or motor problems without a complete understanding of the experiential history probably will fail. A lack of understanding of the underlying structurally based problem can be disastrous because it is the foundational issue of his overall feeding difficulty and must be considered in the overall management of his feeding issues.

Feeding Problem Foundation and Developed or Compensatory Feeding Problem

As the therapist looks at the basis for feeding difficulties, it is important to determine the basis for the feeding problem as well as the developed or compensatory feeding complications. Table 10.1 on page 194 may help in the examination of the feeding-problem basis and the compensatory or developed feeding problem.

What Works? What Doesn't Work?

One of the simplest ways of organizing information is to look very pragmatically at four interrelated areas:

1. What is working for the child?
2. What is not working for the child?
3. What is working for the parent?
4. What is not working for parent?

The therapist can use informal descriptions of what is happening at the mealtime and focus on the ways in which the four elements can be brought together in a treatment program.

Kevin

Kevin is a severely involved 5-year-old boy who lives with Laura, his single mother. She has been trying diligently to help him move from tube feedings to oral feedings without a great deal of success.

Figure 10.1 on page 195 looks at what is working and what is not from both of their points of view.

Oral Feeding	Feeding Problem Foundation	Compensatory or Developed Feeding Problem(s)
Donald	Donald was born prematurely. He had a tracheoesophageal fistula and esophageal atresia. He had a gastrostomy tube placed shortly after birth.	At 11 months, Donald does not know how to eat orally and has no confidence in his oral skills for eating. He cannot organize his mouth for motorically swallowing around the food. Although he was born with the sucking and swallowing skills to eat, these skills were forgotten through disuse and different experiences. On this basis, Donald has developed an additional motor-based feeding problem.
	He had an oral replogle tube placed to suction secretions for 5 months.	
	He has received all nutrition by gastrostomy tube for 11 months.	
	Donald's esophagus was reconnected surgically when he was 5 months old. Since that time he has had weekly dilatation procedures to stretch out the anastomosis site. Though this has included general anesthesia, it has involved objects such as the anesthesia mask coming toward his face.	Donald now is orally overly sensitive to touch, and to liquid and food textures. He gags when food is presented. Donald's gagging can be considered a compensatory sensory-based feeding problem.
	The surgeon wants Donald to start taking foods orally to help keep the esophagus more open.	Donald's early oral experiences have combined in a negative way for him. He has not had pleasant oral-feeding experiences. The adults in Donald's environment want him to eat orally. They have pushed him to take food orally in an effort to keep the esophagus mobile and open. He is fighting these efforts because of fear and discomfort. His attempts to resist eating would be described as a compensatory experientially based feeding problem.
	His mother and therapist have tried to present tastes orally and really want him to eat.	
	Donald is now 11 months old with no experience sucking and swallowing or eating orally.	
	The structure of Donald's gastrointestinal system did not work for him and still provides primary limitations because of scar tissue and strictures. He has a structurally based feeding problem.	

Table 10.1   Examining Donald's Feeding Problems

What's Working and What's Not Working?

Date

	What's Working?	What's Not Working?
Child	Kevin is interested in how his body moves. He enjoys exploration of movement. When his body is well supported and quiet, he can repeat small movements such as opening and closing his hand as well as opening his mouth to look at his tongue in a mirror. He appears interested in learning to eat. His gastrointestinal system works well and supports a comfortable intake of 14–16 ounces of food and liquid by tube during each bolus feeding. He has a rhythmical suckle-swallow in swallowing his saliva and small amounts of food and liquid when the nasogastric tube is removed.	Kevin has extremes of flexion, extension and asymmetry in involuntary movements. Movement often is very disorganized. This pattern is worse when he sits in a chair. He has breathing incoordination at rest, during movement, and during oral feeding. His nonverbal communication skills are inconsistent and difficult to understand. Sensory input (touch, taste, and texture) triggers disorganized movements. He is afraid of fingers, spoons, and cups jabbing his mouth. The nasogastric tube reduces his comfort in sucking and swallowing while the tube is in. Oral-feeding practice occurs only ½ day per week when the NG-tube is changed and is out of the nasopharyngeal area.
Parent	Laura has supported her son's health and wellness by preparing a highly nutritious blenderized formula of organic food and supplements. Since starting this formula, Kevin has moved from a state of chronic illness to wellness. He has good energy and is rarely ill. This is very important to her. Laura has developed a sensitive, supportive style with her son that encourages Kevin to develop acceptance in areas that have been difficult or frightening. Laura has been a strong advocate for Kevin in finding medical, diet, and care alternatives that support his health and well-being.	Laura would like for Kevin to move more rapidly toward oral feeding so that she can return to work. Progress in this area has been very slow. She holds Kevin on her lap for most oral feedings. As the result of a back injury several years ago, Laura experiences pain in her neck and shoulder girdle when she holds him during the lengthy feedings. Kevin does not trust anyone else to feed him during oral-feeding meals. It is very difficult for other people to understand Kevin's communication signals at mealtimes. Laura does not like the idea of moving Kevin from a nasogastric tube to a gastrostomy tube because of her concerns about surgery and potential reflux with a G-tube. This is the only alternative suggested by professionals.

Figure 10.1   **Views on Kevin's Feeding Progress**

Shared Directions for Kevin and Laura

A general picture emerges from this figure that shows a mother who has been a strong advocate for her son's health and well-being, and who wants him to be able to eat by mouth. She sees strong signs of his ability to learn to do so on the day that she changes the NG-tube and it is out of Kevin's nose and throat. She is fearful of the recommended change to a G-tube because she sees this as potentially causing more health problems for Kevin. At the same time, she feels very stuck because Kevin is not comfortable eating by mouth with the NG-tube in place. As a single parent, her personal support system is limited and she would like to return to work, at least part time. She has had difficulty finding respite support for Kevin because of his feeding tube. Her own physical limitations of residual pain from her back injury and Kevin's difficulty being fed by anyone else increase the complexity of moving him toward oral feeding.

From Kevin's perspective, eating by mouth is both interesting and frustrating. He loves the new tastes and tries to cooperate with his mother on the days she feeds him by mouth. He knows how to make sucking movements and is delighted when he can control his body well enough to get a good suck started. When this happens, it is easier to feel the spoon in his mouth, and he doesn't feel scared that he will bite down on it. He doesn't like the feeling of a tube in his nose, especially when it wiggles around. Several years ago, he figured out that it felt better if he didn't move his mouth or swallow when the tube was in.

The common direction for both Kevin and Laura lies in their shared desire for him to eat by mouth. The common frustration lies in the type of feeding tube that supports his current need for tube feeding to sustain his nutrition. Laura is not happy about the limitations posed by the NG-tube and Kevin does not like the way it feels in his body. Both perceive this type of tube as limiting Kevin's ability to move toward oral feeding. However, it is unclear whether Kevin could learn to eat and improve his feeding coordination with the NG-tube in place. How much of Kevin's poorer coordination in eating with the tube is related to chronic discomfort with movement of the feeding tube? How much is related to a lack of experience because his mother rarely offers him tastes on the days when he has the NG-tube in? Laura's uneasiness with moving to a G-tube enables her to stay with an option that is unsatisfactory yet known.

Laura's neck and shoulder-girdle pain limit her ability to explore different supported-feeding positions and alternatives for Kevin on her lap. Kevin's current difficulties with movement and breathing control make it impossible to feed him in a chair or custom seating system.

Based on these observations, treatment might move in the following directions.

- Find ways in which Laura's body can be well supported during tube-feeding and oral-feeding sessions with Kevin. Limit the length of oral feedings to 15 minutes in order to stay within her comfort zone for holding and feeding him.

- Help Kevin increase his comfort and confidence when fed by another knowledgeable adult. Assist Laura in locating a university student who could provide respite child care and feed Kevin one meal a day.

- Set up a daily period of short explorations for taking tastes and small amounts of food with the NG-tube in place. By setting up regular, optimum learning periods, it will be possible to determine whether Kevin can improve his oral-feeding skills enough with his current tube to move gradually toward exclusive oral feeding.

- Provide Laura with written literature and opportunities to discuss the options for different types of G-tube surgery and tube maintenance with physicians and other parents. This will enable her to make a more informed decision about future tube and feeding options.

Pattern Clusters

Therapists become lost in the forest of detail when they focus on single elements. When therapists become familiar with elements that are associated with each other, they can begin to obtain a broader perspective on the child and his problems. In many ways, this is similar to the connect-the-dots books from childhood. When a therapist begins to observe the child and parent, she may begin with the individual elements and see small things that go together. For example, the clinician may notice that when the mother's arm becomes tired, her child's head flops back more into extension. The therapist may observe that when the phone rings that the child becomes stiffer and the mother becomes very frustrated and angry with him. From these small observations, a set of patterns emerges that influences the overall mealtime relationship between the child and parent. Gradually, the therapist connects more pieces of the picture and a total pattern emerges.

Describing the Patterns

In terms of treatment planning, the summary of the child's basic problems enables the therapist to focus on those needs that are the most far-reaching rather than the isolated needs of a leg, an arm, or a tongue. The summary of the child's strengths and assets identifies the key to a successful beginning. In following a guideline for easy learning, the therapist will always begin with what the child knows and enjoys, and use current strengths to build the bridge to new knowledge. Learning is not the mastery of isolated bits of information but, rather, a set of interconnections that enhance current knowledge by creating a rich network of connections between previously learned materials and new facts, ideas, and concepts. When therapists begin with knowledge and skills that are well established, they create the opportunity to develop new connections. With a clear idea of the child's needs, a destination is created for the newly developed connections.

The initial component of any mealtime or feeding summary is a description of the child's mealtime environment. This includes an overview of the adult-child interaction that is part of every meal. It identifies the roles, responsibilities, and responses of the feeder and child to the larger umbrella called the mealtime. The second component of the summary is a description of the child's basic abilities, problems, and needs with postural tone and movement patterns. These patterns form the foundation for specific feeding movements and problems that directly involve the oral, respiratory, and communication systems. The relationship of sensory acuity and processing abilities to the motor system is considered next. Tone and movement patterns are initiated and monitored by the sensory system. When sensation is not processed efficiently, motor control and skill diminish. Difficulties in the sorting of sensory information and regulating the sensory threshold reduce the child's ability to process the multisensory information of a mealtime. Major effects can be observed in all aspects of the feeding system.

A similar summary is created from a description of the child's feeding and communication skills. Problems should be described in greater detail than *feeding difficulties* or *poor breathing patterns*. The use of descriptive language will assist others in picturing the behaviors that the child is using. Examples of different types of language are provided in the following section.

Creating the Plan

After carefully delineating the issues in mealtime interaction, postural tone and movement, sensation, communication, and feeding movements, the therapist can describe appropriate preliminary treatment goals. These are directly related to the basic assets and needs that have been formulated. The therapist should think about these goals as a set of directions in which therapy could move and the order in which they would be approached in therapy.

In addition to short-term treatment goals, the therapist should consider the long-range goals and perspectives. Success in estimating long-term goals increases with personal experience. When the therapist can approach each child as a source of his or her own learning, she begins to develop a personal data bank. Although children with the same overt characteristics will differ in their long-range accomplishments, there are some similarities that can give an initial perspective of the final goal. It can be an interesting challenge to develop a "best guess" that could be labeled as a long-range prognosis. From this, a set of long-range goals can be developed for 1 year. At the end of that period, the therapist should review the changes the child has made. How do these changes relate to the long-range goals? Are there changes that support the therapist's initial impressions? What changes would indicate that the initial set of goals is no longer accurate or appropriate? The therapist should review the year with a sense of detachment. When taking on the role of an outside observer, the therapist's perceptions become more accurate. Learning is clearer because information is not biased by emotion.

John

The following single observations were made of John, a 4-year-old:

- His legs are turned inward and extended with a scissors pattern when he lies on his back.
- He cannot bend fully at the hips when brought into a sitting position.
- His shoulders are retracted.
- He cannot bring his arms forward to play with toys or put his hands in his mouth.
- His tongue thrusts out of the mouth when his head extends.

Each of these observations provides potentially important information about John. However, the basic feature that underlies each single observation is that each is a part of an extensor pattern of movement. Thus, rather than listing and planning to work on each element separately in treatment, the therapist might simply state, "There are strong patterns of extension throughout the body."

John also shows the following patterns:

- strong protraction of the shoulders in sitting
- hip flexion when lying on his stomach
- inability to lift the head and turn it to the side from tummy lying

With this additional information, the therapist could revise the initial statement to, "John shows total patterns of extension or flexion, depending upon the position of the head in space."

This search for patterns enables the therapist to identify the initial clusters of information with which she can work. It narrows the field by grouping areas and issues that are related or have a common set of roots.

Describing John's Patterns

The use of descriptive language will help others understand the patterns that John is actually using. A summary sentence such as "John uses a strong tongue thrust combined with a jaw thrust" has meaning for those who know and use the terms *tongue thrust* and *jaw thrust* in the same way as the therapist. However, it describes neither the uniqueness of John's thrusting patterns nor the situations in which they occur. The sentence creates an entirely different picture for the individual who is unfamiliar with the terms or has different associations connected with them. John's feeding behaviors can be described in a way that makes them clear to everyone: "John pushes his tongue out of the mouth whenever the spoon is presented. This thrusting forward of the tongue occurs with a bunched, thick configuration that prevents the entry of the spoon. A strong downward opening of the jaw occurs approximately 50% of the time when he sees the spoon. Movement is sudden, and the jaw occasionally becomes stuck in the open position. During this thrusting of the jaw, John's tongue is pulled to the back of the mouth, in a pattern therapists call 'tongue retraction.' The feeder is able to place food in the mouth when John is using the jaw-thrust and tongue-retraction patterns. However, food in the mouth generally triggers the tongue thrust that was described above. Food is then pushed from the mouth as the tongue moves forward. John often uses the tongue-thrust and jaw-thrust patterns to let his feeder know he is hungry and ready for the next spoonful."

This description uses many more words than a simple statement or sentence about John. It describes his behavior in a way that each reader can visualize in a similar way. It also creates the definition for terms such as jaw thrust, tongue thrust, and tongue retraction as they relate to John's feeding patterns. These terms can be used later in the report or treatment plan without misunderstanding. A summary statement can be derived from the lengthier description. John's feeding behavior might be summarized in this way: "John's feeding problems are characterized by major difficulties in the areas of jaw and tongue control. Patterns of jaw and tongue thrusting and retraction interfere with his ability to handle foods and liquids. These limiting patterns are used to signal his readiness for food."

John also shows strong reactions of sensory defensiveness and hyperreaction to the face and mouth when touched with the spoon. Touch causes him to startle and whine. He dislikes lumpy food but will accept blenderized food that has been thickened with cereal. This behavioral description could be summarized as: "John's ability to take food from the spoon and cup is limited by oral and facial sensory defensiveness. A strong startle reaction and personal discomfort are communicated to touch on the face or lumps in food."

Patterns and Plans for John

Three summary patterns have been identified for John:

- John shows total patterns of extension or flexion, depending upon the position of his head in space.
- John's feeding problems are characterized by major difficulties in the areas of jaw and tongue control. Patterns of jaw and tongue thrusting and retraction interfere with his ability to handle foods and liquids. These limiting patterns are used to signal his readiness for food.
- John's ability to take food from the spoon and cup is limited by oral and facial sensory defensiveness. A strong startle reaction and personal discomfort are communicated to touch on the face or lumps in food.

The following treatment directions might be set for a 3-month period:

- The therapist will explore movement and touch with John and discover three positions for work on sensory stimulation and feeding in which the limiting patterns of extension and flexion can be controlled or inhibited. John will eat lunch in one of these positions 50% of the time without the presence of limiting extensor and flexor patterns of the neck, shoulder girdle, and hips.
- The therapist will explore ways of providing sensory stimulation to the face in a way that is pleasurable and interactive for John, who will mouth his own fingers and two rubber squeaky toys with different shapes and textures. John's oral exploration will occur 75% of the time without startle, jaw thrust, tongue thrust, or personal discomfort. Assistance will be given to John in getting his hands and toys to the mouth.
- The therapist and John's parents will discover the specific movements and sounds that John uses to communicate during the meal. An observation form will be developed and John's communication behaviors will be observed for 1 month.

■ Setting Priorities

Identifying the Key Issues

The therapist can appreciate the complexity of learning to eat and participate in the mealtime, which is a shared partnership between a child and others in the family or community group. Beliefs, hopes, expectations, and cultural guidelines form the foundation and the glue that connects the child with others at the mealtime. In addition, the child's ability to eat comfortably and competently is influenced by far more than sensorimotor skills of the mouth. Children move toward or away from eating as they attach meaning to levels of comfort (or discomfort), and experience different degrees of ease (or difficulty), while dealing with the motor, sensory, structural, gastrointestinal, cardiac, and respiratory challenges that they face. Their temperament and feelings of being loved and supported (or alienated) move them toward or away from expanding their eating and drinking skills.

Therapists and parents face the challenge of using their personal and financial resources in the most efficient ways. This can occur only when therapists develop the ability to identify the key issues for a child and family. As the therapist evaluates a child's mealtime and feeding skills, she often confronts a very complex intermingling of needs in multiple areas. The challenge is to get to the root of what is going on, and to consider each area and decide how it relates to other areas. Ultimately, the therapist identifies the areas that are the most important to focus on in the child's program. These are areas that strongly influence most of the other areas. If the clinician places a programmatic emphasis in these areas, he will influence multiple other areas. For example, if a child has severe motor control issues of the entire body, more progress will be made in oral control for eating if the therapist addresses the child's problems with postural tone and movement. However, the therapist might realize that the child's postural tone and movement become most disorganized and nonfunctional as a response to pressures to eat at mealtimes and chaotic mealtimes. In this case, the overall difficulties surrounding the mealtime become the most important area to address. The therapist will not make significant progress in motor control with a child who is upset and out of control. These are called key areas because they hold the key to progress in multiple areas. They also can be conceived of as the foundation areas for the child's program. Following is a look at how this process works.

Shannon

Shannon is one of twins. She and her 4-year-old sister lead an active life with their parents and 2-year-old brother. Shannon's muscle tone is low, and she has a great deal of postural instability when she stands and walks. She has some fine motor difficulties that reduce her coordination for finger feeding and spoon feeding. She was born prematurely and developed with multiple medical issues that required management through surgery, medication, and supplemental oxygen. Most significantly she has bronchopulmonary dysplasia (BPD) and received supplemental oxygen for her first 2 years. She has been tube-fed since birth. Her early months were dominated by reflux and vomiting, and at 6 months a Nissen fundoplication was done. At that time, her nasogastric tube was shifted to a gastrostomy tube. Shortly after these procedures, she began to gag, retch, and experience severe gas bloat during and following tube feedings. During this period she was able to take 20–30cc of liquid from the bottle and eat small amounts of pureed food from a spoon. Her eating skills were very unpredictable and erratic, depending on the comfort of her breathing and gastrointestinal systems. In addition, a videofluoroscopic swallowing study showed that she was at high risk for aspiration with thin liquids. Because of the risk to her lungs, she was taken off of all food and liquid orally until she was 15 months old.

When she began to eat again, Shannon seemed more uncomfortable with the nipple and spoon. She gagged more when something came into her mouth. She totally rejected the bottle but seemed marginally interested in small amounts of a few smooth pureed foods from the spoon. Her parents put her in the high chair for meals and offered her food three times a day. They were frustrated by the tiny amounts that she could take in and deeply concerned about the amount of gagging and retching that she did during the meal. On days when she ate more, they became very excited and always pushed her to take a couple of more bites. Shannon generally clamped her mouth closed and turned away after 2 or 3 spoonfuls. However, they persisted, keeping the spoon on her lips until she would open her mouth. The gagging and retching persisted, interfering with her ability to enjoy tube feedings and oral feedings. She gagged up thick mucous and seemed nauseated even when she was not retching. Her gastroenterologist did multiple diagnostic tests. Some tests pointed to delayed gastric emptying; others indicated that gastric emptying was normal. Some suggested problems in esophageal motility; others showed no problems in this area. All agreed that progress in eating was affected by physiological difficulties with retching and gagging. Other than prescribing more medication for reflux and gastric emptying, her physicians were stumped and there seemed to be no way of identifying what was going on or helping Shannon become more physically comfortable. Nothing anyone did seemed to make much difference. During her second year, the number of instances of retching gradually reduced, but their severity did not change.

Shannon's parents became deeply discouraged with her slow progress toward oral feeding. Her therapists saw the feeding issues predominantly as a behavioral problem and set up a series of contingencies to reinforce Shannon whenever she opened her mouth for the spoon. This involved primarily letting Shannon watch short segments of a favorite videotape or allowing her to play with a musical toy when she took a bite. She began to open her mouth somewhat more frequently but continued to take very little food. She was totally uninterested in the food and ate intermittently so that she could play. Finally her parents and therapists decided to enroll Shannon in an intensive, 8-hour-per-day, behavioral feeding program. Reinforcers were made more attractive to Shannon and every spoon was cued with "Shannon open your mouth." Shannon initially kept her mouth closed for the spoon but eventually learned to comply more frequently in order to watch the video. Because of her oral sensory and gastrointestinal discomfort, she learned to open her mouth a very small amount and keep her tongue stiffly bunched in the front of the mouth to limit access of the spoon. Food often was deposited under her tongue where it was more comfortable for her. Over the 8-week program, Shannon gradually took more food until she was eating about 6 ounces of pureed or ground consistency food at each meal. Every bite was still paired with turning the video on and off, and the small mouth-opening and limited entry of the spoon continued to be a challenge. During the next 5 months, Shannon's family continued to apply the principles of the program at each meal at home, and Shannon continued to eat erratically. Everyone was exhausted and her parents' discouragement mounted as they realized that Shannon basically had no interest in eating. They also noticed that Shannon no longer showed preferences for tastes and was totally disconnected from any aspect of the meal except her videotape. They acknowledged that Shannon was really not eating but simply complying by opening her mouth slightly to keep the video going. Shannon and the parent feeding her ate in a separate room and were not part of the family mealtime to avoid the disruption and distraction created by the other two children.

Identifying Shannon's Key Issues and Setting Priorities

A look at the multiple issues that impact Shannon's eating will enable clinicians to consider how they might identify the key issues. Shannon's difficulties initially could be clustered into the following areas:

Motor Issues

- mild low tone and postural instability
- poorly graded movement during self-feeding
- reduced physical coordination of the mouth for efficient eating

Sensory Issues

- mild tactile defensiveness on the body, face and hands
- moderate oral defensiveness
- compensations of small mouth opening and tense tongue posturing to protect the mouth from sensory discomfort as the food comes in
- comfort with drinking small amounts of clear water

Gastrointestinal Issues

- uncomfortable associations between tube and oral feedings and mealtimes
- retching during and after meals (tube feeding and oral feeding)
- changes in stomach structure and physiology after the Nissen fundoplication
- questions about gastric motility and gastric emptying
- lack of hunger and appetite to guide food and liquid intake

Mealtime and Experiential Issues

- parents feel extremely discouraged about Shannon's slow progress in learning to eat
- strong pressure to eat more, no matter how much Shannon eats
- behavior modification program to get Shannon to eat (i.e., comply by opening her mouth and accepting food from the spoon)
- lack of trust in her ability to eat and in others who want her to eat

- high levels of stress and anxiety at meals for Shannon and her family
- dependence on other people for feelings of success

Historical Issues

- respiratory distress and BPD
- risk of silent aspiration as an infant

The therapist who reviews these area clusters should ask which of these areas plays the biggest role in Shannon's current eating difficulties.

Shannon's *motor issues* play a role, but a very small one in relationship to the other areas. Her mild postural instability, limitations in self-feeding, and slight reduction in oral motor coordination are not the main reasons that she is not eating. A therapeutic program should ensure that she is fed in a well-supported position, is given opportunities to feed herself, and is given foods that she is able to handle physically. However, work to fine-tune tongue movement and improve chewing coordination are not appropriate at this time.

Shannon's *sensory issues* play a much more significant role. They reduce her physical comfort with food in the mouth and on her face. They also limit her comfort during self-feeding because she is not comfortable with typical early eating behaviors such as sticking a finger in a taste of new food or getting food on the hands during self-feeding. Her sensory issues also play a major role in determining her perceptual experience of discomfort during periods of gagging, retching, and nausea. Many children who experience sensory defensiveness seem to experience these events more intensely and with a more long-lasting memory of the discomfort than other children. A child without sensory issues may be uncomfortable with eating and choose not to eat only when reflux is active or when experiencing heavy periods of retching. Children with sensory-processing issues frequently remember that this type of discomfort could happen. They refuse to eat or eat only a small amount in order to protect themselves from the discomfort that they predict will occur.

Sensory discomfort usually increases with physical tension. Shannon uses a great deal of physical tension in her jaw and tongue to prevent food from entering and touching her tongue. She clenches her jaw and allows a very tiny opening as the spoon approaches. She tenses and bunches her tongue in a slightly retracted position as a response to her discomfort. However, these strategies actually increase the amount of sensory discomfort that she perceives and decrease her desire to eat. The resulting lack of movement in the tongue limits her ability to chew and makes it more difficult to collect a bolus of food for swallowing softer food. Food tends to scatter on the tongue and trigger random gagging, followed by retching. Shannon seems comfortable only when drinking small sips of clear water. Although she does not like the feeling of water dripping onto her lips or chin, she will initiate some drinking without adult prompting.

Shannon's *gastrointestinal issues* play a highly significant role. She has never experienced the association of comfort with eating or drinking. She felt the pain of gastroesophageal reflux as an infant and developed severe gagging and retching several months after the Nissen fundoplication. Retching and nausea have accompanied nearly every meal she has eaten (whether by tube or orally). These episodes appear randomly throughout the meal and day, and they seem to be out of her conscious control. The timing of her meals and the amount of food given bear no relationship to potential shifts in hunger or appetite. In addition, diagnostic tests of gastrointestinal function have been unclear and have not led to an understanding of ways to manage her discomfort medically. Shannon constantly deals with very unpleasant associations between eating and discomfort that strongly reduce her desire to eat.

At this time, Shannon's *mealtime and experiential issues* appear to play the most significant role in her current feeding situation. These also are the areas that have the strongest impact on her level of comfort or discomfort in the sensory and gastrointestinal areas. When she was an infant, it was difficult for others to understand why Shannon ate more on some days than others. Because she ate better on some days and not at all on others, they thought this meant that Shannon had the ability to eat but was not using this skill. They felt that she was holding back and acting out. They recognized that the retching and nausea reduced her desire to eat, but they felt that the major issues were behavioral. They felt Shannon could eat if she wanted to. She just needed an extra push and encouragement to eat. They also were deeply discouraged by her lack of progress and wanted her to eat very badly. As Shannon began to eat by mouth, they assumed both the parent and the child roles at mealtime. They decided on the type of food as well as the place and time of eating, which are appropriate adult roles in feeding a toddler. However, they also took on the child's role. They attempted to decide what and how much Shannon would eat. She often refused by clamping her mouth closed. They persisted, trying to get her to take just one more bite. The Mealtime Dance described in Chapter 3 did not exist.

Behavioral psychologists and feeding therapists intervened with strategies designed to reinforce and shape eating behaviors such as opening the mouth and accepting the spoon. Shannon tried very hard to please them. However, she was very uncomfortable with eating because of her unresolved issues with sensory defensiveness and gastrointestinal discomfort. She developed strategies to increase her physical comfort such as the small opening of her jaw and the tension in her tongue, both of which blocked the entrance of the spoon. Although quantitative progress toward eating could be measured by an increase in the amount of food that she ate, each mouthful increased stress and anxiety levels for Shannon and her family. Moreover, if the strength of external reinforcers was not increased continually, Shannon refused to open her mouth for the spoon. Gradually the amount of food she would take went down and her refusal behaviors went up. Shannon's parents were concerned about the impact of the program on their relationship with their daughter and with the other children. Shannon and the parent who was feeding her were separated from the rest of the family at mealtimes. Both were stressed and unhappy during the meal. Her parents continued to want her to eat, but began to feel that this would never happen. Their relationship with her seemed to be built around whether she would or would not eat. They sometimes felt that they were neglecting the other children because Shannon needed so much attention.

Both gastrointestinal discomfort and sensory defensiveness create stress at mealtimes. When additional external stress is added, a child's overall level of distress increases. As distress increases, most children increase their resistance to eating. It is probable that the pressures Shannon feels to eat and her negative associations between mealtimes and discomfort trigger a portion of her physiological discomfort from retching and gagging. The degree of sensory defensiveness also increases under conditions of anxiety and stress. Although Shannon clearly showed overall characteristics of a child with mild tactile and oral defensiveness, it was difficult to determine where the defensiveness ended and Shannon's defendedness began. Many of the fight-or-flight behaviors seen in a child with sensory defensiveness can increase as the child attempts to defend the mouth from external invasion.

Shannon was highly dependent on other people for feelings of success. Unlike Sharla, her twin sister, Shannon waited for adults to help her with everything. She did not initiate imaginative play or go to find a desired toy on her own. When food was present, she showed no curiosity about it and did not play or explore—even when assured that the food was for playing, not for eating. Although she was a friendly child who enjoyed people, she was immediately suspicious of anyone who approached her mouth or brought out food or utensils.

Goal Directions for Shannon

Three key issues were identified for Shannon:

1. fear, anxiety, and lack of trust at mealtime
2. gastrointestinal discomfort
3. oral sensory discomfort and lack of positive experience

The three main goal directions and their overall strategies for Shannon's program included:

1. confidence and trust
   — showing respect for Shannon's needs and choices
   — building self-awareness
   — supporting self-empowerment and positive choices

2. gastrointestinal comfort
   — awareness of levels of comfort and discomfort
   — self-pacing and control of the meal
   — prevention of escalation
   — conscious breathing to modify discomfort levels
3. oral sensory comfort and experience
   — reduction of sensory defensiveness
   — discrimination of taste and texture

Shannon's parents and therapists decided to remove the mealtime demands for her to eat. They showed more respect for her needs and choices. Shannon joined her brother and sister at the table for meals and was offered small amounts of the same foods they were served. Her mother made sure there was always a food that met Shannon's physical and sensory needs. They stopped reminding her to take bites, chew, and swallow. Because the other children were expected to take at least two bites of a new food at meals, they decided to include Shannon in this family tradition. They included quiet organizing music and other activities to help organize her sensory system before and during the meals.

A primary emphasis was placed on Shannon's tube-feeding meals. With guidance, she became aware of the initial physical signals of gastrointestinal discomfort. She learned that she had control to tell her mother or father that her tummy needed a short break. When she felt more comfortable, she told them that her tummy was ready for more food. As she felt more empowered to regulate the flow of the formula herself, she had a positive way of controlling her food intake. No one can know the internal needs and readiness level of another person. Shannon's program honored this knowledge and gave her a way of getting in touch with an internal system for guiding the timing or pacing of eating. This strategy also prevented the escalation of gastrointestinal discomfort. The autonomic nervous system was not constantly bombarded by more food coming in during periods of discomfort. This prevented the escalation that usually took Shannon's system past the point of no return into severe retching and gagging. Small amounts of nausea, gagging, or coughing could usually be managed through deep breathing and conscious relaxation. When uncontrolled gagging and retching occurred, Shannon learned how to breathe into the discomfort and not fight it. Many of the techniques used in childbirth and chronic pain control were helpful in giving her a new way of controlling her experience as well as reducing the actual pain she experienced.

Play periods also focused on sensory awareness, discrimination, and discovery. Shannon had an underlying sense of adventure and curiosity as well as a love of imitation. These became focal points in her program to build her self-confidence and inner desire to make discoveries. Gradually, she began to trust that adults would listen and not push her beyond what she felt she could do. As she developed greater trust, she was more willing to risk exploring her mouth, tastes, and the feeling of food pieces on her tongue. Many strategies were incorporated into this part of her program to reduce her sensory defensiveness. She learned how to increase her lip control during cup and straw drinking so that she didn't dribble as much liquid down her chin. However, at the same time, she experienced the types of sensory input to her body and mouth that reduced the feelings of discomfort and need to constantly wipe her wet chin. Through imitation, she discovered the fun of tapping her tongue with her fingers while making funny sounds or listening to rhythmical music. For Shannon, this was fun and play; for her therapist, this was a way to reduce the intensity of the gag reflex and oral defensiveness.

The overall program gradually reduced Shannon's gastrointestinal and sensory discomfort. She had more confidence that she could take care of herself at mealtime and that others would honor her decisions without pushing her. Shannon's need to say "no" to eating as a way of defending herself slowly disappeared and she began to enjoy meals. Although she continued to have periods of physiological discomfort in her gastrointestinal system, this was balanced by periods of pleasure and liking to eat. When she went through periods of discomfort, she did not push herself to eat. When she felt better or was comfortable, she naturally ate more or was drawn to foods with a higher caloric or nutrient level—signs that her eating was becoming internally regulated.

Problem Solving

Each time there is a change or lack of change when therapists design and implement a treatment program, they are challenged to understand the child and themselves at a deeper level. Problem solving is an essential part of the bridge between assessment and treatment. It is the link between the two that enables the therapist to use the observational tools and strategies of the assessment as a way of identifying changes that are needed in the approach to the child or changes that have occurred as part of the intervention. Problem solving is a frame of mind—a way that we view the world and the challenges that come our way. The therapist's attitudes, beliefs, and perspectives play a major role when considering problem solving in the context of the child with a feeding disorder. Even the word *problem* may carry the connotation of difficulty for many people, and difficulty frequently implies effort. Thus, the therapist may carry all of the beliefs she has about problems. If the therapist believes that change is impossible or difficult, she will find the evidence for this as her truth. If the therapist believes that she must decide what a child needs, she will create a program that may meet her needs—not the child's needs and wants. If everything the therapist does with a child must be proven and logical, then she denies the intuitive flashes that may unlock the "stuckness" of the approach.

If the clinician believes that problems are opportunities for learning and growth, then no experience with a child is lost or bad. Each is an opportunity to enhance the therapist's understanding of the child and herself. If life is seen as constantly changing, then the therapist could approach the unexpected with a sense of adventure. Change would be sought, and a static approach to treatment would no longer be part of the guiding model. If the therapist believes that the child knows intuitively what will help him grow, develop, and learn, then the therapist no longer will insist on being "the expert." The therapist will learn to trust the child and to read the verbal and physical messages that are a way of communicating and guiding us. If the therapist is willing to acknowledge that she has many ways of knowing and processing information, then she becomes free to follow her hunches even when data is not yet available to support them.

Problem solving involves organizing information, setting priorities, and having a specific set of strategies that lead from the organization to a resolution of the problem or set of difficulties that have been prioritized.

The Big Picture Model

One effective model of problem solving might be described as an interaction between the big picture and the elements that create it. Essentially it is a process for learning how to see both simultaneously. When therapists have the big picture, they can see and appreciate the essence of each child. The clinician perceives what the child enjoys and has learned, and what sensory and communicative modes are most useful at a particular time. The therapist also may perceive those things that the child might like to do and those elements of growth and development that are hindering exploration and learning of new skills.

Strategies the therapist can use to gain the big picture include:

- Observing for activities that the child likes or seeks.
- Observing for sensory avenues that the child handles well or seeks during independent activity.
- Observing the ways in which the child indicates pleasure, interest, curiosity, dislike, unfamiliarity, displeasure, and other emotional messages.
- Summarizing perceptions of what the child wants to do, and the preferred ways to do it.
- Considering ways in which the child's desires could be expanded. For example, would changes in position or the sensory environment enable the child to enjoy the activity more fully?
- Playing with variations on a theme. The child sets the theme by indicating an enjoyable activity. The therapist introduces ways in which this enjoyed activity can be varied, as well as options or choices that increase the child's ability to explore new possibilities.

- Looking for component parts of a new activity in something that the child is doing. The therapist knows that this small part can be expanded and used as a bridge into the new skill or activity.
- Remembering that many of the necessary components for feeding and communication skills are present in play, and that play is a child's way of learning.

Carl

Carl is a 1-year-old child who often is passive and moves very little. His eyes are crossed and dull, and he rarely looks at his mother or others who play with him. He has difficulty coordinating his eyes and moving them smoothly when he attempts to use them to follow a toy. The therapist may notice that his facial expression changes and he becomes more alert when his older sister enters the room. When he moves, he lies on the floor and arches his body into extension and moves his arms and legs. When he is picked up, he likes to be bounced on his mother's lap. The therapist notices that it is difficult for him to sit because of the low tone of his trunk. Although he enjoys the bouncing, his head flops and his arms and legs often become stiff. After 2 or 3 minutes of this vigorous activity, he suddenly begins to cry. There is a brief pause between the moment he is experiencing laughter and the moment he begins to fuss and cry. His mother comments that this behavior is typical. He enjoys physical activity and roughhousing, but often he becomes tired and irritable. He becomes alert and smiles when rhythmical folk music is played. Carl does not like light, stroking touch on his face. He has not enjoyed having his fingers or toys brought to his mouth. When firm touch is given in rhythm to the folk music, Carl smiles and appears to accept and enjoy it.

When his mother, Paula, feeds him, Carl moves his head toward the breast and then away several times before he is able to draw the nipple into his mouth. At times, his mouth comes open widely and snaps closed, resulting in biting of his mother's breast. He comes off the breast each time there is a sound in the room or when his mother speaks to him or touches him. Although he has difficulty engaging the breast and initiating an organized, rhythmical suck, he eventually shifts toward a sustained sucking pattern with good coordination of breathing and swallowing. This is poorly sustained, and he comes off the breast again to attend to sounds in the room. His mother comments that his sucking is more easily initiated and is well sustained when he awakes during the night and she lies in bed and nurses him. For nutritional reasons, his mother would like to have him learn to eat cereals, fruits, and vegetables. At times when she has tried to give him food by spoon or on her finger, he has cried, fussed, and refused to eat. Carl has had one seizure and recently was placed on phenobarbital three times a day. The seizure medication is the first substance besides breast milk that he has taken by mouth. He cries and fusses whenever it is given.

Identifying Carl's Big Pictures and Developing Treatment Directions

From this brief observation, the therapist might create three big pictures.

The first big picture is one of the essence of Carl. This is the ***child's big picture***. The clinician looks at the things he enjoys and seeks to do for himself and with others, and his responses to different individuals and events. From the elements of this observation, the therapist can create the following picture:

- Carl likes vigorous bouncing for brief periods.
- He is interested in the sound of the voice and music.
- He wants to move and is able to do so by himself through arching into extension and thrusting his arms and legs.
- He shows expression in his eyes, but he does not seek visual activities.
- The difficulty that he experiences with breast-feeding appears to be related to a combination of sensory disorganization as the mouth and face contact the breast and his interest in (or distraction by) sounds and activities going on in the room where he is being fed.
- The crying and fussing that occur after movement or extended periods of touch appear to express discomfort and inner disorganization rather than unhappiness.

- It is possible that the sudden crying also is his response to sensory disorganization or overload when the vigorous bouncing that he seeks and enjoys crosses the threshold of integration and becomes confusing or uncomfortable.
- The need to give the seizure medication by mouth creates aversive input to the mouth at a time when the clinician would like to help him use his mouth pleasurably for eating.

The second big picture is built around his mother's knowledge of her son and her desires for Carl. This is the **parent's big picture**. The therapist looks at the things his mother has found work or don't work and what she would like to work on. From the elements of the clinician's observation, the following picture can be created:

- Paula is able to breast-feed Carl. She enjoys these periods of closeness and would like to continue giving Carl a portion of his meals through breast-feeding.
- She has found that Carl eats best in a quiet room when he is very sleepy.
- She is frustrated by his distractibility during breast-feeding and would like to find a way to reduce this.
- She would like for him to accept pureed consistency foods from the spoon.

The third big picture is the therapist's perception of components that could lead to wider possibilities for movement and feeding. This is the **therapist's big picture**. Through a knowledge of mealtime behaviors, developmental sequences, and his or her observation of the sensory and movement patterns that are limiting Carl's ability to interact with all aspects of his environment, the clinician can create a possible big picture of what needs to be explored with Carl. The therapist incorporates Carl's mother's observations and desires into this big picture. This could include:

- Working toward a higher level of postural tone in the trunk that would provide greater stability and become the basis for additional types of movement.
- Supporting a level of sensory organization and integration that would enable Carl to appreciate all aspects of his environment without becoming overloaded and disorganized.
- Building Carl's awareness that his movements and sounds have communicative value to a listener and can be used for feedback before the threshold of tolerance has been crossed.
- Finding greater ease in organizing sensation and movement with touch to the face and mouth, leading toward a greater enjoyment of breast-feeding and an interest in the taste and texture sensations of other foods.

This third big picture is derived initially from a sense of the child's and parent's desires; that is, Carl seems to want to move, interact with people and the environment, communicate his desires and needs, and eat. His mother wants to be able to feed him more comfortably and introduce a wider variety of eating experiences. This becomes the direction in which the therapist may move with the child during treatment. It is neither a precise agenda nor a set of specific goals that a child must meet in order for a program to be described as successful. It is simply a direction.

The big pictures of the child, parent, and therapist are blended into the therapy program. The therapist derived the direction of therapy from a combination of knowing or sensing what the child and parent would like to do or learn, as well as from a knowledge of activities or sequences that are likely to make learning easy and effortless. Ideas for specific activities or explorations are derived from the child and family, not from a list of what is supposed to work.

Carl's delight with bouncing and vigorous movement through the spine is a clue that he is seeking an activity that will build tone in the trunk and that he likes certain types of strong sensory input. He is unable to communicate to the adult moving him that the amount of stimulation is exceeding his tolerance level. He communicates through crying and fussing when his threshold of enjoyment has been surpassed and he is no longer able to deal with the stimulation. Because he shifts from laughter to tears in less than a minute, Carl's adult playmate usually does not realize that his confusion and irritability are related to the activity they've both so fully enjoyed.

As an alternative, the therapist or parent might explore stimulating Carl by bouncing him on his bottom in a way that provides better support and alignment than in sitting. Thus, possibilities emerge for Carl to experience the same type of stimulation through the spine when he is lying on his side on the therapist's lap or lying on his back with his head elevated and his knees bent. Bumping his bottom or creating a rocking movement through the spine would provide sensations similar to those he experienced as he bounced on his mother's lap. Because these movements are gentler and more organized, it is possible that Carl will enjoy them for a longer time and without the crying and irritability that follow many of Carl's movement activities. This activity could be explored using a background of rhythmical folk music or classical music that could assist Carl's development of slow, sustained, rhythmical movement in his body. The therapist would be following Carl's lead, as he has shown increased attention and calming when quietly listening to music.

Although visual and tactile stimulation would be included in therapy sessions, the sensory channels of hearing and movement would be emphasized. All the activities that Carl enjoys feature this type of input. He experiences difficulty coordinating the movements of his eyes, and often responds in a disorganized fashion to touch, especially touch to the face and mouth. Ways of building on and expanding the means by which sound and movement can be used for play and learning would be explored in therapy. For example, feeding might be easier while rocking on his mother's lap or with soft, organizing music playing during the meal.

Carl clearly wants to let others know when he is interested, happy, excited, hungry, tired, or confused. His communication consists primarily of a broad smile and crying. The therapist can begin to watch for slight changes in muscle tone, alterations in facial expression, and variations in sound, which could be used to express other messages. With this knowledge, the therapist will be able to sense when Carl wishes to stop or change an activity, or the therapist can stop before Carl is ready for the activity to end and observe for small signals that indicate he is saying "more!"

Carl has already told his mother through his physical actions that it is easier for him to initiate and sustain a nursing pattern when he is fed during the night. His mother and the therapist could examine the physical and sensory characteristics of the nighttime feedings and compare them with the daytime meals. At night, Carl is fed in sidelying. He is physically more relaxed after sleep. The room is quiet and darkened. During the day, he is nursed in a semi-sitting position. Before these feedings, he is active and involved in vigorous physical play. Usually there is talking and other activity going on in the room as he is being fed. Carl and Paula know that he will be able to nurse with better coordination if the room is quiet or there is a soft musical background that masks intermittent talking and environmental noises. The sidelying position may allow for better alignment of his head, neck, and trunk, as well as a more normal tucking of the chin instead of his typical hyperextension of the neck. This better alignment creates the possibility of better jaw, tongue, and lip movement.

Although Paula wants Carl to learn to take food from the spoon, Carl has strongly indicated that he is not ready for this step. He does not like intermittent touch to the face, which a spoon repeatedly creates. He does not like the feeling created by touch and texture in the mouth. He does not enjoy mouthing toys or his own hands. Sucking the breast creates a rhythmic flow of milk that is swallowed as part of a coordinated suckle-swallow pattern. The rapid flow of liquid from a cup or a glob of cereal from the spoon often chokes and frightens him. Carl knows at this point that he is not ready to deal with this type of stimulation, so he cries and fights it. By working with activities that child and adult know are appropriate, it is possible to create the readiness for solid foods. Improvement of head and trunk control, enjoyment of touch around the mouth in play with sounds and toys, and the introduction of different smells and tastes can introduce him to the possibility that eating something besides breast milk could be interesting and exciting.

When an open environment for learning and an accepting attitude are present, Carl will take the step toward eating cereals, fruits, and vegetables. He will not need to be pushed or manipulated by the feeder, but will accept these foods because he wants and likes them.

The Component Skills Model

After exploring the broad structures involved in problem solving using a big picture model, the next step is to look at a more detailed approach using the component skills model. This model helps the therapist analyze the parts or components that comprise the feeding skill he is teaching the child. Although the broader approaches to organizing assessment information are critical to determining a direction and set of strategies for therapy, approaches that target specific skills also are helpful. The therapist uses new or pre-existing component charts to break down a larger skill, such as efficient oral feeding, spoon feeding lumpy solids, or biting and chewing, into the smaller abilities or skills that contribute to the final feeding skill (Morris 1999a, 1999b). The therapist organizes the child's abilities and needs in relationship to these components and develops specific treatment directions or goals to enhance the child's competence in each component.

Identifying the Target Components

It is beneficial to look at how this type of system would help a child develop early, efficient oral-feeding skills. Infants and children with severe feeding difficulties pose a physical and philosophical challenge to their parents and therapists. The most frequent questions asked are "Where do I begin to help this child become an oral feeder?" and "How can I help this child eat more easily and more quickly?" It is helpful to analyze efficient oral feeding in order to identify its components. This enables the therapist to examine the child's behaviors that support or limit development of each component of efficient oral feeding.

The ability to take food and liquids orally can be divided into four component groups: eating awareness and desire, sensory awareness and discrimination, postural support, and sucking-swallowing-breathing control. It is helpful to examine the rationale for each grouping of components and consider the specific components that are included in the chart.

Eating Awareness and Desire

An infant or child who has received all nourishment by tube may have little awareness that others eat differently. If the child has received continuous drip feedings, there may be no opportunity to experience physiological signals associated with thirst, hunger, or satiation. The desire to eat and drink is created from a blending of social awareness and participation, physiological cueing, and feelings of pleasure and success. Desire is reduced when any of the following components are absent or when fear and coercion are associated with the presentation of food or liquid.

1. Is aware of the connection between mouth movements and eating.
2. Experiences hunger and satiation. Recognizes these sensations and associates them with tube feedings or eating food.
3. Experiences thirst. Recognizes this sensation and associates it with the ability to drink liquids.
4. Has the desire to learn to eat and drink orally.

Sensory Awareness and Discrimination

Sensory reception, awareness, discrimination, and regulation play a major role in the acceptance and enjoyment of the sensations associated with eating. Sensory input plays a major role in creating the desire to eat and enjoy new foods and liquids. The development of sensory discrimination skills contributes to the guidance of oral movement in handling more complex foods.

5. Enjoys exploring the hands, fingers, toys, and nonfood objects with the mouth.
6. Enjoys taking small tastes of food or liquid.
7. Uses the mouth to discover specific sensory properties of hands, fingers, toys, objects, and food. Discriminates sensory differences in temperature, shape, weight, texture, and taste.

Postural Support

Trunk and head control provide the stable foundation upon which the muscle systems supporting feeding and breathing can act efficiently. Stability initially is provided by the support of others, and gradually, is assumed by the child he develops postural responses against gravity. As movement is refined, it is initiated and sustained without effort, allowing the tongue, lips, and jaw to function efficiently.

8. Holds the shoulder girdle, trunk, and pelvic girdle steady in sitting when supported in a lap or chair. Adjusts position by shifting weight or an integrated movement through the spine. Moves without effort.

9. Holds the head steady and in midline in sitting when supported in a lap or chair. Adjusts the head and maintains head control when tipped slightly backward or forward. Uses a chin-tuck head position during oral play and eating. Moves without effort.

Sucking-Swallowing-Breathing Control

An efficient suck-swallow-breathe synergy is supported by an appropriate degree of resting tension or muscle tone and a regular rhythm. Food is moved rhythmically from the front to the back of the mouth through the activation of a series of valves that direct it through the mouth, pharynx, and esophagus. The valves also inhibit breathing and prevent the entry of food or liquid into the airway. Once the food reaches the stomach, it is prepared for transport through the intestines and into the bloodstream.

10. Tone in the tongue, cheeks, and lips is within the normal range. This allows food to be drawn into the mouth, kept out of lip and cheek pockets and moved efficiently in the mouth.

11. Moves the tongue, lips, and jaw with good rhythm and coordination when taking food or liquid into the mouth in preparation for swallowing. This is done with easy, effortless movement.

12. Uses a slow, deep, and regular breathing pattern. Coordinates sucking and swallowing with breathing.

13. Moves the lips, tongue, and soft palate with efficient coordination while moving food from the front to the back of the mouth during the oral stage of the swallow.

14. Controls the bolus of food or liquid and propels it safely down the pharynx (throat). Does not choke or aspirate food or liquid.

15. Gastroesophageal reflux is not present. This allows a child to experience the satisfaction of eating without the aftermath of heartburn and other esophageal pain or discomfort. Moves food through the esophagus to the stomach with good esophageal motility. Gastric emptying is efficient and intestinal motility functions normally.

Observation and Charting of Component Skills

Following an evaluation of a child's pre-feeding skills, the therapist can organize information according to the fundamental component skills. Three categories of information are helpful in viewing the child's current status and setting treatment goals: supporting abilities, limiting factors, and unknowns.

Supporting Abilities

List the child's abilities or experiences that relate positively to complete acquisition of the component. Although mastery of the skill may not be complete, evidence that the child has learned some or many parts of the component indicates that he is moving toward complete mastery of the feeding skill.

Limiting Behaviors

List the child's problem areas or experiences that relate negatively to complete acquisition of the component. These factors provide a partial explanation of the lack of progress or mastery of the skill.

Unknowns

List questions or areas in which there is incomplete information.

The completed chart provides an organized way of setting goals and directions that can move the child toward efficient oral feeding. The following guidelines can be used in a treatment program.

- The therapist can create a component skill chart at any point to gain an overview of a child's readiness to transition from tube feedings to oral feedings.

- The therapist can set directions for change or specific goals for each component skill. Treatment is not linear. The focus is not placed on reaching the completion of the first goal before approaching the second. The clinician can use a global model that introduces appropriate activities to influence every component during the same time period.

- Component skills in the first three areas—eating awareness and desire, sensory awareness and discrimination, and postural support—provide the foundation for the development of sucking-swallowing-breathing control. Therefore, goals for component skills 10–15 (i.e., sucking-swallowing-breathing control) may be approached initially without food or liquid through the influence of goals in the first nine components.

- The therapist can set goals to increase or expand upon the supporting abilities, reduce the influence of limiting factors, and gain greater understanding in the unknown areas.

Marty

Following is an example of one component in each of the four areas for one child and the bridge to treatment created from the clinician's careful analysis of each component.

Marty is 29 months old. She was born prematurely at 25 weeks and remained hospitalized for 2 years because of severe respiratory complications. Her respiratory system was exceptionally vulnerable, and she remained on a ventilator until she was 25 months old. She has lived at home with her parents for 4 months. Her mother provides her care during the daytime, and she has skilled nursing care at night. Marty's oral motor treatment program began when she was 18 months old. During the past 11 months, she has moved gradually from vomiting brought on by a touch to her lips and an inability to organize a suck-swallow-breathe pattern to enjoying oral play and taking small amounts of food and liquid by mouth.

---

2. Experiences hunger and satiation. Recognizes these sensations and associates them with tube feedings or eating food.

Supporting Abilities	Limiting Behaviors	Unknowns
Marty receives 7-ounce bolus feedings through her gastrostomy tube.	Marty does not fuss or indicate any discomfort if a meal is late. Because of her medical problems, Marty has not missed meals and all tube feedings are the same volume, so she has had little opportunity to discover extremes of hunger or satiation.	Is Marty consciously aware of hunger? Does she relate any physiological feelings of hunger to the act of tube feeding? Does she confuse physiological feelings of hunger or satiation with mild gastric discomfort?

Figure 10.2

Marty's therapist worked closely with her gastroenterologist and pulmonologist to maintain her comfort with bolus tube feedings as the volume of formula was slowly increased and her nutritional and caloric needs grew. Words such as "hungry" and "full" were introduced at appropriate times during the meal. No attempt was made to reduce the current limiting behaviors because of their association with her medical needs. However, at a later time, meal size and time interval may be varied slightly to provide opportunities for appreciating shifts in hunger and satiation.

6. Enjoys taking small tastes of food or liquid.

Supporting Abilities	Limiting Behaviors	Unknowns
Marty will accept some diluted juices and foods with taste, when given in very small amounts.	Marty experiences a strongly aversive response to taste. Although foods with a diluted taste have been presented for the past 9 months, she makes noxious faces, shudders, and refuses to take more than 2–3 spoonfuls.	Does Marty have a specific chemical hypersensitivity to taste? Is this related to low or even low-normal zinc levels?

Figure 10.3

Increasing the variety of diluted tastes that she would accept expanded Marty's supporting abilities. Pureed fruits and vegetables were frozen in ice cube trays to make tiny cubes that could be defrosted and added to water to create diluted juices. Increasing the intensity of taste very slowly reduced limiting behaviors. Her therapist collected a series of articles on marginal zinc deficiency and its relationship to taste and appetite levels to discuss with Marty's pediatrician. Although Marty's zinc levels were normal, they were within the low end of the range. The doctor was willing to add an additional zinc supplement to her diet, which positively influenced her acceptance of stronger tastes and increased her interest in eating by mouth.

9. Holds the head steady and in midline in sitting when supported in a lap or chair. Adjusts the head and maintains head control when tipped slightly backward or forward. Uses a chin-tuck head position during oral play and eating. Moves without effort.

Supporting Abilities	Limiting Behaviors	Unknowns
Marty is able to maintain a midline position of the head in supine, hold her head up in prone, and is beginning to sit with a chin-tuck during feeding.	Marty elevates her shoulders to assist with head control. She initiates all movement with strong head-neck extension.	None

Figure 10.4

Activities to expand Marty's head and trunk control continued. An emphasis was placed on obtaining stronger flexor activity to balance the strong extension.

14. Controls the bolus or liquid and propels it safely down the pharynx (throat). Does not choke or aspirate food or liquid.

Supporting Abilities	Limiting Behaviors	Unknowns
With small spoonfuls of water or diluted juice, Marty uses an easy suckle-swallow pattern. There is minimal loss of liquid. The hyoid and larynx elevate quickly for the swallow.	There is some coughing and choking with larger amounts of liquid. Swallowing of the pureed food is less well coordinated than liquids. The food remains longer in the front of the mouth and is not organized into a cohesive bolus for the pharyngeal stage of the swallow.	Would a videofluoroscopic swallow study show any silent aspiration or pooling in the valleculae or pyriform sinuses prior to the swallow? Is the coughing with larger amounts of liquid due to the normal learning curve experienced by children learning to drink from a cup?

Figure 10.5

Marty loved to drink small amounts of water and diluted juices from the spoon. She was much less skilled and enthusiastic about taking pureed consistency foods. Her program continued to emphasize sucking and swallowing of the thinner liquids with low levels of taste and texture. Gradually, the therapist gave her larger spoonfuls until she could handle a full tablespoon of liquid at one time without coughing or choking. A thickener was added to the diluted juices to give them a pureed consistency. This reduced the negative impact of strong taste on Marty's ability to handle this consistency food, and it helped her learn to organize a more solid bolus for the pharyngeal swallow. As Marty was able to take larger amounts of liquid and pureed consistency foods, her therapist prepared her for a videofluoroscopic swallowing study. During the study, Marty's swallow was initiated rapidly and she showed no risk factors for aspiration. There was no difference in her ability to handle small or large amounts of food or liquid.

Building Bridges

An effective treatment program is based on an in-depth understanding of the child's strengths and needs. This requires a partnership between the feeding therapist, parents, child, and consulting professionals. It calls for an understanding of how different pieces of information fit together. It necessitates building bridges that connect diagnostic information, interpreting information, setting priorities, and linking assessment information to the problem-solving process of therapy. Good planning initially is time consuming. The feeding therapist frequently feels pressure to spend the entire time in direct contact service to the child. As a result, he may give formal planning of the child's program a low time priority. Time for planning is seldom built into the schedule. Treatment sessions become a conglomeration of activities that may be generally therapeutic or educational but lack depth, organization, and relevance to the child's basic needs and wants. An initial investment in a thorough evaluation of needs and assets, a carefully conceived treatment plan, and a regular reassessment of changes are critical to a good program. Without it, the child may receive a token therapy or educational program that is not focused on current needs and abilities. Treatment programs evolve. They should not be set as an arbitrary group of goals at the beginning of the school year. Although the concept of the Individual Educational Plan (IEP) may be an appropriate way of defining a direction for the child's treatment program, it should not become a static track or set of pigeonholes into which the child must fit. Children and their interests and abilities change, and any written program must be flexible enough to accommodate unexpected change. Ultimately, the child will set the direction for the therapy program. The therapist's role is to be sensitive to the child's desires and directions, offer new possibilities, and assist the child in what she wishes to do. When professionals are open to new possibilities and changes, they can blend their perception of what is needed with the child's desires.

Many feeding program administrators and therapists insist that there is no time to develop this type of program. Funding is being cut, therapists spend less time on individualized assessments, and less treatment time is available. Yet, each of these constraints means that it is *more* important to find the correct treatment questions and answers more quickly and efficiently. There is no time or money to waste on best-guesses or non-individualized treatment programs. To the administrator or feeding therapist who says, "We cannot afford to spend time on an individualized approach," the response would be, "You cannot afford *not* to spend this time. You no longer can afford the luxury of working in a trial-and-error approach that may waste time and jeopardize children's trust and comfort levels."

What's Working and What's Not Working?

Date _____

	What's Working?	What's Not Working?
Child		
Parent		

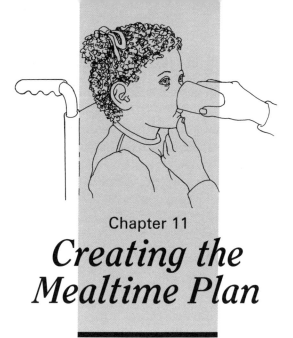

Chapter 11
Creating the Mealtime Plan

The therapist has completed observations of the child's abilities and assets in movement, feeding, breathing, and communication. She also has identified the areas of difficulty and pinpointed the underlying reasons for the child's problems. Additionally, she has examined the relative importance of each problem, set priorities for treatment, and created an initial set of goal-directions. Where does the therapist go from here? How does she create a mealtime plan that is likely to be effective in making the necessary changes?

Although specific mealtime plans differ for different problems and different children, a number of guiding principles can clarify the process of identifying short-term and long-term treatment goals.

■ Setting Goals

When considering setting goals for a child, many therapists think initially about the specific, measurable goals that they plan to write. They may think in terms of movement of the top lip onto the spoon or the number of chewing cycles per mouthful. This is counterintuitive to what we do when we think about decision making in our personal lives.

If I am going to take a vacation trip, my first decision is a much broader decision. What kind of vacation am I seeking? What satisfies my personal needs for this trip? Do I want to be in a city, at the beach, or in the mountains? Basically, where do I want to go? If I decide that I want to go from Wisconsin to the beach and sit in the warm sand and sun for a week, I probably will not decide to travel north. There aren't many warm beaches in the northern United States. The specific direction that I travel will depend on where I begin the trip. Indeed, if I am living in the South or in the Southern Hemisphere (e.g. Arizona, Florida, Australia), I may head north to find a beach. If I live in other parts of the United States, I could head east, west or south. The specific direction would depend on whether I was driving or flying, how much time and money I had for my vacation, and my personal preference for the type and location of the beach. Once I have made the basic decision of where I'm going, then I can address the smaller details. I decide on the form of transportation, where I will be staying, and how I will spend my time when I am there.

This is essentially the process that we need to follow when we begin to set goals for therapy. We decide first on the bigger picture. Where do I want to go with this child and family? What are the priorities and the overall direction that I should take with the therapy program? We come to this decision through the process of organizing assessment information and setting priorities and engaging in the problem solving process described in the previous chapter. From this process, we can clearly answer the questions "Where am I going in therapy?" and "Which direction am I going?" If we don't know where we are going and the general direction we must take to get there, we will never know when we have arrived!

Once we have decided on our goal directions, we can begin to create specific goals for a specific time period. There are many variations in both the specificity and the wording of goals. These depend on many factors such as whether the goals are being written for parents, the agency, insurance provider, etc. Most goals are written as a series of expectations that objectively define specific skills or behaviors that the child will acquire during the period of therapy.

Short-term goals should contain three related components. They include the following:

- What will the child do?
(Marty will taste four new full-strength fruit juices.)
- Under what circumstances will the child do it?
(She will do this during regular therapy sessions while sitting upright on the therapist's lap. Two different juices will be offered at each of two therapy sessions.)
- With what degree of proficiency will the child do it?
(She will use an easy opening of her mouth and will accept 1 teaspoonful of each juice.)

The final 6-month goal for Marty could be written:

> "Marty will accept 1 teaspoonful of four new full-strength fruit juices given by spoon while sitting in an upright position on her therapist's lap. She will open her mouth easily and take two different juices during two different therapy sessions."

The goal is clearly defined and measurable. Measurable goals define the goal-direction and confirm the arrival at a specific destination. In the vacation-planning analogy, this would be similar to saying "I am traveling east and south to Wrightsville Beach, North Carolina" and "I will arrive there on Monday afternoon."

In some circumstances, the therapist needs only to define the goal-direction. Thus, if the therapist were writing a general goal for a longer period of time or a goal written primarily for Marty's parents, she could use a more general wording, such as "Marty will accept four or more new full-strength fruit juices."

It will be helpful to look at goals and formats that were written for two other children. In the first example, the therapist has differentiated between the long-term behavioral goals and short-term objectives. The long-term behavioral goals are general goal-directions for Dylan. The short-term objectives have specific, measurable components for a 3-month period of therapy. A brief summary of Dylan's mealtime issues is included at the beginning, and a general discussion of treatment strategies is provided at the end of each goal section.

Dylan, Age 12 Months

Dylan has moderately low postural tone and substantial postural instability. He pushes back into extension when he sits for meals and is very unsteady and uncomfortable in a sitting position because of poor flexor activity in his abdominal-pelvic girdle. This prevents him from coming forward to the spoon when he is ready for the food. He often is overstimulated and overwhelmed by the multiple sensory input at mealtime. He begins to rock, flap his hands, and withdraw from the situation by cutting out eye contact with others and tuning out. His overall communication skills are limited to smiling and screeching. He communicates an overall dislike for eating pureed consistency foods by spitting them out. He responds to his bottle by smiling and shows some preferences for solid finger foods that stick together and do not become scattered in the mouth.

Long-Term Behavioral Goal 1

Dylan will be able to sustain and use postural tone within the mildly hypotonic range, and will show adequate trunk stability for normal patterns of sitting unsupported, rolling from prone to supine and back, and moving from prone and supine to sitting.

Short-Term Objective A

Dylan will develop sustained activity of the abdominal muscles in a flexor pattern of pelvic elevation and hands-to-knees when lying on his back.

- During play and diaper-changing activities, Dylan will lift his pelvis 2 to 5 inches off the floor while playing with his knees or feet. He will do this at a criterion level of 8 out of 10 times.

Short-Term Objective B

Dylan will develop sustained greater activation of the abdominal muscles while sitting in a supported on-lap position. Muscle activity will be present when he is tipped backward and laterally.

- During play, Dylan will exhibit righting and equilibrium reactions of the head and trunk when his weight is shifted slowly backward and to the right and left sides. He will do this at a criterion level of 8 out of 10 times in each direction.

Treatment Strategies

Movement activities to increase postural stability will be incorporated in all therapy and home-care sessions. An emphasis will be placed on developing the flexor component of movement, which often is overpowered by extensor components in Dylan's spontaneous movement patterns. Dylan's tendency toward sensory overload will be taken into consideration during all movement activities.

Long-Term Behavioral Goal 2

Dylan will show improved sensory organization and integration during therapy and quiet home activities. This will be measured by an increase in sustained eye contact and a reduction in rocking, spinning, hand flapping, screeching, and other behaviors indicating sensory overload.

Short-Term Objective A

Dylan will show a measurable reduction in rocking, flapping, and other withdrawal behaviors during treatment sessions that use auditory and vestibular stimulation to assist sensory integration.

- During play sessions in which music with a 60-beats-per-minute tempo or containing Hemi-Sync sounds is played, Dylan will show rocking, flapping, and reduction of eye contact no more than 25% of the time.

Short-Term Objective B

Dylan will show an increase in his acceptance of toys and textured foods in the mouth.

- During therapy sessions, Dylan will reach spontaneously for toys and put them in his mouth at a criterion level of 8 out of 10 times that they are offered. He will reach for a solid finger food such as banana bread or diced vegetables and put it in his mouth six times during a feeding session.

Sensory input that helps organize sensory processing (vestibular, proprioceptive, deep touch-pressure, auditory) will be used during all therapy sessions and for a minimum of 1 hour a day when Dylan is at home. Dylan's withdrawal behaviors will be interpreted as a signal of sensory defensiveness, sensory overload, or both, and will be responded to by quieting and stopping the activity. Whenever possible, these patterns will be anticipated and avoided by shifting to an activity that is more organizing and integrating for Dylan. Mouth toys will be offered throughout the session. Food will be presented at the end of the therapy session after much preparation of the sensory-processing system. Because Dylan seems more comfortable with solid finger foods, these will be used initially rather than following developmental sequences that begin with pureed food.

Long-Term Behavioral Goal 3

Dylan will show an increase in initiating and responding to communication behaviors during therapy and at home. These will include simple gestures or signs, vocalization and simple words, and pointing to pictures in children's books.

Short-Term Objective A

Dylan will show an increase in positive communicative messages given to his feeder during meals in therapy and at home. These will include eye contact, smiling, and appropriate mouth opening.

- During therapy sessions, Dylan will accept a solid finger food such as banana bread or vegetable dices offered by an adult at a criterion level of 8 out of 10 times. Acceptance will be indicted by opening the mouth, looking at the feeder, smiling, or vocalizing.

Short-Term Objective B

Dylan will choose preferred foods during a meal in therapy and at home. He will use reaching, smiling, or pointing to indicate his preference when given two foods from which to select.

- During therapy, Dylan will indicate *yes* by reaching, smiling, or pointing to one of two foods. He will do this at a criterion level of 8 out of 10 times.
- During meals at home, Dylan will indicate *yes* by reaching, smiling, or pointing to one of two foods when fed in a quiet room by his mother. He will do this at a criterion level of 6 out of 10 times.

Treatment Strategies

Music that helps organize the sensory system will be used during mealtimes. Activities to prepare the sensory comfort of Dylan's mouth will precede all mealtime sessions. The focus of each session will be on Dylan's mealtime interaction and communication with the person playing with him or feeding him. His nonverbal signals will be acknowledged and honored. A solid finger food and a pureed fruit or vegetable will be offered at each session. Foods will be compatible in taste.

This second example was written as part of an assessment report by a private therapist who wanted to help Tyrone's school therapists gain a clearer understanding of the link between assessment findings and treatment directions. The assessment report is broken down into subsections that are followed by specific treatment goal-directions. One segment follows.

Tyrone, Age 5 Years

Oral Motor Support for Feeding

▨ Tyrone's oral movements during feeding and speech vary in their precision and skill. Oral skill-fulness is based on the stability in his head, neck, and trunk. The jaw provides the stability upon which the tongue and lips develop independence, skill, and precision.

During drinking, Tyrone uses a wide up-down, unstabilized movement of the jaw. He chokes when drinking long consecutive drinks. There is drooling and a loss of liquid as he drinks. Tyrone tends to pull the lips back into retraction after the glass is removed from the mouth. He also uses a wide jaw opening when biting off a piece of food. He does not grade or adjust the size of the opening to the thickness of the food. This slows him down and reduces precision.

1. *Tyrone will decrease the amount of unstabilized jaw excursion he uses when drinking liquids from a glass.*

2. *Tyrone will stabilize his jaw during drinking by biting gently on the rim of the glass while sequencing four consecutive suck-swallows.*

3. *Tyrone will drink an 8-ounce glass of liquid with no loss of liquid or saliva.*

4. *Tyrone will exhibit awareness of three different amounts of jaw opening when preparing to bite off a piece of food. He will use a small jaw opening for rapid, repeated bites of long, thin foods such as pretzels and french fries.*

▨ Tyrone's tongue and cheeks are slightly low in muscle tone. This results in a reduction in the normal grooving of the center of the tongue during feeding and reduced precision of tongue and lip movement for chewing. He has a moderate amount of difficulty coordinating movement of the cheeks and tongue to make a bolus (solid, chewed ball of food) for swallowing. Pieces of food become scattered in the mouth and it takes time for him to clear his mouth fully for the next bite. Food that he wishes to spit out becomes stuck on his tongue, and he lacks the coordination to eject it efficiently from the mouth. It takes him a long time to chew more difficult foods such as meat and raw vegetables. Tyrone dislikes chewing meat because of the energy and effort it takes to move it in his mouth and make efficient grinding movements to pulverize it. He is not always aware of small pieces of food left in the mouth.

1. *Tyrone will show an increase in muscle tone in the tongue and will develop greater variability in tongue movement to support greater efficiency in sucking, swallowing, and chewing.*

2. *Tyrone will show an increase in muscle tone in the cheeks and develop the ability of the cheeks to work together with the tongue in gathering food into a bolus for more efficient chewing and swallowing.*

3. *Tyrone will organize semichewed pieces of meat, bagel, or other food of similar consistency and then spit it out of his mouth with efficient organization of movement. He will show greater interest in chewing meat, gum, and other foods that require efficient, sustained chewing.*

▨ Implementing the Plan

There are many options for implementing the mealtime plan in treatment sessions. These options will influence the types of goal-directions that the therapist creates, so it is important that he consider these while developing the plan. Different options fit different children, therapists, and agency environments. Each has its benefits and drawbacks. No system fits every child, family, and therapist. The two most important factors that influence the writing of the treatment plan are the structure and content of the therapy program. These are particularly important when plans and goals are being updated for a child who is already receiving therapy.

Structure

The frequency of therapy sessions is often debated. A common belief is that "more is always better." Parents spend a great deal of time and energy pushing their school systems and insurance providers for more therapy without asking whether the type of therapy or background and working style of the therapist support their child's needs. Treatment may vary in the number of sessions in a given period, the length of each session, the intensity of sessions, and the way in which treatment is integrated with other aspects of the child's life and routine. It is more important to review what is happening during treatment sessions and evaluate the child's response to the sessions than to count the number, length, or intensity of sessions. Lengthy or intensive treatment programs are ineffective if the therapist is working on areas or goals that are inappropriate for the child. Time and full sessions are wasted when children cry and fight against the therapist and program. A great deal of progress can take place in a short time when the therapist, parent, and child agree about the goal-directions of the program and when adults are willing to follow the child's lead.

Sessions

The number of sessions that a child receives often depends on the location and circumstances surrounding the therapy. For example, infants and children who are short-term inpatients in a hospital often receive daily therapy. Children who are in a rehabilitation program or have a low tolerance for handling and input may be seen for two or more very short sessions each day. Weekly therapy seems to be a more common pattern for children who are outpatients in a school system, clinic or home-based parent-infant program. Many children with milder problems may be seen every other week or monthly for maintenance support.

Length

The length of treatment sessions varies a great deal. This is probably a more important variable than the number of sessions. Sessions that are 15 to 20 minutes in length usually are too short to prepare the child's physical and sensory systems for eating. When a child requires more preparation for the meal, longer sessions are much more effective and time efficient. This need may be met by sequencing two therapy sessions so that one prepares for the other. For example, a child requiring a great deal of sensory organization and preparation might spend 30 minutes in occupational therapy engaged in appropriate activities for sensory integration. A feeding or mealtime program with the speech-language pathologist could be scheduled for an additional 30 minutes. The child would benefit from both therapy programs while gaining the equivalent of 60 minutes worth of valuable input in the feeding program because of the time spent preparing for the feeding session.

Intensity

The intensity of treatment is often an important factor when a child is ready to work on a new skill or the overall directions for the treatment program are unclear. Sessions that are scheduled closely together with greater length and number often accelerate the learning curve. Often, it is easier for therapists to see patterns that may be important for the child's program and for children to build on previous successes without other intervening experiences. A therapist may schedule a full day or several days in a row at the child's home. Children may spend a week or more in a therapy or camp program where the focus is on integrated intervention. Therapists in a school or clinical program may reserve several therapy slots each day or week for children who need limited periods of intensive treatment. Children are rotated into these time slots during specific periods when they are likely to benefit from additional therapy. A school district may double the amount of weekly therapy that a group of students receives by using a block-scheduling system. Students may be seen daily for a month and placed on a nontherapy carryover program the following month. For some students, this is much more effective than the same amount of therapy delivered in a regular twice weekly format.

The options are unlimited. Agencies and therapists can develop their creativity in scheduling options to meet the needs of a variety of children.

Integration

All treatment programs must address the integration of new therapy skills into the child's life outside the therapy room. No amount of therapy is enough to make long-lasting changes without specific plans and procedures for skill integration into a child's regular environment. When parents, teachers, and classroom aides are directly involved in program development, it is much easier to integrate new ideas and directions into other settings.

Therapists usually think of integration solely as a process of transferring information and skills to another environment. However, the most important level of integration is internal. When there are changes in a child's body and life, it feels strange or unusual. Even if the child likes and accepts a change, it takes time for that change to feel comfortable. No matter how limiting a movement or sensory pattern may seem to someone else, it is what a child has known and is familiar with. There is always the tendency to move back into the comfort zone, the area of habit and familiarity. Moving slowly into changes and allowing periods in which the child can integrate or stabilize the new change can prevent this. Plateaus can be positive times and spaces for integrating change.

Type

The type of therapy also varies with the child's needs and the resources of the agency. Problems begin only when a single type of therapy is available for all children and families. Not all children are alike, and their needs vary a great deal. Therapists and agencies can offer a variety of options to meet the differing and changing needs of the children and families whom they serve.

Individual

Individual therapy sessions are invaluable to children with more complex mealtime and feeding needs. It is much easier for some children and parents to learn in a quiet environment with the individual hands-on attention of a therapist. Some individual sessions can take place in a classroom setting where a non-pullout model of integrated therapy is used. The therapist comes into the child's class and provides therapeutic intervention while the child is engaged in individual or group activities.

Group

Group sessions frequently take place in a school setting, either in the classroom or in a therapy room. They offer children the opportunity to learn with their peers and provide effective modeling of new skills and behaviors from other children. Because groups can offer a more indirect approach, some children feel less threatened and more comfortable than they would in an individual session. Group "lunch clubs" have been used effectively in the school environment to integrate children with special feeding needs and their non-disabled peers. They also have been used to provide non-pressured peer modeling of mealtimes with small groups of children who have sensory-based and experientially based feeding issues. Small group therapy sessions may also be used in center-based parent-infant programs where the infants in the program have similar therapy issues.

Consultation

In the consultation model, the child usually is not seen for direct therapy. The therapist provides both general and targeted suggestions to the classroom teacher or parent. In some instances, consultation may be combined with a short period of therapy modeling of these alternatives. Consultation works best when the therapist has had direct therapy experience with the child. Many programs seem to be moving to a consultation model in which the therapist observes the child briefly and then offers suggestions to the teacher or parent. This often involves general recommendations for children, with the overall issues demonstrated. It may or may not meet the needs of an individual child.

Education and Support Groups

Education and support groups are developed as an adjunct to therapy. They generally are designed to provide information to parents on specific areas that influence mealtimes and offer a forum for discussion. When all the parents in the group have similar issues, such as tube feeding, the sharing of personal experiences and parent-to-parent support can be extremely helpful.

Content

Therapy goals and the means for attaining these goals are different. This often is a point of confusion for therapists. Some feeding therapists write a series of goals and then sit down and teach the specific skills that the goals measure. Now is a good time to review the comparison of setting goals with planning and taking a personal vacation. I have decided that I am going to drive from Charlottesville, Virginia to Wrightsville Beach, North Carolina.

I could write a measurable goal in the following way. "Suzanne will travel by car from Charlottesville, Virginia, to Wrightsville Beach, North Carolina, on a 2-week vacation. She will return more physically and mentally relaxed, as measured by standard physiological tests and questionnaires measuring stress levels."

My destination, length of vacation and mode of travel are clear. My direction of travel is clear. If I plan to get there in a reasonable amount of time, I will drive toward the southeast. My personal goal of returning with greater physical and mental relaxation and general ways of measuring this are clearly defined. However, the specific roads that I travel, the type of car I select, the amount of time it takes to get there and back, and the way I spend my time are not specified in this goal-direction. I could drive on a series of interstate highways and make the trip in less than a day. I also could take small country roads for the whole journey and arrive later but in a more relaxed frame of mind. I could stop at interesting places en route or drive with a minimal number of breaks. Once I am at the beach, I could spend my entire time sleeping in my hotel room, sitting in the sun, swimming, renting a sailboat, going deep-sea fishing, or going to a series of dances and parties. It all depends upon my personal interests and style and what will meet my needs for becoming more physically, mentally, and emotionally relaxed. I probably would not sit at the beach and ask myself "Am I working on relaxation right now?" or "Would going swimming relax me?" I would focus on doing something that interested me, challenged me, or made me feel better. I would be involved in the process of my vacation, not in the end goal of greater relaxation. What I find relaxing may be quite different from what you find relaxing. We would both do different things on our way to the beach and during our time there; but we both could meet the same goal of returning home in a state of increased physical and mental relaxation.

This analogy applies directly to the therapy process. Therapists set goal-directions and specific descriptions of their destination. They select treatment strategies and specific techniques that will move them toward these goals. The specific content of individual treatment sessions will vary according to the child's interests and needs on a specific day. Therapists do not teach to the goals they have written down. It will be beneficial to look at an example of this concept with Marty, whose assessment is described in the Component Skills Model section for treatment planning on page 208, and whose mealtime goal for taste has been described as:

> "Marty will accept 1 teaspoonful of four new full-strength fruit juices given by spoon while sitting in an upright position on her therapist's lap. She will open her mouth easily and take two different juices during two different therapy sessions."

We hope Marty's therapist will not sit her down and offer her new juices from the spoon throughout each 30-minute treatment session! Marty's overall ability to accept new tastes may depend on her comfort with different types of sensory input. It may depend on her feelings of comfort and stability in sitting or her neurochemical processing of taste sensations. Marty's therapy sessions usually began with more overall physical and sensory activities. On some days, she wanted to move and play with movement for the entire session. Marty's therapist recognized that her specific agenda on those days was extremely important and was critically related to her physical coordination for taking small tastes. On other days, Marty wanted to play with toys in her mouth and discover the differences in the way they felt on her tongue. On still other days, she was interested in smelling things but did not want anything in her mouth. Some days, she wanted to do a bit of everything and was particularly interested in very diluted tastes. On each of these days, Marty was focusing on the part of the whole that she was most ready to learn and incorporate during that session. Her therapist spent time in the library looking for journal articles related to taste because Marty had been taking an unusually long time to get used to diluted tastes. She learned more about the relationship between zinc deficiency and taste, and about sensory defensiveness to taste. She talked to Marty's pediatrician and occupational therapist about additional diagnostic tests and treatment strategies that might be effective. At the end of the 6 months, Marty was taking six different juice tastes and two different pureed tastes. Marty's achievements surpassed her goals because the therapist worked toward the overall goal-direction rather than a specific splinter skill.

The content of therapy sessions varies with the overall approach of the treatment facility, the specific interest and background of the therapist, and the prior experience that the therapist has had with children who have feeding difficulties. As mealtime, oral motor, and feeding programs become more available to families, it is often extremely difficult for parents to understand differences among these programs. They generally assume that therapists who are working with the child's feeding issues have the background to do so, and that the approaches they are using match the needs of their child. Unfortunately, this is not always the case. The philosophy and content presented in this book emphasizes a broad, individualized mealtime approach. Because the mealtime approach incorporates strategies and techniques that relate to oral motor treatment and direct feeding skills, it is also the most complete in its ability to address the total needs of the child. The authors, in their experience, have found that this approach is the most flexible and adaptable to the needs of individual children and families. They also know that other approaches have been effective with individual children. It is important to honor the perspectives and choices of other therapists and families when they differ from one's own.

A second example describes a set of goal-directions accompanied by ideas that will help the child move in these directions as part of a home program. It was written for the child's family. This format shows another integrated way for therapists to look at the interplay between goals, assessment information, and program directions.

Marybeth is a 7-year-old who takes most of her calories orally. However, because of weight loss and a lack of interest in eating, she receives supplemental nutrition at night through a gastrostomy tube. Poor oral coordination and a lack of positive oral-sensory experience due to mild oral tactile defensiveness compromise her eating skills. Mealtimes are stressful for everyone, and Marybeth shows very little interest in eating.

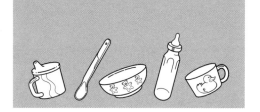

Mealtime Program

Child	*Marybeth*	Age	*7 years*
Therapist	*Marsha K.*	Date	*January 12, 2001*

Part 1: Positive Mealtimes

Goals
To increase Marybeth's interest in eating and drinking, and enable her to become a partner at mealtimes.

Supporting Areas
Marybeth tolerates eating. Over the years, she has gradually accepted a wider variety of foods, but still eats a very limited choice of foods. She will open her mouth for the spoon and usually will continue eating if distracted with a video or favorite toys. Marybeth experiences hunger and sucks on her hand if she has not eaten for a long time. When she no longer wants to eat, she pushes the food away and turns her head away.

Limiting Areas
Marybeth shows very little self-generated interest in eating and drinking. Even if she is hungry, she often will not accept the spoon unless distracted or asked multiple times during the meal. She does not regulate food intake by hunger and a desire to eat.

Possible Activities

1. Engage Marybeth as a full participant in her meals. Share responsibility with her. The role of the feeder in this partnership is to provide food that meets her nutritional needs in a form that she can handle and accept. It is also to create and adjust a sensorimotor environment that enables Marybeth to sit with good support, focus her attention, maintain a functional energy level, and communicate. Marybeth's role is to guide the feeder's selection and timing of the presentation of the food, and to determine what and how much she eats.

2. Prepare for a meal by helping Marybeth organize her body and her response to sensory stimulation. Use swinging or dancing to music before a meal to support sensory organization. Help her "wake up" her mouth by playing with her fingers and hands on her face and mouth or by toothbrushing before a meal. Use a mirror during meals and invite Marybeth to watch herself eat and drink.

3. Play a Hemi-Sync Metamusic™ tape such as Metamusic Masterworks in a stereo boom box placed directly behind her chair. This will help her relax physically and emotionally, and will reduce some of the discomfort of her sensory defensiveness.

4. Wait for Marybeth to let you know she is ready for each bite. Do not offer the spoon when she is clearly not ready. Marybeth often needs time at the beginning of a meal to get her body and mouth ready for the food. She lets you know she is ready by coming forward with her upper body, opening her mouth, or touching your arm and guiding the spoon to her mouth.

5. Set an objective signal for the end of the meal (approximately 20–30 minutes). Let Marybeth help you decide what to use (e.g. timer, end of the music tape). This is set at the beginning of the meal so that both you and Marybeth know when it is time to stop. When the timer goes off, it is time to remove the food. If she has been eating happily during the meal and still wants to continue, you don't have to stop. In this case, let her appetite and desire to eat determine the length of the meal. If she is playing her "yes-no-maybe" game, it is time to stop when the signal goes off.

6. Give her reasonable choices in food, offering no more than three different foods. Serve her very small portions (i.e., 2–3 teaspoons of a food). Place these in a bowl or a divided child's plate. Let her develop a satisfaction with finishing the food, and let her know she can have more if she is still hungry.

(continued)

Figure 11.1

Part 2: Oral Awareness and Discrimination

Goals	To increase Marybeth's acceptance of firm touch to the face.
	To increase Marybeth's interest in, and opportunity for, sensory exploration with the mouth.
Supporting Areas	Marybeth brings her hands and fingers to her cheeks and lips. She accepts feeling a toothbrush in her mouth and is beginning to move the brush on her front teeth. She accepts touch to her face and lips during rhythmical play with music. Marybeth is interested in exploring contrasts in position and movement with her own body. She loves looking into a mirror and finding places on her face that need washing.
Limiting Areas	Marybeth experiences tactile defensiveness in her mouth. This pattern appears to be stronger when she is under stress or distress. She has never put her fingers or toys inside her mouth. She is extremely guarded about others invading her mouth. She has had no real experience with oral-sensory exploration and discrimination.

Possible Activities

1. Prepare Marybeth for successful mouth exploration through work with her body first. Play with bouncing and rhythmical movement to music will help her system become more organized and receptive to playful sensory input. Her use of her hands and mouth together will be easiest in sidelying, where she is more stable and comfortable.

2. Use rhythmical folk music as an invitation to explore and enjoy rhythms on the cheeks and tongue as well as to increase muscle tone in these areas. You can use the rhythms of the music to set a tempo for tapping or patting under the chin (this is on the base or root of the tongue), on the cheeks, or in the mouth on the tongue. The music creates an environment of shared fun. It creates greater access to Marybeth's mouth because the adult is not "doing it to Marybeth." Both are participating in a shared, rhythmical activity.

3. When she is lying or sitting with her hands near her mouth, move them gently toward her mouth or help her play with her cheeks or chin. Explore different ways she can put different parts of her hand in the mouth (e.g., fingers, thumb, wrist, and fist).

4. Approach play and exploration with the mouth with a perspective of fun, adventure, and anticipation. Allow Marybeth the choice of participating with you. Help her develop a trust that you will not force her beyond her desires and perceived abilities. Marybeth often perceives work with her mouth as your attempt to force her to do something she doesn't want. Through trust and experience, she can shift her perception and belief to an enjoyable participation with you in something that is fun.

5. Introduce your finger into Marybeth's mouth and around the face in a game-like fashion, as she becomes comfortable with this. Count her teeth. Sing songs and count or tap to the rhythm of the music. Hunt for different parts of the mouth as in a treasure hunt.

(continued)

Figure 11.1 *(continued)*

Part 3: Rhythmical Suck-Swallow-Breathe

Goals	To help Marybeth develop a rhythmical, strong, sustained suckling pattern before taking small spoonfuls of food.
	To develop Marybeth's ability to draw small amounts of food into the mouth using a rhythmical, suckling movement.
	To help Marybeth develop a suck-swallow-breathe pattern when taking small amounts of food with the head in an upright position.
Supporting Areas	Marybeth has an excellent sense of body rhythm with music. She uses a rhythmical suckle pattern of the tongue when she is sucking small amounts of soft food.
Limiting Areas	Marybeth eats with her head tipped back into hyperextension. Her rhythmical feeding movements are much less efficient when her head is back. Her jaw opens strongly, making it impossible for her to incorporate lip and cheek movement. Her tongue movement is either from a retracted position or with protrusion. Marybeth has a forward protrusion of her upper dental arch and teeth, and an open bite malocclusion of her front teeth.

Possible Activities

1. Work for a more forward head position with a chin-tuck (i.e., with a straight neck and the chin tipped downward toward the chest) to reduce the wide amount of jaw opening and to bring the lips and tongue into a more neutral-forward position. Because she uses the head-back position as a compensation to keep food from falling out of her mouth, your primary focus initially will be on activities for oral awareness and movement, and comfort with her fingers in the mouth.

2. When Marybeth has a very small amount of food in her mouth, help her discover that she can bring her head forward and tip her chin down toward her chest. This is easiest for her when she is completing the final swallow of the food.

3. When she is lying in a supported position on the Boppy™ Pillow for toothbrushing, dip the brush in water and give her a tiny amount of extra liquid to suck and swallow. This will give her an excellent experience with sucking and swallowing with her head and body in proper alignment.

4. When her head is in a more upright position, she can use her lips to help remove the food from the spoon. Encourage her to start out with an open mouth and her head upright. After the food is in her mouth, she can tip it back to keep it from falling out. Gradually, as her lips and cheeks become more active, she will find other ways of keeping the food in her mouth.

5. As she becomes more comfortable and skillful with lip, teeth, and tongue movements, she can draw her lower lip inward and scrape food off her lip to prevent it from falling out. A second alternative is to use her finger to push the food back into her mouth.

6. Marybeth should always have support for her feet when she is eating. She is also more stable when she is wearing shoes. Stamping or marching movements of her feet and legs on the footrest can increase the stability of her body and support rhythmical movements in the mouth.

Figure 11.1 *(continued)*

The third example on page 227 describes a format in which the therapist wishes to provide a general description of mealtime recommendations for a child in the classroom or home setting.

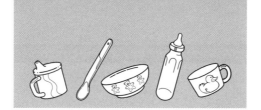

Individual Mealtime Plan

Child	*Carlos*	Age	*5 years*
Therapist	*Suzanne M.*	Date	*January 12, 2001*

Supporting and Limiting Mealtime Skills

Carlos enjoys eating when he can focus on what he is doing. He is severely visually impaired, and often becomes distracted and overwhelmed by a noisy environment. When he is unfocused, he rocks in his chair and refuses to eat foods with texture or to chew. He has a mild hypersensitivity in his mouth for textured foods. It is unclear how much of this is related to his visual problems and lack of early mouthing experiences. It also is unclear how much is a physiological discomfort from oral tactile defensiveness. Carlos shows very poor awareness of his mouth. He often holds food in his mouth for a long time before swallowing it and does not always clear food pieces from his tongue.

Carlos can open his mouth appropriately for the spoon and bite through thin cookies and french fries. He is just beginning to repeat an open-close bite pattern with adult guidance. He has started to lateralize his tongue when food is placed toward the side of the mouth. He also is beginning to move food from the center to the side of his mouth. This is accompanied by a normal movement of the jaw to the side and specific tightening of the lips and cheek on the side of food placement. Carlos' control for biting is better if an adult places the food on the side of his mouth. He prefers to do this himself and usually places the food in the center. Organization of a bolus is emerging as Carlos obtains greater lateral movements of his tongue and better coordination of the tongue and cheeks. Oral defensiveness to scattered pieces of food often reduces Carlos' interest and willingness to bite and chew new foods.

Short-Term Mealtime Focus and Objectives

- To develop the ability to bite small pieces of food from a larger piece of food when Carlos is in a quiet environment for eating.

- To develop a rhythmical chewing pattern with tongue lateralization when food is placed between the biting surfaces of the side teeth and Carlos is in a quiet environment for eating.

Mealtime Suggestions

Environmental Setting for the Meal

Whenever possible, give Carlos his meals at home in a quiet environment and support his focus of attention by using quiet, organizing music. Create a quiet learning environment for lunch at school. The noisy cafeteria shifts Carlos from a learning mode to a survival mode because of his sensory-processing difficulties. Consider feeding him in the classroom or a smaller lunchroom environment with one or two other students.

Preparation for Mealtime

Provide sensory activities that help Carlos become better organized for about 30 minutes before each meal at home or in the classroom. This can include listening to a Hemi-Sync Metamusic tape, swinging in a net hammock in the gym, or bouncing on a green therapy ball. This will increase Carlos' openness to new food experiences and reduce the influence of his sensory difficulties on eating.

(continued)

Figure 11.2

Physical Position

Provide a chair that gives Carlos good physical support for his body and his feet. When he lacks support, he increases tension in his shoulders, arms, and neck. This makes it harder for him to have the fine motor skills for self-feeding and the oral motor skills for swallowing and chewing.

Food Texture, Temperature, and Taste

Continue to give him some of the pureed consistency foods that he prefers, but include some foods at each meal that require biting and chewing as well as foods that build on his love of crunchy foods.

Systematically introduce Carlos to new foods that are somewhat similar in sensory properties to foods that he is already accepting. Build on what he knows and likes, then gradually move toward foods that are more unfamiliar. Use a baby-food grinder to give him experience with many of the same table foods the rest of the family is eating at the meal.

Include a binder or clearing food with each meal that requires biting and chewing. Help Carlos focus on the food remaining in his mouth and his ability to clear it with a bite of smooth pureed food or a spoonful of water.

Don't introduce new or difficult foods when he is tired or appears to be having trouble with sensory regulation. If he is in a challenging sensory environment (i.e., restaurant, school cafeteria), offer him softer pureed foods, which reduce the sensory challenge from the food.

Utensils

Use a regular tablespoon when feeding him. Because he is becoming interested in feeding himself, give him a shorter spoon that has a thicker handle and a large, firm plastic bowl. This will make it easier for him to hold onto the spoon and get it into his mouth comfortably. Let him help with finger feeding by letting him hold the french fry or pretzel and guiding it to the side of his mouth.

(continued)

Figure 11.2 *(continued)*

Assistance Provided During the Meal

Offer spoonfuls of ice water during regular meals. This will alert his mouth and build more awareness. It also will help him clear the residue of remaining food particles from his tongue and create more comfort during eating. Carlos swallows water rapidly. When he is given food after a quick water swallow, Carlos is more likely to use a more rapid swallow with the food.

Offer a crisp, crunchy food, such as a chip or crisp french fry, between spoonfuls of pureed foods. This will alert the mouth and prevent habituation of sensation from holding the softer food in the mouth. In addition, Carlos loves this type of food, and it offers a powerful internal motivation to swallow so that he can have a french fry!

Give him small enough spoonfuls of lumpy food that he can move around in his mouth for chewing. The larger spoonfuls do not give him enough learning opportunities for tongue lateralization in chewing. When he has a large amount of food in his mouth, he mashes it up and down in a munching pattern or sucks it to the back of the mouth for swallowing.

The development of tongue lateralization in chewing will be much easier when placement is on the side of the mouth, rather than in the center. Work for chewing movements of the jaw and tongue by placing the food on the side between the biting surfaces of the teeth. Guide him in alternating sides for food placement so that both sides take a turn at biting. Initially, use foods that dissolve or break easily into small pieces. This can include cheese cubes, graham crackers, shortbread cookies, Cheese Curls™, Veggie Stix™, and thin pretzels.

Have him practice biting a long, thin piece of food with rapid, repetitive bites. Foods such as pretzels, Cheese Curls, french fries, long cookies, and pieces of graham cracker are ideal for this activity. The ability to make many rapid bites is dependent on control of a very small amount of jaw opening. The repetition of the biting pattern introduces the sustained rhythm of chewing.

Support Carlos' desire to stamp his feet while he is chewing. Help him do this in a more coordinated way and make a game of it. This will help him develop better rhythm for chewing and a stronger chewing pattern. The footrest of his chair can be padded or a thin pillow placed on it at home or at school if the noise becomes a problem for others at the table.

Communication and Interaction at Meals

Talk to Carlos about what he is eating and will be given next on the spoon. This will help him anticipate what will happen, because he does not get this information visually.

Figure 11.2 *(continued)*

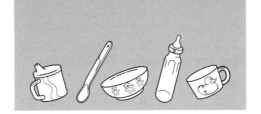

Mealtime Program

Child _____ Age _____

Therapist _____ Date _____

Part ___ :

Goals

_____

Supporting Areas

_____

Limiting Areas

_____

Possible Activities

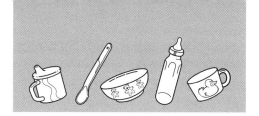

Individual Mealtime Plan

Child _____   Age _____

Therapist _____   Date _____

Supporting and Limiting Mealtime Skills

Short-Term Mealtime Focus and Objectives

Mealtime Suggestions

Environmental Setting for the Meal

Preparation for Mealtime

(continued)

Physical Position

Food Texture, Temperature, and Taste

Utensils

(continued)

Assistance Provided During the Meal

Communication and Interaction at Meals

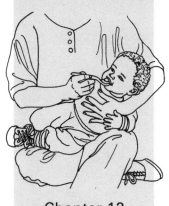

Chapter 12

Treatment Principles and Perspectives

▦ The Concept of Mealtime Programs

Mealtime Circles of Influence

This overview of treatment begins with a broad view that encompasses a total program. This may be likened to the type of view that we achieve by looking through the lens of a camera as it moves from a wide-angle setting to a zoom setting. Within our view is the breadth and depth of the landscape as far as the eye can see. We take in a broad overview of the picture that enables us to understand the smaller segments and how they fit into the landscape. We see the total surroundings that give us a frame of reference for understanding the smaller environments and details that make up this whole. Because our camera lens is adjustable, we may choose to zoom it slowly to different parts of the landscape. We look specifically at other parts of this environment and appreciate the details. We begin to notice and appreciate the related details of these smaller environments. Soon we see an additional set of relationships among the parts in each environment. All is interconnected.

Imagine you are sitting on the porch of a small cottage embedded in the woods. Before you is spread a peaceful blue lake surrounded by the colors of a beautiful autumn day. The colors are blended in a palette that mixes soft yellows and oranges with deep copper, blazing red and dark green. You hear and see the scampering squirrels and hear the call of late fall songbirds and the more brazen call of a hawk circling overhead. Fish jump on the lake, and you notice a small boat with two people fishing. You take in this scene with one glance and appreciate its totality. Your attention is drawn to an area on the shore of the lake where you notice an especially colorful maple tree. You are drawn to the color variations of the leaves as they shade from pale yellow to gold to rich orange. Some have dropped to the ground, creating a colorful carpet on the grass. Others float in a small bay of the lake and mix among the abundant pads of the water lily. Your gaze shifts from the tree to the lake itself as you notice the lily pads in greater detail and the shifting reflections from the tree and sky on the surface of the water. The jumping of a fish and the overhead reflection of the hawk preparing to dive for its supper disturb the quiet surface. Sounds of wildlife now enter your awareness. Your attention moves to two squirrels that chatter as they scurry up a nearby tree, carrying acorns to store for winter. You hear the call of a small bird and the rhythmical tap of a woodpecker coming from the woods. Slowly you are conscious of human voices and shift your eyes to the fishermen in the small rowboat. One has just caught a fish and they pull the fishing line toward the boat and scoop the fish into a small net to bring it aboard. You become simultaneously aware of the total scene that encompasses this autumn

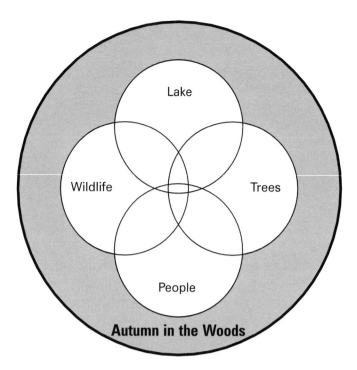

Figure 12.1   **Autumn in the Woods**

day in the woods and the details of each part of the scene. You see and understand the complex inter-relationships among these parts.

We are familiar with our ability to appreciate the whole and then shift our attention to each part. With greater awareness, we notice how the parts are interconnected. Figure 12.1 reflects these relationships in our view of this autumn day in the woods. The lake mirrors the trees and accepts its leaves, which float on the surface. The reflection of the hawk and the presence of the fish remind us of the connection between the wildlife and the lake. The fishermen in their boat admire the beautiful fall colors of the trees as they catch the fish and pull it from the lake. The squirrels gather the acorns that have fallen from trees to the lakeshore and take them to their nest in a nearby tree.

We can destroy the balance and harmony of this scene by losing sight of the interconnections. People can pollute the lake, causing the death of the fish. Its shoreline can be changed by beavers who cut down the maple tree for a dam or by people in motor boats that indirectly increase the growth of swamplands on the lakeshore.

We can take the same familiar concept and use it to represent the foundation for our underlying concept of mealtime programs in Figure 12.2. The broad, wide-angle view is the totality of the meal-time. This allows us to appreciate the interplay of mealtime relationships as they are expressed and influenced by the mealtime, communication, learning, physical, and sensory circle environments.

Every mealtime or treatment session is simultaneously composed of each of these circles. It is impossible, for example, to say, "I'm not going to include a communication environment today." All the circle environments are continuously present. The therapist always has the choice of deciding how to create or influence an environment, but does not have the choice to eliminate it. These circles of influence include developmental skills and progressions as well as limitations that get in the way of development. Each includes the mouth and details of oral feeding as well as the broader influences that support and surround oral feeding.

The **_Mealtime_** circle represents the total interactions and influences on the child's mealtime. It includes all aspects of the four circles that it encloses. In addition, it incorporates the broader aspect of the child's relationship to the family and community at meals. Thus, it relates to aspects such as

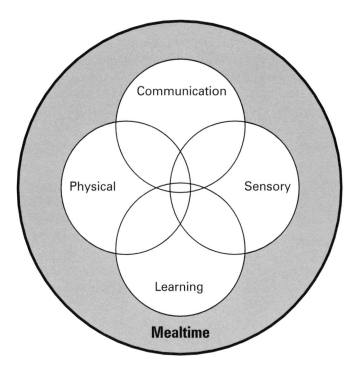

Figure 12.2   **Mealtime Circles**

beliefs, cultural values, health, and socioeconomic issues that have an impact on a child's ability to eat and a family's ability to provide different levels of nourishment.

The ***Communication*** circle encompasses all the verbal and nonverbal mealtime interactions that take place. These include the manner in which the child communicates information that guides or regulates the meal. Infants and children let others know when they are hungry and want to eat or are full and want to stop. They indicate their need for a pause or desire for a bite of a different food. They regulate the speed with which adults offer the food and let them know which foods they like and don't like. Adults respond to the child's messages and offer their own verbal and nonverbal comments about the meal and the feeding relationship. Communication encompasses other children and adults who share the meal, and it includes conversational topics that are unrelated to feeding.

The ***Learning*** circle incorporates the many aspects of learning that are part of the mealtime. Children learn about food and eating skills. They master their mouths, hands, and utensils as they learn to handle more challenging foods and liquids and to feed themselves. They learn what behavioral choices are acceptable to their family and those that are not. They learn about celebrations and family traditions. Every child and parent has a learning style and preferred ways of learning. Some individuals learn more by listening. Others learn by watching. Still others need to feel, move, and physically manipulate things to understand them.

The ***Physical*** circle encompasses the many aspects of the physical relationships at the meal. This involves the way in which the infant or child is held for feeding or the type of chair used for supported or independent sitting. It includes the child's postural tone and stability, body movements, and oral-movement control for eating. Other aspects of the physical environment include the physical position and comfort of the feeder as well as the types of feeding utensils that are used.

The ***Sensory*** circle incorporates the myriad of sensory inputs that are part of every meal—the tastes, smells, sights, textures, temperatures, and sounds that are part of the room and the food. It includes each individual's ability to receive, process, and integrate the sensory input as well as specific physical and emotional responses to these sensations.

It is vitally important to remember that these areas interact and are interdependent. Each environmental circle touches and includes part of every other circle. For example, Kyle's communication skills are strongly influenced by the physical environment. When he is seated in a chair or on a lap in a way that increases his muscle tone, he is unable to coordinate his eyes to look at a specific food or guide his mother who is feeding him. The tension in his body often increases his sensitivity to unexpected sounds or touch so that the feeling of the spoon in the mouth triggers a strong biting reflex. His ability to learn under these conditions is reduced. He and his mother become frustrated and easily angered because of his biting. The mealtime relationship deteriorates, and his mother tries to feed him faster just to bring it to completion. Kyle becomes stiffer and more upset, increasing the limitations in all of these environmental circles.

If the feeder changes an element in one of the circles, it will influence each of the other circles. Kyle's mother initially focuses on the ***physical*** environment. When she shifts Kyle's position so that his hips are more flexed and his head is more forward, his eye gaze and communication skills improve, and he can guide the meal more successfully. He is less sensitive to sounds and touch, and accepts the spoon without biting. He is available for learning new skills. Even if it is not possible to change his physical position, his mother may choose to focus on the ***sensory*** environment. She notices that he is more jumpy when there are loud sounds or when the feeling of the spoon surprises him. She may choose to feed him in a very quiet room or use a plastic-coated spoon instead of a metal spoon. With these changes in the sensory area, his body is less stiff and Kyle eats better. With a quieter, softer body, he is able to guide his mother with mouth cues for eating readiness. He opens his mouth easily and makes suckling movements when he is ready for the spoon. He no longer has a bite reflex on the spoon. Both he and his mother have learned that he can use his mouth as well as his eyes to signal readiness.

In a third example, his mother chooses to focus on the ***communication*** environment. Kyle is still stiff and jumpy because of his position and noises in the room. She begins to talk to him, telling him what is happening and letting him know that the spoon is coming. Her voice provides a calming sensory focus for Kyle, and he relaxes in her arms. His body is less stiff. Because he knows when to expect the spoon, he is less emotionally tense. He trusts his mother and feels her communicative support. The sound of her voice also blocks out some of the environmental sounds that bother him. He learns that he does not have to become tight and upset when his head is back and he is being fed in a noisy room. His mother also has learned another alternative for feeding him when the physical and sensory environments are less ideal.

In another scenario, Kyle's mother focuses on the ***learning*** environment. She thinks about what she has learned in the past about her son's mealtime needs and quickly reviews what is possible or impossible to change in the current setting. Many of the alternatives she has used in the past are unavailable to her. She is sitting in a waiting room of the doctor's office and the only chair available does not support her body well. It is noisy, and other children are crying and running around. She feels stressed by the long wait and her hungry son. She takes time before the meal to relax her mind and body before picking up Kyle. She begins to sing a rhythmical melody softly in Kyle's ear, remembering how well he responds to rhythm. She shifts to a rhythmical tapping on his chest. She tells him that she knows it is noisy in this room and harder to be partners in eating. She suggests that they can pretend that they are having lunch in a special place they both like. She talks to him about the imaginary place where they will be eating and describes it as she offers Kyle the food. Kyle settles down and begins to eat with a soft, controlled body and mouth. He feels like a partner with his mother as they explore this imaginary place together.

In the final example, Kyle's mother reflects on an aspect of the overall ***mealtime*** environment. She is aware of her perception that Kyle is acting out and being a brat. She reflects on her deep-seated beliefs that he pushes back and is messy to get his own way. She and the feeding therapist have been talking about different ways to look at what he does at mealtimes and different ways in which she might perceive his actions. She knows that Kyle sometimes finds eating scary and is fearful that he will choke. She is always aware that she was raised in a family that expected total obedience to parental wishes. When Kyle pushes against her body, she automatically feels that he is fighting her or confronting her desire for an easy, neat meal. She takes a deep breath and suddenly realizes that Kyle is feeling some of the same stresses that she is experiencing. He is hungry. She is in a less-than-ideal environment. She wants things to go well, and they are not. Kyle wants to get the food down and he is very hungry, but he can't achieve the body and mouth coordination to do this. As she lets go of her feeling that he is trying to make things difficult for her, they both relax and feel better about their mutual situation. Kyle begins to eat with greater coordination, and she lets go of her need to be in control of a perfect meal.

The most important concept underlying the mealtime program is that everything is connected. Every area influences every other area. This concept permeates every chapter of this book. The therapist cannot sit back and say, "My job is the mouth!" The development of stability in the pelvis influences trunk control, which influences head and neck control, which influences how the mouth handles food. Tactile defensiveness in the hands reduces the child's comfort in picking up toys for mouthing or food pieces for initial self-feeding. These issues, in turn, influence the oral experiences that the child brings to learning to bite and chew solid foods. Gastrointestinal discomfort during tube feedings influences the child's beliefs about eating and may increase resistance to eating by mouth. Lack of control over his life because of multiple medical problems may increase the child's discovery that saying "no" to eating is a powerful way to be in control. Nothing is disconnected. Success in treatment is linked directly to the therapist's awareness of these connections and her realization that a decision made in one area has the potential to affect many other areas.

Feeding Programs, Oral Motor Treatment Programs, and Mealtime Programs

Many different terms are used to describe a type of program that focuses on improving a child's ability to eat and drink. For many years, these programs were referred to as *feeding programs*. This term is still commonly used today. Often, it is too narrow for the therapist's purposes because it implies that the immediate goal is to get children to eat. Many therapists continue to focus on the narrow goal of getting children to eat a specific quantity of food or a more advanced texture, with minimal attention to the underlying physical, sensory, and oral motor skills that would make this process easier for everyone.

When the first edition of this book was published, the authors chose *Pre-Feeding Skills* as the title to emphasize that there were so many aspects of feeding that preceded the actual use of food and liquid for eating and drinking. The focus was on the importance of preparing the child for success. The terms *oral motor treatment* and *oral motor skills* were used interchangeably to focus on the broad range of communication, learning, physical, and sensory skills that surround and support the feeding process. The term oral motor treatment also has become narrowed by groups of therapists who seem to emphasize specific stimulation and movements of the jaw, tongue, and lips. They often forget that these oral parts and movements are connected to all other areas of the body and influence the entire mealtime interactions. Most important, they often place the movement of the mouth above the interactive participation of the child. These often become programs that "do to children" rather than "participate with children." This is a critically important distinction.

The bias today is toward using the broader term *mealtime programs* to remind therapists of the tremendous importance of the mealtime for the child and family and all that it implies for therapy. If programs are to be successful today, they absolutely must encompass an understanding of the child's feeding and oral motor issues within the broader context of the family. They must honor the fact that some children who can benefit from a mealtime program may never be candidates for oral feeding or have high-level, oral motor skills because of the dangers of aspiration or the presence of severe sensory or motor disabilities. They must provide a model for therapists who are working with tube-fed children whose journey toward oral feeding must provide them with the full range and context of the mealtime. These goals often go unmet in the more limited context of feeding or oral motor programs.

Therapists may conceptualize the three terms as a set of concentric circles that progressively expands the concepts and experiences with which they work.

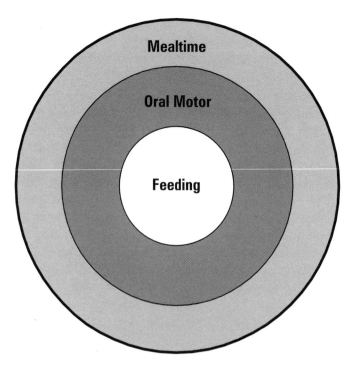

Figure 12.3 **Mealtime Programs**

Therapists continue to use all three terms but acknowledge that even when they are focused on the innermost circle of feeding, they are alerted to the child's oral motor and mealtime needs. Indeed, therapists may be focused most strongly on the direct feeding elements for some children. However, if they work to help a child learn to drink from a cup without the awareness of oral motor skill prerequisites, they will fail. The therapist may focus on the oral motor skills that the child needs to be successful in drinking from the cup, but if he acts as if it is the mouth alone that learns to drink, the therapist will fail. If the therapist maintains a child-centered, family-centered, process-centered approach, he will succeed. The therapist needs the details and the focus supplied by oral motor treatment and by the narrower focus on feeding, but the context must be that of a mealtime program if he is to be truly successful.

Interplay of Assessment and Treatment

In many facilities there is an artificial separation of the assessment and treatment components of intervention. In this book, the guideline used is that assessment and treatment are inseparably intertwined. They are two sides of the same coin, two branches of the same tree. They have common roots and a common vision. Both seek to find out more about the child and gain a greater understanding of the strengths and needs that the child brings to the mealtime. Many people have conceived of assessment and treatment in a linear fashion in which a detailed assessment is completed. This evaluation may or may not be followed by a period of treatment. Often, there is minimal relationship between the findings of the assessment and the treatment program that is developed. The assessment may be done under circumstances that mask or distort the child's feeding abilities and needs. Many parents have told therapists that they do not even recognize their child from the description provided in the assessment report. Children often respond differently in an assessment than they do at home. Some are frightened and exhausted, and they shut down. Others refuse to participate. Still others feel they must be on their best behavior. Some children show a deterioration of eating skills; others seem to eat more skillfully for an unfamiliar therapist.

Many evaluations are done without treatment probes or trials. Suggestions are offered to the family or other therapists based on a computerized list of treatment techniques that are supposed to be effective for children with the diagnostic label or description given to the child.

In a similar fashion, many treatment programs see assessment as something that takes place every 3 to 12 months. An assessment is scheduled to measure progress or revise program goals. During the interim, the therapist does therapy. Goals, strategies, or techniques may be continued during this period whether or not the child is responding or making progress. This is the child's program, based on the assessment. It will continue until the next assessment.

When therapists view assessment and treatment as integral parts of the same process, they are always involved in both components. The clinician simply emphasizes one or the other at a given moment. The therapist may choose to focus on the discovery process of assessment. This is where energy is focused, but treatment enters into the process. The therapist may notice that Carlos becomes agitated when his mother brings out lumpy food. He shuts his eyes and makes a face. When she puts the spoonful in his mouth, he begins to gag. Rather than simply noting his limiting response to this type of food on the assessment form, the therapist can explore some treatment options. The therapist may be unsure of whether Carlos' defensive and gagging response is related to the discomfort of oral tactile defensiveness or because food pieces scatter over his tongue. The clinician could explore a number of therapy options at this point. She could invite Carlos to play with mouth toys that have texture, and notice any overall reticence or discomfort with Carlos' fingers or toys in the mouth. The therapist could explore a variety of strategies designed to prepare the nervous system to integrate sensory information more effectively. She also could introduce more solid pieces of food in a gauze or net bag to prevent food scatter on the tongue. As the therapist explores a variety of therapy strategies, she gains insight about the nature of Carlos' gagging problems. She also gains a clearer sense of therapy directions that would be effective.

Children are different at each treatment session. Their sensory processing and motor coordination skills vary, depending upon a wide number of variables. The therapist cannot make the assumption that treatment will begin at the point where it ended at the previous session. If she can begin with a challenge that is just-right for the child, learning will take place. If the clinician begins with an activity that poses no challenge, the child may become bored or progress that might have been possible during the session is not achieved. If the therapist begins at a level that is too difficult, the child may become discouraged and refuse to participate, or may move into distracting or disruptive behaviors. The child may arrive with a very different agenda or set of interests than those of the therapist, and a session may deteriorate into a contest of whose agenda will be addressed. The only way that these pitfalls can be avoided is to begin each treatment session with a mini-assessment.

Treatment can be guided at each moment by diagnostic observations that evaluate the child's response to what the therapist has just done. These observations tell the therapist whether to continue in the same direction, adjust the challenge of the activity slightly upward or downward, or shift to another activity altogether.

Guiding Principles

Although there are many approaches or models that can be used for problem solving, each functions best when built upon a set of guidelines that becomes a working model for the therapist's interaction with the child. The authors value the following guidelines and use them in all sessions.

The Dance of Mealtime

Mealtimes and therapy sessions that address mealtime and feeding skills are viewed as a dance between the child and the adult. As in any harmonious dance, there is a partnership in which the skills of one person blend with the skills of the other. The dance flows as communication flows between the partners in a give-and-take relationship. The mealtime dance has a division of responsibility and roles within the dance. The responsibility of the therapist or parent is to prepare the child and environment for success in the oral motor or eating activity. The feeding therapist introduces physical and sensory activities that get the body and mouth ready for eating. Food and utensils that are appropriate for the child's developmental and skill level are introduced. Communication and learning preparation are provided. A good therapist learns to be a good salesperson by knowing what the child wants and how to blend the child's desires with the therapist's desires. The child's responsibility is to guide the therapist's selection of activities by letting the adult know verbally or nonverbally what types of activity or input fit at that moment. He gives the therapist feedback that moves the session in a direction that will be more successful. When food is involved, the child is solely responsible for deciding whether to eat, what to eat, and how much to eat.

Developing Trust and Respect

Trusting Ourselves and Others

Trust is the essential element in any interaction between two people. Children know our attitude from our approach. They know when they are being pushed and if their wants are understood and respected. When children know we trust them and are not there to shove them into a new experience, they become free to venture forth. In an atmosphere of trust, children learn when they are invited to explore and discover something new. When they do not trust us and fear they will be forced to change, they learn to shut us out and develop what we label as behavior problems.

In addition, when we do not trust our own abilities, we tend to push ourselves and children to somehow prove that we know what we are doing. We use more effort than we need and often try to move faster than the child is willing or able to go. Life and movement do not have to be effortful. Each flows with its own speed and beauty. Our job is to find the flow and move with it, not against it.

Judgments and Acceptance

When we refuse to judge ourselves, knowing that at every moment we are doing the best we can, everything is possible. Then we see possibilities in every interaction with a child rather than perceiving our limitations (Kaufman, 1975; Kaufman & Kaufman, 1987).

Getting the Child's Permission

The mouth is a very personal and private space for each child and adult. When the mouth is invaded, individuals feel very vulnerable and uncomfortable. When they feel vulnerable, they erect protective barriers. Barriers prevent the development of trusting relationships. When adults ask children for permission to bring a toy to the mouth or to give a new food, children know that they can let down the barriers because the adults will not try to trick them. Adults always must ask for permission. Even if the child refuses, you are building long-term trust and respect. These are the ingredients that enable children to take risks and try something that is new or fear provoking.

Following the Child's Lead

Observing the Child's Response

Our fullest understanding of each child comes from careful observations. These observations then are explored with the full range of our information-processing abilities. When we view information in both sequential and global ways, in analytical and intuitive fashions, and through each sensory modality, the process reveals the fertility of the mind, and answers and insights are possible without effort. When teaching is directed toward something that interests children or matches their focus of attention, learning is faster and more efficient (Watson, 1998; Yoder, Kaiser, Alpert, & Fischer, 1993).

Inner Wisdom

Children know what they want and need. If we learn to observe the messages in the body, eyes, face, and voice, we, too, can know (Kaufman, 1975). What a child wants usually contains a part or component of what we might want for the child.

Children who have sensory and motor problems find ways of responding, moving, and interacting with the world that provide them with what they want and need. They achieve this in the best way they know how. Because of their neurological problems, they often become stuck, and the ways they discover and develop may be effortful or limiting. Our challenge is to explore with the child and find other ways of meeting these needs that allow wider opportunities for learning and development.

The Treatment Partnership

When the feeding partner follows a child's lead, she is not abdicating responsibility as a therapist or parent. Some adults think that this means giving the children their own way all the time. They envision their children turning into rude tyrants and want to prevent this. They are afraid to respond to what the child wants and honor the child's choices because of their fear of the future. Following a child's lead means that therapists or parents are willing to trust that the child knows intuitively what he needs and what will help at that moment.

Nora, for example, wanted to spend the entire treatment session closing doors in her house. She loved doors and loved to push her hands against them and feel them closing. Nora had fluctuating postural tone and tended to move with greater coordination on one side of her body. She had very poor coordination of her breathing and voicing, and was only able to put two words together in one breath. She became disorganized and distractible with visual and auditory sensory input. She had a great deal of difficulty sitting down for an activity and was moving around constantly. Sitting in a chair to work on feeding and language skills was almost impossible. Her therapist accompanied Nora around the house on the adventure of finding doors to close. She followed her lead, creating a partnership in which she introduced slight variations in the basic door-closing activity. Nora could use one hand or two hands. She could push with her hands above her head or at waist level. Some doors required more pressure or strength to close than others. She could make loud sounds with her voice while closing one door and close the next one silently.

When the therapist left, she realized that the activity that Nora had selected contained all of the strategies that she would choose for her. The activity required Nora to stand with her weight more evenly over her two feet. She usually used both hands together, which provided symmetrical weight bearing through her arms and shoulder girdle. This built better postural stability and reduced the fluctuating muscle tone. It also provided strong proprioceptive input into her joints. This is a type of sensory input that helps many children organize or integrate their sensory-processing systems. With better tone and stability, Nora's attention improved and she was less distractible. When Nora pushed on the door, her voice became louder and longer, and her speech improved. Pushing to close doors was exactly what Nora needed! Nora continued to close doors for two more therapy sessions. Toward the end of each session, her therapist suggested that they sit down in the kitchen and have a snack. Nora was able to sit quietly with good postural stability. Her oral skills improved substantially, and her therapist trusted her and followed her lead in the door-closing activity. Her skills also improved because the therapist recognized the benefit of the activity and its interconnections with her own goals and desires for Nora. Each session with a child becomes an opportunity for shared learning. The adult learns from the child and the child learns from the adult.

Building on the Child's Assets

Programs that are built upon what a child does well and enjoys are more likely to lead to changes and growth. They provide more pleasure and enjoyment for the child and the therapist. When an individual feels love and enjoyment with another person, there is greater learning. When the therapist works from the child's abilities, the child perceives himself as able. When the therapist adopts a deficit model of therapy and works only on things the child cannot do and *needs to learn,* the child becomes discouraged and sees only his disability.

Approaches, Strategies, and Techniques

A major concern with any approach to treatment is the way in which it is implemented. Parents and therapists need to address programs and therapies as consumers, in the same way they would address the salesperson who wishes to sell them a car or home. For example, if I want to buy a new car, my first step is to decide on the type of car that meets my needs. What is the overall **approach** to automobile transportation that I am looking for? Do I want a small, fuel-efficient car; a large luxury car; a sports car; a van; or a sport-utility vehicle (SUV)? This decision usually is made on the basis of my personal beliefs and philosophy as well as my current needs. For example, if there are eight people in my family, I will not choose a small sports car as the only form of family transportation. I probably will be drawn toward some type of van or station wagon. On the other hand, if I have a small family and believe strongly in supporting the environment, a small, fuel-efficient car will be at the top of my list.

Once I have decided on the type of car that meets my needs, I can begin to look at the **strategies** that different manufacturers have used within the car type. Some of these strategies are linked closely with the type of car selected. For example, nearly all SUVs feature 4-wheel drive and an open cargo space that is accessed through a rear door. By definition, these cars are designed for some off-road or heavy-duty travel and to carry larger amounts of off-size materials. Yet different car manufacturers approach these strategies in different ways. There are different types of 4-wheel drive systems and different configurations of the cargo space. They also use strategies that are specific to their brand or model of automobile that relate to the engine, transmission, fuel, and brake systems. As a potential buyer, I look at how these strategies fit with what I know about the overall approach to this type of vehicle. I may reject one manufacturer's vehicles because they have introduced a car body that is very low to the ground, yet they have advertised it as a sport-utility vehicle. If I want to take this car on a rutted gravel road or across a field, the strategy of the low body frame doesn't fit with the overall approach to the car. I am drawn to another with a very large cargo space, a body frame that is high to the ground, and a 4-wheel drive system that is extremely easy to activate. Each of these strategies fits with the overall theme or approach to an SUV that I am looking for.

My third level of decision making lies in the specific details I would like in the SUV. What specific **techniques** did the manufacturer incorporate in the overall design that I have selected? For example, there are many ways to access the rear cargo area. Do I want a model in which the rear door opens outward or upward? Do I want one in which the rear window opens separately, allowing the placement of items inside without opening the main door?

Some of the strategies and specific techniques that are common to the SUV also fit with other cars. Many mid-size or smaller cars with a sedan body now have 4-wheel drive. Compact cars with a hatchback design also feature a rear-access door.

When I purchase a car, I ask myself the following questions.

- What style or overall approach to transportation fits my beliefs, personality, and needs?
- Do the strategies selected by the manufacturer for this vehicle fit the overall approach or philosophical design of the car?
- Are there a variety of choices or specific techniques available in different models and features to meet my specific individual needs and desires?

This also is the type of thinking and analysis we can do as we select the type of treatment program we wish to implement or the type of program we seek for our child.

Approach or Philosophy

The approach or philosophy of a program is its overall organizing framework. Every strategy and technique selected should fit into this framework or concept. The framework of the mealtime approach is strongly child centered and family centered. It focuses on nourishment and nurturance. It incorporates diverse aspects of a mealtime such as communication, socialization, health, sensory exploration, and celebration. The mealtime approach incorporates specific work on feeding and oral motor skills into this broader foundation. It utilizes a series of five interlocking, interconnected circles to represent its major areas of focus: mealtime, communication, learning, physical, and sensory.

Strategies

Strategies used in the program reflect ways of implementing the overall approach or framework. They are the overall picture or series of pictures that fit in the frame. There are specific strategies that are used when working within the communication circle or environment. These might include strategies for identifying how the child communicates at mealtime, or strategies for increasing the accuracy and consistency of nonverbal messages. In the physical circle, the therapist would include strategies for normalizing postural tone as well as obtaining movement awareness and control. In both of these examples, the strategies would be in harmony with the overall philosophy or approach to the program. For example, the therapist might ask a child directly how he lets someone know he wants the food, then carefully observe for changes in the child's response. The therapist initially would look for something the child is already doing well and build or expand a communication response on this movement rather than imposing an outside communication system or signal that is foreign to the child. In the physical area, the therapist also would make the child a partner by selecting movement approaches that involve the child's input. The therapist would not select strategies that impose therapeutic exercise on an unhappy or unwilling child because she perceives that it is good for the child's muscles. The therapist would find strategies that engage the child in activating the muscles as part of something that interests him or builds a cooperative partnership between the child and therapist.

Techniques

Techniques consist of the many smaller details and choices that are available to implement a strategy that the therapist has selected. They offer the individualized choices that enable the therapist to customize a strategy for a specific child or developmental need. The technique must fit the approach and the strategy. When a technique involves the use of a specific piece of equipment, it always describes how and when that equipment is used. For example, the NUK Massage Brush™ (see page 436) can be used in a wide variety of ways that fit different strategies in the mealtime approach. In each of the strategies described, its use will be interactive with the child. Its stimulation will never be imposed on the child's mouth. The technique must fit the overall approach. The massage brush can be used as a mouth exploration tool within the strategy of oral exploration of toys. It can be used as a textured spoon in strategies to build greater mouth awareness during feeding. It can be used in a broader technique of tapping on the tongue or stroking the center of the tongue to increase muscle tone and obtain a more central groove during sucking. The massage brush is not the technique. It is a therapy tool that is incorporated within a technique designed to implement a specific strategy.

Techniques are used to express and implement the approach and strategies the clinician has selected. An extensive listing of treatment strategies and techniques is included in Chapter 17 for reference. Techniques, however, should never be used as the approach itself. Some therapists describe what they do as implementing a NUK massage brush program, a ball program, or a brushing program, as if the technique were the program itself. Programs with this type of focus really have no focus and no cohesive direction. Often, they are a hodge-podge of techniques that bear no relationship to what the child needs.

Alternative Pathways

Many programs for children with mealtime, oral motor, and feeding needs are not built with a clear philosophical foundation. Many are a collection of the latest techniques that the therapist has seen in a book or learned about at a workshop. Many are applied randomly to all children to find out in a trial-and-error fashion what will work. Some are continued despite lack of progress or active resistance by the child because someone has assured the therapist that "if you do it long enough, it will work."

Cookbook collections of the "50 best oral motor techniques" for the tongue and other such workshop-generated handouts make the rounds of therapy programs and often become the core of a child's program. These appeal strongly to therapists who feel the pressures of time and the need to have ready-made programs for the children with whom they work.

The concept of critical pathways is quite seductive as a means of increasing quality care and reducing the costs of medical and rehabilitation services (Hofmann, 1993; Neidig, Megel, & Koehler, 1992). It implies that for a given disorder or diagnostic label, the therapist can define a set of steps or landmarks along the path from the beginning to the end of a treatment sequence. It implies that there is one accepted approach to treating the disorder and that every individual with this disorder will fit in somewhere along the path. Theoretically, any therapist should be able to identify where a child or adult is on the pathway and implement subsequent treatment steps that would lead toward successful eating. This concept is still in its infancy and has been primarily applied to acquired adult disorders such as in the hospital management of adults who have had a stroke (Falconer, Roth, Sutin, Strasser, & Chang, 1993). Although the model has been discussed in the management of adult swallowing disorders (Sonies, 1997), its application to a condition as diverse as pediatric mealtime and feeding disorders seems quite limited.

The What and How of Therapy

Therapy itself is a blend of two equal aspects: what therapists do and how they do it. We have found the following thoughts and guidelines extremely helpful as we create therapy programs that make a positive difference in children's lives.

What We Do

- Obtain a broad overview of children's mealtimes and the mealtime and feeding relationships as the starting point in any treatment program. What values, beliefs, and desires motivate the family to seek therapy for the child? What do the family and child want?

- Reduce or eliminate the factors that create limits in the five mealtime circles of mealtime, learning, communication, physical, and sensory influences. Initially, look at these circles of influence in their broadest mealtime perspective. Move from this point to their impact on specific oral motor and feeding components in each area. Always address the limiting factors in the body as a whole before focusing on mouth for feeding.

- Mealtime circles influence each other. Changes in one will influence changes in each of the others. Addressing the mealtime, communication, and learning environments first will have the strongest impact on the child's program. The learning of a motor skill is primarily sensory learning. If the child shows limiting responses to sensory input, learning will be affected. Problems of hyperreaction, hyporeaction, sensory overload, sensory defensiveness, and sensory disorganization must be reduced in order to create an internal sensorimotor environment in which children are able to learn. Therefore, techniques to normalize a child's ability to accept and integrate visual, auditory, tactile, vestibular, taste, and temperature information should be selected before directly facilitating a new oral feeding pattern.

- There is a general order of influence in the area of physical limitations and function. When observing the child's body, the therapist should start at the bottom and work upward. What is happening in the feet, legs, and pelvis will influence what happens in the trunk. Tone and movement in the trunk will affect function in the shoulder girdle. The function of the shoulder girdle influences head and neck control. Head and neck control influences jaw control. Control of tone and movement in the jaw determines control of the lips and cheeks, which in turn influence control of tongue movement. Always explore total body changes before implementing specific changes to the oral mechanism. Create changes in feeding through changes in body position and movement.

- Use the developmental progressions of feeding as a guide for therapy sequences. These sequences and progressions create many answers to the question "What do I want?" Remember that this is a guide, not a fixed recipe. Some stages and progressions can be skipped. Remember that development is a series of overlapping sequences. Infants do not perfect sitting before moving on to crawling. Cup drinking skills continue to evolve as babies begin to chew. Changes in one area often can influence changes in other areas.

- Work for improved quality of movement—not just the quantity of developmental milestones. Movement should occur without effort and with efficiency and speed.

How We Do It

- Acknowledge and respect children's knowledge and follow their lead or direction. This can occur through observing behaviors that give clues to a child's interests and activities, sensory choices, and learning style.

- Help children do what they want to do more successfully, with less effort, more completely, and with more variation.

- Consider the possibility that all activities are connected like a giant spider web. Create bridges from the child's interests and current abilities into something new.

- Make changes slowly. Change is difficult or threatening for many children and adults. Introduce change through small variations in what the child is already able to accept. Variations create small acceptable changes.

- Be aware of opportunities to introduce a variation or activity that will interest the child. Introduce opportunities as ways of enjoying the activity in a new or special way. Create possibilities for greater function. Offer these opportunities as a gift. Do not be unhappy or discouraged if the gift is not accepted initially.

- Create an environment of unconditional love—for the child, parent, and yourself. With unconditional love, people grow toward their greatest potential.

- There is no such thing as a mistake. What therapists call mistakes create *opportunities* for learning.

These principles and perspectives on treatment will be illustrated in the subsequent chapters in this book. Use them as guidelines and return to this chapter often when creating specific therapy and home programs for children and families.

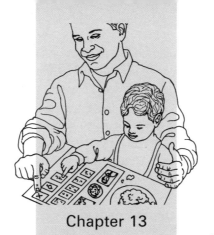

Chapter 13

Learning and Communication at Mealtimes

Maximizing the Ability to Learn

Many influences on the mealtime are described in this book. These include the independent, yet interconnected, impact of normal developmental skills, limiting factors in the body and mouth, sensory processing, and physical positioning and movement. Each of these influences affects learning at every meal.

Factors that influence mealtime learning for the child, parent, and therapist can be described as **internal** and **external** factors. Internal factors for the child include how the child feels during the meal, the motor skills that are available, appetite, desire, and motivation. External factors, which are equally important for the child's learning, include the teaching styles used by adults, the way in which food is offered, the learning environment, and the use of reward and punishment.

Mealtimes also are affected by the internal and external factors that influence the feeder. Feeders are internally guided by how they are feeling, their experiences and beliefs about feeding, and their understanding of the child's nutritional and developmental needs. Externally they are influenced by their physical comfort with the position used for feeding the child and the nature of the sensory environment in which the meal occurs.

Each of these factors influences what the child chooses to do and how the feeder chooses to respond. These choices, in turn, affect the feeding partnership, the mealtime relationship, and learning. Learning at the meal defines another mealtime relationship—the learning relationship.

Principles of Learning

Eating consists of a combination of inborn and learned behaviors. At birth, babies innately know how to eat. A newborn placed on the mother's abdomen will scoot upward to find the breast, latch on, and begin to nurse. Beyond that initial moment, internally guided feeding skills become intermingled with environmental aspects that result in the ongoing journey of learning to eat. Many of the traditional principles of learning easily relate to the learning of eating skills. Infants improve their sucking skills and learn to eat more maturely in developmentally appropriate ways as they are given opportunities and encouragement to eat. Alternatively, they learn not to eat or to eat in less constructive ways because of negative influences on their mealtimes.

Infants and children are influenced by the internal and external experiences that follow eating. When food tastes good and feels good in the mouth and tummy, infants generally continue to eat.

When both the reduction of hunger and feelings of satiation are comfortable, they usually eat until they begin to feel full. The act of eating is followed by something that creates pleasure for the infant. It is reinforced in a positive way. Learning takes place.

Children also learn positive behaviors from negative reinforcement. For example, children who retract the tongue into the airway experience respiratory distress and discomfort. They may learn an alternate forward resting posture of the tongue very quickly because the new strategy stops something that they experience as very noxious. In this instance, learning a new behavior (i.e., forward resting posture of the tongue) is reinforced because it removes the negative consequence (i.e., labored breathing) caused by retracting the tongue.

However, babies also can learn that eating is no fun, scary, or uncomfortable. If infants eat and then choke or frequently vomit, they may learn to eat less. In this case, the act of eating is followed by something unpleasant and, therefore, the behavior is punished. Likewise, when an older child sucks from a straw for the first time, the glee and encouragement of the parent may positively reinforce the learning of straw drinking so that the child wants to do it again. If an adult yells at the child who attempts to drink from a straw because some liquid spills on the table, less learning (or slower learning) will be seen. The punishment of yelling can dampen the child's desire to experiment with the new developmental skill of straw drinking. Children who already are discouraged by repeated criticism or failure may learn quickly that they do not want to use the straw for drinking. These positive and negative actions that follow attempts to learn new mealtime skills can strongly influence how children learn.

Events that precede or occur simultaneously with feeding also can strongly influence how children learn. When children are nauseated or feel pain after drinking a bottle, formula becomes associated with discomfort. Even though the baby may have previously enjoyed the smell, sight, and taste of milk, this food now becomes noxious and the infant may push it away. Gradually, these infants and children broaden their associations and learn to associate pain, discomfort, or nauseousness with all food. This is a common experience for children who experience gastroesophageal reflux or take medications that cause nausea as a side effect.

The impact of learned associations with sucking and swallowing is stronger as infants move from an eating pattern that is more automatic to one that is more volitional. For example, during the first 3 to 4 months, the suck-swallow-breathe pattern is more automatic or reflexive. Many infants struggle to eat despite incoordination, sensory discomfort, or the presence of gastroesophageal reflux. However, as they mature neurologically, the initiation of sucking and swallowing becomes more volitional. At this point, a large number of these infants refuse the bottle or breast. It is as if, in perceiving the association between discomfort and eating, the baby considers eating to be no longer worth the effort. Feeding tubes often are introduced at this point to provide the nutrition that the child needs. Some children initially continue to take a small amount orally, but then stop eating by mouth. Often, this is confusing to parents, who may blame themselves or the feeding tube for the child's loss of oral feeding skills and desire. When this is viewed from a learning perspective, the infant's choice is much easier to understand.

Both parents and children move beyond the simple associations and reinforcement paradigms that shape feeding behavior. Over time, they adopt a series of personal beliefs based on their own experiences and those of others. These beliefs serve as filters through which they interpret experiences and make learning decisions about eating and mealtimes. One child who chokes intermittently on lumpy food may incorporate his mother's loving concern for his well-being and continue to eat. Another child with the same physical response and similar parental reactions will use coughing and choking to end the meal and to gain additional parental attention. A third child under similar circumstances may refuse to eat any solid foods.

These three children arrived at different conclusions from the same experiences and formed different beliefs about eating solid foods. The first child feels safe and supported through the difficult experience of choking and concludes that mealtimes are safe if he has a helping partner. His mother's attention does not reinforce his coughing behavior and cause it to increase. The second child believes that no one pays attention to her unless she is in trouble. Her mother's solicitous and supportive attention to her coughing supports or reinforces this belief, and the child may learn to cough more often to gain attention or bring the meal to a close. The third child has learned to see the world of solid food as a dangerous place. He feels fear and uncertainty when he thinks about prior coughing episodes. He chooses to avoid eating these types of food because they threaten his well-being.

Most infants are born with the desire to eat. Feeding therapists must look at each child and examine the big picture of mealtime learning. They can gain insight into why a child does not eat or does not eat enough only when they understand the internal and external factors that influenced the development of the child's eating patterns. In order to fully understand a child's mealtime behaviors, adults must try to understand how the child learned not to eat or learned to eat in an inefficient manner. They must look at the internal and external factors that influence current mealtimes and recognize how these have an impact on the child, family, and therapists who are involved.

Therapists have the opportunity to guide children and their parents in positive directions for new mealtime learning. They have the challenge of helping many children move from unpleasant associations with meals to more positive expectations. This involves creating and re-creating the external learning environment to provide repeated positive experiences. These experiences can help children develop a new eating history. It also involves helping children and their parents explore their beliefs about eating and mealtimes, and build an internal learning environment that supports a more positive way of developing eating skills.

Making Changes: The Learning Environment

Many parents and therapists assume that change in learning to eat will come primarily from specific techniques and exercises that relate to the physical body and the mouth. The myth has been perpetuated that knowledge of the oral-motor system and techniques for altering the way in which muscles function will provide therapists with the primary answers. This is untrue. Knowledge of the physical system is important; without it, feeding therapists would stumble and have inadequate data for their personal problem-solving computer. However, the primary factors for success do not lie in this area. Therapists are engaged with a child and family in a personal contract to explore the possibility of change. Parents do not seek evaluation or therapy for their child if they are assured that all is well and development is proceeding normally. Even when the parents say that they feel the child has no problem, they have responded to the doubts or questions of others by bringing the child to the evaluation. These spoken or unspoken questions form the basis for potential learning.

> The primary focus of every feeding and mealtime program is to help the child
> and family learn to change the current situation.

Each contact that a parent and child has with a therapist creates the possibility for enhanced learning and understanding. The learning environment can be rich and filled with possibilities for new insights and connections, or it can be the repository for cultural beliefs of limitation and difficulty that impede the easy flow of learning and growth. Learning occurs for everyone involved. It is not solely the parent and child who must learn what the therapist is teaching; the therapist also must learn, grow, and discover new concepts taught by the child and parent. This two-way learning is a must for optimum interaction and essential to the success of the feeding and mealtime program.

The Power of Beliefs and Expectations

A powerful internal aspect of the learning environment is the set of attitudes and beliefs that the therapist and family communicate to the child. The expectations and beliefs of parents and professionals can limit or promote the learning potential of a child with a developmental disability. When therapists hold positive beliefs and do not act judgmentally, they are free to help children learn to eat and succeed in ways that might seem impossible to others. When parents release their fears and beliefs in limitation and no longer see their children's feeding problem as tragic, they communicate a loving intent that provides positive fuel for change in mealtime and feeding skills (Kaufman, 1975). The role played by beliefs at mealtimes is discussed in greater detail in Chapter 2.

The diagnosis of a disability can be traumatic for the family. Professionals often focus on the difficulties that the child will experience in learning and movement. The fear of creating unrealistic positive expectations motivates many therapists and physicians to push for parental acceptance of the child's limitations. Frequently, this is presented as a form of realism to prevent parental denial of the problem. There is a sense that it is better for parents to expect little of the child and be pleasantly surprised if performance is better than predicted. This may reflect a caution on the part of professionals and a fear of erring on the side of disappointing the family later if the child shows greater limitations than originally foreseen.

Each landmark of normalcy is searched for and amplified as the family passes through the process of mourning for the lost dream of a normal child. Professional statements of future limitation in the development of eating skills may be temporarily ignored while confronting the baby's differences. As delays and differences in feeding become more apparent, the infant may be pushed to produce hoped-for milestones. The infant may try to please important adults or he may develop a sense of personal failure when his effort fails to achieve a desired result. Some families find it easier to give up hope and accept the professional edict of limitation; this protects them from further disappointment as the infant develops. This is particularly true when the child is given non-oral feedings through a feeding tube. With either a sense of giving up or a sense of pressure, the child is unable to develop the knowledge of being loved and accepted unconditionally by the family. Negative fears and beliefs can create barriers to the child's full learning capacity.

Students have been shown to progress in classroom learning in harmony with their teachers' expectations. When a teacher was informed that a child of normal intelligence was mentally slow, the child made limited progress in learning and responded as a limited child (Rosenthal & Jacobson, 1968). When the same child was exposed to a teacher who was told she was gifted, the child showed a greater than normal amount of learning. In another study, a litter of rats was bred for a high level of homogeneity (Rosenthal, 1974). The litter was divided into two groups for a maze learning study. Group A was described as a group bred for maze-running intelligence; Group B was described as coming from a long line of slow-learning rats. Under identical learning situations, Group A learned rapidly; Group B completed the task in a delayed manner. The uncontrolled variable was the mental set or expectation of the psychologist taking the rats through the maze.

This impact of beliefs, known as the Pygmalion Effect, also has been applied to infants and geriatric patients. Adults used more negative behavioral descriptors when typically developing infants were described as being prenatally exposed to cocaine than when this label was not used (Woods, Eyler, Conlon, Behnke, & Wobie, 1998). Older nursing home residents received a comprehensive assessment of cognitive, functional, and emotional status. They were randomly assigned to a high expectancy or average expectancy group. Nurses and aides were told that, in comparison with other residents with similar difficulties, residents in the high expectancy group would perform above average in their rehabilitation program. When the assessment was repeated 3 months later, individuals in the high expectancy group showed fewer symptoms of depression, had a lower incidence of severe illness, and improved mental status (Learman, Avorn, Everitt, & Rosenthal, 1990).

Developmentally disabled infants and children often accept and adopt a belief system of limitations. Personal experience with movement and feeding difficulties may reinforce an attitude that life is difficult. This reduces the ability to tap the child's true potential and accelerate learning.

The words *expectation* and *expectancy* are derived from the same root verb, *expect*. Both reflect attitudes and actions that are valuable in designing an optimum environment for learning mealtime skills. Expectation defines the destination, while expectancy describes the journey.

Expectations are goal oriented, with the focus on the end product. Yet, as discussed in Chapter 11, the process of setting goals is directed primarily toward defining the goal directions. These directions enable therapists to define where they are going during therapy sessions and set measurable long-range landmarks that define whether they have arrived at the destination. Having a series of goal-oriented expectations enables adults to recognize opportunities that support the child's learning of appropriate skills.

Learning is enhanced when treatment sessions also include a sense of expectancy—a feeling of excitement and anticipation that something wonderful will occur or be discovered. Expectancy is goal free. One takes a path moving in the desired direction, yet the final goal is not clearly defined. The general direction may lead to a wide variety of skills and knowledge. The process becomes the focus of treatment. The anticipation that the journey will be pleasant and adventurous allows for unexpected discoveries and learning along the way. The teacher or therapist becomes free to enjoy the child and mutual discoveries about the world.

When approaches that guide and lead the child into new responses or beliefs are incorporated into the session, the child discovers options (Morris, 1991). Facilitation of new reactions and sensorimotor behaviors expands the realm of possibilities. It enables the child to discover new ways of being. When this process is combined with an environment that constantly suggests that the child can learn, communicate clearly, and move and eat with greater coordination and skill, the child begins to believe that these new patterns are possible.

For many children and families, providing an environment that is rich in positive suggestions creates an adequate foundation for learning. Others have more complex needs. An individual's deep inner beliefs (mental set) can create selective filters that do not allow positive suggestions for learning to be believed and integrated. The therapist does not work directly for a change in the mental set because logical arguments presenting another view will be rejected and the current view may become stronger. However, a skilled therapist may incorporate nonjudgmental questions to stimulate awareness of belief systems and the possibility of discarding those that are no longer useful (Kaufman, 1975, 1991).

Shifts in the mental set also occur when all aspects of the external learning environment are orchestrated in a relaxed fashion. The use of music, guided imagery, and other learning tools that bypass the more critical information-processing style of the left hemisphere are intended to produce a relaxed, receptive state of mind. As the individual is guided into experiencing acceleration in learning, the inner mind-set of personal limitations often changes.

A nonverbal approach to developing a positive mind-set can be used with young children. A set of new or unfamiliar experiences is created in an atmosphere of warm anticipation. Techniques that facilitate new movement, feeding, or cognitive patterns enable the child to repeat an experience. There is no longer a search for an unfamiliar pattern in a sea of effort and uncertainty because the child does not have to figure out how to move from visual and auditory information alone. Patterns can be matched and compared within the same sensory system rather than across senses. A child who experiences the inner sensations of mouth closure as righting reactions are facilitated for head control will find it much easier to repeat the closing movement. It will be more difficult if the learning takes place by following only verbal instructions or imitating the visual pattern in a mirror. Facilitation techniques for improving feeding and oral motor skills can use sensory input from all areas. Ideas for incorporating tactile, vestibular, proprioceptive, smell, taste, visual, and auditory senses are explored in Chapter 14.

The Power of Suggestion

The power of suggestion is one of the most important external factors in the learning environment. Almost every feature of the sensory environment carries suggestions (Lozanov, 1978; Prichard & Taylor, 1980). The physical environment of a hospital or clinic suggests illness or impairment. A therapy room or classroom that resembles a home rather than an institution promotes the concept of learning and wholeness. Therapy space that includes rooms similar to those found in the child's home suggests that what is being discovered or learned can be used at home. Isolated space within a school or clinic suggests that what is learned has little to do with everyday life. The positive effects of a physical environment can be enhanced through the use of art, color, music, flowers, and natural light.

The therapist or teacher provides numerous indirect suggestions to the child through the rhythm and intonation of the voice and through a sense of authenticity (Campbell, 1992). Children are attuned to adults' nonverbal communication. Facial expression, body movement, and vocal tones carry clear messages of the adult's feelings and intent. As the child develops language skills, he becomes aware of discrepancies between what the adult says and believes. Suggestions become more effective when the teacher's statements are in harmony with what she believes. A sense of authenticity, love, and concern carries a very strong message to the learner about the teacher's belief that changes will occur.

Openness, receptivity, acceptance, playfulness, and exploration enhance the learning experience for both the child and the teacher. As in early childhood, the learning of a new skill becomes a theme with many variations. Infants and young children explore and create hundreds of modifications of a single concept or movement. This weaving and reweaving of the same ideas and patterns is characteristic of a positive learning environment. Learning becomes rich through interconnections among experience, knowledge, and connections with future skills.

The Power of Music

Music can be highly effective in facilitating improved physical movement, feeding, communication, and language skills for a child who has a developmental disability. When used in a therapy program, music becomes a powerful facilitator of change and learning. A regular rhythm and appropriate musical tempo can increase the control of a rhythmic gait in walking (Staum, 1983; Thaut, McIntosh, & Rice, 1997; Thaut, Miltner, Range, Hurt, & Hoemberg, 1999), decrease the amount of muscle tension and assist relaxation (Scartelli, 1982), change the regularity of firing of electrical information to the muscles (Safranek, Koshland, & Raymond, 1982), and increase the amount of muscle co-contraction in muscles that provide postural stability. Appropriately selected music also can contribute to a reduction in hyperactivity (Scott, 1980), an increase in body awareness (Knill, 1983), and improvement in cognitive and communication development (Michel & May, 1984; Miller & Toca, 1979).

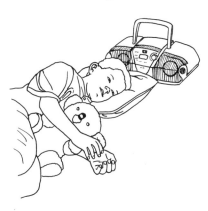

Within the therapy setting, music can be selected to facilitate movement and communication (Morris, 1991). Rhythmical folk music with a clear beat can become the interactive focus for the child and therapist. The rhythm can provide additional facilitation of sustained muscle contraction and rhythmical movement. Vocalization can be increased as the child sings along. A tempo of one-beat-per-second can be quieting and calming. Children who experience difficulty filtering out extraneous sensory input appear to deal with sensory information more appropriately as slower baroque music is played in the background. When quiet music is played at mealtime, a child with a feeding disorder often eats with better coordination. The sucking rhythm is approximately one suck-swallow per second. Music with a similar tempo and a regular rhythm can be combined with rhythmical rocking and stroking of the tongue. With these kinds of auditory and vestibular facilitation, an infant with a poor sucking reflex frequently begins to suck more rhythmically.

A number of research studies have addressed the specific effect of background music on mealtime behaviors (Ayres, 1987; Denney, 1997; Ragneskog, Brane, Karlsson, & Kihlgren, 1996; Ragneskog, Kihlgren, Karlsson, & Norberg, 1996). During sessions in which soothing background music was played, patients ate more food, were calmer, and had reductions in agitation, anxiety, fear, and depression during the meal. They spent more time at the dinner table and ate more calmly.

Music containing carefully blended sound frequencies called Hemi-Sync™ signals has been particularly effective in mealtime programs with children with sensorimotor challenges (Morris, 1997c). Hemi-Sync is a state-of-the-art audio technology that encourages a more synchronized or coherent brainwave activity that is associated with different mental states. It is based on the use of sound to stimulate binaural beats in the brain. The specific Hemi-Sync signals invite the brain to produce specific patterns of activity that may be associated with rest and relaxation, deep sleep, openness for learning, or active thinking. Music containing Hemi-Sync (i.e., Metamusic™) can be played through properly placed stereo speakers or stereo headphones to enhance learning in a variety of ways.

Hemi-Sync is an extremely versatile tool that has an extensive range of applications that support physical, mental, and emotional development. In addition to many anecdotal reports (Russell, 1993), a growing body of research has identified measurable positive changes in focus of attention (Guilfoyle & Carbone, 1996), memory (Kennerly, 1994), openness to suggestion (Brady, 1997), pain management (Kliempt, Ruta, Ogston, Landeck, & Martay, 1999), and vigilance performance and mood (Lane, Kasian, Owens, & Marsh, 1998) in response to the binaural beats created by Hemi-Sync.

Clinical studies by Morris (1996) and Varney (1988) addressed the use of Hemi-Sync's binaural beats with children with developmental disabilities. Morris found that 15 of the 20 children in the study showed positive changes with Hemi-Sync, including improved focus of attention, reduction in tactile defensiveness and overall improvement in sensory organization, increased physical relaxation, improved motor coordination, and reduction in fearfulness. All the children exhibited a greater openness and enthusiasm for learning. Varney reported that five of the six children in the study showed more rapid learning and attainment of specific educational goals, including imitation of gestures, facial expressions, two-word phrases, and spontaneous use of two-word phrases. Significant increases in attending behaviors and child-initiated interactions also were observed.

During mealtime programs, Hemi-Sync Metamusic recordings can provide an auditory background for the use of positive feedback and suggestions about ease and success of learning (Morris, 1997c). Children are in a focused state and frequently are more accepting of new possibilities. In addition, heightened mental awareness and alertness is combined with physical relaxation and a higher level of organization and integration of responses to sensory information. These features support easier, less stressful learning for everyone. Many children whose problems with sensory defensiveness and sensory overload interfere with eating appear to have better sensory organization and fewer sensory problems when Metamusic recordings are played before and during the meal.

Fear and anxiety are extremely common mealtime emotions among children with feeding difficulties. Children with sensory defensiveness live in a mealtime world of *fight or flight*. Children with a history of gastrointestinal discomfort must deal with their anticipation that the meal will be painful or make them feel ill. Children with severe physical disabilities often cope with the fear that the food will disappear while they are still hungry. In each instance, anxiety interferes with the ability to eat, digest food, and enjoy the social and communicative interaction of the mealtime.

The power of quieting music and Hemi-Sync Metamusic to reduce anxiety and create calm is extremely significant. Caine (1991) studied the effects of music on stress behaviors, weight, caloric and formula intake, and length of hospital stay in 52 medically stable preterm and low birthweight infants. Music was played in the infant's Isolette® for two 30-minute periods during the infant's stay in the neonatal intensive care unit (NICU). When compared with a matched control group, the infants who had listened to music significantly reduced their initial weight loss, increased their average daily weight, increased their formula and caloric intake, reduced stress behaviors, and had a shorter hospital stay. Analysis of the data suggested that the length of hospital stay was correlated with the amount of stress that they experienced.

Although Kaminski and Hall (1996) did not specifically look at feeding-related behaviors, they also found that when soothing lyrical music was played in the infant's bed, newborns showed fewer high arousal states and fewer fluctuations in their state. Marley (1984) charted the stress-related behaviors (e.g., crying, throwing objects, absence of vocalization, lethargy, body tension) of hospitalized infants and toddlers. When these children were involved in a program of music and interaction with a music therapist, their stress-related behaviors were reduced. Morris (1996) described greater openness to new experience and reduced anxiety during feeding programs in her pilot study examining the impact of music containing Hemi-Sync on children with developmental disabilities. Other studies have showed measurable reduction in stress and anxiety in a situations as diverse as mechanical ventilation (Chlan, 1995), preoperative surgery (Augustin & Hains, 1996), and general studies of the effect of music on mood (Augustin & Hains, 1996; McCraty, Barrios-Choplin, Atkinson, &

Tomasino, 1998). These studies plus the authors' clinical experience with thousands of children supports the view that music can play a powerful and noninvasive role in enhancing the feeding and mealtime learning skills of children and their parents.

The Power of Imagination

The imagination provides another rich source for learning in the mealtime program. Young children engage in an abundance of pretending that involves creating images for being and doing whatever they think about. Fantasy and imagination thrive in the nonverbal world of the young child and then become verbalized as language skills develop. One of the challenges for parents is to help their children distinguish between *real* and *pretend* events. For many children there is no difference. The mind creates a reality based on images that are as present and meaningful to children as those that take place in the physical space of their lives. Imagery has been incorporated extensively in learning and training programs in education (Bagley, 1984; Murdock, 1987), business (Lawlor, Handley, & Lawlor, 1997) and athletics (Garfield & Bennett, 1984). It has become a powerful adjunct to healing for many individuals (Achterberg, 1985; Epstein, 1989; Porter & Norris, 1985) and has been used in combination with music to support problem solving in psychotherapy and personal growth programs (Bonny & Savary, 1983; Merritt, 1990).

The combination of imagery and suggestion has been used very successfully to reduce postoperative pain in children (Lambert, 1996), increase naming behaviors in aphasic patients (Thompson, Hall, & Sison, 1986), and reduce fear and food refusal in a child with a history of choking on food (Elinoff, 1993). Torem (1992) reviewed the history of using imagery as a vehicle for change and healing in medicine and psychiatry. He discussed the increased effectiveness of imagery when it is combined with the changes in consciousness that are supported by clinical hypnosis. Studies of brainwave patterns show a strong correlation between the ability to respond to hypnotic suggestion and the presence of theta brainwaves (Brady, 1997; Sabourin, Cutcomb, Crawford, & Pribram, 1990). Interestingly, these slower theta brainwaves are stimulated by the binaural beat sound patterns used in Hemi-Sync Metamusic tapes.

The imagination can be harnessed in a variety of ways during feeding and mealtime programs. It is most powerful in helping children create an internal image of what is possible for them. Children who have experienced periods in which their body is quiet or their mouth is moving in a coordinated manner can be asked to practice these same experiences or movements in their minds. The therapist may take children on an imaginary journey in which the body and mouth move well, and the child is eating by mouth or chewing a new food. The child is guided into a state of physical, mental, and emotional relaxation, and the journey usually is presented as an interesting story. The child becomes a character in the story, mentally and emotionally experiencing the new skills or sense of empowerment created by the script. The combination of Hemi-Sync Metamusic and positive suggestion increases the effectiveness of the activity, and many children show greater emotional and physical control during mealtime activities that are related to the content of the story. The use of imagery and positive suggestion is very effective with young children who have developed feeding aversions rooted in fearful past experiences.

The power of the imagination can help therapists and parents understand areas of feeding and mealtime that are difficult to reenact physically. When an adult learner participates experientially in a mealtime activity, intellectual or academic knowledge and understanding are deepened. Imagining oneself as an infant at different stages of feeding development engages not only visual and descriptive memories but also early personal memories and impressions. The learner becomes part of the experience in a way that cannot be duplicated by watching a videotape or listening to a lecture on feeding development. In a similar fashion, parents can be guided through an imagination experience that enables them to re-experience the familiar feeling of reduced oral sensation after receiving Novocaine at the dentist. These parents have a very different level of understanding their child who experiences low oral sensory awareness during eating. Klein and Morris included 44 Imagination Mealtime

Experiences in *Mealtime Participation Guide* (Klein & Morris, 1999). One of them, an experience story related to sensory defensiveness to touch in the mouth, is included in Appendix C on page 751.

Concepts of Change

Therapy is the process of assisting a person with the concept of change. It increases the options or choices available to the child or adult in a given area. Children with feeding and mealtime issues may have a limited repertoire of choices that are comfortable for them and their families. Therapy helps expand those choices, introducing the family to the functional advantages of different options. Therapy does not guarantee that the family's choices will be the ones proposed by the therapist. In order for specific approaches, strategies, and techniques to be considered and accepted, children and their families must be engaged as active participants in treatment.

Therapists and parents can begin to think about making changes by using their own experiences and knowledge as frames of reference. Think for a moment about a change that you made successfully. Perhaps this was a change of jobs, a move away from an abusive marriage, the loss or gain of weight. Ask yourself what made the change possible. Now think about a change that you were unable to make. How was that situation different from the first?

When you think about these two situations, you may become aware that your successful changes usually are ones that *you* wanted. The move toward change came from an internal desire, rather than an externally imposed desire. For example, you personally made a commitment to lose weight. The desire was not initiated and pushed by your spouse or partner. You felt totally supported by others as you were in the process of making the change and probably felt that others loved and accepted you whether or not you were successful. Most important, you set and achieved small steps of change such as setting your goal at losing 1 pound per month instead of 20 pounds.

A therapy program that acknowledges and builds on an understanding of change, communication, and learning will be more successful than one that does not. The following concepts contribute to a therapy program that works well for most children and therapists. These principles have an impact on the learning of therapists as well as children. In an interactive therapy session, the therapist and child are simultaneously teachers and learners.

Learning and communication are partners in change. All children communicate, and they communicate at every moment. When children's messages are received, understood, and respected, their level of trust deepens and their learning ability is enhanced. Trust is built on a base of authenticity and honesty. The child knows that the therapist's communication is honest. When therapists say one thing and do another, trust does not develop. A child who trusts a therapist is more willing to risk and learns more easily. Physical handling by the therapist is a powerful system of communication. A therapist's hands learn to *read* the child's message and move intuitively to provide the support, stability, and movement that are needed.

Communication takes many forms. A child can say *yes, no,* or *maybe* through alterations in muscle tone; changes in body rhythms, facial expression, crying, or vocalizing; or movement with or against the therapist. Movement toward or away from specific activities or interests communicates a child's learning style or sensory preferences. A child who knows that the therapist listens increases the frequency or consistency of expression. Active listening provides empathy, encouragement, and a feeling of acceptance. When children feel respected and understood, they are more willing to challenge the unknown. With a greater willingness to let go of the familiar and explore change, the child discovers more options for function.

> When Martin's therapist brought her hand under his chin to help reduce the excursion of his jaw, a worried look appeared in his eyes. She asked him if he was a bit frightened. As Martin realized that she understood, his body relaxed. Together they explored other ways of moving his jaw.

> As the therapist presented the spoon of peaches, John closed his eyes and turned his head to the left. The therapist asked him if he wanted a drink instead. John brought his

head back to midline and smiled. After the drink, he looked directly at the bowl of fruit and opened his mouth.

Children are their own best experts. Children have an intuitive knowledge of their readiness for what a therapist might introduce. When the therapist moves ***with*** children and in harmony with children's knowledge of themselves, children learn more rapidly.

Observing a child's emotional and physical reaction to an activity is the best feedback of its appropriateness at each moment. Adults can observe a child's interests, and note which activities delight and which sensory areas are pleasing or threatening. From these observations, the therapist can choose activities or techniques that fit with knowledge of the child's developmental readiness. When a child is uninterested or actively opposes an activity, it is a strong cue that the therapist needs to make changes. The activity may be inappropriate for the child or presented in a way that is threatening, uncomfortable, or unfamiliar. Therapy that follows a child's lead and is built on the expertise of the child is more successful than therapy built on the agenda of the therapist.

> Missy sought the rocking chair and tape recorder at the beginning of each therapy session. As she rocked and listened to music, her breathing became more regular, and she began to sing softly with the music.

> David clamped his mouth closed as the therapist gave him liquid from a spoon. He swallowed pureed foods relatively easily. The therapist believed David must learn to swallow liquids as well as solids in order to transition from the gastrostomy tube. When she thickened the liquid, he accepted it.

Change that is gradual and slow is less threatening and more acceptable than change that is rapid. Each child has a sensory feedback system that constantly compares what is familiar and normal with what is unfamiliar and strange. When change occurs in small steps that are related to what is already known and accepted, the child moves more easily and more comfortably in a new direction. The therapist can expand a child's repertoire through subtle variations of familiar patterns.

> Eric's abdominal muscles were inactive as his weight was shifted to the side. With movement away from midline, he was scared and clung to the therapist. His therapist reduced the amount of weight shift, moving him almost imperceptibly to the side. Together they worked within a comfortable range, gradually increasing the amount of movement.

> Robert had always been fed with his head in hyperextension. He fought the therapist's attempt to bring his head into a midline position with a chin tuck. When the therapist slowly explored slight variations of head extension and flexion, he relaxed and worked with her. Within a month, he actively moved into a chin tuck position as the spoon was presented.

Learning occurs more rapidly in an atmosphere of playfulness and fun. Play makes learning accessible to the young child. Eliciting enjoyment and interest in movement, sensory exploration, oral-motor play, and sound play can motivate children. Joyful learning contributes to discovery and desire. Working simply for toleration of handling, oral motor exploration, or any specific desire of the therapist omits this concept. As a result, children become reluctant learners without a real sense of desire and commitment.

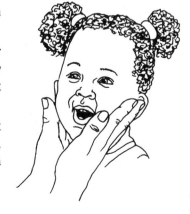

> Ashley began to laugh and coo as she was bounced gently on her mother's lap to the rhythm of nursery rhymes. Together they explored movement, rhythm, and gentle compression to build trunk stability.

> Melissa was reluctant to have her face touched as her therapist worked to build up tone in the cheeks. Using rhythmical folk music, the therapist introduced tapping as a way of playing with the face as a drum. Melissa smiled and enjoyed the new game.

Learning occurs more rapidly when therapy builds upon interests and abilities rather than focusing on disabilities and deficits. Children learn more easily in the areas that interest them (Yoder et al., 1993). They learn more rapidly when they feel capable and competent. When a therapist focuses on a child's deficits, she communicates her beliefs in limitations and a perception of the child's inability to function well. The child learns to depend upon the therapist to fix what goes wrong and is deprived of a joy in accomplishment and participation. Through effective therapy, the child is encouraged to be a full participant in his change. Therapy becomes a dialogue between the therapist and the child.

> Alec wanted to push the vacuum cleaner. The pushing movement and vibration provided strong proprioceptive input and helped him organize sensory information. His therapist introduced chewing activities while pushing to reduce his drooling. Both he and the vacuum *ate* pieces of cereal.

> Nathan's low postural tone resulted in instability and poor respiratory-phonatory control for cup drinking and speech. All he wanted to do was jump and sing in therapy. As his therapist built therapy around these two activities, she noticed that his respiratory control improved and that he was able to obtain better coordination of breathing and swallowing and use a louder, more sustained voice.

Learning is easier and faster in a nonjudgmental atmosphere. When children are judged in their performance, they quickly learn to judge themselves—shifting the emphasis from learning to self-praise or self-condemnation. Therapy that labels movement, sensory responses, or feeding patterns as *good* or *bad* teaches children nonacceptance of themselves. In contrast, a specific movement might be explored as interfering with or assisting a functional activity the child desires. For example, a child can discover and choose a new relaxed or differentiated arm movement because it makes it easier to turn pages in a book. The more familiar, tense movement pattern may be discarded, not because it is a *bad* way, but because it doesn't work as well in obtaining a goal.

> Chrissy's pelvis tilted backward and her shoulders rounded when she sat to turn pages in the book. As her therapist assisted her with an anterior pelvic tilt, she pointed out that this moved Chrissy closer to the book. As Chrissy reached in her old way, the therapist exaggerated the posterior tilt and allowed her to discover that it was harder to reach the pages.

> Justin's mother continued to feed him with his head turned to the side. She and the therapist took turns, feeding him with his head in different positions. They focused on discovering if there were any differences in eye contact and mouth opening with each position. With the self-discovery of a helpful position, she began to feed Justin with his head in the middle.

Awareness increases self-knowledge and enhances the ability to carry over a new concept or movement into daily life. When therapists help children focus their awareness on sensations accompanying a movement, children become more able to repeat that movement pattern independently. Knowledge and learning occur through contrasts. Children understand flexion through its contrast with extension. As children increase their awareness of movement and sensation, they are better able to move toward what they wish. They are less dependent upon the guidance of another person.

> Carla began to suckle and thrust her tongue forward as soon as she was ready for another spoonful. Her therapist suggested that she keep her mouth quiet and use her voice to tell her mother she was ready. Carla's tongue thrust disappeared as she became aware of other ways to communicate.

Children learn to adapt to their anatomical structure and physiological abilities to function. Therapists can observe functional changes that the child has discovered and attempt to understand how a specific movement pattern or adaptation supports function. In the process of change, some children may temporarily need adaptations such as neck hyperextension to assist breathing or a specific head position to protect the airway during swallowing. With this understanding, a therapist can explore treatment options that contribute to greater functional abilities. If these are introduced slowly, the child may discover a better or easier way.

> Nathan experienced respiratory distress and kept his head in hyperextension to enlarge the pharyngeal airway. When his head was brought forward, it was more difficult for him to breathe. His therapist understood his need for this compensation until his respiratory patterns stabilized.

> As food entered Martha's mouth, she tipped her head back into hyperextension. All attempts to help her bring it forward were met with protest. Martha's lips and cheeks were hypotonic and food fell out of her mouth if her head was upright. Head extension was a compensation for poor lip-cheek control.

Mealtime Communication

The communication environment is a part of the learning environment. Like the learning environment, the communication environment deals with external and internal factors and messages. Adults and children never cease communicating. Every body movement, facial expression, or unspoken thought communicates the essence of personal beliefs, expectations, and intent for the therapy session. A nonverbal child is not a noncommunicating child. Even a person in a deep coma communicates responsiveness to the environment and individuals in that environment through changes in blood pressure, heart rate, and breathing rate and rhythms. Newborns communicate their physical condition, emotions, and needs through changes in respiratory rate, color, state, and other physiological cues (Als, 1982, 1986). The mother of a 4-year-old who had been in a near drowning accident described very predictable changes in her daughter's respiratory and cardiac responses to specific people in her hospital room. When her father and grandfather began to speak, her respiratory and cardiac rates slowed and became very regular. When the doctor, who had been very negative about the child's prognosis, came in to talk to the parents, the child's respiratory pattern and heartbeat became very rapid and irregular. She clearly communicated her emotional awareness and responses to those around her even though she appeared to be in a deep coma.

Observation and Discovery

Communication at mealtimes can be observed carefully to learn more about how the child is communicating and how the clarity and consistency of the communicative message can be enhanced. Communication requires that both the listener and the sender use a set of signals that are mutually accepted and understood. When one person speaks a different language, using a different set of signals, a communication breakdown is likely to occur with the other person. Humans communicate verbally and nonverbally. Body language and tone of voice carry 90% of the total message. Some nonverbal signals and symbols are intentional, such as shaking the head for yes and no. Others occur automatically as a reflection of inner thoughts and attitudes. Most adults have communicated their embarrassment through blushing or their fear of walking down a dark street through breathing more rapidly.

Because of the frequency with which communication signals are issued and received through body movement, a child who has difficulty with movement is more likely to send and receive messages that are hard for the listener to understand. Many people believe that children who cannot talk are unable to communicate. They do not look for other means of communication and generally do not acknowledge that the movements produced by a nonverbal child may have communicative value. For example, when a child arches into extension or turns the head to the side, triggering an asymmetrical tonic neck reflex, a therapist may say, "Aha! I need to help this child achieve a better position for feeding. Extension or asymmetry in the body may increase the limiting movements I see in the mouth." This can be a correct observation and interpretation of the physical events, but the trigger of the limiting physical patterns and the child's underlying intent also must be identified. Children use whatever means they have available for communication. A child who is not physically able to climb out of a high chair or verbally able to say "I don't want any more" may deliver the message by arching into extension and turning away from the food.

It is possible to misinterpret a physical response such as arching and pulling away. The mother of a 5-month-old felt that her baby was refusing the breast and rejecting her as a mother when he began pulling off the breast and fussing. She had noted that in other infants, pulling away from an activity or object meant that they were unhappy or did not want to continue the interaction. During the initial months, she and her son had developed a mutually satisfying nursing partnership. Although the baby had low postural tone, he could cuddle and suck efficiently. At 4 months, his postural tone increased, and he developed a tactile hypersensitivity of the face. It became physically difficult for him to maintain the sustained skin contact of his face on his mother's breast for nursing because of this combination of a limiting sensory response and the extensor movement patterns. His message was one of physical discomfort. It was not the message of dislike and rejection that his mother felt she was receiving.

It is important to help feeders learn to observe the child's behaviors and reactions during a meal and develop an understanding of the child's way of communicating (Morris, 1981). In many ways, it is similar to learning a second language. If you are living with people who don't speak your language, you can learn a great deal through careful observation. You can notice what they do or say when you know or suspect they are hungry. You can observe how they indicate that they would like to have you pass the mashed potatoes at the dinner table. Adults can use this general approach successfully when they are learning the child's language. It is important simply to observe the child's mealtime patterns, make some preliminary guesses, and finally to check out these guesses.

For example, the parent and therapist want to know how the child communicates likes or dislikes for a particular food. If they have spent a lot of time feeding the child, they already have an intuitive knowledge of the child's likes and dislikes based on observations of the child's reactions as the food was presented. This time, when the adult observes, this stored knowledge can be brought to a conscious level.

The following activity will help adults develop their ability to observe and interpret new communicative behaviors.

1. Select three foods for a meal with a child whom you know well. Select one food that you sense the child does not like, one that is a favorite food, and one that is neutral.

2. Observe the child as you present each food. What reactions do you see in the child's eyes? What reactions do you see around the child's face and mouth? What body reactions do you see? What kinds of sounds does the child make?

3. Write your observations.

4. As you feed other foods you are less sure of, watch for some of the reactions you saw when you were sure.

5. Repeat the activity several days later. Notice whether the child's responses are the same as when you first noted his likes and dislikes. If they are not, note the differences. Continue to explore and fine-tune your observations.

6. Continue this type of observation while asking the following questions about the child:
   - How does the child indicate he wants to eat if food is present or it is a regular mealtime?
   - How does the child indicate he wants to eat if food is not present or it is a time when a regular meal isn't scheduled?
   - How does the child indicate he needs a slower pace for feeding or a brief pause?
   - How does the child indicate he wants you to speed up the pace of feeding?
   - How does the child indicate readiness for the next spoonful?
   - How does the child indicate a choice of which food or liquid to eat next?
   - How does the child indicate hunger and the desire to continue eating?
   - How does the child indicate he is finished with the meal?

Make notes of each observation and begin to discover the sensorimotor language the child uses to communicate. While observing and repeating these observations, ask whether you think the child is actually communicating a message. In some instances, children may not seem to attempt to communicate a particular message or thought. For example, some children will respond when food is present. It reminds them that they are hungry, and that if they make noise or wiggle someone will bring them food. However, the same child may not associate the inner signals of hunger with the memory of food or the knowledge that another person could do something to relieve the hunger. Thus, if food is not present, there may be no effort to communicate the inner discomfort. The child may sit passively until someone notices what time it is and offers food.

Observe also whether the child usually has the opportunity to communicate a message. When a child must be fed, the feeder often makes all decisions as to which foods are offered and the order in which they appear. It may not occur to the child to indicate to the feeder, "I am tired of applesauce and would like a drink."

How easy is it to understand each message? Some messages may be communicated easily. Others may leave the feeder wondering if there really was a message at all. If the message is not easily understood, it may be related to the clarity of the child's signals or the consistency with which the child uses a particular signal to indicate a particular need. Look at each of these factors and decide which of the messages are clear, consistent, and easily understood. Which messages are unclear, inconsistent, and poorly understood?

Determine which type of behavioral response (e.g., vocalization or speech, face and mouth movements, gestures or body movements, eye signals) the child uses most frequently in communicating. Some children use the eyes very strongly in signaling a message to the feeder. Other children use minimal eye gaze signals, and instead use arm and body movements to let the feeder know their needs.

Observe how sophisticated the child's messages are. One child may indicate hunger by crying. Another child might sit in front of the refrigerator and point. A third child might call his mother, nod his head to the refrigerator, and make sucking noises while looking from his mother to the refrigerator. Each of these messages shows an increasing level of sophistication of the message and expanding communicative intent.

Enhancing the Mealtime Environment

Once adults have completed their observations, they are ready to help the child expand and enhance the mealtime environment. The first step in any change is to identify the place to begin. The mealtime observations provide this information. The second step is to decide if the existing communication-interaction can become more effective. The final step is to identify new possibilities or ways to change elements of the behavior that may improve the interaction. It is helpful to organize observations and recommendations based on concepts of the physical, sensory, and communication environments.

Physical Environment

The way in which children are seated or positioned during mealtimes strongly influences the type of movement they have available for communication. When they are positioned with the head in midline and the body comfortably supported, more normal movements are available for looking, reaching, and vocalizing. For older babies, a fully supported position, reclining on the lap and facing the feeder, can provide the opportunity for eye contact and positive interaction.

If it is easier or more appropriate for the feeder to sit next to the child, nonvisual ways of interacting should be provided. Turning the head to look at the feeder may cause a postural asymmetry that would increase muscle tone and limiting movement patterns. This type of communication would make feeding more difficult. The feeder could look for and respond to other signals. When the child's mouth opens for the spoon, the feeder might comment, "Your open mouth lets me know you are ready," and give a small hug or other physical acknowledgment of the message. If the child continues to desire a visual confirmation that the message was sent and received, the feeder could use a mirror placed in front of the child, so that visual feedback could be obtained without turning the head.

Many ideas for providing comfortable physical support for both the child and the feeder are in Chapter 15.

Sensory Environment

The sensory environment can support good interaction and communication or it can create serious problems. Vocal signals may become lost in the noise of a busy school cafeteria. If the child tries to use a louder voice in this environment, the increased effort could trigger limiting movement patterns in the mouth. This, in turn, would make the physical act of eating more difficult. A child who is easily overstimulated or overwhelmed in a noisy or confusing environment will communicate discomfort during the meal. This communication may take the form of withdrawal, increased rocking or screeching, throwing food, running around, or becoming more physically tense. Teachers and therapists often label this as negative behavior, and they institute programs to reduce or eliminate it. For many children, the behavior is a form of communication that expresses sensory overload, frustration, or anxiety. To eliminate the communication without dealing with the underlying issues does a disservice to children.

The environmental considerations provided in Chapter 14 will help feeders create sensory environmental aspects that support a different type of communication. When the child no longer needs to communicate distress, other messages can be developed.

Communication Environment

Mealtime is the finest natural environment for working on communication strategies. Mealtime occurs frequently. It provides a high level of need and motivation for communication. Increased skill in communication can improve the child's physical abilities to eat. This connection between improved oral motor ability and communication effectiveness is critical.

Pragmatic communication skills, such as requesting, indicating, and describing, occur naturally during a meal. If the feeder is aware of the value and opportunities for supporting basic communication skills, communication skills will increase. An effective communicator can assume the roles of initiator and responder, and is familiar with the concept of alternating the roles of listener and speaker (Manolson, 1992). These are important concepts to be built into the meal.

The feeder can wait for a signal before putting the spoon in the child's mouth. Signals for a pause or a different food indicate that the child is initiating an interaction. When food is placed in front of the child, eye gaze can signal the child's choice of which food to eat next. When food is placed in different small dishes rather than lumped together on the same plate, children have greater opportunity for selection.

The communication environment at mealtime includes the nonverbal communication of adult attitudes and expectations. Many parents feel that they are not forcing their children to eat and that they give their children mealtime choices. Yet, during the meal, they are tense and anxious about every bite that the child takes or does not take. They clench their jaws as if they are trying to swallow reminders to the child. When the child refuses the spoonful, they may frown or abruptly leave the room. Children get the message and respond accordingly. Children, however, also may use their sensitivity to nonverbal messages to assume that the adult is upset with them. A parent or therapist simply may be having a bad day or be worried about something unrelated to the child. Yet many children will interpret the message in a personal way. The key is that the adult's verbal and nonverbal messages are out of sync. When verbal and nonverbal messages match, it is much easier for children to understand and deal with what is going on. When there is a mismatch, the child usually responds to the truth of the nonverbal message. It can be helpful for the adult to tell a child, "I've had a bad day and feel a bit grumpy inside. It doesn't have anything to do with how I feel about you." Or he might say, "I'm really feeling inside that I'd like for you to eat more food. It's taking me a while to know that you are the one who needs to make that decision."

Messages From Within

Hunger and Satiation

It is traditional to think of communication as taking place only externally. The sender and receiver of the message are two different individuals. Yet communication also takes place between different parts of the same person. The most important set of messages from within are connected with hunger and satiation. The body puts out a set of physiological signals to the conscious mind that indicates a need for food. Higher levels of conscious awareness recognize these signals and correctly interpret them as hunger signals. The individual receives this message that says, "I'm hungry. I need food," and responds by moving toward sources of food (e.g., the refrigerator, cupboard, restaurant) or by communicating this need to another person who is responsible for distributing food. At some point while the individual is eating, the body puts out a message of satiation that says, "I'm full. That is enough food." Once again, the message is sent, perceived, and interpreted, and the individual stops eating.

Children or adults may fail to receive, perceive, or correctly interpret these messages for widely different reasons. A small number of children lack the physiological mechanism in the hypothalamus of the brain that sends the message of hunger or satiation. Because the message is not sent or does not get through to the conscious mind, the child does not experience the signals of hunger or satiation. Most children with this type of dysfunction also experience other areas of malfunction in areas controlled by the hypothalamus, such as poor temperature regulation.

Hunger signals usually get through. However, the child may fail to recognize them, may misinterpret them, or may override them. These are more common situations when children do not respond to situations that should stimulate hunger. The mind recognizes and attaches meaning to information more readily when it appears in patterns. This is true of the sensory information associated with hunger. Hunger signals appear at regular intervals throughout the day. The interval for an infant is about every 3 to 4 hours. The uncomfortable sensations occur and are relieved by taking milk from the breast or bottle. This regular pattern of discomfort and comfort helps the baby notice and recognize the physiological signals. Some babies begin to fuss and cry as soon as the signals occur while others wait until the signals are stronger.

The baby's awareness of hunger signals and their relationship to eating can become distorted when the patterns are missing or do not support a positive recognition. For example, some infants and children who receive food through a feeding tube eat a single meal over a 12- to 24-hour period of time. Their formula is delivered by a pump that drips the food into the gastrointestinal system at a very slow rate. These children typically do not experience either hunger or satiation. Their bodies are satisfied enough with the slow feeding that the brain does not send out the signals saying "feed me" or "stop feeding me." They have never experienced a pattern of hunger, followed by comfort. They have never experienced a pattern of fullness, followed by comfort.

Some of these children may be interested in taking small tastes of food or liquid, but lack any internal desire to eat enough to support their nutritional needs orally. Reducing the volume of food received through tube feeding seems to make no difference in the amount that the child eats. The appropriate body communication patterns are missing, and the child either does not notice the hunger signals or does not associate them with the need to increase the amount of food eaten by mouth.

This situation becomes extremely complicated when eating is not associated with comfort. Many children who have gastroesophageal reflux, gagging, or retching experience extreme discomfort when they eat. See Chapter 22 for a full discussion of these issues. When these children begin to perceive and recognize hunger signals, they discover a pattern of hunger followed by increased discomfort. The pattern of the inner message may tell them to eat a few mouthfuls to satisfy the immediate hunger signals and then to stop eating to prevent discomfort. The child may ignore the hunger message because acknowledging it does not lead toward a desired response.

Hunger is a very subtle signal when compared with the pain and discomfort of gastroesophageal reflux, esophagitis, or retching. The child may be focused only on the more intense gastrointestinal signals and may not perceive the softer signals of hunger. When hunger becomes intense and begins to compete in the arena of strong signals, it may join the pattern of uncomfortable sensations associated with eating or mealtime. Some children have developed a conditioned response that associates eating and the process of learning to eat with pain and discomfort. As children with a history of gastrointestinal distress experience hunger signals, they may respond with fearful anticipation of pain, may not notice the signals, or may ignore them.

Children often receive mixed messages from their bodies that interfere with their ability to regulate food intake. Signals of fullness, like those of hunger, initially are subtle. For most people, the perception is one of slight discomfort, with the signals increasing in intensity. This discomfort motivates most children and adults to stop eating so that they will be comfortable. However, children who have a history of gastrointestinal discomfort have learned that these subtle signals lead to more intense discomfort. The similarity between the early sensations caused by the stomach filling and the discomfort of nausea and reflux can lead to confusion and inner conflict. The child still may be hungry, but misinterprets the inner message as one of fullness. These children often stop eating as soon as they feel the sensations that come from stretching the walls of stomach. Children who have sensory-based feeding problems may continue to confuse these hunger signals and actively move away from feeding because they have strong memories of gastrointestinal discomfort even when the original gastrointestinal problems have been resolved.

A large number of children have learned to ignore signals of hunger and satiation because they have discovered that these messages are meaningless. Adults have taken full responsibility for when they eat and how much they eat. Infants whose hunger level varies or who need to eat more often than every 4 hours experience frustration and long periods of unresolved discomfort when they are fed on a 4-hour schedule. Children who must eat a specific amount determined by a parent must override the inner message that says "I'm not hungry right now" or "I am really full and should stop eating." A demand-feeding schedule for infants and toddlers supports children's discovery of the internal messages of hunger and fullness. The division of mealtime responsibility that has been discussed throughout this book enables children to listen to the messages from within and honor the needs of their own bodies. Children who are taught to ignore these messages have difficulty regulating the amount of food that they eat and may develop problems with obesity (Johnson & Birch, 1994; Satter, 1991).

Enhancing Inner Messages

The goal for all children is to build and support their ability to guide eating through inner messages. When children do not eat enough, parents and professionals often attempt to increase their intake through medication that stimulates the appetite, behavior modification, or constant reminders to eat more. It is more effective in the long run to develop a program that focuses on the learning and communication aspects of eating. The program includes these five related stages.

Provide the opportunity for the child to:

- experience hunger and satiation signals
- experience comfort following eating
- recognize the pattern of hunger and satiation signals
- associate these signals with eating or stopping eating
- control the amount of food eaten and guide intake through internal messages

A child who experiences active gastrointestinal discomfort or is on continuous drip feedings does not have the internal ability to receive positive messages about hunger and its connection with eating by mouth. The mealtime program should focus on increasing the child's experience with taste and expanding oral sensorimotor comfort and skills. At this stage, it is inappropriate to reduce the amount of the tube feeding in hopes that the child becomes hungry enough to eat.

As gastrointestinal problems begin to resolve, the feeding therapist can help the child build patterns that lead toward awareness and recognition of hunger. Bolus feedings help a child experience the contrast of a full stomach and an empty stomach. When these bolus feedings are offered at regular meal and snack times throughout the day, the child's body begins to associate the inner signals of hunger with the routine of being fed. It is critically important to keep the size of the bolus feedings within the child's comfort zone. The partnership among the feeding therapist, gastroenterologist, and pediatrician is essential. If the child is pushed to take a greater volume of food, discomfort will become a learned part of the mealtime pattern. Many physicians have not been introduced to the concept that gastrointestinal discomfort with tube feedings can lead to the rejection of oral feedings and long-term tube feedings.

Many children experience comfort with bolus tube feedings of water long before they are comfortable with bolus feedings of formula. This concept and the procedures for implementing it are discussed in Chapters 16 and 23. The feeding therapist can gradually increase the amount of water that the child takes at one time and reduce the amount of time needed for this drink. Because water passes through an empty stomach relatively rapidly, this process offers the opportunity to help the child experience a comfortable feeling of filling and emptying of the stomach. It also offers the opportunity to talk about the sensations and the feelings of being hungry and full.

Over time, bolus feedings of formula and small oral feedings are offered at regularly scheduled mealtimes. The child gradually learns to associate a positive inner message with comfort after the meal. Parents can observe their child and begin to notice changes in the child's mood, facial expression, or mouth movements as the time for the next meal approaches. Some children become slightly fussy or begin to drool or swallow more frequently. At these times, an adult can tell the child, "Your tummy is saying that it is time to eat. I think your mouth is telling me that you are hungry." This can be combined with gently touching the child's abdomen and bringing the attention to the part of the body that is giving hunger signals.

As food is offered at the meal, the child is given the responsibility of deciding what and how much to eat. When children reach this point in the mealtime program, inner messages of hunger and fullness can become powerful guides for regulating the amount of food that the child eats orally.

At this point in the program, the child is ready to listen to hunger signals, interpret them as the body's message that it is time to eat, and continue eating until signals of fullness are experienced.

Behavior as Communication

Children express their feelings, beliefs, and needs through their behaviors. Donnellan, Mirenda, Fassbender, and Fassbender (1984) describe the importance of looking carefully at the communicative function of aberrant or acting-out behaviors in children with severe multiple disabilities. Kaufman (1991) emphasizes that every individual takes care of himself or herself by choosing behaviors that reflect their beliefs. Hirama (1989) describes the self-injurious and abusive behaviors of many institutionalized children and adults as a reflection of inadequate levels of somatosensory stimulation. Hirama hypothesizes that many of these behaviors began as an individual's attempt to communicate the need for sensory input and control. When these behavioral communication signals are responded to, the behaviors stop or are sharply reduced.

Children who refuse to eat, engage in mealtime tantrums, or show other maladaptive responses at mealtimes usually are attempting to communicate that something is wrong. They may be uncomfortable, frightened, feel out of control, have a stomachache, or feel overwhelmed by the mealtime environment. They may be telling adults that they do not feel valued or important, or that they feel disempowered or deeply discouraged (Dreikurs & Stoltz, 1964). Adults usually are uncomfortable with this type of communication and perceive it as a child's inappropriate behavior. They focus on eliminating the behavior rather than on what the child is communicating through the behavior (Kohn, 1993).

Children and adults learn to respond to the actions or inactions of others with additional behaviors. For example, children with the primary respiratory difficulties of bronchopulmonary dysplasia (BPD) experience physical and emotional challenges in learning to eat and drink orally. A rapid respiratory rate initially may make it very challenging to coordinate the timing of sucking, swallowing, and breathing. The need to inhibit breathing briefly during swallowing may increase anxiety and create reminders of being unable to breathe and survive. Many children with BPD also have a history of gastroesophageal reflux. When oral feedings are introduced, many of them are overly cautious and reluctant to accept a bottle, cup, or spoon. They may push the utensil away, close the mouth, and turn the head; in effect, saying, "This doesn't feel right. I'm frightened. I don't like it when I can't breathe." Feeders who recognize and acknowledge this message offer the child the opportunity to learn. The adult might say, "Your body is telling me that you don't want to do this right now. I think it feels scary to have the food in your mouth." When children feel they are understood, they are much more willing to trust and to risk.

Feeders who see the child's refusal of the food strictly as a behavior that must be eliminated never stop to figure out why the child might have selected the specific behavior in the first place. They often refer the child for diagnostic testing to rule out aspiration and severe gastroesophageal reflux. When these tests come back negative, they assume that the child has no reason to refuse the food. They begin to push the child to eat. The child responds with verbal and non-verbal behaviors that say "I don't like it when you push me; I want to be in control of what I eat." Rather than turning away and closing the mouth, the child throws the bowl, screams, and spits out any food that gets into the mouth. The focus continues to be placed on the child's negative behaviors, and the vicious cycle continues.

Mealtime Communication Tools

Learning and communication at mealtimes are enhanced when children can express their needs and when adults can understand them. A number of tools are available to help in this process and provide the external support for learning new mealtime skills.

Mealtime Communication Board

The child and therapist can use a mealtime communication board to send and receive messages throughout the meal.

When it is easier for the food to be placed on a table at the child's side (rather than in front), pictures can be placed in a clear plastic photo pocket that is hung around the feeder's neck. This pocket can contain pictures of three or four of the foods at the meal. If the child has other ways of indicating the food selection, the photo pocket can contain symbols for a more complex meal message that the child would like to communicate.

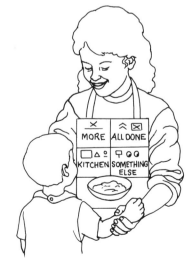

The child can point to the appropriate message with the eyes or hands, or use a light pointer strapped to the head. When the child can turn the head to one side without triggering limiting body movements, word cards—or the food itself—can be placed to the side for pointing.

Careful consideration should be given to the words or pictures selected for this mealtime communication board. The board should be developed solely for the mealtime and be different from other more general communication boards that the child uses. The words should be important to the child and important for communication at the meal. It would be redundant, for example, to use pictures of the food when the child can point to the food itself. A requirement that the child point to the picture of the food rather than the food itself does not support the overall goals of communication.

When a communication board is used at the meal, the feeder models its use in conversation with the child. For example, if the board contains a picture or symbols for the word ***more***, the feeder might point to the picture and then to the sandwich on the table, and ask, "Do you want more sandwich?"

This places communication in an interactive context and reduces the demands placed on the child. When people are interested and excited about an idea or an activity and invited to participate, they become more readily involved than if there is pressure to participate.

Mealtime Place Mat

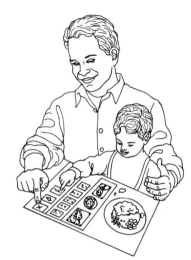

Another type of mealtime communication board is the mealtime place mat. The mat is created from poster board and covered with a clear plastic case or laminated to make it waterproof. One side of the mat is blank or has a drawing of a plate. The other side contains a small communication board with pictures and symbols that are appropriate to the child and the meal. This type of place mat is particularly appropriate for the child who has pointing skills. The communication board can be placed on the side of the mat nearest the child's dominant hand to make pointing easier. The mat can be used by a child who is a self-feeder or a child who is fed by an adult.

The place mat is easy to construct, and new versions can be created as the child's physical abilities or vocabulary needs change.

Making a Mealtime Place Mat

1. Cut a cardboard mat the size of a typical table mat.

2. On one-third of the mat, draw or paste pictures with the messages you wish to include. The side chosen for messages depends on the child's best visual field and hand used for pointing.

3. Leave the remaining two-thirds clear for placement of the child's plate, food, and utensils.

4. Sew clear, flexible plastic into a case that can be fastened by a Velcro® strip. The case enables feeders to change the mat as needed.

5. The place mat also can be covered permanently with clear adhesive plastic or laminated.

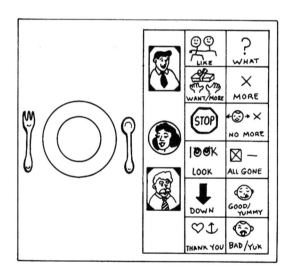

Mealtime Book

Successful carryover of a feeding program requires a partnership between the child and the feeder. When one person feeds the child every meal, it becomes relatively easy to develop a consistent understanding of the child's signals and the ways of feeding that will make the meal easier and more pleasant for everyone. When there are many feeders or the child is fed in various settings, it requires more effort to provide a consistent way of working together.

A mealtime book can help each feeder learn the communication method and ways to feed that will make the meal easier. The book is designed and constructed for each child and is written in the first person, as if the child were speaking. Photographs of the child demonstrating each point are provided to inform the feeder of needs and procedures. The book can be taken to school or to the baby-sitter. The child will enjoy looking at the photographs and sharing the book with others. When ideas are given to feeders in this way, they become an invitation to enjoy the meal with the child. This communicates a very different message than the typical instruction list of how to feed the child, which is often perceived as creating demands and restrictions on the feeder.

Making a Mealtime Book

1. Plan the book to meet the individual child's needs and specifications. It is important to emphasize ways of feeding that work well and those that do not. Develop a tentative script or format for the book.
2. Take Polaroid pictures to illustrate the ideas you wish to communicate in the book.
3. Express the ideas for each picture in a first-person script. Create the impression that the child is telling the reader about the idea in the picture. Use language and expressions that are appropriate to the child's age and personality.
4. Insert the pictures and their typed descriptions into plastic photo pockets or a photo album.
5. Revise the mealtime book periodically as changes or updates are needed.

The following information was included in one child's book:

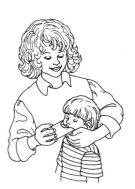

Place your hand gently under my chin to steady my jaw. Use a small, folded washcloth to keep both of us from getting wet.

Tip the glass slowly. Please wait until I let you know that I am ready to drink. I will make sucking sounds with my tongue. Then, please tip the cup a bit more so I can drink.

I keep my eyes looking at the glass as long as I want to drink.

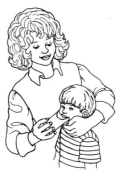

When I look up with my eyes, I am telling you to stop tipping the cup.

When I shake my head and say "uhn-uh," I don't want any more.

The Interplay of Communication and Learning

Messages and Belief Systems

Guidelines for most of the therapeutic decisions that professionals face are created from a series of personal and cultural beliefs. Everything therapists and parents do carries a message that reflects some aspect of their belief system. Adults may nonverbally communicate something different from what they consciously intended when they are unclear about what they believe and feel about an issue, or when they have not given it adequate consideration.

The use of gloves in therapy is a familiar example for professionals. Most therapists have always held the well-being of their clients as a high priority. Thorough washing of hands and cleaning of toys and equipment has been standard practice for many years. When awareness of the potential impact of viruses triggering diseases such as HIV, cytomegalic inclusion virus (CMV), and hepatitis C increased, most hospitals and clinics issued a ruling that stated that all therapists working in or near children's mouths must wear gloves. For many therapists, this created no conflict. Gloves were issued and worn without question.

Because very little thought was given to the underlying communication of this procedure and its potential impact on feeding and oral motor programs, gloves became a negative or limiting feature in many programs. Hospitals often provided the same powdered latex gloves for changing diapers as for stimulating the mouth. Many of these gloves tasted bitter and felt extremely aversive in a child's mouth. Because many therapists were constantly reminded that children's mouths could be carriers of serious disease organisms, they inadvertently communicated this concept to the children with whom they were working. The therapist might be playing interactively with the child with ungloved hands and then prepare to move into mouth play or feeding activities. At this point, the adult put on gloves. The nonverbal message told children that their mouths were dirty or unsafe. The aversive taste further distanced the child from the therapist and confirmed the child's interpretation that there was something wrong with the mouth. If the therapist resented having to wear gloves but did it to remain employed in the current setting, the child received many mixed messages about gloves and why they were being used.

Therapists who understood or explored the beliefs behind the regulations often communicated the need to wear gloves differently to their children. Through greater awareness, they considered the possibility of negative associations between gloves and mouth activities, and consciously sought to reverse this communication. Rather than seeing gloves as a necessary means of protecting themselves from the child, they shifted their belief about gloves and perceived them as simply a necessary part of the hospital's use of universal precautions. They looked for ways of associating play and building positive associations with gloves.

Before using any gloves with children, these therapists put the gloves in their own mouths and chewed on them. If the gloves were aversive in any way, they asked the agency to purchase gloves that were orally acceptable. For example, gloves that are marketed to dentists generally do not taste bad. Some therapists initially blew up the fingers of the gloves to create balloons. Others drew faces on a pair of gloves and used them as finger puppets. When the therapist put on other gloves for oral or feeding therapy, the child already had positive associations with them. Some therapists told children that they used gloves because their own hands get too dirty to put into the child's mouth rather than implying that it was the child's mouth that is dirty. Honesty and playfulness go a long way in creating a positive communication and learning environment for therapy and mealtimes.

Many hospitals and agencies are adamant that the mandatory use of gloves is the only way to protect children and staff. Others allow alternatives to gloves as long as the part of the therapist's hand that enters the child's mouth is covered. Still others allow the individual therapist to decide how much and what type of protection is used. The important feature is that the child and adult require the most positive support for health and wellness that is possible. When therapists work in an environment that does not mandate the use of gloves, they have a wider variety of choices for honoring their own health needs and those of their clients. Some choose to use gloves. Others find that a finger cot or Infa-Dent™ Finger Toothbrush provides covering for the finger that enters the child's mouth but leaves the rest of the hand free. Still others use a soft washcloth over a soft plastic bag or over the type of clear plastic glove used by people who handle food in restaurants.

One of the by-products of using a single guideline (i.e., latex gloves worn by everyone at all times) is the increasing number of latex allergies that are being identified in professionals and children as a result of constant exposure to latex. Although vinyl gloves also are available, they are not ideal for a variety of reasons and they expose children to phthalate chemicals that soften the vinyl and make it pliable. The decision to use gloves or not is less important than the way in which that decision is carried out. Learning and communication play major roles in determining whether the decision supports feeding and mealtime programs or whether it becomes an additional limiting factor.

The purpose of this discussion is not to make a case for or against the use of gloves in therapy, but to point out that every decision is rooted in the beliefs of an individual, agency, or culture. In this example, the challenge of universal precautions interacts with the beliefs of the therapist and agency. Different scientists view even something that seems as objective as protecting children and adults from germs in different ways. Some people believe that bacteria and viruses cause diseases and that exposure to these germs automatically causes illness. Others believe that illness is caused by the interplay between the virus or bacteria and the mental and physical health of the individual. Most individuals carry billions of unfriendly germs in their bodies, yet they do not become ill (Justice, 1987). However, a sleepless night or period of physical or emotional stress can weaken the immune system, contributing to the onset of a cold or the flu. Even when the physical system becomes severely stressed, the individual's beliefs can prevent immediate illness. For example, it is extremely common for the mother of young children to spend long periods of time with limited sleep or personal time when her family is ill. She may become the one who is there to nurse the others back to health. She does not get sick despite massive exposure to bacteria or viruses. Her intention is to stay well so that she can meet the needs of her children. However, weeks later when everyone else is well, she may suddenly fall ill with the same flu or cold.

Therapists who believe that viruses do not automatically cause illness may select different options for using appropriate protection when this does not conflict with the guidelines set by an employer. The adult may choose to use gloves or not work inside a child's mouth if the child is unwell or going through a stressful period. The same guidelines also might be selected if the therapist is under stress or has a cut or abrasion on the hands. At other times, gloves may be unnecessary. Honoring the need for cleanliness with careful attention to washing the hands may be all that is needed.

Occasionally, therapists' beliefs differ from the agencies' beliefs. Therapists may acknowledge that these are the agency's regulations and abide by them with a less emotionally charged understanding. Others may shift employers and find a work environment that is in greater harmony with their underlying beliefs.

Behavior and Learning

Behavior Modification Programs

A child's innate desire to eat often becomes modified by the internal and external environments of the mealtime. Events that are positive for the child can increase his desire to eat and enhance the development of feeding skills. Negative events that are associated with mealtimes may reduce the child's desire to eat and develop more advanced feeding skills.

The most frequent approach to children's feeding behaviors that is cited in the research literature is that of traditional behavior modification (Babbitt et al., 1994; Kedesdy & Budd, 1998). This model of learning is based on B. F. Skinner's work on operant conditioning in animal learning. Tasks or skills are broken down into their component parts and a series of desired and undesired behaviors is identified. The focus is then placed on how each behavior can be increased or decreased, depending on the stimulus that comes after it. When a reinforcer or reward follows the behavior, the animal or person is more likely to repeat the behavior. When the behavior is ignored or not reinforced, it is less likely to reoccur.

When this approach is applied to children with feeding disorders. the therapist or parent positively reinforces behaviors that are compatible with learning to eat and ignores or punishes those that are not in accord with eating. The reinforcer or reward can be anything that interests or motivates the child. This could include playing with a favorite toy, watching a brief segment of a video, having a drink of a preferred liquid, receiving a special treat or privilege at the end of the meal, or receiving social attention. Change is achieved by means of successive approximations or shaping in which the small steps toward the final goal are modified through reinforcement contingencies. Reinforcers gradually are faded or reduced so that the final behavior is maintained without the need for external rewards.

In some of these traditional programs, physical or verbal guidance such as pressure to the jaw or requests to open the mouth may be paired with the presentation of the food to guide the child toward the desired behavior. If the child opens the mouth and takes a bite of food, a reward is given. The feeding therapist monitors the child's progress by recording the number of successful and unsuccessful trials for the target behavior. When the child reaches a specified percentage of positive responses, the behavior is presumed to be established, and the therapist advances the program through successive approximations toward the final eating goal.

The idea of using positive reinforcement to change behavior is a common feature of many programs that address learning and performance. These programs generally reward a behavior that is desired by the therapist or parent. The concept rarely is questioned, and many people believe that this is the most effective way to help children learn. Parents are advised to lavish praise when their children behave according to family rules or standards. Teachers give gold stars or draw a happy face when children complete their assignments. School districts offer special treats such as free pizza to students who read a specified number of books during the summer. Employers offer incentive or pay-for-performance programs to entice their employees to do a better job. As a result, many therapists believe that principles of reinforcement and behavior management are the best ways of changing children's behaviors and teaching them to eat.

The results of behavior modification programs frequently are cited as proof that these principles effectively teach children desired eating skills (Handen, Mandell, & Russo, 1986; Kedesdy & Budd, 1998; Stark, Powers, Jelalian, Rape, & Miller, 1994; Thompson, Palmer, & Linscheid, 1977; Wolff & Lierman, 1994). It is important to ask specifically what these programs communicate to children and what children are learning in the programs. What impact does a behavior modification program have on the broadest aspects of children's lives?

In his book, *Punished by Rewards,* Kohn (1993) critically evaluates both the underlying premises of behavior modification and the role played by rewards in this system. He cites hundreds of studies that support the following observations.

Rewards support short-term changes in behavior.

Although short-term changes in behavior occur frequently when rewards are used, most people return to their original behaviors shortly after a study has been completed. In order to keep the behavior going, rewards must continue. In many instances, the reinforcer or reward must become larger or stronger to maintain the behavior.

Rewards and punishments are effective primarily in inducing compliance.

Reinforcement does not change the attitudes, beliefs, or emotional commitments that underlie behavior. If the objective is to get the person to obey or comply with the will of another person, reinforcers can be effective. If the goal is to support children's development of values or encourage self-directed learning, rewards are ineffective.

Rewards may improve the quantity of simple tasks, but they do not change the quality of the task or activity.

Research shows that reinforcement can increase the rate of simple, mindless tasks such as pressing a lever or sealing envelopes. However, when the task is interesting or open-ended, incentives have a detrimental effect. Qualitative changes and changes that require thinking do not occur spontaneously with rewards.

Rewards and punishment are two sides of the same coin.

Both rewards and punishment involve controlling others. Retracting a promised or implied reward for noncompliant behavior and enacting a punishment for that behavior are essentially the same thing.

Rewards and punishment work best in relationships where one person has most of the power.

This asymmetry of the power relationship is created and worsened by behavioral programs that use reward and punishment to support learning. Behavioral programs do not nourish cooperative learning and problem solving.

Kohn (1993) comments that …

"Someone who is raising or teaching children, for example, probably wants to create a caring alliance with each child, to help him or her feel safe enough to ask for help when problems develop. This is very possibly the single most fundamental requirement for helping a child to grow up healthy and develop a set of good values … This is precisely what rewards and punishments kill. If your parent or teacher or manager is sitting in judgment of what you do, and if that judgment will determine whether good things or bad things happen to you, this cannot help but warp your relationship with that person. You will not be working collaboratively in order to learn or grow; you will be trying to get him or her to approve of what you are doing so you can get the goodies." (page 57)

Rewards ignore reasons.

Children develop and enact behaviors for very specific reasons. Rewards simply address the behavior and pay no attention to the reasons why the problem developed. Reinforcers are used primarily when children are not behaving how adults want them to or are not motivated to learn. No one asks why the child refuses to eat or is uninterested in learning. Behaviorists do not have to ask "why?" to implement their programs.

Rewards discourage risk-taking and reduce creativity.

When rewards become the prime motivator of behavior, children and adults develop the behavior that is rewarded (Pearlman, 1984). They tend to do what is necessary to get the reward and no more. Children who concentrate on getting a good grade in school or receiving a reward for reading a specific number of books tend to do exactly what is required to receive the desired prize. They are unwilling to take intellectual risks or to attempt more difficult books. Risk and unconventional thinking are prerequisites for creativity. Studies support the idea that reinforcements actually interfere with the creative process, and reduce the skill and performance of subjects who are rewarded (Amabile, 1998; Amabile, Hennessey, & Grossman, 1986).

Rewards reduce the learner's intrinsic interest in the activity.

Rewards do not increase a person's interest in continuing the activity once the rewards have been withdrawn. A number of studies have shown that rewards actually interfere with the development of intrinsic interest and motivation. The use of rewards and bribes tells children that the activity isn't worth doing for its own sake. Two studies relating to children's food preferences are particularly applicable to the learning of mealtime behaviors.

Birch, Marlin, and Rotter's (1984) classic study of food preferences rewarded children for eating a new food. Some of the children in the group were praised while others received a movie ticket when they tried the food. Those in the control group did not receive any reward. When they studied the children's preferences for the same food a week later, children who had been rewarded with praise or a movie ticket liked the food less than they had the previous week. Those who had not been reinforced for eating it liked it as much or more than they did when they first tried it.

Newman and Taylor (1992) examined the effect of using one food as a reinforcer for eating another food. Although both foods were equally attractive to the children at the beginning of the study, the food that was rewarded had much less appeal at the end of the study. Rewarding the child for eating the food actually decreased how much the child liked it.

Praise can have a negative effect on learning.

Although praise is less controlling than other reinforcers, it often increases the pressure that the individual feels to live up to the compliment. The resulting stress can contribute to lower performance and learning. Some children learn to avoid difficult tasks because of fear of failure. Other children become hooked on praise and become dependent on the evaluations of others.

When praise is offered as a judgment of children's behavior or with a calculated goal of changing behavior, it can have a detrimental effect on learning. However, praise is not intrinsically harmful to children and their development. It can be given as a spontaneous appreciation of something that a child has done, provide informational feedback, be offered in a way that supports children's control over their lives, and support self-motivation.

Changing Children's Feeding Behavior Through Behavior Modification

Researchers are not in agreement about the effects of modifying behaviors through a reward system (Reitman, 1998). Many behavioral therapists argue that changes in feeding behaviors are well documented through research and clinical experience. Programs have focused primarily on increasing the amount of food eaten, reducing selective eating patterns, eliminating food refusals and food phobias, expanding food tastes and textures, and eliminating disruptive behaviors.

The impact of Kohn's critique of behavior modification must be considered in evaluating the effectiveness of these programs on children's mealtime behaviors. The majority of the behavioral studies of children's feeding development report only the short-term gains achieved while the child attended the program or participated in the research study (Babbitt et al., 1994). A number of studies have included a follow-up component to document that the gains achieved in the program were maintained for periods varying from 1 month to 1 year (Hoch, Babbitt, Coe, Ducan, & Trusty, 1995). Informal inquiry and clinical experience supports the observation that many children who participate in intensive behavioral feeding programs do not maintain the gains they initially achieved. Many are readmitted to inpatient feeding programs, and many parents are blamed for the child's failure to achieve long-term changes in eating behaviors.

The studies that report improvement in children's feeding address only the quantitative features of eating that can be objectively documented, such as the amount of food eaten, the number of different foods accepted, and the transition from tube feedings to oral feedings. None describe the qualitative aspects of feeding such as the adequacy of oral motor skills used during eating or drinking, the child's enjoyment of the mealtime, the child's intrinsic motivation to eat, or the quality of mealtime interactions.

Many children whose program was considered successful continue to need reminders and extrinsic rewards to maintain their eating abilities. They do not eat because they want to participate or because they enjoy food. They eat to please adults or to watch a favorite videotape during the meal. The father of one child asked how his daughter would learn to enjoy eating as a result of the program. He was told that enjoyment was not the goal. The behavioral psychologist emphasized that the child must learn to approach eating in the same way that many adults approach a job that they do not like. They go to work each day because it is a job and they need the money. In his belief system enjoyment was irrelevant to work and eating.

Behavior modification programs rarely explore or honor the child's nonverbal or behavioral communication. They do not ask why a specific child is not eating or why he is using the behaviors that are observed. It is assumed that the behavioral patterns exist because they are reinforced by the environment or are conditioned responses to an event in the child's past. Many children with ongoing sensory integration difficulties, mild dysphagia, and gastrointestinal problems have reasons for the mealtime behaviors that they use. Their behavioral communication of discomfort or fear frequently is ignored, and they are expected to comply with the adult-controlled feeding program. Some of these children do not comply. Others learn to put up with the discomfort and survive the program, only to go back to food-refusal patterns after they return home.

Many children with feeding refusals and aversions have survived severe medical complications because of their indomitable spirit. Some behavioral feeding programs attack the spirit of these children. Some children dig in their heels and refuse to eat for long periods. Others gradually give up and submit to adult wishes because they are hungry or desire the social interaction.

This is not to say that feeding programs based on behavior modification do not work. They help many children move toward more adequate diets and transition from tube feedings to oral feedings. The financial and personal cost of these programs can be substantial for some children and families. Most programs have not addressed the qualitative personal ramifications for children and their families.

Incorporating Behavioral Principles of Learning in Mealtime Programs

Although the more rigid structure of formal behavior modification programs is incompatible with a child-guided mealtime program, many underlying behavioral strategies fit in well. Most of these involve understanding the sequential progressions within the new skill and creating ways of providing greater success for the child in the learning program. The following learning guidelines can be helpful in mealtime programs.

Examples are provided for Brianna, a 2-year-old who takes her meals from a gastrostomy tube. Brianna has many unpleasant associations with food because of her history of sensory defensiveness and gastroesophageal reflux. Her reflux appears to be under control with medication, and she is able to take bolus feedings when she is preparing to go to sleep. Her sensory processing skills have improved. Signs of sensory defensiveness appear primarily when she is in emotionally stressful situations. However, Brianna retains many negative associations between feeding utensils and discomfort. She fusses when she is placed in her high chair, gags when she sees the spoon, and retches when she sees the tube-feeding syringe.

Break down larger skills or behaviors into smaller steps or components.

Children and parents learn more easily and rapidly when changes are small than when they are large. When therapists break down a larger skill into its component parts, it is easier to understand the child's strengths and limitations.

Brianna's mother and therapist developed a series of small steps that they used to help her accept a spoon without gagging. They noticed that she loved to play with water and adored bath time. Their first step was to include spoons and cups in the bath for water play. Because other toys for stirring and pouring also were present, Brianna did not feel that the spoons were there to make her eat. Once Brianna was comfortable with the spoons, her mother and therapist introduced a game of giving drinks of water to different bath toys. Initially, this was done in the tub. Later, the activity was transferred to a small basin of water in the playroom. Eventually, Brianna began to put the spoon in her own mouth and drink small amounts of water.

Build positive associations between feeding and something the child enjoys.

If a therapist wants to help change the child's negative response to the mealtime environment and food, it is important to change the stimulus that usually triggers the negative response.

Brianna had strong negative associations with the spoon because it meant that someone would make her eat. Eating caused discomfort in her mouth and then in her tummy. The sight of the spoon reminded her that eating was uncomfortable. She developed a strong belief that spoons were dangerous because they caused her severe discomfort. When her mother began to pair the spoon with a new stimulus (i.e., the bathtub and water play), the association became less strong. She built many new associations between spoons and play and imagination. Spoons developed positive associations as long as they did not have food on them.

Brianna did not enjoy sitting in her high chair for tube feedings. Because the high chair also was used for oral feedings, it was negatively associated with eating—including eating by tube. In addition, the emotional stress of this association contributed to an upset stomach and increased sensory defensiveness. As a result, Brianna frequently retched as soon as she saw the feeding tube and syringe. Brianna had a special table and chair that she and her mother used for doing puzzles, her favorite activity. Tube feedings were introduced during puzzle play. The syringe was kept out of sight, and Brianna's attention was focused on the puzzle. Calming music was played during the activity to increase her emotional comfort. She began to build a positive association between play and comfortable filling of her tummy.

■ **Change the stimulus that triggers the negative response.**

When children have built strong negative associations with a stimulus that is common at mealtime, it often is difficult to help them discover that the original situation may have changed. At one time, eating may have caused reflux or oral discomfort. However, with therapy and maturation, the child's negative physical or sensory response may have diminished or been resolved. Often, simply telling the child that there is no longer pain or discomfort is useless. The child has built the association into a firm belief (i.e., "When I eat, I hurt"). When the child gags in response to the memory of the discomfort, the gagging and emotional stress can trigger the old physical discomforts. It is as if the child says, "See, I told you it hurts when I eat!"

The initial step in changing the association for Brianna began in the bathtub. The triggering stimulus of the spoon took on other associations. She no longer had to be on guard to protect herself when she saw the spoon. She accepted water from the spoon during play. However, when food was presented on the spoon, her old gagging behaviors returned. Her therapist introduced diluted tastes of juice into the water play. He encouraged Brianna to stick her fingers in the water and then the diluted juice, and then put them into her mouth. Gradually, he increased the strength of the taste and then thickened the liquid. Brianna now had a new association of fingers and food that was positive. Her therapist introduced the small bath toys into the food-tasting game. These animals had ears, feet, and tails that became covered with food tastes. He began to lick the food off with his tongue to model what he wanted Brianna to do. Soon Brianna was feeding herself small amounts of food from the toys. Eventually, the therapist incorporated the spoon into the food play, and Brianna dipped the spoon into food and put it into her mouth.

Learning Alternatives in Teaching Feeding and Mealtime Skills

There are many alternatives to behavior modification programs for children with feeding difficulties. Programs that emphasize the intrinsic wisdom of children to guide their own feeding therapy are self-empowering. They return responsibility and control of eating to children and relinquish the need for adults to make all the decisions. They offer choices and teach children how to choose wisely. Tools such as music, imagery, and enhanced communication skills assist children who are fearful or resistant to change. Behavioral strategies that break down a task and build positive associations with meals may be incorporated. These programs focus strongly on building the child's inner desire to eat and discover the sensory and social pleasures that accompany mealtimes. Curiosity, a sense of adventure, and shared participation are accentuated and valued. The emphasis is placed on the quality of eating as well as the quantity. The mealtime environment is addressed and modified in a way that supports physical, sensory, communication, and learning abilities. Parents and therapists become partners who facilitate the child's desire and ability to make mealtime changes.

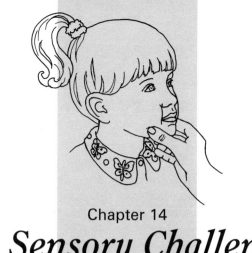

Chapter 14

The Sensory Challenges of Mealtime

Mealtimes challenge all the senses in many ways. The tastes, smells, and textures of different foods affect the enjoyment of them. The lighting, sounds, visual presentation of the meal, and comfortable chairs all become part of the mealtime ambiance. Having a delicious meal in an unpleasant environment will change the meal participant's opinion of that meal. In the same way, having a poorly cooked meal in a fine restaurant may ruin the entire mealtime experience. An enjoyable mealtime is based upon positive experiences through all of the senses. One sensory aspect of the meal can affect the whole meal. As this book explores mealtimes for children with sensory difficulties, it also will reveal each individual's need to be aware of the powerful personal effect sensations have on a meal. Therapists will need to look beyond the mouth to the entire sensory environment and notice how changing one sensory aspect of the meal can affect the whole meal.

The Senses and Mealtimes

Personal Nature of the Senses

The information a person receives from the vestibular, proprioceptive, tactile, visual, auditory, olfactory, and gustatory senses powerfully influences her ability to eat and enjoy mealtimes. Everyone receives this sensory information, but how each individual interprets and reacts to it is very personal. Some people love the flavor of peppermint and others avoid it. Some enjoy the smell of coffee while others hate it. Some crave the texture of custard while others stay far away from it. There are as many variations in the interpretation of sensations that surround mealtimes as there are individuals! What people like, they really like, and what they don't, they **don't!** Children are the same way. They can have strong sensory preferences. Many children have sensory systems that, for one reason or another, are not functioning optimally. Their creative sensory responses to mealtime sensations can be quite a challenge for feeding.

Beyond the Mouth

Many traditional feeding programs have focused on the mouth. Tastes and textures have been studied and changed without looking at the whole mealtime environment. Looking at the meal in the context of a child's complete day helps therapists look at the sensory variables before, during, and after the meal. It helps to look beyond the mouth to the preparation of the environment for feeding, the sensory preparation of the child, the sensory preparation of the feeder, the sensory aspects of the meal, and the sensory information the child may need in transitioning to the next activity of the day.

Understanding Sensory Variables

Because of the powerful nature of the sensory components of eating, therapists must be careful in offering suggestions for sensory change. Sensory input should be carefully understood, with changes made in a planned and prescriptive fashion. Changes made to the sensory features of a meal should be positive in a manner that facilitates improved eating skills and enjoyment. Children are their own best experts. If a child is offered a sensory change and the change fits that child's needs, therapists will know and recognize the change through the child's response to the meal. This is a signal to adults to continue to incorporate this type of sensory change. If the child lets the therapist know that the change was not needed or effective, the type and degree of sensory input must be modified.

To understand the child's sensory responses at mealtime and begin to make thoughtful decisions about the sensory variables that surround and include the meal, therapists need to understand each sensory variable and how these variables can affect the total sensory environment of the meal. Children take in sensory information from the environment, process that information, and make an adaptive response. They will attend to the sensory variables that are the strongest or most alerting before responding to neutral or calming sensory variables. When mealtime occurs in homes or classrooms that are filled with sensory stimuli, therapists need to analyze the total input that the child is receiving. They can create an environment in which the child is alerted to the feeding process rather than to environmental sensory variables. For example, ideally the child focuses attention on the food, the spoon, or the feeder. When there are distracters such as a soiled diaper, loud music, or bright lights, the child may focus on the distractions in the room instead of the meal.

Following is a look at each of seven sensory variables and an analysis of its alerting, calming, or neutral features. Therapists and parents can use this knowledge to create an optimum mealtime environment.

Vestibular Sensory Information (Balance and Equilibrium)

The vestibular system picks up sensory information relating to pull of gravity on the central axis of the body. It lets a person know when he is falling or moving, and how fast the movement occurs.

Movement can occur in any direction—up and down, back and forth, side to side, rotational, or any combination of these directions. It can be fast or slow, predictable or unpredictable, even or uneven, rhythmical, or absent.

Try these movement experiences with a partner. Focus on the feelings of the movement. Are some more alerting or attention getting than others are? Are some more predictable? Which movements most likely have a calming effect?

- Rock slowly in a rocking chair.
- Rock fast in a rocking chair.
- Stand and turn slowly in one direction.
- Stand and spin rapidly around one spot on the floor.
- Stand up and down slowly, and then fast.
- Sway from side to side slowly and evenly, and then fast.
- Move your partner slowly and rhythmically.
- Move your partner suddenly from behind.

Be aware of your reactions. Probably at first you were more alerted to the contrast of movement versus no movement; that is, if you moved, you noticed movement, and if you did not move, you did not notice movement. However, some movements alerted you more than others. It is likely that you noticed movement more if it was fast, unexpected, arrhythmic, or uneven. Movement that is slow, predictable, even, or rhythmic usually can be less noticeable. Did you find spinning more alerting than up-down or side-to-side movement? People tend to pay rapid attention to the aspects of movement that are associated with falling.

How can these observations be applied to mealtime? Think for a moment about what should be emphasized at the meal. Should the child's attention be directed toward movement? Is it important for the child to be constantly alerted to position in space? How much attention should be paid to feelings of falling? How much emphasis should be given to postural stability? In most cases, the therapist wants the child to attend to the meal, the food, the eating process, and the mealtime interaction. Direct attention to vestibular information can distract from the meal. Vestibular input can create changes in muscle tone or tension. In most people, this contributes to adjustments to the pull of gravity. In a child with a neurological disorder, it can result in strong and predictable patterns of changes in tone throughout the body. When the child sits sloppily in the chair with the head and body tilted toward one side and feet dangling, the vestibular system demands attention and the child is less able to focus on the more important eating and social aspects of the meal. A child who is positioned in any vestibularly alerting posture must primarily attend to the vestibular input and only secondarily attend to the meal.

Therefore, the therapist should make sure that the child is positioned in a stable, well-supported position. In most cases, this is a stationary, comfortable position in a chair or on a lap. At times, a more dynamic positioning is desirable. This involves gentle stimulation or activation of the vestibular system in a way that integrates it with other sensory input. For example, if the child's postural tone is in a normal range, a slight tipping movement in a backward direction could bring the chin into a tucked position. This head and chin position could make jaw, tongue, and lip movement easier. In this case, the vestibular information does not compete for attention. Sometimes, vestibular stimulation in the form of gentle movement is given prescriptively during a meal to help a child become more organized for the meal. This might be done in a rocking chair or in the parent's arms. Another child may require bouncing or swinging during treatment to help alert her to the meal or to increase postural tone and stability. This might be done with the child on a lap or on a ball, with gentle bouncing done between bites. However vestibular sensory information is used, the focus should be the postural, movement, and attentional needs of the child.

There are general variables that can help calm a child's excessive vestibular input so that the focus is on the meal. Some children find slow vestibular stimulation very calming and organizing to their ability to relax and attend to the meal. In the previous participation activity, did you find that slow rocking in the rocking chair was calming? It may have reminded you of ways in which your mother helped you calm down and become better organized when you were a child. The vestibular system also helps the nervous system integrate or organize other sensory information (Ayres, 1972). Many children who are hyperactive or become overwhelmed by the sensory environment will benefit from slow rocking, gentle up-down bouncing movements, and some swinging. Generally, this is done before a meal, although feeding while sitting on a lap in a rocking chair also may be helpful.

Each child's vestibular system has different needs and should be considered individually. Based on these needs, determine if you need to alert or calm the child's vestibular system before or during a meal. Make the appropriate adjustments to maximize the mealtime interaction.

Proprioceptive Sensory Information (Inner-Muscle and Joint Awareness)

Proprioceptive sensory information is collected in the joints, muscles, and tendons. It consists of the internal feedback received from muscles that lets a person know what his muscles are doing at any given moment. Proprioceptive information is necessary to make the constant postural adjustments that occur as an individual moves and to maintain normal muscle tone. Adequate proprioceptive information is needed to create a smooth motor plan for any motoric activity, be it walking, writing, chewing, or drinking.

Try these movements. While standing, hold one arm out to the side of your body parallel with the floor. Close your eyes. Feel the position of the arm. Hold out your other arm and make it match the exact position of the first arm. Notice how easily you were able to do this. This was possible with the help of your internal muscle awareness or proprioceptive input.

The muscles respond to many types of movement, just as the vestibular system does. Different information is provided when muscle movements are fast, slow, even, uneven, tight, loose, or made against resistance.

The proprioceptive information a person receives constantly from the joints and muscles helps her function smoothly in the environment. Too much muscle tension or high muscle tone will work against an activity, while too little tension or low tone serves as a poor foundation for movement. An individual can have a reasonable amount of muscle tone, yet have poor or inconsistent proprioceptive feedback. When this happens, she is unable to interpret how and where the body is moving. Therapists can use proprioceptive techniques to increase children's awareness of their muscles. Some children create constant motion for their arms, legs, or head as a way of providing the proprioceptive input they need to *find* these body parts. Giving deep-pressure proprioceptive input can calm these children and help them focus on the information that will help them develop a smoothly executed movement pattern.

Here is another activity for you to try. Tighten the muscles of your arm by flexing your elbow tightly near your trunk. Reach for a cookie. Is your attention on the tightness in your arm or on the cookie? Now lift a piece of paper while keeping the same amount of tension in your arm muscles. Notice how much you feel these tense muscles. Now lift a large dictionary. With the weight of the dictionary, was your attention on your arm or the book?

Now is a good time to relate these abstract concepts to mealtime. It is important to consider the child's muscle tone and motor-planning abilities when developing a mealtime program. If muscle tension is too tight or too loose or fluctuates rapidly, the child can become frustrated because it is difficult to perform the desired movements. Attention becomes focused on how difficult it is to move. These abnormalities in postural tone and movement are a response to vestibular and proprioceptive input. To obtain the most normal muscle tone possible, the therapist needs to prepare the child before and during the meal. With this environmental support, the child will be able to focus on mealtime successes, not frustration. There will be a discussion in the following chapter on handling and positioning techniques to facilitate more normalized tone.

Think about your experience in lifting a piece of paper and compare it with lifting the dictionary. When you lifted a heavier object, you probably were more aware of it. This observation has implications for several mealtime situations. A child may continually have difficulty planning the smooth motor movement needed to bring the food into the mouth. A heavier spoon would increase the proprioceptive feedback and may make the child more aware and alert to the task. Another child, who is learning to drink from a cup, may have difficulty with the runny liquid moving rapidly all over the mouth and face. It may be moving so quickly that the child is not getting sufficient sensory-weight feedback to let the tongue adjust its configuration to collect the liquid more efficiently. Drinking skills may improve with a heavier liquid, such as a milkshake or a mixture of juice and applesauce, which could give enough proprioceptive feedback to start a smooth, suck-swallow drinking response.

Another child may be having a hard time focusing on the mealtime process and is diverting energy and attention to extraneous arm, head, and foot movements. Seating the child in a beanbag chair or a seat that provides deep pressure at the shoulder and hip joints may help increase awareness of the body in space. As awareness increases, extraneous movements may be reduced. The child no longer needs to move to become aware of the body. In this way, proprioceptive information can be very calming.

Tactile Sensory Information (Touch)

The sense of touch has many components. For purposes of this mealtime discussion, it is defined as the sensory system that interprets texture and consistency, light touch, deep pressure touch, pain, temperature, and vibration.

Choose a partner to help you with this activity. Experience each of these sensations. If you prefer, close your eyes and concentrate on imagining the feeling of these experiences:

- the texture of baby-food strained pears in your mouth
- the texture of applesauce with raisins
- the feeling of water in your mouth, compared with the feeling of freshly squeezed orange juice
- the feeling of a pin prick on your finger, compared with the feeling of a pinch on your arm
- the feeling you have when someone walks up behind you and lightly touches your shoulder
- the feeling of ice water versus warm water versus hot water
- the feeling of a firm hug
- the feeling of a feather brushed lightly over your arm
- the feeling of clothes on your body
- the feeling of a regular toothbrush in your mouth, compared with the feeling of an electric vibrating toothbrush

Which touch did you notice more? Which ones alerted you? Which sensations did you not notice or gradually ignore as they continued?

Think again about which feelings were more alerting and which were more calming or even neutral. For most people, uneven or rough textures are more alerting or noticeable than smooth, even textures. The extremes of hot and cold are more alerting than neutral, warm temperatures. Pain is always alerting because of its primary role in survival. Feathers and light ticklish touch seem to be more alerting or noticeable than deep-pressure touch. It appears that deep pressure initially is noticeable or alerting, but when it is continued, it becomes a calming or quieting sensory input as the person gets used to the touch. Vibration, such as that found with the electric toothbrush, tends to be noticeable or alerting. Other vibrational frequencies may be calming to the system.

In general, touch draws attention to or away from an activity. The therapist should consider the reactions a child may have to different types of touch and how the tactile environment that gains the child's attention for the mealtime can be created. If the child's diaper is wet, the coldness that results when the dampness interacts with air will create discomfort and draw the child's attention away from the meal. Uncomfortable clothing or seating positions will have the same effect. Textured foods that are cold may help draw attention and be alerting. This can be one of the therapist's goals for a child with low muscle tone or low sensory awareness. A deep-pressure hug may create the inner calming that a child needs in preparation for a meal. Used prescriptively, touch can prepare a child for a meal and help focus attention on the desired interaction.

Gustatory Sensory Information (Taste)

Gustatory sensory information is received and interpreted through the taste buds on the tongue. They interpret sweet, sour, bitter, and salty. Mixtures of these four primary tastes, in combination with smell, create many other taste combinations. The gustatory system works in close contact with the olfactory system to finely interpret taste.

Try this gustatory sensory participation activity. Blindfold yourself. Have your partner place various tastes on your tongue. Explore the following foods and become aware of your responses to them. Notice which are the more alerting flavors.

- pickle
- saltine cracker
- water
- baby-food strained pears
- baby-food strained squash
- chili powder mixed with a small amount of water
- a hot creamed wheat cereal
- lemon juice
- chocolate
- cheese
- vinegar
- flour and water paste
- potato chip
- a crushed aspirin mixed with a small amount of water

Did you notice that the strong flavors in the primary senses of sweet, sour, bitter, and salty tend to get your attention immediately? The more bland flavors, such as hot creamed wheat cereal and flour and water paste, were less effective in getting your attention. A neutral or almost tasteless substance such as water was easy to ignore. Children often respond differently to taste than adults. Older children and adults make automatic comparisons and judgments in taste with what is familiar. Many parents notice that children who had been reared on a diet of artificially flavored foods found that the natural foods were too bland and tasteless. Thus, the children preferred ice cream with artificially flavored and colored strawberries to a strawberry ice cream made of natural ingredients. Because adults lose taste buds as they age, they require a stronger taste input to build awareness than children. At one time, commercial baby foods were filled with sugar and salt additives to make them taste better to the mothers who purchased them. This taught many children to crave sweet and salty tastes in food—a habit that contributed to poor health. Today, baby foods generally are free of most additives. In most instances, the bland flavors are more appropriate for young infants. They may not be as appropriate, however, for older infants and children who have feeding difficulties. Homemade blended foods prepared from fresh fruits, vegetables, and meats usually have a fuller, richer flavor than their commercially prepared counterparts.

Children who are poorly alerted to food or unmotivated to eat may respond and eat better when herbs or spices are added. In contrast, some children have difficulty organizing and integrating sensory information. These children may be more accepting of food and use better feeding movements when less alerting foods, such as those with sour or bitter tastes, are eliminated from the diet. Certain medical conditions, medications, and even a mild deficiency of zinc can cause distortions in taste and cause the child to refuse food (Alpers, 1994). Although infants are readily alerted to sweet tastes (Lawless, 1985), it is wise to offer foods in the feeding therapy program in which a sweet taste does not predominate. Because of the power that sweetness holds in the body's taste system, it is easy for people to become addicted to sweets. Such addiction can easily begin in a therapy program if the therapist is not aware of the importance of using other types of food.

Olfactory Sensory Information (Smell)

Try to think of a smell that does not get your attention—one that is **not** alerting. Smells are **always** alerting initially. Whether you like a smell or not, you **are** aware of it. We tend to accommodate to smell in several minutes. A smell that initially was alerting quickly becomes not noticed. Have you ever been painting in a closed room and not noticed the paint smell until someone walking into the room brought it to your attention? Yet, after being in the room for a few minutes, that person no longer noticed the smell.

Smell perception occurs when the chemicals stimulate the olfactory receptors in the nasal cavity. Smell can reach the nasal cavity from the air breathed in through the nostrils as well as from the nasopharynx upward towards the roof of the nasal cavity. Smell that is interpreted through the nostrils is described as coming through the oronasal route. Smell that is interpreted through the nasopharynx upward takes the retronasal route. The retronasal route includes suckling in infants and chewing and swallowing in older children and adults (Mennella & Beauchamp, 1993a). Without the sense of smell, many of the subtleties of flavor are missed.

Flavor perception, therefore, requires a combination of the olfactory and gustatory systems. Most people recall their response to food when they have a cold, remembering how nose congestion interfered with the ability to taste foods. Food flavors needed to be quite strong to be tasted.

Try it! Pick several foods. Try tasting them first with your nose plugged and then without. Notice the difference in your flavor perception. Notice how much more alerting or full the flavor is with the sense of smell paired with the sense of taste!

Therapists need to consider this factor when working with children who are chronically congested with a stuffy nose. These children are losing not only smell but also taste information. Food choices for these children are extremely important. Stronger or spicier flavors may make the difference in motivation level and appreciation of a meal. Children who are dependent on a ventilator or a tracheostomy for breathing do not appreciate smells because the major flow of air for breathing bypasses the olfactory receptors in the nose. When foods are introduced orally, they may taste very strong or unpleasant because the blending and softening of taste that occurs with smell is missing. Often, this is a major difficulty for a child who has acquired a feeding disorder and tracheostomy after developing normal taste associations.

Smells are picked up in the nasal cavity and interpreted in the brain. Because the olfactory centers in the brain are associated with the limbic system, smell has a strong emotional component and a strong association with memory storage. Smells are very memorable! Have you ever smelled a particular fragrance or odor and immediately remembered a time and place when you previously experienced that smell? A perfume or cologne may bring back memories of a high school sweetheart; the smell of home-baked bread may bring back memories of grandmother's kitchen. Conversely, a smell may have unpleasant connotations. A child may remember an uncomfortable experience with a particular food or feeder, and that negative memory may be contributing to the child's current difficulty in accepting or handling that specific food.

Smell becomes an important part of every meal. The therapist should carefully consider its contribution to the total mealtime. Smell of the food usually is a child's first hint that the meal is forthcoming. Are other strong smells in the environment competing with the food smells? In settings where many dependent children or adults are fed at one time, diaper odors or the smell of a disinfectant can compete with the smell of the food, making it difficult for both the feeder and the child to attend to the meal. Adults who are feeding children should be aware of the powerful influence of smell and notice each child's reaction to mealtime smells.

Visual Sensory Information (Sight)

The eyes work together to give visual information. They focus on objects near and far; track in vertical, horizontal, diagonal, and circular directions; and can diverge and converge focus. People have central (front) vision as well as peripheral (side) vision. The brain divides the vision of each eye into four quadrants. Full vision requires that a person be able to receive information from all four quadrants. When there is brain damage or damage to a portion of the eye, the person may not be capable of receiving a full range of visual information.

Consider this participatory activity. Look at a palette of colors. Which ones draw your attention most rapidly? Look around the room and through several magazines or children's books that have colored pictures. Become aware of your reaction to color and shape. Notice where your eyes stop.

- Does the shape of an object or its color attract you more?
- What effect does the level and type of light in a room have on your attention?
- Do you attend more rapidly to moving or nonmoving objects?
- Which gets your attention most quickly—movement in the center or on the periphery of your vision?

Brighter primary colors tend to get a person's attention more than pale, neutral colors. Shiny objects tend to get one's attention more rapidly than those with a dull finish. Detailed or unusual pictures get people's attention more than those that are familiar. The unexpected is alerting. Moving objects usually elicit a rapid, alerting response, especially if the movement is unexpected. Peripheral movements alert one more rapidly than movements occurring in the center of vision. Contrasts in color, shape, or movement are more alerting than blends of color and form.

Here is another color participatory activity that may provide insight. Explore your personal and inner reactions to color. Make a pile of 12-inch fabric squares in each of the following colors: red, pink, orange, white, yellow, black, green, violet or purple, indigo or purplish blue, and light or royal blue. With each color,

- place the cloth on a table in front of you and look at it.
- hold the cloth up to your eyes and look through it.
- close your eyes and feel the cloth with your hands. Sense the color through the vibrations received by your touch sense.

Notice how each color makes you feel. Which colors calm you? Which ones are energizing? Are you aware of any other feelings? Can you recognize a color just by feeling it?

Color is created through different light vibration patterns. Through the sense of touch, a blind person can learn to recognize the different vibrations and learn the color names associated with each vibratory category (Ostrander & Schroeder, 1979). When these color vibrations reach the body, a person responds to them at an inner level as well as an outer level of color recognition (Ackerman, 1991). Green, blue, indigo, violet, and pink evoke calm feelings. Often, people choose these colors for a bedroom or other area where they like to relax. Red, orange, and yellow tend to be very energizing colors. These might be selected for an office, kitchen, or work area. Color choices in clothing or colors that predominate in the paint or fabric of a room can influence a person's feelings and energy level.

To use this information at mealtime, the therapist should think about where she wants to focus the child's attention. Should it be on the other children in the room, the brightly decorated walls, the plate, the table, or the feeder? If the therapist wants to increase the child's ability to focus on the spoon, she could use a shiny spoon or one that is coated with a contrasting color. She also could create a colored or lighted handle for the spoon, or attach a pom-pom, small plastic face, or a ponytail popbead to the handle. The clinician must be sure that the plate contrasts with the table or the place mat, and select food that contrasts with the plate. Minimizing environmental movements also is advisable, as they can be very distracting to a child who is sensitive to peripheral motion. Using color can calm a child and reduce distractibility and hyperactivity. The therapist could make a set of laminated, solid-color place mats in a wide variety of colors that are alert or calming. Then, she could let the children choose the color of place mat that they would like to use.

It is best for the therapist to work with each child's ophthalmologist, optometrist, or functional vision specialist to determine the child's optimum field of vision. Food should be presented within the child's best visual field quadrants. Occasionally, children who are described as distractible, hyperactive, or indifferent to food and objects respond in these ways because of a visual field deficit. They fail to respond consistently because food or an object may be presented in a field in which they have no vision. At other times, they respond appropriately because the object is within a visual quadrant where there is usable vision. Constant head movements or a particular tilt of the head may be used as a compensation to improve functional vision.

Auditory information has been described as *touch from a distance* because sound is transmitted as sound waves touching the eardrum, causing it to vibrate. When hearing is intact, a person can localize the direction of a sound and discriminate between a wide variety of environmental and speech sounds.

Try this participatory activity. Listen to sounds in your home and outdoors. Which sounds did you notice most? Which ones were less noticeable? Remember sounds in your daily life. Which ones wake you up? Which ones put you to sleep? Which sounds do you usually ignore? Which sounds always or usually get your attention? Listen to music on the radio, tapes, or CDs. Find music that is quieting or relaxing to you. Find music that energizes you. Find music that makes you feel irritable. Notice your reaction to the rhythm, loudness, melody, and harmony in the music.

Loud, unexpected, intermittent, and high-pitched sounds tend to get a person's attention more rapidly. Soft, repetitive, familiar, sustained, and low-pitched sounds may be ignored. People often quiet their behavior when these sounds are in the background. They respond a great deal to their personal preferences in music. Familiar music often is selected out of habit. Basic characteristics of music influence the functioning of the body and mind (Campbell, 1997). Music with a slow tempo and a regular, sustained rhythm slows down breathing and heart rhythms, contributing to greater relaxation.

Sound plays a major role at mealtime. Children who are fed in a school cafeteria or institutional dining room often must deal with the loud, intermittent noise of talking, kitchen sounds, and sounds reverberating off cement walls and floors. At times, the sounds of television, rock music, and the chatter of feeders who are focused on each other rather than the children predominates. Children can ignore intense visual stimulation by shutting their eyes or looking away from the feeder and the meal. Auditory stimulation is always there. It cannot be ignored peripherally. Some children attempt to deal with the overload and confusion by engaging in rhythmical stereotyped movements such as flapping the hands or rocking. Others appear to be deaf by shutting out the noise at an inner level. Distracting sounds should be eliminated or reduced from the mealtime area whenever possible. This often provides a creative challenge for parents and staff, but it is well worth any effort it involves. Once the overall noise level is reduced, sound can be used directly to quiet the child, help him focus attention, and create more appropriate feeding rhythms. The use of sound and music as part of the learning environment was discussed in Chapter 13.

Sensory Preparation and Mealtimes

Listening to the Child

Where do therapists begin to incorporate all this information about the different sensory variables and their qualities? What step is next? How do clinicians begin to apply these concepts to their work with children? As the therapist focuses on the sensory needs of children, she needs to look to them for the answers and listen to what they tell us. Children tell adults a great deal about the kinds of sensory input they are drawn to or need. The child who moves rapidly, crashes into furniture, and bumps and tumbles into everything may be telling adults about a strong need for movement and proprioceptive input. The therapist may introduce more challenging foods to this child in a rocking chair or while sitting on a bouncy ball. Children who mouth everything in sight, from toys to fingers to clothing, may be reminding adults that they need tactile input to the mouth. Textured toys, electric toothbrushes, and small vibrating facial massagers might be used to prepare the mouth for the meal. These children also might remove food from one of these toys.

The therapist needs to take the information collected about the child's sensory needs and handling of sensory information and use it to help prepare the environment, the child, and the feeder for the meal. Then, the therapist can transition the child into the next activity.

Sensory Preparation of the Environment

As therapists learn about children's sensory systems, they begin to understand what works for them. They can create a mealtime environment that is sensorially prescriptive for each child. The therapist can take the information she knows about the child's ability to interpret stimuli from each of the senses to prepare the environment before the meal. The clinician can minimize distractions with changes in light and sounds. Incorporating quiet background music helps focus attention. She can increase the ability to focus on the meal with attention to plates, cups, and place mats. The therapist can help the child attend to the food by creating variations in smell, taste, texture, and temperature. Food and equipment should be prepared ahead of time and be available in the dining room when the child comes to the table. The first step is to prepare an environment that optimizes the child's individual learning style and mealtime focus.

Clinicians can observe and record the sensory features of the child's mealtime environment using the Environmental Sensory Variable Analysis form on page 291. They can write down alerting and calming variables, along with ideas for adjusting each sensory component to meet an individual child's needs.

Sensory Preparation of the Child

When adults think about preparing a child for the meal, they consider what can be done just before the meal to ready the child for the approach of the spoon or the food. They may ask what facial exercises or tongue "wake-up" activities are right for this child. Therapists know that if they prepare the child only during the moments just before the food is presented, they miss an important part of the preparation process. The most effective preparation for the transition to mealtime occurs throughout the day with a special focus on the hour before the meal.

It would be helpful to think about a familiar analogy with the bedtime ritual. Many parents establish a regular bedtime routine to help their child ease gently into sleep at night. First, they give the child a warm bath and then put on warm pajamas. A parent reads several favorite stories as the child is unwinding and his muscles are relaxing. There may be a goodnight song followed by reassuring goodnight kisses. The lights are turned out, and immediately the child goes to sleep. Changing the scenario a bit, imagine that the family has been out for the day, perhaps on an adventure to the amusement park or the zoo. They have all had a very exciting day. The child gets home late after the big day and needs to forego the usual bedtime routine and go immediately to bed. It is not surprising then, that the child cannot get right to sleep. Sleep does not come easily because the child did not have enough transition time to calm the sensory system before bed.

The same types of sensory transition preparation may be necessary for some children as they move into a mealtime. Preparation that helps the child transition from one activity level to another can be very important in helping the child focus and maximally enjoy the meal. Some babies need to be rocked or have a complete massage before they are organized enough to eat well. Some children need time to bounce on a ball or jump on a trampoline to wake up their system to a ready, alert state before a meal. For others, bouncing and jumping would be too disorganizing. Still other children may need to quietly sit with headphones or open speakers and a Hemi-Sync Metamusic tape to help them relax and focus (Morris, 1997c). Others need the entire day to be filled with their own special sensory diet (Wilbarger & Wilbarger, 1991). This concept is based on the idea that each person needs a certain level of sensory information or input to be most alert, adaptable, and skillful in everyday activities. Sensory diets can include activities that provide sensory information to all the senses, with emphasis on the specific input needed most by that child.

Individual children also may need a time of personal sensory preparation in addition to the more general period of sensory transition. This preparation specifically focuses on the child's immediate sensory needs at the beginning of the meal (Frick et al., 1996). Some children need a facial massage focused on relaxing tight retraction of the lips. One child may need specific tongue activities that alert the mouth and help the tongue move more actively at the beginning of the meal.

Another will begin the meal by sucking or chewing pickles because sour tastes may make it easier for the cheeks and tongue to move together. Still others may begin the meal with resistive sucking through a straw to create a more general focus of attention. The personal sensory preparation focuses on preparing the oral motor system for optimum handling of the food through sucking, swallowing, biting, and chewing.

Sensory Preparation for the Adult

Therapists are trained to think about preparing the environment and the child for the meal. They often forget that the adult who is feeding the child also needs sensory preparation for the meal. Special consideration should be given to the physical support provided by a comfortable chair or couch. The chair should be close enough to the child so that the feeder doesn't experience physical strain. The adult's position should encourage good eye contact and interaction. Parents need to be very aware that feeding a child with complicated problems can be a strain on them physically and emotionally. Any adult feeding a child needs to take the time to locate comfortable pillow supports for the arm or back. Meals will be easier and less stressful for everyone if the feeder takes a few moments before the meal to breathe deeply, listen to calming music, or talk quietly with the child. It is easy to get stuck in the complications of feeding a child and sometimes lose track of the social and interactional components of meals.

Sensory Variables During the Meal

Sensory information is an integral part of all mealtimes. The mealtime for many children starts with the transition preparation and personal preparation previously discussed. The meal does not begin with presentation of food. But now that the child is prepared, it is a good idea to explore how specific sensory information can be used in a prescriptive fashion **during** the meal.

Food has multiple sensory properties. It has a unique appearance. It has a smell, a taste, a temperature, often more than one texture, and sometimes a sound. Each of these bits of information can affect the child positively or negatively. For the purposes of looking prescriptively at the variables, it will help to look at a continuum of sensations. For example, food does not just taste spicy. It can be a little spicy or a lot spicy. There can be a hint of cinnamon or lots of cinnamon flavor! Textures are not just smooth and rough. Smooth foods can be more like liquid, pudding, or mashed potatoes. All can be described as smooth, and yet each is different. Liking one texture does not necessarily mean liking the next.

When children have a narrow range of food interests, the minute increments in the continuum of taste, temperature, and texture are important in considering what foods and drinks to offer.

Grading of the Sensory Continuum of Food

Taste

Tastes can be sweet, sour, bitter, or salty. They can be strong or weak, concentrated or diluted. They can be slightly sweet or slightly salty. They can be combinations of flavors. Milder, dilute tastes may be easier to handle for a child who is very sensitive to tastes and changes. Introducing a very diluted juice may provide an easier taste transition than concentrated juice. For example, an extremely taste-sensitive child may have major difficulty transitioning from water to juice. However, if the therapist makes an ice cube of juice that gradually melts into the water, the taste of juice emerges slowly. Because this is not a sensory surprise, the child may find it much easier to make the transition. The juice flavor might have been immediately rejected if the flavor had not started out mixed with the water. The gradual melting provided a very dilute, slowly changing taste experience.

The therapist should remember that smell strongly influences taste. Some children interpret flavor information more strongly with a stronger sense of smell. Others have chronic congestion or are mouth breathers with less olfactory influence on flavor. To prepare for a new taste, the therapist should let the child smell the food. Having time to smell the food can begin to prepare the child for the flavor that follows. Conversely, for a very smell-sensitive child, the therapist may need to provide the taste, such as a new juice, in a lidded cup with a straw, to reduce the smell and an immediate rejection based on smell alone, before it is tasted.

Temperature

On the temperature continuum, foods can be hot or cold and many different degrees in between. Children will let adults know if they need hot or cold, warm or room-temperature foods. Some children do not care about the temperature variations while others notice the smallest change. The therapist should notice food temperature and its influence on the child.

Texture

The texture continuum is more complicated because of the variations available. For people who enjoy foods, the variations in texture add to the pleasure of tasting and eating. For those who have difficulty with textures or experience oral defensiveness, the many texture variations can be a source of discomfort and stress.

There are many ways to describe variations in food texture. Thinking of descriptors leads one to realize that most foods are a combination of these texture words. Foods can be described as liquid or solid, hard or soft, thin or thick, smooth or rough, wet or dry, lumpy or smooth, even or uneven, pointed or round, or scattered or stuck together. Some foods are very smooth while others are thin like a liquid. Some are scattered and dry while others are scattered and wet. Some have hard lumps, while others have soft lumps. The contrasts and combinations are infinite. To be comfortable and skillful with eating, people need a system that can adjust to all variables. When therapists are responsible for offering children food, it is important that they begin to look at food textures carefully and offer foods that provide thoughtful, slow, and graded change in each characteristic.

Just as there are flavor variations from dilute to concentrate and temperature changes by degree, texture changes in tiny increments along a continuum. Liquids can be thin to thick. Purees can be smooth to lumpy. Hard foods can be crumbs to solids. Pieces can be small to large. Shapes can be round to sharp. Scatter-foods can be stuck together with a binder or drier and more separate. For every variable in food consistency, there can be an incremental grading of the texture.

Some children make these texture transitions easily with curiosity and enthusiasm. Sensitive children, however, may need to make these transitions slowly, cautiously and in tiny increments, inching along this continuum.

Sensory Preparation for Transition to the Next Activity

Just as therapists need to prepare children to move into the mealtime environment, they may need to prepare them to move on to the next activity after a meal. A child who becomes deeply relaxed during the meal may need an alerting activity before going back to the classroom. The child may need to march from the cafeteria to the classroom or bounce on the parent's lap before going off to play. If the meal has created tension or stress, or if the child has gastrointestinal difficulties, something that supports generalized relaxation would be appropriate before the next activity. Such a child may need a bit of rocking or an extended hug before leaving the mealtime environment.

Helping Children Handle the New Sensory Challenges of Mealtimes

The following general strategies have been found to be helpful when guiding the sensory-sensitive child to explore and enjoy mealtime sensations.

Listen to Children

Children will let adults know what they like and don't like, what is working and not working. They will set the pace of the meal and show the feeder their sensory needs.

Prepare for the Meal

The child and the feeder need to be prepared for the meal. The therapist must prepare the environment, the child's whole body and face, and the feeder. He also should prepare the food and the sensory experiences most likely to be successful for the mealtime.

Preferences are Personal

Sensory interpretations are personal, and these personal preferences can change within the day, with developmental stages, and with experience. Just because a child enjoyed a certain taste, texture, or temperature yesterday, does not guarantee that he will enjoy it today. Just because the therapist likes the flavor, does not mean the child likes it!

Seek Foods Most Likely to Elicit Favorable Responses

For mealtime to be nourishing to the whole child, it must be pleasurable. When possible, the therapist should allow the child to help choose foods that work for her. When the child has oversensitivities, the therapist should be sure to pick foods along the sensory continuum with tiny changes in sensation. He should watch for the child's responses and adapt the presentation accordingly. For other less sensitive children, the favorable response is more likely with stronger, wake-up flavors.

Get Permission

The clinician should remember that children usually do best when they are in charge of what goes into their mouth. It is a good idea to wait for the child to open her mouth or lean forward to grant this permission. The therapist also can give the child a sense of control by allowing the child to hold the spoon or therapist's hand as the food is presented.

Start With the Familiar

For sensitive children, the therapist can start with familiar foods and expand from there. Routine helps with acceptance of new sensations. The therapist also should consider using a familiar place mat, plate, cup, and fork. A positive way to approach each meal is to begin with a food the child enjoys. Trying gradually to make taste, texture, or temperature changes is wise. For example, the therapist might prepare a bowl of pureed food that the child enjoys. She can thicken some of the food and add increased texture, crumbs, or lumps to part of it. The therapist should start with the familiar and gradually add a bit more of the new texture. If the child likes it, the therapist can try again; if not, she can go back to the puree texture and try less of the new texture for the next spoonful. The therapist should proceed cautiously and slowly.

One Thing at a Time

Overly sensitive children can be so tightly wired that they respond quickly and emotionally to changes. Whereas one child may spit out an unpleasant food or wipe his mouth, an overly sensitive child may gag or vomit. That quick reaction is right there near the surface. Such a child needs to trust that the therapist will do her best to provide gradual changes with only one variable at a time. Changing the texture or a couple of the textures, the taste, and the temperature all at once could much more easily push the child to the point of overload and hyperactive response.

Mouthing Helps

New food tastes and textures do not need to be given on the old familiar spoon. The therapist can try to help the child prepare his mouth before introducing the new sensory mealtime experience. The child can put favorite mouthing toys, fingers, toes, and vibrators into the mouth. Each could be coated with food flavors or textures. By providing the child with the opportunity to put these items in the mouth, get used to them, and enjoy them *before* the introduction of the food, the therapist is helping the child relax and get used to a mouthing sensation to ready himself for the food. When the child then brings the mouthing toy to the mouth with food, he is more ready.

Be Aware of Sensory Surprises

The feeder can help a meal be more predictable. A sensory surprise can end the meal quickly! Children should be prepared for changes that are to be presented. The parent can talk about the food, show it to the child, and let her explore it. The child's nose and the lips can check out the food before it even touches the tongue. Sensory change can be small so as not to elicit a large response.

One way to predictably prepare for a new flavor or texture is by pairing the presentation with a song or a movement experience. The therapist should consider singing a song with the child tapping her body for emphasis throughout. The therapist also could try tapping the wrist, forearm, upper arm, shoulder, chin, and mouth. When the touch rhythmically and predictably gets to the face and mouth area, the child usually is more prepared. With the rhythmic presentation, the child knows the touch is coming and can prepare for its sensory components. She also knows when the approaching touch will end and can plan accordingly. The swing also can be used to present predictable touches. The therapist can try having the child swing on a swing. Each time the child swings toward the therapist, he can touch the child's head, face, or mouth, if the child allows. The child then knows the touch is coming and that as the swing moves away, the touch will end. Of course, permission should be given for the touch.

Environmental Sensory Variable Analysis

Mealtime Environment _____ Date _____

Sensory System	Alerting Variables	Calming Variables	Adjustments Needed
Vestibular			
Proprioceptive			
Touch			
Taste			
Smell			
Vision			
Hearing			

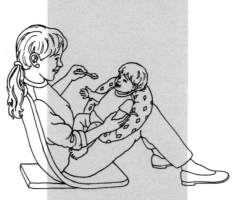

Chapter 15

Positioning and Handling Influences on the Mealtime

Handling and Movement

Although the focus of this book is on the role of positioning and handling at mealtimes, the impact of postural tone and movement impacts every aspect of the child's life. Children with difficulties in motor control and coordination require specific treatment programs to help them develop overall sensorimotor control. A discussion of different programs and specific guidelines for helping children develop this coordination clearly goes beyond the scope of this book. Treatment approaches and systems change over the years as knowledge and understanding of movement and motor control grows. Some approaches to physical development and movement are clearly in harmony with the overall philosophy of working with children expressed in this book (Bly, 1999; Bly & Whiteside, 1997; Boehme, 1988; Finnie, Bavin, Bax, Browne, & Gardiner, 1997; Rywerant & Feldenkrais, 1991; Shafarman, 1997). Others impose uncomfortable manipulations on children and do not allow them to become active co-creators of the physical therapy program. In providing an overall approach to the physical and emotional development of children's mealtime and eating skills, movement programs should meet the following general criteria.

A compatible program for handling and movement skill development:

- listens to children and does not impose an adult agenda on a protesting child
- takes the child's interests and current abilities into consideration and helps children do what ***they*** want to do
- focuses on the tone and movement patterns that underlie function while simultaneously helping children obtain better function in daily life
- builds children's awareness of how they move and might move in different ways
- helps children learn to move efficiently and without effort
- focuses on the quality of movement as well as the child's developmental skills

Considerations for Positioning at Mealtimes

Mealtimes are for nurturing the body and emotions. In selecting the positions for feeding an infant and eating with an older child, the therapist or caregiver needs to consider both of these very important aspects of the meal. A position chosen solely for the ease of food intake may not help nurture the

---

valuable social and emotional aspects of mealtime communications. A position chosen purely for social interaction may not facilitate the physical and physiological needs of the child. A position chosen for the child may not address the needs of the feeder, and a position chosen for the feeder may not facilitate the needs of the child. Therapists must look at the big picture. Positioning must consider the feeding relationship and mealtime communication. It must support the socialization that comes from inclusion in the family mealtime; the child's developmental feeding skills; and the gastrointestinal, respiratory, and neurological needs of the child. It must reflect the child's physical safety and needs for postural support, as well as the feeder's physical and comfort needs. Each child has a unique combination of influences that need to be considered in developing the optimum seating position for feeding.

Mealtime Communication

Any position chosen for feeding a child must take into consideration the communication give-and-take that occurs at the mealtime. Children need to be positioned so they can let their feeders know what they need. They need to let their feeders know when they are ready for the nipple or a spoonful, what food they prefer next, whether they want food presented more slowly or rapidly, and what they want next. They communicate when they are full and when the meal should end. The feeders need to listen to those cues and proceed accordingly.

The feeding relationship is built on this reciprocal communication and trust. In order to develop the trust and nurturing bond that grows into a feeding relationship, the baby must feel secure and comfortable during feedings. The mother's arms naturally are the first feeding support position for babies. The bodies of the infant and mother have been designed to fit together in such a way as to provide the position, support, and comfort for ideal infant feeding. The mother's body supports the infant's body and head securely as the baby becomes more skilled with sucking and swallowing. The body-to-body contact provides a closeness and warmth that sends messages of love and caring. The position allows for direct eye-to-eye contact for that "I love you!" look. As the baby grows older, the position allows for smiles and social pauses that further deepen that mother-infant bond. The position provides an easy way for the baby to reach for and hold the bottle or breast, enabling the infant gradually to take a more active role in the mealtime process.

To encourage mealtime communication and interaction, the child and feeder need to be in positions that support interaction with each other and the meal. Children communicate by many methods. Positioning needs to reflect those methods. Children use body language and eye contact, facial expression, sounds, words, pointing, or some other adaptive communication method. If pointing to pictures, symbols, or words is used, the angle of the chair seat and any chair modifications should enable the child to use weight bearing on the elbows or forearms. The child needs to be able to send these messages, and the feeder needs to be able to read and respond.

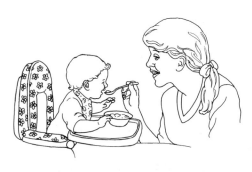

To optimize positioning and seating, the therapist must observe the interactional aspects of positioning. Does the position chosen support a positive feeding relationship? Does it maximize the opportunities for interacting and communicating? What must the child and feeder do to see each other's faces? Is the child given control over choices in the mealtime process? Are there possibilities for the child to make those choices? Are those choices understood and honored? What options does the child have to indicate discomfort or desire for a change in position or activity?

Mealtime Socialization

Socialization is an important aspect of mealtime that must be considered when positioning and seating is determined. From early infancy, babies take pauses in feeding to socialize with their mothers or fathers. These smiles, coos, facial expressions, and pauses enable babies not only to pace the meal, but also to socialize as they and their parent "fall in love." As children gain more skills and communication strategies, the socialization expands. The child who is included at the family mealtime learns the give-and-take of family communication and many of the refined social aspects of the meal through incidental and direct learning. The child may learn which end of the fork to use, and the importance of replacing the cup on the tray after drinking. Cultural guidelines such as the use of a napkin, how to serve food, chewing with the mouth closed, and not talking with the mouth full are some of the mealtime manners that are learned by participating in regular meals with the family.

To optimize socialization opportunities, care must be taken in choosing positions and seating for children. Socialization requires communication and interaction. Is every effort made to support the social aspects of the meal in addition to the nutritional aspects? Is the child included at the family mealtime? Are there other people present during the child's meal? Children with feeding problems often have been excluded from the family mealtime in an effort to make it easier for the child and family. Yet the therapist must remember that the social aspects of the meal are important and that eating in isolation does not allow the child the learning and socialization provided by participation in a family mealtime. Some children, for example, are tube-fed and are not able to orally eat the food the family eats. These children, however, can be given their bolus feeding while in a high chair at the table with the rest of the family. Children who receive slow-drip tube feedings at night can still sit with the family and engage in the discussions and socialization of the meal although they receive no tube feedings or oral feedings during the day. Mealtimes provide the unique experiences of food smells, sounds, routines, and socialization.

Developmental Feeding Skills

Mealtime positions and seating options must support the child's changing developmental needs. Babies initially are very dependent on their feeders as they take breast-feedings or bottle-feedings. Gradually, they learn to sit and show interest in pureed foods, finger foods, and solid foods. Babies move from the feeders' arms to other seating options. Infant seats provide support as babies try out pureed foods. These seats support the whole body so that the baby needs to focus only on the changing sensations and experiences of the mouth. As foods become more of a challenge, babies also begin to experiment with autonomy. Finger foods, high chairs, and independence seem to go together. The high chair provides the support young children need as they begin to explore solid foods as well as the containment that both children and parents need for their overall comfort. This seating option allows the child mastery opportunities for food exploration and self-feeding. The high chair tray is necessary initially for extra trunk support and stability as the infant tries to manage new foods and learns to lean into the spoon as it approaches the mouth. The tray gives the extra trunk stability needed as a solid foundation for the fine motor skills of eating. The tray provides a place for forearms and elbows to lean in early self-feeding attempts. Gradually, as trunk control and balance skills improve, the tray becomes a playground of exploration and refinement of self-feeding skills.

As the child develops independence with spoons, forks, cups, and straws, there is usually a move toward the table for eating with the rest of the family. At this point, the child has many options including booster seats, regular chairs, picnic table benches, and sitting on the floor. The more sensorimotor control that children have in their bodies, the more choices they have for seating positions at mealtimes.

It is important that seating options change with the child's changing developmental needs. Continuing to feed a child in an infant seat, for example, when he is interested in sitting up and finger-feeding, can frustrate the child and the feeder, as well as delay the mastery of the finger-feeding skill. Feeding a child who has poor trunk control in an unsupported upright position may make it difficult or impossible for her to develop a refined chewing pattern or self-feeding.

Feeding Methods

Children are fed using different feeding methods, depending on their developmental stage and medical needs. Infants are breast- or bottle-fed, requiring different positioning considerations. Older babies are spoon-fed and introduced to more complex foods for finger-feeding. Gradually, the feeding method moves from being fed by another person to independent feeding. Success with self-feeding may require a backward chaining method that requires the adult to sit next to or behind the child as the hand and spoon are brought to the mouth and the food is removed. Many medically fragile children are tube-fed. The tube feeding can be by bolus or continuous drip. It can be dependent on the adult or rely on a pump that the child wears in a backpack. Some children are fed by parenteral nutrition where nutrition bypasses the alimentary canal and enters the circulatory system directly. These total parenteral nutrition (TPN) feedings are given by peripheral intravenous lines or central lines. There would be unique positioning considerations with TPN feedings.

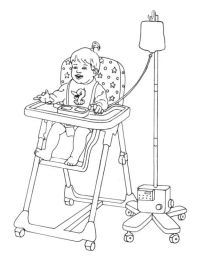

Oral Motor Skills

Children learn the skills of eating through experience with liquids and foods. When all goes well, they suck, swallow, then bite, and chew. They suck from a breast or bottle, then drink from a cup or straw. Many children who have feeding issues get stuck somewhere along this sequence and need additional help to learn specific oral motor skills. They may need extra support at the cheeks in nippling or special support at the jaw for cup drinking. They may need help with lip closure during adaptive straw drinking. When specific therapeutic support is necessary for oral motor skill development, it influences the positions of the child and the feeder. The feeding therapist needs to find the positioning relationship that is easiest and most efficient for the adult and the child.

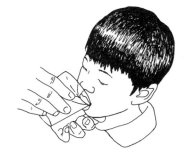

Gastrointestinal, Oral-Facial, Respiratory, and Neurological Positioning Needs

Gastrointestinal, oral-facial, respiratory and neurological conditions influence the feedings of many children. These issues must be considered when feeding positions and seating options are considered.

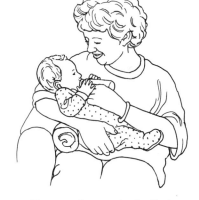

Gastrointestinal issues, such as gastroesophageal reflux (GER) or esophageal motility disorders, require positioning considerations during and after feeding. The infant who has GER may need to be positioned more upright during feeding to decrease the tendency for upward flow of gastric contents. The semi-reclined feeding position used more typically to feed infants may make reflux worse. The typical trunk flexion bend of many older children seems to aggravate the GER. Many parents use a pillow or towel roll with bottle-feeding to straighten the back in an attempt to reduce reflux episodes. Some babies with severe GER who are tube-fed may need to be placed on the tummy or lying on the right side for the fewest reflux symptoms. Many children with esophageal motility disorders need to be fed upright to allow the maximum help from gravity.

The therapist also must consider sensitive gastrointestinal systems when contemplating straps and seat belts. The therapist should notice where the straps are resting on the child and be sure that the lower esophageal sphincter area is avoided, as it may negatively influence reflux. Sometimes there

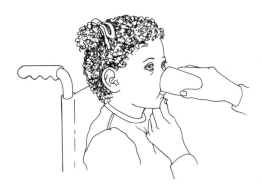

can be so many straps that the stomach is unintentionally compressed. This can influence the child's comfort and appetite. Seat belts or shoulder straps, if necessary, can be used in combinations that avoid pressure on the stomach. There usually are creative ways to provide the supportive guidance of seat belts without creating a negative impact on the gastrointestinal system.

Oral facial anomalies also are affected by the feeding position. Babies who have cleft palates, for example, seem to eat best in a more upright position. This seems to reduce the amount of upward flow of food and liquid through the open palate and into the nasopharynx. As a result, this upright positioning reduces the chronic ear infections that these children develop when they continually are seated in a more reclining position.

The respiratory system should be considered in positioning and seating choices. Many children have chronic respiratory conditions that have led to an elevated rib cage, tightening of the intercostal muscles between the ribs, diaphragmatic or belly breathing instead of thoracic breathing, and generally more shallow breathing patterns. Positions and straps that apply pressure to the chest may interfere with depth of excursions for breathing. Too much pressure on the abdomen may make breathing much more difficult for children who use primarily a diaphragmatic movement pattern.

The position in which the child's head rests will influence swallowing and breathing. Though most children seem to eat better in a tucked chin position, some actually have increased breathing difficulties in this position. Head positioning for feeding should be considered on an individual basis for each child. It is very important to understand each child's respiratory needs before changing head position.

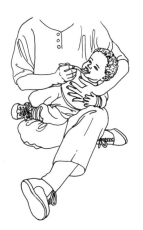

Neurologically involved children often have significant physical challenges that influence feeding. Their physical position is strongly influenced by primary and compensatory changes in muscle tone throughout the body. These variations in tone and movement influence their ability to relax and obtain the appropriate foundational support and stability for feeding. Additionally, some neurologically involved children have seizure disorders. The seizures may lead to choking during a meal. Seizure activity may require a change of position during feeding. Seating options should allow for easy removal of the child from the chair if it becomes necessary during a mealtime. Too many belts and straps may make this very difficult.

■ Physical Needs and Seating Choices

The Child's Individual Needs

A child's efficient use of the mouth for eating depends heavily on the steadiness or stability of the trunk, neck, and head. This stability is provided by the support surface of a lap, infant seat, or seating system. Many children with neurological or postural difficulties are not able to independently assume or maintain good positions for optimum eating. Their muscle tone, postural asymmetries, and overall motor control may not provide the foundational support and stability needed for the refined motor skills of sucking, swallowing, chewing, or self-feeding. The therapist may need to consider supportive or adaptive seating (Trefler, 1993).

To determine the optimum physical components of a seating system for a child with special physical challenges, the therapist needs to understand every aspect of the child's postural control system. He must observe and determine the child's postural strengths and needs, looking at the specific aspects of the child's posture. In what position is the trunk? How are the shoulders held? What type of head control does the child have? What type of foundational support do the hips provide?

Before changing a child's feeding position, the therapist must look at the general or global aspects of the child's posture. Does the child have excess movements or minimal movements? Does the child tend to slouch forward in flexion or extend the whole body into extension? The therapist needs to remember that each part of the body influences other parts and that one aspect of posture cannot be changed without influencing the total posture.

Following are the various aspects of posture that can influence the decision for specific seating recommendations during therapy and at mealtime, and some seating options that can meet children's needs. First is a look at body alignment and its influences on eating.

Observing Body Alignment

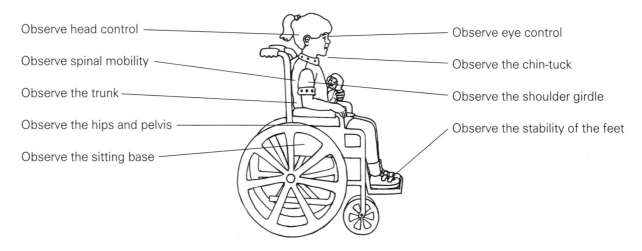

Observe head control

Observe spinal mobility

Observe the trunk

Observe the hips and pelvis

Observe the sitting base

Observe eye control

Observe the chin-tuck

Observe the shoulder girdle

Observe the stability of the feet

How Do All of These Components Interact?

Hips and Pelvis

It has been said that control at the top begins at the bottom. In order to look at the skills of the head and mouth for feeding, the therapist must begin by looking at the way the hips and pelvis are positioned. They provide the base foundation of support in the chair—a foundation upon which the trunk, shoulder, and head provide further support for the mouth and eating. Anterior or posterior tilting of the pelvis in sitting or standing can influence head control, breathing, voicing, and mouth control. This occurs through action on the spine and the child's attempt to compensate for the imposed spinal curve or position. Full extensor spasms of the spine often begin with thrusting back of the pelvis. This creates major problems in the shoulders, head, and mouth while the child is sitting.

The position of the child's pelvis should be viewed in a variety of different seating options. Would a rolled towel or foam under the knees increase the posterior pelvic tilt? Would a roll or wedge of foam in the lumbar spine area facilitate a better anterior pelvic tilt? Seat depth, width, and the angle created by the chair seat and back influence the type of pelvic tilt that the child experiences.

Sitting Base

Observe the sitting base. After observing the width of the child's support base and how he uses it, you must determine whether it provides a stable base for the oral and fine motor control needed for eating. If the sitting base is narrow, the child will need a greater amount of trunk control. Children who lack adequate trunk control will have greater problems if their legs are adducted (brought closely together) when sitting on the floor or in a chair. Using an abduction wedge or pommel to separate the legs can widen the sitting base, enabling the child to use a more limited amount of trunk control while eating. Sometimes the sitting base is too wide. If a narrower sitting base is needed, or if the thighs turn or pull outward in a frog-legged position, you can use hip adductor cushions to bring the knees closer together.

Feet

Observe the feet. Are they resting on the floor or on a stable surface? Do they support the legs and provide a foundation for the stability and balance needed for good oral motor skills? The feet can serve as anchors that enable the legs to be still during feeding. Dangling feet in a chair that is too high can work against your best efforts to provide the child with stability in the hips, pelvis, trunk, and head. Lowering the chair so that the feet touch the floor or providing adequate footrests can make a significant difference when improved balance and stability is the goal. Remember, however, that every child is an individual. For some children, foot support may serve as a trigger for pushing into extension of the body. In this case, it may be more effective to remove foot support instead of add it.

Trunk

Observe the trunk by feeling it. What is its tone? Does it provide stability for other parts of the body? Is there symmetry or does the trunk pull down more on one side? Problems with the trunk can lead to compensations and tension in other parts of the body. Poor trunk control leads to poor head control because the neck needs a stable foundation for precise control.

Consider seating options that provide adequate trunk supports. These may need to be bilateral or unilateral supports. The side supports work best for some children when they are lower and near the hips; others may need supports in the mid-chest region. Be sure that the child's feet have a firm basis of support.

Shoulder Girdle

Observe the shoulder girdle. If the scapulae are adducted, the shoulders will pull back into a retracted position. This retraction causes a tension that often pulls the neck into hyperextension and influences the pattern of lip, tongue, and jaw retraction. If there is scapular adduction, the child will have difficulty getting the hands to the mouth, putting the hands together, and reaching for a spoon or finger food.

The shoulders also can be held with too much forward rounding or protraction. This position influences the position of the neck and changes oral motor patterns. Think of the shoulders as the base or floor upon which the neck and head sit. If a balance does not occur, with the shoulders providing a stable base for the head and neck, it is impossible for the child to develop the graded fine motor control required for oral motor skills.

Once you have determined the child's typical shoulder posture, you can make the necessary alterations in seating arrangements. Too much shoulder retraction may require a softer chair (such as a beanbag chair), the placement of softer material (such as foam or soft towel rolls) behind the shoulders, or more firm backing (such as a corner chair or a molded seating system). Too much shoulder protraction can be reduced by using a vest attached to the chair or placing a roll of foam or towels on the table for the child to lean on. If the roll is high enough, the child can lean forward from the pelvis, using the roll under the arms. When working to improve the position of the shoulder girdle, it is essential to make the initial changes in the pelvis. Once pelvic alignment is appropriate and the child is sitting with equal weight on both sides of the buttocks, the therapist can consider some shoulder supports. Sometimes the only shoulder support needed is the tray or tabletop. Leaning forearms or elbows on the surface can provide extra trunk and shoulder stability.

Relationship of the Head and Spine

Observe the relationship of head control and spinal mobility. Head control is mediated through the entire spine. An active, flexible spine enables the entire vertebral column to do the work of head control. When the spine is rigid or fails to respond as a coordinated unit, the neck must support the head independently. The muscles of the cervical spine are not strong, and they fatigue easily when they must take full responsibility for maintaining the head in an upright position. When a child is positioned or strapped into a chair or corset so tightly that spinal movement is impossible, the full spine cannot assist in head control. If such positioning is necessary to provide trunk control in school or for transportation, therapy should include activities that will develop mobility and control through the entire spine.

The position of the head must be observed in relationship to the hips, pelvis, trunk, and shoulder girdle. Often, changes in these key areas enable the head to assume a more normal posture without special head-control changes in the seating system. A variety of headrests are available to help the child maintain a more normal head and neck posture. These cannot be considered in isolation from the rest of the child's chair. The angle formed by the chair back and seat influence head position. The more upright the child is sitting in the chair, the more the head and neck need to work. When control is poor, the effort required to remain upright often elicits a dysfunctional head position. A slightly reclining position in the seating system can give the child better support and reduce the amount of effort involved. Many chairs have a "tilt-in-space" feature that allows for variable levels of reclining (tilting backward) of the entire chair. This provides a great deal of flexibility for children whose need for support varies throughout the day.

Abdominal-Pelvic Girdle

Observe and feel the abdominal muscles. The abdominal wall is composed of a series of muscle groups whose fibers run vertically, horizontally, and diagonally. These muscles connect to the ribcage, pelvis, and spine. Together they create an abdominal-pelvic girdle below the ribcage in the same way that we have a shoulder girdle at the top of the ribcage. The abdominal muscle system provides a major contribution to developing trunk control. As control of the abdominal muscles emerges at 5 to 6 months of age, babies include lateral trunk movements and the diagonal movements needed for rotation in sitting and rolling. Activating these muscles creates a retaining wall to support the abdominal contents. This reduces the stress on the infant's lower esophageal sphincter and can decrease the number of reflux episodes. The abdominal muscles also hold down the lower border of the rib cage, enabling greater activity of the intercostal muscles and deeper chest breathing. Controlled activation of the abdominal muscles is required for vocalization that is loud and sustained. Activation of the abdominal muscles is paired with a coordinated relaxation of the muscles of the lower back and pelvis. It is this balance of flexor activation and extensor relaxation that provides an increasing amount of graded control for refined movement and vocalization. The treatment program should include activities to activate and coordinate the abdominal-pelvic girdle. The muscles may be stimulated by touch or pressure and by slow movement in all directions.

It is difficult to change tone in this part of the body during static positioning in a chair. Building more appropriate muscle tone and control of the abdominal muscles should be a part of the overall treatment program. Preparation of abdominal control before a meal can assist the child with trunk control as well as improve breathing and postural adjustments during mealtime. Careful positioning that does not intrude on abdominal control or function is necessary, however.

Freedom of Movement

Observe the child's ability to move around the body axis. Freedom of movement implies the ability to combine and integrate both flexor and extensor components of movement. This ability enables smoothly graded movement with small steps and transitions. In a static piece of equipment, it is difficult to create a seating option for feeding that allows a great deal of freedom of spinal movement or changes in movement around the body axis. These needs must be facilitated dynamically during therapy sessions. Feeding activities that focus on rotation can be incorporated into therapy sessions. During mealtime, give the child as much support as needed to create a stable base for eating, but not so much that movement adjustments that are possible cannot occur. A seating system must be modified constantly to acknowledge the child's changing needs and abilities.

Vision

Observe eye-control skills. Can the child maintain focused eye contact with an object or face? How easily does the child change focus or communicate visually? How quickly or slowly can the child track movement? Can the child track in all directions? In which quadrants does the child use vision most functionally? Problems with eye-movement control and limitations in the visual field can influence how children hold their heads. Tilting the head into extension or to one side may be the child's way of compensating for inadequate focus, field of vision, or movement of the eyes in one or more directions.

Functional vision should be considered when seating systems are designed. The head control supports should not interfere with usable vision. The placement and size of trays will be influenced by the optimum visual field of the child. Tracking and focusing activities can be incorporated into mealtimes by carefully considering where a feeder sits and how the meal is presented.

Compensating Patterns of Movement

Observe original tone, primary movement patterns, and compensatory patterns. The movement behavior that therapists see in neurologically involved older infants or children usually is a mixture of the original pattern imposed by the brain damage and the child's response to that pattern. It is never successful to take away a compensation without providing a better movement or control pattern.

Any modification to the child's seating system for feeding should be directed at the underlying or basic issues or problems. When creating chair modifications, therapists tend to provide a strap or restraint for every deviant or limiting movement pattern the child produces. This is not necessary when the original, primary patterns are identified and worked with in treatment. Modifications to a seating system that focus primarily on these patterns will have far-reaching effects. Older children and those with severe physical limitations may develop muscle contractures and deformities of the bones. These also must be considered in creating an effective positioning system for feeding.

The key points of physical positioning have been discussed individually to help therapists analyze the process of looking at postural tone and movement. However, the child must be observed as a whole child, not as a collection of shoulders, pelvic tilts, and trunk control. No position changes occur in isolation. Positioning changes made in one part of the body will affect all other parts of the body.

As therapists look at the hips and pelvis, sitting base, feet, trunk, shoulders, head and neck control, spine, and abdomen, as well as their foundational stability, freedom of movement and compensatory patterns, they have information to begin to make changes in positions and seating for feeding. Any changes that are made, however, must be done slowly and carefully. Therapists must remember to move children gradually, and without force, into new feeding positions. Each child learns to accept food in a particular posture that feels normal. It is part of the child's mind-set and body-set associated with eating and having hunger needs met. When adults make changes too quickly, the child doesn't know what to expect, and the sensory feedback is one of abnormality. Although a therapist may see a child's typical feeding position as quite limited, this is the child's normal frame of reference. Changes from that position initially feel very strange and limiting to children, and they often will attempt to move back to the "normal" pattern with which they are familiar. If a therapist gradually changes the accustomed position, the feeder and the child will experience more success and less stress.

Recording Information

During or following the observation of the child's body alignment at mealtime, the therapist can record the information on the Body Alignment for Seating and Positioning Checklist on pages 309–310.

Comfort

A mechanically correct seating system can be designed for a child. On paper it looks wonderful. In theory it makes sense. However, the child may act extremely uncomfortable in it. Perhaps she arches and pulls away from the chair. Perhaps she has greatly increased tension. This may be because too many positional changes were imposed at once. However, it may be because the chair is not right for this child. The seating position may be appropriate for the trunk, but stressful on the respiratory system. It may provide a stable base for the hips and pelvis but have a negative impact on the digestive system. Think back to the feeding position of the baby in the mother's arms. Not only was that position *right*, but it also was comfortable, safe, and secure. It allowed for intimate mother-infant interaction. Building toward the total comfort of the child is the bottom-line consideration in developing the details of any seating system.

Straps and Belts

Therapists and professionals who fit seating systems often have a tendency to strap, belt, and cushion a child into a chair so that the body alignment looks perfect. Before you know it, there is a head strap, a chest strap, lateral trunk cushions, a seat belt, thigh straps, and foot straps. Imagine you are the child in that chair. Would you want to eat? The child may *look* perfect but lose her appetite! The therapist must consider the feeding situation. Does the child need all of the straps? Perhaps this level of support is necessary to satisfy the need for physical safety when riding the school bus; however, it may be totally inappropriate for mealtimes. Would it be possible to keep the seat belt, but relax the chest straps? If the chair were reclined slightly, could the head straps be removed? The therapist should look at each strap and belt creatively to see if any can be removed safely while still supporting the child's posture as a proper foundation for feeding.

Safety

All decisions about seating for meals must consider the child's safety. From the seat belt in the high chair to the headrest in the adapted wheelchair, safety must come first. Feeding sometimes brings a risk of choking and aspirating. Be sure there is an easy and quick option for removing the child from a chair, should a choking episode occur.

Feeder's Position

The therapist should observe how different feeders use their bodies. The therapist, educator, and parent should become aware of their use of movement. They should explore various possibilities for creating their personal comfort when feeding the child. Feeder tension or lack of comfort influences the child's eating and drinking skills. Well-meaning feeders can easily become tense during the feeding process without even realizing it.

Many severely involved children continue to be on-lap feeders into the preschool years. Feeding these children often is easier on the lap; although extended use of this position can take its toll on the adult body. The strength of the child's pushing from extensor tone or the amount of total support needed for the child with low tone can make holding him difficult. A lengthy mealtime may make any position uncomfortable without proper supports.

When efforts are made to carefully support the adult posture during feeding, mealtimes can be presented comfortably for the adult and the child. Efficient, gentle, and rhythmical movement from the adult can increase the likelihood of easy movement from the child. Where holding the child is effortful or tense, the child receives the message that the activity is difficult and that effort is appropriate. Adults who are physically uncomfortable tend to rush through the meal. This gives the child the sense that the adult, not the child, is in control. Rushing may not allow the child sufficient time to take in sufficient calories. Problems with growth can then develop.

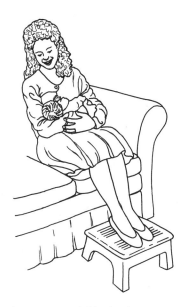

The first step in making any change in the physical position of the feeder is to help the adult develop an awareness of feedback from his body. The therapist should notice when the position is awkward and change it before it becomes a chronic problem. The feeder's chair should be at a height that enables the adult to help the child without reaching and straining the arms, neck, shoulders, and back. A variety of straight-backed chairs, stools, and benches are available for home or school. Many office chairs have a hydraulic feature that makes it easy to make small adjustments in the height of the chair. Therapists can explore these systematically to discover the most comfortable seating arrangement for the feeder. Feet should be flat on the floor or on a stool with an angled surface. This can be done by using a chair of a lower height or using a footrest. A small box or stool under the feeder's feet can create different lap angles when the child is held. The back should be supported. This can be done by picking the right high-backed chair or by leaning against a wall. Pillows or similar supports may increase the adult's comfort. A simple chair made from a tubular frame with a firm, foam cushion and canvas back (e.g., the BackJack™ chair) can provide excellent support when the adult is sitting on the floor.

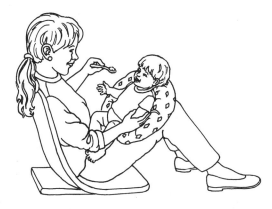

When the adult uses her arms to hold the child, she may need an arm rest or pillow support. The arm end of a couch or comfortable chair may be all that is necessary. Some people prefer the arm supports of an office chair. This can have the added advantage of height adjustability. When armrests are used, each feeder needs to explore the comfortable height for the adult and the child.

Some feeders feel as if they need one more hand! They can creatively position the child with physical support, which takes the place of the extra hand. A pillow may give extra support to the child's back, and a crescent pillow may give extra support to the head and neck.

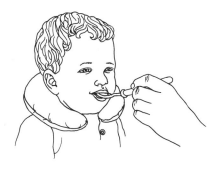

If the child is in a larger adapted chair, the feeder should sit as close to the child as possible to avoid awkward forward or sideways leaning during the presentation of the meal.

Recording Information

During or following the observation of the child's seating arrangements at mealtime, the therapist can record the information. This can provide a valuable resource for planning changes that will support the mealtime. Use the form, Seating and Positioning Considerations for Mealtime Support, on page 307.

Active Therapy, Positioning for Meals and Equipment

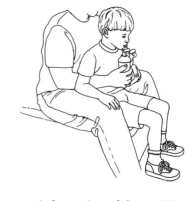

Equipment should be used to maintain a movement pattern or posture with which the child is familiar and comfortable. It should not be used to create or achieve a new movement pattern. Thus, the child should be prepared for sitting in a specific chair through therapeutic handling during treatment sessions and before a meal. If the seating position or equipment is new, the child may spend the meal focusing on the new sensory information of the position rather than the meal. With preparation and an interactive approach to learning, the child can learn to work with a chair as a supportive and guiding friend, rather than fight it as a restraining enemy.

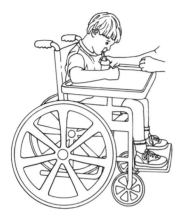

Therapeutic facilitation can prepare a child before a meal, and it can help optimize tone and functioning after a meal. It should become a focus of regular direct therapy to maximize the child's function. Static seating systems may be necessary at meals. Daily life for most children is active. Between meals, the use of special seating systems should be monitored, giving the child as much time and experience with active movement as possible.

Helping Children Handle the Physical Challenges of Mealtimes

The following general strategies are helpful when guiding the child with physical challenges in participating comfortably in the mealtime.

Listen to Children

Children will let therapists know what they like and don't like, what is working and what is not. They will set the pace of the meal and show their physical needs. They will let therapists know when change is too great or they are not comfortable.

Prepare for the Meal

The child and the feeder need to be prepared physically for the meal. The therapist should work with ideas from the child's overall movement therapy program to obtain more normal postural tone and postural stability before positioning the child on the lap or in a chair for the meal. If the therapist is working on specific feeding and oral motor skills in a therapy session, he should begin the session with movement activities that prepare the rest of the body first.

Direct Treatment at Primary Patterns, Not Compensatory Patterns

As the therapist observes the child's responses during handling and positioning, she should distinguish between primary and compensatory patterns of tone and movement. Children develop compensatory patterns as their best way of dealing with the limitations created by the primary patterns. The therapist should always direct treatment at reducing the impact of the primary patterns. This enables children to let go of compensatory patterns they no longer need. Children will not release compensatory patterns that they still need to function. Children who push the head into hyperextension when the therapist offers the spoon may do this for many reasons. They may do this as part of a total extension pattern of the body that is triggered by sensory input. But they also may use the same pattern because they are trying to communicate that they want to stop eating. Look for the underlying reasons and patterns.

Help Children and Adults Develop Body Awareness

Children and adults generally move habitually with very little awareness of tone and movement in their bodies. The way they move feels normal, and they will always come back to what feels familiar—even if they have been introduced to an easier or more functional way of moving. The therapist's goal is to help them develop a different frame of reference to which they can return. They need to know what it feels like to be tight or stiff and to be soft and easy. They need to understand from feedback when they are using excessive effort to move and do what they want to do.

There is Always More Than One Way

Therapists should introduce children and parents to the concept that there is always more than one way to do something. We tend to become stuck in what we know or the way we have always done something. When we are introduced to change as a variation of something we already know, it is easier to make the change. Think of therapy as having a series of central themes and hundreds and thousands of variations on each theme. This creates mental and physical flexibility in the nervous system.

Introduce Very Small Changes

The therapist should introduce very small changes in the child's position on her lap or in a chair. She should not try to do everything at once. The body often can integrate changes when they are small, yet reject these same changes if they are too great. For example, if a child typically eats with the head back in hyperextension, the therapist should not immediately move to a forward chin-tuck position. She should explore the gradations of extension that are slightly more forward and gradually move toward the most optimum position.

Start at the Bottom

Physical control begins with the hips, pelvis, legs, and feet. These provide a solid foundation for building control in the rest of the body. Even if the therapist is most interested in the jaw or lips, he should begin observation and movement exploration with the lower part of the body. Even tension in a child's toes can strongly influence the mouth!

Children Learn to Move by Moving

Although seating systems may give children more optimum function for eating, transportation and classroom learning, they do not help children learn to move more efficiently. Children learn to move by moving. They need lots of time out of their chairs and on the floor, especially when they are younger.

Help Children Work With Their Special Chairs

When special chairs or seating systems are introduced too rapidly to children, they often respond by fighting them with their bodies. They do not know how to relax into the chair and let it really support them. The therapist should spend time in therapy using her body or lap to prepare the child for the type of movement control that is needed in the chair. She should move the child into the chair initially without special straps or restraints so that the child can feel the control of his own body. The therapist should gradually add the straps or restraints that are absolutely necessary.

Identify a Series of Seating Options That Fit the Child

Children's physical needs can change from day to day. At times, they have better postural stability and control; at other times, their control is poorer. They may need more support from a chair or the feeder's body, depending upon the sensory environment or their degree of fatigue or wellness. There is no such thing as the *best position* for a child. The positioning that is best will vary according to the child's needs at each moment.

Position at Mealtime Addresses the Child's Physical and Emotional Needs

The best positioning options for mealtimes nurture both the child's physical and emotional needs. Communication and socialization are vital parts of every mealtime. The child's position should support full interaction with others as well as provide a solid foundation of physical support for eating.

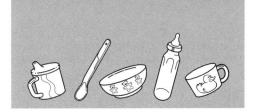

Seating and Positioning Considerations for Mealtime Support

Child _____ Date _____

Therapist _____

Communication Considerations

How do the baby and feeder communicate? How can positioning support this communication?

Socialization Considerations

What are the child's socialization needs (e.g., baby and one-to-one or family meal)?

Developmental Considerations

In what developmental stage is the child (e.g., bottle-feeding, spoon feeding, finger-feeding, independent feeding)?

Feeding Method Considerations

How is the child fed (e.g., by bottle, spoon, by tube)?

Oral Motor Considerations

Is the child learning to suck and swallow, chew, drink from a bottle, cup, straw? Are there considerations in the way the feeder presents the food to support emerging oral motor skills (e.g., cup support, jaw support, self-feeding support)?

Digestive Considerations

Does the child have any digestive issues that should be considered in seating and positioning (e.g., gastro-esophageal reflux, esophageal motility)?

Respiratory Considerations

Does the child have any respiratory issues that should be considered in the seating and positioning (e.g., shallow breathing, unpredictable breathing that may call for a quick removal from the chair)?

(continued)

Oral-Facial Considerations

Does the child have any oral-facial issues that should be considered in positioning and seating?

Neurological Considerations

Does the child have any neurological issues that should be considered in the seating and positioning?

Physical Positioning Considerations

Are there considerations in body alignment, posture, and muscle tone that influence feeding positioning (e.g., hips and pelvis, sitting base, trunk, shoulder girdle, head control, abdominal muscles, mobility around the body axis, functional vision)?

Are there considerations for straps and belts? What is necessary? What is not?

Is the positioning or seating comfortable for the child?

Feeder Positioning Considerations

Is the feeder comfortable? Are there considerations in body alignment or support that influence feeder comfort throughout the meal?

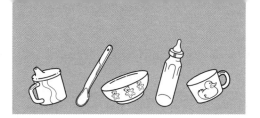

Body Alignment
for Seating and Positioning Checklist

Child _____ Date _____

Therapist _____

Area	Comments/Changes Needed
Hips and pelvis	
Sitting base	
Feet	
Trunk	
Shoulder girdle	
Head control	
Abdominal-pelvic girdle	

(continued)

Area	Comments/Changes Needed
Freedom of movement	
Functional vision	
Position for interaction with feeder	
Position for interaction with family	

Additional observations

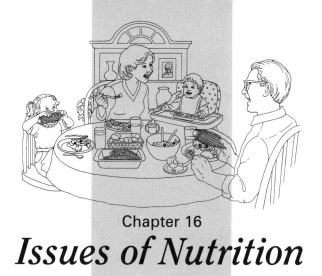

Chapter 16
Issues of Nutrition

This chapter does not include a complete overview of nutrition. It focuses on the nutritional issues that relate to feeding programs and provides a foundation of information and questions that enable the feeding therapist to work in partnership with the dietitian. A dietitian is a key member of the feeding team who works with therapists and parents regarding food decisions for each child.

Three major components are involved in children's nutritional status:

- **intake,** which consists of the calories and nutrients in the foods that the child eats
- **utilization,** which describes the assimilation and use of these nutrients by the body
- **output,** which defines the amount of energy that the body uses

Each of these components plays a significant role in determining a child's nutritional needs and the role played by dietitians and feeding therapists. Weight, age, and activity level determine the amount of energy a child needs. Children at the same age who weigh more burn more calories and need more energy than children who weigh less. Because their energy needs are higher, their intake must be greater. Infants who are experiencing rapid rates of growth require more calories per pound than toddlers whose rate of growth is decelerating. When a child's activity level is low, the number of calories and nutrients needed is lower when compared to a child of the same age who is very active. Children with high muscle tone or fluctuating tone burn many calories despite not having good movement control. With a high need for energy, their intake requirements may be higher than those for children with low tone.

Utilization of calories and nutrients is the bridge that describes how efficiently the body uses the fuel it is given. If the body is inefficient in its processing and assimilation, it will need more fuel to provide the needed output of energy. Likewise, efficient processing means the body requires less fuel to provide the needed energy. A child with a high metabolic rate uses up a great deal of energy supporting basic cardiac, respiratory, and digestive functions. Because the "engine" is running at a high rate, the child may be more physically active. A higher level of intake is required to maintain the child's growth and physical development. In contrast, when the metabolic rate is low, the body needs to do less work and the child's intake may need to be reduced to prevent obesity. Some infants do not assimilate specific nutrients and may require a higher intake of foods with these nutrients or supplements.

Assessment of Nutrition

Children with feeding difficulties benefit from a dietitian's specialized knowledge and input. Nutritional problems are more prevalent in this group of children than in children who have the same diagnosis but do not have feeding issues (Kovar, 1997; Krick & Van Duyn, 1984; Thommessen, Kase, et al., 1991). Therefore, assessment of nutritional status should become a routine part of the child's care and feeding program (Baer & Harris, 1997; Bartz & Deubler, 1990; Wodarski, 1990).

The ultimate physical goal of any feeding program is to enable the child to take in and utilize the nutrients that support health and well-being. The feeding therapist works to remove the physical, sensory, and experiential limits that interfere with the child's intake of food and liquid. She plays a role in selecting the food that is given to the child and in suggesting various food alternatives to the family. Although this can be accomplished in general terms by using the guidelines recommended for infants and children of specific ages and weights, this is not always appropriate for children with the disabilities that accompany feeding issues. Nutritional needs change over time. Growth patterns, reduction in dietary variety, specific stressors in the child's life, and the amount and type of physical activity influence a child's dietary needs. Unfortunately, a dietitian sees many children only when they initially are diagnosed with a medical or feeding problem. Although the dietitian makes appropriate dietary recommendations at that time, the child may not return for a follow-up assessment unless problems in growth are observed. Many children whose general growth parameters of height and weight are within the normal range may not receive the type and amount of specific nutrients that they need because of limitations in their dietary intake or utilization. Therefore, children who have feeding difficulties require dietary consultations on an ongoing basis.

The assessment of the child's nutrition may consist of a variety of measures, including a history, dietary records, and anthropometric measurements.

History

The initial evaluation includes a history of the child's medical and feeding issues. The child's diagnosis and medical history may increase the risk factors for certain types of dietary deficiencies. Certain genetic disorders such as Down syndrome, Noonan syndrome, Prader-Willi syndrome, and Turner syndrome have predictable variations in growth patterns (Giordano, 1992). Also, the pattern of growth of children who have a history of prematurity is different from the pattern seen in full-term infants (Guo et al., 1996, 1997; Hack et al., 1996). Growth patterns of children with cerebral palsy appear to be related both to nutritional and non-nutritional factors (Stevenson et al., 1994, 1995). In addition, medications may increase the need for specific nutrients (Epstein et al., 2000).

The evaluation also includes information on the child's family because genetics determines many aspects of a child's growth (Perusse & Bouchard, 1999; Towne et al., 1993). Tall parents are more likely to have tall children than short parents. Children whose parents and siblings are overweight tend to gain weight more rapidly than those who have parents with weight in the normal range. A propensity toward obesity interacts with environmental influences to produce children who also may be overweight.

Dietary Records

The family is asked for specific information on the type and amount of food that the child eats in a typical day. Because food intake varies among young children, parents usually are asked to keep a detailed record of the food a child eats for either a 3- or 7-day period. This information is analyzed for the presence and adequacy of calories and a wide variety of different vitamins, minerals, and amino acids. Because children with feeding difficulties often lose a great deal of food as they eat, it may be difficult to measure the specific amounts of each food that the child actually swallows. Children with reflux may eat a measurable amount of each food and then vomit a portion of the meal. Although the amount vomited may be measured, it is impossible to say which foods and nutrients actually remain in the body and which are lost.

Anthropometric Measures

Nutritional status frequently is evaluated by measuring the body. Measurements usually include height, weight, head circumference, and height-to-weight ratio. Specific features generally are plotted on special growth charts at regular intervals. The chart enables the physician or dietitian to compare the child's growth with other children and to observe the child's rate of growth over time. Specialized growth charts have been developed for children with Down syndrome (Toledo et al., 1999), Turner syndrome (Lyon et al., 1985), quadriplegic cerebral palsy (Krick et al., 1996) and prematurity (Guo et al., 1996, 1997).

Other measurements also may be used. Measures of skin-fold thickness provide information on total body fat. Measurement of arm circumference assesses muscle mass in the body and may identify protein-energy malnutrition. Length of the tibia or upper arm or knee height can be used when a child has contractures and cannot straighten a limb for accurate measure of height (Kong et al., 1999; Stevenson, 1995).

Measures such as height and weight must be examined very carefully in determining whether a child's growth patterns are cause for concern. Chapter 24 contains a discussion of growth charts and their interpretation.

Intake

Feeding Skills

The initial concern of dietitians and feeding therapists should be the adequacy of the child's food intake. A child's feeding skills play a large role in the type and amount of food that is eaten at each meal. When sensorimotor coordination for eating is easy, children can take in an amount guided by their appetite and eat a wide variety of foods to supply the calories and nutrients needed by their bodies. When coordination is poor or sensory comfort is lacking or variable, children may take in far less food than they need for growth and wellness. Gisel and her colleagues observed that the primary cause of malnutrition in feeding impaired children is their mechanical inefficiency in feeding (Gisel, Applegate-Ferrante, Benson, & Bosma, 1995; Patrick & Gisel, 1990). They found that children often experience their major nutritional difficulties as they move into adolescence and require larger amounts of food at each meal than their feeding coordination can support. Researchers examined the effect of feeding problems on the nutrient intake of 221 children with disabilities (Thommessen, Riis et al., 1991). They found that children who had feeding problems due to oral motor dysfunction showed reduced caloric and nutrient intake in the food they ate. They also found that the effect of reduced food intake was lessened by therapeutic feeding strategies used by parents and therapists.

Many children with limiting motor patterns have severe difficulties with oral motor coordination for eating. This reduced eating efficiency typically results in longer meals. Gisel and Patrick (1988) compared the eating efficiency of seven children with cerebral palsy and growth failure with typically developing children at the same weight. The children with cerebral palsy took up to 12 times longer to eat a standard amount of pureed food and up to 15 times longer to chew solid food than did children in the matched control group. Although no published research has compared a child's eating skill and efficiency at the beginning and end of a meal, many parents and clinicians have observed that children eat more poorly toward the end of the meal. An increased time devoted to meals does not always improve nutritional adequacy. The feeder and the child become more fatigued and frustrated as eating time expands. It may become physically impossible for many children to take in enough calories and nutrients although they are capable of eating smaller amounts by mouth.

Often, tube feedings are recommended to prevent or treat malnutrition and poor growth in children whose feeding skills do not support full oral nutrition. In a study of caregiver perceptions of gastrostomy tube feedings, Tawfik et al. (1997) cited weight gain and a shorter feeding time as benefits of tube feedings. Corwin et al. (1996) observed catch-up growth in weight and length during the first 18 months after receiving a gastrostomy tube in a group of 75 children with failure to thrive (ages birth to 6½ years). The amount of growth did not depend on when tube feedings were initiated.

The results of other studies have suggested that it is easier to reverse nutritional deficits in children with severe cerebral palsy when adequate nutritional management is initiated early in the child's life. Isaacs et al. (1994) evaluated weight gain and skin-fold fat mass in 22 nonambulatory children (ages 1–12 years) with neurological impairment who received at least 50% of their calories by gastrostomy feedings. Measurements were made three different times after the children received gastrostomy tubes. Ten of the 22 children made improvements, with the researchers noting that undernutrition before tube feedings may limit growth in some children. Rempel et al. (1988) studied changes in weight and length after beginning gastrostomy tube feedings for a group of 57 children with severe cerebral palsy. The majority of the children remained at less than the 5th percentile for both weight and height. Improvements in height were less common than improvements in weight. Children who received the gastrostomy during the first year of life were more likely to exceed the 5th percentile. The researchers concluded that gastrostomy feedings could improve nutritional status in children with cerebral palsy but did not eliminate the child's growth retardation. Sanders et al. (1990) compared the influence of the time period in which tube feedings were initiated in 51 children with cerebral palsy. Children whose tube feedings were begun within the first year after their neurological condition was identified initially showed fewer signs of undernutrition and normalized both their weight and length after 6 months of tube feedings. Children whose tube feedings were started later were more malnourished and made fewer gains in weight and height with the support of tube feedings. When tube feedings were initiated more than 8 years after the onset of the neurological insult, children were able to make some improvements in weight-for-age and weight-for-length but showed no change in length-for-age.

Food

Food provides energy and nutrients. It is the most important variable in determining the nutritional status of children. At different ages and weights, children and adults require different amounts and types of food to provide the energy and nutrients needed for growth and health. The recommended dietary allowances (RDA) published by the National Research Council (National Academy of Sciences, 1995) provides a set of standards for healthy, typically developing children. These guidelines specify the number of calories and amount of nutrients needed by the body at each age level. Many people consider these amounts to be the minimum needed. Others believe that the RDA is the dietary equivalent of the minimum wage (i.e., enough to stay well, but not enough for many people to thrive) (Sears & Sears, 1999). Many people require substantially higher nutrient levels. Some children have different biological needs based on genetics, lifestyle, and activity levels. Others have increased needs for specific nutrients related to medications or medical diagnosis.

Although there are recommended dietary allowances at each age level, the amount of food that the child needs to eat depends upon two features of food—caloric density and nutrient density. ***Caloric density*** refers to the number of calories in a given volume of food. For example, most vegetables and fruits have a relatively low caloric density. One ounce of pureed carrots contains 8 calories. Meat, poultry, and other foods with high levels of protein and fat have a much higher caloric density. One ounce of pureed chicken contains 43 calories, and 1 ounce of a chocolate candy bar contains 140 calories. ***Nutrient density*** refers to the amount and type of nutrients in a given volume of food. Green and yellow vegetables, for example, are rich in vitamins, minerals, and phytochemicals needed by the body for health. Grains and other complex carbohydrates are also full of these types of nutrients and considered to have a high nutrient density. Many snack foods, such as chocolate, potato chips, and soda pop, contain very few nutrients that the body needs and are foods with a low nutrient density.

Many children with feeding difficulties eat a small amount of food at mealtime because of difficulties with physical coordination or sensory processing. The ideal foods for these youngsters are high in nutrient and caloric density. This enables them to eat less food yet still receive the calories and nutrients that they need. Problems develop when either the nutrient or caloric intake in food is inadequate.

Parents and therapists typically do not memorize the caloric or nutrient values of specific foods. They rely on a translation of the RDAs into the number of servings per day of specific types of food. The Food Guide Pyramid visually describes the ideal number of servings per day of different food groups (U.S. Department of Agriculture & U.S. Department of Health and Human Services, 1995). The pyramid shows foods that should be eaten more frequently and in larger quantities (such as bread and grains) on the bottom. Fruits and vegetables should be the next most frequently eaten food groups and are at the second level. Layered on top of this is a protein group that contains milk, yogurt, cheese, meat, poultry, fish, legumes, eggs, and nuts. Fats and sugars crown the pyramid, indicating they should be eaten sparingly. Specific information on caloric and nutrient recommendations for children of different ages and weights is available in books that focus on pediatric nutrition (Klein & Delaney, 1994; Tamborlane, 1997; Trahms & Pipes, 1997).

Calories

Calories provide the fuel that gives the body energy for support and physical activity. The average number of calories that a child needs each day depends on many factors, including the stage of growth and level of activity. Infants need more calories per pound than toddlers because they grow very rapidly during the first 6–12 months. However, toddlers and preschoolers eat a larger total number of calories because their body weight is greater. During growth spurts, most children have a larger appetite and take in more calories. The child's appetite should determine the number of calories eaten during the meal. This will vary from meal to meal throughout the day and even from day to day. Birch and her colleagues found that young children were highly unpredictable in the amount of food and calories consumed at a single meal (Birch et al., 1991). A child might eat very little at one meal and make up for it later in the day. The researchers also found that children's intake at specific meals was influenced directly by calories and nutrients eaten at prior meals (Birch et al., 1993).

Macronutrients

Macronutrients are the major components of foods: carbohydrates, fats, and protein. All food consists of one or more of these large nutrient groups.

Carbohydrates

The largest percentage of calories in a healthy diet is derived from carbohydrates. Each gram of carbohydrate provides 4 calories of energy. **Simple carbohydrates** are the sugars that occur in whole foods and give a sweet taste to fruits, certain vegetables, and honey. Sugars also are refined and concentrated so that they can be added to other foods. Refined sugar (e.g., cane, beet) and syrup (e.g., maple, corn, rice, molasses) are added to various prepared foods. Many food labels list a variety of simple carbohydrates by their specific biochemical names such as glucose, fructose, lactose, galactose, and xylose. Simple carbohydrates pass through the digestive tract and into the bloodstream relatively quickly, resulting in rapid and uneven bursts of energy. The term **complex carbohydrates** is used to describe the starches found in foods such as whole-grain breads, cereals, rice, pasta, vegetables, legumes, potatoes, and yams. Complex carbohydrates require more digestion than simple carbohydrates. They remain in the stomach longer and provide a more even energy source.

Fruits, vegetables, and grains consist primarily of carbohydrates. They provide the best nutrition for the body when they are eaten as whole foods. Modern society has created the technology to extract portions of foods and refine them in a variety of ways. For example, the grain used to make whole-grain bread includes the fiber-rich outer bran layer and the nutritious inner germ of the kernel that contains most of the grain's nutritional content. Whole-grain bread is brown, relatively dense, and very nutritious. White bread and many lighter brown breads are made from refined wheat flour that has eliminated the bran and germ portions. Although these breads are quite popular, they have much less nutritional value than whole-grain breads. Whole juices can be extracted from fruits and vegetables, or they can be processed with the addition of other sugars.

Many whole foods that are rich in carbohydrates also contain fiber that cannot be digested. Fiber provides the bulk that is needed to move waste materials efficiently through the large intestine and reduce toxins in the intestinal tract. It is extremely important in preventing constipation. Breast milk and infant formulas do not contain fiber because infants and young children lack the digestive enzymes that help break down the fiber. Too much fiber can cause gastrointestinal distress in children under the age of 2 and can fill them up, leaving inadequate room for foods that provide calories.

Fats

Fats are a very important part of every diet, especially for infants and young children. Each gram of fat provides 9 calories of energy, more than double the caloric content of equivalent grams of carbohydrate or protein. In addition to supplying a high level of energy, fats provide the major nutritional building block for the brain and central nervous system (Farquharson et al., 1992). They also provide body fat for insulation and protecting vital organs. Fats are required for the assimilation of fat-soluble vitamins such as vitamins E, A, D, and K. Although excess consumption of fat can lead to health problems in older children and adults, a low-fat diet is inappropriate for infants and children under the age of 2. Fat accounts for approximately 50% of the calories in breast milk and 30% to 54% of the calories in typical infant formulas (Cunningham & McLaughlin, 1999). Although adults should get only 20% to 30% of their calories from fat, children require a higher percentage. The fat content of the infant's diet is reduced somewhat as complex carbohydrates are added in solid foods. However, this level does not go below 35% until the child is 2 to 3 years old (Roberts et al., 1999).

All fats are not created equal. Some fats contribute to growth and health while others do not. Saturated fats are solid at room temperature. They are found in most meats, eggs, and dairy foods. Monounsaturated and polyunsaturated fats are found in oils that are liquid at room temperature. Saturated fats contribute to heart disease and obesity in older children and adults. Although present in many health-promoting foods, they do not provide the consistently high nutritional benefits of most polyunsaturated fats. Polyunsaturated fats supply a very important group of essential fatty acids (EFAs) that support brain development and visual, cardiac, and immune system function (Pitchford, 1993; Uauy, Mena, & Valenzuela, 1999; Uauy et al., 1996). Two basic fatty acids are omega 6 (linoleic acid) and omega 3 (alpha-linolenic acid). Although both are required for brain development and function, omega 3 is the more important of the two (Holman, 1998; Uauy et al., 1996). Omega 3 fatty acids are converted into two acid components called docosahexaenoic acid (DHA) and eicosapentaenoic acid (EPA), which appear to provide the most essential components of brain cell development and ongoing support of neurotransmitters. The brain of the young infant is 60% fat. During the baby's first year, the brain grows rapidly and uses 60% of the total calories that are consumed (Sears & Sears, 1999). Infants who are breast-fed typically receive an adequate intake of all of the omega 3 fatty acids; some of the essential fatty acids now are added to cow's milk formulas. The fat content of breast milk varies during the meal. The foremilk at the beginning is low in fat. Gradually, the fat content increases as the baby takes the rich hindmilk toward the end of the feeding. When infants nurse for brief periods, they may not stay on the breast long enough to get the hindmilk. Their diet may become deficient in fatty acids, and they may fail to gain adequate weight because they are missing the most calorically dense portion of the meal (Thompson, 1998).

Dietary insufficiencies can begin after the infant moves to a solid food diet and no longer obtains essential fatty acids through breast milk or formula. The typical American diet is lacking in omega 3 fatty acids (Sears & Sears, 1999). Deficiencies have been identified in children with attention deficit/hyperactivity disorders (ADHD), and supplements of these fatty acids have improved their behavioral function (Aman et al., 1987; Burgess, Stevens, Zhang, & Peck, 2000; Stevens et al., 1995). A preliminary study by Stordy (2000) identified improvements in dark adaptation in young adults with dyslexia and improvements in movement coordination in children with motor planning disorders (dyspraxia) when they received supplements of one or more of the omega 3 fatty acids.

Essential fatty acids are provided primarily in vegetable oils, nuts, seeds, and fish. The richest sources of omega 3 are flax oil, canola oil, soy products, walnuts, and cold water fish (e.g., salmon, tuna, mackerel, lake trout, halibut, sardines, herring). If canned rather than fresh fish is included in the diet, children should be given the natural oil-packed fish. When tuna is packed in water instead of its own fatty oil, most of the omega 3 oils are lost.

Liquid polyunsaturated oils tend to turn rancid and have a short shelf life. To counteract this problem, manufacturers use a process called hydrogenation that makes the fat more solid. Hydrogenated and partially hydrogenated oils are used regularly in the production of margarine, cookies, and other baked goods. However, hydrogenation creates a trans-fatty acid that inhibits the conversion of essential fatty acids for brain growth and development. Researchers have suggested that the amount of trans-fatty acids be identified on food labels and that intake should be limited in young children (Decsi & Koletzko, 1995; Demmelmair et al., 1996).

Often, these fat facts leave parents and therapists very confused because it is unclear how much of each type of fat is acceptable in the diet for infants and young children. In addition, current labeling laws do not require manufacturers to list the amount of trans-fatty acids in a product.

Protein

Proteins provide the building blocks for tissue formation and repair throughout every system in the body. They provide an energy supply of 4 calories per gram. Most children get an abundant amount of protein in their diet because it is found in meat, fish, eggs, milk, poultry, vegetables, grains, and legumes. Protein foods provide 20 amino acids that are the cellular building blocks of the body. The body can manufacture some amino acids if they are not available in the diet; however, nine essential amino acids must come from food. Many people assume that protein is available only in meat, poultry, fish, and dairy products. However, vegetables and grains also contain an abundant amount of protein. Animal foods contain complete protein that includes all of the essential amino acids. With the exception of soy (which is a complete protein), nonmeat sources of protein do not contain all nine essential amino acids. However, when two or more vegetables, grains, or legumes are eaten during the day, their amino acids can complement each other and provide the body with all of the amino acids required.

Protein must be added very carefully to the diet of an infant or young child. If the diet contains too much protein, the kidneys will excrete too much water, resulting in dehydration.

Micronutrients

Food also contains an extensive and complex mixture of micronutrients, which include the vitamins and minerals that are essential to the body in very small amounts. Inclusive lists of these nutrients, their specific functions in the body, symptoms of deficiency and toxicity, and recommended daily allowances are available in most books that focus exclusively on nutrition (Murray, 1996; Trahms & Pipes, 1997). Following is a simple overview of the topic. Greater detail is provided for nutrients that have specific relevance in the development of feeding and mealtime programs.

Vitamins

Vitamins are essential for the health and repair of the body and for ongoing metabolism. In most cases, they must come from outside the body, primarily through food. There are two major groups of vitamins: fat soluble and water soluble. Water-soluble vitamins include vitamin C and the B-complex vitamins. Because they dissolve in the water of the body, they are excreted in urine if the vitamin level is too high. For this reason, it is very difficult to overdose on water-soluble vitamins. Fat-soluble vitamins include vitamins A, D, E, and K. These vitamins are drawn into solution with fats that are taken into the digestive tract and absorbed into the body. Therefore, it is important to eat foods that provide some fat during a meal that includes fat-soluble vitamins. These vitamins are retained when fat is stored in the body. As a result, they can build to a toxic level when their intake is too high. Some fats, such as mineral oil, are indigestible and pass rapidly through the intestines. If mineral oil is given for constipation when food is still in the upper portion of the digestive tract, the fat-soluble vitamins in the meal will not be absorbed because they pass out of the body with the mineral oil and feces. This can contribute to a deficiency of vitamins A, D, E, and K in the body.

Vitamins act synergistically with each other and with minerals. When they are consumed as part of a balanced diet of foods, vitamins and minerals complement and support each other. For example, vitamin D is required for the absorption of calcium, while vitamin C enhances the absorption of iron. Vitamins in the B-complex group (e.g., thiamin, riboflavin, niacin, pyridoxine, and B-12) must be consumed in a specific balance. As part of a natural diet, a complementary balance is usually attained. However, problems can occur when supplements are taken of a single B vitamin because it disrupts the balance and can cause deficiencies in other B-complex vitamins. People who eat a vegan diet (i.e., containing no meat, poultry, eggs, fish, or dairy products) may need supplements of vitamin B-12 because it is available only through animal sources. Vitamin C supports immune system function and acts as a natural antihistamine, making it particularly effective in the treatment of allergies and cold symptoms (Rapp, 1991).

Table 16.1	**Food Sources of Vitamins in Children's Diets**
Vitamin A	liver, sweet potatoes, carrots, spinach, cantaloupe, winter squash, pumpkin, apricots, green leafy vegetables, tuna
Beta Carotene (precursor of vitamin A)	apricots, mangos, peaches, cantaloupe, carrots, sweet potatoes, kale, winter squash
B Complex	tofu; pork; wheat germ; legumes; whole-grain breads; milk; liver; green, leafy vegetables; eggs; poultry; fish; peanuts; brewer's yeast; potatoes; bananas; oatmeal; shellfish; eggs; yogurt; soybeans; nuts
Vitamin C	citrus fruits; tomatoes; papaya; raw, leafy vegetables; broccoli; strawberries; cantaloupe; cabbage; green and yellow peppers; potatoes
Vitamin D	vitamin D-fortified milk, salmon, sardines, liver, herring
Vitamin E	milk, avocado, wheat germ oil, corn oil, soybean oil, sunflower oil
Vitamin K	green, leafy vegetables; broccoli; onions
Folic Acid (F)	lentils, spinach, kidney beans, pinto beans, wheat germ, chickpeas, avocados

Minerals

The body needs a wide variety of minerals, including calcium, phosphorus, sodium, magnesium, iron, zinc, selenium, copper, iodine, fluoride, molybdenum, chromium, sulfur, and manganese. Some minerals, such as calcium and phosphorus, are needed in relatively large quantities; while others such as copper, selenium, and molybdenum are required in trace amounts.

Although all minerals are important in nutrition, several play key roles in areas that support feeding. Calcium (along with phosphorus, magnesium, and vitamin D) is essential in building strong bones and teeth (Koo & Tsang, 1984). Calcium and magnesium also contribute to the proper balance of muscle contraction and relaxation. Deficiencies or imbalances of these minerals prenatally or postnatally contribute to poor development of tooth enamel and can cause oral pain during eating. Although rare in healthy children, deficiencies of magnesium can cause central nervous system symptoms that affect attention, muscle tone, coordination and the development of seizures (Kozielec & Starobrat-Hermelin, 1997; Langley & Mann, 1991; Lynch & Rust, 1994). Preterm infants are born before their bodies have been able to build up a normal storage level of magnesium (Stigson & Kjellmer, 1997). Magnesium sulfate is given to many women just before a premature birth to prevent the intraventricular hemorrhage that often causes cerebral palsy (Hirtz & Nelson, 1998). Studies have shown that adding magnesium supplements to the diet reduces symptoms of ADHD (Kozielec & Starobrat-Hermelin, 1997) and autism (Martineau et al., 1985).

Iron is essential to the manufacture of hemoglobin, the portion of the red blood cells that carries oxygen to the cells. Infants and children who have an iron deficiency can develop cognitive and motor delays, weakness, fatigue, and shortness of breath (Lozoff & Brittenham, 1987; Wasantwisut, 1997). The healthy, full-term infant is born with a storage of iron in the liver that lasts 4 to 6 months. Because these iron stores are accumulated during the last trimester of the pregnancy, premature infants have a smaller reserve and, therefore, a higher risk for iron deficiency than full-term infants. Breast milk provides an additional small amount of iron that is more easily assimilated than the iron in cow's milk. Most infant formulas are fortified with iron. Problems with iron deficiency can develop between 6 and 12 months of age as the baby requires more iron due to growth and the depletion of the inborn reserve of iron. For this reason, infant cereals are fortified with iron, and the American Academy of Pediatrics (1992) has recommended that infants remain on breast milk or iron-fortified infant formula until they are 12 months old. The introduction of whole cow's milk before 12 months can cause iron deficiency (Tunnessen & Oski, 1987; Udall & Suskind, 1999).

The body absorbs iron from meat sources more efficiently than from vegetable and grain sources. However, vitamin C enhances absorption of iron, especially from non-animal sources (Fashakin & Oladimeji, 1986). Iron deficiency often is difficult to detect, but it is common in toddlers and older infants. This occurs primarily when the baby is shifted to cow's milk before 12 months and when toddlers stop eating iron-fortified cereals. Low intake of foods containing vitamin C also can contribute to an iron deficiency during this period.

Reduction in gastric acid can impair the body's ability to absorb iron from grain or vegetable sources. Skikne et al. (1981) measured a 28% reduction in iron absorption from a meal that was preceded by administration of 300 mg of cimetidine (an H2 blocker that reduces gastric acid production) in a small group of adults. Antacids caused a 52% decrease in iron absorption. The researchers concluded that cimetidine in the doses usually recommended would not have a major effect on iron nutrition; however, when combined with antacids, cimetidine would significantly impair iron absorption.

These issues may become magnified when infants and children have feeding problems. Many infants with feeding difficulties experience delays in moving to supplemental feedings of pureed foods. They may remain exclusively on breast-feeding or bottle-feeding until they are well past their first birthday. This is particularly true for infants with sensory-based feeding difficulties who experience greater comfort and sensory organization during breast-feeding. These infants often are extremely resistant to accepting iron-fortified cereals in their diet. A number of toddlers and older children in this group continue to resist foods that are smooth and soft in favor of crunchy or salty foods. Calories in their diet are provided primarily by cow's milk and foods such as crackers, chips, and french fries. None of these foods contain the iron that they need. Most children with gastroesophageal reflux are given medications, such as cimetidine, that reduce their output of hydrochloric acid. Some are given more than one of these medications and many receive a combination of acid-reduction medications and antacids. These medications may contribute to reduced absorption of iron.

Zinc is needed in more than 100 enzymes involved in digestion and metabolism (Dietz & Stern, 1999). It supports appetite, dietary intake, growth, taste, and immunity (Chandra, 1997b; Friel et al., 1985; Russell et al., 1983; Shankar & Prasad 1998). Although present in both breast milk and infant formulas, zinc is more easily absorbed from breast milk. Children who don't receive a balanced diet containing foods that are high in zinc may not obtain an adequate amount. Skinner and her colleagues (Skinner, Carruth, Houck, Coletta, et al., 1997; Skinner, Carruth, Houck, et al., 1999) studied the longitudinal dietary records of children between 2 months and 5 years. Low dietary intake of zinc was evident consistently. Mild deficiencies of zinc can contribute to a reduced appetite, poor growth, difficulties with taste perception, and a greater propensity to infection (Alpers, 1994; Gibson et al., 1989; Ploysangam et al., 1997; Solomons et al., 1976). Zinc supplements have been effective in improving appetite and growth. Zinc, like other vitamins and minerals, acts in a balance with other minerals in the diet. Elevated levels of calcium or iron, for example, can reduce zinc absorption.

Gastric acid increases zinc absorption. Low acid levels can contribute to poor utilization of zinc. Sturniolo et al. (1991) evaluated the effect of cimetidine and ranitidine (medications used to inhibit acid production in gastroesophageal reflux) on zinc absorption. They concluded that gastric acid secretion played a role in the regulation of zinc absorption. Serfaty-Lacrosniere et al. (1995) examined the effect of omeprazole, another medication that inhibits hydrochloric acid in the stomach. When given before a meal, it reduced acid but did not interfere with the absorption of calcium, phosphorus, magnesium, or zinc. Neither of these studies examined the long-term effects of reduced gastric acid on zinc absorption. This raises important questions for children who take these medications for many years.

Because of its negative impact on children's appetites and dietary intake, feeding therapists should have a high awareness of the role of zinc deficiency in nutrition. When the reasons for a child's reduced appetite are unclear or taste aversions persist despite treatment, it is appropriate to recommend evaluation of the child's zinc levels. In many instances, even when zinc levels are in the low normal range, children's appetite and interest in eating have improved with zinc supplementation. This should always be done under the guidance of a dietitian or a physician with special training in nutrition. This helps avoid problems resulting from too high a dose of zinc, which can create a deficiency in copper (Sandstead, 1994; Solomons, 1985).

Selenium is another trace mineral that may play an important role in the health of children with feeding problems. It is involved in immune system support (Beck, 1999; Dhur et al., 1990; McKenzie et al., 1998). Deficiencies may result in a higher incidence of bacterial and viral illnesses and allergies (Galland, 1987; Kadrabova et al., 1996). Selenium may have a positive impact on improving mood (Benton & Cook, 1991) and play a major role in brain development and cognition (Wasantwisut, 1997). Numerous studies have found selenium deficiencies in children on tube feedings, particularly those receiving parenteral nutrition (Abrams et al., 1992; Gramm et al., 1995; Saito et al., 1998; Van Caillie-Bertrand et al., 1984). Supplemental vitamin C increases the bioavailability of natural selenium in foods (Mutanen & Mykkanen, 1985).

Table 16.2	**Food Sources of Selected Minerals in Children's Diets**
Calcium	milk and dairy products; tofu; green, leafy vegetables; calcium-fortified orange juice; shellfish; almonds; broccoli
Copper	nuts, legumes, cereals, poultry, dried fruit, shellfish, organ meats
Iron	iron-fortified cereal; fortified breakfast cereals; chicken; red meat; tofu; eggs; whole-grain breads; green, leafy vegetables; prune juice; chickpeas
Magnesium	soybeans, tofu, beans, whole grains, almonds, cashews, sesame seeds
Selenium	brazil nuts, seafood, organ meats, meat, poultry, garlic, sunflower seeds
Zinc	whole-grain cereal, dry beans, nuts, meat, fish, poultry, dairy products, shellfish

Beyond Vitamins and Minerals

Phytonutrients

The traditional emphasis in nutrition has been placed on the role of carbohydrates, protein, fat, vitamins, and minerals in the diet. However, thousands of other nutrients are found in fresh fruits and vegetables that are vital to good health. These phytonutrients (i.e., nutrients from plants) are designed primarily to keep plants healthy by protecting them from the sun's rays and a wide variety of diseases. Hundreds of scientific studies have shown that these phytonutrients play a crucial role in the human immune system function and in repairing or rebuilding damaged cells. Many produce substances that prevent cancer (American Dietetic Association, 1995).

Recommendations on the Food Guide Pyramid include at least 2 to 4 servings of fruits and 3 to 5 servings of vegetables per day for optimum health. Research indicates that people who exceed the recommended daily servings tend to have fewer risks for disease and improved overall health. A recent study (Joshipura et al., 1999) showed that in a population of more than 100,000 people, the risk of stroke was reduced by 30% in those who ate more than five servings of fruits and vegetables per day. However, most people do not come close to even the minimum recommended number of servings (Kant et al., 1991; Muñoz, Krebs-Smith, Ballard-Barbash, & Cleveland, 1997). Patterson et al. (1990) found that only 9% of the adults surveyed ate the minimum 5 servings per day of fruits and vegetables.

Children with feeding problems often eat a diet that is limited in the variety and quantity of foods necessary for optimal health. Their diets typically consist of highly processed foods and formulas that do not contain the phytonutrients present in fresh fruits and vegetables. Food supplements of high quality freeze-dried fruits and vegetables can provide a valuable addition to the diets of children (Dykman & Dykman, 1998; Nisinzweig, 1999).

Glyconutrients

Healthy bodies comprised of many components working together in harmony must have accurate internal communication to function optimally. In its most basic form this communication occurs at the cellular level as cell-to-cell communication. Cells communicate their needs to be fed, regulated, cleansed, repaired, defended, and recognized.

The energy value of carbohydrates has been recognized for a long time; however, it is only in recent years that scientists have recognized their vital contribution to cellular function. Simple carbohydrate molecules known as monosaccharides attach to protein molecules through a process called glycoconjugate synthesis. These become the glycoproteins that facilitate cellular communication. Eight simple sugar molecules (the *glyco* part of glycoprotein) have been identified as necessary to cell-to-cell communication (Murray, 1996; See et al., 1998). They are glucose, galactose, mannose, fucose, xylose, n-acetyl-glucosamine, n-acetyle-galatosamine, n-acetyl-neuraminic acid-sialic acid. The average diet is deficient in all but glucose and galactose. Galactose is lacking in people who do not consume dairy products containing lactose. Although the body efficiently absorbs all eight monosaccharides through the intestines, glucose can be converted to the other seven carbohydrates (Gardiner, 2000a, 2000b). However, this process can take up to 15 steps, requiring time and energy, and each step creates a larger margin for error. Elements such as toxins, stress, drugs, viruses, and other invaders can interfere in the conversion process. When the intricate language of the cell is garbled so that the message is no longer clear, health problems can occur.

Glyconutritionals are dietary supplements that shortcut this enzymatic conversion process by making the full range of monosaccharides available directly to the cells in larger quantity and more rapidly. Research has identified the role played by these glyconutrients in improving immune system function, reducing inflammation, and protecting against cancer (Gardiner, 2000a, 2000b). The addition of glyconutrients to the blood cells of patients with chronic fatigue syndrome enhanced natural killer cells and improved other aspects of immune system function (See et al., 1998). The addition of supplemental glyconutrients to the diet has shown promising initial results in the long-term reduction of symptoms in adults with fibromyalgia and chronic fatigue syndrome (Dykman et al., 1998), and in improving function in children with ADHD (Dykman & Dykman, 1998), autism (Nisinzweig, 1999), and carbohydrate-deficient glycoprotein syndrome type I (Alton et al., 1997). Research in this area is expanding exponentially, and use of glyconutritional supplements to improve underlying nutrition and health can play a major role in building health and wellness.

Dietary Diversity

The nutrients needed by the human body are contained in a highly diverse group of plant and animal products. Children's dietary needs are satisfied only when they eat many different foods because each food provides a unique variety of nutrients. From birth, the human body is biased toward receiving a diversified diet. The breast-fed infant is exposed to dietary diversity at each meal. The taste of food eaten by the mother passes into the breast milk, giving the baby a great deal of taste variety (Mennella, 1995). The fat content of the milk varies from the beginning to the end of the meal—again, offering change and nutritional variety during the meal (Lawrence & Lawrence, 1999). By 6 months, the diet of the typical infant is expanded to include cereals, fruits, and vegetables. Anecdotal reports about bottle-fed infants suggest that there is both a greater eagerness to transition to supplemental foods and a greater difficulty in making the transition to new tastes. Perhaps this occurs because of an inner drive and need for dietary diversity, as well as a lack of preparation for the shift to greater diversity because of the single taste of the infant formula. Continued diversity in infant feeding is encouraged during the first year to provide a strong foundation for the variety that will support a nutritious diet later. A study by Capdevila, Vizmanos, and Marti-Henneberg (1998) of 120 normally developing, bottle-fed infants showed that as babies are weaned during the first year, their increased energy requirements for growth came from an increase in caloric density rather than through increasing the volume of the foods eaten.

The phenomenon of sensory-specific satiety also biases children toward a more diverse diet (Rolls, 1986). Research indicates that people become satiated and less interested in eating foods that they have just eaten. When a variety of foods is available at the meal, individuals tend to switch from one food to another as they get tired of eating a single food. Pleasure associated with eating appears to increase as the person samples the sensory properties of the new food. Typically, when a meal has more sensory variety and more foods available, children will eat a larger quantity of food as well as a larger variety of nutrients.

Ideally, all nutrients should be available through the foods that children eat. However, this often is not the case. Children's diets can vary substantially depending upon the types of foods their parents offer (Skinner, Carruth, Moran, Houck, Schmidhammer, et al., 1998) and by the level and types of nutrients in the foods that are eaten. Cox et al. (1997) developed a Variety Index for Toddlers (VIT) to assess variety within and among food groups based on the number of servings in each of the food groups in the Food Guide Pyramid. A longitudinal profile was created for 124 toddlers between 24 and 36 months. VIT scores were computed for intake adequacy for each of the food groups. Bread groups received the highest scores, while vegetable and meat groups received the lowest. Skinner, Carruth, Houck, Coletta, et al. (1997) followed a group of 98 mother-infant pairs from 2 months to 24 months. They compared the child's actual dietary intake for calories and nutrients with the RDA, then asked the mothers about the child's typical food intake and food likes and dislikes. The children ate a variety of foods, but vegetables were their least favorite foods. They also ate a large number of dairy products that were not fortified with vitamin D. Overall low intakes of zinc, vitamin D, and vitamin E were observed. The dietitians were very concerned about low fat intake from the use of reduced-fat milks and dislike of vegetables during the second year. The same researchers conducted a second longitudinal study of a group of 72 preschool children at targeted ages between 24 and 60 months old (Skinner, Carruth, Houck, et al., 1999). Using 3-day dietary records they examined the children's intake of calories and nutrients, identified the percentage of children consuming specific foods, and looked at the variety of foods eaten. The foods most commonly eaten by this group included fruit drinks, carbonated beverages, 2% milk, and french fries. Vegetables were at the top of the least favorite foods list. As a group, these children were not getting an adequate amount of zinc, folate, and vitamins D and E. Hampl et al. (1999) evaluated the level of vitamin C in the diets of 2,258 children between the ages of 7 and 18. Between 12% and 20% of the children had intake levels below the RDA. Stallings (1997) cites national survey data that showed that dietary calcium intake was variable in children and adolescents, with approximately 50% consuming less than the RDA intake. Muñoz et al. (1997) evaluated the mean number of servings per day of each recommended food group for 3,307 children between the ages of 2 and 19 years. Only 1% met all dietary recommendations. Sixteen percent did not meet any recommendations; 30% met the recommendations for fruits, grains, meat and dairy; and 36% met the recommendations for vegetables. The researchers concluded that children and teens in the United States follow eating patterns that do not meet national recommendations. Vitamin and mineral supplements may be needed when dietary intake is inadequate.

Infants and children who have feeding difficulties often have major difficulties obtaining a diet that contains a large enough number of different foods to provide the nutrients that are needed for health and growth. When children have sensory issues that increase selective eating patterns, they often resist the introduction of new foods. Most parents and therapists assume that the child doesn't like the new food and stop offering it. They desperately offer one food after another and are relieved when the child begins to eat a larger amount of a familiar food. Gradually the diet becomes more and more restricted. Children with motor-based feeding difficulties may experience a similar restriction in diet because of their coordination problems. Many of these youngsters eat very slowly and handle certain foods more easily than others. It may take them longer to organize sensation and movement to accept new foods. The dietary focus may be placed more on caloric intake than foods that provide a balance of nutrients. Parents and therapists of children who are transitioning from tube feedings to oral feedings typically measure progress in terms of the amount, rather than the variety, of food eaten. In the early stages of weaning from the tube, dietary adequacy is provided by the child's enteral formula. However, if diversity is not emphasized during the early stages of oral feeding, the child may not be willing to take the variety of foods required to actually transition to an age-appropriate diet. Many of these children end up learning to drink the same formula that supported them during tube feedings.

Developmental Guidelines

Dietary guidelines for infants and children are based on the child's energy and nutrient needs, the maturity of the gastrointestinal and urinary systems, and the oral motor coordination available for eating and drinking. Chapter 5 contains an in-depth discussion of the roles played by sensorimotor and gastrointestinal systems and the amount and types of foods in the diet during the infant's first year. Nutritional recommendations for children of various ages have varied over the years. Many research studies are based on a small group of children or on animals, making it difficult to generalize the results to a larger population of children. Cultural biases and beliefs, as well as shifts in the knowledge base, contribute to changes in professional recommendations. For example, before the 1920s, most infants were not given solid foods and got their full nutrition from breast milk or formula until they were 12 months old. In the 1950s, this trend shifted radically, and parents were advised to introduce supplemental foods early. For the next 20 years, it was common for infants to be given cereal and other pureed foods during the first 1 to 2 months. This trend was fueled by a belief that offering supplemental foods early would help infants sleep through the night. In the late 1970s the American Academy of Pediatrics Committee on Nutrition (1980) strongly recommended that infants take only breast milk or formula until they are 4 to 6 months old. A subsequent study showed that giving infants cereal at 5 weeks of age did not influence their sleeping patterns (Macknin et al., 1989). Despite these shifts in recommendation and research, many mothers continue to give their infants cereal at 2 to 3 months of age (Skinner, Carruth, Houck, Moran, et al., 1997). General guidelines for age of introducing specific foods do not address every infant. In all areas of development there is a range of readiness and skill development. Adults can offer children new dietary or developmental experiences at the beginning of a recommended age range, but should take into consideration individual readiness factors and the child's interest level. Children are their own best experts.

Many dietary guidelines for the timing of introducing specific foods, however, do fit most children. Adults must remember that children decide which foods and how much of each food to eat. Their appetites vary extensively from meal to meal and day to day. The body of a healthy child maintains a store of most nutrients and extra fat that can be burned for energy to support physical and mental processes during low-eating periods.

Birth to 6 Months

- Between birth and 6 months of age, infants obtain all of their energy and nutrient needs from breast milk or an infant formula.
- Thin, pureed cereal, fruits, and vegetables can be introduced when a child is between 4 and 6 months of age. During this period, the amount of these supplemental foods is small and is not needed for nutritional purposes. The purpose of adding these foods before 6 months is to provide exposure to tastes and the opportunity to develop the oral motor coordination for solid foods.

6 to 12 Months

- The infant should remain on breast milk or infant formula. Cow's milk should not be offered.

- Supplemental foods play a larger role in providing calories and nutrients in the infant's diet. An emphasis should be placed on dietary variety in introducing cereals, fruits, vegetables, meats, and other protein sources. Offer very small servings of new foods to help the baby develop familiarity and comfort with changes in smell, color, taste, and texture.

- Iron-fortified cereals are recommended for children from 6 to 18 months of age.

- Avoid offering high-allergen foods (e.g., cow's milk, egg whites, wheat, citrus, peanuts, tree nuts).

- Introduce one food at a time, allowing three to four days before adding another new food. This allows parents to watch for allergic reactions to the new food.

- Because of the risk of botulism poisoning and the immaturity of the digestive system, honey should not be offered before the baby is 12 months old.

1 Year and Beyond

- Use the Food Guide Pyramid as a guideline for the types of foods and number of servings to include in the child's diet. Serving sizes will be smaller for young children than for adults, but the number of servings in each food group is the same.

- Use a serving size guideline of 1 tablespoon for each year of the child's age. For example, a 1-year-old child would be offered a single serving of 1 tablespoon of the food, a 2-year-old would receive 2 tablespoons, and a 3-year-old would eat 3 tablespoons. For foods such as breads or pieces of fruit or cheese, the toddler should be offered one-quarter of the adult serving size.

- Wean the child from an infant formula to either whole milk or a toddler formula. Do not offer fat-reduced milk until the child is at least 2 years old.

- Use the following general guidelines in selecting food choices for meals in each age period (Dietz & Stern, 1999, page 92).

Helping Children Improve Dietary Intake

The following general strategies support children's ability to improve their dietary intake and receive meals that provide appropriate calories, macronutrients, and micronutrients. A registered dietitian should regularly monitor the diets of children with feeding difficulties.

- **Improve the child's oral sensorimotor skills for feeding.** Reduce the child's sensory and physical limitations that interfere with the ability to eat an age-appropriate diet. Make adjustments in taste and texture to support the child's current sensorimotor skills and reduce sensorimotor limitations. Refer to Chapters 14, 15, and 17.

- **Support a partnership between oral feedings and tube feedings for children who have difficulty sustaining their nutrition solely through oral feedings.** Children's nutritional status is the most important aspect of any feeding program. Inadequate calories and nutrients reduce the energy children have available for learning, impair their physical and cognitive development, and make them more vulnerable to illness. Tube feedings can provide nutrition while reducing the stress on parents, children, and therapists to get children to take in an adequate diet orally. Tube feedings may trigger gastrointestinal difficulties in a few children. However, they enable most children to develop feeding skills at their own pace without compromising nutrition. Refer to Chapter 23.

- **Make every bite count.** In order to reduce the amount of food that the child must eat, offer foods that are both calorie- and nutrient-dense. High-quality foods that appeal to children include avocados, broccoli, brown rice and other whole grains, cheese, eggs, fish, kidney beans, yogurt, pasta, peanut butter, potatoes, poultry, squash, sweet potatoes, and tofu (Sears & Sears, 1999). Read labels and select alternatives that have gone through the least amount of processing and have the fewest additives. Consider adding concentrated foods such as soluble whole-grain rice

Table 16.3   **Serving Sizes for Food Groups**

Food Group	1 to 3 years 1 serving	4 to 6 years 1 serving	7 to 10 years 1 serving
Grains 6 to 11 servings per day	1/2 slice bread 1/4 cup cooked cereal, rice, pasta, 1/3 cup dry cereal 2 to 3 crackers	1/2 slice bread 1/3 cup cooked cereal, rice, pasta, 1/2 cup dry cereal 3 to 4 crackers	1 slice bread 1/2 cup cooked cereal, rice, pasta, 3/4 to 1 cup dry cereal 4 to 5 crackers
Vegetables 2 to 3 servings per day	1/4 cup cooked vegetables	1/4 cup cooked vegetables 1/2 cup salad	1/4 cup cooked vegetables 1/2 cup salad
Fruits 2 to 3 servings per day	1/4 cup cooked or canned fruit 1/2 piece fresh fruit 1/4 cup juice	1/4 cup cooked or canned fruit 1/2 piece fresh fruit 1/3 cup juice	1/3 cup cooked or canned fruit 1 piece fresh fruit 1/2 cup juice
Dairy 2 to 3 servings per day	1/2 cup milk 1/2 ounce cheese 1/3 cup yogurt	1/2 cup milk 1 ounce cheese 1/2 cup yogurt	1 cup milk 1 ounce cheese 3/4 to 1 cup yogurt
Protein 2 servings per day	1 ounce, 1-inch cubes meat, fish, poultry, tofu 1/4 cup dried, cooked beans 1/2 egg	1 ounce, 1-inch cubes meat, fish, poultry, tofu 1/3 cup dried, cooked beans 1 egg	2 to 3 ounces meat, fish, poultry, tofu 1/2 cup dried, cooked beans 1 to 2 eggs

From *American Academy of Pediatrics Guide to Your Child's Nutrition* by W. H. Dietz and L. Stern. Copyright © 1998 by American Academy of Pediatrics. Reprinted by permission of Villard Books, a Division of Random House Inc.

or dehydrated fruits and vegetables to the diet. See Meeting the Child's Nutritional Needs on page 333 for specific food suggestions.

■ **Create happy mealtimes.** No one enjoys eating when mealtimes are stressful and unhappy. When children are under pressure to eat and parents are under pressure to feed them, everyone loses. Meals become a battleground, and children rarely get enough to eat of the right foods. When mealtimes are happy, children are more likely to become curious about food and more open to eating a larger amount of a wider variety of foods.

■ **Emphasize food variety more than food volume.** Children need to eat enough food to satisfy their caloric needs. However, for long-term dietary adequacy, it is more important to introduce children to a wide variety of foods than it is to emphasize eating larger amounts of one or two foods. Small tastes of new foods should be offered at least 10 times to allow children to increase familiarity without pressure (Birch, 1989; Sullivan & Birch, 1994).

■ **Provide opportunities for children to learn about nutritional foods and build positive associations.** Include activities at home and in therapy that offer children opportunities to build positive associations with a variety of nutritional foods. Planting a garden, then harvesting and preparing vegetables that the child has grown provides a strong incentive for eating the vegetables. Children who live in apartments can create small salad and herb gardens in flowerpots that fit on a windowsill. Trips to the produce department of the grocery store or a visit to a farm or orchard offer opportunities to talk about foods that support good growth. Helping to prepare foods or entire meals can provide many positive associations that invite children to take tastes. Use imagination when presenting food to children at mealtimes. String cereal on a necklace or fill an ice cream cone with cottage cheese instead of ice cream. Alternating pieces of fruit on a kabob stick emerge as amusing fruit caterpillars. Sandwiches take on an added allure when they are cut into interesting shapes with cookie cutters or decorated as faces with vegetables or cheese. Creative names also build interest. Children are enticed by avocado boats, broccoli trees, and banana wheels.

■ **Guide parents in providing appropriate foods and opportunities for their children to try nutritious foods.** Parents often feel stuck without a plan for introducing their children to appropriate foods and feeding opportunities. Often, the path taken with other children in the family doesn't work because the special child lacks the feeding skills or refuses to eat foods that are developmentally appropriate. Children are more likely to eat foods that they see others eating. Parents do not usually offer foods that they do not include in their own diets (Contento et al., 1993; Fisher & Birch, 1995; Rozin & Millman, 1987; Skinner, Carruth, Moran, Houck, Schmidhammer, et al., 1998). If the rest of the family lives on fast food hamburgers, white bread, french fries, and diet soda, this is the diet that may become most appealing to the child with a feeding difficulty. The overall feeding program should include informal discussions of food choices for the whole family and how these foods may be modified for the child with a feeding problem (e.g., increasing or decreasing taste intensity, adjusting textures). Although the dietitian makes appropriate dietary recommendations, it often is the feeding therapist who knows the child and family more intimately and can adjust these recommendations to family and cultural patterns and to the child's special physical or sensory needs.

■ Utilization

Eating is the first step in a complex process. Whether food provides the nutrients and calories that the child needs depends on how available these nutrients are and how well the body utilizes them. Digestive enzymes, mixture of food with water and gastric acids, gastric emptying time, pH levels in different regions of the gastrointestinal system, contributions of friendly bacteria in the intestinal tract, and peristalsis through the gut all contribute to the digestive process. If one or more of these processes are inefficient, the body's ability to digest and assimilate food for growth will be compromised.

Digestion

The process of digestion is described in detail in Chapter 4. As food passes through the mouth and digestive tract, it gradually is broken down by a series of enzymes and acids that reduce it to a nutrient-rich liquid that can be absorbed into the bloodstream through the walls of the small intestine (Gershon, 1998; Phillips & Wingate, 1998). Difficulties with this digestive process can result in the loss or malabsorption of nutrients. Children with gastroesophageal reflux may vomit food and fail to thrive because they cannot keep food in the stomach long enough for it to pass into the intestines (Borowitz & Borowitz, 1997; Fonkalsrud & Ament, 1996). Structural or neurological dysfunction of the intestinal tract can interfere with the absorption of nutrients (Borowitz & Borowitz, 1997; Fonkalsrud & Ament, 1996; Phillips & Wingate, 1998). The body may require a larger amount of specific nutrients or may inadequately metabolize nutrients, resulting in poor growth. This can occur when the digestive system is compromised by lack of specific digestive enzymes (Howell, 1985), allergy (Rapp, 1991), or increased intestinal permeability (Chaitow & Trenev, 1990). Please refer to Chapters 6 and 22 for more detailed discussions of these digestive issues.

Enzymes and the Breakdown of Food

Metabolic enzymes are the molecules that speed up the chemical reactions that are required for function of all systems of the body. Most enzymes are made up of a protein combined with an essential mineral and vitamin. If the enzyme lacks the mineral or vitamin, it cannot function optimally. Zinc, for example, is needed by the enzyme that activates vitamin A for vision. Without it, vitamin A is not converted properly, leading to poor night vision (M. T. Murray, 1996).

Digestive enzymes are directly related to digestion and the breakdown and absorption of food. They are present externally in raw or uncooked foods and internally in the digestive tract (Prochaska & Piekutowski, 1994). *Amylase* breaks down starch molecules into simple sugars; *protease* splits protein molecules into single amino acids; *lipase* helps to digest fat. These three enzymes are produced in the pancreas and act upon food as it enters the small intestine. The digestion of starch begins in the mouth when amylase in saliva is mixed with food (Valdez & Fox, 1991). Enzymes in food begin digestion in the upper portion of the stomach before the food is mixed with acid (Howell, 1985). Breast milk contains the necessary enzymes for its digestion, supporting the infant's immature digestive system and production of pancreatic enzymes (Heitlinger, 1983). In early human history, the enzymes from raw foods provided the major raw materials for digestion, allowing the pancreas to produce supportive enzymes. As the diet evolved to include more cooked and processed foods, this balance shifted. The high heat used in cooking destroys food enzymes, causing a complete reliance on the body to produce the enzymes needed for digestion. Some believe that this places a heavy stress on the body, which can create greater susceptibility to illness (Howell, 1985).

Often, children with feeding issues are unable to breast-feed and rely on processed formulas for early nutrition. Many must rely on formulas that are predigested because of allergies or digestive difficulty breaking down the milk protein (Billeaud, Guillet, & Sandler, 1990). Raw foods require skilled chewing, which is difficult or impossible for many children. Pasteurization of juices and dairy products subject them to heat and destroy food enzymes. Unless supplemental digestive enzymes are added to their diet, children must depend totally upon enzymes produced by the body. Children with cystic fibrosis have pancreatic insufficiency and must take pancreatic enzymes with meals.

Water and Digestion

The human body depends heavily on water for survival. The body of an infant is 70% to 85% water, while that of the adult is 60% to 70% water (Tamborlane, 1997). Water is also contained in the cells of foods in the diet. Fruits and vegetables consist of 80% to 90% water; meats are 50% water. Infants need 1½ ounces of liquid intake per pound each day, while adults need ½ to ¾ ounces of liquid per pound each day. Water is essential for digestion, absorption of nutrients, growth and repair of tissues, removal of waste products in the urine, and temperature control. The body also needs free water that is not bound in food (Batmanghelidj, 1995). The digestive system is heavily dependent upon water for efficient function. Children and adults who lack adequate water intake may experience a chronic subclinical dehydration that can contribute to reflux and other gastrointestinal problems. Water is recommended for all children and adults (Kleiner, 1999). The optimum amount of water varies with the age range and weight of the person. Infants who are on a total formula or breast milk diet do not need additional water in their diet. Although physicians frequently state this, researchers found that ¼ of a group of well-educated mothers gave their infants additional water at least three times a week during their first month (Scariati, Grummer-Strawn, & Fein, 1997). If too much water is given or the formula is diluted with water, the baby's body can release too much sodium in the urine, leading to seizures and brain damage (Borowitz & Rocco, 1986). Water should be added by age 6 months when the baby begins to eat solid foods (Tamborlane, 1997) and has a more mature urinary system. Children need the number of ounces equivalent to two-thirds of their body weight (Batmanghelidj, personal communication, 1996). For example, a child weighing 36 pounds needs 24 ounces of water, the equivalent of four 6-ounce glasses. When children reach the age of 10 to 12 years, their water needs approach that of adults. They need the number of ounces equivalent to half of their body weight. For example, an older child weighing 60 pounds needs 30 ounces of water). It is commonly stated that adults need a minimum of six to eight 8-ounce glasses of water per day. Juice, milk, tea, and soda do not count toward the daily allotment of water. The body needs clear fluid that is not a food requiring digestion (Batmanghelidj, 1995). Salt regulates the amount of water that is held in the area around the cells. When the individual doesn't drink enough water, the nervous system tries to keep sodium in the body to prevent additional fluid loss.

Batmanghelidj also suggests adding a pinch of salt on the tongue when giving water to older children and adults to stimulate the body's retention of water in the extra cellular tissues rather than its release by the kidneys. He says, "A pinch of salt on the tongue after drinking water fools the brain into thinking a lot of salt has arrived in the body" (1995).

In his book, *Your Body's Many Cries for Water,* Batmanghelidj (1995) makes a strong case for gastroesophageal reflux as a symptom of inadequate water intake. The stomach needs copious amounts of water for digestion. When the individual drinks a glass of water 30 minutes before a meal, it rapidly passes through the stomach and is absorbed by the intestine (Murray, Eddy, Bartoli, & Paul, 1994). As food is eaten a half hour later, the stomach wall secretes the same amount of water to mix with acids and enzymes and assist with digestion. Water is also essential in creating the watery bicarbonate solution that is secreted by the pancreas as the pyloric valve opens and moves the acid food solution from the stomach into the small intestines. If the body is chronically dehydrated, there may be inadequate production and release of this alkaline solution. In order to protect the delicate lining of the small intestine from acid, the pyloric valve may not open until enough of the bicarbonate solution has been manufactured and released. With the delay in gastric emptying, the lower esophageal sphincter may relax, allowing acid stomach contents to reflux into the esophagus.

It is commonly believed that the body requires a specific level of liquid intake—rather than a specific level of water intake—for health and well-being (Batmanghelidj, 1995). Because children with feeding problems usually receive the bulk of their nutrition through formula or pureed consistency foods, it often is assumed that they do not need additional water. It is also assumed that water will fill them up and reduce their desire to eat or their tolerance for tube feedings. Thus, fear of reduced caloric intake may contribute to the failure to give needed water. Formula is a food, which like most milks, fruits, and vegetables, has a high percentage of water. However, this does not replace the body's cellular need for clear water to provide optimum function of all cells and systems.

Stress and Digestion

Stress interferes with digestion. Stressors trigger a fight-or-flight sequence that pours adrenaline from the adrenal glands into the bloodstream, enabling the body to prepare for an emergency. Blood is directed toward the muscles of the extremities and away from the digestive system. With less focus on the gastrointestinal system, digestion slows down and becomes incomplete or inefficient. When stress is chronic, the digestive system is unable to operate at peak efficiency.

There are many stressors in the lives of children with feeding problems. They are asked to adapt to many unfamiliar adults in health care, education, and rehabilitation. Frequent hospitalizations for illness and surgery may be part of their life. Medications create added stresses by creating side effects and imbalances in bodily systems as they are directed at specific problems or diagnoses. Children who experience a noxious, defensiveness response to environmental sensations (such as touch, movement, sound, light) are constantly triggering the fight-or-flight reaction and accompanying stress (Wilbarger & Wilbarger, 1991). In addition, feeding itself can be stressful. Physical tension may interfere with the child's ability to move the mouth efficiently or coordinate breathing with sucking and swallowing. Anxiety and fear of choking can be part of the mealtime experience for many children. Tastes and textures may trigger oral sensory defensiveness and high levels of stress. Children are usually very sensitive to the moods and emotions of their parents and the people who feed them. When the feeder is anxious because the child is not eating, the child shares this anxiety. If children feel that they are being pushed or forced to eat, they may respond with strong emotions that reduce digestive comfort for eating. Children whose lives are stressed may not utilize food nutrients adequately for growth.

Eating foods with an appropriate amount of each vitamin and mineral does not guarantee that the body can use the nutrients. All nutrients are not available to the body in the same way. Breast milk contains a low level of iron and zinc. Yet the body utilizes these minerals in breast milk more efficiently than the same level in cow's milk or soy formulas (Lonnerdal, 1985). For this reason, iron, zinc, and other trace minerals have been added to infant formulas to increase their bioavailability. Foods that are eaten at the same time influence each other, either supporting or interfering with the level of specific nutrients that the body can use. High amounts of fiber and substances known as phytates found in cereal products reduce the absorption of minerals such as calcium, magnesium, zinc, and manganese (Greger, 1999; Solomons, 1982). Lactose in milk increases the absorption of calcium and other minerals (Ziegler & Fomon, 1983). High levels of zinc inhibit the intestinal absorption of copper, resulting in a potential copper deficiency (Sandstead, 1995b). Many other interactions among specific vitamins and minerals in food are widely accepted (Sears & Sears, 1999). Vitamin C improves the absorption of calcium and iron. Iron from animal sources is more easily absorbed than iron from plants. The body absorbs fat-soluble vitamins (A, D, E, and K) only when meals contain fat. Soft drinks such as soda pop that contain citric or phosphoric acid decrease absorption of calcium. Foods high in phosphorus (e.g., meat, poultry, corn, potatoes) also interfere with calcium absorption. Oxalic acid in spinach reduces the amount of iron absorbed, but this effect is reduced when vitamin C is present in the meal. Stress can reduce the absorption of calcium.

These interactions are extremely complex yet they can provide guidelines for maximizing the body's ability to absorb nutrients. This is particularly critical for children with feeding difficulties who have trouble eating larger amounts or a sufficient variety of foods. It makes sense to serve iron-fortified orange juice or fruits and vegetables that contain high levels of vitamin C (e.g., broccoli, tomatoes, peppers, potatoes, papaya, strawberries, cantaloupe) with plant foods containing iron (e.g., iron-fortified breakfast cereals, whole grain bread, tofu). Meat, poultry, and fish also increase the iron absorption from plants. Combining meat and vegetables in the same meal will increase iron absorption more than eating either alone. The absorption of iron from cereal or toast will be increased when orange or papaya juice is included in the same breakfast. Because vitamin C also increases calcium absorption, a breakfast of cereal, milk, and a citrus juice is a nutritional powerhouse for increasing bioavailability.

The issues of bioavailability and nutrient interaction strongly support the widely accepted perspective that it is preferable to get the required nutrients from a wise selection of foods than through vitamin and mineral supplements. Many children are not getting the needed nutrients through their diet or require higher levels of specific nutrients. Children with feeding difficulties and erratic eating patterns may be at particularly high risk for being unable to take in and absorb all that they need from the diet. Medications that the child receives may reduce the absorption of specific nutrients. In these instances, a dietitian or physician may recommend the use of a balanced vitamin and mineral supplement or the addition of specific nutrient supplements. Special health needs are discussed on pages 341–350.

Metabolism

Once food is digested and nutrients are absorbed into the bloodstream, the body goes through a series of physical and chemical processes known as metabolism. This complex series of conversions enables the body to utilize the nutrients for energy and the growth and functioning of all its systems. Metabolism takes place through an intricate set of biochemical interactions that are influenced by the genes, the individual's stage of development, and the environment. Inherited enzyme abnormalities, diseases of endocrine organs, or liver failure cause a series of diseases and abnormalities (Wharton & Scott, 1996). Many metabolic disorders include feeding difficulties because of their negative impact on neurological function, sensory processing, and gastrointestinal function. These children require complex nutritional interventions to sustain their life and well-being (Giovannini, Biasucci, Luotti,

Fiori, & Riva, 1995). Some children lack an enzyme that enables them to utilize specific nutritional components. For example, children with phenylketonuria (PKU) are born without the enzyme that enables them to metabolize the amino acid phenylalanine (Start, 1998). When this amino acid is not utilized, it builds up in the blood and causes mental retardation and other abnormalities. Screening tests for PKU are required at birth so that children with this metabolic disorder can be placed immediately on a formula that does not contain phenylalanine. A diet excluding foods such as meat, fish, eggs, milk, cheese, legumes, and nuts is continued at least through adolescence. Many vegetables and fruits are allowed in very small amounts. Special low-protein breads and pastas are used to supplement the diet. The diets of children with metabolic disorders must be monitored carefully and additional supplements may be provided to prevent nutritional deficiencies that can result from an unbalanced intake of food nutrients (Kishnani, Boney, & Chen, 1999; Krasnewich & Gahl, 1997; Scheinberg & Sternlieb, 1996; Yannicelli, Rohr, & Warman, 1994).

Many children and adults experience abdominal pain, gas, and diarrhea as the result of a deficiency in lactase, an enzyme responsible for the absorption of lactose, the predominant sugar in milk (Rings, Grand, & Buller, 1994). Lactose intolerance reduces the ability of the body to digest and metabolize milk. The amount of lactase in the body is dependent upon racial, ethnic, age, and gastrointestinal factors. Humans gradually lose the lactase enzyme after infancy, beginning by age 2 with resultant difficulties in digesting milk in later childhood and adulthood (Wang et al., 1998). Genetic mutations in prehistory resulted in a preservation of lactase activity in the majority of the adult population in Northern and Central Europe. "In North American adults lactose maldigestion is found in approximately 79% of Native Americans, 75% of blacks, 51% of Hispanics, and 21% of Caucasians. In Africa, Asia, and Latin America prevalence rates range from 15% to 100% depending on the population studied" (Scrimshaw & Murray, 1988, p. 1,079). A secondary lactase deficiency occurs when the intestinal mucosa is damaged during influenza and other gastrointestinal illnesses (Boudraa et al., 1990; Sears & Sears, 1999). Treatment for lactose intolerance includes the use of soy and other formulas that do not contain lactose, reduction in milk intake, and the use of yogurt and other fermented dairy products, and the addition of a lactase supplement (Sinden & Sutphen, 1991; Suarez, Savaiano, & Levitt, 1995; Varela-Moreiras, Antoine, Ruiz-Roso, & Varela, 1992).

A child's basal metabolic rate (BMR) plays a significant role in determining the number of calories needed in the diet. The BMR is the energy (measured in calories) that the body expends in maintaining normal resting body functions such as heart rate, respiration, muscle tone, and regulation of body temperature. BMR is influenced by age, weight, height, gender, environmental temperature, dieting, and exercise. Infants and children have a higher or faster metabolic rate than adolescents or adults because of the additional energy needed for cellular growth. Restrictive dieting slows down the metabolic rate to conserve energy. Metabolic rate is also influenced by thyroid hormones. When there is an inadequate level of thyroid hormones in the system, the metabolic rate is reduced. When thyroid hormone levels are too high, the metabolic rate is increased. Basal metabolism accounts for approximately 75% of the calories that are burned each day to provide energy. In addition to the energy baseline determined by the BMR, the body needs calories to support different levels of activity. A child who is very active has a higher metabolic rate than a child who is sedentary. Metabolism is essentially the speed at which the body's motor is running. A child with a rapid metabolism burns calories more quickly and needs more calories in the diet than a child who has a slow metabolic rate.

Helping Children Utilize the Foods They Eat

The following general strategies can help children's bodies use the foods that they eat more effectively and efficiently.

- **Reduce stress surrounding mealtimes.** Be aware of stressors that surround mealtime for the child and parents. Incorporate strategies to enhance the learning and communication environments that are discussed in Chapter 12. These may include exploring belief systems that contribute to stress; enhancing the child's mealtime communication skills; finding alternatives to forcing children to eat; and the inclusion of music, imagery, and playfulness to reduce stress.

- **Be aware of the child's medical needs and their impact on nutrition.** Every feeding therapist should have a thorough knowledge of the child's underlying medical condition and special nutritional needs that are associated with the diagnosis or medications that the child is taking. If feeding therapists do not read food labels carefully, they may inadvertently introduce foods in therapy or at home that contain substances that may be harmful to the child.

- **Provide support for efficient digestion.** Evaluate the amount of water in the child's diet and gradually increase the intake of clear water to support digestion. Discuss safe levels of water intake with the pediatrician or dietitian, especially for infants with immature kidney function or children with cardiac or kidney disorders that may reduce the ability to excrete fluid in the urine. Consider the use of supplemental digestive enzymes such as freeze-dried green papaya (containing papain) or pineapple (containing bromelain), which enhance the breakdown of food and increase absorption. Be aware of food combinations that are physically comfortable for individual children and those that are not. Some children, for example, seem to produce gas and experience gastrointestinal discomfort when they eat fruits with or following meats. When fruits are given alone at the beginning of a meal, the child does not experience these symptoms. These patterns can be unique to a specific child. They should be honored in creating mealtime suggestions for that child even if there is no research that indicates that the combination pattern applies to larger groups of children. See Maximizing Nutrition for Children with Special Health Needs on pages 350–351 for specific guidelines for supporting digestion.

- **Provide parents with meal suggestions to increase the bioavailability of nutrients.** Help families create meals that contain food combinations that increase the bioavailability of fat-soluble vitamins, calcium, iron, and zinc. Because vitamin C strongly increases the bioavailability of calcium and iron, foods high in vitamin C or a powdered vitamin C supplement should be included at all meals.

Output

Input is Defined by the Output Required

The number of calories and specific levels of nutrients required by children depend on a number of interrelated factors that are considered by dietitians who make dietary recommendations.

The amount and type of growth differ according to the child's age. Infants grow very rapidly during the first 6 to 12 months. They typically double their birthweight during their first 4 to 6 months. Between 12 and 18 months of age, toddlers show a strong drop in growth along with a marked reduction in appetite and caloric intake. The requirements for different macronutrients and micronutrients are also age related. For example, infants and toddlers require a higher percentage of fat in the diet than older children.

Caloric needs also are defined by body weight. Between 6 and 12 months of age, infants need 50 calories per pound each day (i.e., 850 calories for a 17-pound child). The per-pound amount drops to 46 calories between 1 and 3 years of age (i.e., 900–1,800 calories) and to 41 calories between 4 and 6 years of age (i.e., 1,300–2,300 calories) (Tamborlane, 1997). Additional calories usually are recommended to provide catch-up growth when children experience growth failure (Krick, Murphy, Markham, & Shapiro, 1992; Maggioni & Lifshitz, 1995).

The child's activity level strongly influences the BMR and the speed with which the body burns calories. Physical activity stimulates a higher BMR, which requires more energy in the form of calories to support the resting functions of the body. When children are sedentary because of a physical disability or an addiction to television and potato chips, they burn calories more slowly. They often take in more calories than their bodies need, which can result in obesity.

This interplay among age, weight, and physical activity creates many challenges for dietitians and physicians in recommending an appropriate diet for children with special needs. Many children with feeding problems weigh less and are smaller than other children of the same chronological age. Their activity level may differ from typically developing children. Because of their smaller size, their caloric needs may be closer to those of a younger child, while their nutrient needs are defined by their chronological age. They may be sedentary because of problems with postural tone and movement, yet have greater caloric needs because of chronic muscle contractions that burn calories.

Many children with motor-based feeding difficulties due to athetoid cerebral palsy become physically tense during meals or increase their involuntary movements. These limiting motor patterns increase their difficulty with oral motor coordination for eating and result in a reduction in food intake. Calories supply the energy for respiration, digestion, and other body functions during the meal. However, when a child's muscles are contracting and the body is moving during the meal, additional calories are burned (Johnson, Goran, Ferrara, & Poehlman, 1996). Some children appear to burn almost as many calories as they take in during meals.

Although the focal problem for most children with feeding problems is inadequate growth and weight gain, the opposite problem can occur when children are placed on feeding tubes. When the child is already undernourished or is at risk of failure-to-thrive, calories are added to the diet to support catch-up growth. In their enthusiasm to help the child gain weight, professionals may base the child's dietary intake on chronological age. However, many of these children have increased or decreased postural tone and are less active than other children (Stallings, Zemel, Davies, Cronk, & Charney, 1996). Many of these children become obese and experience greater difficulties with movement because of their weight gain. Other children who have genetic disorders that are associated with a lower activity level or metabolic rate can gain too much weight on a diet based primarily on their age and weight (Chad, Jobling, & Frail, 1990; Giordano, 1992; Jun Tze, Dunn, & Rothstein, 1981).

The level of nutrients in the diet is closely correlated with the number of calories eaten. When large amounts of different foods are eaten, it is much easier to get the amount and diversity of nutrients that are required for health and growth. When individuals restrict their caloric intake either through dieting or feeding difficulties, it is extremely difficult for them to support their nutritional needs through the concept of a balanced diet. For this reason, many children with feeding difficulties require dietary supplements to support their nutritional needs.

Helping Children Balance Intake With Energy Output

The following general strategies can help parents and professionals provide appropriate recommendations for calories in the child's diet based on activity level.

- **Reduce muscle tone and extraneous movement that burns calories at mealtimes.** Information in Chapter 14 stressed the importance of body tone and movement on the oral mechanism and feeding. Because increased tone and involuntary movement also burn calories, it is important to help children develop quiet, relaxed bodies during mealtimes. When children burn fewer calories at mealtime, their overall caloric needs are somewhat reduced. This can make a big difference for children who are not able to take in larger amounts of food.

- **Identify ways to encourage more pleasurable physical activity in children with low tone or low activity levels.** Low tone or low activity levels often influence children's low appetites and low caloric intake. Greater physical activity can stimulate a higher metabolic rate and increase the body's internal signals for taking in more food.

- **Provide feedback to physicians and dietitians on children's activity levels that influence caloric needs.** It is often difficult for physicians and dietitians to identify children's activity levels. Different children with the same diagnosis may have very different activity levels. Children may be more withdrawn or more agitated than normal when they visit the dietitian. Activity levels and corresponding nutrient and caloric needs often change and require changes in the child's diet. Children typically see feeding therapists more frequently than they see dietitians. Clinicians can provide feedback to physicians and dietitians that results in more appropriate dietary recommendations as changes occur.

Meeting the Child's Nutritional Needs

The initial sections of this chapter have addressed the theoretical and practical issues involved in providing an appropriate diet for children. Implications for children with special needs have been discussed in general terms. The remainder of the chapter includes specific strategies and suggestions for addressing the nutritional needs of children with special feeding needs.

Increasing Calories

Many children who have oral motor difficulties or feeding problems have difficulty gaining weight. Feeding therapists need to work with dietitians, physicians, and families to determine ways to supplement the diet and improve the child's chances of growing properly.

The goal is to add calories and nutrients, not bulk, to the diet. Typically, these children have a tiny stomach with limited space for food. Feeding may take a long time, and usually the children become tired of eating before adequate nutrition is consumed. Rather than filling the available space and time with empty calories or food that is low in nutritional value, we want every ounce of intake to count. This can be done by adding foods that increase both the caloric and nutrient density of the meal.

Three meals a day may not be adequate for underweight children. Many mini-meals may provide a more consistent source of calories. All meals should be high in nutrition, high in calories, and as low in volume as possible. Calories should come from protein, fat, and unrefined carbohydrates. Refined carbohydrates such as sugar may add calories but are not as helpful for lasting growth and development.

Increasing caloric density should be done carefully and with the guidance and feedback of a dietitian, especially when working with infants. The term ***osmolality*** is used to describe the level of concentration in a liquid formula. When the level of concentration is too high, the kidneys may draw too much water into the urine, depleting the body of water and causing dehydration. This occurs primarily when the diet includes too much salt or protein. Because the kidneys of infants under 6 months of age have more trouble concentrating and retaining urine, the risk of water loss and dehydration from a diet that is too concentrated is increased.

Protein Calories

Protein foods such as milk, eggs, beans, legumes, meat, poultry, fish, seeds, and nuts are important for growth. Extra protein calories can be added to meals in some of these ways:

- Add ¼ cup powdered nonfat milk to 1 cup fluid milk; 2 cups mashed potatoes; 1 cup uncooked cereal; 2 cups flour (in recipes for cornbread, pancakes, etc.); 2 cups gravy, cream sauce, or pudding; milk shakes; or juice drinks.
- Add an instant breakfast powder to milk.
- Serve beans or peas in sauces made with cheese and milk.
- Give frequent snacks of crackers, tortillas, or bread spread with cream cheese, peanut butter, cashew butter, almond butter, liverwurst and other soft meats, or egg salad.
- Mix tuna fish with cream cheese. Use oil-packed tuna, which has more calories per ounce than water-packed tuna.
- Add an extra whole egg to raw foods that are to be cooked, such as puddings, macaroni and cheese, ground meats, and pancakes.
- Sprinkle Parmesan cheese on meats and vegetables.
- Add ground sunflower seeds, sesame seeds, or almonds to cereals or vegetables.

Adding more fat to the diet will increase calories without adding bulk. Remember that fat has 9 calories per gram, while protein and carbohydrates have 4 calories per gram.

- Emphasize vegetable oils such as flaxseed or canola and cold water fish that supply high levels of the essential fatty acids (omega-3 and omega-6). Avoid or reduce the use of foods with hydrogenated or partially hydrogenated oils that create trans-fatty acids that interfere with the body's ability to utilize the essential fatty acids.
- Medium chain triglicerides (MCT) oil is frequently recommended for infants and children with vulnerable digestive systems because it is easy to digest. It can be used as an energy supplement to boost calories but should not be the child's main fat source because it provides no essential fatty acids.
- Add butter or oil to meats, vegetables, hot cereals, and cooked desserts.
- Mayonnaise, sour cream, and salad dressings can be served on vegetables, meats, sandwiches, and fruit salads.
- Include peanut butter and other nut butters that are high in oil.
- Cream and ice cream have a high fat content.
- Add heavy cream to puddings.
- Mix fruit-sweetened ketchup or yogurt with 1 to 3 teaspoons of flax oil to get rid of the oily taste and make it more palatable to children.
- Avocados are high in fat and calories. They are excellent for softer diets.

Increasing the amount of fat in the diet can increase the child's exposure to pesticides and chemicals. These substances are fat-soluble and are more likely to accumulate in fatty or oily food. Pesticides are more harmful to children than to adults because of a child's smaller size and more rapid metabolism. Maximum acceptable levels of pesticides and chemicals defined by the government have been based on adult weights and eating patterns. Children eat proportionately more of a contaminated food on a volume-per-weight basis (Sears & Sears, 1999). This is particularly true when additional fats are added to the diet to increase weight gain. Many fish that are high in essential fatty acids (e.g., tuna, salmon) may have high levels of toxic minerals such as mercury that come from the environmentally polluted plants they eat. These toxins are stored in the fish oil and passed on to children and adults who eat the fish. Research has been mixed in this area, with some studies showing little or no impact on children's mercury levels and development while others have indicated a potential risk (Davidson et al., 1998; Knobeloch, Ziarnik, Anderson, & Dodson, 1995; Myers et al., 1997). Some individuals are more sensitive than others, and some fish carry higher levels of environmental pollutants. Thus, it is extremely difficult to predict the risk for a given child. Foods such as canned tuna and salmon are favorite foods for many children with feeding problems. Their beneficial role in the diet (i.e., easy to eat, high in calories and essential fatty acids) must be balanced with the potential risk of mercury pollution when eaten in large amounts. Parents can be encouraged to purchase "certified organic" vegetable and dairy foods that are high in fats such as oils, peanuts, butter, and nuts. Because of the more stringent restrictions on pesticide use in the United States than in other countries, imported produce usually contains a higher level of pesticides than American-grown foods.

Increased amounts of fat can be problematic for some children with feeding problems. It takes the digestive system longer to process fats, which slows down gastric emptying. This may cause or increase gastroesophageal reflux for some children, especially those who already have a problem with delayed gastric emptying. Children who are at risk of aspiration also will have more problems when lipids (fats) enter the lungs. Some children whose appetite is poor may become less interested in eating because fats stay with them for a longer period of time.

Caloric Values of Specific High Nutritional Foods

The foods in Table 16.4 can be added to a child's diet without substantially increasing the volume of food taken.

Table 16.4 **High Nutritional Foods**

Food	Amount	Calories
Ground sunflower seeds	1 oz. (1/4 cup)	159
Ground sesame seeds	1 oz. (1/4 cup)	155
Ground almonds	1 oz. (1/4 cup)	170
Flax oil	1 Tbsp.	150
Dried powdered milk	1/4 cup	182
Untoasted wheat germ	1 oz. (1/4 cup)	110
Ground raisins	1/4 cup	190
Honey*	1 Tbsp.	61
Natural maple syrup	1 Tbsp.	50
Soluble rice bran	3 Tbsp.	83
Grated Parmesan cheese	1 oz.	143

* Because of the danger of botulism, honey should not be given to an infant under 12 months of age.

The foods in Table 16.5 can be used as a base for a meal. They are high in calories and nutrition, and children usually enjoy them. The nut butters may be served alone or mixed in a blender with cream cheese, ricotta or cottage cheese, or tofu. Mixing tuna with a binder such as cream cheese may make it easier for the child who has difficulty handling foods that separate or have lumps.

Table 16.5 **Food Sources Used as a Base for a Meal**

Food	Amount	Calories
Peanut butter	1 Tbsp.	100
Cashew butter	1 Tbsp.	105
Almond butter	1 Tbsp.	105
Cream cheese	1 oz.	100
All cheeses except "low fat"	1 oz.	100
Mashed avocado	1/2 cup	194
Sweet potato or yam	4 oz.	155
Tuna packed in oil	3.5 oz.	268

Some foods increase their protein value when they are combined with other foods. The following combinations create a complete vegetable protein needed for full utilization by the body. These foods do not have to be served at the same meal.

- Grains and dairy products
- Grains and legumes (including peanuts)
- Legumes and dairy products
- Grains and seeds

All nuts and seeds should be finely ground and refrigerated. Because of their high fat content, they can become rancid if stored in an open, warm environment. Rancidity destroys vitamins in the body. Salted products should never be given.

Increasing Dietary Diversity

The concept of dietary diversity is at the core of creating a balanced diet that will support children's health and well-being. It emerges from an understanding of its importance for all children and should be at the heart of every feeding program. Guiding or changing a child's diet requires an understanding of dietary choices for the entire family. The foods selected for a family diet vary considerably, depending upon family values, culture, socioeconomic factors, and the time available for preparing meals. In addition, advertising accompanying children's television programs encourages children to ask for specific food brands associated with their favorite television personalities. Cereals with high levels of refined sugar and artificial coloring may be chosen for the child with a feeding problem primarily because they are eaten by other children in the family. A daily trip to a fast food restaurant for hamburgers, french fries, and a special toy may be part of the family culture.

Toddler's food preferences mirror the preferences of other family members (Skinner, Carruth, Moran, Houck, Schmidhammer, et al., 1998). The adult diet is markedly deficient in vegetables. Many children never see adults eating and liking vegetables. Yet parents often are confused and concerned because their children don't like vegetables. Children need and use adult models in setting their life-long eating patterns. Children develop a taste for the types of foods to which they are introduced. Many families are unaware of dietary guidelines or incorrectly feel that preparing meals with fresh foods requires too much time or money (Satter, 1999). Feeding therapists can become gentle guides in educating parents and children about food choices.

Many youngsters who are just learning to eat discover cookies, candy, chips, and fast food restaurants through their therapy programs. When these are offered as the first choice and the children accept them because of their high levels of salt and sugar, it may be very difficult to help children transition to healthier foods. Questionable food choices may not make a lot of difference in the early period if children are supported nutritionally by formula or tube feeding. However, if a wide variety of healthy choices is not introduced early, it may interfere with children's ability to move to oral feeding. Suggestions for offering a variety of health-promoting foods should be introduced gradually throughout the feeding program. From the beginning, tastes of new foods can be introduced and parents can be guided and supported in offering all children in the family a wider variety of foods. Dietary diversity can be supported in children who are eating very small amounts of food by preparing larger amounts of food and freezing it into meal-size portions. Either homemade or commercial pureed or lumpy food can be frozen in ice cube trays and covered with clear plastic. The frozen cubes then can be removed from the tray and placed in airtight freezer bags. Parents can thaw out small amounts for meals or tasting sessions.

Many therapists and parents believe that the amount of food eaten by the child is more important than the type of food, especially if the child is receiving a tube feeding formula. Children can become stuck in eating only sweet foods, such as pudding or ice cream, or limit their eating to a single food category, such as dairy foods. Once these habits are established, it is difficult to change them. It is more time efficient to focus on a wider variety of foods from all food groups and build good eating habits from the very beginning. In encouraging children to eat a wider variety of foods, it is important not to use desserts or other sweet foods as a reward for eating other foods. This strategy teaches children that these sweet foods are highly valued and encourages them to want more of them. Children often think that if you have to bribe them to eat a specific food, there must be something wrong with it! Several research studies have shown that rewarding children for eating a specific food actually decreased their liking for the food (Birch et al., 1984; Newman & Taylor, 1992).

Specific suggestions for increasing dietary diversity in children who are picky eaters are incorporated in Chapters 16 and 23. These include ideas for reducing the impact of limiting sensorimotor problems that interfere with the acceptance of taste and texture, providing opportunities for children to explore new foods and the frequent reintroduction of foods that have been refused.

Breast-fed infants are introduced to many aspects of a diversified diet shortly after birth. The fat content of the mother's milk varies at different points in the meal (Wagner, Anderson, & Pittard, 1996) and the milk takes on the taste of foods that the mother has included in her diet (Mennella, 1995). Infants and young children who are unable to take nutrients by mouth usually are limited in receiving a diversified diet. Like the bottle-fed infant, the baby who receives tube feedings generally is given a single formula during the first 6 months. However, this singular dietary formula is continued, and the body receives none of the normal variation found in whole foods that are associated with typical growth and development. The formula usually is changed as the child grows and requires a higher level of nutrients and calories; however, a formula similar to the infant formula generally is recommended. For example, if babies have been on a soy formula, a standard soy formula often is introduced when they are ready for a higher calorie formula.

Because of swallowing and gastrointestinal problems, many of these infants are not introduced to oral feeding until they are toddlers. Often, there is a strong resistance to accepting pureed foods by mouth. Some of this resistance may be due to a lack of familiarity with dietary diversity in the gastrointestinal tract as well as in the mouth. Theoretically and clinically, there is a strong advantage to creating diversity within the tube-feeding diet, beginning at 6 months when other infants would be experiencing a wider variety of foods. This can be done through the rotation of formulas; the addition of tiny amounts of different grains, fruits, vegetables, and meats to the child's formula; or the use of homemade formulas. In addition to providing gastrointestinal diversity, small changes in smell and taste are added as the infant experiences the odor of different formulas during burps.

Commercial Formulas

Most physicians and dietitians recommend commercial formulas for a number of reasons. Ingredients are standardized, and calories, macronutrients, and micronutrients are targeted for children of a given weight and age range. In addition, cans of a processed formula are easier for parents to give their children because no food preparation is involved. However, these formulas lack dietary diversity and a multiplicity of micronutrients that are present in whole foods. Hundreds of phytonutrients that are present in fruits and vegetables are not included in any processed formula, no matter how good the formula may be in other respects (see page 320).

The easiest way to introduce a tube-fed child to greater dietary diversity is to mix small amounts of a wide variety of pureed foods into the child's formula. The initial amounts should be very tiny (i.e., ⅛ teaspoon) and gradually increased as the child shows no adverse reactions to the new food. New foods can be added gradually, with different foods offered at each meal. The amount added to the formula will depend upon the child's gastrointestinal system and the volume of liquid that can be taken comfortably into the stomach. These small amounts of food are an addition to the tube-feeding formula, not a replacement for it.

Formulas can be rotated on a 3- or 4-day cycle so that a child receives a formula with different nutritional protein and carbohydrate components each day of the period. This is an important option for some children who have food allergies or sensitivities. Unless the child has been identified with a clear allergy to specific foods (which should be eliminated), formulas with cow's milk, soy, casein, and beef can be selected and rotated. Formula rotation should be introduced gradually. One formula at a time can be added in order to identify formulas that may not agree with the child. The new formula initially should be diluted and gradually increased to full strength. When two formulas are accepted well, a third one can be added. Children with food sensitivities may show a withdrawal reaction when the food is eliminated from the diet. If this is not recognized, a caregiver may assume that the negative response is to the new formula, rather than to the elimination of an addictive formula. Formulas should be rotated on a daily basis, not on a meal basis. Any changes in formula should be made under the direction of a dietitian or physician.

Homemade Formulas

Many older infants and children are much better off eating a pureed whole food diet instead of a commercial enteral formula. There is greater gastrointestinal comfort for some children and reduced gastroesophageal reflux. This may be related to greater dietary diversity or to the heavier weight of food that enters the stomach and stays there with greater ease. Some children seem to be sensitive to chemicals or other additives used during the processing of commercial formulas. They can handle similar food ingredients without a problem. When processed formulas are stopped or reduced, these children feel better and have more energy, less congestion, and less gastrointestinal discomfort. Clinically, it often is easier to help children move from tube feedings to oral feedings when their systems have had experience with different foods. Children who have been on the same set of formulas all of their lives seem to have more resistance to moving into a varied food diet orally, providing they are ready to make the transition.

Homemade tube-feeding formulas provide the answer for many children and families. Their preparation and use requires a commitment from parents and collaboration between the parents and dietitian. Simply blenderizing food does not guarantee an adequate diet. High quality foods should be selected and given in accordance with serving recommendations from the Food Guide Pyramid.

The major challenges in creating a workable homemade formula include:

- selecting, combining, and blenderizing ingredients so that they will pass through the tube without clogging it
- providing the appropriate calorie and nutrient levels in as small a volume as possible

Some foods require a great deal of liquid to blenderize them enough to go through the tube. If too much liquid is used, the volume of food may exceed the child's stomach capacity. This can result in an inadequate intake of calories and nutrients or more frequent meals. Often, parents must experiment with food alternatives recommended by the dietitian until the right combination is discovered for their child.

Many parents have found that the easiest homemade formulas are created by blending prepared baby foods with milk or formula, then adding oils or specific food supplements that can increase calories and nutrients. Often, this is the best alternative for older infants and toddlers whose diets generally include these types of food. Commercial baby foods are convenient, and fruits and vegetables are grown with fewer pesticides than are used for fresh nonorganic foods available in the supermarket. In some instances, commercially prepared baby foods actually are better choices than home-prepared foods. For example, home-prepared spinach, beets, turnips, and collard greens contain high levels of nitrates that can interfere with the body's use of iron. Commercially prepared baby foods of these vegetables are safe because the manufacturers must test for nitrates.

Homemade baby foods or formulas created from fresh foods are closest to the diet eaten by other children. Locally grown fruits and vegetables that are vine-ripened before picking offer high levels of nutrients. Many families live in areas where a selection of organically grown fruits and vegetables are available. Meat, poultry, and fish also may be available from animals raised without antibiotics.

Increasing Nutrients

The focus on dietary diversity is a simple way to provide children with the variety of nutrients needed by their bodies. However, this by itself may not be enough for many children. In making every bite count, parents and therapists must learn to make wise choices among foods in the grocery store. In many instances, food supplements may be needed to provide the full array and amount of nutrients needed by the child.

Food Supplements

Many dietitians and physicians support the use of targeted nutritional supplements for all children in a given age range. In some instances, specific vitamins or minerals are added to commercially available foods for infants and children. For example, vitamin D is added to cow's milk, and iron is added to infant cereals. In other cases, a general multivitamin and mineral supplement for infants or children may be recommended. In still other situations, specific supplements of vitamins A and C, zinc, selenium, or iron may be recommended (Bendich & Langseth, 1995; Curtis, 1990; Sandstead, 1995a; Wasantwisut, 1997).

Special nutritional needs or deficiencies as a result of eating patterns, medications, or medical diagnosis also must be considered. The addition of nutritional supplements such as zinc may have a positive impact on the child's feeding program by increasing appetite even if zinc levels are only marginally low (Krebs, Hambidge, & Walravens, 1984).

Identifying nutritional deficiencies and recommending specific vitamin and mineral supplements requires the specialized knowledge of a skilled dietitian. An excess of some nutrients can contribute to secondary deficits in others. High levels of some nutrients can lead to severe toxicity and even death (McGuire et al., 2000).

Feeding therapists, however, can play a major role in modeling healthy food choices in therapy and creating treatment directions and goals that increase the nutritional value of foods that children eat. In addition, they can inform parents about special food supplements with high nutritional content. These supplements are foods, not isolated vitamin or mineral supplements. The specific foods, manufacturers, and distributors change over time. Please refer to Chapter 17.

Choices at the Supermarket and in Therapy

Feeding therapists and parents face a barrage of choices at the supermarket. Different variations of the same category of food can make a major difference in the nutritional quality of a child's diet. Differences in brands may reflect different ingredients or methods of preparation. The following ideas contribute to developing healthy food choices in the feeding program:

- Read labels and understand what they tell you about the food ingredients and processing.

- Select whole wheat bread instead of white bread or generic wheat bread. Read labels and look for 100% whole wheat as the first ingredient listed. Whole wheat contains the outer bran layer and the inner germ of the wheat kernel. The bran layer adds fiber to the diet, while the germ delivers vitamins B6 and E, folic acid, copper, magnesium, manganese, and zinc. Wheat bread is made from refined wheat flour with the bran and germ removed.

- Include the following nutrient-rich foods in the child's diet whenever possible: avocado; chickpeas; eggs; fish; flax seeds and oil; kidney beans; lentils; sweet potatoes; tofu; tomatoes; whole grains; plain, nonfat yogurt; almonds; artichokes; broccoli; cantaloupe; garlic; orange; papaya; peanut butter; peppers; pink grapefruit; sunflower seeds; and turkey. Sears and Sears (1999) include these in the "Top Twelve Foods" for a child's diet.

- Avoid the following junk foods whenever possible: beef jerky; colored, sweetened cereals; doughnuts; potato chips; gelatin desserts; candies; punch; sodas; juice drinks; and marshmallows. Sears and Sears (1999) call these "The Terrible Ten Junk Foods."

- Think natural color when choosing foods. Build on children's interest in bright colors and let them know that foods that have strong natural coloring (red, pink, orange, yellow, dark green, blue, dark purple, and dark red) are health-building foods.

- Avoid foods that have high levels of sugar, white flour, saturated fat, hydrogenated oils, food dyes (yellow No. 6, red No. 40, blue No. 2, blue No. 1), salt, and caffeine.

- Hard cheeses, such as Parmesan, are higher in calcium but lower in fat and calories than soft cheeses.

- Offer a wide variety of fresh fruits, which can satisfy a child's desire for sweetness as well as provide important nutrients. Fruits should be washed in a mild detergent and peeled to remove pesticides. Raspberries and strawberries cannot be peeled, often retain high pesticide levels, and are difficult to clean because of their rough texture. The avocado has the highest nutritional value of all fruits. It is high in protein, fiber, vitamin E, niacin, thiamin, riboflavin, folic acid, and zinc. Most of its calories come from monosaturated fat with a trace of essential fatty acids (omega-3). For this reason, it is very high in calories. Bananas are high in potassium and are excellent for children who must take a diuretic for cardiac problems because diuretics deplete potassium in the body. Papaya is high in calcium, folic acid, vitamin C, and fiber. It is a very low-acid fruit, containing digestive enzymes that are well tolerated by children with gastroesophageal reflux. Pineapple also contains digestive enzymes and is the highest fruit for manganese. Oranges and grapefruits are very high in vitamin C.

- Infants and young children are genetically programmed to prefer sweet foods. Therefore, fruits often are easier to introduce than vegetables. Vegetables with a sweeter taste, such as carrots, sweet potatoes and yams, are good choices for a child's first vegetables. Sweet potatoes are more nutrient-dense than white potatoes and provide higher amounts of fiber, beta-carotene, folic acid, and calcium.

- Buy locally grown fruits and vegetables whenever possible. Many **fresh** foods are picked before they are ripe and spend a great deal of time in shipment and sitting at the grocery store. These fruits and vegetables have lost many nutrients by the time they are eaten.

- Buy only **natural** fruit and vegetable juices. Avoid juice drinks (i.e., juice cocktails, juice punch) that are mostly sugar. Juices such as white grape, orange, grapefruit, lemon, pineapple, strawberry, raspberry, and blackberry are friendlier to the intestines. Juices such as prune, pear, cherry, peach, and apple ferment more easily and fill the large intestine with gas. This can result in abdominal pain and diarrhea if children drink large amounts of them.

- Fruit nectars (e.g., papaya, mango, apricot, peach, pear, prune) contain more fiber and are more nutrient dense than thin juices. Their greater thickness can be important for children with swallowing problems. Vegetable juices such as carrot and tomato juice are more nutrient dense than fruit juice. Mixing small amounts of vegetable juice with sweeter fruit juices can help children learn to like and accept the taste of vegetables.

- Include soy foods such as tofu and soy beverages as a foundation for fruit smoothies. The blend of soy and fruit creates a high-powered, nutritional breakfast or lunch. Tofu is very bland and absorbs the taste of foods with which it is mixed. It also can be mixed with spaghetti sauce in pasta dishes. Tofu is a nutrient-dense food that is high in protein, calcium, iron, and zinc. It is the only plant food that contains all of the amino acids, making it a complete protein.

- Include yogurt that has retained significant levels of live and active bacterial cultures. Yogurt is basically milk plus a bacterial culture that changes the lactose, proteins, and minerals into more digestible forms. The intestine-friendly bacterial cultures continue to support digestion, boost immunity, and decrease the risk of yeast infections. Unfortunately, the pasteurization of yogurt kills the bacteria. However, if pasteurization of the milk occurs before the addition of the bacteria that turn it into yogurt, the bacteria remain active. Look for brands that have significant levels of live and active bacterial cultures. Avoid brands that say, "heat treated after culturing." Look for brands that have a minimum number of ingredients. Many manufacturers add sweeteners and artificial colors and flavors to their products. Consider buying plain yogurt and adding fruit to control the type and amount of sweetening.

- Nut butters are highly nutritious and can provide a major contribution to a diet that is nutrient and calorie dense. Most parents think immediately of peanut butter and jelly sandwiches, but many other nut butters (e.g., almond, cashew, soy) are available.

- Chips and crackers of all kinds (potato, rice, corn, wheat) appeal to children who need stronger sensory input to organize oral movements. This often poses a challenge to therapists and parents who want to provide nutritious foods. Many of these foods by themselves are highly nutritious. However, the use of additives and the method of processing can reduce their nutritional value. Therapists can identify healthier alternatives by reading labels. Limit the use of products that contain artificial colors and flavors, chemical sweeteners, and hydrogenated or partially hydrogenated oils.

Balance is the key in all areas of therapy. This also applies to nutrition and the selection of food for children and families. It is important to move toward a healthier diet and encourage wise eating choices for children with feeding difficulties. However, this is not always immediately possible. Therapists begin where children and families are at the moment. They can introduce new foods slowly and model alternative choices. They look at the family diet and explore alternative foods that bring it into a better nutritional balance. Foods with empty calories (i.e., junk foods) can be included in the program in small amounts to provide the intense sensory input that the child seeks and convenience for parents. However, healthier foods with similar sensory impact also can be incorporated.

Special Health Needs and Nutrition

Medications

Medications often can benefit children by reducing seizures and heart and respiratory stress, and helping to fight infection. However, many of the medicines that appear necessary to support life can interfere with nutrition or have side effects that make eating uncomfortable or decrease the child's desire to eat (Graedon & Graedon, 1995; *Physicians Desk Reference,* 1998). Let's look at a few examples.

Food and Medication Interactions

Many seizure medications interfere with the absorption of folic acid, other B vitamins, vitamin D, and calcium. Dilantin, an anticonvulsant, causes hypertrophy of the gums with accompanying discomfort in the mouth for many children. This may reduce the child's desire to eat certain types of food. Mineral oil, which still may be recommended for constipation, can reduce the body's ability to absorb vitamins A, E, and D, leaving the child more vulnerable to infection. Diuretics such as Lasix, which often are given to reduce cardiac and respiratory stress, can cause excess excretion of calcium, potassium, and other minerals. Antibiotics such as tetracycline, cortisone medications, and diuretics all decrease zinc absorption or increase its excretion from the body. Deficiencies of zinc can contribute to a reduced appetite and hypersensitivity or hyposensitivity of taste. Appetite reduction, anorexia, and nausea also can occur as a side effect of drug therapy. It is extremely important to know what role medications may play in the child's approach to food and in the body's ability to be nurtured by the food that is eaten.

Our knowledge of nutrient-drug interactions is constantly changing. If a child is on any regular medication, it is important for the feeding therapist to consult with the physician and dietitian to learn about possible side effects and interactions of the medication with food. The answers are not simple. Some foods interact with medications and decrease their bioavailability (Williams, Davis, & Lowenthal, 1993). The absorption of tetracycline group of antibiotics is decreased when taken with milk or other dairy products (Yamreudeewong, Henann, Fazio, Lower, & Cassidy, 1995). Tetracycline also binds calcium and iron and prevents absorption. Theophylline is a major drug for children with asthma. Its side effects are increased when it is taken with high-fat foods.

Vitamin and mineral supplementation may be very important for some children. For others, supplements must be given only under medical supervision. Unfortunately, supplements of certain vitamins and minerals can interfere with the body's ability to absorb a medication that is critical to the child's survival or well-being. For example, even moderate doses of vitamin B6 can sharply reduce the amount of phenobarbitol or Dilantin in the blood, interfering with medical treatment for seizures.

Some medications given for hyperactivity (e.g., Ritalin, Prozac) or seizures (e.g., Depakote, Klonopin) may cause reduced appetite or anorexia. Other medications for muscle relaxation (e.g., Valium, baclofen), seizures (e.g., Dilantin, Depakote, Klonopin), and gastroesophageal reflux (e.g., Tegretol, Zantac) may cause nausea, vomiting, and constipation. Children who experience side effects from their medications may be uninterested in eating or actively avoid food because of the associated discomfort.

Antibiotics and the Gastrointestinal System

Antibiotics reduce the intestinal production of biotin, pantothenic acid (B5), and vitamin K. They speed the passage of food through the intestines, decreasing the overall absorption of nutrients.

Antibiotics frequently are prescribed for children with developmental disabilities. This is a reflection of the high use of antibiotic in general medical practice as well as the higher incidence of life-threatening situations in the histories of children with disabilities. However, many articles in medical textbooks and peer review journals support the view that antibiotics are overprescribed and inappropriately prescribed for viral infections (Schmidt et al., 1994). Schmidt et al. (1994) cite a large study of preschoolers, in which antibiotics were prescribed to 49% of children with upper respiratory tract infections. Many parents believe that antibiotics are needed to help their children get well. Physicians respond to the parental expectation that they will prescribe an antibiotic (Mangione-Smith, McGlynn, Elliott, Krogstad, & Brook, 1999; Watson et al., 1999). The study by Mangione-Smith and colleagues found that physicians' perception of parental expectations for antibiotics was the only significant predictor of actual prescribing of these medications for upper respiratory symptoms caused by a virus.

There is a high incidence of middle ear infections (otitis media) in infants and young children. Many children experience multiple bouts of otitis media each year for which they receive antibiotics. The increasing incidence of otitis media in children may be related to the increase in the use of child care, a higher prevalence of allergies in children, and the routine use of antibiotics (Cantekin, McGuire, & Griffith, 1991; Lanphear, Byrd, Auinger, & Hall 1997; Schmidt et al., 1994). Many children who receive multiple courses of antibiotics for repeated otitis media do not have a bacterial infection. They develop fluid in the middle ear and pain as a result of chronic closure of the Eustachian tube and a generalized swelling and inflammation related to an allergy to milk. When dairy products are removed from their diet, the ear infections stop (Fireman, 1988; Nsouli et al., 1994; Schmidt, 1990).

Antibiotics can save lives when given for a severe bacterial infection. However, their overuse has resulted in the development of strains of bacteria that are highly resistant to all or most antibiotics, and the massive destruction of the friendly bacteria in the intestines (Klein, 1999).

The intestinal tract is colonized shortly after birth by billions of bacteria that live in a cooperative relationship with the body (Chaitow & Trenev, 1990). More than 400 species of friendly bacteria assist with digestion and health. These bacteria make a wide variety of contributions to health. Some manufacture B vitamins such as biotin, niacin, pyridoxine, and folic acid. Others provide the enzyme lactase, which enables the digestion of milk-based foods and calcium for people who cannot digest milk. When bacteria are present in yogurt or cultured milk, these bacteria enhance protein digestion and absorption. Some bacteria demonstrate antibiotic properties by altering the acidity of the gut so that harmful bacteria cannot survive or actively producing antibiotic substances. They control potentially harmful yeasts such as *candida albicans*. They enhance bowel function by increasing peristalsis and reducing the time needed for food to pass through the gastrointestinal system. They play a vital role in the development of a healthy gastrointestinal tract in infants.

The balance of friendly intestinal flora in the gastrointestinal tract can be altered by antibiotics, low levels of hydrochloric acid in the digestive juices, and stress (Schmidt et al., 1994; Chaitow & Trenev, 1990). Anything that changes the degree of acidity in the gut changes the habitat for these bacteria. This changes the type and number of the microorganisms—typically killing large numbers of these friendly intestinal residents and allowing for an overgrowth of unfriendly bacteria and yeasts. These three factors—antibiotics, reduced hydrochloric acid, and stress—often are chronic companions for the child with a feeding disorder. Medications that alter the pH by reducing stomach acidity are commonly given if the child has gastroesophageal reflux. These include antacids as well as medications such as H-2 blockers (e.g., Zantac, Tagamet) and proton pump inhibitors (e.g., Prevacid, Prilosec), which reduce the amount of hydrochloric acid secreted by the stomach. These negatively influence the survival of friendly bacteria that require an acidic environment. Antibiotics kill bacteria contributing to illness; however, most of them kill the friendly bacteria as well. This is particularly true of broad-spectrum antibiotics (e.g., Bactrim, Ceclor) that are not targeted at a specific bacteria group. When children are chronically ill or have reduced immune function, they often are given this type of antibiotic over a long period to prevent further illness.

The most serious gastrointestinal consequence from the use of antibiotics is the uncontrolled growth of the **candida albicans** yeast (Schmidt et al., 1994; Trowbridge & Walker, 1986). Candida is present in every gastrointestinal tract to some degree. Friendly bacteria keep it in balance and prevent it from colonizing in the wall of the intestine. When the balance is upset, the candida yeast grows rapidly and changes into a fungal form that produces long root-like structures that penetrate the mucosal walls of the intestines. Chaitow and Trenev (1990) state that "Penetration of the gastrointestinal mucosa breaks down the boundary between the intestinal tract and the rest of the circulation allowing introduction into the bloodstream of many substances which are antigenic (i.e., stimulate the immune system to defend itself), possibly resulting in allergic reactions" (p. 87). This condition of increased intestinal permeability (often referred to as **leaky gut syndrome**) is associated with allergies in children (Akinbami, Brown, & McNeish,1989) and is also found in some children with autism (D'Eufemia et al., 1996). Yeast infections can express themselves locally through oral thrush, urethral or vaginal infections, or severe diaper rash. They can also occur systemically with widespread involvement of all systems of the body, causing fatigue, increased infections, gastrointestinal discomfort, depression, and a general sense of feeling ill (Trowbridge & Walker, 1986).

Just as antibiotics act against the bacteria in the intestinal tract, probiotics help to repopulate the gastrointestinal system with friendly bacteria. Cultured foods such as yogurt or food supplements containing high levels of bacteria can be added to the child's diet. If the child has been on frequent antibiotics, feeding therapists can work with a physician or dietitian to develop a daily program in which probiotic supplements are used.

There are many different categories of these bacteria. The specific supplemental bacteria chosen will depend upon the child's age. **Bifidobacteria** are used exclusively with children under the age of 2 years. Older children may receive a mixture of lactobacilli including **Bifidobacteria, Lactobacillus acidophilus, Lactobacillus bulgaricus,** and **Lactobacillus casei**. A special food for bacteria called fructo-oligosaccarides (FOS) can be added to the diet to promote the growth of friendly bacteria such as the Bifidobacteria. Chaitow and Trenev (1990) suggest in their book, *Probiotics,* that for supplements to be valuable and take up residence in the gastrointestinal tract, there have to be billions of organisms, and they have to be of strains that will survive digestion. They state that not all probiotic supplements meet these criteria. Buyers should check that the number of viable organisms is several billion per gram. Because the organisms have a limited survival period, buyers should check to see that the label shows an expiration date. Products that have been refrigerated are more likely to remain potent and stable. Powdered products are more stable and have a slower deterioration than liquid products. The product label should always indicate which strains of bacteria are present.

Parents and therapists can support the child's development of a strong immune system and reduce the overall incidence and severity of illness through a strong wellness program. Working with health-care providers, they can seek alternatives to antibiotics and use these when the child has a viral illness or a nonlethal bacterial infection (Schmidt et al., 1994; Zand, Walton, & Roundtree, 1994). They can reserve antibiotics for the serious bacterial infections for which they are effective (Schmidt et al., 1994). Options that can be considered are homeopathy, dietary modifications, herbal medicine, massage, acupressure, phytonutritionals, and glyconutritionals.

Allergies and Food Sensitivities

In implementing any feeding program, the feeding therapist must be alert to both the signs of allergic reactions and ways in which food sensitivities can be prevented. Allergy is an adaptive response of the immune system designed to protect the individual from a substance that the body perceives as dangerous to its welfare. As the body mounts its warfare against the foreign substance, symptoms are produced. We tend to think of runny nose, red eyes, sneezing, wheezing, hives, rashes, and other symptoms produced by the skin and respiratory system when someone mentions allergy; but allergic symptoms can be created by every system of the body (Rapp, 1991). Increases or decreases in muscle tone or spasticity, or increases in incoordination, irritability, hyperactivity, sleep disorders, headaches, fatigue, and depression can occur when the brain and nervous system react to the irritating substance. Gastrointestinal symptoms can include indigestion, cramps, reflux, and colic. Swelling of the eustachian tubes can interfere with middle ear function and lead to chronic ear infections. People with allergies frequently develop dark circles or "bags" under the eyes. These circles are sometimes called ***allergic shiners.***

There are many types of adverse reactions to food; however, to be defined as an allergy, the immune system must produce an allergy antibody (IgE). This type of response is present in a small percentage of the general population. The pattern of giving cereals and other foods to infants during the first 3 months can provoke allergic reaction. The gastrointestinal system is not prepared to handle these food molecules, and they pass into the blood. Identifying them as invaders, the body mounts a defense. Although the early introduction of solids was common 10 years ago, cereals, fruits, and vegetables now are delayed until the infant is 4 to 6 months old. Many allergists now recognize that an individual may produce the same type of bodily reaction without the classical immune system response that has been used to measure and define allergy (Rapp, 1991). It is important to consider any maladaptive reaction to a food or chemical. Food and chemical sensitivities occur more frequently than traditional allergies.

Some children have a genetic predisposition to developing food allergies (Chandra, 1997a). If a child's parents or sibling has an allergy or asthma, there is a higher risk that the child also will have an allergy. Some children become sensitized to foods in utero if the mother eats them during her pregnancy (Frank, Marian, Visser, Weinberg, & Potter, 1999; Vandenplas, 1993). Infants with a predisposition to allergy also can develop specific allergies to foods in the mother's diet during breast-feeding (de Boissieu, Matarazzo, Rocchiccioli, & Dupont, 1997; Machtinger & Moss, 1986). The tendency toward allergy can be increased by severe stress. Some allergists point to the increased stress produced by modern society (Mandell, 1976; Randolph & Moss, 1990). They perceive that pollution of air, food, and water sources has severely taxed the body's ability to maintain a balance and cope with other stresses in the environment. The stresses produced by intrauterine complications during pregnancy or a traumatic birth can reduce the infant's ability to deal with the stress of living in a polluted environment.

Up to 8% of children under the age of 3 experience food allergies to a limited number of foods (Sampson, 1999). The foods that most commonly cause allergic reactions in children are milk, eggs, peanuts, soy, wheat, citrus, tree nuts, fish, and shellfish (Rapp, 1991; Sicherer, 1999). Allergy to cow's milk is most common in infants under 12 months (Host, Jacobsen, Halken, & Holmenlund, 1995); however, some children retain the allergy into early childhood and express it in different ways as they get older (Cavataio, Iacono, Montalto, Soresi, Tumminello, Campagna, et al., 1996). Peanuts and tree nuts can trigger strong anaphylactic responses in children who are allergic to them (Burks, Bannon, Sicherer, & Sampson, 1999).

Some allergies can be prevented by careful attention to the foods that infants are given during their first year. This is particularly important if there is any history of allergy in the baby's family. Breast-feeding enables the allergy-prone infant to remain as long as possible on a diet of human milk and eliminates the early adjustment to cow's milk. The use of soy formulas and predigested hydrosalate formulas provide less allergenic choices for the bottle-fed infant. Foods with a lower risk of allergy should be introduced one at a time into the child's diet. For example, most infants can handle rice cereal, which does not contain gluten, and most fruits and vegetables between 4 and 6 months of age. Foods such as wheat, eggs, fish, and citrus fruits should be added closer to 12 months of age because they are more likely to cause an allergic response in sensitive children (Chandra, 1997a). Frank et al. (1999) found that children whose mothers ate peanuts more than once a week during pregnancy were more likely to have an allergic response to them. They found that these children also had an increased risk of sensitization to other foods as they were introduced into the diet. Rance and Dutau (1999) describe peanut as the major allergen in the United States. In their study, 54% of the 132 children with an identified peanut allergy were allergic to other foods, and 63% were allergic to airborne allergens. Because of their high allergy potential, peanuts should be introduced very cautiously into the child's diet during the toddler years. Unlike allergies to other foods in infancy and early childhood, peanut and tree nut allergies rarely are outgrown (Bock & Atkins, 1989; Sicherer, Burks, & Sampson, 1998).

Allergies and sensitivities to foods can serve as triggers that increase a child's sensory and motor difficulties. The following personal clinical examples illustrate these interconnections. Jason used a strong tongue thrust during feeding, combined with extensor patterns of movement in the arms, head, and pelvis. He was constantly congested with a thick, stringy mucous. When milk products were eliminated from his diet, his congestion decreased and mucous was thinner and easier to get rid of. The tongue thrust was reduced by approximately 75% of the frequency observed during the original diet that included milk and milk products. He was able to eat with greater skill and proficiency. Annie showed periods of increased muscle tone followed by severe autistic withdrawal during which she frequently did not eat. After 4 or 5 days, her postural tone became more normal and she was more in contact with her surroundings. Allergy testing showed a severe reaction to milk, sugar, beef, and wheat. When these substances were eliminated from her diet, she improved in the ability to integrate sensory information from the environment and establish eye contact. What is significant is that the symptoms produced by both children had been attributed to their diagnosis of cerebral palsy. Carol's mother was told that her child's projectile vomiting of milk as an infant was simply a part of the expected motor behavior of a child with cerebral palsy. Andy's physician refused to look at the possibility of an allergy to cow's milk as the trigger for his gastroesophageal reflux. He told Andy's parents that prematurity could explain the problem and placed Andy on medications, which did not reduce his vomiting. Finally, fundoplication surgery was performed to stop the reflux. Two years later, an allergist diagnosed Andy's multiple food and environmental allergies. It is probable that the surgery could have been avoided if his allergy to cow's milk had been diagnosed earlier (Cavataio, Iacono, Montalto, Soresi, Tumminello, Campagna, et al., 1996).

Because physicians often see sensorimotor behaviors that are associated with the primary diagnosis, they may fail to consider the possibility that an allergy or sensitivity to something in the child's environment could compound the original problem. In a pilot study of the allergic responses of 29 children and adults who had cerebral palsy, 90% of these individuals showed an allergic reaction to one or more of the food, chemical, or inhalant substances that were tested (Mandell, 1982). Among the symptoms observed were those affecting the coordination of movement and presence of muscle spasms. It is conceivable that children with neurological disorders may experience fluctuations in muscle tone as well as muscle spasms of the body and gastrointestinal tract as a response to an increased sensitivity to food, chemicals, or inhalants (Mandell, 1979).

Allergic sensitivities can be developed in any person with this tendency by repeated exposure to a substance (Rapp, 1991, 1996). Allergists with a strong interest in environmental medicine emphasize the tendency for a person to have the greatest sensitivities to foods that are eaten every day. Cravings or an intense liking for specific foods, tastes, or smells can indicate foods and chemicals to which the person is sensitive or allergic. This has been described as an allergic addiction. When foods are involved, the individual repeatedly eats the same food and a sensitivity may develop. Because the body experiences the beginning of a withdrawal reaction when the food is not eaten, the person eats more to relieve the symptoms. Many people are familiar with the withdrawal symptoms they experience when they cannot have their morning cup of coffee or indulge in a chocolate binge. When the upper stress level is reached, often the person becomes ill. During these periods of flu, colds, muscle aches, or indigestion, the exposure to the food goes down and the body is given a brief rest. Then the cycle begins again.

How do these observations and perceptions relate to the development of a feeding program? We are dealing with infants and children who have experienced significant stress in their lives. Because of feeding difficulties, the variety of foods and liquids they can eat is limited. There is a tendency to give the child the same foods repeatedly because they allow for success in feeding. This pattern can trigger food allergies or sensitivities in some children. Because of this possibility, it is a good idea to aim for as much food variety as possible in the feeding program. The effects of a food can remain in the body for 3 to 4 days. When the food is repeated, the body is never given a rest. The effects can build up. If foods are rotated so that the same one is not given more often than every 4 days, the system may not have to deal with the cumulative effects (Rapp, 1991). Many individuals who are sensitive to a particular food can add it to their diet occasionally. One goal in a feeding program is to develop the child's ability to eat five vegetables, five fruits, five cereal grains, and five meats. Many children benefit from eating a different set of foods every day in 4- or 5-day cycles. This can be particularly important when there is a history of allergy in the family.

If a child is showing symptoms such as excessive mucus, persistent vomiting, chronic colds, extreme variability in sensorimotor abilities, or irritability, an allergy consultation is appropriate. Before visiting the allergist, the family can explore differences in the child's symptoms and behaviors by eliminating specific foods from the diet for 7 to 14 days. Suggestions for creating the elimination diet and charting the child's behavior are provided in *Tracking Down Hidden Food Allergy* (Crook, 1980).

Children who are tube fed may be highly vulnerable to the development of an allergy or sensitivity. A single formula is usually prescribed, and the child receives the same formula at each meal until oral feedings are established. The implications of this system are significant when one considers the theory that a vulnerable individual can develop an allergy or sensitivity to a food that is eaten daily. Although it is more difficult and more expensive for parents to purchase and use several different formulas, it may be to the child's benefit to rotate tube-feeding formulas. Commercial formulas designed to supply full nutrition contain many of the same vitamins, minerals, and additives. Their basic protein supply, however, is derived from different food sources. Some formulas use a cow's milk base, others use a soy base, and still others are derived from meat. There are also hydrolyzed formulas that eliminate lactose and pre-digest the protein source. These four types of formula could be rotated so that the child's system is never bombarded with a single formula food. This option is important to consider when the child experiences severe gastroesophageal reflux. It should be discussed during the consultation with the child's physician and dietitian.

Dietary Aspects of Attention Deficit and Learning Disabilities

Approximately 5% of young children have been diagnosed with attention deficit/hyperactivity disorder (ADHD) (Roberts et al., 1999). The criteria for diagnosis of ADHD is not standard, and the exact percentage of children with the disorder varies among studies; however, trends indicate that increasingly more children are diagnosed and treated for the disorder. A recent study found that 18% to 20% of fifth-grade Caucasian boys in two Virginia cities were diagnosed with ADHD and given stimulant drugs. Frequently, stimulant medications such as Ritalin (methylphenidate) are prescribed to correct an underlying disorder of the brain neurotransmitter dopamine and reduce the symptoms that interfere with the child's ability to learn and function at home and in school.

When children have coexisting problems of ADHD and a feeding disorder, pharmacological alternatives (e.g., methylphenidate, dexamphetamine) may increase the impact of the feeding problem by causing side effects of nausea and appetite suppression (Efron, Jarman, & Barker, 1997). Alternative approaches to the management of ADHD symptoms become very important for this group of children. Dietary management is an option for some children. A number of well-conceived double-blind research studies have identified children with ADHD who are sensitive to various food ingredients (Boris & Mandel, 1994; Carter et al., 1993; Rowe & Rowe, 1994). These have included sensitivities to food dyes and other additives as well as specific high-allergen foods such as citrus fruits, milk, wheat, eggs, beet sugar, and chocolate. Children's behavior improved when they were on a diet that eliminated foods and additives to which they were sensitive. Kaplan, McNicol, Conte, and Moghadam (1989) conducted a 10-week single-subject design crossover study of 24 hyperactive preschool boys. When the children were placed on an experimental diet that eliminated artificial colors and flavors, chocolate, monosodium glutamate, preservatives, and caffeine, more than 50% of the children showed reliable improvement in their behavior. Other double-blind studies have shown no effect of changes in the diet. However, most of the negative studies eliminated only a single additive, which may have had a limited impact on the behavior of children with multiple sensitivities (Jacobson & Schardt, 1999).

Dietary deficiencies also have been identified in research on children with learning challenges related to ADHD, dyslexia, and dyspraxia. Kozielec and Starobrat-Hermelin (1997) found a deficiency of magnesium in 95% of a group of 116 children (9–12 years old) with a diagnosis of ADHD. There was a positive correlation between the levels of magnesium and the child's degree of distractibility. Bekaroglu and colleagues (1996) identified zinc deficiencies in a group of 48 children with ADHD. They suggest that a primary zinc deficiency plays a role in the etiology of attention deficit disorders.

Dykman and Dykman (1998) found that the addition of a glyconutritional supplement of eight essential carbohydrate sugars to the diet of 17 children with ADHD decreased the number and severity of symptoms by the second week of the 6-week study.

Children with ADHD may be deficient in essential fatty acids (EFAs), especially arachidonic acid and docosahexaenoic acid, which are derived from omega 6 and omega 3 fatty acids (Burgess et al., 2000; Stevens et al., 1995). Burgess and colleagues (2000) found that children with lower levels of omega 3 fatty acids had significantly more behavior problems, temper tantrums, and problems with learning, health, and sleep than did children with higher omega 3 levels. Stordy (2000) identified similar low levels of essential fatty acids in small groups of adults with dyslexia and children with dyspraxia. Fifteen adults with reading difficulties attributable to dyslexia experienced difficulty with the visual-retinal skill of dark adaptation. Dark adaptation improved in 50% of the group after taking a docosahexaenoic acid (DHA)-rich fish oil for 1 month. Movement skills involving manual dexterity and dynamic and static balance improved in a group of 15 children with the motor-planning disorder of dyspraxia after receiving supplements high in DHA.

These studies are too small to draw firm conclusions about the role played by fatty acid deficiencies in children with attention and learning disorders. However, many parents have increased the amount of essential fatty acids in their children's diets with anecdotal reports of positive gains in attention and motor coordination.

Gastroesophageal Reflux

The challenge of gastroesophageal reflux and its impact on children's desire to eat are discussed in depth in Chapter 22. It is important to remember that reflux can be triggered by foods that lower the resting pressure of the lower esophageal sphincter (LES) or irritate an inflamed esophagus. These foods may include chocolate, orange and other citrus fruit and juice, tomato, fried or fatty foods, peppermint, spearmint, pineapple, and coffee and other caffeinated beverages. Fatty foods take longer to digest and remain longer in the stomach. The resulting delay in gastric emptying also contributes to gastroesophageal reflux.

Food allergies or sensitivities can trigger or aggravate reflux for some infants and children (Iacono et al., 1996; Cavataio, Iacono, Montalto, Soresi, Tumminello, Campagna, et al., 1996). Eliminating the offending foods from the diet often reduces the frequency and intensity of reflux or eliminates it altogether.

Mucous Congestion

Problems with thick or excess mucus contribute heavily to feeding difficulties. When mucus creates nasal congestion, the sense of smell is reduced and taste perception is affected. When mucous congestion is chronic, children often lose interest in eating. Thick mucus in the pharynx may trigger gagging, choking, and retching in vulnerable children. It also may contribute to incoordination of the suck-swallow-breathe synergy, increasing the risk of aspiration.

The lubricatory functions of mucus have been well described in Western medicine. The body produces mucus primarily as a functional strategy to moisten membrane surfaces in order to support movement of body structures without excess friction. Excessive production of mucus has been viewed primarily as an inconvenient symptom of a cold or allergy, and medications have been designed to dry up secretions or inhibit further output. Eastern medical traditions, however, have honored production of mucus as the body's practical way of ridding itself of substances that do not contribute to health (Ballentine, 1978). By understanding this excretory function of mucous production, we have an expanded awareness of the etiology of this symptom. The body increases production of mucus during a respiratory illness to entrap bacteria, viruses, and dead cells and to move them out of the body. Allergies increase toxins and dead cells as the immune system fights a perceived invader. Mucus is produced to eliminate this material. The lungs produce mucus to help move aspirated food out of the respiratory tract. Even constipation can contribute to increased mucus production. If the body is not removing the toxins produced by accumulated fecal waste through the bowels, it may increase the production of mucus throughout the body to assist in an overall cleansing of the system. Clinical experience supports the concept that improving bowel movements and reducing constipation solves the problem of excess mucus for many children who have feeding problems.

Thick mucus also is related to subclinical chronic dehydration (Batmanghelidj, 1995). The body uses sodium to increase water retention. Sodium also breaks up mucus, thinning it so that it can be moved from the body more efficiently. When chronic dehydration is present, the body retains salt and does not use it to loosen mucus. Increasing water in the diet can effectively thin and loosen mucus because the body no longer has to hoard cellular water by retaining salt.

Constipation

Chronic constipation is common among children with neuromuscular disorders. Its multiple causes, impact on eating, and treatment are discussed in Chapter 22. Two of the most common contributors to constipation are insufficient water intake and insufficient fiber in the diet. Children with feeding difficulties may have greater difficulty getting enough liquid in the diet than other children. When skill with drinking liquids is not as developed or controlled as in other children, the child may be given less liquid during the day. The major function of the large intestine is to remove excess water from the waste material of digestion and form solid stools that can be excreted. When there is chronic dehydration, the residue lacks the water needed to allow it to pass easily through the bowels. In addition, the body may try to conserve water and extract it from the intestines for delivery to other parts of the body. Inadequate water intake, therefore, contributes heavily to constipation.

Indigestible carbohydrates from solid food provide the major source of digestive residue that is excreted in the child's stools. Fiber increases peristaltic movement of the intestines and the movement of waste products through the digestive system. Children with impaired oral motor function may eat a diet that provides an inadequate amount of fiber.

In designing feeding and oral motor treatment programs, the feeding therapist needs to maintain contact with the child's dietitian and physician, and consider dietary contributions to constipation. The treatment program can prevent constipation by improving eating and drinking skills that enable the child to increase the daily intake of fluid and fiber in the diet and by increasing the amount of water given to children with feeding tubes.

The following foods may be added to the diet to increase fiber content:

- high-fiber cereals
- whole grain bread
- uncooked vegetables
- nuts
- uncooked fruits
- cooked vegetables such as sweet potato, cabbage, spinach, broccoli, dried peas, and beans
- unprocessed bran (no more than 3 teaspoons daily, sprinkled in food or in milk shakes)

For children who have difficulty chewing or handling lumpy solid foods, a mixture of raisins, prunes, dates, figs, and prune juice may be processed to a smooth paste in the blender. A commercial version of this substance also is available. Many children enjoy eating it as a spread on crackers or mixed with yogurt. Prune juice also can be given to children who are fed by a tube.

Mineral oil often is recommended to soften and lubricate stools, making it easier for them to pass through the colon. However, it is important to remember that mineral oil can contribute to deficiencies in fat-soluble vitamins. Also, aspiration of mineral oil in children with swallowing difficulties or chronic gastroesophageal reflux has been linked to a severe type of pneumonia (Bandla et al., 1999; Sears & Sears, 1999; Wolfson, 1989). However, flaxseed oil also has laxative properties (Sears & Sears, 1999). Unlike mineral oil, it is a valuable source of nutrition that facilitates the absorption of fat-soluble vitamins.

Diet and Dental Health

Dental problems complicate the oral motor issues of children with feeding difficulties. Feeding therapists and parents must give a high priority to oral and dental health and preventing dental problems. Diet plays a large role in programs to support dental health (Tamborlane, 1997). A nutritionally adequate diet that includes appropriate levels of vitamins, calcium, phosphorus, and protein is essential for well-formed, decay-resistant teeth and healthy gums. Tooth decay is the major dental problem of children. Sugar consumption and the frequency with which it is eaten play the primary role in the development of cavities. Bacteria in the mouth attach to the teeth and form a sticky coating called dental plaque. When these bacteria interact with carbohydrates in food, they produce acid that attacks the teeth and demineralizes their surfaces, increasing the risk of dental decay. The acid may remain in the mouth for 20 minutes or longer. Saliva counteracts the acid and reduces the amount of demineralization (Kaplan & Baum, 1993). However, minimal saliva is produced at night when children are asleep. For this reason, teeth are more vulnerable to decay when children eat before bedtime or go to sleep nursing at the breast or sucking a bottle of milk or juice (Nowak, 1993). When children eat frequently throughout the day, acid is produced more often and there is less time for saliva to create its buffering action. Sticky foods (e.g., honey, molasses, candy) remain on the teeth longer and are more difficult for the saliva to remove.

Children with feeding disorders are particularly vulnerable to developing cavities and other dental diseases (Boyd, Palmer, & Dwyer, 1998; Hennequin, Faulks, Veyrune, & Bourdiol, 1999; Judd & Kenny, 1990). Inefficient oral movements contribute to poor bolus formation and scatter and retention of food pieces in cavities that are in contact with the surfaces of the teeth. A dry mouth with inadequate saliva to cleanse the teeth and counteract acid buildup occurs in many children with oral motor difficulties. This can be caused as a side effect of common medications, surgery to reroute salivary ducts to reduce profuse drooling, dehydration, and mouth breathing (Astor, Hanft, & Ciocon, 1999; Ship, Fox, & Baum, 1991).

Gastroesophageal reflux also contributes to dental erosion and decay (Jarvinen, Meurman, Hyvarinen, Rytomaa, & Murtomaa, 1988; Shaw, Weatherill, & Smith, 1998). This appears to be more severe in children who reflux acid materials into the mouth than in those whose reflux is limited to the esophagus (O'Sullivan, Curzon, Roberts, Milla, & Stringer, 1998).

Sensorimotor difficulties contribute to more frequent small meals throughout the day for many children. Because of the calming effect of sucking, a large percentage of infants who experience difficulties with sensory modulation self-calm primarily when they are sucking at the bottle or breast. These babies typically go to sleep at the breast and nurse through the night or become frantic if they cannot rely on their bottles to calm themselves for sleep. They may remain on the bottle or breast long past the 12-month time of weaning recommended by dentists. The oral sensory issues experienced by children with sensory-based feeding problems also contribute to difficulties with toothbrushing and other oral care. Dental appointments can be extremely traumatic for a child with oral sensory defensiveness, and parents often postpone formal dental care.

Some children with feeding difficulties have coexisting disorders that necessitate a special diet. These include restriction of specific foods (e.g., phenylketonuria, lactase deficiency, ketogenic diet for seizure control), a need for medications timed with the meal (e.g., diabetes, cystic fibrosis), or high caloric requirements (e.g., bronchopulmonary dysplasia, cystic fibrosis). A child's dietary needs can influence the mealtime and create pressures on the child to eat. When children resist eating or stop eating before taking in enough calories, parents become very worried. If dietary guidelines are not followed, the child may become ill or even die. This places major stresses on the mealtime relationship and interferes with an appropriate division of responsibility.

Maximizing Nutrition for Children With Special Health Needs

The following general therapy strategies can maximize nutrition for children with special health needs:

- **Support mothers who wish to breast-feed their infants.** Breast milk provides the highest level of nutrition for infants. It contributes to improved immune and gastrointestinal function and prevents the development of allergies. Many mothers of infants who have initial difficulty nursing would prefer to breast-feed. Although many hospitals encourage mothers to express their milk and give it to the baby through the bottle or feeding tube, support for breast-feeding infants with special feeding needs often is lacking. Feeding therapists working in hospitals and clinics with young infants can become strong advocates for mothers who wish to breast-feed. They can collaborate with lactation consultants to identify strategies and special equipment that will support the infant's ability to nurse.

- **Be knowledgeable about the medications that the child receives and become aware of potential food and medication interactions.** Our health-care system has become fragmented by the number of specialists who are involved with infants and children with complex medical needs. Children with feeding disorders may receive simultaneous care and medications from pediatricians, gastroenterologists, pulmonologists, allergists, neurologists, urologists, orthopedists, psychiatrists, and many other medical professionals. The pharmacist often becomes the key professional in identifying deadly drug interactions. Although a dietitian may be involved at key points in the child's treatment, often nutritional consultations are infrequent and medications are added or stopped without reference to the child's dietary needs. Feeding therapists are in a position to provide an informal monitoring of changes in the child's medications and diet. Side effects of medications and dietary deficiencies can have a profound impact on the child's desire and ability to eat. Through awareness of medications that increase the need for specific nutrients and a routine check of potential interactions, the feeding therapist can encourage parents to raise questions and discuss problem areas with a dietitian or physician.

- **Influence children's tone and movement patterns, and provide nutritional alternatives to reduce constipation.** Constipation plays a major role in reducing mealtime comfort for many children. Feeding therapists often ignore difficulties with the lower digestive tract, assuming that their responsibility primarily is getting the child to eat and swallow food safely. Constipation must be addressed within the feeding program. Increasing the amount of water and fiber in the child's diet can be critical in reducing constipation. When this is combined with movement and sensory activities to support easier bowel movements, problems with constipation can be eliminated for many children.

■ **Encourage families to consider dietary exploration and management before resorting to medication and surgical alternatives.** When children experience symptoms of gastroesophageal reflux, nausea, appetite reduction, mucous congestion, and constipation, physicians typically prescribe medication or surgery to reduce the discomfort. In many instances, this is similar to disconnecting the warning light in the car that tells a driver that there is a problem with oil pressure. Symptoms are the body's way of communicating that there is something wrong. Suppressing or preventing them through medication or surgery does not address the underlying cause of the problem. In many instances, the symptoms that interfere with learning to eat have dietary roots. Dietary exploration and management may take more time and energy than giving another pill, but it is in the child's best interest. Medications are expensive and have many side effects. The complex interactions that arise when children take multiple medications are virtually unknown. Anti-reflux surgical procedures such as a fundoplication and pyloroplasty have a high incidence of complications (e.g., dysphagia, gagging, retching and dumping syndrome) that interfere with a child's desire and ability to eat by mouth.

Exploration of elimination and rotational diets, increasing water in the diet, and using food and other dietary supplements can reduce the need for complex medical procedures and multiple medications.

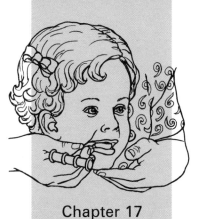

Chapter 17

Specifics of Oral Motor Treatment

It is helpful to have a clear sense of options for some of the more common problems and guidelines for selecting the most appropriate possibilities. This chapter provides a discussion of some common oral motor and feeding problems, treatment directions, treatment strategies, and possible activities.

An understanding of the big picture of the mealtime is essential for the success of a treatment program. What is working for the child and the parent at mealtime? What is not working for them? What developmental and physical skills are available upon which to build a feeding program? How do the child's structural, physiological, wellness, experiential, and environmental limitations influence the mealtime? Therapists may know a great idea about an oral motor treatment technique that previously worked with many other children, but it may or may not be appropriate for another child. Even when the treatment idea is appropriate, if it is not integrated into the big picture for that child and family, it probably will not work. It certainly will not work as effectively as if the therapist had looked more carefully at the whole situation.

Success also depends upon the therapist's abilities to determine and treat the child's abilities and needs within the big picture context, and to communicate treatment strategies and activities that caregivers can implement at home. There will be a constant challenge to discuss, describe, demonstrate, and photograph treatment techniques and activities that incorporate those techniques. Therapists are in a position to teach specific techniques and activities to parents in a multisensory way that supports easy learning. They have opportunities to demonstrate the procedure, draw pictures, and take photographs to provide visual input. When giving verbal suggestions, they can describe what they are doing and describe how the child should respond. They can demonstrate the activity directly with the parent in a way that provides tactile, kinesthetic, and vestibular information. Each parent can be encouraged to feel the limiting pattern and experientially understand the therapist's approach to facilitating a more normal response. Thus, sensory information can become integrated and understanding occur. With understanding, the parent will be able to incorporate these ideas into the natural routines of the family.

Some participatory experiences were presented in earlier chapters and many more are available through the *Mealtime Participation Guide* (Klein & Morris, 1999). These enable feeding therapists and parents to feel and experience the sensory and motor

Table 17.1	**Oral Motor Treatment Guidelines**
	Look at the Big Picture of the mealtime.
	Work with other team members to determine the child's feeding needs.
	Rule out medical complications that potentially influence a feeding disorder.
	Look at the feeding relationship.
	Build a program on the foundation of what works with the child and parent, taking into account what is not working for them.
	Develop the steps of the feeding program, working from the proximal to the distal parts of the body.
	Work to normalize muscle tone and reduce the influence of limiting reflexes and movement patterns.
	Work developmentally from the child's present abilities.
	Introduce one change at a time (position, temperature, texture, or utensil).
	Listen to the child.
	Introduce changes at home that have been well established in therapy.

patterns that form the basis for an understanding of treatment. Ideas coming from a base of understanding and personal knowledge are implemented more readily and consistently than suggestions that come from another person's experience.

The first portion of this chapter discusses the oral motor challenges that are encountered most frequently in children with feeding difficulties. Sections include problems with the function of individual oral structures, problems with sensory processes, problems with feeding processes, and the role of food in therapy. Each section presents a description of the problem as well as a series of treatment considerations and directions that includes a discussion of possible causes and relationships and overall treatment strategies. The final portion of the chapter is a detailed compendium of treatment strategies and possible activities for implementing each strategy. The purpose is to point out common causes and suggest appropriate treatment strategies and activities to address the problem. This is not a finite list that would describe and meet the needs of every child.

Each suggestion must be weighed against the big picture of mealtime, medical knowledge of the child, observation of and interaction with the child, and personal mealtime experiences. The chapter is not intended to become a cookbook of cures. It is not a Band-Aid for therapy. It simply provides a list of options and possible activities to inspire the creativity of both therapists and parents. Movement and handling suggestions should be discussed with the occupational and physical therapists on the team or with other team members who have experience with specialized movement and handling. The strategies and possible activities are not given in order of priority. Therapists should read all of them and choose the strategies and activities that most closely relate to the particular child's medical and therapeutic needs. Suggestions given in one section of this chapter may be appropriate for a child who has difficulties described in another section. Therapists should play detective and be selective.

No child is a separate collection of jaw, tongue, lips, cheeks, bodily and oral sensations, and behaviors. No feeding problem is due to a single factor. The process of feeding is a complex, interconnected, and flowing event. Each child is engaged in a dance of growth and development. The feeding therapist becomes the choreographer of the learning experience, assisting the child and family in developing the flow and efficiency that allows feeding to become effortless.

For ease of organization and learning, the chapter has been broken into artificial divisions. For example, the initial section on problems with individual oral structures focuses primarily on issues of deviations in tone and movement in each oral structure. These are patterns that interfere with the flow of normal development. The treatment directions and strategies that are suggested explore ways in which the oral reflexive behavior can be diminished or inhibited, and the ways overall control of oral movement can be enhanced. The second section focuses on the feeding processes that are developed by the normal child during the first 2 years of life. In that section, the flow and transitions from suckling to sucking to chewing, as well as the many variations within each, are considered. Although the influence of problems of the jaw, tongue, lips, and cheeks is discussed in relation to the feeding process, this is primarily a section on developing new feeding behaviors. These two sections are related. In real life, the therapist constantly moves between ways of diminishing undesirable events in the mouth and ways of encouraging new and productive feeding movements and behaviors.

Treatment goals and activities are created from a series of interrelated concepts and specific techniques. Each technique that is incorporated into the treatment program has elements of timing that are related to the child's and parent's learning styles and needs. A therapist selects the set of elements that are appropriate for a given child. These will lead to learning and success if they are brought into the session in a sequence that allows growth and change to occur as a series of small, interdependent steps. The timing of the activity creates the flow. When to remain with an activity, when to expand it, and when to stop it are critical decisions. This sense of timing and flow comes from within. It is primarily a reflection of acute observational skills and openness to intuitively knowing what the child needs next. It comes from listening to the child. Although specific criteria can be set to represent mastery of the skill, the flow of treatment that leads to this mastery is not well described by linear data collection. The therapist will learn to use and trust the analytical and intuitive knowledge that is available when the mind becomes versatile in its ability to process information.

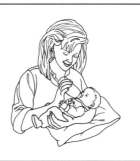

Interconnections

The child and the process are not separate.

The child and the feeder are not separate.

The child and learning are not separate.

They are one.

Throughout this treatment chapter, references are made to different types of treatment materials. Chapter 18 includes considerations for selection of treatment materials and resource information on many useful feeding materials.

This chapter does not repeat the general principles of treatment that apply to all children or the specific directions and treatment strategies that relate to specific groups of children. When therapists seek appropriate treatment strategies and activities for a child, they initially should review the chapters that relate directly to that child. For example, a child with feeding problems as a result of cerebral palsy typically has many difficulties with movement and motor control. Chapter 15 offers guidelines for evaluating children with movement problems, as well as suggestions for positioning and handling these children. The same child may experience discomfort at mealtime related to gastroesophageal reflux. The issues of reflux and their impact on feeding are discussed in Chapter 22. The feeding therapist should consult these chapters first, knowing that they will contain important directions and specific treatment strategies and activities that are not repeated in this chapter.

Oral Motor Problems and Treatment Directions

Problems With Function of Individual Oral Structures

Jaw

Jaw Thrust

Problem

The jaw moves open suddenly and with force, or the jaw moves up and down with force.

Treatment Considerations and Directions

Consultation

If the child's teeth are decayed or infected, closing the mouth may be extremely painful because of the contact of the teeth and gums. The child may respond with a strong thrusting open of the jaw. Consultation with a dentist can rule out this contribution to a jaw thrust and may be the primary treatment involved.

Some children have poorly formed or poorly functioning temporomandibular joints, which can cause pain with jaw movement. Some children move the jaw to a certain point and then have pain or a "catching" of the bones. They may respond to the pain with a wide-open jaw excursion. Consultation with a dentist, physician, or physical therapist who specializes in TMJ treatment may be necessary.

Physical Issues

Increased patterns of muscle tone can influence overall extensor patterns of movement throughout the body. A poor sitting position with too much hip extension and posterior pelvic tilt can contribute to an overall increase in forceful body extension. Neck hyperextension may be present with the head tipped back on the neck in a pattern of capital extension rather than the normal pattern of capital flexion. Both patterns of physical hyperextension frequently include other strong extensor movements such as the jaw thrust.

Breathing patterns may be limited or stressed because of physical tension in the ribcage, shoulder girdle, and pelvic-abdominal girdle. The airway may become blocked by the retraction of the tongue. Because the pharyngeal airway is physiologically enlarged by slightly hyperextending the neck, some children will use this strategy to improve their stridorous breathing pattern. Strong jaw thrusting may accompany this maneuver because of the combination of neck hyperextension and severe respiratory stress.

When the jaw thrust is part of a total pattern of hypertonicity and extension of the body, treatment strategies initially must be directed at changing appropriate aspects of the overall physical environment. Treatment strategies must focus on physical handling and positioning. These will involve reducing the extent and impact of limiting extensor patterns of the body as a key in reducing the strength and frequency of the jaw thrust.

Sensory Issues

An overstimulating sensory environment may cause the child to react with limiting jaw movements. Some children may thrust the jaw because of hyperreaction to the sensory input from the teeth contacting each other or from contact of the teeth and gums with a toy, feeding utensil, or finger. This sensory input elicits a strong avoidance response that moves the child into a jaw thrust.

When the jaw thrust is a response to sensory input, treatment strategies initially must be directed at changing appropriate aspects of the overall sensory environment. This may involve reducing the overall level of sensory stimulation present in the child's mealtime environment or helping the child adjust to small amounts of sensory input to the mouth without triggering an avoidance response.

Interaction Issues

Opening the mouth for food is one of the strongest natural signs of readiness for eating. When a child has poor control of jaw opening and an underlying tendency toward a jaw thrust, this pattern of thrusting may become a communication signal. The feeder recognizes the jaw thrust as the child's way of indicating readiness for another mouthful of food. A child may continue to use the jaw thrust to let the feeder know he needs another bite, even when his head is in good alignment and sensory input is appropriate. Jaw thrusting also can be used to express excitement or pleasure with the food and mealtime.

As long as children think that a jaw thrust is the only way of communicating readiness to the feeder, they will continue to use this type of limiting jaw movement at mealtime. Treatment strategies must focus on finding other ways of communicating the message that don't involve limiting tone and movement patterns.

Oral Control Issues

Oral control issues in a child with a jaw thrust usually are secondary to the medical, physical, sensory, and interactional triggers that elicit the thrusting pattern.

Treatment strategies to improve oral control will center primarily on reducing the frequency and strength of the jaw thrust itself and then on strategies to develop greater control of jaw movement.

Specific Feeding-Skill Issues

The jaw thrust can be a strong deterrent in the development of sucking, swallowing, biting, and chewing. The suddenness and force of the movement pattern breaks the underlying rhythm and flow of feeding. Children may have difficulty initiating or sustaining the appropriate movement patterns for eating and drinking. The amount of interference will depend upon the frequency and strength of the jaw thrust pattern.

Work on a specific feeding skill must always address limiting oral patterns such as the jaw thrust in the initial phases of the feeding program.

Experiential Issues

For some children who regularly thrust the jaw during mealtimes, the frustration of not having control can be strong. These children can develop stressed emotional responses in anticipation of the presentation of the meal. The stress can lead to increased muscle tone throughout the body and the triggering of a jaw thrust. Over time, the child may learn to thrust the jaw in anticipation of the presentation of food.

Treatment strategies for these children must include rebuilding trust in the child's own body and the ability to influence movement patterns. They may include helping the child adjust to small amounts of sensory input in the mouth without triggering an anticipatory emotional hyperreaction.

Exaggerated Jaw Excursions

Problem

The jaw moves open with wide, exaggerated excursions. Unlike the jaw thrust, it is *not* a forceful opening.

Treatment Considerations and Directions

Consultation

The teeth and gums may be decayed or infected. Closing the mouth, causing contact of the teeth and gums, may be painful and result in an exaggerated excursion of the jaw. Consultation with a dentist can rule out this contribution to wide jaw excursions.

Physical Issues

Fluctuations in muscle tone can cause wide ranges of movement in joints. In the jaw, these athetoid-like fluctuations frequently cause exaggerations in jaw opening. Children with fluctuating tone frequently move from a closed position to a widely exaggerated jaw opening, with little control in between.

Some children have decreased muscle tone and poor ability to control the closing of the jaw or to maintain its closure during gross motor or fine motor activities. The exaggerated jaw opening can be an overflow or organizing movement as the child fixes the jaw into an open position.

When increased tone, decreased tone, or fluctuating tone influences exaggerated excursions of the jaw, treatment strategies must be directed toward changing appropriate aspects of the overall physical environment. These will include strategies for reducing the impact of the tone changes on oral skills before and during the mealtime.

Sensory Issues

Oral hypersensitivity may be present. The contact of the teeth against each other, the gums, the spoon, cup, or the food texture can elicit an exaggerated jaw opening response. The jaw may touch the food or utensil and then open widely to avoid the sensory contact. This oral sensory overreaction may cause the child to avoid bringing toys or other objects to the mouth for exploration. This can cause children to have decreased mouthing, jaw holding, and biting experiences.

When oral hypersensitivity and the resultant overprotectiveness leads to exaggerated excursions of the jaw with presentation of foods, treatment strategies initially must be directed at changing appropriate aspects of the sensory environment. This may involve carefully selecting sensory variables in the presentation of the meal and helping the child adjust to small amounts of sensory input to the mouth without triggering exaggerated jaw excursions as an avoidance response.

Interaction Issues

Opening the mouth for food is one of the strongest natural signs of readiness for feeding. When the child has poor control of jaw opening, it can send confusing communication signals to the feeder. For many children with fluctuations in tone, the exaggerated opening often is followed with an exaggerated closing as compensation.

When exaggerated jaw excursions interfere with clear communication between the child and the feeder, treatment strategies should focus on clear mealtime communication.

Oral Control Issues

The child may have poor ability to sustain a contraction of the muscles involved in jaw closing. Jaw instability and lack of the needed co-contraction at the temporomandibular joint can contribute to the poorly graded, wide-opening pattern. Low or fluctuating muscle tone can reduce the overall stability needed for graded, controlled jaw movements.

When there are exaggerated jaw excursions because of low or fluctuating tone, poor cocontraction of the TMJ, and poor jaw stability, treatment strategies must include methods of improving jaw grading and stability, the child's internal awareness of the jaw, and the ability to move and control the jaw in isolation of the movement of the whole body.

Specific Feeding-Skill Issues

Wide excursions of the jaw can interfere with the foundational stability necessary to support efficient bottle drinking, food removal from a spoon, cup drinking, biting and chewing, and straw drinking. The lack of jaw stability and holding influences jaw closure and leads to less efficient swallowing and excess spillage in all areas of eating.

Treatment strategies may include improving the child's control of jaw movements during bottle drinking, removing food from a spoon, cup drinking, biting and chewing, and straw drinking. Treatment may include experiences that involve swallowing with jaw and lips closed.

Experiential Issues

Some children with wide excursions of the jaw have not had the opportunity to mouth toys. They have not experienced holding toys with different sizes, shapes, and textures in the mouth while simultaneously learning to move the tongue separately from the jaw.

When lack of oral experiences influences jaw control, treatment strategies must include opportunities for mouthing and oral exploration following activities to reduce the extent of the exaggerated opening of the jaw.

Jaw Instability

Problem

The jaw slips and shifts to the side or forward because of insufficient tone and control at the temporomandibular joint. The instability may be seen as the child opens or closes the mouth. There can be asymmetries in these positions. Some children will try to stabilize by holding the mouth in a tense, open position or in a closed, biting position.

Treatment Considerations and Directions

Consultation

Jaw instability occasionally is caused by extreme laxity of the temporomandibular joint, which may cause dislocation and subluxation. Specific delays or deviations in the development of stability at the temporomandibular joint may be related to overall hypotonia or to specific deviations of development of the joint. If structural problems are suspected, a referral to a dentist or physician who specializes in TMJ treatment may be necessary.

Physical Issues

Generalized hypotonia in the face and body can cause a poor foundation for building good jaw control for feeding. The low muscle tone provides an insufficient basis of muscle co-contraction, strength, and control to allow for smoothly graded opening and closing of the jaw. Gravity biases the low tone jaw toward an open position. Movements of the jaw can be inconsistent.

When jaw instability is part of a total pattern of hypotonia, treatment strategies initially must be directed at changing appropriate aspects of the overall physical environment. Treatment strategies must focus on physical handling and positioning. Strategies can include determining what can be done before or during the meal to prepare the child's muscle tone for feeding. Activities should include ways to provide physical feedback to the child regarding the proper resting position and functioning of the jaw.

Oral Control Issues

The child may have poor ability to sustain contraction of the muscles involved in keeping the jaw in alignment. Jaw instability and lack of the needed co-contraction at the temporomandibular joint can contribute to the poorly graded, unstable movement pattern. Low or fluctuating muscle tone can reduce the overall stability needed for graded, controlled jaw movements.

Treatment strategies must include methods of improving jaw grading and stability, increasing the child's internal awareness of the jaw, and controlling the ability to move the jaw in isolation of movement of the whole body.

Specific Feeding-Skill Issues

Jaw instability can affect all the skills involved with eating and drinking. The jaw must provide a stable foundation upon which the cheeks, lips, and tongue perform their coordinated efforts at sucking, swallowing, biting, chewing, and bolus formation. Treatment efforts to develop specific feeding skills must focus on developing or assisting jaw control as this foundational skill.

Problem

The jaw moves upward into a tightly clenched posture as a part of a total body pattern of movement, making it difficult for the child to open the mouth. The tightness of the closure and the force of the jaw closure are what separate jaw clenching from stability biting. The external sensory input of touch to the gums or teeth is not necessary to elicit a jaw clenching, which differentiates it from a tonic bite response.

Treatment Considerations and Directions

Consultation

Some children who have a chronic jaw-clenching pattern can develop problems with the structure and functioning of the temporomandibular joint. Shortening of the jaw-closing muscles can occur, with resulting contractures. This may result in the anatomical inability to open the mouth adequately or contractures of the muscles around the temporomandibular joint. Consultation with a dentist, physician or therapist who specializes in TMJ problems would be appropriate.

Physical Issues

Jaw clenching can be a part of all overall flexion pattern. A poor sitting position with too much hip flexion and posterior pelvic tilt can contribute to an overall increase in body flexion. This increases the probability that jaw clenching will be elicited.

When jaw clenching is part of a total pattern of flexion of the body, treatment strategies initially must be directed at changing appropriate aspects of the overall physical environment. Treatment strategies must focus on physical handling and positioning. These will involve reducing the extent and impact of limiting flexor patterns of the body as a key to reducing the strength and frequency of jaw clenching.

Sensory Issues

An overstimulating environment can cause the child to react with limiting increased flexor movement patterns, which may include jaw-clenching movements.

When jaw clenching is a response to sensory input of the environment, treatment strategies initially must be directed at changing appropriate aspects of the overall sensory environment.

Interaction Issues

Opening the mouth for food is one of the strongest natural signs of readiness for eating. When a child has poor control of jaw opening and closing and an underlying tendency toward jaw clenching, this pattern of clenching may become a confusing communication signal. The child may use the clenching to slow the pace or refuse the food. The child, however, may not mean to communicate that message at all. The feeder may misinterpret the jaw clenching as an indication that the child does not want the food, is not ready for the next bite, or is full and wants to end the meal. These may not be what the child is saying at all, and the feeder may end the meal before the child has had enough to eat.

As long as children think that jaw clenching is the only way to communicate that they need to pause or end the meal, they will continue to use this type of limiting jaw movement at mealtime. Treatment strategies must focus on finding ways to communicate these messages that don't involve limiting tone and movement patterns. Treatment also should focus on relaxing the child so the jaw clenching becomes less of a potentially confusing message to the feeder.

Oral Control Issues

Oral control issues in a child with a jaw-clenching pattern usually are secondary to the physical, sensory, and interactional triggers that elicit the clenching response.

Treatment strategies to improve oral control will center primarily on reducing the frequency and strength of the jaw clenching, and then on strategies to develop greater control of jaw movement.

Specific Feeding-Skill Issues

Jaw clenching can be a strong deterrent in the development of sucking, swallowing, biting, and chewing. The force of the movement pattern breaks the underlying rhythm and flow of feeding. Children may have difficulty initiating or sustaining the appropriate movement patterns for eating and drinking. The amount of interference will depend on the frequency and strength of the jaw-clenching pattern.

Work on a specific feeding skill must always address limiting oral patterns, such as the jaw clenching, in the initial phases of the feeding program.

Experiential Issues

Some children who regularly clench the jaw at mealtimes experience a great deal of frustration at not having control of jaw opening. These children can develop stressed emotional responses and, over time, learn to clench the jaw in anticipation of the presentation of the meal. Continued stress can lead to increased muscle tone throughout the body and more jaw clenching.

Treatment strategies must include ways for the child to rebuild trust in his body and the ability to have some influence over oral movement patterns. They may include helping the child adjust to small amounts of sensory input to the mouth without triggering an anticipatory emotional hyperreaction.

Tooth Grinding

Problem

The teeth slide together, making a tense grinding noise.

Treatment Considerations and Directions

Consultation

Sometimes, chronic grinding causes teeth to wear down, reducing the child's dental alignment for biting and chewing and resulting in pain. A consultation with a dentist may be necessary to support optimum dental care.

Physical Issues

For some children with severe extremes of muscle tone, the contact of the teeth against each other can trigger a sustained tonic bite reflex. Slight shifts of tone in the overall picture of flexor hypertonicity create the noises associated with tooth grinding.

When a tonic bite response is part of a total pattern of hypertonicity with extremes of flexion or extension of the body, treatment strategies initially must be directed at changing appropriate aspects of the overall physical environment. Treatment strategies must focus on physical handling and positioning. These strategies involve reducing the extent and impact of limiting flexor and extensor patterns of the body as a key in reducing the strength and frequency of the tonic bite.

Sensory Issues

Many children discover interesting tactile and auditory sensations from the eruption and growth of the teeth. Grinding noises are used for exploration, play, and self-entertainment.

Some children are old enough to be biting and chewing solid foods, but remain on liquids and pureed food. Their jaws do not regularly receive the proprioceptive experiences other children their age receive from biting and chewing hard foods. When children have missed the developmentally appropriate stimulation received from holding, biting, and chewing a variety of objects and foods, they may grind their teeth to provide their own internal proprioceptive stimulation.

Treatment strategies for children who grind their teeth to provide proprioceptive stimulation should include strong proprioceptive input to the jaw.

Interaction Issues

Tooth grinding can create an uncomfortable and irritating sound for adults in the environment. Their continued attention to this behavior enables the child to discover an arena for attention and control.

Treatment strategies may need to include exploring the reactions of the adults in the child's environment in an effort to determine how the adults are reinforcing this behavior. Once the relationship between tooth grinding and the people in the environment is discovered, appropriate interactive strategies can be implemented.

Oral Control Issues

Some children who grind their teeth have poor stability and grading in the movements of the jaw. They often fluctuate between resting their jaws in an open position or grinding the teeth in a closed position. The in-between movements are not well controlled.

For children who have poor jaw stability and grading of jaw movements as an influencing factor in toothgrinding, treatment strategies should include ways to develop graded jaw control.

Stability Bite

Problem

The jaw closes to bite on the spoon, cup, or straw for added stability. This is generally not done with force. It has a voluntary quality. Children usually can open the mouth easily as they regain some of the stability needed for the task. This is not the same jaw closure that is a voluntary communication of "Stay out of my mouth, I do not want any more!"

Treatment Considerations and Directions

Physical Issues

Low muscle tone can influence posture throughout the body as well as muscle tone around the mouth. The influence of gravity on a low-toned body can cause postural rounding and movement into the supporting surface. With rounding at the pelvis and back, the shoulders often compensate by coming forward and the neck then compensates with hyperextension. The head is tipped back in a pattern of capital extension rather than the normal pattern of capital flexion. This biases the mouth toward an open posture. This low tone in the trunk and postural instability can create a need for the child to bite in reaction to the open mouth. This stability biting can be an effort to close the open jaw or recruit muscle tone in a poorly graded jaw.

Fluctuations in muscle tone can cause wide ranges of movement in joints. In the jaw, these athetoid-like fluctuations often can cause wide ranges of movements from exaggerations in jaw opening to biting for stability. Children with these problems often use a closed or a widely exaggerated jaw opening with little control in between.

When low muscle tone or fluctuations in tone influence stability biting of the jaw, treatment strategies must be directed at changing appropriate aspects of the overall physical environment. They also should focus on aspects of overall tone and movement control that can be used before and during mealtimes. These will include strategies for reducing the impact of the tone changes on oral skills before and during mealtimes.

Sensory Issues

Some children use a stability bite as they move the jaw toward a closed position because they are receiving poor or inconsistent proprioceptive feedback from the muscles and joints that surround the jaw. They may feel unstable or in need of clearer sensory feedback that tells them what the jaw is doing.

When sensory issues contribute to stability biting, the therapist should select strategies and activities that increase the child's sensory awareness, discrimination, and feedback.

Oral Control Issues

Children who bite briefly on the spoon or cup for stability generally have not developed graded control of jaw movement. There may be poor graded control of jaw opening or closing through the midranges of movement. When children use stability biting but have poor ability to control the opening and closing of the jaw through midranges of movement, treatment strategies should include activities to improve jaw control and movement.

Specific Feeding-Skill Issues

Although stability biting can interfere with the smooth presentation and rhythm of a meal, children often use it to compensate for jaw stability problems. This helps children be more successful at mealtimes. Spoon feeding, cup drinking, and straw drinking can be much more efficient without the extra biting. Some biting on the edge of a cup for stability is part of the normal developmental sequence. Stability biting becomes a problem only when it actively interferes with the child's ability to take in food in a rhythmical fashion or when a pattern of internal jaw stability does not develop.

Strategies to improve jaw control during feeding skills should be explored in treatment so that the child can develop the internal stability needed for efficient feeding, rather than the external stability provided by stability biting. The child will not reduce stability biting until some internal stability is developed.

Experiential Issues

Many children have lacked the early childhood mouthing and oral exploration experiences that can provide a foundation for jaw stability and control. In addition, some families delay the presentation of bitable foods for a variety of reasons. Children who continually receive spooned foods or tiny pieces of solid foods may lack jaw grading and control that is influenced by biting through different textured foods.

Treatment strategies can encourage mouthing and oral exploration opportunities. They can explore parental experiences and beliefs about when and how to introduce safe bitable foods.

Tonic Bite

Problem

The jaw moves upward into a *tightly* clenched posture when the teeth are stimulated by a finger, spoon, or other object, making it difficult for the child to open the mouth.

The child has difficulty releasing the tonic bite once it has been stimulated.

Treatment Considerations and Directions

Consultation

Some children have poorly formed or poorly functioning temporomandibular joints, which can cause pain with movement of the jaw. Some children move the jaw to a certain point and then have pain or a "catching" of the bones. They may respond to the pain with clenching of the jaw. Stimulation of the teeth can cause more pain in the joint and what appears to be a tonic bite. Consultation with a dentist, physician, or therapist who specializes in TMJ treatment may be necessary.

Physical Issues

Increased patterns of muscle tone can influence overall flexor and extensor patterns of movement throughout the body. A tonic bite can be a part of an overall flexor pattern or a compensatory pattern of movement associated with an extreme extensor pattern of movement.

A poor sitting position can contribute to an overall increase in body tension toward flexion or extension. This increases the probability that a tonic bite will be elicited in a child who has a tendency toward this type of bite.

When a tonic bite response is part of a total pattern of hypertonicity with extremes of flexion or extension of the body, treatment strategies initially must be directed at changing appropriate aspects of the overall physical environment. Treatment strategies must focus on physical handling and positioning. These strategies will involve reducing the extent and impact of limiting flexor and extensor patterns of the body as a key in reducing the strength and frequency of the tonic bite.

Sensory Issues

An overstimulating environment can cause the child to react with strong jaw closing movements. For some children, such an environment can trigger the extremes of flexor and extensor movement patterns that can contribute to a tonic bite response.

Oral hypersensitivity can be present, resulting in a tonic bite when the teeth are touched. This may be more pronounced when the child has engaged in few normal oral motor experiences. The contact of the teeth against each other also can trigger a sustained tonic bite reflex.

When the tonic bite is seen as a response to sensory input, treatment strategies initially must be directed toward changing appropriate aspects of the overall sensory environment. This may involve reducing the overall level of sensory stimulation in the child's mealtime environment or helping the child adjust to small amounts of input without triggering a tonic bite response.

Interaction Issues

Opening the mouth for food is one of the strongest natural signs of readiness for eating. When a child has poor control of jaw opening and closing and an underlying tendency toward a tonic bite, this pattern of biting may become a confusing communication signal. The tonic bite may tell the feeder that the child doesn't want the food or is trying to keep the spoon out of the mouth. Because of the miscommunication, the feeder may end the meal before the child has had enough to eat. In other instances, the child may want to stop the meal. Because of poor control of the jaw and an increase in tension and oral hypersensitivity with anticipation and emotion, the bite occurs as the spoon reaches the mouth. If adults see this as an uncontrolled reflex pattern, rather than the child's attempt to say "no more" or "I need a pause," they will continue to offer the food.

Treatment also should focus on relaxing the child and finding alternative ways to communicate at mealtime so that the tonic bite becomes less of a potentially confusing message.

Oral Control Issues

Oral control issues in a child with a tonic bite pattern usually are secondary to the physical, sensory, and interactional triggers that elicit the biting response.

Treatment strategies to improve oral control will center primarily on reducing the frequency and strength of the tonic bite and then on strategies to develop greater control of jaw movement.

Specific Feeding-Skill Issues

A tonic bite can be a strong deterrent in the development of sucking, swallowing, biting, and chewing. The force of the biting pattern breaks the underlying rhythm and flow of feeding. Children may have difficulty initiating or sustaining the appropriate movement patterns for eating and drinking. The amount of interference will depend upon the frequency and strength of the tonic bite pattern.

Work on a specific feeding skill must always address limiting oral patterns such as the tonic bite in the initial phases of the feeding program. The feeder can change the way in which spoons, cups, and finger foods are presented so that they don't constantly trigger a tonic bite reflex.

Experiential Issues

A tonic bite can be a frightening or even painful experience for children, especially if they have inadvertently bitten their own hand or finger, the feeder's hand, or a metal spoon. For some children, the memory of the tonic bite can cause tension as they see the approaching spoon. The tension then can elicit the tonic bite, and the cycle continues with an added emotional component. Because of a fear of biting their own fingers or an adult's fingers, many infants and young children avoid putting their hands in their mouths or resist oral stimulation by an adult.

Strategies for treatment can include relaxation strategies that help the children learn to prepare for the approach of the spoon and to trust their ability to work with a partner to release the bite should it occur. Therapists must select feeding equipment that reduces the risk of pain or injury during a tonic bite. Strategies may include helping the child adjust to small amounts of sensory input to the mouth without triggering an anticipatory emotional hyperreaction and bite reflex.

Jaw Retraction

Problem

The jaw is pulled in a backward direction by muscle tension.

Treatment Considerations and Directions

Physical Issues

Increased patterns of muscle tone can influence overall extensor patterns of movement throughout the body. Poor sitting position with too much hip extension and posterior pelvic tilt can contribute to an overall increase in forceful body extension. Neck hyperextension may be present with the head tipped back in a pattern of capital extension rather than the normal pattern of capital flexion. Both patterns of physical hyperextension frequently include other strong extensor movements such as shoulder girdle retraction and jaw retraction.

Micrognathia describes the small jaw structure seen in some infants and children. Because of the disproportionate relationship between the lower jaw and the rest of the face, the jaw often appears to be retracted. It may not be functionally retracted by muscle tension that limits the range and extent of movement.

When jaw retraction is present as part of a total pattern of hypertonicity and extension of the body, treatment strategies initially must be directed at changing appropriate aspects of the overall physical environment. They must focus on physical handling and positioning. Strategies involve reducing the extent and impact of limiting extensor patterns of the body as a key in reducing the strength and frequency of the jaw retraction.

Sensory Issues

An overstimulating sensory environment may cause the child to pull the jaw into a retracted pattern. Jaw retraction may be a physical response to the sensory environment of mealtime. This pattern also is seen in some children as a response to the sensory experience of food or liquid falling from the mouth.

When jaw retraction is a response to sensory input, treatment strategies initially must be directed at changing appropriate aspects of the overall sensory environment. This may involve reducing the overall level of sensory stimulation in the child's mealtime environment or helping the child adjust to small amounts of sensory input to the mouth without triggering an avoidance response.

Interaction Issues

Some children use jaw retraction for communication. It can be used as part of a general pullback from the food to tell the feeder to stop or change the way that food is presented. For some children, the jaw retraction is seen with excitement or as an overflow movement. Under these circumstances, it can become part of the total communication strategy.

When children begin to use limiting patterns of movement to communicate, other methods must be investigated. As long as children use jaw retraction to communicate, they will continue to use limiting jaw movement at mealtime. Treatment strategies must focus on finding other ways of communicating that don't involve limiting tone and movement patterns. Treatment also should focus on relaxing the child so that jaw retraction becomes less of a potentially confusing message to the feeder.

Oral Control Issues

Oral control issues in a child with a jaw retraction usually are secondary to the medical, physical, sensory, and interactional triggers that elicit the retraction pattern.

Treatment strategies to improve oral control will center primarily on reducing the frequency, strength, and duration of the jaw retraction and then on strategies to develop greater control of jaw movement.

Specific Feeding-Skill Issues

Jaw retraction can be a strong deterrent in the development of sucking, swallowing, biting, and chewing. The tension of the movement pattern and position of the jaw can break the underlying rhythm and flow of feeding and provide a less functional base. Children may have difficulty initiating or sustaining the appropriate movement patterns for eating and drinking. The amount of interference will depend upon the frequency, duration, and strength of the jaw-retraction pattern.

Retraction of the jaw can move the base of the tongue into the pharyngeal airway, causing noisy breathing and poor coordination of sucking, swallowing, and breathing.

Treatment strategies will focus on methods of eating that promote optimum jaw usage without stimulating the jaw retraction pattern.

Tongue

Tongue Retraction

Problem

The tongue pulls back into the oral cavity so that the tip lies in the posterior three-quarters of the cavity. The tongue may press against the hard palate for stability or intrude into the pharyngeal airway, creating a noisy, stressed breathing pattern.

Treatment Considerations and Directions

Consultation

Infants with a diagnosis such as Pierre Robin sequence have a small lower jaw (micrognathia) and a tongue that is retracted into the pharyngeal airway. As the tongue falls back into the unstable airway, it often causes airway obstruction. Treatment involves medical consultation with the physicians who are managing the craniofacial and airway difficulties.

Physical Issues

Low or high tone in an infant can create exaggeration of early, normal extensor movements. Tongue retraction can accompany these movements. Tongue retraction can be seen in combination with jaw retraction.

Neck hyperextension or an appearance of shortening of the neck (capital extension) frequently is combined with shoulder girdle retraction (scapular adduction). This movement pattern tends to pull the tongue into retraction.

The infant with a cleft of the posterior two-thirds of the hard palate may learn to maintain the tongue in a retracted resting posture. There is a tendency for the tongue to elevate and rest in the open space of the cleft. Because the cleft provides a posterior resting orientation, the retracted tongue position becomes habitual. Once the cleft is repaired, the tongue may find a new resting place.

When tongue retraction is part of a pattern of low or high tone of the body, treatment strategies initially must be directed at changing appropriate aspects of the overall physical environment, focusing on physical handling and positioning.

Sensory Issues

Some children retract their tongues in response to the various sensory properties of food. The texture, taste, or temperature of the food can cause tongue retraction as somewhat of an avoidance reaction. Children find that by retracting the tongue, they often can reduce the contact of textured food with the surface of the tongue or prevent textured food from being swallowed.

When tongue retraction is a response to sensory input, treatment strategies initially must be directed at changing appropriate aspects of the overall sensory environment. This may involve an overall program to reduce sensory defensiveness, careful selection of food according to its sensory properties, and careful sensory preparation of the mouth before the meal.

Interaction Issues

When children are fed against their will, they often figure out ways to avoid discomfort or to reduce the amount of food that is swallowed. In some instances, the child discovers that a retracted tongue acts like a cork in the back of the mouth, effectively preventing the accidental swallowing of food. This becomes the child's volitional statement that no one can make him swallow or that he can hold food in the mouth for a long time and only swallow when he decides to.

This pattern only emerges as an interaction issue when children are being forced to eat or when the adult takes over the child's responsibility for the timing of spoonfuls of food. The treatment program must focus on the mealtime relationship and on reading the child's communicative cues of readiness for a mouthful of food.

Oral Control Issues

Tongue retraction influences the freedom of movement of the tongue and reduces tongue-tip elevation.

Treatment should focus on facilitating a more forward resting position of the tongue. Up and down tongue movements and tongue-tip elevation should be promoted.

Specific Feeding-Skill Issues

The tongue is actively involved in sucking, swallowing, chewing, and bolus formation. Tongue retraction limits the mobility and freedom of the tongue to assist in eating and drinking.

Treatment efforts must focus on reducing tongue retraction so that the tongue can function from a more normal, forward-resting position.

Exaggerated Tongue Protrusion

Problem

Exaggerated tongue protrusion maintains the easy flow of movement seen in the normal suckle pattern. However, the protrusive movement is exaggerated. On the outward portion of the in-out movement, the tongue moves forward beyond the border of the gums and may stick out between the lips. This is contrasted with a tongue thrust by the gentle protrusion in the exaggerated protrusion and the forceful pushing out of the tongue thrust. This also is contrasted with a purposive spitting out of food in which the tongue may move in an exaggerated forward direction.

Treatment Considerations and Directions

Consultation

Children who maintain the tongue in a more forward position and use an exaggerated tongue-protrusion pattern during swallowing frequently develop misalignment of the teeth (i.e., dental malocclusions). Treatment may involve consultation with orthodontists or other dentists specializing in the use of dental prostheses to retrain tongue and lip patterns or consultation with a myofunctional therapist.

Physical Issues

A constant open mouth position, oral structural defect, or significant open-bite position of the teeth can make lip closure difficult or impossible during food manipulation and swallowing. Without adequate lip closure and the dental barrier formed by good tooth alignment, the tongue may protrude in an effort to find a place of stability for swallowing. The development of an open-bite malocclusion of the teeth is usually the result of the forward-resting position of the tongue between the teeth as they are erupting. The open bite then provides an easy hole for further exaggerated protrusion of the tongue.

Low muscle tone can influence the quality of jaw, cheek, lip, and tongue movements. Low tone in all of these areas allows the tongue to be much less active and push forward during food manipulation and swallowing. High muscle tone in the tongue can cause the tongue to extend or gently push forward during use.

Stressed breathing patterns can contribute to tongue protrusion. The infant or child positions the tongue forward to enlarge the pharyngeal airway and increase respiratory capacity. The child may hold the tongue between the gums with the teeth to keep it in a forward position. This frequently is seen in children with a history of bronchopulmonary dysplasia and other primary respiratory disorders. It also may be seen in children with Down syndrome, who are prone to upper respiratory congestion.

Neck hyperextension or an appearance of shortening of the neck (capital extension) often is seen as a low-tone compensation. This movement pattern often creates an exaggeration of extensor patterns in the mouth, such as exaggerated jaw opening and exaggerated tongue protrusion.

When exaggerated tongue protrusion is part of a total pattern of low or high tone, treatment strategies must be directed at changing the overall physical environment, focusing on physical handling and positioning, or mealtime seating. Therapists first must consider safety of the airway and improvement of breathing patterns.

Oral Control Issues

Control of the jaw and lips and maturation of tongue skills influences tongue protrusion. Poor jaw stability provides a poor base for tongue movements. When a child has poor jaw stability, tongue protrusion is an increased possibility. Poor lip closure makes it more difficult for the tongue to find a closed environment to practice up-down and tongue-tip elevation movements. Lack of tongue lateralization and mobility can lead to an exaggerated protrusion to move food from the front to the back of the tongue. A child may discover that lumpy food stuck on the front of the tongue automatically is scraped toward the back of the tongue by the teeth if the tongue is moved forward. Delay in development of tongue-tip elevation may necessitate a more active forward movement in an effort to find stability during the swallowing process. As children with low tone in the tongue develop greater control and movement, they may exaggerate the forward and backward movement of the tongue.

When delayed or limiting oral skills influence an exaggerated tongue protrusion, treatment strategies must focus on improving overall jaw, lip, cheek, and tongue control in biting, chewing, and swallowing.

Specific Feeding-Skill Issues

The tongue is actively involved in sucking, swallowing, chewing, and bolus formation. Tongue protrusion limits the mobility and freedom of the tongue to assist in eating and drinking. It can get in the way in cup drinking. It can push the spoon out during spoon feeding and expel the food once it is in the mouth. It may limit the textures that the child can eat because the movement interferes with tongue lateralization and chewing. It also influences the development of a mature swallowing pattern because the protrusion pattern is incompatible with tongue-tip elevation.

Treatment must focus on reducing the protrusion so that the tongue can move from a more normal position in the mouth. Activities to promote jaw stability and lip closure will support improved tongue movement.

Tongue Thrust

Problem

Tongue thrust describes a very forceful protrusion of the tongue from the mouth. It is a stronger movement than the extension-retraction movements seen in either the infantile suckling pattern or the mildly limiting, exaggerated tongue protrusion. Frequently, movement is arrhythmical, and its intermittent occurrence can break a previously sustained rhythm. The thrusting makes it difficult to insert the nipple or spoon, and may cause food and liquid to be pushed out of the mouth.

Treatment Considerations and Directions

Physical Issues

Low tone can create exaggeration of early normal extensor movements of the body. Tongue retraction may be associated with these early movements. As ***stronger*** extensor tone develops, the infant develops the ability to push the tongue farther forward during the in-out suckle. When muscle tone continues to be low, the forward push may become stronger, resulting in a more powerful tongue thrust.

Neck hyperextension or an appearance of shortening of the neck (capital extension) frequently is combined with shoulder girdle retraction (scapular adduction). This movement pattern often creates an exaggeration of extensor patterns in the mouth. Tongue thrust is an extensor movement that often is triggered by extensor patterns of the shoulders and pelvis.

When the tongue thrust is part of a total pattern of hypertonicity and extension of the body, treatment strategies initially must be directed at changing appropriate aspects of the overall physical environment.

Sensory Issues

Oral hypersensitivity may be present. The contact of the food or spoon on the tongue can elicit a tongue-thrusting response. Sometimes, an overstimulating environment can cause the child to react with limiting extensor patterns and tongue thrusting.

When tongue thrusting is a response to the sensory input of the environment or oral hypersensitivity, treatment strategies initially must be directed at changing appropriate aspects of the overall sensory environment and the sensory aspects of the food and utensils presented.

Interaction Issues

Some children who have a tongue thrust learn to use it as a method of communicating with the feeder. When the child has poor control of the tongue and an underlying tendency toward a tongue thrust, this pattern of thrusting may become a communication signal. The feeder may recognize the thrust as an indication of whether the child wants to eat. Children may continue to use the tongue thrust to let the feeder know they need another bite or want the meal to stop, even when their heads are in good alignment and the sensory input is appropriate.

As long as children think that a tongue thrust is the only way to communicate readiness to the feeder, they will continue to use this limiting tongue movement at mealtimes. Treatment strategies must focus on finding other ways to communicate that don't involve limiting tone and movement patterns.

Oral Control Issues

Sometimes, a tongue thrust is seen as a compensatory tongue movement for a child with significant tongue retraction. The tongue thrusting is the powerful attempt to move out of the retraction.

Treatment strategies should include treating the causes of the tongue retraction and improving controlled tongue movements.

Specific Feeding-Skill Issues

The tongue is actively involved in sucking, swallowing, chewing, and bolus formation. Tongue thrusting severely limits the mobility and freedom of the tongue to assist in eating and drinking. It can get in the way in cup drinking. It can strongly push the spoon out in spoon feeding and push the food out once it is in the mouth. It can limit the textures the child can eat because of the restrictions in lateralization. It may reduce a child's development of mature swallowing patterns because of limitations in tongue-tip elevation.

Treatment efforts to develop specific feeding skills must focus on reducing the tongue thrust so that the tongue can function within the mouth. Activities to help the child develop greater overall tongue control in the mouth can give the child an alternative to pushing the tongue out of the mouth.

Low Tone With Unusual Tongue Configuration

Problem

Hypotonia in the tongue reduces the strength and skill with which the tongue can move during feeding and speech activities.

When tone is low, the tongue frequently lacks the normal, thin, cupped, or grooved configuration that assists efficient sucking. The tongue may be thick and humped. Food entering the mouth falls over the edges into the buccal cavity or becomes scattered. Bolus collection is inefficient.

Treatment Considerations and Directions

Consultation

Damage to cranial nerve XII (hypoglossus) can result in a bulbar paralysis of the intrinsic muscles of the tongue. Damage to cranial nerve VII (facial) interferes with the sensory innervation of the tongue. This can be reflected in low muscle tone, weakness, and an unusual tongue configuration. For many children who have cranial nerve involvement, the damage usually is incomplete, leaving a partial function of the damaged cranial nerve. Therapists should consult with medical personnel to rule out cranial nerve dysfunction or paralysis.

Physical Issues

Low tone can be reflected in the mouth as well as the rest of the body. It can be seen in unusual tongue configurations when it is asymmetrical or when there is fluctuating tone in the tongue.

When low muscle tone influences the configuration of the tongue, treatment strategies focus on physical positioning and handling to improve the foundational tone upon which the mouth gains its stability.

Sensory Issues

Poor sensory awareness and feedback also can result in reduced tone and an unusual configuration of the tongue.

When sensory issues influence tone and configuration, treatment strategies can include building oral awareness, discrimination, and feedback.

Oral Control Issues

The damage to cranial nerves XII and VII, as described under Consultation, can be reflected in low muscle tone, weakness, and an unusual tongue configuration with limitations in tongue control. This damage usually is incomplete, leaving a partial function of the damaged cranial nerve. Treatment can focus on maximizing tongue control and the movements available to the child, and providing normal bilateral and unilateral motor and sensory experiences.

Specific Feeding-Skill Issues

Low tone in the tongue with a flat or humped configuration reduces the child's overall skill in organizing a bolus and directing it toward the pharynx for swallowing. During early bottle drinking or spoon feeding, food and liquid may fall over the sides of the tongue into the buccal cavity or fall out of the mouth. Tongue movements during chewing may be weak and unsustained, increasing the overall effort and energy that must be expended to chew more complex foods. Many children with low tone in the tongue dislike eating meats or other foods that require a stronger, more sustained chewing pattern.

Treatment strategies should include treating the causes of the low tone in the face and mouth, increasing tone in the tongue, and improving controlled tongue movements.

Tongue Asymmetry

Problem

Uneven muscle strength and coordination on the sides of the tongue can cause it to deviate in one direction when it is protruded. The tongue does not move equally well to both sides during chewing.

Treatment Considerations and Directions

Consultation

Damage to the cervical spine or rotation of the cervical spine can cause a pinching of the cervical nerves, which can result in asymmetry. A referral to a neurologist may be necessary.

Physical Issues

Postural asymmetry because of an asymmetrical tonic neck reflex (ATNR) can result in the tongue pulling to the side toward which the head is turned.

Anytime asymmetry is a result of limiting movement patterns in the body, treatment strategies must be directed at changing appropriate aspects of the overall physical environment. Treatment strategies must focus on physical handling and positioning, and involve reducing the impact of the asymmetrical tonic neck reflex.

Oral Control Issues

A child may have experienced greater damage on one side of the brain than the other, resulting in better function on one side of the body and poorer function on the other. This is described as a hemiplegia or a double hemiplegia, if there is unequal damage to both sides. Weakness on one side of the tongue will cause it to deviate or pull toward the stronger side. Damage to the right cortex of the brain will cause dysfunction on the left side of the body because the nerve fibers to the limbs cross and innervate the opposite side of the body. Nerve fibers from the cranial nerves in the brain stem do not cross on their way to the tongue. Thus, damage to the right side of the brain and brain stem (cranial nerve XII, the hypoglossus) affects the muscles of the right side of the tongue and the left side of the body. The stronger, more normal movement of the left side of the tongue would pull it to the left, creating a deviation and better function on the hemiplegic side. For many children who have cranial nerve involvement, the damage usually is incomplete, leaving a partial function of the damaged cranial nerve.

When cranial nerve damage influences the tongue, often it is incomplete. Treatment strategies should be aimed at maximizing the tongue skills the child has and can recruit from intact neural structures. Bilateral oral activities can provide the symmetry that children do not usually receive independently.

Specific Feeding-Skill Issues

Tongue asymmetry may affect where the food is placed in the mouth and on what side of the mouth the child bites food. If one side of the tongue is more active, the food will be better controlled on that side.

Treatment will focus on feeding opportunities that promote symmetry, such as cup drinking and straw drinking, along with food placement to both sides for biting and chewing.

Limited Tongue Movement

Problem

Tongue movement is minimal when food is placed in the mouth. Tongue movement is reduced when mouthing toys or making different vowel or consonant sounds.

Treatment Considerations and Directions
Physical Issues

The tongue can be stiff because of hypertonicity. Forward-back, up-down, and side-to-side movement can be limited because of increased tension in the tongue. The tongue also can be floppy because of hypotonicity. Movement is limited because of insufficient tension in the tongue.

When tongue movements are limited because of hypertonicity or hypotonicity, treatment strategies initially should be directed at changing appropriate aspects of the overall physical environment. Positioning and handling are important. The emphasis should be on reducing the impact of the limiting patterns of movement on tongue movements.

Sensory Issues

The tongue can be underreactive to sensation. It may take stronger sensations of taste, temperature, or touch to elicit a motor response from the tongue.

When tongue movements are severely limited because of hyporeaction to sensation, treatment strategies must focus on changing appropriate aspects of the overall sensory environment, with a careful look at the sensory properties of the food and utensils presented.

Oral Control Issues

The tongue can be flaccid because of damage to cranial nerve XII.

When cranial nerve damage influences the tongue, often it is incomplete. Treatment strategies should be aimed at maximizing the tongue skills the child has and can recruit.

Specific Feeding-Skill Issues

The tongue is actively involved in sucking, swallowing, chewing, and bolus formation. Tongue limitations influence the mobility and skill of the tongue in eating and drinking. This can limit the textures the child can eat because of the restrictions in lateralization and influence swallowing because of limitations in tongue-tip elevation.

Treatment efforts must focus on improving the mobility and activity level of the tongue. Food can be offered after oral preparation, with utensils and food placement that provide the degree of stimulation required to obtain better tongue movement.

Lips and Cheeks

Lip Retraction and Pursing

Problem

If muscle tone is too high, there is a tendency for the lips and cheeks to be pulled into a tightly retracted position. Lip retraction occurs when the lips are drawn back so that they form a tight horizontal line over the mouth.

It becomes difficult for the retracted lips and cheeks to assist in sucking from the bottle or breast, in removing food or liquid from the spoon or cup, and in the chewing, transfer, and retention of food in the mouth.

Lip pursing is seen when the child attempts to counteract the effects of lip retraction. When the lips are pulled forward from a tightly retracted position, it appears as though the lip muscles are being drawn closed in the puckered way as when a drawstring pulls a cloth laundry bag closed.

Treatment Considerations and Directions
Physical Issues

A poor sitting position with too much hip extension can contribute to an overall increase in body extension. This increases the probability that lip retraction will be elicited.

Neck hyperextension may be present. The head may be tipped back with a pattern of capital extension rather than the normal pattern of capital flexion. The hyperextended pattern frequently includes other extensor movements, such as lip and cheek retraction. The use of effort to speak or eat in spite of the lip retraction can result in lip pursing.

When the lip retraction and pursing are part of a total pattern of hypertonicity and extension of the body, treatment strategies initially must be directed at changing appropriate aspects of the overall physical environment. Treatment strategies must focus on physical handling and positioning, and involve reducing the extent and impact of limiting extensor patterns of the body on the lip retraction and lip pursing.

Sensory Issues

An overstimulating environment can cause the child to react with limiting patterns of lip and cheek retraction and pursing.

When lip pursing and retraction are a response to sensory input, treatment strategies initially must be directed at changing appropriate aspects of the overall sensory environment. This may involve reducing the overall level of sensory stimulation present in the child's mealtime environment or helping the child adjust to small amounts of sensory input to the mouth without triggering an avoidance response.

Interaction Issues

Some children use lip retraction and pursing to tell the feeder to stop or change the feeding presentation. For some children, lip retraction and pursing are seen with excitement, as an overflow movement, which quickly becomes a communication signal.

When children begin to use limiting patterns of movement to communicate, other methods of communication must be investigated. As long as children use lip retraction, pursing, or both to communicate, they will continue to use limiting lip movements at mealtime. Treatment strategies must focus on finding other ways of communication that don't involve limiting tone and movement patterns. Treatment also should focus on relaxing the child so the retraction and pursing becomes less of a potentially confusing message to the feeder.

Oral Control Issues

Oral control issues in a child with a lip retraction and lip pursing usually are secondary to the medical, physical, sensory, and interactional triggers that elicit the retraction pattern.

Treatment strategies to improve oral control will center primarily on reducing the frequency, strength, and duration of the lip retraction and pursing, and then on strategies to develop greater control of lip and cheek movement.

Specific Feeding-Skill Issues

Lip retraction and pursing can be a strong deterrent in the development of sucking, swallowing, biting, and chewing. Children may have difficulty initiating or sustaining the appropriate movement patterns for eating and drinking. The amount of interference depends on the frequency, duration, and strength of the lip retraction and pursing patterns. Considerable liquid and food is lost during eating. Some children will tip the head into hyperextension as a compensation to prevent the loss of food and saliva.

Treatment strategies should focus on feeding methods that optimize the normal usage of the lips and minimize the need for lip retraction and pursing.

Low Tone in the Cheeks

Problem

Hypotonia in the cheeks reduces the strength and skill with which the lips and cheeks can move during feeding and speech. When tone is low, the cheeks and lips frequently lack the control and flexibility that assist efficient sucking. Food entering the mouth falls into the buccal cavity. Bolus collection is inefficient. This problem is increased when the tongue has a low-tone, humped configuration. Low tone can cause the mouth to hang open, and the child may drool excessively.

Treatment Considerations and Directions

Consultation

Damage to cranial nerve VII (facial) can result in a bulbar paralysis of the facial muscles. Damage to cranial nerve V (trigeminal) interferes with the sensory innervation of the face and the motor innervation of the jaw muscles that open and close the mouth. When cranial nerve involvement is suspected, a referral to a neurologist may be indicated.

Physical Issues

Low tone in the body can be reflected in the mouth. Often, low tone in the jaw is seen in conjunction with low tone in the cheeks and lips. The resulting instability makes it more challenging for the child to develop control of the lips and cheeks.

When low tone in the cheeks is a reflection of decreased muscle tone throughout the body, treatment strategies initially must be directed at changing appropriate aspects of the overall physical environment. Treatment strategies must focus on physical handling and positioning that improve foundational muscle tone, working from the body to the jaw, cheeks, and lips.

Sensory Issues

Poor sensory awareness and feedback also can result in reduced tone and movement in the lips and cheeks.

When sensory issues influence muscle tone, treatment strategies should include building oral awareness, discrimination, and feedback.

Interaction Issues

Low tone in the cheeks and lips typically results in reduced facial movement and facial expression. With the lack of expected affect, many children can give the impression that they do not understand what others are saying or that they are cognitively delayed. Adults may reduce their level of interaction and language input with the child. The lack of facial expression and affect may be confusing to the feeder. Although children with low facial tone usually find other ways to express their basic feeding needs, they may have difficulty expressing subtler mealtime messages. For example, a child might turn away or fuss if he did not want the food on the spoon. However, the lack of facial expression could limit the same child's ability to use a questioning expression or express a very mild dislike of the food.

Oral Control Issues

Damage to cranial nerve VII (facial) can result in a bulbar paralysis of the facial muscles. Damage to cranial nerve V (trigeminal) interferes with the sensory innervation of the face and the motor innervation of the jaw muscles that open and close the mouth. This can be reflected in low muscle tone, weakness, and facial asymmetry if there is greater damage to one side. For many children with cranial nerve involvement, the damage is incomplete, leaving a partial function of the damaged cranial nerves. Poor sensory awareness and motoric function in the face and mouth can result in incomplete contraction of the cheek and lip muscles. The cheeks can sag and become much less active in the eating process. The cheeks may not be able to provide the sustained contraction needed for sucking and swallowing. They may not provide the drawing-in support needed to help keep food over the grinding surface of the teeth during chewing.

When the low tone in the cheeks interferes with efficient oral skills, treatment should be focused on improving cheek and lip control, and improving the jaw skills as a foundational basis for cheek control.

Specific Feeding-Skill Issues

Low tone in the cheeks can interfere with the development of sucking and swallowing skills, as well as efficient biting and chewing. The level of interference depends on the degree of decreased tone and the child's responsiveness to therapeutic interventions to prepare cheeks for these eating skills.

Work on specific feeding skills must address ways to prepare the cheeks for active involvement in the eating process.

Problem

Upper lip movement is minimal when food is introduced by spoon or placed in the mouth. It is reduced when mouthing toys or producing sound. The upper lip may not assist efficiently in lip closure during swallowing.

Treatment Considerations and Directions

Consultation

Many children develop an overbite malocclusion of the teeth because of a lack of inward pressure from the upper lip. Once this has developed, the child may find it difficult to involve the upper lip actively in feeding and speech movements. Treatment may involve consultation with an orthodontist or other dentist specializing in the use of dental prostheses to retrain tongue and lip patterns, or consultation with a myofunctional therapist.

Physical Issues

The lips and cheeks may be floppy because of hypotonicity. Movement may be limited because of insufficient tension in the face. The lips and cheeks may be stiff because of hypertonicity and retraction. Movement may be limited because of the increased tension in the face.

When hypotonicity or hypertonicity influence movements of the upper lip, therapy must deal with the underlying tone issues. Treatment strategies must be directed at changing the appropriate aspects of the overall physical environment. Physical handling and positioning will be important during treatment. The aim is to normalize foundational tone of the body, jaw, and lips in an effort to increase the activity and readiness of the lips.

Sensory Issues

Sometimes, the upper lip is limited in its involvement because of increased sensory defensiveness. The lip pulls away from tactile contact with the spoon, cup, or finger food.

When upper lip movement is decreased because of a sensory hyperreaction or sensory defensiveness, treatment should focus on decreasing the limiting sensory patterns and increasing the oral exploration possibilities available to the child.

Oral Control Issues

Damage to cranial nerve VII (facial) can result in a bulbar paralysis of the facial muscles. Damage to cranial nerve V (trigeminal) interferes with the sensory innervation of the face. This can be reflected in low muscle tone, weakness, and facial asymmetry, if there is greater damage to one side. For many children with cranial nerve involvement, the damage usually is incomplete, leaving a partial function of the damaged cranial nerves.

When limited upper lip activity interferes with oral skills, treatment should focus on increasing the range of motion and controlled activity level of the upper lip.

Specific Feeding-Skill Issues

Limited upper lip movement can interfere with the development of sucking and swallowing skills, food removal from the spoon, and efficient biting and chewing. The amount of interference depends on the degree of upper lip limitations and on the child's ability to compensate with strong cheek and lower lip movement.

Many children do not use upper lip movement during cup drinking or in helping to remove food from the spoon because they have not developed a stable pattern of jaw opening and closing. When the spoon is presented, the mouth moves in a total suckle pattern. Without the quieting of the tongue and the stability provided by the jaw, the upper lip cannot develop differentiated movement control.

Work on specific feeding skills must address ways to promote the most active and controlled upper lip involvement possible. These strategies always include a focus on the development of the stability and graded movement control of the jaw.

Palate

Nasal Reflux

Problem

Food or liquid taken into the mouth refluxes upward into the nasal cavity rather than being swallowed efficiently.

Treatment Considerations and Directions

Consultation

Infants with a cleft of the hard or soft palate lack the anatomical closure to keep food and liquid out of the nasal cavity. Sometimes, nasal reflux is an indication of an undiagnosed submucous cleft of the palate. A referral to a physician specializing in craniofacial disorders may be indicated to rule this out.

Physical Issues

Neck hyperextension or an appearance of shortening of the neck (capital extension) frequently is combined with shoulder girdle retraction (scapular adduction). This movement pattern tends to increase tension in the jaw, tongue, and pharynx. The increased tone often leads to incoordination of timing for palatal elevation during the swallow.

Gravity increases the amount of nasal reflux when a child is fed in supine or with the head in hyperextension. When this extended pattern is combined with increased tension, the probability of incoordination and nasal reflux increases.

When nasal reflux occurs because of neck hypertension or shortening, treatment strategies should focus on changing appropriate aspects of the overall physical environment. Treatment strategies will include handling and positioning to reduce the extent and impact of the limiting neck patterns of movement that influence the tension and shortening. When nasal reflux is increased with gravity, more upright position and seating changes will be important.

Oral Control Issues

Insufficient length of the soft palate (velopharyngeal insufficiency) can reduce its ability to contact the pharyngeal wall as the palate elevates for the swallow, causing a portion of the bolus to reflux into the open nasal cavity. In addition, incoordination in swallowing can create timing problems that leave the nasal cavity open to food and liquid before or during the swallow.

Treatment strategies to improve oral control will focus on the organization and timing of swallowing.

Specific Feeding-Skill Issues

Nasal reflux can be disconcerting and uncomfortable, and can affect the timing and coordination of sucking and swallowing liquids and solids. Nasal reflux during feeding also can trigger apnea and bradycardia in infants.

Work on specific feeding skills must include careful food selection and presentation to minimize the nasal reflux.

Structural Deformities of the Mouth

Problem

The hard palate is high and narrow, and the dental arches have failed to spread. When children have poor tongue movements, solid food can become lodged in the high palatal arch. Other structural deformities of the dental arches and teeth may be present. The child may have a cleft of the lip or palate.

Treatment Considerations and Directions
Consultation

Children with clefts of the lip or palate generally have been seen by medical specialists in craniofacial disorders before referral to the feeding specialist. The specialized issues and treatment strategies involved with clefting are discussed in Chapter 25.

Physical Issues

Structural deformities of the mouth can be present at birth or can develop during infancy or childhood. Disruptions in midline development during the fetal period when the palate is formed can result in a highly arched palate. Infants with low tone often receive a sustained pressure to the cheeks and lateral dental arches from the support surface when they are in sidelying. This can move the dental arches inward toward the midline and contribute to a high palatal vault. A high narrow hard palate also can result from the sustained pressure of an endotrachial tube.

Oral Control Issues

In normal development, the dental arches are spread and the palate remains broad and flat because the tongue spreads and presses gently against the upper dental arch. When the tongue is hypotonic, the pressure against the arch and palate often is insufficient to promote and sustain the outward movement that results in a wide, flat palate. When the tongue is hypertonic, it often is thick and bunched, with a lack of sustained spreading. Both situations contribute to the postnatal development of a high narrow palate.

Specific Feeding-Skill Issues

A high narrow palate usually does not interfere with the development of feeding skills if a child has relatively normal movement control of the tongue, lips, and cheeks. When tongue movement is poor, solid pieces of food can be pushed into the palatal vault, where they become stuck. This can create discomfort for the child and difficulty getting the food unstuck. Many children end the meal with a substantial amount of food packed into the narrow palatal vault. This causes additional problems removing the food and keeping the mouth clean.

■ Problems With Sensory Processes

Hyposensitivity

Hyporeaction

Problem

The child may have milder reactions to a specific sensation than would be expected. For some children, elevation in the sensory threshold results in a smaller amount of information reaching the child's awareness.

Reduction in the acuity of taste, smell, and touch-pressure receptors in the mouth can cause severe motor-feeding disorders or indifference to eating. Severe visual impairment reduces the child's ability to anticipate and prepare the mouth for the next bite when the feeder gives only visual cues that the food is coming. A tracheostomy prevents airborne smells from reaching olfactory receptors in the nose, reducing both the senses of smell and taste at mealtimes.

Treatment Considerations and Directions
Consultation

High levels of anticonvulsant medication can elevate a child's sensory threshold and reduce overall responsiveness. The therapist may need to consult with the neurologist if the medication severely reduces the child's response to sensation.

Problems with acuity resulting in impairment in the visual, auditory, tactile, kinesthetic, vestibular, taste, and smell senses can be considered an organ hyposensitivity. This includes disorders resulting from dysfunction of the cranial and peripheral nerve supply, as well as those of the organ receptors. If organ dysfunction is suspected, referral to an appropriate specialist should be considered.

Neurological damage can result in a raised threshold and underresponsiveness to sensory information. When neurological changes affect sensory responsiveness, a referral to a neurologist may be appropriate.

Physical Issues

Decreases in postural tone can raise the sensory threshold to all stimulation so that the child's ability to perceive small amounts of sensory information may be reduced.

When decreased muscle tone influences hyporeactions to stimuli, treatment should focus on changing appropriate aspects of the overall physical environment. Physical handling and positioning will work to increase the child's postural tone and overall physical responsiveness to sensory input.

Sensory Issues

The child may experience major difficulty in filtering out unnecessary sensory input. Problems with foreground-background information interfere with the ability to function in a multisensory environment. Because of a high level of sensory overload, the child's nervous system protects itself by increasing the sensory threshold, or sometimes, shutting down completely.

When the hyporeaction is a response to sensory input, treatment strategies initially must be directed at changing the appropriate aspects of the overall sensory environment. This may involve reducing the overall level of sensory stimulation in the child's mealtime environment.

Interaction Issues

At times, feeders misinterpret hyporeactions to mealtime stimuli as a lack of interest in the meal or the food. The child's responses may be slow or relatively undifferentiated. The feeder may not wait for the child's response or may misinterpret it.

Hyporeactions to mealtime stimuli can be confusing. Treatment should focus on helping the feeder clearly understand the child's cues.

Oral Control Issues

Oral control can be slow and inefficient in a child with a low level of response to sensory information. This can affect the ability to sustain the movements necessary for efficient eating. Children may tire more rapidly or lose interest in eating more challenging food.

Treatment strategies to increase oral control will center primarily on finding the sensory components of the meal that facilitate the most efficient and normalized response.

Specific Feeding-Skill Issues

Hyporeaction to mealtime stimuli can interfere with the development of sucking, swallowing, biting, and chewing. The amount of interference will depend on the degree of hyporesponsiveness to the mealtime information. Children may have difficulty initiating or sustaining the appropriate movement patterns and control for eating and drinking. They may be unaware of food in the mouth and stuff the mouth to increase the amount of sensory information. Pieces of food may become scattered and remain in the mouth for many hours after the meal is completed.

Treatment strategies will focus on ways to increase sensory awareness, discrimination, and feedback while promoting developmental feeding skills.

Hypersensitivity

Hyperreaction

Problem

The child has stronger reactions to a specific sensation than would be expected. The excessive reaction to stimulation can trigger hypertonicity and limiting movement patterns in the body. Touch to the teeth can trigger a tonic bite reflex. The child may have a hypersensitive or easily elicited gag reflex.

The child becomes overly excited by sensory stimuli associated with eating. The sound of the refrigerator opening can cause the mouth to fly open in full anticipation of being fed. The approach of a spoon can trigger limiting oral patterns, interfering with the child's ability to take the food.

Treatment Considerations and Directions

Consultation

Gastrointestinal issues can contribute to gagging as a hyperreaction to sensory input. When gastrointestinal issues are suspected, a referral to the primary care physician or gastroenterologist may be indicated.

Neurological damage can result in a lowered threshold and overresponsiveness to sensory information. When neurological changes affect sensory responsiveness, a referral to a neurologist may be appropriate.

Physical Issues

Increases in postural tone and obligatory reflex patterns may reduce the sensory threshold to touch and movement.

When hyperreactions to sensory stimuli are influenced by patterns of total body hypertonicity, treatment strategies should include changing appropriate aspects of the overall physical environment. Treatment strategies must focus on physical handling and positioning that involve reducing the extent and impact of limiting tension patterns of the body as a key to reducing the hyperreactive responses.

Sensory Issues

A hyperreaction can occur to any sensory stimuli (e.g., sight, smell, taste, touch, hearing, proprioception, and movement). All of these can affect the meal. For some children, the gag reflex may not have diminished or normalized. It is as easily activated from the front of the tongue as it is in early infancy. This may be because of a lack of normal oral sensory experiences.

Because hyperreactions are seen predominantly and initially as responses to sensory input, treatment strategies must be directed at changing appropriate aspects of the overall sensory environment of the meal. When hyperreactive gag reactions are influenced by lack of normal oral sensory experiences, treatment should focus on grading sensory input and providing normal oral exploratory and mouthing experiences.

Interaction Issues

Some children have hyperreactive responses to the presentation of a meal, resulting in a strong emotional response such as excitement or distress. Simply thinking about eating or seeing the feeder can trigger a strong hyperreaction. For other children, mealtime interactions may have been stressful, affecting the feeding relationship. Children can learn to use a hyperreactive response to the presentation of food to communicate that they want to eat, that the meal is finished, or that they do not want the particular food being offered.

When stressful mealtime interactions have contributed to hyperreactive responses, treatment should focus on rebuilding trust in the relationship, and improving the mealtime interactions and feeding relationship. When anticipation and excitement are the main triggers for a hyperreaction to the feeder, treatment can include activities that use a graded approach to social stimuli and imagery.

When children use hyperreaction as a method of communication, efforts need to be made to help the child learn other, more positive methods to communicate with the feeder, as well as to help the feeder be more consistently responsive to the child's communication.

Oral Control Issues

Oral control issues in a child with hyperreactions to sensory information usually are secondary to the sensory triggers that elicit these responses.

Treatment strategies to increase oral control will center primarily on finding the sensory components of the meal that promote the most mature oral patterns of movement.

Specific Feeding-Skill Issues

Hyperreaction to mealtime stimuli can strongly interfere with the development of sucking, swallowing, biting, and chewing. The level of interference depends on the strength and frequency of the hyperreaction. Children may have difficulty initiating or sustaining the appropriate movement patterns and control for eating and drinking.

Treatment strategies will focus on ways to limit the child's hyperreaction, while promoting developmental feeding skills.

Experiential Issues

Reduction of oral stimulation because of tube feedings may cause a child to experience all oral sensations as excessively strong when food is introduced. Taste, touch, and temperature changes can elicit dramatic overreactions.

When a lack of oral experience influences hyperreactive responses, treatment should focus on providing developmentally appropriate, safe, and trusting positive oral experiences.

Sensory Defensiveness

Problem

The child has strong reactions to a specific sensation that is perceived as unpleasant or negative, often triggering a "fight-or-flight" response.

The child has intense dislikes of specific sensory properties of food such as texture, taste, spiciness, acidity, and smell. These responses are developed on the basis of a sensory discomfort rather than simple dislike. The transition to solid foods may be unsuccessful. The child can be a very picky eater who creates many frustrations for the parent who wishes to provide a balanced diet.

Because of discomfort with sensory stimulation, the infant often may resist being held. It may be difficult to give a bottle or the breast because the baby pulls away from the sensory stimulation of the nipple and of being held.

The excessive reaction to stimulation may trigger many limiting tone and movement patterns, primarily as the child attempts to escape from the stimulus.

The baby may reject softer toys for play and mouthing because they create a light, tickling touch that is uncomfortable. The child may dislike certain types of clothing or bibs because of the light contact they create with the skin. Wiping or washing the face and hands after meals may be extremely uncomfortable, particularly if this is done with a fast swiping movement.

Treatment Considerations and Directions

Sensory Issues

In sensory defensiveness, the child's response to sensory information occurs at a phylogenetically older level, where the primary distinction or reaction is one of safety or danger. The nervous system may not have developed the phylogenetically newer ability to discriminate additional properties of the stimulus.

The child may have difficulty integrating sensory input from many different channels.

Because light touch is more stimulating than firm touch, the child with tactile defensiveness is more uncomfortable and rejecting of light and caressing touch.

When sensory defensiveness is a response to common sensory input, treatment strategies initially must be directed at changing appropriate aspects of the overall sensory environment to minimize the possibilities for overreaction. Each sensory channel needs to be reviewed to identify those that are involved in sensory defensiveness. Because feeding involves a great deal of tactile input, it is particularly important to help the child learn to respond appropriately to all manner of touch, from deep pressure and massage touch to light touch and texture variations. This may involve helping the child adjust to small amounts of sensory input to the hands and mouth, without triggering defensive responses.

Interaction Issues

A child who has sensory defensive responses can provide confusing communication messages to a feeder. The defensive reaction to the sensory input may be misinterpreted as a lack of hunger or interest in the meal when the child may be quite hungry, but unable to eat within the available sensory environment. Because defensive responses can be intermittent and unpredictable, the child may experience sudden negative reactions to a bite of food or the way in which a utensil is placed in the mouth. Sometimes, the child who has had many extreme defensive responses learns to use those responses to communicate a dislike of the meal or foods presented, or a wish to end the meal.

When the sensory defensive reactions interfere with clear communication at the mealtime, treatment strategies must focus on finding other ways of communicating clear mealtime messages that do not involve the sudden defensive responses.

Oral Control Issues

Oral control issues are secondary to the sensory triggers that elicit the sensory defensive pattern. Treatment strategies to improve oral control will center on determining which sensory variables promote the most organized and controlled oral responses.

Specific Feeding-Skill Issues

Sensory defensiveness can strongly influence the acquisition of mature feeding skills. The extremes of responses can interfere with controlled sucking, swallowing, biting, and chewing, and thereby influence the quality of eating and drinking responses.

Work on specific feeding skills must be done with sensitivity to the specific sensory thresholds of the child and with prior and simultaneous preparation to reduce sensory defensiveness.

Experiential Issues

Many children with a history of oral or tactile defensiveness have had inadequate experience with oral stimulation. Tactile defensiveness of the hands reduces the child's desire to pick up toys and bring them to the mouth. Tube feedings can reduce the overall amount of sensory input that the child has experienced in the mouth. Oral experiences may have been negative for the child and may have contributed to a powerful sensory defensiveness as emotions complicate the underlying physical and sensory interactions.

Treatment for children who have not had adequate or positive sensory-oral experiences must focus on a slow rebuilding of trust and reintroduction of positive oral interactions.

Sensory Overload

Problem

The child experiences major difficulty in filtering out unnecessary sensory input. Problems with foreground-background information can interfere with the ability to function in a multisensory environment.

Because of poor sensory modulation, the child's system becomes bombarded in situations that other children deal with successfully. When the amount of sensory input becomes too great, the child may fall apart emotionally (i.e., go into "meltdown"), tune-out all input and become nonresponsive to environmental stimuli, or be unable to eat in restaurants or other stimulation environments.

The child may have difficulty focusing attention and may show hyperactive behaviors. There may be acting-out behaviors, such as hitting, biting, screaming, and head banging, as the child communicates frustration and confusion.

There can be poor eye contact. The child actively averts his gaze as a functional means of reducing sensory input.

The overstimulated child may engage in rhythmical self-stimulation activities, such as rocking, spinning, and flapping the fingers in front of the eyes. These stereotypic behaviors may be the child's attempt to provide some type of rhythmical input to the nervous system to deal with the overload.

The child with a sensory overload can be withdrawn and appear to have profound retardation, autism, or deafness. More appropriate responses are observed in situations with a minimum of sensory input. For example, a child who appears to be profoundly hearing impaired may respond inconsistently to the quiet opening of a door.

Treatment Considerations and Directions

Sensory Issues

The reticular formation of the brain does not function adequately to filter background stimuli or inhibit reactions to stimulation. The child's system can become bombarded by stimuli from all channels that compete for attention. The child may have difficulty integrating sensory input from many different channels. It may be particularly difficult to integrate and understand movement and touch. Because these inner senses are distracting and uncomfortable, the child may not learn sensory-discrimination activities that focus on vision and hearing.

When sensory overload is seen as an extreme response to common sensory input, treatment strategies initially must be directed at changing appropriate aspects of the overall sensory environment to minimize the possibilities for such overreaction. Each sensory channel needs to be reviewed to identify those most vulnerable to sensory overload. It will be important to help the child and family identify situations that trigger sensory overload, and develop strategies for preventing it, as well as strategies to increase the overall ability to regulate sensory input.

Interaction Issues

Often, a child who regularly responds with sensory overload is confusing to the feeder. Sensory overload may be misinterpreted as a lack of hunger or interest in the meal when the child may be quite hungry, but unable to eat within the available sensory environment. Sometimes, a child who has experienced many extremes of sensory overload learns to use those responses to communicate a dislike of the meal or foods presented, or a wish to end the meal.

When the overload response interferes with clear communication at the mealtime, treatment strategies must focus on finding other ways of communicating mealtime messages that do not involve overload responses.

Oral Control Issues

Oral control issues are secondary to the sensory triggers that elicit the periods of strong sensory overload. Treatment strategies to improve oral control will center on determining which sensory variables promote the most organized and controlled oral responses.

Specific Feeding-Skill Issues

Sensory overload responses can strongly influence the acquisition of mature feeding skills. The extremes of responses can interfere with controlled sucking, swallowing, biting, and chewing, and even the ability to participate in a mealtime. They influence the quality of eating and drinking responses.

Work on specific feeding skills must be done with sensitivity to the child's specific sensory thresholds. Feeding skills can be worked on only in an environment that supports the child's sensory needs.

Experiential Issues

Sensory overload is a common experience for infants and children fed in extremely noisy or complex environments. The school cafeteria or a fast-food restaurant can contribute to major feeding issues for some children. The common practice of forcing all children to eat with their classmates in the school cafeteria for purposes of mainstreaming can be highly detrimental.

Work on specific feeding skills must be done with sensitivity to the child's specific sensory thresholds. Feeding skills can be worked on only in an environment that supports the child's sensory needs.

Problems With Feeding Processes

Sucking

Facilitating a Normal Suckling Pattern

Problem

The infant or child may have difficulty initiating a suckle pattern. The suckle pattern may be arrhythmical or disorganized, poorly sustained, or weak. It may be inefficient, taking an extensive amount of time for a minimal amount of liquid. A nonnutritive suck may be substituted for the nutritive sucking pattern. The infant may have difficulty coordinating suckling, swallowing, and breathing.

Treatment Considerations and Directions

Consultation

When breast-feeding techniques are not working for the child who otherwise seems healthy, a referral to a lactation consultant may be necessary to support the baby and the mother through the process.

When cardiac issues are suspected as a cause for poor endurance and timing with suckling, a referral to a pediatric cardiac specialist may be necessary.

When neurological issues are suspected as a cause for tone and alertness difficulties with suckling, a referral to a pediatric neurologist may be necessary.

When gastrointestinal issues are suspected as a cause of timing issues with suckling, a referral to a pediatric gastroenterologist may be necessary.

When pulmonary issues are suspected as a cause for timing and coordination difficulties with suckling, a referral to a pediatric pulmonologist may be necessary.

Because infant suckling issues can be a first symptom of other system problems, it is important that they be viewed as a team issue. Treatment may involve multiple specialists.

Physical Issues

The child's breast-feeding or bottle-feeding position may not be conducive to good suckling. There may be too much total body extension, insufficient body support, or too much extension in the neck and head. Because suckling and sucking are flexion skills, the extensor biased positioning can interfere with the mechanics of good suckling.

Decreased postural tone interferes with the ability to use a suckle pattern that is easily initiated, rhythmical, sustained, strong, and efficient. Increased postural tone with limiting reflexes and movement patterns interferes with the ability to use a suckle pattern that is easily initiated, rhythmical, sustained, strong, and efficient.

Neck hyperextension may be present. The head is tipped back with a pattern of capital extension rather than the normal pattern of capital flexion. The hyperextended pattern increases tongue and jaw retraction, increases the up-down excursion of the jaw, and reduces the strength and efficiency with which an infant can suck. Oral sucking movements and their coordination with swallowing and breathing become disorganized when liquid is introduced to the nonnutritive suck.

When muscle tone and movement difficulties interfere with the ability to develop efficient sucking, treatment initially should be directed at reducing the impact of limiting physical patterns and facilitating more normal movement through physical handling and positioning.

Sensory Issues

Oral sucking movements can become disorganized with touch on the tongue.

The environment may be overstimulating, causing reactions from disorganization to shutdown to limitations with jaw, lip, and tongue movements. These responses interfere with the suckling pattern.

Some infants have oral hypersensitivity. This may be related to neurological difficulties or negatively perceived oral experiences. In extreme situations, the contact of the nipple with the gums or lips may trigger refusals; gagging; vomiting; or jaw opening, thrusting or clenching. These responses interfere with the suckle pattern and break its rhythm.

When sensory-processing difficulties interfere with the ability to develop efficient sucking, treatment initially should be directed at reducing the impact of limiting responses to sensation and developing more normal responses to the sensory environment.

Oral Control Issues

The infant may have difficulty with timing and coordination of the suck-swallow-breathe synergy of breast-feeding and bottle-feeding. The child may cough, choke, and sputter as he sucks. Some infants retract the tongue as the nipple is inserted. Some are unable to cup the tongue around the nipple to help direct the bolus of liquid to the back of the mouth for swallowing.

All oral skills are influenced by extremes of muscle tone from low to high. These tone issues must be dealt with as a part of any treatment for improving oral control.

Treatment strategies will focus on developing a suckle pattern that is easily initiated, rhythmical, strong, sustained, and efficient.

Facilitating the Transition From Suckling to Sucking

Problem

The child has a strong in-out suckle pattern. A spontaneous shift to a more up-down sucking pattern has not occurred.

Treatment Considerations and Directions

Physical Issues

The child's breast- or bottle-feeding position may not be conducive to good sucking. There may be too much total body extension, insufficient body support, or too much extension in the neck and head. Because sucking is a flexion skill, the extensor-biased positioning can interfere with the mechanics of good suckling.

Some children continue to move the tongue in and out in a more immature suckle-like action rather than a more mature up and down sucking action because of a total body tendency toward extensor posturing.

When muscle tone and movement difficulties interfere with the ability to move toward efficient sucking, treatment initially should be directed at reducing the impact of limiting physical patterns and facilitating more normal movement through physical handling and positioning. The transition to sucking is easier when the child uses the chin-tuck position of capital flexion.

Interaction Issues

Some infants develop an in-out pushing of the tongue as a communication strategy to let the feeder know they do not want the nipple in the mouth. If the feeder is unaware of this message, the child may continue using an in-out pattern because she perceives no alternative.

Treatment strategies need to include helping the feeder become more sensitive to the infant's communication and developing communicative strategies for mealtime that do not involve the in-out movement of the tongue.

Oral Control Issues

The child may show poor control of the lips and cheeks, with either low tone and relative inactivity or high tone and lip retraction. Because the lips do not create a proper seal, the child has difficulty shifting to a sucking pattern that requires greater intraoral pressure.

The child may remain stuck in an early primitive suckle pattern and not know how to move to the more mature suck.

Treatment should focus on strategies to help the child develop up-down movements of the tongue and improved lip closure.

Specific Feeding-Skill Issues

The child may not have reached the developmental age of 6 to 9 months, when the shift from suckling to sucking pattern usually begins. A predominant in-out suckle pattern can interfere with the transition to spoon feeding and cup drinking. Treatment should follow the developmental sequence from the more in-out suckling motions of the tongue to the more up-down sucking pattern as the child matures. Activities used to facilitate the more mature suck pattern should be incorporated into work on bottle, spoon, and cup skills.

Facilitating Mature Oral Movements During Spoon Feeding of Soft Foods

Problem

The child uses limiting movements of the jaw, tongue, lips, and cheeks when taking food from the spoon.

The child continues to use early primitive patterns of spoon feeding. An in-out tongue movement may predominate. The upper lip does not come forward and down to remove food from the spoon. The lower lip does not draw inward to be cleaned by the upper incisors.

Treatment Considerations and Directions

Physical Issues

The child may show poor control of the lips and cheeks, with either low tone and relative inactivity or high tone and lip retraction. These patterns usually are related to overall problems of tone and movement in the body.

When muscle tone and movement difficulties interfere with the ability to develop efficient spoon-feeding skills, treatment initially should be directed at reducing the impact of limiting physical patterns and facilitating more normal movement through physical handling and positioning.

Sensory Issues

Some children become extremely uncomfortable when the spoon touches the lips or tongue. To avoid the sensory contact as the spoon enters the mouth, they will elevate or retract the lips. They may pull the tongue into retraction or elevate it so that food is placed under the tongue rather than on top of it.

When sensory processing difficulties interfere with the ability to develop efficient spoon feeding, treatment initially should be directed at reducing the impact of limiting responses to sensation and developing more normal responses to the sensory environment. Spoons must be selected carefully so that their shape and texture do not contribute to sensory discomfort.

Interaction Issues

Children who have been forced or pressured to eat specific foods or amounts may learn to pocket the food under the tongue or in the cheek cavity to delay or prevent eating it. This situation may deteriorate into a power contest with the feeder.

Treatment strategies will include helping the feeder become more sensitive to the child's need to make choices during the meal, developing an appropriate mealtime partnership, and avoiding power contests.

Oral Control Issues

The child may not have reached the developmental age of 6 to 8 months, when the upper lip moves forward and downward to clean the spoon. The child may not have reached the developmental age of 10 to 15 months, when the cleaning of the lower lip develops. The child may not have developed the ability to use the lips together to support the spoon as well as remove the food from the bowl of the spoon. The child may not have developed the ability to separate upper lip from lower lip movement. Refinement of upper lip skills with the ability to move the lip forward and downward may not be present. The upper lip may move as a whole, instead of having stability at the lateral borders with mobility of the central portion of the lips. The child may not have developed the stability of the lower jaw in an open position that would enable upper lip mobility and separation of movement to develop for removing food from the spoon.

Treatment strategies to improve oral control need to focus on improving stability and control of the jaw and lips.

Specific Feeding-Skill Issues

Treatment of specific feeding skills would focus on helping the child learn to take soft foods from a spoon. Strategies may include oral exploration with a variety of different shaped and textured toys, as well as practice taking foods from spoons with different shapes and depths.

Facilitating Mature Oral Movements During Cup Drinking

Problem

The child uses limiting movements of the jaw, tongue, lips, and cheeks when taking liquid from the cup.

The child continues to use early primitive patterns associated with bottle-feeding or breast-feeding with the cup. An in-out tongue movement may predominate. The upper lip may not come forward and down on the rim of the cup. The tongue may protrude beneath the cup. The jaw may move up and down with the presentation of the cup, thereby spilling liquids. The child may choke and gag with liquids presented from a cup.

Treatment Considerations and Directions

Physical Issues

The child may show poor control of the lips and cheeks, with either low tone and relative inactivity or high tone and lip retraction. These patterns usually are related to overall problems of tone and movement in the body.

When muscle tone and movement difficulties interfere with the ability to develop efficient cup-drinking skills, treatment initially should be directed at reducing the impact of limiting physical patterns and facilitating more normal movement through physical handling and positioning.

Sensory Issues

The intermittent touch of the cup as it is placed on the lips may trigger limiting reactions related to oral hyperreaction or sensory defensiveness. The child may turn the head or close the lips to avoid the touch of the cup.

When sensory processing difficulties interfere with the ability to develop efficient cup drinking, treatment initially should be directed at reducing the impact of limiting responses to sensation and developing more normal responses to the sensory environment. This may involve helping the child adjust to small amounts of sensory input to the mouth, without triggering the hypersensitivy response. Cups must be selected carefully so that their shape and texture do not contribute to sensory discomfort.

Interaction Issues

Children who have been forced or pressured to take liquids from the cup may clamp their mouths closed and refuse to let the liquid enter. They may allow the liquid to enter the mouth but then let it dribble or flow out without swallowing. They may actively spit liquid at the feeder. These resistive behaviors may deteriorate into a power contest with the feeder.

Treatment strategies should include helping the feeder become more sensitive to the child's need to make choices during the meal, developing an appropriate mealtime partnership, and avoiding power contests.

Oral Control Issues

The child may not have reached the developmental age of 6 to 9 months, when cup-drinking skills evolve. The child may not have developed the stability of the lower jaw that enables skilled activity of the lips and tongue to develop during drinking. The child may not have the lateral stability provided by the corners of the lips to support the cup. This stability is necessary for keeping liquid in the mouth. The timing of drinking coordination may be too slow to handle thin liquid. The child may have difficulty with the transition from a nipple to the cup. Bolus formation may be more difficult when thin liquid enters the front of the mouth.

Treatment strategies to improve oral control must focus on improving stability and control of the jaw and lips and on strategies for improving bolus control.

Specific Feeding-Skill Issues

Some children can drink only if a specific cup is used. They lack the ability to generalize the sensorimotor aspects of drinking coordination with different utensils. Treatment should include experiences with a variety of different open and spouted cups.

Swallowing

Facilitating a Normal Swallowing Pattern: Aspiration

Problem

The child chokes and aspirates food and liquid. The swallow reflex may be absent or delayed.

Treatment Considerations and Directions

Consultation

The child may have structural or physiological limitations such as asymmetrical movement in the pharynx, a tracheostomy, or gastroesophageal reflux that influence the ability to protect the airway. Referrals to appropriate otolaryngology, pulmonary, or gastroenterology specialists may be necessary.

When a child is suspected of being at high risk for aspiration, the therapist may need to consider a videofluoroscopic swallowing study as a part of the overall treatment planning for the child.

Physical Issues

High or low postural tone, limiting postural reflexes, and restrictive movement patterns may interfere with the ability to coordinate and time the oral and pharyngeal phases of the swallow. Severe respiratory dysfunction can cause the swallow reflex to be inhibited for survival. It often returns with improvements in respiratory function.

When muscle tone and movement difficulties contribute to poor swallowing with the risk of aspiration, treatment initially should be directed at reducing the impact of limiting physical patterns and facilitating more normal movement through physical handling and positioning.

Sensory Issues

Some children have very poor sensory awareness in the mouth. This may interfere with their ability to recognize when food or liquid remains in the mouth or with their ability to form a bolus for safe swallowing. Food can slip over the back of the tongue and into the airway without triggering a swallow reflex.

When sensory-processing difficulties interfere with the ability to swallow safely, treatment initially should be directed at reducing the impact of limiting responses to sensation and developing more normal responses to the sensory environment. Activities to build sensory awareness and develop a stronger sensory feedback system will be particularly important.

Oral Control Issues

Damage to cranial nerve X (vagus) can result in a paralysis of the laryngeal muscles, reducing protection of the airway during the swallow. Damage to cranial nerves V, VII, IX, X, and XII interferes with sensation and movement to the jaw, tongue, face, or palate. This can be reflected in low muscle tone, weakness, and asymmetry if there is greater damage to one side. For many children with cranial nerve involvement, the damage usually is incomplete, leaving a partial function of the damaged cranial nerves.

The child may be unable to coordinate sucking and swallowing with breathing. The child may be unable to form a bolus and move it to the back of the mouth to initiate the pharyngeal phase of the swallow.

Treatment strategies must focus on improving the timing of the sucking, swallowing, breathing, and bolus formation. For children with cranial nerve involvement, this will involve optimizing whatever function the child has available and teaching compensatory strategies.

Specific Feeding-Skill Issues

Safe swallowing is critical when food and liquids are used in the treatment program.

Treatment for the development of a safe swallow focuses on increasing the strength and coordination of the child's rhythmical suck or suckle pattern and using it as a trigger for a more efficient swallow. The overall goal may be to develop the child's ability to take repeated amounts of food of approximately ⅛ teaspoon in size, so that a videofluoroscopic swallowing study can be used to help identify safe food consistencies, amounts, and timing of presentation. Treatment may include exploring different ways of presenting food and liquid, and different utensils to see which ones promote the best head position and sucking patterns for swallowing.

Experiential Issues

Emotional stress often causes physical tension that can inhibit the ability to protect the airway. Children who have had negative swallowing experiences may tense the body in anticipation of the presentation of the bottle, cup, or spoon. Children who cannot swallow safely usually receive their nutrition from a feeding tube and lack the overall oral sensorimotor experiences that build associations among swallowing, hunger, and satiation.

When fearful emotional responses lead to tension that limits the ability to protect the airway, treatment strategies must include ways of building relaxation and trust during therapy and at mealtimes. When children receive non-oral feedings, treatment should focus on helping the child develop the appropriate mealtime associations during tube feeding.

Problem

The child gags on pureed foods or on solid foods with lumps. The child may swallow the food and then gag. Gagging may occur as the food touches the lips, tongue, palate, pharynx, or esophagus. It may occur in response to the sight, smell, or presentation of food.

Treatment Considerations and Directions

Consultation

The child may have gastroesophageal reflux, causing increased gagging. A referral to the primary care physician or gastroenterologist may be necessary.

The child may have structural problems, such as an esophageal stricture or tumor, that lead to structural-based gagging. A referral to the gastroenterologist or pediatric surgeon may be necessary.

Physical Issues

Problems with hypertonic, hypotonic, or fluctuating muscle tone can influence the timing and efficiency of bolus formation. This can cause food to slip into the pharynx before a proper swallow has been triggered, causing a motor-based gag. Sometimes, the child is able to swallow efficiently without a gag only if the whole body is stable rather than moving.

When muscle tone and movement difficulties contribute to the child's problem with gagging, treatment initially should be directed at reducing the impact of limiting physical patterns and facilitating more normal movement through physical handling and positioning.

Sensory Issues

A sensory-based gag may occur when the child has difficulty handling changes in food texture because of increased intraoral sensitivity or defensiveness. The area for eliciting a gag reflex may have moved forward. Touch or food on the front of the tongue or lips may trigger the hyperactive gag reflex.

When sensory-processing difficulties contribute to gagging, treatment initially should be directed at reducing the impact of limiting responses to sensation and developing more normal responses to the sensory environment. This may involve helping the child adjust to small amounts of sensory input to the mouth and lips, without stimulating a gag response. It may include increased oral exploration and mouthing.

Interaction Issues

A communication-based gag may occur when the child does not like the food or feels pressured to eat. This type of gagging strongly communicates, "I don't want this."

When children use gagging to communicate, treatment should focus on finding other ways of communicating that don't involve gagging. It may involve helping the feeder understand earlier communication cues before the child resorts to gagging.

Oral Control Issues

The child may be unable to clear all the food from the mouth. A portion may remain on the back of the tongue in the area that triggers a gag reflex. Difficulty with timing and coordination of bolus formation and swallowing can cause motor-based gagging. The bolus may not be well collected. A partially chewed bolus or part of the bolus can pass over the back or sides of the tongue before the child is ready to swallow. The gagging is a motoric effort to keep a piece of food that is not the appropriate size for swallowing from being swallowed.

Treatment strategies should focus on the child's ability to coordinate bolus formation and the timing of the swallow.

Specific Feeding-Skill Issues

Gagging can influence the way a child responds to food or liquid. Treatment strategies will identify the underlying issues and explore ways to reduce the impact of gagging on the meal.

Some children gag as a way of protecting themselves from food that is too large or inappropriate for their developmental age. When this is a factor, treatment will be directed at educating the feeder in selecting foods appropriate for the child's developmental age.

Experiential Issues

The child gags when oral stimulation or feeding reminds him of emotional reactions from a prior negative intraoral experience such as intubation, nasogastric, or orogastric feedings.

Treatment should focus on rebuilding trust in the feeding relationship and helping the child establish newer positive oral experiences.

Facilitating a Normal Swallowing Pattern: Drooling

Problem

The child drools saliva. This may occur during or immediately following a meal, during fine motor activities, or throughout the day.

Treatment Considerations and Directions

Consultation

Drooling can result from a constant open mouth position that does not allow saliva to collect and provide the pressure cues needed to trigger the swallow. This mouth position may be related to nasal congestion and chronic upper respiratory infections. Increased saliva production can be a side effect of some medications or an allergic reaction. Gastroesophageal reflux or aspiration can cause excessive saliva production. Drooling can be caused by neurological changes. In any of these situations, a referral to a primary care physician or specialist may be indicated.

Physical Issues

Although teething often causes children to increase saliva production and drool, no action to reduce drooling is required. This type of drooling is a normal part of the teething process and usually disappears after the eruption of the teeth.

Increased or decreased tone in the cheeks and lips may lead to inefficiency in swallowing and increased drooling. Many children experience poorer saliva control when they are engaged in motor activities that require balance or fine motor coordination. Some children have inadequate head and trunk control to support efficient swallowing.

When muscle tone and movement difficulties contribute to drooling, treatment initially should be directed at reducing the impact of limiting physical patterns and facilitating more normal movement through physical handling and positioning.

Sensory Issues

Some children lack the sensory awareness that there is saliva to be swallowed. Saliva accumulates in the mouth because of a reduced frequency of swallowing and causes drooling. A constantly wet face from drooling can reduce the sensory cues needed to trigger a proper swallow.

Sweet foods often increase saliva production. If a child lacks the sensory awareness to handle an excess amount of saliva, drooling may occur more frequently when the child eats sweet foods.

When drooling is influenced by poor or inconsistent sensory awareness, treatment should be directed at increasing the child's sensory awareness in and around the mouth. This can be combined with strategies to improve cognitive and visual awareness of drooling as a way to associate the loss of saliva with the associated sensations.

Interaction Issues

Drooling can be used as a means of obtaining attention or power. Many children know that adults find drooling unpleasant. Often, adults show discomfort or displeasure when the child drools or constantly remind the child to swallow.

When drooling becomes a focal point for attention or a power struggle with adults, the adult-child relationship must be reexamined.

Oral Control Issues

Drooling can result from a constant open mouth position that does not allow saliva to collect and provide the pressure cues needed to trigger the swallow. This mouth position may be related to either poor muscle control or poor coordination. Inadequate jaw stability makes efficient swallowing difficult and can cause drooling. Poor lip closure allows saliva to drool out of the mouth. Inefficient swallowing may lead to excessive drooling.

When oral control issues influence drooling, treatment will focus on increasing control and stability in the jaw, lips, cheeks, and tongue for food and liquid intake and swallowing.

Facilitating a Mature Swallowing Pattern

Problem

The child uses the early suckle-swallow pattern and does not separate the suck and swallow stages of the pattern.

The child uses the primitive pattern of protruding the tongue between the gums during the swallow. A mature swallow pattern has not developed.

Treatment Considerations and Directions
Consultation

Children who maintain the tongue in a more forward position and use the less mature tongue protrusion pattern during swallowing frequently develop misalignment of the teeth (i.e., dental malocclusions). Treatment may involve consultation with orthodontists or other dentists specializing in the use of dental prostheses to retrain tongue and lip patterns, or consultation with a myofunctional therapist.

Physical Issues

Hypertonicity and hypotonicity can influence the child's ability to control the jaw, lips, and tongue for swallowing. Low muscle tone can influence the quality of jaw, cheek, lip, and tongue movements. Low tone in these areas allows the tongue to be much less active and push slightly forward during swallowing. High muscle tone in the tongue can cause the tongue to extend or gently push forward during swallowing.

When muscle tone and movement difficulties interfere with the ability to develop an efficient swallow, treatment initially should be directed at reducing the impact of limiting physical patterns and facilitating more normal movement through physical handling and positioning.

Sensory Issues

Some children lack the fine-tuned sensory awareness within the mouth and pharynx that is needed to provide sufficient feedback during bolus formation and swallowing.

When sensory-processing difficulties interfere with the ability to develop efficient swallowing, treatment initially should be directed at reducing the impact of limiting responses to sensation and developing more normal responses to the sensory environment. Specific treatment strategies should focus on the sensory aspects of the food and liquid.

Oral Control Issues

The child may not have developed the stability of the lower jaw that enables skilled lip activity and tongue-tip elevation to develop during swallowing. When a child has poor jaw stability, the probability of tongue protrusion during the swallow increases. Poor lip closure makes it more difficult for the tongue to find a closed environment to practice up-down and tongue-tip elevation movements.

When delayed or limiting oral skills influence the development of tongue elevation during swallowing, treatment strategies must focus on improving overall jaw, lip, cheek, and tongue control in biting, chewing, and swallowing. Treatment would include work on improving jaw stability, the ability to close the lips during swallowing, and improved bolus formation.

Specific Feeding-Skill Issues

Some children who continue to use a slight tongue protrusion during swallowing lose small amounts of food or liquid when they swallow. Others use the immature swallow pattern with no discernable effect on their feeding skills

Treatment should be directed at the underlying issues that influence food or liquid loss that is related to tongue movements during swallowing. Strategies for helping the child wipe the lips and reduce the social impact of messy eating are important.

Coordination of Sucking, Swallowing, and Breathing: Breast-Feeding or Bottle-Feeding

Problem

The baby nurses without pausing for breath. There is a tendency for the infant to turn blue or gasp for breath while nursing.

The baby uses a gasping inspiration during nursing that draws unswallowed liquid into the airway.

The coordination of breathing and feeding is stressful, resulting in increased muscle tone during feeding and an increase in limiting movement patterns in the body and mouth.

Treatment Considerations and Directions

Consultation

If the child has a primary respiratory disorder, such as respiratory distress syndrome or bronchopulmonary dysplasia related to prematurity, feeding decisions should be made in partnership with the child's pulmonologist. If the baby has problems with low or high muscle tone a referral to a neurologist may be indicated.

Physical Issues

Dysfunction of the respiratory control center of the brain may interfere with the timing and coordination required for sucking, swallowing, and breathing. Rapid breathing rates seen in infants with primary respiratory disorders make it extremely difficult for them to coordinate breathing and swallowing.

Fluctuations of tone and movement in the body can create a general incoordination for feeding. Each part of the process may function adequately, but the timing and coordination are inadequate.

When muscle tone and movement difficulties influence the coordination of sucking, swallowing, and breathing, treatment initially should be directed at reducing the impact of limiting physical patterns and facilitating more normal movement through physical handling and positioning. Additional treatment strategies must focus on exploring and guiding the timing relationship between breathing and feeding.

Sensory Issues

Some infants have a decreased sensory awareness of liquid in the mouth. Timing problems with swallowing can result, causing difficulty with feeding and breathing coordination. The infant may fail to clear liquid from the mouth and then breathe it into the airway.

When sensory-processing difficulties interfere with the ability to develop efficient coordination of sucking, swallowing, and breathing, treatment initially should be directed at reducing the impact of limiting responses to sensation and developing more normal responses to the sensory environment. Specific treatment strategies would focus on increasing oral sensory awareness of the liquid.

Interaction Issues

Stress influences respiratory patterns. When feeding difficulties arise between the infant and parent at mealtime, the resulting stress can increase the baby's problems with respiratory coordination. This, in turn, can create more stress for the parent and an escalation of the infant's feeding difficulties.

Treatment programs should include strategies that support the physical and emotional relaxation of the infant and the feeder at mealtimes. Many parents need the opportunity to discuss their concerns about the baby's breathing and feeding problems to reduce their own anxiety.

Oral Control Issues

Some infants use an excessive amount of effort in nursing. The resulting increase in tension interferes with feeding and breathing coordination. Often, this effort is accompanied by unusual sounds and periods of breath-holding. The child may retract the tongue into the airway during feeding, making it difficult to suck efficiently and coordinate breathing with swallowing.

Treatment must help the infant develop a strong, efficient sucking and swallowing pattern and reduce physical stress on the respiratory system.

Specific Feeding-Skill Issues

Problems with sucking or swallowing can affect the overall coordination required for safe and efficient breast- or bottle-feeding. Treatment strategies may include removing the nipple intermittently to give the baby more frequent breathing pauses.

Experiential Issues

The poor coordination of sucking, swallowing, and breathing may result in feeding refusal for some infants. These babies discover that eating takes too much effort, and they are too fatigued to eat.

Coordination of Sucking, Swallowing, and Breathing: Cup Drinking

Problem

The child drinks without pausing for breath. There may be a tendency for the infant to turn blue, gasp for breath, or choke while drinking.

The child may use a gasping inspiration during cup drinking that draws unswallowed liquid into the airway.

The coordination of breathing and feeding may be stressful, resulting in increased muscle tone during cup drinking and an increase in limiting movement patterns in the body and mouth.

The child may be able to take two or three sucks without coughing and choking, but the child may not be able handle drinks of 1 ounce or more without gasping, coughing, and choking.

Treatment Considerations and Directions
Consultation

If the child has a primary respiratory disorder that includes lung damage such as bronchopulmonary dysplasia, it may be appropriate to refer the child for a videofluoroscopic swallowing study if there are continued difficulties coordinating swallowing and breathing during cup drinking.

Physical Issues

Dysfunction of the respiratory control center of the brain may interfere with the timing and coordination required for feeding. The child may use an excessive amount of effort during drinking. The resulting increase in tension can interfere with feeding and breathing coordination. Tension also can be caused by hypertonicity throughout the body. Sometimes, hypotonicity can influence the ability to efficiently coordinate feeding and breathing.

A child with poor hand-to-mouth coordination may have difficulty drinking during self-feeding. He may pour liquid into the mouth too rapidly because he has insufficient physical control when bringing the cup to the mouth.

When muscle tone and movement difficulties influence the coordination of sucking, swallowing, and breathing, treatment initially should be directed at reducing the impact of limiting physical patterns and facilitating more normal movement through physical handling and positioning. When self-feeding is involved, the physical environment must be created for optimum hand-to-mouth success.

Sensory Issues

Some children have a decreased sensory awareness of liquid in the mouth. Timing problems with swallowing can result, causing difficulty with feeding and breathing coordination. The child may fail to clear liquid from the mouth and then breathe it into the airway.

When sensory-processing difficulties interfere with the ability to develop efficient coordination of sucking, swallowing, and breathing, treatment initially should be directed at reducing the impact of limiting responses to sensation and developing more normal responses to the sensory environment. Specific treatment strategies would focus on increasing oral sensory awareness of the liquid.

Interaction Issues

The child's timing of drinking and pausing differ from the rhythm and timing set by the feeder. If the child is unable to communicate timing needs, respiratory incoordination and choking can result.

When breathing and drinking coordination difficulties result from misinterpreted communication between the child and the feeder, treatment strategies should include helping the child communicate in a clear and consistent fashion and helping the feeder be sensitive to that communication.

Oral Control Issues

The child may not have reached the developmental age of 12 months, when long, coordinated drinks of liquid from a cup are controlled. She may take drinks one sip at a time. The ability to control the jaw, lips, cheeks, and tongue will influence the ability to coordinate feeding and breathing while drinking from a cup.

Treatment would focus on improving control of the jaw, tongue, lips, and cheeks, and on increasing the child's ability and confidence in taking more than one sip at a time when drinking liquid from a cup.

Biting and Chewing

Facilitation of a Normal Controlled Biting Pattern

Problem

The child is unable to bite through soft or hard food efficiently. The bite may be weak with insufficient force to bite through the food. Biting may be absent, and the child sucks or suckles all food that enters the mouth. Biting may be present but the child uses a rapid, phasic bite pattern instead of a controlled bite. The child may react with jaw thrust, jaw clenching, or a tonic bite when foods are presented.

Treatment Considerations and Directions
Consultation

If the child's teeth are decayed or infected, biting on food may be extremely painful because of the contact of the teeth and gums. Consultation with a dentist can rule out this contribution to poor biting and chewing.

Physical Issues

The child may not have teeth to support advanced levels of biting. A child usually has enough strength in the jaw alone to bite through soft foods without teeth, but needs teeth for more advanced biting. Adults should wait to offer foods that require greater cutting or tearing until the child has teeth.

Decreased postural tone can interfere with the ability to use a strong, sustained biting pattern. Increased postural tone with obligatory reflexes and limiting movement patterns also interferes with the ability to use a controlled biting pattern.

When muscle tone and movement difficulties interfere with the ability to develop a sustained and controlled biting pattern, treatment initially should be directed at reducing the impact of limiting physical patterns and facilitating more normal movement through physical handling and positioning.

Sensory Issues

Oral hyperreaction can interfere with a controlled biting pattern. The contact of the food with the gums or teeth may trigger jaw opening, jaw clenching, or lip retraction.

An overstimulating environment may contribute to increased tension and movement disorganization of the entire body, causing the child to react with limiting jaw, lip, and tongue movements. These reflexive patterns interfere with the controlled biting pattern.

Children who experience oral sensory defensiveness often avoid biting pieces of food if they are uncomfortable with lumpy food or scattered pieces of food on the tongue. In most instances, biting reduces solid foods to this lumpy consistency. If children cannot handle the resulting texture, they often resist learning to bite off pieces of food.

Some children seek strong proprioceptive input through their teeth and will overgeneralize a biting response. Because they like the sensory input, they may bite adults or other children.

When sensory processing difficulties contribute to difficulties in developing a controlled biting pattern, treatment initially should be directed at reducing the impact of limiting responses to sensation and developing more normal responses to the sensory environment.

Interaction Issues

Some children discover the power of biting others and continue to do so for attention, power, or revenge. Adults must understand the roots of the child's behavior. Is this child simply biting for the sensory input? Has biting become a way for the child to feel important or powerful? Treatment will be directed at resolving the underlying issues rather than punishing the biting behavior.

Oral Control Issues

The child might not have reached the developmental age of 9 to 12 months, when controlled biting patterns are developing. Some children have difficulty inhibiting tongue movement and stabilizing the jaw in an open position for biting.

Treatment strategies should include work on increasing control of the jaw, tongue, and lips for controlled and sustained biting.

Specific Feeding-Skill Issues

Failure to develop a controlled biting pattern can limit the child's development of chewing skills.

Facilitation of Munching, the Earliest Stage of Chewing

Problem

The child is unable to chew food. Chewing may be absent, and the child sucks or suckles all food that enters the mouth. The child may react with limiting oral patterns such as a jaw thrust, tongue thrust, tongue retraction, lip retraction, or a tonic bite when foods are placed in the mouth for chewing. Chewing may trigger associated movements and tension in the rest of the body. The child may gag and choke when foods that require chewing are presented.

Treatment Considerations and Directions

Consultation

If the child's teeth are decayed or infected, chewing food may be extremely painful because of the contact of the teeth and gums. Consultation with a dentist can rule out this contribution to poor chewing.

Physical Issues

For some children, increased postural tone with retained reflexes and limiting movement patterns may interfere with the ability to munch in a relaxed fashion. There may be too much or too little muscle tone to support the coordinated up-down movement of the jaw and tongue.

When muscle tone and movement difficulties interfere with the ability to develop a munching pattern, treatment initially should be directed at reducing the impact of limiting physical patterns and facilitating more normal movement through physical handling and positioning.

Sensory Issues

Children who experience oral sensory defensiveness often avoid foods that require chewing if they are uncomfortable with lumpy food or scattered pieces of food on the tongue.

An overstimulating environment may contribute to increased tension and to movement disorganization of the entire body, causing the child to react with limiting jaw, lip, and tongue movements. These reflexive patterns interfere with the development of chewing.

Oral hyperreaction can interfere with the development of a munching-chewing pattern. The contact of the food with the gums or teeth may trigger jaw opening or jaw clenching.

When sensory-processing difficulties interfere with the ability to handle textured solids and the development of a munching pattern, treatment initially should be directed at reducing the impact of limiting responses to sensation and developing more normal responses to the sensory environment. This may involve reducing the overall level of stimulation in the child's mealtime environment or helping the child adjust to small amounts of sensory input into the mouth, without triggering sensory defensiveness or hyperreaction.

Oral Control Issues

Some children do not chew because they have not have reached the developmental age of 6 months, when early munching-chewing patterns are developed.

Some children have difficulty inhibiting tongue movement and stabilizing the jaw in an open position as the food is placed in the mouth. The lack of graded control of the jaw also can reduce the effectiveness of a munching pattern.

Treatment strategies should include work on increasing control of the jaw, tongue, and lips for the coordinated movements needed for munching.

Facilitation of Lateralization in Chewing

Problem

The child lacks the full development of lateralization patterns in chewing. An up-down munching pattern of the jaw and tongue is present. Lateral tongue and jaw movements do not occur or are limited in frequency or extent. The child may be unable to move food from the side to the center of the tongue for swallowing or from the center of the tongue to the side for chewing. Food transfer across midline and use of a grinding rotary jaw pattern during chewing may be absent. The asymmetrical tightening of the lips and cheeks needed to keep food in the mouth and to assist in food transfers may be absent. The child may be able to transfer food to one side of the mouth but not the other, or there may be major differences in skill between the two sides. Food may be swallowed whole if the child does not chew sufficiently.

Treatment Considerations and Directions

Consultation

A short lingual frenulum can interfere with tongue lateralization in some children. If this interferes with chewing development, a consultation should be scheduled with the child's primary physician or an oral surgeon.

If the child's teeth are decayed or infected, chewing food may be extremely painful because of the contact of the teeth and gums. Consultation with a dentist can rule out this contribution to poor chewing.

Physical Issues

Mild or intermittent degrees of hypotonicity or hypertonicity, or asymmetries in the jaw, lips, cheeks, and tongue may interfere with skilled transfer movements.

When muscle tone and movement difficulties interfere with the ability to develop tongue lateralization skills for chewing, treatment initially should be directed at reducing the impact of limiting physical patterns and facilitating more normal movement through physical handling and positioning.

Sensory Issues

Oral sensory defensiveness may be present. Sensory contact of the food with the tongue or teeth may be uncomfortable. The child may do very little chewing and may swallow the food to get rid of it as quickly as possible.

Mild acuity or perceptual difficulties in the mouth interfere with the child's ability to perceive the location and texture of food in the mouth. As a result, food is not completely chewed or remains in the mouth after swallowing.

When sensory-processing difficulties interfere with the ability to handle textured solids and develop a mature chewing pattern with tongue lateralization, treatment initially should be directed at reducing the impact of limiting responses to sensation and developing more normal responses to the sensory environment. This may involve focusing on sensory awareness and discrimination of food in the mouth.

Oral Control Issues

The child may not have reached the developmental age of 6 to 9 months, when tongue lateralization in chewing develops. The child may not have reached the developmental age of 24 months, when children develop circular-rotary chewing patterns with smoothly integrated transfer of food across the midline. The child may have insufficient jaw stability to provide a foundation from which to lateralize the tongue. This might be seen in a child who has athetoid or ataxic cerebral palsy. Some children can lateralize the tongue, but are unable to sustain the lateralization throughout the chewing of an entire mouthful of food.

Treatment should include work on oral control issues to increase jaw stability, increase tongue mobility, and sustain lateral tongue movements.

Specific Feeding-Skill Issues

Children learn to lateralize the tongue for chewing when they are given foods that require more sustained placement of the food between the teeth for chewing. Some children have had very limited experience with firmer foods requiring this type of chewing.

If the child simply lacks experience with more solid foods, these foods should be introduced into the diet gradually so that more advanced feeding skills can develop.

The Role of Food in Therapy

Food Transitions

Moving From Liquids to Smooth Solids

Problem

The child may accept liquids, but rejects smooth solids such as pureed consistency cereal, fruits, and vegetables. The addition of smooth solids may trigger hypertonicity and limiting movement patterns.

Treatment Considerations and Directions

Consultation

If the child has experienced allergies when taking formula or breast milk and is resistant or uncomfortable with the transition to smooth solids, it may be appropriate to consult the child's pediatrician or an allergist.

Physical Issues

Hypertonicity and limiting movement patterns may influence the child's ability to comfortably make the transition from liquids to solids. These patterns can influence all stages of sucking and swallowing.

When muscle tone and movement difficulties affect the child's ability to make a texture transition, treatment initially should be directed at reducing the impact of limiting physical patterns and facilitating more normal movement through physical handling and positioning.

Sensory Issues

The gag reflex may not have diminished or normalized. It may be activated from the front of the tongue as easily as in early infancy. Gagging also can be triggered by oral sensory defensiveness. The child may experience oral defensiveness to the increased variety of taste, smell, texture, and temperature of smooth solids.

When sensory-processing difficulties interfere with the child's ability to take smooth solids, treatment initially should be directed at reducing the impact of limiting responses to sensation and developing more normal responses to the sensory environment. This may involve focusing on a very gradual change in the sensory properties of the food and on reducing the gag reflex.

Interaction Issues

When children are fed against their will, they often figure out ways to avoid discomfort or to reduce the amount of food that they take into the mouth and swallow. They may clamp the lips closed and turn the head or push the spoon away. They may take food into the mouth and then choke or gag to let the feeder know that they do not want to eat the new food.

This pattern only emerges as an interaction issue when children are being forced to eat or when the adult takes over the child's responsibility for the timing of spoonfuls of food. The treatment program must focus on the mealtime relationship and on reading the child's readiness cues for a mouthful of food.

Oral Control Issues

Foods presented by spoon do not create the rhythm and continuous flow experienced with the bottle or breast. This break in rhythm reduces the child's ability to handle food. Food may become scattered in the mouth, and the child has difficulty collecting a bolus for swallowing

Treatment would focus on helping the child develop bolus control of the new food.

Specific Feeding-Skill Issues

Smooth, solid foods generally are given to children by spoon. When children refuse to eat this type of food, they may not develop the overall feeding skills associated with spoon feeding.

Experiential Issues

Some children have had very limited experience with smooth, solid foods and still take only liquids by bottle- or breast-feeding. Many of these children were introduced to smooth solids before they were ready and rejected them. They and their parents may have been reluctant to attempt the transition again.

If the child simply lacks experience with smooth foods, these foods should be introduced gradually into the diet in a way that is comfortable for the parent and the child.

Moving From Smooth Solids to Lumpy Solids

Problem

The child may accept smooth solids but reject lumpy solids such as commercially available third-stage foods and ground food. The addition of lumpy solids may trigger hypertonicity or limiting movement patterns.

The addition of lumpy solids may trigger gagging or choking.

Treatment Considerations and Directions

Physical Issues

Hypertonicity and limiting movement patterns may influence the child's ability to comfortably make the transition from smooth solids to lumpy foods.

When muscle tone and movement difficulties affect the child's ability to make a texture transition, treatment initially should be directed at reducing the impact of limiting physical patterns and facilitating more normal movement through physical handling and positioning.

Sensory Issues

The child may experience oral defensiveness to the texture of lumpy solids. The gag reflex may not have diminished or normalized. Scattered lumps may trigger gagging.

When sensory-processing difficulties interfere with the child's ability to take lumpy solids, treatment initially should be directed at reducing the impact of limiting responses to sensation and developing more normal responses to the sensory environment. It should focus on careful attention to a gradual introduction of texture changes in foods. Treatment also may involve helping the child control the gag reflex.

Interaction Issues

When children are fed against their will, they often figure out ways to avoid discomfort or to reduce the amount of lumpy food that they take into the mouth and swallow. They may clamp the lips closed and turn the head or push the spoon away. They may take food into the mouth and then choke or gag to let the feeder know that they do not want to eat the new food.

This pattern only emerges as an interaction issue when children are being forced to eat or when the adult takes over the child's responsibility for the timing of spoonfuls of food. The treatment program must focus on the mealtime relationship and on reading the child's readiness cues for a mouthful of food.

Oral Control Issues

Food pieces may become scattered in the mouth, causing the child difficulty in collecting a bolus for swallowing.

Treatment should focus on helping the child develop bolus control of the new, textured food.

Specific Feeding-Skill Issues

Chewing requires the ability to handle lumpy pieces of food. When children have difficulty handling lumpy solids, they may not develop the overall feeding prerequisites needed for chewing.

Treatment should focus on helping the child develop the oral sensorimotor skills needed to eat this type of food.

Experiential Issues

Previous uncomfortable experience with lumpy solids may have convinced the child or parent that these are dangerous and should be avoided.

Treatment should focus on careful selection of textures to rebuild trust and confidence in the child's ability to handle these texture changes.

Moving From Lumpy Solids to Chewy Solids

Problem

The child accepts lumpy solids but rejects solids that require chewing. The child may accept some chewy solids, but swallows them whole or with minimal chewing. The child might be able to chew, but chokes or drools with food that consists of combined textures. The child chews food partially and spits it out or stores it in the cheek pockets without completely swallowing it.

Treatment Considerations and Directions

Physical Issues

Hypertonicity, hypotonicity, or limiting movement patterns may influence the child's ability to comfortably make the transition from lumpy solids to chewy foods.

When muscle tone and movement difficulties affect the child's ability to make a texture transition, treatment initially should be directed at reducing the impact of limiting physical patterns and facilitating more normal movement through physical handling and positioning.

Sensory Issues

The child may experience oral defensiveness to the texture of chewy solids. Because of oral hypersensitivity, the child gets rid of the food as quickly as possible by swallowing it whole. Scattered lumps may trigger gagging.

When sensory-processing difficulties interfere with the child's ability to take chewy solids, treatment initially should be directed at reducing the impact of limiting responses to sensation and developing more normal responses to the sensory environment. It should focus on careful attention to a gradual introduction of texture changes in foods. Treatment also may involve helping the child control the gag reflex.

Interaction Issues

When children are fed against their will, they often figure out ways to avoid discomfort or to reduce the amount of chewy food that they take into the mouth and swallow. They may clamp the lips closed and turn the head or push the spoon away. They may take food into the mouth and then choke or gag to let the feeder know that they do not want to eat the new food.

This pattern only emerges as an interaction issue when children are being forced to eat or when the adult takes over the child's responsibility for the timing of spoonfuls of food. The treatment program must focus on the mealtime relationship and on reading the child's cues of readiness for a mouthful of food.

Oral Control Issues

The child may lack the precise coordination required to swallow the liquid portion of the bolus while simultaneously chewing the solid portion.

Chewing movements may be weak, unsustained, or inadequate for complete chewing. The child may either spit out or horde partially chewed food that is not pulverized adequately for swallowing. The child may have only a munching-chewing pattern without the lateralization required to efficiently chew more difficult foods.

Treatment should focus on improving jaw control and grading necessary for good chewing. It should promote efficient tongue lateralization and cheek control to keep the food over the grinding surfaces of the teeth as well as good lip control to keep the food in the mouth and assist with bolus formation for swallowing.

Specific Feeding-Skill Issues

The ability to handle larger, chewy, solid foods is required for chewing. When children have difficulty handling chewy solids, they may not develop the overall feeding prerequisites needed for more chewing with tongue lateralization.

Treatment should focus on helping the child develop the oral sensorimotor skills needed to eat this type of food.

Experiential Issues

Previous uncomfortable experience with lumpy solids may have convinced the child or parent that these are dangerous and should be avoided.

Treatment should focus on careful selection of textures to rebuild trust and confidence in the child's ability to handle these texture changes.

Treatment Strategies and Activities

This section is designed as a review of common treatment strategies for improving oral motor skills for feeding. Each strategy is followed by activities that can be used in therapy and at home to improve the child's oral motor skills and control. Each child and family is different. Children will be ready for some activities but not for others. Parents may be drawn to some activities but find others distasteful—even if they are physically appropriate for the child. Initially, the therapist should review the challenges faced by the child as described in the preceding section of the chapter. Then he or she should develop a general listing of the treatment directions that are appropriate for the child. Next, the therapist should select the specific treatment strategies he or she wants to include and review the activities that are listed. Selections should be based on the therapist's intimate knowledge of interests and priorities of the child and family.

Strategies and activities are not listed in a specific order of priority or difficulty. The lists include a few activities that address each strategy. Therapists will create many others as they listen to children, families, and their own creative spirit.

In the following section, please note that the ◉ marks a goal, the Ⓐ indicates an activity, the ✛ marks variations of an activity or additional guidelines, and the ▼ indicates a warning or important guidelines.

◼ Physical Issues

Supporting Areas

Postural Alignment

Head, Neck, and Trunk Alignment

◉ Work for better sitting posture on the lap or in a chair.

Possible Activities

Ⓐ The trunk and pelvis should be in good alignment. The shoulder girdle should be forward, with abduction of the scapulae.

Ⓐ The cervical spine (neck) should be elongated, with capital flexion (chin-tuck) as the child can accept it.

Ⓐ Changes in feeding position need to be made gradually. The child needs time to adjust to the changes in sensorimotor feedback that are given by the more appropriate position. Changes that are made too rapidly may be rejected because they are unfamiliar and uncomfortable.

▼ All programs involving positioning and seating for oral motor and feeding treatment must be individualized. Because of physical contractures or other structural deformities, the aligned position just described may be impossible to attain or may be dangerous for the child. The child's physical therapist and physicians should be consulted if major changes or recommendations in postural alignment are considered.

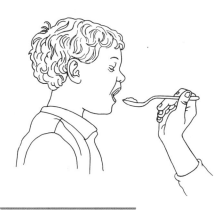
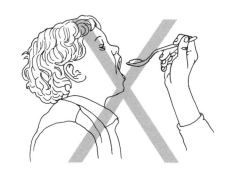

| | |

Capital Flexion

⊙ Work for a relationship between the head and neck in which the neck is elongated or straight and the chin is tipped toward the chest.

Possible Activities

🅰 Position the child in a comfortable supine (back-lying) position with the head resting in your lap. Use pillows or other supports under the child's legs so that his knees are bent and slightly rolled outward. Gently massage the neck, and use a very slight traction to bring it into an elongated position. Help the child explore easy head movement in a head nodding (as for **yes**) and head-shaking pattern (as for **no**). Move the child's head only as far as it moves easily without tension or resistance.

🅰 Use a small, crescent-shaped, neck pillow under the child's head in supine or sitting to encourage an easy chin-tuck position.

🅰 Position the child in a comfortable supine (back-lying) position with the shoulders supported on a Boppy pillow. Use a second Boppy pillow under the child's legs so that his knees are bent and slightly rolled outward. Use a small, crescent-shaped pillow under the child's head to encourage an easy chin-tuck position.

▼ All programs involving positioning and seating for oral motor and feeding treatment must be individualized. Because of physical contractures or other structural deformities, the aligned position just described may be impossible to attain or dangerous to the child's safety. The child's physical therapist and physicians should be consulted if major changes or recommendations in postural alignment are considered.

Symmetry

⊙ Select positions for feeding that encourage the child to keep the head in midline and maintain body symmetry.

Possible Activities

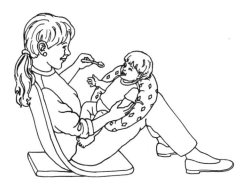

🅰 Position an infant or young child on your lap so that she is facing you. This allows the child to be positioned symmetrically. Eye contact and communication with you encourages the child to maintain the head in a midline position.

  ✥ This can be done while you sit on the floor with bent legs and the child reclines on your thighs. A Boppy pillow can provide additional support for the child.

  ✥ Alternatively, you can sit in a chair and rest the child's body on a firm pillow or wedge pillow that rests against a table.

◢ Use a small, crescent-shaped neck pillow under the child's head in supine or sitting to keep the child's head in midline.

◢ Position the child in a comfortable supine (back-lying) position with a Boppy pillow supporting the shoulders. Use a second Boppy pillow under the child's legs so that his knees are bent and slightly rolled outward. Use a small, crescent-shaped pillow under the child's head to keep his head in midline.

▼ All programs involving positioning and seating for oral motor and feeding treatment must be individualized. Because of physical contractures or other structural deformities, the aligned position just described may be impossible to attain or dangerous to the child's safety. The child's physical therapist and physicians should be consulted if major changes or recommendations in postural alignment are considered.

Stability

Head and Trunk Stability

◉ Work toward the child's ability to achieve and maintain a stable or steady support of the trunk in an upright position with the head vertical and the mouth horizontal in relationship to the pull of gravity.

Possible Activities

◢ Seat the child on your lap with his back against your chest and his pelvis in a neutral position. The back should be straight. Gently bounce your lap up and down to stimulate the contraction of the muscles that contribute to postural stability. This is done only with children who have low tone in the trunk.

◢ Seat the child on a small therapy ball. Support the child's feet on the floor or on your lap if you are seated on the floor in front of the ball. The child's back should be straight and her pelvis in a neutral position. Bounce the ball up and down to stimulate the contraction of the muscles that contribute to postural stability. This is only done with children who have low tone in the trunk.

◢ Engage the child in activities that stimulate normal extensor and flexor patterns of the trunk. Work for the balance between flexion and extension that provides postural stability of the trunk.

◢ If the child can walk independently but has low tone and poor stability, use a mini-trampoline and help her learn to jump. The proprioceptive stimulation through the child's feet and legs, combined with the vestibular input of jumping, can stimulate greater postural stability.

▼ Consult with the child's physical or occupational therapist to determine the level of supported or independent trunk activity that is appropriate.

◉ Work for weight shifting and balance reactions that activate the child's ribcage and abdominal-pelvic girdle.

Possible Activities

◢ Seat the child on your lap with his back straight and the pelvis in a neutral position. Gently shift your lap so that one leg is higher than the other. Slowly alternate legs. This shifts the support surface on which the child is seated and facilitates a weight shift from one buttock to the other. As weight is shifted toward the support buttock, the trunk on that side should elongate while the trunk on the opposite side should shorten.

◢ Seat the child on a small therapy ball. Support the child's feet on the floor or on your lap if you are seated on the floor in front of the ball. The child's back should be straight and the pelvis in a neutral position. Gently move the ball forward, backward, right, or left. Do this slowly so that the child can shift weight in the direction of the ball's movement. Look for the stimulation of trunk and head positions that accompany head righting and equilibrium reactions.

▼ Consult with the child's physical or occupational therapist to determine whether the child has the prerequisite skills for working on weight shift and balance reactions.

Airway Stability

⊙ Increase the sustained opening of the pharyngeal airway to support unobstructed respiratory support.

Possible Activities

🅰 Reduce jaw and tongue retraction and compensatory jaw thrusting that causes pharyngeal airway obstruction. Use the activities described in the Retraction: Jaw and Retraction: Tongue on page 455 and Thrusting: Jaw on page 451.

🅰 Position a small child in prone (on the tummy) on your lap, with her arms forward across your thigh. Position a larger child in the same fashion over a bolster. Angle the support surface of your lap so that the child's shoulders are higher than her hips. This provides better trunk (thoracic) elongation to support breathing, and it stops the forward flexion of the shoulders that reduces air intake. Gravity may cause the tongue and jaw to drop into a more forward position, which enlarges the pharyngeal airway. This can be combined with a therapeutic, gentle rocking movement through the child's spine that may get more movement in the ribcage and loosen tension in the jaw. Gently place your hand under the jaw, using a slight traction forward to further enlarge the airway. Jiggle the jaw gently to reduce thrusting and clenching movements.

▼ This positioning is appropriate only when the child accepts a prone position without getting tight in flexion. The adult must avoid bringing the child's head into hyperextension. Traction on the jaw and base of the tongue must be done very gradually and gently, and stopped immediately if the child resists in any way.

🅰 The same gentle pulling forward on the lower jaw and the base of the tongue can be done with an older child who is positioned appropriately in sitting. Maintain forward traction on the lower jaw as the child listens for changes in breathing sounds that occur when the airway is open and the tongue no longer obstructs the air flow.

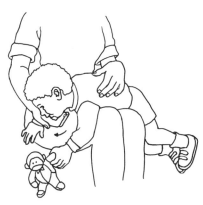

Limiting Areas

Change Tone

Decrease Tone

⊙ Reduce overall high postural tone that accompanies or triggers limiting movement patterns in the jaw, tongue, lips, and cheeks (e.g., jaw and tongue thrust, jaw and tongue retraction, jaw clenching, tonic bite).

Possible Activities

🅰 Consult a physical therapist or other professional who has special training in therapeutic movement to select activities that will alter tone. In general, activities such as slow vestibular stimulation, relaxing music, and positioning to break up total reflexive patterns of movement can be used to reduce tone.

◼ Provide regular massage to reduce tone and promote physical relaxation.

♦ The child should be actively involved in the massage, giving permission for the touch. Perform the massage slowly and cautiously, individualizing the strokes for this child. As the massage progresses, involve the upper body and face. Massage usually is easiest to handle farther away from the mouth, with strokes gradually toward the mouth.

♦ The child should maintain a quiet mouth during the massage. If the mouth is tense or moving during the massage, adapt the positioning or strokes so that mouth tension and movement is reduced.

♦ Use quiet, organizing music during the massage to enhance physical and mental relaxation.

♦ Massage the child after a relaxing bath.

♦ Review Drehobl and Fuhr's *Pediatric Massage for the Child with Special Needs* videotape (1991) and revised manual (2000).

◼ Have the child use his mind to give messages to different parts of his body. When children try to relax, they often increase tension and limiting movements as a result of the effort. The idea that they can simply think of the arm and tell it to let go, or make a picture of the arm in the mind and see it getting soft, involves no effort. With this approach, the child begins to strengthen the inner abilities to direct the body. Sometimes, it is amazing to discover how effective this can be for the child who feels like the victim of a body that doesn't work.

Increase Tone

◉ Reduce overall postural hypotonicity that accompanies or triggers limiting movement patterns in the jaw, tongue, lips, and cheeks (e.g., limited movement, exaggerated jaw movement, exaggerated tongue protrusion, stability bite).

Possible Activities

◼ Consult a physical therapist or other professional who has special training in therapeutic movement to select activities that will alter tone. In general, activities such as bouncing, tapping, and rocking through the spine can be used to build tone and develop better postural stability. This must be done very carefully so that it does not result in hypertonicity.

◼ Use the activities described in Stability: Head and Trunk Stability on page 404.

Stabilize Tone

◉ Stabilize fluctuating postural tone that accompanies or triggers limiting movement patterns in the jaw, tongue, lips, and cheeks (e.g., random involuntary oral movements, combinations of low and high tone oral movement patterns).

Possible Activities

◼ Consult a physical therapist or other professional who has special training in therapeutic movement to select activities that will alter tone.

◼ Provide regular massage of the body to stabilize tone and promote physical relaxation. See the guidelines in Decreased Tone on page 444.

Change Physical Position

Influence Tone

⊙ Use a physical position that does not require the child to maintain an upright position against gravity.

Possible Activities

🅰 Upright positions such as sitting often increase postural tone because of the position of the head in space and the effort used by the child to remain upright. Explore positions in supine or sidelying on the floor or lap that provide good support and allow the child's body to release tone.

🅰 For feeding, use a tilt-in-space wheelchair that allows the entire seat of the chair to tilt backward in varying degrees. This allows the relationship of the angle between the trunk and the pelvis to remain constant as the chair is tipped backward. Explore the amount of reclining that allows the child to release tension.

Change or Break Up a Total Pattern

⊙ Reduce the strength of a total flexion or total extension pattern with movement and positioning that breaks up the total pattern.

Possible Activities

🅰 Position a small child in sidelying on your lap while you sit on the floor. Break up the pattern by extending the child's trunk on your lap and flexing one or both legs. Support the child's head with your arm. Your thigh supports the child's lower arm, which is slightly extended. The child's upper shoulder girdle and arm can be brought forward or toward the mouth for play or bringing toys or food to the mouth. The position expands the ribcage and supports better breathing patterns.

  ⊕ This position can be adapted or adjusted in many ways that can move the child into a more upright position against gravity. This happens when you bend the leg that is supporting the child's trunk and lower arm. Movement can progress toward a fully supported side-sitting position on the lap or the floor.

🅰 While the child is sitting on your lap, bend one of the child's legs and tuck it under her other leg (flexion and abduction). Alternate the leg that you bend.

▼ All programs involving positioning and seating for oral motor and feeding treatment must be individualized. Because of physical contractures or other structural deformities, the aligned position just described may be impossible to attain or dangerous to the child's safety. The child's physical therapist and physicians should be consulted if major changes or recommendations in postural alignment are considered.

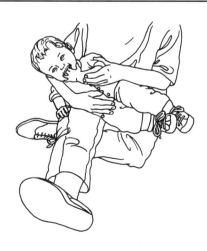

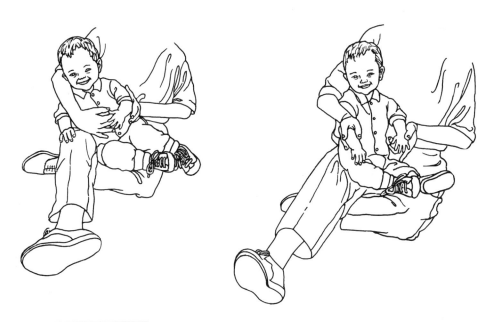

Influence Interaction

⦿ Use a physical position that supports face-to-face communication with the child.

Possible Activities

🅰 Sit directly in front of the child's chair so that the child's head is maintained in midline. If possible, sit slightly lower than the child so that she does not have to tip the head into hyperextension to establish eye contact.

🅰 Position an infant or young child on your lap so that she is facing you. This allows the child to be positioned symmetrically. This can be done while you sit on the floor with bent legs and the child reclines on your thighs. A Boppy pillow can provide additional support for the child. Alternatively, you can sit in a chair and rest the child's body on a firm pillow or wedge that rests against a table.

Influence Digestion

⦿ Use a physical position that supports efficient gastric emptying and reduction of reflux.

Possible Activities

🅰 See Chapter 22 for a discussion of positioning alternatives to reduce reflux and enhance gastric emptying.

Change Sensory Input

Decrease Input

⦿ Reduce the amount of sensory input in the mealtime environment.

Possible Activities

🅰 Feed the child in a quiet room with a limited number of distractions in order to reduce the level of excitement, muscle tone, and sensory arousal.

🅰 Feed the child in the classroom or a small lunchroom rather than the school cafeteria. Gradually incorporate other children into the lunch group to create a more typical mealtime social environment.

🅰 See Chapter 14 for an in-depth discussion on variations among sensory variables.

Increase Input

⊙ Increase the amount of sensory input in the mealtime environment.

Possible Activities

🅰 Feed the child in a room with more physical and sensory stimulation. Some children with low postural tone or low levels of sensory awareness move toward more normal muscle tone and alertness when they share a meal with others or eat in a restaurant or other more active social environment.

🅰 See Chapter 14 for an in-depth discussion on variations among sensory variables.

Increase Sensorimotor Awareness

⊙ Increase the child's awareness and interest in different ways of moving the body, hands, and mouth to discover many variations of doing the same activity.

⊙ Increase the child's awareness of the easiest ways of doing a specific activity.

⊙ Increase the child's ability to monitor stability and movement in the body while simultaneously engaging in another activity.

Possible Activities

🅰 Emphasize the discovery of multiple ways of doing the same activity. Encourage the child to discover differences that make an activity easier or more difficult. Include other activities that build awareness of sensory contrasts and improve sensory organization and discrimination.

🅰 Introduce sensory activities that are gentle and interesting to the child. Give the child feedback to help him discover the difference between stiffness and softness in different parts of the body. Build on the child's sense of curiosity to develop an interest in discoveries about his own body. Build the child's awareness of the connection between a steady body with a more upright head position and easier hand and mouth skills.

🅰 Incorporate sensory activities of the whole body—discovering how things feel and what the child can do to discover different interesting and pleasurable sensations with the body and mouth. Help the child build awareness of different ways of doing an activity to increase movement variations and increase comfort in making small changes.

🅰 Help the child build a stronger awareness of what her body is doing, without judging anything as good or bad. Use words or phrases such as tense/tight, soft/easy, and fingers open/fingers closed. Help her discover what she can and cannot do when tense and when more relaxed. Allow her to discover advantages in altering her body or head position. Use questions such as, "What happens if …" (i.e., your body is quiet?, you move your head slowly?)

🅰 Use a *thinking* approach to help the child monitor what her body is doing. Emphasize using mental checklists such as thinking about whether the feet are flat on the floor for good support, weight is even on both sides of the body, or the arms are quiet on the table. Incorporate this concept in activities such as drinking, eating, vocalizing, and using the hands.

Change Emotional Input and Response

Interaction

⊙ Reduce the frustration and negative emotion that results from poor communication and interaction.

Possible Activities

🅐 Become aware of small changes in body tone and movement, facial expression, eye gaze, mouth movement, and vocalization that the child uses to express needs or wants.

🅐 See Chapter 13 for detailed information on helping children expand their nonverbal communication at mealtimes.

⊙ Reduce the number of tantrums the child throws to communicate feeding needs and preferences.

Possible Activities

🅐 Incorporate activities for enhancing mealtime communication and reducing tantrum behaviors described in the Trust section on page 423, Communication section on page 424, and Negative Interactions section on page 425.

Learning

⊙ Reduce the amount of excess effort (e.g., increased body tension and associated reactions) that is associated with learning a new skill.

Possible Activities

🅐 Break down the components of a skill into small, manageable segments so that the child experiences success more easily.

🅐 Increase the child's sensorimotor awareness of tension or associated movements in the body. Contrast these sensorimotor experiences with movements that are done without tension or unnecessary movement.

🅐 Help the child learn through contrasts in body position and tension. For example, you can emphasize or exaggerate some of the child's patterns of tension. When the child pushes back into extension, ask her if she can push back harder. Can she figure out how to do that? As she becomes more aware of how she gets tight, the contrasting relaxation or softness of the muscles will become clearer.

🅐 See Chapter 13 for a detailed discussion of learning environments and their influence on a child's sensorimotor skills.

Sensory Issues

Sensory Awareness

Overall Sensory System

⊙ Increase overall sensory awareness of the environment.

Possible Activities

🅰 Provide many opportunities for the child to engage in activities with sensory awareness. Point out and comment on different sensory aspects of the child's environment (e.g., the sound of the toilet flushing, a ringing telephone, a bright red ball, fast swinging, firm touch). Physically take the child to objects or people creating sounds (e.g., grandmother's voice in the kitchen, radio in the living room).

🅰 Give the child many opportunities to become aware of body sensations during movement.

✤ When the child's body and arms are soft, guide his hands in touching as many body parts as possible. This might include using the hand to touch the opposite arm and shoulder, the ears, the top of head and hair, the chest, abdomen, legs, and feet.

✤ When guiding the child's movements for rolling or other physical activities, move slowly in order to increase the ability to pay attention to small and subtle differences in how he can move his body. Moving the child rapidly can be fun. However, slow movement and attention to the movement are important elements for learning to take place.

✤ Comment on what the child is doing when the movement is in a positive direction. This can be done in a matter-of-fact way that encourages focus of attention to the movement or degree of tension in the body (e.g., "You turned your head toward Mommy to roll; that was easy. You can turn over by lifting this shoulder").

Face and Mouth

⊙ Increase sensory awareness in the mouth through opportunities to mouth and explore hands, simple environmental objects, and toys.

Possible Activities

🅰 Provide many opportunities for the child to engage in generalized mouthing activities of the hands, simple environmental objects, and toys.

🅰 Provide good postural support of the child's body as a foundation for bringing hands and toys to the mouth and mouthing with easy oral movements.

🅰 Provide assistance with stability at the shoulder, elbow, and wrist when helping a child explore the hands. The attempt to put fingers in the mouth can result in uncomfortable jabbing if the child cannot stabilize the rest of the arm. Many children avoid hand-to-mouth activities because they hurt themselves.

🅰 Cut the child's fingernails if you include activities that encourage moving the hand to the mouth. Scratches and jabs are uncomfortable and discouraging.

🅰 Work on physical activities that reduce shoulder-girdle retraction and elevation, and make it possible for the child to bring the hands and toys to the mouth independently.

🅰 Develop the child's ability to enjoy putting her hands in her mouth and discovering the sensory feelings involved in contrasting movements and body parts. For example, explore the feeling of the thumb in the mouth, contrast this feeling with the feeling of the index finger in the mouth or the whole fist in the mouth.

🄰 Mouthing of body parts provides sensory input and awareness in the child's mouth and in another part of the body. Older children who have had limited mouthing experience can be encouraged to explore their fingers by feeling them with their lips, counting them as they go into the mouth, or licking a taste off of each finger.

🄰 Play with individual fingers in the mouth and gradually place them further back onto the tongue without stimulating a gag reflex.

🄰 Develop the child's ability to enjoy toys in the mouth. Select toys or feeding utensils that have a simple shape and limited surface texture. Encourage the child to feel and become aware of all parts of the toy with the gums, teeth, lips, and tongue. The child can bring the object to the mouth independently or be assisted in doing so.

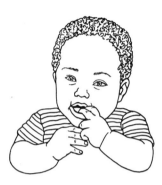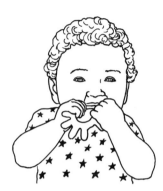

🄰 Place a toy or a Chewy Tube™ between the older child's teeth or gums in the molar region. Encourage the child to make biting or chewing motions on the toy.

◉ Increase sensory awareness in the mouth through vibration.

🄰 Provide the child with vibration experiences in and around the mouth. Many times children show an interest in vibration when they have no interest in other mouthing experiences. Vibration can wake up the mouth when other non-vibratory toys may be less noticed.

🄰 Offer the child fun, vibrating toys to hold or mouth. Play games with the vibration moving closer to the chin, face, or mouth.

🄰 Vibration can be scary at first. Notice the frequency and sound of the vibrating massager. Sometimes, you need to use an old battery so the intensity of the vibration is decreased. Sometimes, the child will handle the vibration more easily if you hold the vibrator and the child feels the vibration through your hand.

🄰 Help the child brush his teeth with a vibrating toothbrush. There are many commercially available electric toothbrushes. Especially good is the DentalMate™, which is a vibrating handle that can be put on a toothbrush. Always start this and any new oral activity by asking for and receiving the child's permission for placement in the mouth. You may need to play games around the chin and lips before the child parts his lips to let the toothbrush in. You initially may need to use the electric brush on the front and side teeth before the child opens his mouth to let the brush near the inside of the teeth and the tongue.

🄰 Put the child in prone on the therapy ball. Roll the ball onto a working vibrator. Encourage the child to place his mouth on the ball so he receives the vibration on the face and through the ball.

🄰 Once the child likes the massager, it can be used to introduce new, scarier flavors and textures. The DentalMate works with Maroon Spoons™ in addition to toothbrushes. This can provide vibration during spoon feeding as a transitional activity for some children.

⊙ Increase sensory awareness in the mouth through foods that have alerting qualities.

Possible Activities

🅰 Different food textures can provide more or less alerting sensory information that can be very important in the quality of oral motor performance and in oral motor challenges. Careful food selection is appropriate. Crunchy or hard foods tend to be more alerting and require more active jaw, tongue, lip, and cheek involvement. It is important that you offer the child safe foods.

🅰 Provide the child with noisy foods that he can hear during biting and chewing. This provides the extra auditory information that tells the child he is biting the food and where it is in his mouth. Foods such as crackers, chips, puffed crackers, and hard fruits such as apples provide nice, noisy biting and chewing feedback.

🅰 Provide the child with foods that are varied in texture so that he needs more active mouth movements for chewing and forming a bolus. Smooth foods such as yogurt or puddings can easily be swallowed with little jaw, tongue, cheek, and lip interactions. Biting sandwiches, raw and cooked fruits and vegetables, crackers, and fruit peels provide more active oral motor involvement for bolus formation. Vary the foods you offer; for example, moving from bread sandwiches to toast sandwiches to cracker sandwiches to bagel sandwiches. Each requires differing amounts of jaw control for biting and chewing. Biting through a banana, for example, is quite different from biting through an apple, and yet both types of biting are important in learning to grade jaw movements.

🅰 Add texture to smooth foods. When there are only smooth foods in the diet, the child may need to have the texture *alerted.* Try adding crushed crumbs or dried cereal to the food. This can help alert the child's attention to the food, and increase the ability to find it and move it around the mouth. When crumbs are added to food, they tend to become soft with the moisture of the food. This adds some texture to the food. Sprinkling crumbs on top of each spoonful will add more alerting quality. This can vary with the type of crumbs chosen. Soda cracker or pretzel crumbs tend to be sharper and more alerting than crushed wafers, graham crackers, or butter cookies.

Sensory Modulation

Overall Sensory System

⊙ Increase the ability to handle an increasing amount of sensory stimulation at a typical mealtime.

Possible Activities

🅰 Begin by reducing the overall amount of ambient sensory stimulation. Work with the child in a quiet room with as little added sensory input as possible. Gradually bring in more input as the child can handle it successfully. This can include sound recordings of the school cafeteria or videotapes of other children eating as precursors to preparing a child for returning to meals in the school cafeteria.

🅰 Use guided imagery activities to experience the thought of a sensation or action while the physical body remains quiet. Many children enjoy imaginative stories in which they play a central role. The child can imagine going to the beach, making muddy footprints on the wall, going on a picnic, driving the car, building with blocks, and running in the meadow. There are no limits to the mind's ability to create. This ability can be used to learn to control overreactions. For example, you can suggest that the child is going to a friend's birthday party. During the party, the child will watch as the cake comes in and the candles are blown out. Guide the child to imagine smelling the frosting and, finally, tasting a piece of cake. As you give each creative description, pause to let the child imagine becoming part of the scene. Provide guidance to "move the mouth in the mind, not your real mouth" or to "think about cutting the cake in your mind. Use the arm in your mind to cut it. Let your real arm be quiet and relaxed."

▣ Teach concentration and centering skills that enable the child to learn to maintain an inner focus without distraction. Many books on centering activities and meditating with children contain ideas that can be incorporated in a therapy or classroom program. It is important to teach a child to quiet the mind as well as the body. As the mind becomes quiet and centered, the body becomes quiet and moves in harmony with the mind. Centering activities can be taught to children who are functioning cognitively at the level of a 3-year-old.

Face and Mouth

⊙ Prepare the child for direct touch to the face and mouth.

Possible Activities

▣ Encourage parents to give lots and lots of kisses all around the child's face. This kiss therapy is fun for both child and parent.

▣ "Teddy bear kisses" can be given, using a favorite stuffed toy or doll. This allows a familiar stuffed toy to move toward the face during a playful, anticipated activity. *Kiss* firmly to avoid eliciting a ticklish, defensive response. The child can learn to respond quietly without triggering hyperreactions.

▣ Use squeak toys, stuffed dolls, or even your own fingers to *walk up* the child's arm, perhaps while you sing a tune, until you get to the child's face and give a kiss.

▣ Some older children enjoy stickers placed on the face. As these are slowly moved toward the face, the child can anticipate and prepare for the touch.

Sensory Discrimination

Overall Sensory System

⊙ Increase sensory discrimination of different aspects of the environment.

Possible Activities

▣ Provide many opportunities for the child to engage in activities that involve sensory discrimination. Create situations in which you vary different sensory aspects of the child's environment (e.g., loudness of music, speed of swinging, brightness of a light, intensity of a vibrating toy).

▣ Full learning of an activity or movement pattern requires the ability to repeat basic movement patterns with many different variations of muscle activity, timing, and coordination. Variations upon a theme also enhance thinking and information-processing abilities for learning. Provide situations and games in which the child discovers many ways of doing the same activity. Variations of the same movements or sensory activities provide more learning value than the rote learning of a single method.

Face and Mouth

⊙ Increase sensory discrimination in the mouth through opportunities to mouth and explore complex environmental objects and toys.

Possible Activities

▣ Provide many opportunities for the child to engage in discriminative mouthing activities of the toys and familiar objects. See specific suggestions listed in the Combined Oral Sensorimotor Control: Mouthing section on page 441.

▣ Provide a variety of age-appropriate objects for the child to mouth. The child can bring the object to the mouth independently or be assisted in doing so. Use objects such as toothbrushes, spoons, cups, water picks, blowers, whistles, and straws when encouraging mouthing in older children.

- Select toys or feeding utensils that have more complex shapes and a distinctive surface textures. Encourage the child to feel and notice sensory contrasts in all parts of the toy with the gums, teeth, lips, and tongue.
- Help the child explore the surface of a toy with a variety of jaw, tongue, and lip movements. For example, use an animal that has different shapes or body parts. Use the teeth, lips, and tongue to discover its feet, tail, nose, and head.

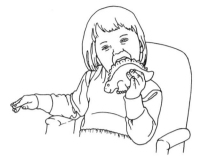

- Children may be interested in mouthing some toys if there is a small taste of food on the toy. Dipping the mouthing toy in a favorite flavor may encourage greater oral exploration with the jaw, tongue, and lips.

Sensory Feedback

Overall Sensory System

◉ Increase sensory feedback of different aspects of the environment.

Possible Activities

- Explore ways of giving feedback that describe what the child is doing or experiencing. For example, say, "You are really figuring out just how much water you need" or "Notice how easily you are moving your arm." Comments like these don't draw children away from what they are experiencing and don't judge the experience as good or bad.

Face and Mouth

◉ Increase sensory input and feedback of the jaw, cheeks, and lips in a relaxed, closed mouth position.

Possible Activities

- Use facial molding.
  - ✥ Begin with a general massage of the child's body and face. Be sure to relax the child first so abnormal tone is not working against you.
  - ✥ Think of the child's face as a piece of clay that you will sculpt. After reducing hypertonicity in the neck and shoulder girdle, gently mold or massage the face toward a closed mouth/closed lip position. Place your fingers on the side of the child's nose and vibrate downward toward the bottom of the upper lip, working toward a closed mouth position slowly and evenly. The emphasis is on the sustained aspect of the stretch and vibration, not on simply stretching the upper lip downward. This vibratory movement and stretch to the side of the nostril provides a long-lasting relaxation of upper lip tightness for many children.

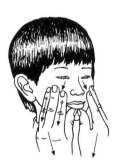

  - ✥ The massage can be done using your palms or with your fingers, either spread apart or together. It can be done with a cloth between the hand and the face, or with the hand directly on the face. It can be done with and without vibration.
  - ✥ Move slowly and with the child's permission. If your massage stresses the child or increases the facial tension, stop or try another approach. You might be moving too fast, giving too much pressure, pushing on a sore tooth or lip, or providing too much overall stimulation.

- For especially retracted lips and cheeks, it often helps to massage toward the closed mouth position and then to hold the mouth closed for a short time so that the child feels the closure and the muscles relax in that position.
- Encourage parents and other caregivers to wipe the child's face before or during the meal, moving the child's face toward a closed mouth position with their hands and the towel. This can be done with extended fingers, flat palms, or a warm cloth. The movement is gradual and sustained.

⊙ Increase sensory feedback of jaw position and movement.

Possible Activities

🅰 Use a snack cap during speech, feeding, and play activities.

- Make a snack cap for each child. Start with a comfortable, familiar cap, such as a baseball cap. Attach a 1-inch wide piece of elastic from one side, under the chin, and to the other side. Some children need a smaller front chin piece for proper positioning on the jaw. Without it, the chinstrap inches its way back toward the throat, becoming uncomfortable. It seems to work best to have at least one side attached by safety pin or Velcro so that the tension can be increased or decreased. The elastic should be tight enough to help the child feel the jaw movements while chewing, talking, or singing. It should not be so tight as to be restrictive nor so loose as to provide no resistance to jaw movement.
- First, help the child become comfortable with the cap during an activity that provides distraction. The child can wear the cap first without the chinstrap and then with it. Initially, have the child do a movement activity such as swinging or a very exciting game activity to draw attention away from the cap.
- As the child becomes comfortable with the cap, give the child a familiar snack to eat while wearing the chinstrap. Chewing with the strap on provides resistance to the jaw movement and increased proprioceptive information. Take the cap off about three-quarters of the way through the snack. Then have the child finish the snack. This gives the child the opportunity to use the increased proprioceptive feedback received with the chinstrap and offers the opportunity for carryover into a non-therapy situation.

⊙ Increase sensory input and feedback of the jaw, tongue, cheeks, and lips during feeding or mouth exploration activities.

Possible Activities

🅰 Use a small table mirror with activities to develop graded control of the jaw, lips, or tongue.

🅰 Use a small table mirror to provide visual feedback during the child's regular meals.

🅰 Provide auditory feedback by having the child bite through noisy foods such as dry crackers, cereals, and other crisp snacks.

🅰 Provide taste and touch feedback by having the child bite into a piece of food, such as a juicy orange or grapefruit slice, that has been wrapped in a gauze bag. (See the Jaw Control: Graded Jaw Movements section on page 432.)

🅰 Have the child bite through textured foods that give differing degrees of resistance.

Hyporeaction

Environmental Sensory Input

⊙ Increase awareness of the sight, sound, and touch sensations that surround mealtimes.

Possible Activities

🅰 Incorporate activities that build postural tone in the trunk. This will help the child develop some proximal stability. With greater stability, there will be more movement that can help increase muscle tone and bring the threshold for sensation to a more normal level. Use the activities to increase postural tone described in Change Tone: Increase Tone on page 406.

🅰 Select the type, intensity, and frequency of sensory stimulation that is appropriate for the specific child. Observe the child carefully for indications of appropriate response to the stimulus and signs that some aspect of the stimulus is inappropriate. Gradually increase the stimulus until an appropriate response level is reached. Decrease the stimulus if the child gives any sign of discomfort or an increase in tone or movement. If the child does not respond to an intense stimulus, consider whether the lack of response is related to severe sensory overload. Gradually identify the level of sensory input that is appropriate when exploring other therapy options to improve the child's feeding skills.

▼ Increasing the sensory stimulation is inappropriate where problems of reduced threshold due to compensation for sensory overload have been identified.

Bodily Sensory Input

⊙ Increase awareness of touch, taste, smell, and temperature sensations before and during mealtimes.

Possible Activities

🅰 Provide the child with oral alerting activities around and in the mouth. (See Chapter 14 for an in-depth discussion of variations among sensory variables.) These alerting experiences may be done before or during a meal, depending on the child and the variable.

  ⊕ Give the child alerting touch experiences.
  ⊕ Give the child alerting texture experiences.
  ⊕ Give the child alerting taste experiences.
  ⊕ Give the child alerting temperature experiences.

🅰 Increase the child's awareness and discrimination of the sensory stimulus. When a low level of awareness is related to cranial nerve dysfunction, frequently there are sensory and motor fibers in the damaged area that are functional. Building awareness through the intact fibers can improve overall function in activities that require participation of the damaged cranial nerve area.

Hyperreaction

◉ Reduce limiting patterns of tone and movement in the body and mouth as you introduce exciting or overstimulating environmental stimuli.

Possible Activities

🄰 Create a physical space that contains a minimum of sensory stimulation. This may consist of a small room with white or pastel-colored walls, devoid of pictures, and open shelves. Dim the lights to reduce the visual input and use carpeting to reduce reverberations and ambient sounds. In a noisy building, sound can be reduced further by carpeting the walls. Soft music with a regular rhythm, slow tempo, and constant volume can create a calming auditory space.

🄰 Enter the quiet room with the child. Allow the child to explore the space. Sit quietly and verbally or nonverbally encourage the child to sit or lie down next to you.

🄰 Following is a very effective position for work with smaller children. However, it should be used only where it is comfortable and accepted willingly by the child. Sit with your back against the wall for support. Stretch out your slightly bent legs, creating a semicircle or oval shape with your body and legs. Have the child lie down on his back in this circular space between your legs. Support the child's head on a pillow or use your feet as a pillow if this is comfortable. Allow the child's legs to separate and rest over your thighs or around your waist.

This position and relationship to the child usually works well. It provides a loose framework of support for the child, allows for face-to-face contact with the child for communication and the monitoring of the child's facial expression, and reduces confusing sensory input from gravity and movement that could occur if the child were sitting or standing.

🄰 Use deep pressure stroking or firm patting on the child's chest in rhythm to music. Stop when you pick up signals from the child that the stimulation is too much. Use speech and eye contact only when you sense that these can be integrated. Add one sensory input at a time.

🄰 Continue to explore touch and movement with the child's body. Contrast in movement or touch increases attention and provides an easier learning situation. For example, explore the kinesthetic contrast of an open hand and a closed hand on the chest, or the tactile contrast of a stroke and a pat on the chest. Give the child time to sense what you are doing and to integrate the sensations and the contrasts. As you repeat the movement contrasts, you may find that the child will anticipate the next movement and will actively join you in initiating the response.

🄰 Explore touch and movement with the face and mouth as you have done with the body. When the child is ready, explore contrasts in the way that different foods or liquids taste or feel in the mouth. Your goal is to present sensory information in a way that makes it possible for the child to respond positively and with interest. You may have to present many variations of the information before the child is ready and able to respond in a new and accepting way. When the child says "no," respect that choice. Observe and evaluate the situation, figure out a new way to present the experience, then offer it again. Know that the child has an inner timetable and understands what is needed before a change and new level of organization is possible.

▼ Each quiet space and physical relationship between the therapist and the child will be somewhat different. The basic principles described for this option are appropriate for most children who have sensory defensiveness or severe sensory overload. The details, the way they are implemented, and the timing will differ among children, depending on their degree of hyperreaction and sensory overload.

🄰 If a child's overreaction to sensory input includes strong limiting patterns of the jaw and tongue, incorporate physical assistance in maintaining the jaw in a closed position. It is important to work for better body movement and positioning before closing the mouth and providing stimulation.

- ▲ Gradually present the stimuli that cause overreaction in a graded, controlled fashion. For example, if the child typically responds with a jaw thrust and head extension when she sees the spoon, use your hands and body to control these reactions as you slowly bring the spoon into view. If the child's physical reactions are difficult to control, this is a signal that the stimulus of the spoon is too much. Perhaps the activity could be repeated as the child watches a doll being fed with a toy spoon. You also could present a spoon of a different shape or material.

- ▲ Stimuli that cause overreaction can be introduced through all sensory channels and in situations that are part of a child's daily experience. Identify all factors and combinations of factors that trigger the child's limiting reactions. Gradually add each of these to the therapy setting while helping the child discover new ways of responding. Although the handling and introduction of sensory stimuli are done very carefully and precisely in the initial stages, the goal is to enable the child to function efficiently in the real world.

- ▲ The amount of handling can be reduced gradually, giving the child a greater responsibility for inner control. Stimuli then can be introduced suddenly and with less initial preparation. As the child's skills improve, you can add complex sensory stimuli, such as tape recordings of lunchroom noise or therapy field trips into environments that typically are overstimulating. Your goal is to increase gradually the degree and complexity of the child's sensory environment while maintaining the child's ability to respond normally.

◉ Reduce jaw thrusting or tongue thrusting, and increase mouth control as a person or object approaches the face.

▼ Direct work to the mouth should be discontinued when the stimulation increases or causes high tone and limiting movement patterns in the rest of the body.

Possible Activities

- ▲ Help maintain the jaw in a closed position. It is important to work for better body movement and positioning before closing the mouth and providing stimulation.

- ▲ Help the child learn to anticipate and trust the movement of people and objects toward the face without becoming overly stimulated or overly reactive. At non-meal times, play games that center on face touching or kissing. Always let the child know what you are going to do. This can be a verbal preparation, rhythm, or game that allows for the anticipation of touch.

- ▲ Have the child lie prone on a therapy ball. As the ball is moved toward you, give a kiss or playful touch to the child's face. Do this slowly and carefully so as not to elicit an overreaction.

◉ Reduce hyperreactive response to all aspects of the mealtime (e.g., thinking about food, seeing food, seeing the feeder).

Possible Activities

- ▲ Create a focused mealtime with calming music, reduced visual and auditory distractions, and a positive and supportive communication environment.

Bodily Sensory Input

◉ Reduce the hyperreaction that occurs when the teeth make contact with a spoon, toy, or finger.

▼ Direct work to the mouth should be discontinued when the stimulation increases or causes high tone and limiting movement patterns in the rest of the body.

Possible Activities

🅐 Use carefully graded, firm pressure to the face, gums, and teeth while maintaining the jaw in a closed position. It is important to work for better body movement and positioning before closing the mouth and using oral stimulation.

🅐 Maintain a firm-pressured, closed jaw position while doing a distracting activity such as singing a song, reading a story, or moving the child on a therapy ball.

🅐 Some children handle touch better if it occurs during swinging. The child can be on a swing independently or with an adult. As the rhythm of the swing is established, touch the child on the face in rhythm with the swing. The movement of the swing provides a pattern for touch that is anticipated.

🅐 Begin activities with the body massage activity described in the Change Tone: Decrease Tone section on page 406.

🅐 Introduce gradations in vibrating massagers and toys by using an old battery so that the intensity of the vibration is decreased. Gradually move to stronger batteries and vibratory stimulation.

🅐 Use the toothbrushing activities described in the Combined Oral Sensorimotor Control: Oral Toothbrushing section on page 439.

◉ Reduce the hyperactive gag that occurs when the gag is elicited from the lips, front, or middle of the tongue.

Possible Activities

🅐 Use your finger, a toy, or a spoon to press down firmly on the front of the tongue. Gradually move this pressure backward until the child begins to gag. Usually you can sense the beginnings of a gag before it occurs. Move forward again, and gradually play back and forth in this reflex zone. Some children respond more positively if stimulation begins with touch-pressure to the hard palate.

🅐 Use folk or classical music to set a rhythm and predictability for the firm touch. This also focuses the activity on the fun and pleasure of the mouth-and-music game rather than on an invasive activity that triggers a gag.

🅐 If a gag is elicited by touch to the tip of the tongue, begin with touch to the lips, cheeks, jaw, and the base of the tongue under the chin. Gradually work into the mouth as the child indicates that this is acceptable.

🅐 Gradually help the child move the gag-sensitive area backward so that the gag is elicited from touch to only the back one-quarter of the tongue.

🅐 If the child continues to gag, reduce the gag's power by flexing the child's head forward so that the chin pushes against the chest. Increase the amount of flexion by pressing against the sternum of the chest with your other hand. Gagging is uncomfortable and anatomically difficult in this position. Use this maneuver to let the child know that it is possible to stop a gag before vomiting. Use warm praise for stopping the gag.

🅐 A gag-distraction approach can be effective. Select a gag distraction such as looking the other way, singing, or showing a toy or book to the child. Use this when the child gags, focusing attention on the distraction rather than the gag. In this way, a child can learn to control the gag independently without undue adult attention directed toward gagging.

◉ Reduce the hyperreaction that occurs to unexpected sensory properties in food.

Possible Activities

🅐 Organize and present new foods on a gradual taste continuum that assures acceptance and success.

Sensory Overload

Mealtime Input

⊙ Reduce environmental sensory input that can overload the child's system, resulting in a reversion to limiting or more immature oral movement patterns.

Possible Activities

🅰 Help the family find appropriate times for feeding the child separate from the main family meal. Suggest finding help for a brother or sister who runs around and vies for attention as the child with disabilities is fed.

🅰 Create a small lunch club for school-age children that can substitute for noisy meals in the school cafeteria. Include children with and without disabilities in the group. Help the child make a gradual transition into the more complex cafeteria environment when ready to graduate from the lunch club.

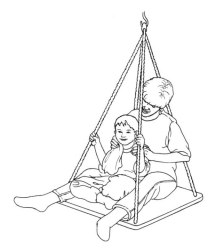

🅰 Movement can be used to organize and calm many children. It can provide an environment from which to provide other stimulation. Sit with the child on the swing and introduce sensations of touch and taste that otherwise might be rejected. The movement can provide a calming distraction to the new input.

🅰 Use music to help the child organize and integrate sensory reactions in the nervous system and create a calm feeding environment. At first, use baroque music with a slow tempo of 60 beats per minute. Hemi-Sync® Metamusic has helped many children respond appropriately to sensory information. The changes that are facilitated through these special sounds appear to remain when the music is no longer present.

　⊕ Observe the child for feedback on the appropriateness of the music. Use changes in respiratory pattern, vocalization, and general activity level as guides for continuing, withdrawing, or changing the music.

🅰 Provide a special quiet place to which the child can retreat when feeling overloaded. This may be a specific room in the house, a pile of pillows, or a small enclosed space such as a box or tent. It may contain pillows, books, music, or any calming and quieting sensory input that helps the child. Help the child recognize internal feelings of impending overload and learn to seek the quiet place before falling apart.

Food Input

⊙ Reduce direct sensory input from food that can overload the child's system, resulting in a reversion to limiting or more immature oral movement patterns.

Possible Activities

🅰 Incorporate suggestions for reducing sensory overload from overall mealtime input (see above).

🅰 Evaluate the child's responses to sensory features of the food and offer food selections that do not overstimulate the child.

⊙ Reduce sensory defensiveness that interferes with the child's ability to eat and participate in a mealtime.

Possible Activities

🅰 Use activities that introduce slow vestibular stimulation. This type of input to the sensory nervous system helps the child to integrate multiple pieces of sensory information. Let the child provide feedback to regulate the appropriate amount of stimulation. Observe carefully for any adverse reactions during or following swinging activities. These activities are particularly effective in integrating tactile information. Include these activities before or during the mealtime:

   ⊕ Rock with the child on your lap in a rocking chair.

   ⊕ Hold the child and walk rhythmically up and down stairs.

   ⊕ Swing the child on a swing or in a chair swing.

   ⊕ Roll or bounce with the child on a large ball.

   ⊕ Swing the child slowly in a net hammock.

▼ Activities that involve swinging, spinning, or bouncing work most effectively when done in consultation with a therapist who has a background in movement and sensory integration.

Some children may show an increase in seizure activity with vestibular stimulation. These activities are inappropriate if the frequency or severity of seizures is increased.

🅰 Use activities that provide firm proprioceptive input into the joints and muscles. This type of input to the sensory nervous system helps the child integrate multiple pieces of sensory information. The child will provide feedback to regulate the appropriate amount of stimulation. Include these activities before or during the mealtime:

   ⊕ clapping

   ⊕ marching

   ⊕ pushing a cart or wheelbarrow

   ⊕ jumping

   ⊕ bouncing

🅰 Explore ways in which touch can be used communicatively. Use firm touch that still has a gentle and caring quality. The tendency for light touch to be overstimulating to many children creates a major problem for adults, because light stroking of the head is used in our culture to communicate caring, concern, and personal warmth. When this response is used automatically by a mother, the child may push her away and appear to reject this statement of caring. It is a challenge to find other ways to share these feelings. Firm touch with deep pressure is more easily accepted and integrated. Some children who reject other types of touch enjoy play with vibration.

   ⊕ As you explore touch with the child, note the areas that are most and least hypersensitive. Explore different parts of the body and differences in the amount and timing of touch, using it with warmth and gentleness. Children may more easily accept touch when it is provided to the least sensitive areas of the body first and directed slowly and with deep pressure toward the more sensitive parts. Touch the child as a way of communicating understanding, caring, and love.

   ⊕ Do not use touch mechanically to desensitize the mouth or another part of the body. Even when the child's body can accept this type of touch, it rarely is integrated as well as touch that communicates caring.

🅰 Use music to help the child organize and integrate sensory reactions in the nervous system. At first, use baroque music with a slow tempo of 60 beats per minute. Hemi-Sync Metamusic has helped many children respond appropriately to sensory information. The changes that are facilitated through these special sounds appear to remain when the music is no longer present.

- ✛ Observe the child for feedback on the appropriateness of the music. Use changes in respiratory pattern, vocalization, and general activity level as guides for continuing, withdrawing, or changing the music.
- **A** Incorporate vestibular, proprioceptive, deep touch-pressure, and special music activities at special times throughout the day to create an individualized *sensory diet* for the child. See Chapter 14 for an in-depth discussion on sensory programs for children with sensory defensiveness.
- **A** Be trustworthy and help the child learn to trust you. Incorporate ideas from the Trust section below.

◉ Reduce oral sensory defensiveness.

Possible Activities

- **A** Incorporate vestibular, proprioceptive, deep touch-pressure, and music activities before providing specific sensory input to the mouth.
- **A** Incorporate ideas for developing generalized and discriminative mouthing patterns, which are described in the sections on Sensory Awareness: Face and Mouth on page 411 and Sensory Discrimination: Face and Mouth on page 414.
- **A** Introduce the toothbrushing activities described in the Combined Oral Sensorimotor Control: Toothbrushing section on page 439. Focus on the child's sensory awareness and discrimination skills in this activity.
- **A** Sensory information is accepted and integrated more easily when the child provides the sensory input than when adults attempt to desensitize the child's mouth.

▼ Guide and encourage the child, but **never force** a child to accept oral sensory input.

- **A** Give children time to prepare their sensory systems before dealing with input that may cause a defensive reaction. Sing a song or say certain words (e.g., "Here it comes!" or "Open your mouth"). If the child does not have defensive responses to touch on the hands, consider putting the child's hand on your hand or on the spoon so the child can feel the spoon approaching. A bright spoon or bell on the handle may get and maintain the child's attention to the approaching spoon. Squeak a toy en route to the mouth. This gives a visual and auditory cue. The child who is ready for the spoon approach often can handle its touch more appropriately.

Interaction Issues

Supporting Areas

Trust

◉ Build trust in the feeder so that the child does not need to purposively close or clench the mouth to prevent the entrance of certain foods.

Possible Activities

- **A** Involve the child in all oral interactions. Get permission before putting anything in the child's mouth so that he learns to trust that he can lead the treatment as he is comfortable. If the child is fussing, upset, or scared, he cannot have the optimum learning opportunity from the oral experience offered.
- **A** Be consistent. Do what you say you are going to do. Do not try to trick the child.
- **A** Communicate your caring and trustworthiness through firm but gentle touch that is acceptable to the child. The communicative use of touch should be introduced and explored with all children. When your touch communicates caring and respect, the child is more likely to trust you.

Touch that is given mechanically to placate a dysfunctioning nervous system lacks a personal connection. Often, the child rejects it because she perceives it as invasive.

⊕ You also can communicate love and acceptance by joining the child in creating and selecting movements and sounds. If you rock your body as the child is rocking or flick your fingers in front of your eyes as you join the child's movement, you communicate a special bond with the child. It becomes a way of saying, "I want to understand your world" or "I want to be with you and tell you that you're okay just exactly as you are."

◉ Increase the child's level of self-trust and knowledge that change is possible.

Possible Activities

🅰 Strong interconnections exist between the mind and body. Although the focus has been on getting the child to relax or move parts of the body to learn, it is equally effective to teach a child to imagine participation in the desired movement pattern. As the mind creates the image, the body actually rehearses the movement, using tiny muscle contractions. Because imagery activities and pretending begin by age 2, children who are functioning cognitively at the 2- to 3-year-old level can enjoy participating in imagery activities.

Anticipation

◉ Increase the ability to maintain a quiet body and mouth or use a graded movement response when food and utensils are presented.

Possible Activities

🅰 Engage the child's imagination while listening to a story with the body and mouth quiet. Gradually move into stories about eating and food, and ask the child to pretend to move the hand or mouth to eat as the real body and mouth remain quiet.

🅰 Create predictability by using rhythms, counting, or singing a specific song to cue the child to open the mouth for the food.

Communication

◉ Increase communication alternatives that reduce the use of the jaw thrust, wide jaw excursions, or a suckle as a communication signal at mealtimes.

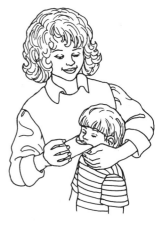

Possible Activities

🅰 Encourage the child to look into the cup to cue the feeder to tip it for drinking. This will bring the head toward a chin-tuck alignment and reduce the use of strong jaw and tongue movements used to signal readiness for drinking.

🅰 Help the child develop a set of signals to indicate readiness to begin drinking and the need to stop. Use signals such as looking down into the cup to signal the feeder to tip the cup for drinking and looking up from the cup to signal the feeder to tip the cup down to stop. Some type of intentional signal can be developed with most children who have reached a developmental level of 8 months, when vegetative signals begin to carry communicative intent.

🅰 See Chapter 13 for a discussion of communication alternatives at mealtime.

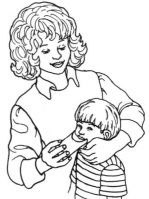

Physical and Sensory

◉ Reduce the use of non-mealtime-related distractions.

Possible Activities

🅰 Use distractions selectively as a therapeutic strategy at mealtimes. Too many distractions can draw the child's attention away from the meal. Lots of toys, videotapes, and books at a meal can teach the child to focus not on the eating, but on the mealtime entertainment. Although these distractions may be started to help a child eat more, they often backfire and cause the child to eat less and to require even more entertainment. However, some distractions can help. They can be important in helping the child focus on a fun aspect of the meal rather than a potentially more stressful new texture or flavor.

🅰 Give a child her own spoon while you are feeding her food from another spoon. This can reduce the number of times she grabs for your spoon. It also provides a distraction while you are getting the spooned food in her! This is an appropriate mealtime-related distraction.

🅰 Dry cereal on the tray can be a distraction while the child is being fed. It is so much fun to chase the tiny pieces around the tray that the child may relax into the spoon process. This is an appropriate mealtime-related distraction.

🅰 Children who are overly sensitive to changes in the meal (i.e., texture, taste, or temperature) may need a distraction to get past their hyperreaction to that sensation. This is the mealtime situation in which a toy distraction or song may be useful. For example, if a new texture is carefully selected to be a small change on the texture continuum and there is anticipation that the child may overreact, it may help to start a song, or distract the child with at toy at the moment the change is presented. This diverts attention to the play activity and not the oral change.

🅰 In some therapy situations, a child may sit on a glider swing with you. At the moment a new texture is tried, you may swing the glider swing and use movement as the distraction from the overreaction.

Negative Interactions

◉ Reduce the number of tantrums the child throws to communicate feeding needs and preferences.

Possible Activities

🅰 Serve food that is appropriate in its sensory characteristics and motor requirements for the child's abilities. Introduce new foods gradually through single changes in the sensory properties or motor requirements.

🅰 Define the role that the temper tantrum plays in the pattern of total communication at mealtime. When most children find something that works, they seldom consider ways of expressing the same message in a fashion that is more acceptable to adults.

🅰 Explore the child's current communication patterns. Observe and discover how the child communicates mealtime needs to the feeder. See Chapter 13 for guidelines for obtaining this information.

🅰 Consider movements or sounds that the child uses for other purposes that he could use to express the feelings and message communicated by a tantrum. Present other possibilities for communicating the basic message.

🅰 Put the child's basic message into words. If you sense that the tantrum means "I don't like this food. It tastes yucky and I won't eat it," use these words and concepts when you observe the beginning signs of the tantrum. For example, as the child begins to arch and grind her teeth, make the emotional statement: "Carol says, 'I hate this food! It feels awful. Don't make me eat it!'" The essence of this message can be repeated while the tantrum is continuing. In this case, make no effort to remove the attention given to the tantrum. You might even help the child use stronger movements and join her in a joint expression of feelings about the food. When the tantrum and the message have been completed, show the child other ways to convey the message that she doesn't like the food.

🅰 Acknowledging how a child feels does not imply that the feeder is giving in to the child's demands. Most people feel more reasonable and willing to negotiate when they know that another person understands. Empathy provides a base of emotional support for change. The child who feels misunderstood and coerced will spend a great deal of energy fighting any change that the feeder wishes to make.

◉ Develop an appropriate division of responsibility at the meal in which the parent is responsible for providing a healthy and varied meal and the child is responsible for determining the foods and amounts eaten.

Possible Activities

🅰 Select foods that are appropriate for the child's physical, sensory, and developmental needs.

🅰 Create an appropriate time and place for meals.

🅰 Offer children new foods repeatedly so that they become more familiar with each exposure.

🅰 Do not push children to eat specific foods or amounts. The choice to eat is the child's responsibility. Some children have tantrums because they feel pushed to eat more than they want or foods they do not like. A tantrum may be their way of saying, "Listen to me! I am full!" or "I do not feel well enough to eat." Reading the child's cues and being sensitive to parent and child roles at mealtimes can reduce the number of tantrums.

◉ Increase the feeder's self-observation and understanding of personal reactions to the child's mealtime behavior.

Possible Activities

🅰 Children are quite aware of others' feelings and reactions, and they will respond according to the feedback given to their behavior. If adults wish to understand the child and to change their own behavior, they need to be aware of what they are feeling and doing when the child's mealtime behavior does not meet expectations.

⊕ Observe your basic inner and outer reactions when the child throws a temper tantrum at the meal or during therapy. How do you feel: angry, irritated, vengeful? What do you do during the tantrum? What do you do after the tantrum? Mealtime is a common battleground for young children in their attempts to defeat a parent. When the child refuses to eat, spits food, or throws a temper tantrum, the parent usually will meet the child's expectations. Mothers who fear that their child will not get enough food or will become malnourished often will do anything to get food into the child. In our culture, a mother whose child doesn't eat well often feels that she is not a good mother.

⊕ When the feeder becomes involved in the child's decision to eat, a power contest can develop. However, if one person refuses to become involved in a power conflict, it is hard for the other person to continue. There is much truth in the old proverb, "You can lead a horse to water, but you can't make him drink." Translating the proverb, there is no way you can force a child to eat. However, any feeder can stop fighting and help the child learn about eating more appropriately through the natural consequences of being hungry.

⊙ Increase the feeder's positive expectations of the child and the mealtime.

Possible Activities

🅰 Set aside a few minutes for yourself before you serve the child a meal. Sit quietly and create a mental picture of a meal in which you and the child work in harmony. Feel the pleasure you experience when you are together. Imagine a situation that involves better communication and shared problem solving. See the child learning something new at this meal. Sense the child's pleasure and pride. Hear yourself telling the child how much you enjoy being together and how proud you are because the child is trying new things. After you have created this image, release it. Let it go. Don't hang onto it for comparison with the meal that follows. You have set your intent that the meal will be harmonious and that the child will enjoy learning.

⊙ Eliminate mealtime power contests. Build the child's interest and cooperation at mealtimes through natural and logical consequences.

Possible Activities

🅰 Serve food that is appropriate in its sensory characteristics and motor requirements for the child's current abilities. Make no comments about eating or not eating. Focus on your expectancy that important learning will occur for both of you during this meal. If the child is a self-feeder, provide assistance only as needed or requested.

  ✛ Set a timer for 30 to 45 minutes, depending on the child's feeding abilities. Tell the child, "The bell will let us know when the meal is over." When the bell goes off, clear away all dishes and any uneaten food. The bell sets an objective cutoff point for the end of the meal. Food is not removed to punish the child for being slow or not eating.

  ✛ Serving small portions makes it easier to let the child know how nice the clean plate looks. This helps the child gain a feeling of success in completing a meal.

  ✛ After the meal, select an activity that you and the child can enjoy together. Talk about topics of interest. Avoid discussing food or future hunger. When you say to a child, "You're going to be hungry later because you didn't eat," or you take away an important time together because food was left, you are letting the child know you are still involved in the power game over food. The child may find it more fun to continue playing the game with you, despite being hungry, than to learn from hunger pangs that it would be better to eat more food at the next meal.

  ✛ If you withdraw from the power struggle and allow nature to take its course, the child probably will be hungrier for the next meal. At the next scheduled meal, serve foods the child likes as well as new ones that he less easily accepts. Let increased hunger provide the motivation for learning to eat. Include liquids at the meal, but offer the solid foods first. Much of the motivation for eating the new solids will be reduced if the child fills up on milk or juice at the beginning of the meal. If the child constantly chooses a liquid at the beginning of the meal, offer water or diluted milk so that calories are reduced. Low-calorie liquids are less likely to satisfy hunger.

  ✛ Children sometimes can go without food for several days without endangering their health. Children who are in good health and not underweight have been known to hold out for 3 or 4 days if they have been used to getting their own way in eating. At first, the child may not understand why the feeder has changed the rules of the game and may refuse to eat as a way of reminding the feeder to play according to the old rules. The feeder must understand the child's purpose in not eating and know that a lowered food intake for several days is acceptable. If the feeder chooses to become upset when the child goes without food, the child has discovered another means of control. Without adult interference, most children will decide to eat when they get hungry enough.

▼ There are a few children with damage or atypical function of the autonomic nervous system or gastrointestinal system who do not have a normal mechanism for regulating hunger. Because they do not experience or recognize normal signals for hunger, this natural consequence will not work for them. The approach still can be effective if the feeder clearly withdraws from the power contest. The adult cannot rely on the child's hunger, and preferred foods will need to be added to the diet in 2 or 3 days if the child has not begun to eat. This type of food deprivation program should be considered only with input from the child's primary physician and after looking at the child's big picture.

🅰 Sometimes a child throws a temper tantrum to force an adult to give another food. The purpose of a tantrum may be to impress the audience. If there is no audience, the tantrum will stop. When the child throws a tantrum, the adults can say nothing and walk out of the room.

✣ If tantrums occur at school or when there are guests, it may not be appropriate for others to leave. In that case, remove the child from the room. The action of removing the child can be done with firmness and love. It is not necessary for the adult to talk or explain why this action is taken. If it is appropriate, the child can be told, "You can scream and throw yourself on the floor in another room, but not in the dining room. When you are quiet, you may come back with the family."

✣ A severely disabled child who is fed by an adult may try to push the spoon away, throw the head back, or try to physically fight the feeder. When this happens, and the food contains the properties that the child can handle, the following procedure may be helpful:

a. Bring the spoon toward the child, stopping half an inch from the mouth. Wait for the child to come forward to actively take the food from the spoon. If the child pushes you away, spits out the food, or tries to keep you from giving the food, turn your face and body away. Do not look at or talk to the child. Ignore the behavior for 5 or 10 seconds. Turn back to the child, and say, "Let's have another bite."

b. If the child chooses to refuse the food a second time, say, "You are telling me that you are not ready to eat, so I will finish something I need to do in the next room." Then get up from the table with the food and leave the room for 5 minutes.

c. Return to the room and offer the food a third time. If the food is refused again, assume that the child is not hungry enough to be tempted by the meal. Quietly take off the child's bib, wash the hands and face, and take the child away from the table. Do this with a feeling of love and respect, knowing that the child is learning something about your unconditional love as well as the relationship between hunger and eating.

✣ Whenever the child is given the opportunity to decide to eat or not eat, offer food only at a regularly scheduled meal. Regularly scheduled snacks can be continued and used as additional opportunities for learning about choices. Refuse demands for food at unscheduled times. Say, "It is not time to eat now," and tell the child when the next meal or snack will be served.

✣ If changes in diet are implemented primarily during snacks and lunch at school, suggest that the parents give the child a very light breakfast to assure a higher level of hunger later in the morning.

▼ These steps are most appropriate when you believe that the child's refusal to eat and temper tantrums are influenced by your involvement in a power contest. It is important first to check out the appropriateness of the food and communication aspects of the meal.

🅰 Parent participation and cooperation with the program will vastly increase its success. If the parents decide to continue scolding the child for not eating or give in to demands for special snacks, the child's response to hunger cues becomes less important and less exciting than playing the power game. Children are very clever and observant, and they know clearly how each adult in their life is likely to react.

- The adult who constantly caters to the child's wants and becomes a short-order cook shows very little self-respect. The adult who forces the child to eat shows very little respect for the child. The best way to show mutual respect is for the adult to serve food that is appropriate to the child's physical abilities and needs, allowing the child to eat it or not, as desired.

- The feeding therapist can increase the long-range effectiveness of the program by accepting the parents' decisions with understanding. At times, our sense of what a child needs may not be in harmony with the needs of the family. When we can offer our suggestions for change in a way that lets the parent feel free to implement them or not, we create an environment of respect. When we put aside our belief that we know what is best for a child and a family, we are free to share new perspectives and help others explore the beliefs that direct their actions. This enables the parents to look at problems and issues in a new way, and creates an atmosphere for implementing changes that will meet everyone's needs. We can invite others to follow a new path, but the final change must come from within.

Reduced Independence

◉ Develop a cooperative partnership between the feeder and the child who is motivated for self-feeding.

◉ Develop a cooperative partnership between the feeding therapist and the child in relationship to direct work with the child's body and mouth.

Possible Activities

🅰 Create choices at each meal. Let the child select which food, spoon, bowl, bib, or plate will be used. When the adult offers reasonable selections, the child's choice is always acceptable. Young children need to select from a limited number of options. A choice between apple juice and grape juice is more meaningful than the open-ended choice of "What do you want to drink?"

- Choices are appropriate for all children who have reached a developmental age of 6 to 8 months. At that age, an infant can make a choice visually or by reach when shown a filled cup or spoon.

🅰 Emphasize turn-taking in all aspects of the program. Preschool children have a basic sense of fairness, and they quickly learn to share in turn-taking games. Even the child who refuses to allow an adult to put food in the mouth may enjoy a game of hiding a raisin in mother's mouth and then having mother hide the raisin in the child's mouth. Help the child discover and use signals to the feeder to regulate the speed of food presentation and the specific food or drink that is given next.

- The rhythm established by the adult who alternates a bite for the child and a bite for the teddy bear develops the basic understanding of sharing an experience. Thus, the concept of turn-taking can begin at an early age.

🅰 Build trust between the feeder and the child so that the child does not need to confront adults to get her needs for independence met. Incorporate ideas described in the Trust section on page 423.

🅰 Find ways that allow the child to take a physical responsibility for assisting with feeding. Choices must be made when using the hands or a spoon independently increases hypertonicity and limiting movement patterns in the mouth or reduces oral feeding skills. It is better to postpone self-feeding for as long as possible for the child with severe oral problems, but being actively involved never has to be postponed. The concept of working in partnership with the feeder appeals to many young children. A partnership can be developed in these ways:

- Suggest that you are the *outside helper* and the child is the *inside helper*.

- Encourage the child to be responsible for holding the mouth open until you put the spoon in or place food for biting between the side teeth.

- Tell the child, "You can hold the top of the cup with your teeth while I hold the bottom of the cup with my hand."
- Suggest that the child hold the top of your hand while the spoon holds the bottom of your hand as it moves from the dish to the mouth.

▼ The concept of partnership is appropriate for children who have reached the developmental age of 12 to 18 months.

🅰 Implement suggestions for teaching the child to be a self-feeder in ways that do not increase tension and limiting movements of the body and mouth. Many suggestions for modifying feeding procedures and teaching the small steps that lead to successful self-feeding are provided in Chapter 19.

▼ Independent feeding is appropriate when it does not contribute to deterioration of oral feeding abilities. Self-feeding procedures can be modified to enable the child to become an active participant in the meal. When these modifications are selected and implemented appropriately, the child's physical participation in self-feeding will not interfere with movements of the mouth.

Lack of Opportunity

◉ Provide developmentally appropriate opportunities for the child to participate in the mealtime.

Possible Activities

🅰 Provide the most appropriate foods and utensils for the child's developmental age and physical and sensory needs. This may require exploration to identify the combination that works most effectively for the specific child.

🅰 Provide assistance and adaptations in positioning and handling that enable the child to participate physically without using excessive effort.

🅰 Provide choices that let children know that they are in control of what they eat and how much they eat at the meal.

▪ Oral Control Issues

Supporting Areas

Jaw Control

Jaw Opening and Closing

◉ Assist controlled downward and upward jaw movement and increase the child's ability to achieve and maintain jaw closure and jaw opening without oral tension.

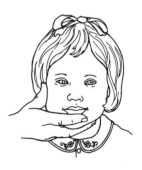

Possible Activities

🅰 Provide assisted oral control (i.e., jaw control) to guide the jaw in upward and downward movement and provide sustained jaw closure or opening as desired.

- Place your hand on the jaw as described in the following table and pictures. This helps the child experience a closed-mouth sensation and provides greater stability for the jaw at the temporomandibular joint.

Table 17.2   **Assisted Oral Control Hand Placement**

Feeder's Position	Finger	Placement	Purpose
To the side or from behind	Middle	Under the jaw just behind the chin	To assist upward jaw movement and reduce tongue protrusion
	Index	a. On the chin	a. To assist downward jaw movement
		b. Below the lower lip	b. To stabilize the lower lip
	Thumb	At the temporomandibular joint	To stabilize the feeder's hand
From in front	Middle	Under the jaw just behind the chin	To assist upward jaw movement and reduce tongue protrusion
	Index	At the temporomandibular joint	To stabilize the feeder's hand
	Thumb	a. On the chin	a. To assist downward jaw movement
		b. Below the lower lip	b. To stabilize the lower lip

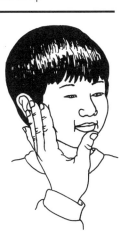

✛ This procedure to provide jaw stability and support can be done in at least two ways: from the side or back and from the front.

🄰 Gradually reduce the amount of control or assistance as the child is able to reduce the amount of jaw thrust.

▼ This strategy should not be used if the child has a strong jaw or tongue thrust or resists facial handling by the adult.

🄰 Use toothbrushing as a functional activity to achieve controlled jaw opening and closing movements. See specific suggestions listed in the Combined Oral Sensorimotor Control: Toothbrushing section on page 439.

Jaw Stability in an Open Position

◉ Sustain a quiet opening of the jaw as food is presented.

Possible Activities

🄰 Provide assisted oral control (i.e., jaw control) to guide jaw movement downward to provide sustained jaw opening. Help the child keep the jaw open for 2 to 3 seconds. Follow the guidelines listed for Jaw Control: Jaw Opening and Closing on page 430.

🄰 Without food present, ask the child to open her mouth and keep it open and quiet as a pretend spoon or piece of food approaches it.

🄰 Ask the child to open his mouth and keep it open and quiet as a real spoon or piece of food approaches and enters it.

🄰 Ask the child to open her mouth and keep it open until you place a piece of food between the side teeth for biting.

Jaw Stability in a Closed Position

⊙ Sustain a graded closure of the jaw on a toy or feeding utensil.

Possible Activities

🅰 Provide the child with objects for oral exploration and mouthing. Objects can include teether toys or toys of different textures, weights, sizes, shapes, and temperatures. Each toy that is explored can be held with the jaw while the tongue and lips further explore its sensory properties.

🅰 Have the child hold a cloth between the teeth, shake the head, and growl like a dog while you gently pull the cloth.

🅰 Have the child pretend to be a cat with whiskers, holding a straw between the teeth and biting in the center of the straw so that the ends protrude from the sides of the mouth.

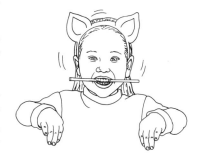

🅰 Offer cups and straws for liquid. Cup and straw drinking can be motivating. They require stability of the jaw as a foundational base. They give the child practice holding the jaw in a controlled position. Some children need to bite the cup or straw to initially hold it.

🅰 Use a stopwatch to time how long the child can hold a thin object gently between the teeth. A Linguistix™ or flavored tongue depressor works well for this activity.

🅰 Place a toy between the child's teeth or gums in the molar region. Encourage the child to hold the toy or a Chewy Tube™ with the teeth.

🅰 Play games with whistles and party blowers.

🅰 Encourage the child to hold on to the edge of the glass or cup with the teeth while drinking. This utilizes a normal strategy in the developmental sequence of acquiring jaw stability during drinking.

   a. Tell the child, "I will hold the bottom of the glass with my hand and you can hold the top of the glass with your teeth." This emphasis on partnership and the suggestion that the child can be a partial self-feeder encourages cooperation and is rewarding.

   b. While the child holds an empty glass or cup between the teeth, pour in a small amount of liquid. Help the child tip the cup to get the liquid while continuing to hold the cup. If you use a small amount of water or juice, the child receives excellent feedback from letting go, and the amount of spilling is inconsequential.

Graded Jaw Movements

⊙ Increase the graded control of jaw movement during mouthing and oral exploration activities.

Possible Activities

🅰 Provide many opportunities for the child to engage in generalized mouthing activities of the hands, simple toys, and familiar objects, using appropriate gradations of jaw movement. See specific suggestions listed in the Sensory Awareness: Face and Mouth section on page 411.

🅰 Provide many opportunities for the child to engage in discriminative mouthing activities of more complex toys and objects, using appropriate gradations of jaw movement. See specific suggestions listed in the Sensory Discrimination: Face and Mouth section on page 414.

🅰 Provide oral exploration activities that promote using appropriate gradations of jaw movement. Normal, pleasant oral experiences can provide meaningful practice for the jaw as it moves in and out of different postures to perform the activity. See specific suggestions listed in the Combined Oral Sensorimotor Control: Oral Exploration section on page 442.

⊙ Increase the graded control of jaw movement during dynamic movement activities.

Possible Activities

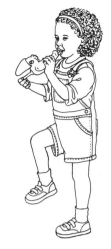

🅐 Incorporate activities that pair more mature jaw closure with other movements of the whole body so that jaw control is not just treated in isolation of other body movements. By activating purposive oral movements with activities that challenge the child's balance or require fine motor skills, the child gains the ability to develop a more dynamic oral control.

🅐 Give small snacks or gum to chew while the child is moving in and out of different positions in play. These snacks keep the jaw active, not allowing the extremes of jaw opening or closing often seen in jaws with poor stability.

🅐 Let the child blow a blower or whistle while doing another movement activity such as swinging on a swing, balancing on a therapy ball, moving prone on a scooter board, or marching.

🅐 Have the child drink from a straw while being tilted on a therapy ball or swinging on a glider swing. This provides jaw closure and oral motor activity while balance reactions are occurring throughout the body.

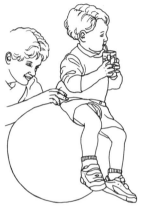

⊙ Increase the graded control of jaw movement when biting through foods that offer different degrees of resistance.

Possible Activities

🅐 Offer the child foods to bite through that are pleasing and safe. Often, we give children small broken off pieces of food so that the child does not overstuff the mouth or choke. This limits practice with biting through textures and resistances.

🅐 Hold the food in the side of the mouth so that the child can bite off a small piece, thereby reducing the amount of food that enters the mouth. Long, thin foods are easiest to place for controlled biting.

🅐 Begin with foods that dissolve quickly in the mouth so that the child can focus on the control he needs for biting without being concerned about food pieces that require additional chewing and bolus organization for swallowing.

🅐 Wrap foods that offer more resistance or require chewing in a thin, porous bag made of gauze, cheesecloth, or nylon organza. You can make this by placing the food on a small square of cloth and tying it with string or dental floss. Hold the cloth bag in the side of the child's mouth and guide the jaw in a graded opening and closing for biting. The Baby Safe Feeder™ is made from a solid plastic handle with a screw-on ring. A small nylon mesh bag is firmly attached to the ring for convenience and safety. Food placed in the bag can be bitten and chewed without food pieces breaking off in the child's mouth. These biting and chewing bags also can hold juicy fruits such as orange or grapefruit slices that often are difficult for children to manage safely.

🅐 Older children with better jaw control skills can bite off pieces of food and then spit them out into a dish. This gives the child practice biting without needing to eat every food provided in therapy. For spitting-out practice, use a particular bowl or cup so that the child voluntarily spits a certain piece out in a certain place. This "all-done dish" also can be used during regular meals to encourage children to sample new foods without making a commitment to chew and swallow them.

🅰 Offer foods that vary slightly in thickness and resistance for biting practice. When these are presented in random order, the child learns to open her mouth the appropriate amount for each food and exert the correct amount of sustained biting pressure as the jaw closes on the food.

🅰 Cut sandwiches in long, thin strips so that they can be placed on the side of the mouth for more efficient biting.

Lip and Cheek Control

Lip Rounding and Spreading

◉ Increase symmetrical lip rounding during play and feeding.

Possible Activities

🅰 Have the child use lips symmetrically to blow. Blowing requires directed airflow and lip coordination. It can be a very organizing activity. Blowing can be done with or without a straw. The straw gives a physical prompt to help the lips coordinate and helps the child more accurately direct the flow of air.

⊕ Have the child use a straw to blow bubbles in a pan of water. As a variation, put colored ice cubes in the water so that the bubbles move them around. Use different colors with the water and ice cubes so the melting ice turns the water a new color.

⊕ Have the child blow a Ping-Pong™ ball across a pan of water. The child may or may not use a straw.

⊕ Have the child blow into a pile of feathers, using a straw. As a variation, put feathers on a piece of paper and ask the child to blow all the feathers off the red paper or onto the yellow paper. This can become more complex as you ask the child to blow the red feathers onto the red paper and the yellow feathers onto the yellow paper. These activities can be done at a table, in prone, or on a scooter board.

⊕ Put tempera paint on a piece of paper and have the child blow it into a design, using a straw.

⊕ Have the child blow the cotton "snowballs" into a pile, using a straw or not.

⊕ Have the child blow pinwheels, using a straw or not.

⊕ Have the child blow party blowers. Use the type of party blowers that unroll to have the child move a balloon dangling by a string or knock plastic blocks off a table.

⊕ Have the child blow air onto a mirror to see the condensation.

⊕ Have the child blow horns and whistles. There are a variety on the market that offer different sounds, shapes, and degrees of difficulty.

🅰 Have the child do oral activities in which both sides of the face are doing the same thing at the same time.

⊕ Have the child drink through a straw and play straw drinking games.

⊕ Use the straw activities described in the Sucking: Straw Drinking section on page 467.

⊕ Play blowing games. (See above.)

⊕ Play symmetrical facial imitation games in front of a mirror such as smiling, frowning, kissing, or making exaggerated *eeeeeee* and *oooooo* sounds.

◉ Increase the amount of appropriate lip closure at rest and during eating.

Possible Activities

🅰 The ability to close the lips and maintain closure depends primarily on the child's jaw control. Incorporate activities that improve jaw stability as described in Jaw Control: Jaw Stability in a Closed Position on page 432.

🅰 Build the child's sensory awareness, discrimination, and feedback in the mouth and face using the sensory activities described in Sensory Awareness: Face and Mouth on page 411, Sensory Discrimination: Face and Mouth on page 414, and Sensory Feedback: Face and Mouth on page 415. Focus primarily on activities involving the jaw, lips, and cheeks.

🅰 Incorporate suggestions for developing lip control during spoon feeding and straw drinking. Specific activities are described in the Sucking: Spoon Feeding section on page 463 and in the Sucking: Straw Drinking section on page 467.

Cheek Compression

◉ Increase the amount of inward movement of the cheeks to assist in bolus formation and transfer of food from the teeth to the center of the mouth.

Possible Activities

🅰 "Hide" pieces of cookie or cheese in the cheek pockets. Encourage the child to find them by pushing the pieces to the center of the mouth with the cheek. If the child has difficulty getting the food out of the cheek pocket, give help by moving the cheek and lip forward with the hidden food.

🅰 Use a cotton swab to place drops of liquid at the corner of the lip or in the cheek pocket. Encourage the child to make a slurping noise while sucking the liquid into the mouth. This activity lends itself to turn-taking, with the child and feeder alternately feeding each other.

🅰 If a reduction in cheek compression is related to high or low tone in the cheeks, incorporate activities that normalize tone in the lips and cheeks. See Increased Tone: Lips and Cheeks on page 443 and Decreased Tone: Lips and Cheeks on page 445.

🅰 Incorporate suggestions for activating the cheeks through early munching-chewing and toothbrushing found in the Chewing: Munching section on page 477 and the Combined Oral Sensorimotor Control: Toothbrushing section on page 439.

Tongue Control

Tongue Shape

◉ Work toward greater *flattening and spreading* of the tongue.

Possible Activities

🅰 Build the child's sensory awareness, discrimination, and feedback in the tongue, using the sensory activities described in the Sensory Awareness: Face and Mouth section on page 411, Sensory Discrimination: Face and Mouth section on page 414, and Sensory Feedback: Face and Mouth section on page 415. Focus primarily on activities involving the jaw and tongue.

🅰 Use a small massager for vibration under the chin, on the base of the tongue, to provide greater stability for movement of the internal or intrinsic muscles of the tongue.

🅰 Use slight downward pressure with the bowl of the spoon during feeding.

▼ Use pressure and vibration on the tongue only with children who have low tone in the tongue or children whose primary problem is low sensory awareness. *Do not* use this type of stimulation with children who have problems with hyperreaction or sensory defensiveness in the mouth.

> 🅰 If a reduction in flattening and spreading is related to high or low tone in the tongue, incorporate activities that normalize tone in the tongue. See Increased Tone: Tongue on page 443 and Decreased Tone: Tongue on page 445.

⊙ Work toward greater *central grooving* of the tongue.

Possible Activities

> 🅰 Build the child's sensory awareness, discrimination and feedback in the tongue using the sensory activities described under Sensory Awareness: Face and Mouth on page 411, Sensory Discrimination: Face and Mouth on page 414 and Sensory Feedback: Face and Mouth on page 415. Focus primarily on activities involving the jaw and tongue.

> 🅰 Use vibration with a small massager under the chin, on the base of the tongue, to provide greater stability for movement of the internal or intrinsic muscles of the tongue.

> 🅰 Invite the child to put a vibrating toy or massager in his mouth so that the surface of his tongue receives vibratory stimuli. This type of stimulation often activates the tongue to curl around the toy, frequently encouraging or enhancing the central groove.

> 🅰 Play with a NUK™ massage brush in the center of the tongue. Encourage the child to move it around or to guide you in the type and amount of stimulation provided by the brush.

▼ Use direct stimulation on the tongue only with children who have low tone in the tongue or children whose primary problem is low sensory awareness. *Do not* use this type of stimulation with children who have problems with hyperreaction or sensory defensiveness in the mouth.

> 🅰 Use the NUK massage brush to give the child small amounts of pureed consistency food. This "textured spoon" provides increased sensory input to the center of the tongue and often stimulates more central grooving.

> 🅰 Have the child drink through a straw and play straw drinking games. Use the straw activities described in Sucking: Straw Drinking on page 467.

> 🅰 If a reduction in central grooving is related to high or low tone in the tongue, incorporate activities that normalize tone in the tongue. See Increased Tone: Tongue on page 443 and Decreased Tone: Tongue on page 445.

Tongue Movement

⊙ Work toward greater *forward-backward* movements of the tongue.

Possible Activities

> 🅰 If a reduction in forward-backward movement is related to high or low tone in the tongue, incorporate activities that normalize tone in the tongue. See Increased Tone: Tongue on page 443 and Decreased Tone: Tongue on page 445.

> 🅰 Work toward a more equal balance of forward and backward movement. Some children tend to have a predominance of one or the other. This is particularly true of children who have had a history of limiting tongue retraction or exaggerated protrusion or thrusting. Even when these patterns no longer influence oral movement, the child can continue to show an imbalance of normal movement.

> 🅰 Use a small massager for vibration under the chin, on the base of the tongue, to provide greater stability for movement of the external muscles of the tongue.

◪ Build the child's sensory awareness and feedback of tongue movement, using the sensory activities described in Sensory Awareness: Face and Mouth on page 411 and Sensory Feedback: Face and Mouth on page 415. Focus primarily on activities involving the jaw and tongue.

  ✤ Explore activities to develop graded forward and backward movement of the tongue. This can be done with a mirror or by asking the child to bring her tongue to your finger or an object placed in different areas on the forward-backward path.

◪ Build a stronger, more rhythmical suckle movement of the tongue in taking food from the bottle, breast, cup, or spoon. Incorporate appropriate activities from Sucking: Suckle Pattern on page 460.

◪ Encourage more active tongue movement in discriminative mouthing and oral exploration. See the activities in Combined Oral Sensorimotor Control: Mouthing on page 441 and Combined Oral Sensorimotor Control: Oral Exploration on page 442.

◉ Work toward greater *elevation-depression* of the tongue

Possible Activities

◪ If a reduction in tongue elevation and depression movements is related to high or low tone in the tongue, incorporate activities that normalize tone in the tongue. See Increased Tone: Tongue on page 443 and Decreased Tone: Tongue on page 445.

◪ Use a small massager for vibration under the chin, on the base of the tongue, to provide greater stability for movement of the external muscles of the tongue.

◪ Build the child's sensory awareness and feedback of tongue movement, using the sensory activities described in Sensory Awareness: Face and Mouth on page 411 and Sensory Feedback: Face and Mouth on page 415. Focus primarily on activities involving the jaw, tongue, and lips.

◪ Work toward more active lip and cheek control. When the lips seal the oral cavity, it is easier to stimulate depression of the body of the tongue to increase intraoral pressure.

◪ Help the child move from a suckle pattern to a more mature sucking pattern. Incorporate appropriate activities described in Sucking: Transition From Suckling to Sucking on page 462.

◪ Use a cotton swab to stimulate rhythmically the tip of the tongue and the center of the alveolar ridge behind the central incisors. This is the area of contact when the tongue tip elevates during the mature swallow and speech.

◪ Encourage tongue clicking and smacking of the tongue against the palate or alveolar ridge. Most children initially make this movement and sound with the tongue and jaw moving up and down together.

◪ Encourage more active tongue movement in discriminative mouthing and oral exploration. See the activities in the Combined Oral Sensorimotor Control: Mouthing section on page 441 and the Combined Oral Sensorimotor Control: Oral Exploration section on page 442.

◉ Work toward greater *lateralization* of the tongue.

Possible Activities

◪ If a reduction in tongue elevation and depression movements is related to high or low tone in the tongue, incorporate activities that normalize tone in the tongue. See Increased Tone: Tongue on page 443 and Decreased Tone: Tongue on page 445.

◪ Provide touch or taste stimulation to the side or lateral border of the tongue during oral play and toothbrushing. This may stimulate the normal, early transverse tongue reflex, which guides the tongue toward the stimulus.

◪ Incorporate activities to increase tongue lateralization as found in Chewing: Lateralization on page 478.

Velopharyngeal Control

⊙ Increase the range of movement of palatal closure.

Possible Activities

🅰 Using firm pressure on the hard palate, move your index finger to the juncture between the hard and soft palates. Build the child's ability to accept this stimulation without gagging.

🅰 Gradually move your finger back onto the muscular tissue of the soft palate. Stimulate the muscles to elevate.

🅰 Repeat the same activities, using firm portions of a toy or the first brush of the NUK Toothbrush Trainer Set™. Provide other sensory stimuli, such as cold or warmth, to the soft palate.

▼ If the muscles are of adequate length but movement is inadequate, this procedure may improve muscle contraction. However, it may be of limited value in transferring the elevation into a coordinated pattern during feeding or speech. Much of the elevation that occurs in this circumstance is related to the gag reflex, which uses a very different type of coordination than the swallow.

🅰 Consult with medical and dental specialists if the child's palate is too short. Recommendations may be made to close a portion of the palate surgically through a pharyngeal flap or to use a palatal prosthesis or obturator. These procedures typically are done only with older children whose oral cavity growth has become more stable.

Timing and Coordination

⊙ Reduce nasal reflux and move toward optimum timing and coordination of the palate with the entire feeding mechanism.

Possible Activities

🅰 The timing of palatal closure is part of a total automatic or semi-automatic pattern of coordination of sucking, swallowing, and breathing. If any portion of this combined pattern lacks coordination, the timing and coordination of palatal closure may be reduced. This is particularly true for children who have had primary issues of palatal control, including a cleft palate or velopharyngeal insufficiency. Activities that improve all aspects of the suck-swallow-breathe synergy can improve the coordination of palatal movement.

🅰 Improve cheek and tongue function so that the child is able to create a more efficient bolus. See the suggestions on how to improve tone and movement of the lips and cheeks and a cupped configuration of the tongue in Lip and Cheek Control: Lip Closure on page 435, Lip and Cheek Control: Cheek Compression on page 435, Tongue Control: Tongue Shape on page 435, and Tongue Control: Tongue Movement on page 436. The development of a rhythmical suckle-swallow with improved bolus formation often reduces the amount of nasal reflux.

🅰 Add cereal to thicken formula for drinking or give pureed consistency foods from a spoon or small cup. Thicker liquids and food often move downward in the pharynx with greater efficiency, while thin liquids are more likely to reflux upward into the nasal cavity. Remember that cereals and other solids usually are not added to the diet until the infant is 4 to 6 months old.

Oral Motor Imitation

Oral-Facial Imitation

⊙ Increase motor-planning skills in the face and mouth.

Possible Activities

🅰 Create a theme with multiple variations and sensory contrasts. For example, how many different ways can the child clap his hands? How many different faces can the child make in a mirror? How many ways can the child move to get a toy? This type of activity can assist children in their ability to motor-plan and learn that there is always more than one way of doing something.

🅰 Develop games such as shared clapping or patting that have variations (e.g., clapping your hands together, clapping the palms of your hands against the child's with your hands horizontal or with your hands vertical, clapping both hands at the same time or alternating right and left hands). Encourage the child to change the way she is clapping so that you can imitate her.

🅰 Play face imitation and sound games. Make different *eeeee* and *ooooo* sounds and exaggerated faces with the jaw closed.

🅰 Pretend to be farm animals making the faces and sounds of the animals.

🅰 Put on a pretend moustache made from paper, cotton, or whipped cream. Have the child wiggle the mustache in the mirror.

🅰 Have the child put shaving cream on his face and *shave* with a wooden craft stick. Make faces as the shaving cream is removed.

🅰 Have the child sit in front of a mirror and put on a clown face with creams or with a brush and cornstarch (i.e., clown face powder). Make funny clown faces once the face is decorated.

🅰 Moisten the child's lips with juice or saliva, and then press crumbs onto the lips, giving *crumb kisses* with your fingers. Children also can do this to themselves. They can wet their lips and put both lips on a plate of cracker crumbs, and then lick them off.

Combined Oral Sensorimotor Control

Toothbrushing

⊙ Develop sensory acceptance, as well as motor control and coordination of the jaw, lips, cheeks, and tongue during toothbrushing.

Possible Activities

🅰 Involve the child in all oral interactions during toothbrushing. Get permission before putting anything in the child's mouth so he learns to trust that he can lead the treatment as he is comfortable. If the child is fussy, upset, or scared, he cannot have the optimum learning opportunity from oral experience offered by toothbrushing.

🅰 Combine work on toothbrushing with handling and positioning that reduces limiting movement patterns in the body. Discontinue or modify direct work to the mouth when stimulation causes increased tone and undesired movement in the rest of the body.

🅰 Use the generalized mouthing and vibration activities described in the specific suggestions listed in the Combined Oral Sensorimotor Control: Mouthing section on page 441 and Sensory Awareness: Face and Mouth section on page 411.

🅰 Develop a sequence for toothbrushing that is appropriate for the child with whom you are working. Although the specific steps will vary with different children, the following progression will be appropriate for many. It is important to involve the child in every step of this progression. Get permission to put any object in the mouth. Children will give permission if they feel safe. They will grant permission with their eyes, by leaning toward the object, or by parting the lips or opening the mouth in a controlled fashion. Listen to the child and let her control the pace at which you proceed.

a. Introduce activities with the fingers or with toys that enable the child to experience touch, taste, and movement in the mouth enjoyably.

b. Encourage the child to explore and play with a beginning toothbrush such as the initial massage brush in the NUK Toothbrush Trainer Set™. Guide the child in discovering the feeling of touch and movement of this brush on the lips, cheeks, tongue, gums, and teeth. Initial safe exploration may not involve the toothbrush in the mouth. It may be on the chin, cheeks, or lips. As the child's comfort level increases, he may move the brush into mouth.

c. Provide sensory input with your finger, a finger toothbrush, or with the child's finger as if it were a toothbrush. One such finger toothbrush is the InfaDent Finger Toothbrush™. Rub it along the outer lips. As the child parts the lips, giving permission to let you put it on the teeth, gently brush the front teeth. Gradually brush the outside of the upper and lower gum ridges, the biting surface of the teeth, and the inside surface of the teeth. The exact locations stimulated and the amount and timing of stimulation will depend on the presence and strength of limiting sensory and motor patterns such as the tonic bite reflex. Proceed slowly and systematically within the child's tolerance and organization level.

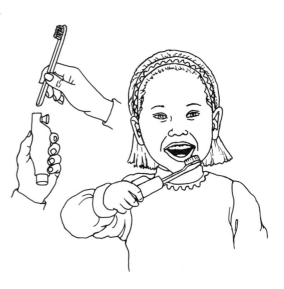

d. Repeat these activities using a small cosmetic sponge, the edge of a terrycloth washcloth, a sponge swab, or the NUK™ toothbrushes dipped in water. If you use the NUK toothbrush set, gradually introduce each of the brushes until the child accepts the sensations of the soft standard child's toothbrush.

e. Explore the sensation of brushing in all parts of the mouth. Brushing the tongue, cheeks, and lips can stimulate muscle tone. Brushing the sides of the tongue will encourage tongue lateralization for better control in chewing. An electric toothbrush or vibrating toothbrush handle with a soft child's toothbrush such as the Dental Mate™ can be used if the child likes and accepts it. Be careful that toothbrushing does not cause overstimulation and disorganization.

f. Introduce taste on the finger, cloths, or toothbrushes. Gradually increase the strength of the taste.

g. When the child is able to enjoy oral stimulation, brushing movements, and taste in the mouth, introduce small amounts of toothpaste on the brush.

h. Use an electric water pick or basting syringe to squirt water into the mouth. If the child leans forward over a basin placed on a table or wheelchair tray, the water will clean the open mouth, reducing the amount of toothpaste that is swallowed. Most young children swallow some toothpaste during the learning stages of toothbrushing. You may wish to use a non-fluoride toothpaste with children who cannot spit or get the paste out of the mouth without your help.

🅰 Use rhythmical cues during toothbrushing so that the child can anticipate short periods of brushing followed by equal periods during which the toothbrush is out of the mouth. For example, count "in–1–2–3, out–1–2–3." Most children can learn to accept short periods of brushing if they know when it will end and are given time to recover.

🅰 Sing a rhythmical song about toothbrushing. Combine this with gentle bouncing of the body or patting. The rhythm and words provide predictability and structure that make it easier for many children to accept the feeling of the toothbrush and paste.

Mouthing

◉ Develop sensory acceptance, motor control, and motor coordination of the jaw, lips, cheeks, and tongue during *generalized mouthing.*

Possible Activities

🅰 Provide many opportunities for the child to engage in generalized mouthing activities of the hands and simple environmental objects and toys with appropriate gradations of oral movement.

🅰 Provide good postural support of the child's body as a foundation for bringing his hands and toys to the mouth to enable mouthing with easy oral movements.

🅰 Provide assistance with stability at the shoulder, elbow, and wrist when helping a child explore her hands. The attempt to put fingers in the mouth can result in uncomfortable jabbing if the child cannot stabilize the rest of the arm. Many children avoid hand-to-mouth activities because they hurt themselves.

🅰 Cut the child's fingernails when you include activities that encourage moving the hand to the mouth. Scratches and jabs are uncomfortable and discouraging.

🅰 Work on physical activities that not only reduce shoulder girdle retraction and elevation, but make it possible for the child to bring his hands and toys to the mouth independently.

🅰 Develop the child's ability to enjoy putting her hands in her mouth and discovering the sensory feelings involved in contrasting movements and body parts. For example, explore the feeling of the thumb in the mouth, contrast this feeling with the feeling of the index finger in the mouth, and create another contrast with the whole fist in the mouth.

🅰 Mouthing of body parts provides sensory input and awareness in both the child's mouth and another part of the body. Older children who have had limited mouthing experience can be encouraged to explore their fingers by feeling them with their lips, counting them as they go into the mouth, or licking a taste off of each finger.

🅰 Play with individual fingers in the mouth and gradually place them farther back on the tongue without stimulating a gag reflex.

🅰 Develop the child's ability to enjoy toys in the mouth. Select toys or feeding utensils that have a simple shape and limited surface texture. Encourage the child to feel and become aware of all parts of the toy with his gums, teeth, lips, and tongue. He can bring the object to the mouth independently or with assistance.

🅰 Place a toy or a Chewy Tube™ between an older child's teeth or gums in the molar region. Encourage the child to make biting or chewing motions on the toy.

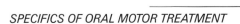

◉ Develop sensory discrimination and motor control and coordination of the jaw, lips, cheeks, and tongue during ***discriminative mouthing.***

Possible Activities

🅰 Provide many opportunities for the child to engage in discriminative mouthing activities of more complex toys and objects, using appropriate gradations of jaw movement.

🅰 Provide a variety of age-appropriate objects for the child to mouth. The child can bring the object to the mouth independently or with assistance. Use objects such as toothbrushes, spoons, cups, water picks, blowers, whistles, and straws when encouraging mouthing in older children.

🅰 Select toys or feeding utensils that have more complex shapes and distinctive surface textures. Encourage the child to feel and notice sensory contrasts in all parts of the toy with the gums, teeth, lips, and tongue.

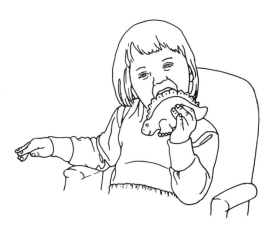

🅰 Help the child explore the surface of a toy with a variety of jaw, tongue, and lip movements. For example, use an animal that has different shapes or body parts. Have the child use her teeth, lips, and tongue to discover its feet, tail, nose, and head.

🅰 Children may be interested in mouthing some toys if there is a taste of food on the toy. Dipping the mouthing toy in a favorite flavor may encourage greater oral exploration with the jaw, tongue, and lips.

Oral Exploration

◉ Increase the variety of oral movements of the jaw, tongue, lips, and cheeks during oral exploration.

Possible Activities

🅰 Give the child food of different sizes, shapes, textures, and temperatures to lick. The child can lick an ice cream cone or Popsicle. He can lick cheese dip off the sides of a pretzel, yogurt off Mardi Gras beads, peanut butter from a spoon, and crumbs from wood craft sticks.

🅰 Give the child favorite foods to eat off a novel object. For example, children love to eat applesauce off a cookie, the foot of an animal toy, plastic keys, or the coil of a telephone cord. The child could eat bean dip off the surface of a rough cracker, corn chip, or bagel.

🅰 Play face imitation and sound games. Have the child open or close the jaw, using the mirror for feedback, if it helps. Make different ***eeee*** and ***ooooo*** sounds and exaggerated faces with the jaw closed.

🅰 Put Chap Stick® on the child's lips. Encourage the child to adjust the jaw to different degrees of opening while applying the lip balm.

Increased Tone

⊙ Influence muscle tone in the face and mouth by increasing muscle tone in the body.

Possible Activities

▲ Work with physical handling techniques that reduce tone in the trunk and provide proximal stability. Reducing tone in the body can reduce tone in the face and mouth. Greater stability in the neck and shoulder girdle area contributes to more normal control and movement patterns of the jaw. Use activities to decrease postural tone as described in the Change Tone: Decrease Tone section on page 406.

▲ Consult a physical therapist or other professional who has special training in therapeutic movement to select activities that will alter tone in the body as a whole.

Face

⊙ Reduce muscle tone in the face to support improved movement control.

Possible Activities

▲ Use the facial molding activity described in the Sensory Feedback: Face and Mouth section on page 415.

Jaw

⊙ Reduce muscle tone in the jaw to support improved movement control.

Possible Activities

▲ Use the facial molding activity described in the Sensory Feedback: Face and Mouth section on page 415.

Tongue

⊙ Reduce muscle tone in the tongue to support improved movement control.

Possible Activities

▲ Use the facial molding activity described in the Sensory Feedback: Face and Mouth section on page 415.

Lips and Cheeks

⊙ Reduce muscle tone in the lips and cheeks to support improved movement control.

Possible Activities

▲ Use the facial molding activity described in the Sensory Feedback: Face and Mouth section on page 415.

Decreased Tone

◉ Influence muscle tone in the face and mouth by increasing muscle tone in the body.

Possible Activities

🅰 Work with physical handling techniques that build tone in the trunk and provide proximal stability. Increasing tone in the body can increase tone in the face and mouth. Greater stability in the neck and shoulder girdle area will contribute to more normal control and movement patterns of the jaw. Use the activities to increase postural tone described in the Change Tone: Increase Tone section on page 406.

🅰 Consult a physical therapist or other professional who has special training in therapeutic movement to select activities that will alter tone in the body as a whole. In general, activities such as bouncing, tapping, and rocking through the spine can be used to build tone and develop better postural stability. This stimulation must be done very carefully so that hypertonicity does not result.

▼ This approach is useful for a child with low tone and severe postural instability. The child must be able to accept and integrate sensory stimulation without excessive and limiting increases in postural tone and movement.

Face

◉ Increase muscle tone in the face to support improved movement control.

Possible Activities

🅰 Use the facial molding activity described in the Sensory Feedback: Face and Mouth section on page 415.

🅰 Use the activities described in the Decreased Tone: Jaw section below and in the Decreased Tone: Lips and Cheeks section on page 439.

Jaw

◉ Increase muscle tone to provide greater stability of the jaw.

Possible Activities

🅰 Play patty-cake, peek-a-boo, and other children's games that enable patting, tapping, stroking, and other types of tactile and proprioceptive stimulation of the muscles that open and close the jaw. Tapping can be done directly around the temporomandibular joint.

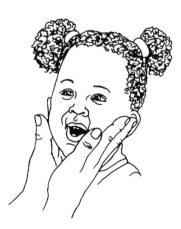

✚ Use folk music with a clear rhythm and regular tempo during tapping or providing other sensory input to the muscles and joint. Children enjoy singing while you touch and tap the face. It is playful and fun, and emphasizes the interaction rather than the facial stimulation.

✚ Play peek-a-boo with extra facial touch. Put a cloth (e.g., washcloth, hand towel, silk scarf) on the child's face and pull it off while simultaneously touching the face and gently drawing it forward with jaw and lip closure.

▼ This approach is useful for a child with low tone in the facial area. Because stimulation is firm and regular in rhythm and predictability, stimulation can be given playfully to a child who also shows some facial hypersensitivity. The child must be able to accept and integrate sensory stimulation without limiting increases in postural tone and movement in the rest of the body.

A Incorporate functional oral motor activities that help increase tone and control of jaw movements. See specific activities in the Jaw Control section, such as Jaw Stability in an Open Position on page 431, Jaw Stability in a Closed Position on page 432, and Graded Jaw Movements on page 432.

Tongue

◉ Increase muscle tone in the tongue to support improved movement control.

Possible Activities

A Keep the child's head in a chin-tucked position, with the neck elongated. Gently tap upward under the chin on the muscular area that is the base of the tongue. This can provide greater tongue stability and give it more tone.

A Use folk music with a clear rhythm and regular tempo while tapping or providing other sensory input directly to the tongue muscles under the chin and within the mouth. Children enjoy singing while you touch and tap the tongue. It is playful and fun, and emphasizes the interaction rather than the stimulation. Use instrumental music from the baroque period with children who become overstimulated with the more active folk music. Because the slow baroque music has a regular rhythm and a tempo similar to the rate of sucking, it can be effective when rhythmically tapping activities are used during a meal.

▼ This approach is appropriate if the tongue feels low in tone and the child is able to accept touch and pressure to the face and neck and within the mouth. The child may accept this approach more readily if it is done playfully or in rhythm to music.

A Incorporate functional oral motor activities that help increase tone and control of tongue movements. See the specific activities in the Tongue Control section, such as Tongue Shape on page 435 and Tongue Movement on page 436.

A Increase sensory input to the tongue through play, food selection, and specific discrimination activities. Explore the different textures and configurations of spicy, tart, or sour foods; ice; body parts; and toys. Challenge the child to identify the specific area of the tongue you have touched or to indicate whether there was one touch or two.

A Use vibration with a small massager or electric toothbrush directly on the tongue or under the chin, on the base of the tongue.

Lips and Cheeks

◉ Increase muscle tone in the face to support improved movement control.

Possible Activities

A Play patty-cake, peek-a-boo, and other children's games that incorporate patting, tapping, stroking, and other types of tactile and proprioceptive stimulation of the cheeks and lips. Tapping can be done directly around the temporomandibular joint to provide better jaw stability for lip and cheek mobility.

A Use folk music with a clear rhythm and regular tempo while tapping or providing other sensory input to the muscles. Children enjoy singing while you touch and tap the face. It is playful and fun, and emphasizes the interaction rather than the stimulation.

A Increase sensory input to lips and cheeks through play, food selection, and specific discrimination activities. Explore the different textures and configurations of spicy, tart, or sour foods; ice; body parts; and toys. Encourage the child to provide vibratory stimulation to the lips and cheeks with a small, battery-operated, hand vibrator. Challenge the child to identify the specific area of the face you have touched or to indicate whether there was one touch or two. These activities are helpful when the child is unclear about sensory information. Low sensory awareness and discrimination often contribute to low muscle tone.

- **A** Use toothbrushing to increase muscle tone in the lips and cheeks. Use the toothbrushing activities described in the Combined Oral Sensorimotor Control: Toothbrushing section on page 439.
- **A** Incorporate functional oral motor activities that help increase tone and control of lip and cheek movements. See the specific activities in the Lip and Cheek Control section such as Lip Rounding and Spreading on page 434, Lip Closure on page 435, and Cheek Compression on page 435.

Clenching and Biting

Jaw Clenching

⊙ Reduce the increased tone in the jaw that keeps the mouth tightly closed in a clenched posture.

Possible Activities

- **A** Use the activities to decrease postural tone described in the Change Tone: Decrease Tone section on page 406.
- **A** Reduce the strength of a total flexion pattern with movement and positioning that breaks up the total pattern. Use the activities described in the Change Physical Position: Change or Break Up a Total Pattern section on page 407.
- **A** Use activities to obtain greater postural alignment as described in the Postural Alignment: Head, Neck, and Trunk Alignment section on page 402. Focus on specific strategies to reduce flexor patterns in the body and shoulder girdle that often accompany jaw clenching related to strong flexion.
- **A** Use the facial molding activity described in Sensory Feedback: Face and Mouth on page 415. Adapt the procedure by using a gentle pressure into the temporomandibular joint to help the child release a strongly clenched jaw pattern.
- **A** If jaw clenching occurs primarily as an attempt to gain stability when the child is engaged in other physical movements, incorporate activities that pair more mature jaw closure with other movements of the whole body as described in the Jaw Control: Graded Jaw Movements section on page 432.

⊙ Reduce the sensory hypersensitivity that triggers a clenched posture of the mouth.

Possible Activities

- **A** If a clenching movement of the jaw is part of the tonic bite response, it may be triggered by touch or pressure on the gums or teeth. Reduce the hypersensitivity that occurs when the teeth contact a spoon, toy, or finger. Use a carefully graded firm pressure to the face, gums, and teeth while maintaining the jaw in a slightly open position. It is important to work for better body movement and positioning before closing the mouth and using oral stimulation.
- **A** Toothbrushing ideas are helpful in reducing the strength and automatic eliciting of a limiting oral movement, such as jaw clenching, for children who are able to accept touch to the face, lips, and the outer surface of the gums. Use the toothbrushing activities described in the Combined Oral Sensorimotor Control: Toothbrushing section on page 439. Combine this work with handling and positioning that reduces limiting movement patterns in the body. Discontinue direct work to the mouth when stimulation causes increased tone and undesired movement in the rest of the body.
- **A** Use the generalized and discriminative mouthing activities described in the Combined Oral Sensorimotor Control: Mouthing section on page 441.

⊙ Increase positive interactive and experiential aspects that allow children to reduce jaw clenching that is used to protect the mouth.

Possible Activities

🅰 Incorporate ideas from the section on Trust on page 423.

🅰 When jaw clenching seems to be part of a learned response, help the child explore mouth movements and oral sensation with a sense of adventure and pleasure. Children often become stuck in a pattern of clenching because they have not experienced other options that would be pleasurable. Children who are physically and psychologically touchy concerning the mouth may keep it clenched as a way of protecting themselves. It is important to build a sense of trust and comfort. Help the child discover other entertainment if tooth grinding is serving this purpose.

🅰 Use the generalized and discriminative mouthing activities described in the Combined Oral Sensorimotor Control: Mouthing section on page 441.

Tonic Bite Reflex

⊙ Reduce the strength and frequency of the tonic bite reflex.

Possible Activities

🅰 Use activities to obtain greater postural alignment as described in the Postural Alignment: Head, Neck, and Trunk Alignment section on page 402.

🅰 Reduce the amount of multisensory information that the child must deal with in the feeding environment. Create a quiet, focused mealtime with calming music, reduced visual and auditory distractions, and a positive and supportive communication environment. Because the tonic bite reflex can be considered a type of tactile hypersensitivity, it is always beneficial to reduce other sensory information that could overload the system.

🅰 Reduce the hypersensitivity that occurs when the teeth contact a finger. Use a carefully graded firm pressure to the face, gums, and teeth while maintaining the jaw in a slightly open position. It is important to work for better body movement and positioning before closing the mouth and using oral stimulation.

🅰 If you are comfortable with your hands and fingers in a child's mouth, use your fingers to provide stimulation rather than a toy, spoon, or other tool. If you are uncomfortable with putting your fingers in the mouth, it is better not to do so. When a child picks up a nonverbal message that is in conflict with the total situation, tension increases. Increased inner tension can change the strength of the tonic bite. Latex or vinyl gloves can help create a more sanitary environment if this is a concern to the adult, is required by the therapist's place of employment, or is necessary because of the child's state of health.

⊕ Slide your index finger (or little finger, if it is a tiny baby) along the outer surface of the upper and lower gums. Use a firm, sustained pressure. Your finger can pick up cues that will tell you whether to continue the stroking, stop and remain in the mouth, or gently remove your finger. If the child is personally comfortable with your finger, it is better to remain in the mouth and pause or stop the movement when you feel slight increases in tension. As tension subsides, begin the stimulation again. If the child objects to having your finger in the mouth, remove it and find ways to make the activity fun and acceptable.

⊕ Slide your finger parallel with the child's gum and roll it in and out along the gum rather than sticking it in perpendicular to the gums and teeth. This is often a faster and safer movement for the therapist.

- Carry out the activity in an atmosphere of mutual exploration. The child has the opportunity to discover ways in which the mouth can receive stimulation without biting. The therapist has the opportunity to discover the amount of pressure, speed of movement, and timing required to obtain a more normal response. Because each mouth is somewhat different, it is impossible to describe a specific way in which the stimulation should be done. When guided by a sense of exploration and discovery, the therapist will provide stimulation responsively and interactively. When recipes for oral stimulation are followed, stimulation often is provided in a very mechanical way.

- Use both hands to provide graded stimulation. The upper and lower gums on one side of the body will be done by one hand, and the other hand will stimulate the gums on the other side of the body. Your hand and index finger will be able to move in a smooth, flowing manner when you alternate the hands. When one hand works on both sides of the mouth, movement may be awkward and jerky as the hand twists to find the back corner on the side closest to it.

A Be clever and playful when you work inside the mouth. Pretend to count the child's teeth or search for an imaginary animal as you stimulate the gums.

A When the child accepts and enjoys firm touch to the gums, introduce stimulation to the upper or biting surface of the gums or the teeth. Because this is the area contacted by a spoon during feeding, it is important to prepare the child directly for work with the spoon. Your finger will move more rapidly and skillfully when you use a rolling movement while it is extended than when you move it back and forth with extension and flexion. Speed and skill enable you to move in and out of vulnerable or sensitive areas without getting bitten. This is important to both you and the child. As you rub the outer surface of the child's gums, gently roll your extended finger inward so that it contacts more of the upper surface of the gums or teeth. Continue this rolling motion, alternating it with the rubbing along the lower gum line that is more familiar to the child.

A When using your fingers in a child's mouth, you may be bitten. You can lower the risk by handling and positioning the child in ways that support more normal postural tone and movement. You lower the risk again when you create a level of stimulation that is adjusted to the child's tolerance level. When you allow yourself to explore slowly and discover the timing of movement and stimulation that is best, you program yourself for success. Your fears and expectations also can play a major role. When you are afraid of being bitten or expect that you will be because of the child's reputation as a biter, you increase the probability that this will occur. Fears create tension in the body, and tension reduces the skillfulness with which you move. The child can sense your anxiety and may become more tense and hypersensitive.

A Occasionally, biting occurs with your finger in the way. It is important to know how to deal with this. Pulling against a tonic bite reflex usually causes the child to increase the strength of the bite. Yanking your finger out of the bite usually increases the discomfort. The child probably is frightened or upset because of accidentally biting you. Panic and unhappiness increase bodily tension and the bite. Your panic will make the situation worse.

- The most important element in solving this uncomfortable problem is your own ability to remain calm. Focus your attention on calming the child. Rock or use gentle vestibular movement to reduce the child's body tension. Adjust the child's head position, bringing it into better alignment with the body. Remember what you know about this child's combination of head and mouth patterns. Does this child usually have the mouth open if the head is extended? (For most children, the mouth will open when the head is hyperextended. However, generalization does not apply to every child.) If another person is with you and the bite does not release with these procedures, have the other individual place her thumbs on both sides of the child's jaw at the temporomandibular joint. Slight pressure inward on the joint can help release the bite. In extreme cases, some children will release the bite when you blow into their face, unexpectedly sprinkle water at their face, or plug their nose. These approaches may be frightening or startling, and should be used only as a last resort.

- Help the child know that you are a trusted partner when the tonic bite occurs. Incorporate ideas from the Trust section on page 423.

◼ Introduce toothbrushing as an activity to provide graded stimulation while assisting the child in controlling the tonic bite reflex. Use the toothbrushing activities in the Combined Oral Sensorimotor Control: Toothbrushing section on page 439.

▼ Direct work to the mouth should be discontinued when the stimulation increases or causes high tone and limiting movement patterns in the rest of the body.

◼ Reduce the hypersensitivity that occurs when the teeth contact a coated spoon during feeding. Use a carefully graded introduction of firm pressure to the face, gums, and teeth while maintaining the jaw in a slightly open position. It is important to work for better body movement and positioning before closing the mouth and using oral stimulation.

◼ Explore the child's response to the presence of a toy or spoon or other firm object against the teeth. Discover the rhythm of touch and removal of touch that enables the child to reduce a biting tendency.

◼ When feeding a child who continues to show a tonic bite reflex, reduce the frequency with which the bite is elicited.

⊕ Develop a clear rhythm of spoon or cup presentation to increase the probability that contact with the utensil will occur when the mouth is in a more open phase.

⊕ Place the cup on the lower lip. Attempts to stabilize the jaw by biting the cup are not appropriate at this point.

⊕ Use a coated spoon so that any biting does not harm the child's teeth or cause discomfort.

⊕ Present the spoon or cup on the lower lip so that the lips, not the teeth, are stimulated. When the child initiates a suckle-swallow from this closed mouth position, the rhythmical pattern is not interfered with by the tonic bite reflex. Sometimes a lateral approach to spoon presentation is helpful.

◼ When feeding a child who continues to show a tonic bite reflex, explore the child's active ability to relax and release the bite after it has been stimulated. Many children feel that they are victims of their bite reflex. Once the bite has occurred, they respond as if there is nothing they can do. Their fear of the bite and injuring themselves often increases the difficulty of releasing it. During a snack or toward the end of a meal, when the child is less hungry, allow the bite to occur. Problem-solve aloud as you work with the child to release the bite. Emphasize the concept of partnership and the positive ability to work together to release the bite on the spoon. By reducing the sense of panic and helplessness that occurs with the reflexive bite, the child does not add further tension to the initial bite.

◼ Use the body massage activity described in the Change Tone: Decrease Tone section on page 406.

◼ Use the facial molding activity described in the Sensory Feedback: Face and Mouth section on page 415. Adapt the activity to place greater upward pressure into the temporomandibular joint.

Stability Bite

◉ Reduce the need to bite for stability by increasing underlying postural stability and jaw stability.

Possible Activities

◼ Use activities to increase postural tone as described in the Change Tone: Increase Tone section on page 406.

◼ Use activities to obtain greater postural alignment as described in the Postural Alignment: Head, Neck, and Trunk Alignment section on page 402.

◼ Use appropriate activities for developing volitional control of jaw movements as described in the Jaw Control section on page 430.

◼ Use the toothbrushing activities described in the Combined Oral Sensorimotor Control: Toothbrushing section on page 439.

A Incorporate activities such as using a snack cap and biting through foods that offer different degrees of resistance as described in the Sensory Feedback: Face and Mouth section on page 415.

Tooth Grinding

⊙ Reduce tooth grinding that is related to postural tone and sensory stimulation.

Possible Activities

A Use activities to decrease postural tone as described in the Change Tone: Decrease Tone section on page 406.

A Use activities to obtain greater postural alignment as described in the Postural Alignment: Head, Neck, and Trunk Alignment section on page 402. Focus on specific strategies to reduce flexor patterns in the body and shoulder girdle that often accompany tooth grinding related to jaw clenching.

A Provide chewable toys and foods that can provide strong proprioceptive information to the jaw. Chewable tubing, such as TheraTubing™, can be given for chewing. Give the child beef jerky, dried fruits, fruit leathers, licorice strings, bubble gum, and other very chewy foods to bite, hold, or chew.

A Provide vibration using vibrating toys and massagers as a form of strong sensory input.

A Increase sensory awareness and feedback with the jaw in a relaxed, closed mouth position to help the child become more aware of the tension being held in the jaw and more relaxed alternatives. Follow this with mouthing activities done with a relaxed mouth.

⊙ Change adult behaviors that may be contributing to tooth grinding that has become part of attention seeking or a power contest.

Possible Activities

A Your reactions to the child will let you know what purpose the behavior serves. When attention is an issue, the adult usually feels irritated at the child. The child may stop the grinding for awhile, but resume as soon as the adult's attention shifts to something else. When power is involved, the adult generally feels angry with the child for the behavior, and the child either will ignore requests to stop the tooth grinding or will stop briefly and then increase the amount of tooth grinding. Explore the reactions of adults in the child's environment. How much attention does the child receive for grinding the teeth? How upset do adults become when the child continues to make the noise? If you suspect that the child is using the behavior to get attention or engage others in a power struggle, try some of the following ideas.

⊕ When the child begins tooth grinding, do not pay attention to him. Adults may leave the room after determining that the child is physically safe. Balance this procedure by finding times to give warmth and attention when the child's mouth is quiet. Use the quiet times for hugs, reading a story, or taking a walk.

⊕ When you feel yourself becoming angry or irritated from tooth grinding noise, tell the child you must leave and go where it is quieter. Say, "You can stay here and make the tooth noises if you like. I am going into the living room to listen to music quietly." Give *I messages* that let the child know what you want and how you are going to find what you want. This is very different from the *you messages* that tell the child what to do. Children who have a disability often feel powerless. Tooth grinding can become a way to assert a normal need to have some control over life. Introduce other possibilities for offering choices and more control in therapy and home activities.

⊕ Explore other ideas for dealing with attention and power behaviors. You can find excellent suggestions in *Children: The Challenge* (Dreikurs & Stoltz, 1964).

Thrusting

Jaw

⊙ Reduce or inhibit a downward jaw thrust to prepare for oral motor and feeding activities that require controlled jaw movements.

Possible Activities

🅰 Use activities to decrease postural tone such as those in the Change Tone: Decrease Tone section on page 406.

🅰 Reduce the strength of a total extension pattern with movement and positioning that breaks up the total pattern. Use the activities in the Change Physical Position: Change or Break Up a Total Pattern section on page 407.

🅰 Use activities to obtain greater postural alignment. Try those described in the Postural Alignment: Head, Neck, and Trunk Alignment section on page 402. Focus on specific strategies to reduce extensor patterns in the body and shoulder girdle that often accompany jaw thrusting related to strong extension.

🅰 Use assisted oral control as described in the Jaw Control: Jaw Opening and Closing section on page 430.

▼ Do not use this strategy if the child has a strong jaw or tongue thrust or resists facial handling.

🅰 Reduce confusing sensory input that might overload the child's system. The stress involved can cause a reversion to limiting movement patterns such as a jaw thrust. To address these issues, include activities to simplify the sensory environment for the meal as described in the Hyperreaction: Environmental Sensory Input section on page 418.

🅰 When a jaw thrust is a hyperreaction to touch to the mouth, incorporate activities as described in the Sensory Feedback: Face and Mouth section on page 415.

🅰 Read Chapter 13 for alternative communication strategies you can use when children use limiting patterns of movement such as a jaw thrust to communicate.

Tongue

⊙ Reduce or inhibit a tongue thrust to prepare for oral motor and feeding activities that require controlled tongue movements.

Possible Activities

🅰 Use activities to decrease postural tone as described in the Change Tone: Decrease Tone section on page 406.

🅰 Reduce the strength of a total extension pattern with movement and positioning that breaks up the total pattern. Use the activities in the Change Physical Position: Change or Break Up a Total Pattern section on page 407.

🅰 Use activities to obtain greater postural alignment as described in the Postural Alignment: Head, Neck, and Trunk Alignment section on page 402. Focus on specific strategies to reduce the extensor patterns in the body and shoulder girdle that often accompany tongue thrusting related to strong extension.

🅰 Help the child achieve and maintain the tongue in the mouth. Use assisted oral control as described in the Jaw Control: Jaw Opening and Closing section on page 430. Placing the middle finger directly under the chin allows you to use firm pressure to reduce the forward movement of the base of the tongue.

▼ Direct assistance with maintaining the tongue in the mouth can be effective after limiting patterns are reduced through handling and positioning. Procedures for helping the child develop better jaw stability and oral control will be ineffective when the thrusting pattern is strong and you must use force to keep the child's tongue in the mouth. It also is inappropriate when tongue protrusion is a compensation for respiratory distress or when the child resists facial handling.

🄰 Work for the easy initiation of a suckling or sucking pattern from the lips rather than the tongue. Use thickened liquids or pureed foods from a clear or cutout cup with a large diameter or a spoon with a flat bowl. Support the jaw as needed to provide greater stability for the base of the tongue. Present the liquid or food horizontally at the lower lip so that the upper lip can come down to assist the lower lip with sucking. When the suck is initiated from the lips rather than from the tongue, the tongue tends to remain behind the lips.

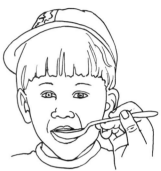

🄰 Presenting the spoon laterally or sideways so that it is parallel to the mouth works well for children who have a tongue thrust when the spoon touches the tongue. With this lateral placement, the feeding therapist can avoid stimulating the tongue while providing increased stability at the lip corners. The placement of the spoon and the option to tip up the outside edge can help keep the tongue in the mouth. For more information, see the Sucking: Spoon Feeding section on page 463.

🄰 Reduce confusing sensory input that might overload the child's system. The stress involved can cause a reversion to limiting movement patterns such as a tongue thrust. To address these issues, include activities to simplify the sensory environment for the meal as described in the Hyperreaction: Enviromental Sensory Input section on page 418.

🄰 When a tongue thrust is a hyperreaction to touch to the mouth, incorporate the activities in the Hyperreaction: Bodily Sensory Input section on page 419.

🄰 Read Chapter 13 for alternative communication strategies you can use when children use limiting patterns of movement such as a tongue thrust to communicate. Incorporate ideas from the Trust section on page 423.

Exaggerated Movement

Jaw (Wide Excursions)

◉ Reduce or inhibit exaggerated jaw movement to prepare for oral motor and feeding activities that require controlled jaw movements.

Possible Activities

🄰 If the wide jaw excursions are related to low tone and postural instability, include activities to increase postural tone such as those in the Change Tone: Increase Tone section on page 406.

🄰 Use activities to obtain greater postural alignment as described in the Postural Alignment: Head, Neck, and Trunk Alignment section on page 402. Focus on specific strategies to reduce the extensor patterns in the body and shoulder girdle that often accompany wide jaw excursions related to hyperextension.

🄰 Use assisted oral control as described in the Jaw Control: Jaw Opening and Closing section on page 430.

▼ Do not use this strategy if the child has a strong jaw or tongue thrust or resists facial handling.

🄰 Incorporate activities as described in the Jaw Control: Jaw Stability in an Open Position section on page 431 and the Jaw Control: Jaw Stability in a Closed Position section on page 432.

- ▲ Reduce confusing sensory input that might overload the child's system. The stress involved can cause a reversion to limiting movement patterns such as exaggerated jaw movement. To address these issues, include activities to simplify the sensory environment for the meal as described in the Hyperreaction: Environmental Sensory Input section on page 418.
- ▲ Use the snack cap described in the Sensory Feedback: Face and Mouth section on page 415.
- ▲ Increase sensory input and feedback of the jaw, tongue, cheeks, and lips during feeding or mouth exploration activities by using activities in the Sensory Feedback: Face and Mouth section on page 415.

Tongue (Protrusion)

◎ Reduce or inhibit exaggerated tongue protrusion to prepare for oral motor and feeding activities that require controlled tongue movements.

Possible Activities

- ▲ If exaggerated tongue protrusion is related to low tone and postural instability, include activities to increase postural tone as described in the Change Tone: Increase Tone section on page 406.
- ▲ Reduce the strength of a total extension pattern with movement and positioning that breaks up the total pattern. Use the activities in the Change Physical Position: Change or Break Up a Total Pattern section on page 407.
- ▲ Use activities to obtain greater postural alignment as described in the Postural Alignment: Head, Neck, and Trunk Alignment section on page 402. Focus on specific strategies to reduce the extensor patterns in the body and shoulder girdle that often accompany exaggerated tongue protrusion related to hyperextension.
- ▲ Help the child achieve and maintain the tongue in the mouth. Use assisted oral control as described in the Jaw Control: Jaw Opening and Closing section on page 430. Placing your middle finger directly under the child's chin enables you to use firm pressure to reduce the forward movement of the base of the tongue.

▼ Direct assistance with maintaining the tongue in the mouth can be effective after limiting patterns are reduced through handling and positioning. Do not use if the child resists facial handling.

- ▲ Work for the easy initiation of a suckling or sucking pattern from the lips rather than the tongue. Use thickened liquids or pureed foods from a clear or cutout cup with a large diameter or a spoon with a flat bowl. Support the jaw as needed to provide greater stability for the base of the tongue. Present the liquid or food horizontally at the lower lip so that the upper lip can come down to assist the lower lip with sucking. When the suck is initiated from the lips rather than from the tongue, the tongue tends to remain behind the lips.
- ▲ Place the flat bowl of the spoon into the child's mouth so that the spoon is parallel with the floor of the mouth. Rest the spoon on the middle of the tongue. Press evenly downward, using a vibratory movement through the spoon. Slowly remove the spoon, encouraging the lips to close and assist with food removal from the spoon. For many children, this pressure on the tongue provides sufficient sensory information to help the child keep the tongue in the mouth. For other children, the pressure on the tongue can cause a worsening of the tongue-thrusting behavior. For this latter group, a sideways or lateral spoon presentation may work better.

▼ This type of pressure and vibration is most effective when there is low tone in the tongue. With a hypotonic tongue, the added stimulation can increase tone and activate the tongue. It will not achieve the desired results if there is tonic bite or hypertonicity in the tongue. Pressure and vibration to the tongue may cause sensory disorganization for some children.

- ▲ Presenting the spoon laterally or sideways so that it is parallel to the mouth works well for children who have an exaggerated protrusion when the spoon touches the tongue. Using this lateral placement, you can avoid stimulating the tongue while providing increased stability at the lip corners. The placement of the spoon and the option to tip up the outside edge can help keep the tongue in the mouth. You can find more information and a drawing of this activity in the Sucking: Spoon Feeding section on page 463.

🅰 Reduce confusing sensory input that might overload the child's system. The stress involved can create a reversion to limiting movement patterns such as exaggerated tongue protrusion. To address these issues, include activities to simplify the sensory environment for the meal as described in the Hyperreaction: Environmental Sensory Input section on page 418.

🅰 When an exaggerated protrusion of the tongue is a hyperreaction to touch to the mouth, incorporate the activities described in Hyperreaction: Bodily Sensory Input on page 419.

🅰 Change the consistency of the child's food so that tongue protrusion is not needed to move it backward. Explore the child's sucking and chewing abilities. If the child has not developed up-down tongue movements for sucking and munching, begin at that level of development. If these movements are present when a less lumpy food is given, help the child to develop the tongue and cheek movements that will allow food to be moved from the center to the side teeth and back. Incorporate appropriate activities as described in the Sucking: Transition From Suckling to Sucking section on page 462 and Chewing: Munching section on page 477.

▼ Food changes and practice on the steps leading to chewing can make a big difference for the child whose lack of tongue lateralization and mobility lead to exaggerated tongue protrusion to move food from the front to the back of the tongue.

🅰 Provide the child with oral alerting activities around and in the mouth. (See Chapter 14 for an in depth discussion on variations among sensory variables.) These alerting experiences may be done before or during a meal, depending on the child and the variable.

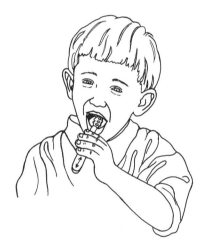

🅰 Feed the child using an alerting texture to wake up the tongue and increase its activity.

⊕ Use a NUK Massage Brush. Dip the brush into a pureed food and roll it onto the tongue. Initially present it by rolling it between the lips. As the child parts the lips and gives you permission to put it on the tongue, place the brush lengthwise along the central groove of the tongue to help it create the natural trough. Let the child suck the food off the Nuk brush and then remove it.

⊕ A vibrating spoon handle also may alert the jaw, cheeks, lips, and tongue in spoon feeding.

▼ This is most effective for the child who has low tone around the mouth and who needs wake-up sensory information to activate more mature oral patterns. It may not work well for a child who becomes easily disorganized during feeding.

🅰 Use the snack cap described in the Sensory Feedback: Face and Mouth section on page 415.

🅰 Increase sensory input and feedback of the jaw, tongue, cheeks, and lips during feeding or mouth exploration activities by using activities from Sensory Awareness: Face and Mouth on page 411, Sensory Feedback: Face and Mouth on page 415, and Combined Oral Sensorimotor Control: Mouthing on page 441.

Retraction

Jaw

⊙ Reduce jaw retraction that is related to postural tone and sensory stimulation.

Possible Activities

A To decrease postural tone, use activities such as body massage described in the Change Tone: Decrease Tone section on page 406 when jaw retraction is associated with increased tone throughout the body.

A Reduce the strength of a total extension pattern with movement and positioning that breaks up the total pattern. Use the activities described in the Change Physical Position: Change or Break Up a Total Pattern section on page 407.

A Use activities to obtain greater postural alignment as described in the Postural Alignment: Head, Neck, and Trunk Alignment section on page 402. Focus on specific strategies to reduce extension and retraction in the body and shoulder girdle that often accompany jaw retraction.

A Reduce confusing sensory input that might overload the child's system The stress involved can cause a reversion to limiting movement patterns such as jaw retraction. To address these issues, include activities to simplify the sensory environment for the meal as described in the Hyperreaction: Environmental Sensory Input section on page 418.

A When jaw retraction is a hyperreaction to touch to the mouth, incorporate activities described in the Hyperreaction: Bodily Sensory Input section on page 419.

A Use the facial molding activity in the Sensory Feedback: Face and Mouth section on page 415.

A When the jaw is retracted, often the child's breathing is affected. The resulting respiratory distress can lead to increased emotional and physical tension, as well as increased jaw retraction. Incorporate activities that encourage a more forward position of the jaw and tongue as described in the Airway Stability section on page 405.

Tongue

⊙ Reduce tongue retraction that is related to postural tone and sensory stimulation.

Possible Activities

A To decrease postural tone, use activities such as body massage described in the Change Tone: Decrease Tone section on page 406 when jaw retraction is associated with increased tone throughout the body.

A Use activities that build and stabilize tone in the trunk, shoulders, and neck, and provide proximal stability when low tone and poor stability are a major main issue. See Change Tone: Increase Tone on page 406 and Change Tone: Stabilize Tone on page 407.

A Use activities to obtain greater postural alignment as described in the Postural Alignment: Head, Neck, and Trunk Alignment section on page 402. Focus on specific strategies to reduce extension and retraction in the body and shoulder girdle that often accompany tongue retraction.

A Reduce confusing sensory input that might overload the child's system. The stress involved can cause a reversion to limiting movement patterns such as tongue retraction. To address these issues, include activities to simplify the sensory environment for the meal as described in the Hyperreaction: Environmental Sensory Input section on page 418.

A When tongue retraction is a hyperreaction to touch to the mouth, incorporate activities as described in the Hyperreaction: Bodily Sensory Input section on page 419.

A Use the facial molding activity described in the Sensory Feedback: Face and Mouth section on page 415.

- ▲ When the tongue is retracted, often the child's breathing is affected. The resulting respiratory distress can lead to increased emotional and physical tension, as well as increased tongue retraction. Incorporate activities that encourage a more forward position of the jaw and tongue as described in the Airway Stability section on page 405.

- ▲ With the child in prone or sidelying, stimulate the lips with your finger. Move into the mouth, stroking the tongue rhythmically and enticing it to follow the tip of your finger as it slides toward the front of the mouth. A taste of food on your finger will make it more interesting for the child.

- ▼ This approach works well when the child can accept prone or sidelying without increasing tension and when there is no oral hypersensitivity. If the child rejects having an adult's finger in the mouth, or if stimulating the tongue increases retraction or disorganization, stimulation of only the lips is appropriate.

- ▲ Keep the child's head in a chin-tucked position, with the neck elongated. Gently tap upward under the chin on the muscular area that is the base of the tongue. This can provide greater tongue stability and give it more tone for moving forward.

- ▼ This approach is appropriate if the tongue feels low in tone and if the child is able to accept touch and pressure to the face and neck. The child may accept this approach more readily if it is done playfully or in rhythm to music.

- ▲ Place the child in prone or face-to-face with you. Make sure that the child's head and trunk are well aligned, with the chin tucked toward the chest. Put a finger in the child's mouth, entering the cheek pouch from the side. Gently work your finger toward the gums and tongue. As your finger reaches the tongue, begin a downward vibration on the center of the tongue to flatten it. You also can use a rapid lateral motion of your finger to vibrate the tongue. Stroke forward on the tongue as your finger comes out of the mouth. When used appropriately, this approach can relax and flatten the tongue.

- ▼ This approach works well when the child has a stiff tongue with increased tone and retraction. This approach is not appropriate if the child rejects an adult's finger in the mouth, has a tonic bite reflex, or if stimulating the tongue increases retraction or disorganization.

- ▲ As the tongue begins to move into a more forward position, incorporate the generalized and discriminative mouthing activities described in the Combined Oral Sensorimotor Control: Mouthing section on page 441.

- ▲ If the tongue retraction is seen with jaw retraction, see the activities in the Retraction: Jaw section on page 455.

Lips and Cheeks

⊙ Reduce lip and cheek retraction that is related to postural tone and sensory stimulation.

Possible Activities

- ▲ To decrease postural tone, use activities such as body massage as described in the Change Tone: Decrease Tone section on page 406 when lip and cheek retraction are associated with increased tone throughout the body.

- ▲ Use activities to obtain greater postural alignment as described in the Postural Alignment: Head, Neck, and Trunk Alignment section on page 402. Focus on specific strategies to reduce extension and retraction in the body and shoulder girdle that often accompany lip and cheek retraction.

- ▲ Reduce confusing sensory input that might overload the child's system. The stress involved can cause a reversion to limiting movement patterns such as lip and cheek retraction. To address these issues, include activities to simplify the sensory environment for the meal as described in the Hyperreaction: Environmental Sensory Input section on page 418.

■ When lip-cheek retraction is a hyperreaction to touch to the mouth, incorporate the activities in the Hyperreaction: Bodily Sensory Input section on page 419.

■ Use the facial molding activity from the Sensory Feedback: Face and Mouth section on page 415. The process of using firm, sustained pressure for gentle facial molding enables children who use lip retraction to feel the more normal, less retracted posture. This approach to releasing facial tension is appropriate for children with high muscle tone and retraction of the upper lip.

■ Create a relaxed environment that will enable the child to use more mature feeding patterns without using effort. Discover possibilities for success that can be done in a relaxed manner. Allow the child to discover that learning and success can occur with ease.

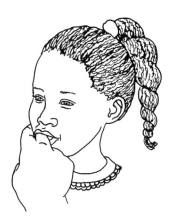

   ⊕ Emphasize ease of learning and success as part of treatment sessions for all children. Many children who have movement disorders have learned to succeed by fighting against tension to achieve a particular goal. Feeding becomes another battle to succeed. The tension that occurs when a child tries very hard to conquer lip and cheek retraction can change the original pattern to one of lip pursing. When this pattern is present, it is helpful to look at the underlying approach and the child's beliefs about trying hard.

■ After reducing hypertonicity in the neck and shoulder girdle, gently grasp the child's cheek scissor-fashion between the index and middle fingers. Use a very rapid or fine vibration or shaking of the fingers on the cheeks as the cheeks are drawn forward. Combine this movement with vocalization or singing.

▼ This rapid vibration and forward movement will reduce hypertonicity in the cheeks if it is combined with appropriate handling techniques in the rest of the body. It is appropriate when the child can accept direct stimulation to the mouth without increasing tone. It is inappropriate when tension or retraction of the cheeks is related to oral sensory defensiveness.

■ After reducing hypertonicity in the neck and shoulder girdle, place your index and middle fingers on the side of the child's nose. Slowly and evenly, vibrate downward to the bottom of the upper lip. The emphasis is on the sustained aspect of the stretch and vibration, not on simply stretching the upper lip downward. This vibratory movement and stretch to the side of the nostril provides a long-lasting relaxation of upper lip tightness for many children. As tone decreases in the cheeks and lips, the upper lip and cheeks have greater opportunity for movement.

Asymmetry

Tongue

◉ Reduce tongue asymmetry that is related to asymmetrical postural tone and movement or poor sensory awareness.

Possible Activities

■ Work with physical-handling techniques that support the child's ability to keep the head in a midline position. Gradually develop the child's ability to move the head slowly in and out of midline to integrate the asymmetrical tonic neck reflex (ATNR) so that it does not influence tone and movement when the head is turned. This approach is appropriate for children older than 6 months whose motor behavior is influenced by the ATNR.

■ Stimulate the less active side of the tongue with a toy, finger, or electric toothbrush.

■ Increase sensory input to the tongue and build sensory awareness and discrimination to a wide variety of sensations on the tongue. Include appropriate activities from Sensory Awareness: Face and Mouth on page 411 and Sensory Discrimination: Face and Mouth on page 414.

A Have the child do oral activities in which both sides of the face and mouth are doing the same thing at the same time.

    ✛ Drink through a straw and play straw drinking games.

    ✛ Use the straw activities in Sucking: Straw Drinking on page 467.

    ✛ Play blowing games. Use the blowing activities in Lip and Cheek Control: Rounding and Spreading on page 434.

A Play symmetrical facial imitation games in front of a mirror (such as making exaggerated *eeeeeee* and *oooooo* sounds) as described in the Oral Motor Imitation section on page 439.

Limited Movement

Jaw

⦿ Increase active movement of the jaw.

Possible Activities

A When limited jaw movement is due to low muscle tone, use activities to increase postural tone as described in the Change Tone: Increase Tone section on page 406 and the Decreased Tone: Jaw section on page 444.

A When limited jaw movement is due to high muscle tone, use activities to decrease postural tone as described in the Change Tone: Decrease Tone section on page 406 and the Increased Tone: Jaw section on page 443.

A Use the generalized and discriminative mouthing activities in the Combined Oral Sensorimotor Control: Mouthing section on page 441.

Tongue

⦿ Increase active movement of the tongue.

Possible Activities

A When limited tongue movement is due to low muscle tone, use activities to increase postural tone as described in the Change Tone: Increase Tone section on page 406 and the Decreased Tone: Tongue section on page 445.

A When limited tongue movement is due to high muscle tone, use activities to decrease postural tone as described in the Change Tone: Decrease Tone section on page 406 and the Increased Tone: Tongue section on page 443.

A Increase sensory input to the tongue and build sensory awareness and discrimination to a wide variety of sensations on the tongue. Include appropriate activities from Sensory Awareness: Face and Mouth on page 411 and Sensory Discrimination: Face and Mouth on page 414.

A Use foods with alerting tastes and textures during mealtimes to increase the amount of movement.

A After reducing hypertonicity in the neck and shoulder girdle, place your index finger directly on the tongue. Use a very rapid or fine vibration or shaking of your finger on the tongue. Combine this movement with vocalization or singing. This rapid vibration can reduce hypertonicity in the tongue if it is combined with appropriate handling techniques in the rest of the body. It is appropriate when the child can accept direct stimulation to the mouth without increasing tone.

A Use the generalized and discriminative mouthing activities in the Combined Oral Sensorimotor Control: Mouthing section on page 441.

A Use the vibration activities from the Sensory Awareness: Face and Mouth section on page 411.

A Use the toothbrushing activities in the Combined Oral Sensorimotor Control: Toothbrushing section on page 439.

Lips and Cheeks

⊙ Increase active movement of the lips and cheeks.

Possible Activities

🅐 When limited lip and cheek movement is due to low muscle tone, use activities to increase postural tone as described in the Change Tone: Increase Tone section on page 406 and the Decreased Tone: Lips and Cheeks section on page 445.

🅐 When limited lip and cheek movement is due to high muscle tone, use activities to decrease postural tone as described in the Change Tone: Decrease Tone section on page 406, Increased Tone: Lips and Cheeks section on page 443, and Retraction: Lips and Cheeks section on page 456.

🅐 When limited lip and cheek movement is due to lip retraction, use the activities in the Retraction: Lips and Cheeks section on page 456.

🅐 Increase sensory input and build sensory awareness and discrimination to a wide variety of sensations on the lips and cheeks. Include appropriate activities from Sensory Awareness: Face and Mouth on page 411 and Sensory Discrimination: Face and Mouth on page 414.

🅐 Use the generalized and discriminative mouthing activities in the Combined Oral Sensorimotor Control: Mouthing section on page 441.

🅐 Use the vibration activities from Sensory Awareness: Face and Mouth on page 405.

🅐 Use spoons with different bowl depths to stimulate greater lip activity during spoon feeding. Specific activities are described in Sucking: Spoon Feeding on page 463.

🅐 Use lateral placement of the spoon to stimulate greater lip activity during spoon feeding. Specific activities are described in Sucking: Spoon Feeding on page 463.

Specific Feeding Skill Issues

Sucking

Suckle Pattern

⊙ Reduce postural, sensory, and oral motor limits that interfere with the development of an efficient suckle pattern.

Possible Activities

🅰 Observe the relationship among the child's lip, cheek, jaw, and tongue movements and the limiting tone and movement patterns of the face and mouth.

🅰 Explore changes in positioning and body movement to discover ways of changing these oral-facial patterns. See Oral Control Issues: Limiting Areas on page 443 for suggestions for influencing tone and movement in the mouth. Work with the child's therapy and medical teams to determine optimum feeding positions.

🅰 When there are increases or decreases in tone and limiting movement patterns of the jaw, tongue, lips, and cheeks, work to reduce or eliminate them must precede any direct work to obtain a more advanced normal pattern. As these patterns diminish, normal movements are facilitated. This can take place within the same therapy session and may seem to occur simultaneously if the child's system is easily changeable.

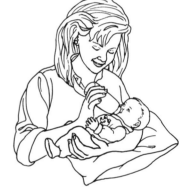

🅰 Work for a better semireclined feeding position on the lap with an infant or on a Boppy pillow with a young child. The trunk and pelvis should be in good alignment. The shoulder girdle should be forward, with abduction of the scapulae. The cervical spine (neck) should be elongated, with capital flexion (chin-tuck). Bring the infant's arms forward or toward the midline.

🅰 Position the older infant with micrognathia or tongue or jaw retraction in prone or on your lap with his arms forward across your thigh. You also may use a sidelying position. Angle the support surface of your lap so that the child's shoulders are higher than the hips. This provides better trunk (thoracic) elongation to support breathing and stops the forward flexion of the shoulders that reduces air intake. Use an angle-necked bottle so that the baby can suck in a prone position. Use your hand to steady the jaw and reduce the amount of downward movement.

▼ The child must be able to comfortably accept prone or sidelying without increasing flexor tone.

If the prone position is used, the feeder must prevent the baby's head from being hyperextended. The angled bottle makes it possible to keep the head in a more neutral position with good alignment with the neck.

🅰 Reduce confusing sensory input that can overload the child's system. The stress involved may cause a reversion to more immature or limiting movement patterns of the body and a more disorganized suckling pattern.

　　⊕ Feed the child in a quiet location away from other children, the television, and other family activities.

　　⊕ Use quiet background music or music with 60 beats per minute to create a calm feeding environment for the child and the feeder.

✤ Swaddle the infant in a cotton receiving blanket to reduce the effects of random touch and movement on the body.

✤ Dim the lights in the feeding environment.

✤ Place a baby blanket on the child's head like a hood to block out extraneous peripheral distractions.

◉ Develop a suckling pattern that is rhythmical, strong, sustained, and efficient.

Possible Activities

🅰 Rule out a neurological, respiratory, or gastrointestinal basis for the feeding difficulty.

🅰 When the child's suck lacks the rhythm and tempo of the nutritive suck, use music with a regular rhythm and tempo of 60 beats per minute. Classical music from the baroque period or a contemporary composition such as "Comfort Zone" by Steven Halpern is appropriate. For older babies, gently tap the child's lips in time with the rhythm. Move into the mouth, stroking the tongue with your finger to the same rhythm and tempo. Move your finger downward and forward. Put tastes of food on your finger to make it more interesting for the older child. Use the rhythmical reminder of touch to the lips to initiate a coordinated suckle pattern. Use this initiating rhythmical touch with drops of liquid on your finger. When the child achieves a rhythmical suck, repeat the procedure using the nipple of a bottle.

🅰 Increase the sensory information by rocking the child in a rocking chair to the rhythm and tempo of the music.

▼ If the child rejects your finger in the mouth, or if stimulation of the tongue increases retraction or disorganization, stimulate the lips only.

🅰 Provide cheek support during suckling to help the infant latch on to the nipple and organize the sucking response. Pair this with a proper chin-tuck position. This can be done with or without jaw support, as needed by the infant.

🅰 Provide an angle-necked bottle or use a short, wide bottle. This enables the infant to maintain a tucked chin during sucking. These bottles come in various styles and sizes.

🅰 Observe bottle nipple size, shape, and rate of flow to determine whether these might be factors in the steady intake of fluid.

🅰 A medicine-pacifier, such as the Numi-Med™, can be used to control liquid flow. This special orthodontic pacifier has a small, hollow container in the handle that can hold liquid. The pacifier end has a small hole to allow the infant to suckle the liquid into the mouth. Use an identical orthodontic pacifier without the hole and attachment. When the infant has a skilled nonnutritive suck on the pacifier, place a small amount of milk or formula into the medicine-pacifier container. Allow the infant to suck the liquid. See Chapter 29 for a list of resources for specialty feeding equipment.

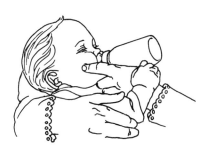
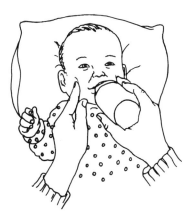

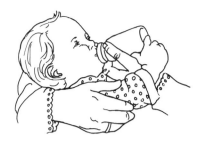

🅰 Help the child to achieve and maintain the tongue in the mouth by placing your hand on her jaw. To reduce forward movement of the base of the tongue, place your finger directly under the child's chin and apply gentle, sustained pressure.

▼ Direct assistance with maintaining the tongue in the mouth can be effective after limiting patterns are reduced through handling and positioning. Do not use oral control procedures when the thrusting pattern is strong and the child must use force to contain the tongue in the mouth. These procedures also are inappropriate when tongue protrusion is a compensation for respiratory distress.

🅰 Use drops of liquid on your finger or on a cotton swab to tap and stroke the lips outward and with a circular motion to initiate the suckle from the lips. As the suckle becomes easily initiated from the lips, place a spoon or medicine cup on the lower lip. Encourage the child to suckle the liquid from the spoon or cup. Facilitating a suckle or sucking pattern from the lips works well when the child's suckling becomes disorganized from touch to the tongue. Because the nipple provides this type of touch, the child may move directly to a cup, bypassing the bottle or breast. Initiating the suck from the lips enables the child to regulate the amount of liquid or food taken into the mouth at one time.

🅰 Contact a lactation specialist for support in breast-feeding techniques.

🅰 Some women who wish to breast-feed and have worked with a lactation consultant to refine the breast-feeding process still may have difficulty because of the infant's inability to initiate and sustain a strong sucking pattern. For some of these situations, a supplemental nursing device such as Medela's Supplementary Nursing System™ or Lact-Aid International's Lact-Aid™ can be used.

 ✛ This type of supplemental nursing device uses a small tube attached to a bag or plastic container, which the mother hangs around her neck. The container is filled with expressed breast milk. The free end of the tube is taped to the mother's breast and extends about ¼-inch beyond the nipple. The milk provides an initiating flow of milk as the infant moves the mouth to nurse. This enables the baby to receive breast milk simultaneously through the breast and the supplemental device. Many infants with sucking difficulties who are nursed without the assistive device will stop sucking or suck inefficiently when they are not rewarded with milk for their efforts. The supplemental nursing system provides an easy, slow source of milk that can help the infant become more organized and use less effort while learning to suck.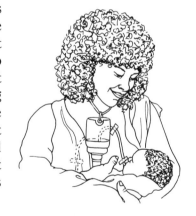

Transition From Suckling to Sucking

◉ Reduce postural, sensory, and oral motor limits that interfere with the transition from a suckling to a sucking pattern.

Possible Activities

🅰 Observe the relationship among the child's lip, cheek, jaw, and tongue movements and the limiting tone and movement patterns of the face and mouth.

🅰 Explore changes in positioning and body movement to discover ways of changing these oral-facial patterns. See Oral Control Issues: Limiting Areas on page 443 for suggestions for influencing tone and movement in the mouth. Work with the child's therapy treatment and medical teams to determine optimum feeding positions.

▲ When there are increases or decreases in tone and limiting movement patterns of the jaw, tongue, lips, and cheeks, work to reduce or eliminate them must precede any direct work to obtain a more advanced normal pattern. As these patterns diminish, normal movements are facilitated. This can take place within the same therapy session and may seem to occur simultaneously if the child's system is easily changeable.

◉ Develop a sucking pattern that has a more predominant up-down movement pattern and a reduced backward-forward movement pattern of the tongue.

Possible Activities

▲ Use music with a regular rhythm and a tempo of 60 beats per minute (e.g., classical music from the baroque period, a contemporary composition such as *Comfort Zone* by Steven Halpern). Tap the tongue with your finger to the rhythm and tempo of the music. Move your finger upward and downward. This is the direction you want to teach the tongue to move as it learns the pattern for the suck. This also can be done with food on your finger while you are feeding the child.

▼ This approach is inappropriate if the child rejects your finger in the mouth or if stimulation of the tongue causes retraction or thrusting.

▲ Develop greater normal activity in the cheeks and upper lip during sucking and swallowing. It is easier to begin teaching this activity using a spoon and pureed or blenderized foods rather than liquids from a bottle or cup. This approach is appropriate for the child who shows poor control of the lips and cheeks, with either low tone and relative inactivity or high tone and lip retraction. Developing a better seal improves the child's ability to create greater intraoral pressure in the mouth. This is required for the up-down sucking pattern.

▲ Give the child a drink from a cup containing a thick liquid such as pureed or blenderized pears or peaches. A clear cup with a wide mouth, a medicine cup, or a cutout cup works well. Provide jaw and cheek support as needed. Gently rest the cup on the lower lip. Tip it so the liquid moves slowly toward the mouth as the child begins a suckle-swallow pattern. Position the cup and provide jaw support so the tongue does not come out of the mouth. The thickened drink provides strong proprioceptive and tactile feedback. When combined with jaw and cheek support, a more mature up-down sucking pattern often will emerge. It is important for the sucking pattern to be initiated from the lips rather than from the tongue. This approach is appropriate for the child who shows beginning control of the lips and cheeks and a consistent suckle pattern of the tongue.

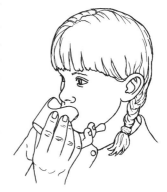

Spoon Feeding

◉ Reduce postural, sensory, and oral motor limits that interfere with the development of efficient spoon feeding of soft smooth foods.

Possible Activities

▲ Observe the relationship among the child's lip, cheek, jaw, and tongue movements and the limiting tone and movement patterns of the face and mouth.

▲ Explore changes in positioning and body movement to discover ways of changing these oral-facial patterns. See Oral Control Issues: Limiting Areas on page 443 for suggestions for influencing tone and movement in the mouth. Work with the child's therapy and medical teams to determine optimum feeding positions.

▲ When there are increases or decreases in tone and limiting movement patterns of the jaw, tongue, lips, and cheeks, work to reduce or eliminate them must precede any direct work to obtain a more advanced normal pattern. As these patterns diminish, the normal movements are facilitated. This can take place within the same therapy session and may seem to occur simultaneously if the child's system is easily changeable.

🅰 Use the facial molding activity in the Sensory Feedback: Face and Mouth section on page 415.

◉ Develop an organized rhythmical pattern of suckling or sucking in removing soft smooth foods from the spoon.

Possible Activities

🅰 Select a spoon whose depth and sensory properties fit the child's skill level.

🅰 Present the spoon from within the child's vision and at the level of the lower lip. A spoon presented at too high a level will cause the child to lift the head into capital extension and can bias the jaw toward opening and the tongue toward extension.

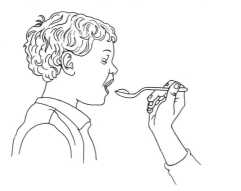 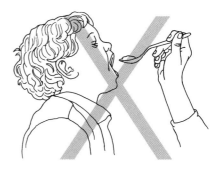

🅰 Stimulate an active suckle or sucking movement of the lips and tongue through sucking on a finger, nipple, or pacifier, or by stroking the child's lips. Place the spoon and food in the mouth during the active sucking movement.

◉ Develop a mature pattern of removing soft smooth foods from the spoon that includes upper lip movement to remove food from the spoon and drawing in of the lower lip for cleaning by the upper incisors.

Possible Activities

🅰 Pause with the spoon at the lips or on the tongue so that the child has time to close the lips around the spoon for food removal. Too rapid a removal of the spoon allows the child to depend on the feeder to scrape the food on the upper lip to get the food in the mouth.

🅰 Develop the child's ability to quiet the jaw and tongue as the spoon enters the mouth. Precise mobility of the lips requires stability and quieting of the other parts of the system. This step should be taught initially to any child who has not developed jaw stability in an open position.

🅰 Using assistance with jaw control, help the child develop the concept that the mouth can be quiet and ready before the spoon enters. Initial work with this concept can be done with the mouth closed if this is easier for the child. Work for a maintained open-mouth position and a quiet tongue as the child observes the spoon.

   ✛ If it is difficult for the child to keep the mouth quiet as food approaches, begin the activity by touching the child's mouth with a toy, then moving the toy away. Continue until the child can remain completely quiet during the activity.

   ✛ Use a tongue depressor, cotton swab, or other spoonlike object for the touch-and-go activity.

   ✛ Use an empty spoon. Ask the child to look at the spoon and stay very quiet. Show the child that there is no food on the spoon. Use pretend activities to imagine the kind of food on the spoon or smelling it.

- ✛ Tell the child, "Now there is food on the spoon, but it is not time to eat it. This is a time to practice keeping the mouth quiet and ready." Repeat the activity of bringing a filled spoon to the mouth, touching the lips, and moving away.
- ✛ Tell the child, "I will bring the food to your mouth while it is quiet and ready. When I touch your lips, you may eat the food."

🄰 Present the spoon laterally instead of directly placing it straight into the mouth and on the tongue. Rest it gently on the lower lip, with the spoon bowl resting on the lip corners. The contact with the lip corners provides extra stability for the upper central lip to be more active in food removal. Pause with the spoon in this position to enable the child to use the upper lip to remove the food from the spoon. If needed, you can gently tip the outside edge of the spoon upward to encourage the upper lip to actively come down to remove the food. This sideways presentation enables the child to use the lips to remove the food and begin the easy suck-swallow process. It also helps keep the tongue in the mouth. A flat-bowled spoon (e.g., Maroon™ spoon) works well for this activity.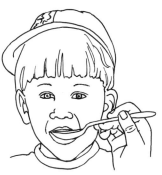

🄰 Use spoons with different bowl depths to stimulate greater lip activity during spoon feeding.
- ✛ Food removal from the spoon provides the opportunity to use upper lip to clean the spoon. Different spoons have different spoon bowl depths. Deeper bowls require more upper lip activity and more shallow bowls require less upper lip activity during food removal.
- ✛ Use different sizes and shapes of spoons when presenting spooned foods. This challenges the central upper lip to become more and more active as it has to reach into the spoon bowl for the food.
- ✛ Different food provides varying degrees of resistance during food removal. Liquids require little effort as they can be poured into the mouth. Often, yogurt or pudding are favorite foods and work well with this task because of their smoothness and limited resistance. Honey, jam, and peanut butter provide strong resistance, challenging the upper lip to maximum work.
- ✛ Sometimes the lips need a little alerting to find the depth of the spoon bowl. Put a sticky substance such as a thin coating of jam on the spoon. Sprinkle crumbs on the substance. The crumbs can **wake up** the lip to more actively search for the bottom of the spoon bowl.
- ✛ Play with the different texture combinations. For example, the child first may be able to remove smooth pudding, then pudding with crumbs, then jam, and finally peanut butter. Or, a child may move through the progression with one food, such as pudding, but with increasing challenges in spoon depth.

🄰 Use the spoon to create gentle downward pressure on the tongue as you enter the mouth. This stimulation often activates a downward movement of the upper lip. This technique is effective only after the child has developed some ability to stabilize the jaw and quiet the tongue as the spoon enters the mouth. This approach often is effective for a child who has limited movement because of low tone.

▼ This activity is not appropriate when the stimulation triggers increased sensory distress or limiting patterns such as jaw or tongue retraction or thrusting.

🄰 Feed the child with a slight degree of sloppiness, allowing extra food to get on the lower lip. Call the child's attention to the remaining food. This can be done verbally, with a mirror, or by touching the lip. Move the lower lip under the upper teeth and help the child remove the food. This technique is effective only after the child has developed some ability to stabilize the jaw and quiet the tongue as the spoon enters the mouth.

▼ This activity is not appropriate when the stimulation of the extra food triggers increased sensory distress or limiting patterns such as jaw or tongue retraction or thrusting.

⊙ Reduce postural, sensory, and oral motor limits that interfere with the development of efficient cup drinking.

Possible Activities

🅰 Observe the relationship among the child's lip, cheek, jaw, and tongue movements and the limiting tone and movement patterns of the face and mouth.

🅰 Explore changes in positioning and body movement to discover ways of changing these oral-facial patterns. See Oral Control Issues: Limiting Areas on page 443 for suggestions for influencing tone and movement in the mouth. Work with the child's therapy and medical teams to determine optimum feeding positions.

🅰 When there are increases or decreases in tone and limiting movement patterns of the jaw, tongue, lips, and cheeks, work to reduce or eliminate them must precede any direct work to obtain a more advanced normal pattern. As these patterns diminish, normal movements are facilitated. This can take place within the same therapy session and may seem to occur simultaneously if the child's system is easily changeable.

⊙ Develop an organized rhythmical pattern of sucking and swallowing when drinking liquids from a cup.

Possible Activities

🅰 Using a thickened liquid greatly facilitates the learning of cup-drinking skills. The child receives more sensory information from the thicker liquid, and it does not run into and around the mouth as quickly as thin liquids. A thicker liquid also is easier for the feeder to control. Use a liquid the child likes. Strained fruits or vegetables mixed with a small amount of liquid can be used for cup drinking with an infant who is familiar with the foods and likes them. Older infants and children will enjoy milk shakes, blended smoothies, applesauce diluted with other liquids, gazpacho, or blenderized fruits and vegetables.

🅰 Identify a cup that works well for the child and the feeder. Cutout cups and those with a wide or flared shape enable the feeder to see the liquid as it approaches the child's mouth. This makes it easier for the feeder to see the liquid and adjust the flow rate as she tips the cup to the child's lips. Some cups have lids that control the flow for the child, but still allow the child to feel the lip of the cup.

🅰 Maintain constant contact of the cup and lower lip. Tip the cup up for drinking and down for pauses rather than taking it away from the child's mouth. Use a constant, predictable rhythm to help the child organize the drink-pause sequence. This approach is essential when the child becomes disorganized with the intermittent contact of a cup or spoon. When hypersensitivity is present, the repeated on-off nature of the cup-lip contact can trigger repeated restrictive and aversive reactions. The sustained tactile contact helps the child organize the drinking sequence.

⊙ Develop a quiet, stabilized jaw position when drinking liquids from a cup.

Possible Activities

🅰 Place your hand on the child's jaw to help him achieve and maintain a stable degree of jaw opening and closing during drinking. This helps the child experience a sensation of greater stability and the knowledge of what drinking without up-down jaw movement can be like. Using assistance with oral control, you can help the child develop the concept

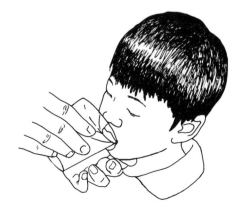

that the mouth can be quiet and ready as the cup approaches. Work with this concept is done with the mouth closed. The same progression that was outlined for obtaining quiet stability of the jaw and tongue during spoon feeding can be introduced with the cup. The goal is to enable the child to begin drinking from a quiet, neutral position of the mouth. This step is essential in the initial stage of cup drinking. Use assisted oral control as described in the Jaw Control: Jaw Opening and Closing section on page 430 and the Sucking: Spoon Feeding section on page 463.

A Help the child develop greater jaw stability in the opening and closing positions, as well as improved sensory awareness and feedback of jaw position and movement. These include the following options.

  ⊕ Use the generalized and discriminative mouthing activities in the Mouthing section on page 441.

  ⊕ Use the activities for sustaining graded jaw closure on a toy or feeding utensil and developing oral exploration described in Jaw Control: Jaw Stability in a Closed Position on page 432.

  ⊕ Use the snack cap described in Sensory Feedback: Face and Mouth on page 415.

  ⊕ Use activities that increase the graded control of jaw movement when biting through foods that offer different degrees of resistance. See Jaw Control: Graded Jaw Movements on page 432.

A Encourage the child use her teeth to hold on to the edge of the glass or cup while drinking. This uses a normal strategy in the developmental sequence of acquiring jaw stability during drinking.

  ⊕ Tell the child, "I will hold the bottom of the glass with my hand, and you can hold the top of the glass with your teeth." This emphasis on partnership and the suggestion that the child can be a partial self-feeder encourages cooperation and is rewarding to many children.

  ⊕ While the child holds an empty glass or cup between the teeth, pour in a small amount of liquid. Help the child tip the cup to get the liquid while continuing to hold the cup. If you use a small amount of water or juice, the child receives excellent feedback from letting go, and the amount of spilling is inconsequential.

▼ Do not use this activity if the child has a tonic bite reflex or an opening avoidance response when the teeth are stimulated.

Straw Drinking

◉ Reduce postural, sensory, and oral motor limits that interfere with the development of efficient straw drinking.

Possible Activities

A Observe the relationship among the child's lip, cheek, jaw, and tongue movements and the limiting tone and movement patterns of the face and mouth.

A Explore changes in positioning and body movement to discover ways of changing these oral-facial patterns. See Oral Control Issues: Limiting Areas on page 443 for suggestions for influencing tone and movement in the mouth. Work with the child's therapy and medical teams to determine optimum feeding positions.

A When there are increases or decreases in tone and limiting movement patterns of the jaw, tongue, lips, and cheeks, work to reduce or eliminate them must precede any direct work to obtain a more advanced normal pattern. As these patterns diminish, normal movements are facilitated. This can take place within the same therapy session and may seem to occur simultaneously if the child's system is easily changeable.

⊙ Use physical and sensory adaptations to teach straw drinking skills.

Possible Activities

🄰 Teach the child to drink from a straw. This provides a symmetrical oral activity that helps the child mature his oral skills for liquid intake. It provides an alternative to bottle drinking for toddlers and young children. It seems to have an organizing quality as an activity. It can increase movement and control of the upper lip.

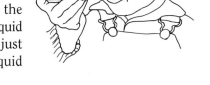

   ✛ Many children learn to drink from a straw just by having it placed in the mouth. A variation of the natural sucking pattern infants use with bottles is adapted for straw drinking with the slightly protruding tongue cupping the straw and the use of an up-down sucking action.

   ✛ Some children need a little more help. Put a straw in a glass of liquid. Put your finger over the top end of the straw, keeping the liquid in the straw. With the straw slightly greater that horizontal, put the straw to the child's lips. As the child closes her mouth around the straw, take your finger off the straw end and let the liquid move into the mouth. Gradually move the straw to just below horizontal to enable the child to suck the liquid through the straw.

   ✛ Gently squeeze a juice box; soft, plastic bottle; or sports bottle to bring the liquid up the straw to the child's mouth.

🄰 See Chapter 19 for an in-depth discussion on teaching straw drinking, using adapted equipment and procedures.

⊙ Expand straw drinking skills through games that reinforce basic oral motor skills used with the straw.

Possible Activities

🄰 Have the child suck different thicknesses of liquids and purees and puddings from a straw. Consistencies from water to juice to applesauce, pudding, and yogurt can be pulled up through a straw, requiring varying degrees of effort.

🄰 Have the child drink from short straws, long straws, wide straws, and narrow straws. Use colored straws, straight straws, and crazy bent straws.

🄰 Have the child suck from the straws from different positions on the lips: the center, side, and in between.

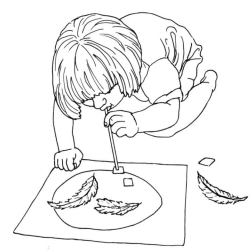

🄰 Have the child suck a piece of paper up to a straw and carry it to a designated place and then let it go. The pieces of paper can be fun shapes such as hearts for Valentine's Day, flowers for a bouquet picture, or animals for a farm theme. At first, have the child suck the shape to the straw and carry it a short distance to put it on the page. As the child's skills and ability to maintain the suction for longer times increases, move the page farther from the pile of shapes so the child must maintain the suction longer.

Swallowing

⊙ Reduce postural, sensory, and oral motor limits that interfere with the development of safe and efficient swallowing.

Possible Activities

🅰 Observe the relationship among the child's lip, cheek, jaw, and tongue movements and the limiting tone and movement patterns of the face and mouth.

🅰 Explore changes in positioning and body movement to discover ways of changing these patterns for better bolus formation and swallowing. See Oral Control Issues: Limiting Areas on page 443 for suggestions for influencing tone and movement in the mouth. Work with the child's therapy treatment and medical teams to determine optimum feeding positions.

🅰 When there are increases or decreases in tone and limiting movement patterns of the jaw, tongue, lips, and cheeks, work to reduce or eliminate them must precede any direct work to obtain a more advanced normal pattern. As these patterns diminish, normal movements are facilitated. This can take place within the same therapy session and may seem to occur simultaneously if the child's system is easily changeable.

Safe and Efficient Suckle-Swallow

⊙ Identify the presence or absence of a swallowing reflex and of risk factors for aspiration.

Possible Activities

🅰 It is critical to determine whether a swallowing reflex is present before food and liquid are used in the child's program. If the swallowing reflex is absent, food and liquid are inappropriate. See Chapter 23 for a discussion of treatment priorities for children who are fed by tube and suggestions for a total program of oral motor treatment.

✥ Using a straw or other pipette, place small drops of water on the back of the child's tongue. Observe for signs of swallowing.

✥ Notice whether the child can control saliva and use a spontaneous swallowing pattern.

✥ Feel for the elevation of the larynx-hyoid complex in the neck and elevation of the root or base of the tongue.

✥ Notice whether the child coughs and chokes when fed.

✥ Review the child's records. A history of recurrent pneumonias may be related to repeated aspiration.

🅰 You may consider videofluoroscopy to determine the timing and components of the swallowing response during a modified barium swallow procedure. This provides more information on which to base the treatment program. See Chapter 8 for an in-depth discussion of videofluoroscopic swallowing studies and strategies for preparing the child for the evaluation.

⊙ Develop a safe and efficient suckle-swallow.

Possible Activities

🅰 Work to increase the strength, duration, and timing of the suckle pattern that often results in the triggering of an appropriate swallow. Use activities for developing a normal suckle pattern as described in the Sucking: Suckle Pattern section on page 460.

🅰 Cold liquids or purees can be used therapeutically to try to stimulate a faster and more organized swallow. With some children, you can apply cold stimulation to the anterior fauceal arches in the back of the mouth. Stimulating this area with an object at a very cold temperature can increase responsiveness of the area that is activated by the intent to swallow. There are many ways to provide cold to this area. Some tools you can use include:

- Chilled liquid or pureed food.
- A very small laryngeal mirror dipped in ice water. The glass portion of the mirror should be removed or dipped in latex if the child has a tonic bite reflex.
- Cotton swabs dipped in water and frozen.
- An ice stick created by freezing water in a plastic straw. Before using, run the straw under warm water to loosen the ice. Push out an inch of ice. Keep the remainder within the straw to prevent it from breaking off in the mouth and to create a handle.
- Small amounts of lemon or grapefruit sherbet on a cotton swab or small spoon. The combination of the cold temperature and sour taste often provide an excellent stimulus for swallowing.
- Because the cold stimulus prepares the area for a more rapid swallow, have small amounts of liquid or soft food available immediately. Observe for elevation of the larynx and hyoid bone that indicate a swallow has occurred.
- Repeat the cold application for 10 to 15 minutes three or four times a day when the child will accept this activity.
- For this approach to be effective, the child must be able to hold the mouth open while the stimulation is applied. Present the activity as a game or explain why the activity is important.

▼ Good preparation is essential if you decide to explore this option. Include cold touch to the back of the mouth as part of a touching activity that prepares the child for touch in other parts of the mouth. Cold presented to the fauceal area without preparation might startle the child, causing the throat to be jabbed or the palate to be punctured by a tool.

These techniques may not be helpful and could be dangerous with children who have severe hypertonicity and hypersensitivity of the body and mouth, a strong tonic bite reflex, or severe problems of sensory defensiveness or sensory overload. It is critical to evaluate the child's total response and prepare carefully for this activity.

🅐 Determine whether the child swallows thin or thickened liquids most safely. Sometimes this information can be observed clinically. Sometimes a videofluoroscopic swallow study is necessary. Often, the thickened liquids are heavier and slower, and therefore easier to organize before and during swallowing. However, children who can swallow their saliva without choking or drooling already are swallowing small amounts of a thin liquid. They may do better with thinner liquids.

🅐 Use pushing activities to increase the amount of laryngeal closure. Have the child push against a wall or against your hands while you provide slight resistance; or have the child lift the buttocks while pushing the hands down against the seat of a chair. Where possible, these activities can be done as the child produces a sound. Any activity that increases the volume and sustained control of the voice simultaneously improves the strength and control of the vocal folds for closure during swallowing. Use this technique only when active pushing does not create hypertonicity and limiting movement patterns in the body. Because active cooperation is required, the child must be able to imitate or follow instructions.

🅐 If swallowing activities are included in the program for a child who has a tracheostomy, place your finger over the tracheostomy when the child swallows. This improves the pressure for swallowing and reduces the possibility of aspiration. If the child depends on the tracheostomy for taking in air, be sure to remove your finger after the swallow. A speaking valve is extremely helpful when vocalization and swallowing work are part of the program. A valve cap covers the end of the tracheostomy tube. It opens during inspiration, but remains closed the rest of the time. If the child uses a cuffed tracheostomy, it should be deflated during swallowing activities.

Some people suggest adding a blue food coloring to the liquid or puree to enable the parent or clinician to see if there is leakage through the tracheostomy, which might indicate penetration of food into the airway during the swallow.

▼ Consult medical personnel to determine the appropriateness of oral feeding and precautions or contraindications for a child with a tracheostomy.

△ Use a pacifier modification such as the medicine-pacifier (e.g., Numi-Med™) to help control liquid flow. Incorporate activities for using a medicine-pacifier as described in the Sucking: Suckle Pattern section on page 460.

△ Let the child practice holding a small plastic medicine dropper between the side teeth or gums.

    ⊕ Gradually draw a few drops of water or a thin or thickened liquid into the dropper. Slowly squeeze the liquid into the child's mouth. The jaw stabilization provided by biting and holding the dropper reduces oral disorganization for some children, resulting in a more efficient suck and swallow.

Mature Swallow

◎ Increase the ability to swallow, using tongue-tip elevation with food and liquid.

Possible Activities

△ Introduce activities that will help the child develop jaw stability in the open position when the spoon or a cookie is presented and stability in the closed position during biting. Incorporate the activities in the Jaw Control: Jaw Stability in an Open Position section on page 431 and Jaw Control: Jaw Stability in a Closed Position section on page 432.

△ Help the child organize liquids or purees presented by bottle, spoon, or cup into an efficient bolus before swallowing. Include appropriate strategies and activities from the following sections: Transition From Suckling to Sucking on page 462, Spoon Feeding on page 463, and Cup Drinking on page 466.

△ Place your hand on the child's jaw to help him achieve and maintain the jaw closed with the tongue in the mouth. Use assisted oral control as described in Jaw Control: Jaw Opening and Closing on page 430. To reduce forward movement on the base of the tongue, place your finger directly under the child's chin and apply firm pressure.

△ Use a cotton swab or finger to touch sequentially the tip of the tongue and a spot on the hard palate just behind the central incisors to remind the child where the elevated tongue should contact. Repeat this paired contact and remind the child to swallow.

△ Provide oral and sensory support to help the child use tongue-tip elevation while swallowing liquids and foods. Elevation of the tongue in contact with the palate provides stability for the wave-like tongue movement needed to move the bolus from the mouth to the pharynx for swallowing.

    ⊕ Support the child in closing the jaw during swallowing. Closing the mouth puts the tongue in proximity with the palate.

    ⊕ Help the child close the lips during swallowing. Closing the mouth area allows for the intra-oral pressure changes needed for efficient bolus movement during swallowing.

    ⊕ Thickening the liquids is sometimes all that is necessary to provide additional weight, viscosity, and proprioceptive pressure to activate the tongue toward elevation.

△ Press tongue with an up-down action with a NUK Massage Brush, InfaDent™ finger toothbrush, or small child's toothbrush. Maintain contact with the tongue. As the child has collected saliva, remove the brush while touching the top of the palate where the tongue should be placed during tongue-tip elevation. This activity seems to wake up the tongue and point out where you want it to be placed.

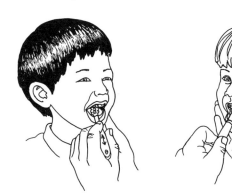

◪ Vary the use of these massage toothbrushes by dipping them in pureed food or crumbs. As you remove them, the tastes stimulate tongue activity.

◪ Encourage the child to use her teeth to hold onto the edge of the glass while drinking. This uses a normal strategy in the developmental sequence of acquiring jaw stability during drinking. Do not use this technique if the child also shows a tonic bite reflex or an opening avoidance response when the teeth are stimulated.

◪ Build proprioceptive awareness and control of the midranges of jaw control. Use the snack cap described in Sensory Feedback: Face and Mouth on page 415.

Saliva Control—Drooling

◉ Increase swallowing coordination to reduce the amount and frequency of drooling.

Possible Activities

◪ Work for improvements in head and trunk control. This may be very subtle if the child's physical impairments are minimal. Head control provides the basis for developing oral control for swallowing and control of drooling. Work with head and trunk control is appropriate to consider for every child who drools, but critical for children who have pronounced disabilities with physical control of the body.

◪ Work for improvements in sensory awareness on the face and within the mouth. It is important for children to develop an awareness of pressure cues in the mouth and wetness and dryness cues on the face. Children who drool so that the face is always wet need to experience the contrast with dryness that would make them want to swallow. These ideas are appropriate for children who do not monitor their own swallowing and seem to be unaware that the face is wet.

⊕ Increase general sensory awareness and discrimination by varying temperature, taste, pressure, and texture of food and objects in the mouth. Help the child play with a small, battery-operated, hand vibrator around the face to build sensory awareness.

⊕ Build an awareness of the language concepts *wet* and *dry*. Explore these concepts in games and activities with all parts of the body. Help the child discover what can make the face wet and dry. Play with the different perceptions of a hair dryer blowing air on a wet body part and a dry body part.

⊕ In all activities, emphasize the sense of discovery. Minimize negative associations with a wet face and the command for the child to swallow and keep a dry face.

⊕ Play *waking up the face* games with wiping, brushing, and tapping the face. Include these stimuli before starting activities that require specific awareness and perception.

⊕ Use the vibration activities described in Sensory Awareness: Face and Mouth on page 411.

⊕ Use the generalized and discriminative mouthing activities described in the Combined Oral Sensorimotor Control: Mouthing section on page 441.

⊕ Use the snack cap described in Sensory Feedback: Face and Mouth on page 415.

■ Work for improvements in jaw, lip, and cheek control. Activities that reduce jaw thrusting, a passive open mouth, and inactive or retracted lips and cheeks provide the child with greater opportunities to swallow and control drooling. Drooling is a function of infrequent swallowing and inadequate oral movement during the swallow. The quality of movement during the swallow is the most important factor. Use a mirror or other visual or nonverbal auditory feedback to let the child know as soon as loss of saliva occurs. With awareness comes the option to swallow and control drooling.

   ✛ Incorporate activities described in Jaw Control: Jaw Stability in an Open Position on page 431 and Jaw Control: Jaw Stability in a Closed Position on page 432.

   ✛ Use the oral exploration activities in the Jaw Control: Graded Jaw Movements on page 432 and Combined Oral Sensorimotor Control: Oral Exploration section on page 442.

   ✛ Use activities that increase the graded control of jaw movement when biting through foods that offer different degrees of resistance. See Jaw Control: Graded Jaw Movements on page 432.

   ✛ Incorporate activities that pair more mature jaw closure with other movements of the whole body as described in Jaw Control: Graded Jaw Movements on page 432.

   ✛ Have the child drink through a straw and play straw drinking games. Provide adaptations for securing better lip closure and tongue position. Use the straw activities in Sucking: Straw Drinking on page 467.

   ✛ Use blowing activities to improve the child's movement coordination of the face with breathing as described in theLip and Cheek Control section on page 434.

   ✛ Incorporate activities that increase motor-planning skills in the face and mouth as described in the Oral Motor Imitation section on page 439.

■ Obtain medical consultation for any child whose open mouth posture is related to congestion and frequent upper respiratory infections. Although decongestants may reduce the nasal stoppage, side effects can be more negative than the original symptoms. You also can use diet, food supplements, vitamin and mineral supplements, and other approaches to increase the child's general level of wellness.

■ When you place the emphasis on dryness, you focus attention on the end goal and its potential value for the child. Often, when a child drools, we emphasize the negative aspects of drooling and the inconvenience it causes. However, in the daily management of drooling, very little attention should be directed to the drooling itself or to the child's wetness. The child can receive quiet, warm recognition when the face is dry rather than comments or criticism when everything is wet.

■ Once dryness has become recognizable and desirable, the child can be given the responsibility for maintaining a dry face. Various alternatives include voluntary swallowing or using a handkerchief or terry cloth wristband.

Coordination of Sucking, Swallowing, and Breathing

   ◎ Reduce postural, sensory, and oral motor limits that interfere with the development of the coordination of sucking, swallowing, and breathing.

Possible Activities

■ Observe the relationship among the child's lip, cheek, jaw, and tongue movements and the limiting tone and movement patterns of the face and mouth.

■ Explore changes in positioning and body movement to discover ways of changing these oral-facial patterns. See Oral Control Issues: Limiting Areas on page 443 for suggestions for influencing tone and movement in the mouth.

■ When there are increases or decreases in tone and limiting movement patterns of the jaw, tongue, lips, and cheeks, work to reduce or eliminate them must precede any direct work to obtain a more advanced normal pattern. As these patterns diminish, the normal movements are facilitated. This can take place within the same therapy session and may seem to occur simultaneously if the child's system is easily changeable.

Bottle-Feeding or Breast-Feeding

◉ Develop a well-coordinated suck-swallow-breathe pattern during bottle-feeding or breast-feeding.

Possible Activities

🅰 Select a position for bottle-feeding or breast-feeding that reduces stress on the respiratory system. Often, sidelying or prone over the lap will create a better opportunity for chest expansion and reduce shoulder girdle protraction, retraction, and elevation that interfere with efficient breathing. Often, gravity will cause the tongue and jaw to drop into a more forward position, enlarging the pharyngeal airway. Gently place your hand under the child's jaw, using a slight traction forward to further expand the airway.

🅰 Explore the timing the baby requires for breathing and feeding. Allow the infant to suck briefly. Notice any changes in muscle tone or movement patterns during nursing that might indicate the baby is stressed for air. When you see these signals, remove the nipple or lower the bottle to slow the liquid flow. Allow the child time to breathe. Notice whether the need to breathe occurs in any predictable pattern or interval. Find the infant's personal rhythm of breathing and sucking. Support this rhythm by removing the nipple at specific intervals.

🅰 Observe the child's respiratory patterns at rest and with activity. Notice rapid, irregular breathing patterns. Notice any tendency to hold the breath and suddenly gasp air. These behaviors can interfere with the coordination of feeding and breathing. Explore ways to influence the type, depth, regularity, and rate of breathing. This can include the use of quiet calming music or Hemi-Sync Metamusic to slow down and regularize the breathing pattern. See Chapter 13 for a discussion on the use of music in feeding programs.

Cup Drinking

◉ Develop a well-coordinated suck-swallow-breathe pattern during cup drinking.

Possible Activities

🅰 Using a thickened liquid during cup drinking greatly facilitates the learning of a coordinated feeding and breathing pattern. The child receives more sensory information from the thicker liquid, which does not run into and around the mouth as quickly as thin liquids. A thicker liquid also is easier for the feeder to control, placing less stress on the child and feeder.

🅰 Select a cup that enables the feeder or child to control the flow of liquid easily. A cutout cup or clear plastic cup enables the feeder to see the liquid as it approaches the child's lips. Children who are learning to hold the cup and give themselves a drink usually need a cup with a lid. For some children, the cup may include a spout. Other children drink more easily from a cup that has small holes in a depressed lid. With some cups, it is possible to alter the rate and amount of liquid flow by varying the number of holes through which the liquid flows.

🅰 Some children need more stability in the upper trunk and shoulder girdle as they attempt to bring the cup to the mouth independently. Provide a surface on which the child can lean (e.g., table, wheelchair tray). As the child leans on her elbows, her control of cup-to-mouth movements may improve. This increases the predictability of liquid flow into the mouth, making it easier for the child to coordinate sucking and swallowing with breathing.

🅰 Help the child develop signals to indicate readiness to begin drinking and the need to stop. The child can look into the cup to signal the feeder to tip the cup up for drinking and look up from the cup to signal the feeder to tip the cup down. See Chapter 13 for a discussion of communication signals at mealtimes.

A Observe the child's respiratory patterns at rest and with activity. Does the child have rapid, irregular breathing patterns? Notice any tendency toward holding the breath and sudden gasping of air. Explore ways of influencing the type, depth, regularity, and rate of breathing. These can include:

⊹ Consistently following the child's cues and waiting for permission to start the flow of liquid into the mouth establishes an environment of trust for the presentation of liquid from the cup. This enables the child to relax and improve the timing and coordination of drinking.

⊹ Calming music to slow the breathing rate.

⊹ Hemi-Sync Metamusic to slow down and regularize the breathing pattern.

⊹ Blowing activities to develop greater control of inspiration and expiration. Incorporate activities for blowing as described in the Lip and Cheek Control section on page 434.

⊹ Singing and extended vocalization to develop greater control of respiratory-phonatory patterns.

A Establish a rhythm of drinking and stopping when choking occurs during cup drinking. Observe how many sucks and swallows the child can take before coughing and choking. Tip the cup down before the child takes too much liquid. For example, if the child runs out of air and breathes in air and liquid after three or four sucks, tip the cup down after every two sucks. Set up a clear rhythm to teach a new pattern of drinking and breathing. Gradually increase the number of sucks that the child can take without choking.

A Help the child develop the ability to stop and start drinking on command. Give the older child cues of *go* and ***stop***. This can encourage the child to develop the internal controls for stopping to breathe before running out of breath. Gradually fade out the verbal reminders and encourage the child to stop to breathe regularly.

Biting

◉ Reduce postural, sensory, and oral motor limits that interfere with the development of biting.

Possible Activities

A Observe the relationship among the child's lip, cheek, jaw, and tongue movements and the limiting tone and movement patterns of the face and mouth. See Oral Control Issues: Limiting Areas on page 443 for suggestions for influencing tone and movement in the mouth.

A Explore changes in positioning and body movement to discover ways of reducing tonic and stabilizing bite patterns. Use activities to decrease postural tone as described in Change Tone: Decrease Tone on page 406 and activities to obtain greater postural alignment as described in Postural Alignment: Head, Neck, and Trunk Alignment on page 402.

A When there are increases or decreases in tone and limiting movement patterns of the jaw, tongue, lips, and cheeks, work to reduce or eliminate them must precede any direct work to obtain a more advanced normal pattern. As these patterns diminish, the normal movements are facilitated. This can take place within the same therapy session and may seem to occur simultaneously if the child's system is easily changeable.

Controlled Bite

⊙ Increase the child's ability to use a controlled bite with foods that provide different amounts of resistance.

Possible Activities

🅰 Reduce environmental sensory input that can overload the child's system, resulting in a reversion to limiting or more immature oral movement patterns that interfere with learning a controlled bite. This approach is most effective with a child who shows signs of poor sensory integration and sensory overload such as poor eye contact, rhythmical self-stimulation, and hyperactivity.

🅰 Help the child develop the concept that the mouth can be quiet and ready before the food enters for biting. Begin with assisted oral control as described in Jaw Control: Jaw Opening and Closing on page 430. Initial work with this concept can be done with the mouth closed if this is easier for the child. Work to have the child maintain an open mouth and quiet tongue as he observes the food.

    a. If it is difficult for the child to keep the mouth quiet with the approach of food, begin the activity by touching the child's mouth with a toy, then moving the toy away. Continue until the child can remain completely quiet during the activity.

    b. Use a tongue depressor, cotton swab, or foodlike object for the touch-and-go activity.

    c. Tell the child, "Now the cookie will touch your mouth, but it is not time to eat it. This is a time to practice keeping the mouth quiet and ready." Repeat the activity of bringing the cookie to the mouth, touching the lips, and moving it away.

    d. Tell the child, "I will bring the food to your mouth while it is quiet and ready. When I touch your lips, you may open your mouth and take a bite of the food."

    e. Repeat this sequence with the child's mouth in an open, quiet, and ready position for the cookie. A similar sequence for spoon feeding, described on page 431, is appropriate to work on for developing a controlled biting pattern.

🅰 Ask the child to hold a soft cookie between the teeth or gums. Say, "I will break off the outside piece while you hold the part that is in your mouth." The ability to stabilize the jaw in a closed position while holding an object or food occurs in normal development before the ability to use a controlled bite through the food. Teach this step if the child does not have a tonic bite reflex and is able to quiet or inhibit movement as food enters the mouth.

🅰 Help the child develop the ability to sustain a holding pressure for a bite. This is particularly important when the child has low tone in the jaw or jaw instability.

    ✤ Play patty-cake, peek-a-boo, and other children's games that incorporate patting, tapping, stroking, and other types of tactile and proprioceptive stimulation of the jaw opening and closing muscles. Tapping can be done directly around the temporomandibular joint.

    ✤ Use folk music with a clear rhythm and regular tempo to provide tapping and other sensory input to the muscles and joint. Children enjoy singing while you touch and tap the face. It is playful and fun, and emphasizes the interaction rather than the stimulation.

▼ The child must be able to accept and integrate sensory stimulation without developing hypertonicity and limiting movement patterns in the rest of the body.

🅰 Help the child achieve and maintain a stable degree of jaw opening and closing by placing your hand on the child's jaw during biting. This enables the child to experience a sensation of greater stability and the knowledge of what an easy up-down movement can be like. See the section on assisted oral control described in Jaw Control: Jaw Opening and Closing on page 430 for instructions and illustrations for hand placement. Emphasize the pressure of your finger directly under the chin to help the child focus on the feeling of holding the food and biting through it. Vary the amount of pressure and the thickness and resistance of the food. Follow this or combine it with tapping and playful activities that require the child to sustain a stable closure of the jaw.

▼ Oral-control techniques are useful only after reducing limiting movement patterns in the body through handling and positioning. They are of limited value when discomfort or a response such as a jaw thrust is triggered by touch to the face. They often provide too high a level of psychological control for the child who is dealing with issues of independence. Activities that encourage the child to hold something between the teeth are useful only when the child does not have a bite reflex.

> 🅰 Build the child's awareness and feedback of jaw movement by using the snack cap described in Sensory Feedback: Face and Mouth on page 415.

> 🅰 Introduce long, thin toys or other nonfood biting materials that can be held between the molars. Vary the diameter and resistance of the object (e.g., different sizes of Chewy Tubes™). Initially, have the child hold the object between the teeth for increasing lengths of time. When the child is able to do this, invite the child to open and close the jaw on the object in a repeated biting movement.

Chewing

◉ Reduce postural, sensory, and oral motor limits that interfere with the development of chewing.

Possible Activities

> 🅰 Observe the relationships among the child's lip, cheek, jaw, and tongue movements and the limiting tone and movement patterns of the face and mouth. See Oral Control Issues: Limiting Areas on page 443 for suggestions for influencing tone and movement in the mouth.

> 🅰 Explore changes in positioning and body movement to discover ways of reducing tonic and stabilizing bite patterns that interfere with chewing. Use activities to decrease postural tone as described in Change Tone: Decrease Tone on page 406 and activities to obtain greater postural alignment as described in Postural Alignment: Head, Neck, and Trunk Alignment on page 402.

> 🅰 When there are increases or decreases in tone and limiting movement patterns of the jaw, tongue, lips, and cheeks, work to reduce or eliminate them must precede any direct work to obtain a more advanced normal pattern. As these patterns diminish, the normal movements are facilitated. This can take place within the same therapy session and may seem to occur simultaneously if the child's system is easily changeable.

> 🅰 Reduce environmental sensory input that can overload the child's system, resulting in a reversion to limiting or more immature oral movement patterns that interfere with learning to chew. This approach is most effective with a child who shows signs of poor sensory integration and sensory overload such as poor eye contact, rhythmical self-stimulation, and hyperactivity.

Munching

◉ Develop an early munching pattern of chewing.

Possible Activities

> 🅰 Add thickened and lumpy soft foods to the child's diet. Ground foods, commercial third stage foods, and thick, lumpy cereal do not require chewing. The child usually sucks these foods and experiences the new textures. This experience with lumps and bumps in food is a prerequisite skill to chewing. Chewing does not blenderize food; it cuts and pulverizes it to the consistency of a ground food. The child must be comfortable with this consistency before chewing can be expected.

> 🅰 Teach the child to move from an in-out suckle pattern with softer foods to the up-down sucking pattern. The up-down tongue movement is part of munching, the earliest chewing pattern. See Sucking: Transition From Suckling to Sucking on page 462 for suggestions.

◬ An intermittent, rhythmical contact of the gums or teeth is part of the early phasic biting pattern. To chew, the child must be able to bring the teeth together around the food and release the contact. This pattern is repeated hundreds of times during a meal. Help the child develop a heightened awareness of the teeth and the sensation of biting.

⊕ Give the child sturdy toys that she can bite during play. Some of the firm rubber bones and tug-toys made for dogs can be used appropriately. Chicken legs with the meat removed are wonderful for biting practice. Select activities from the Combined Oral Sensorimotor Control: Mouthing section on page 441.

⊕ Click the child's teeth together by rhythmically jiggling or tapping under the chin. Children enjoy the sound this makes and the new sensations with the teeth.

⊕ Use a battery-operated vibrating massager. Encourage the child to explore the vibrations with the lips and teeth. Many children will discover pleasurable sensations from the teeth when the vibrator is placed in the mouth.

▼ This approach is most effective with a child who shows no awareness of the teeth and has not used them for exploration biting. It should not be used with a child who has a tonic bite reflex.

◬ Reduce the probability that pieces of food will be bitten off when the child is practicing a chewing motion. Wrap foods in a thin, porous bag made of gauze, cheesecloth, or nylon organza, then tie them with a string or dental floss. This food ball can be used between the front or sides teeth to stimulate munching. The child does not have to simultaneously learn how to organize and swallow lumpy pieces that come off in the chewing process. The Baby Safe Feeder™ is made from a solid plastic handle with a screw-on ring (see the picture on page 433). A small, nylon mesh bag is firmly attached to the ring for convenience and safety. Food placed in the bag can be bitten and chewed without coming off in the child's mouth. These bags also can hold juicy fruits such as orange or grapefruit slices that often are difficult for children to manage safely.

Lateralization

◎ Develop tongue lateralization in chewing when food is placed on the side of the mouth.

Possible Activities

◬ Increase sensory input to the tongue and build sensory awareness and discrimination of a wide variety of sensations on the tongue. Include appropriate activities from Sensory Awareness: Face and Mouth on page 411 and Sensory Discrimination: Face and Mouth on page 414.

◬ Use foods with alerting tastes and textures during mealtimes to increase the amount of tongue movement.

◬ Encourage a wide array of tongue movements during discriminative mouthing and oral exploration activities. See Combined Oral Sensorimotor Control: Mouthing on page 441 and Combined Oral Sensorimotor Control: Oral Exploration on page 442.

◬ Using assistance with jaw control, help the child develop the concept that the mouth can be quiet and ready before food is placed between the teeth for chewing. For the feeder to be able to place the food precisely between the teeth and on the side of the mouth where it will be handled most efficiently, the child must be able to open the mouth and keep the tongue quiet. A moving mouth and a tendency toward reflexive biting encourages a feeder to move in and out of the mouth hastily. Speed and panic reduce efficiency of placement. Without precise placement, the moving tongue immediately pushes the food out of the mouth. Incorporate activities from Jaw Control: Jaw Stability in an Open Position on page 431 and Jaw Control: Jaw Stability in a Closed Position on page 432.

◬ Place food between the biting surfaces of the teeth on the side of the mouth. Encourage the child to take several bites to develop a simple chewing pattern with lateral movements of the jaw and tongue toward the side of food placement. Work to tighten the cheeks and the corner of the lip on that side. See activities in Lip and Cheek Control: Cheek Compression on page 435. Use foods that are relatively soft and dissolve easily. Graham crackers, crackers, small pieces of cheese, and cereal bits work well.

🅰 Take turns hiding food in the child's cheek pockets and having the child hide food in your mouth. Do this in a playful game of hide-and-seek. Place food pieces in areas that the child can handle and gradually work toward areas that require more tongue lateralization or cheek compression. Observe for tightening in the cheeks and the corner of the lip on the side of food placement. The child should be able to use the cheek to bring the food to the center of the mouth. Children who are reluctant to have an adult place food in the mouth usually will join in a turn-taking game. This is a particularly effective technique for a self-feeder who will not allow an adult to interfere during a regular meal.

⊕ At first, use foods that are relatively soft and dissolve easily. Graham crackers, crackers, small pieces of cheese, and cereal bits work well. As the child's skill improves, use food that is smaller and provides clear sensory input. Grape-Nuts™, granola, and raisins are effective. Alternate the side of the mouth for food placement.

🅰 Reduce the chance that pieces of food will be bitten off when the child is practicing a chewing motion. Wrap foods in a thin, porous bag made of gauze, cheesecloth, or nylon organza, then tie them with a string or dental floss, or use the Baby SafeFeeder. This food ball can be used between the teeth to stimulate chewing. The child does not have to simultaneously learn how to organize and swallow lumpy pieces that come off in the chewing process. The rough texture of the fabric bag facilitates greater tongue movement to the side. Change the food bag when it shows signs of tearing.

🅰 As the child's chewing ability improves, use food that has a long, thin shape. Food in this shape allows continued biting and chewing as it is slowly moved into the mouth between the teeth. This "bite-chew" activity emphasizes a rhythmical chewing pattern and provides constant lateral stimulation to remind the tongue to stay in the lateral position during the entire chewing process. The prolonged lateral tongue position develops improved carryover of tongue lateralization at other times.

⊕ Foods that work well include thin pretzels, bread sticks, French fries, graham crackers cut lengthwise, and sandwiches cut in inch-wide strips. For higher nutrition, use strips of partially cooked broccoli, potato, turnip, and cauliflower. The degree of cooking depends on the child's skill. Begin with soft vegetables and increase the texture by decreasing cooking time as the child improves.

🅰 Present the food to only one side at a time until lateralization begins. Alternate food placement as lateralization becomes more consistent.

🅰 Teach the self-feeder how to place food on the side of the mouth during a meal. Encourage the child to let both sides have a chewing turn. The child can do this at mealtime when finger-feeding pieces of fruit, vegetable, or meat.

🅰 Help the child achieve and maintain a stable degree of jaw opening and closing by placing your hand on the child's jaw during chewing. Use assisted oral control as described in Jaw Control: Jaw Opening and Closing on page 430. This helps the child experience a sensation of greater stability and the knowledge of what rhythmical chewing with lateral movements of the jaw feels like. Press your finger directly under the chin to emphasize the feeling of holding the food and biting through it. Your hand can help the jaw swing or move toward the side of food placement. Vary the amount of pressure used as the child's skill increases.

▼ Jaw control or oral-control techniques are useful only after reducing limiting patterns of the movement in the body through handling and positioning. They are of limited value when discomfort or a jaw thrust is triggered by touch to the face. They often provide too high a level of psychological control for a child who is dealing with issues of independence.

- ⓐ Use the snack cap described in Sensory Feedback: Face and Mouth on page 415 to give the child greater sensory awareness of jaw movement in chewing.
- ⓐ Use an adult's finger, a toy, cotton swab, pretzel, or electric toothbrush to stimulate the lateral borders of the tongue. Stimulate the child's tongue to move to the side.
- ⓐ Use toothbrushing activities as described in Combined Oral Sensorimotor Control: Toothbrushing on page 439 to increase muscle tone in the tongue, lips, and cheeks, and to increase tongue lateralization for chewing.

◉ Develop tongue lateralization in chewing when food is placed in the center of the mouth.
- ⓐ When the child can lateralize the tongue to food placed between the side teeth, begin to place food in the center of the tongue. Press down slightly on the tongue as the food enters the child's mouth. This alerts the tongue to the presence of food and helps it move the food to the side.
- ⓐ Notice toward which side the child habitually transfers the food. If one side is preferred over the other, place the food slightly to the right or left of center on the nonpreferred side.
- ⓐ Create a game of transferring food. Place food on the center of the tongue and let the child choose the side for food transfer. Alternate this with hiding the food on the side or in the cheek pouches. Pretend that a raisin is a jumping animal or someone on ice skates who will move to the side of the mouth pond.
- ⓐ When the child can lateralize the tongue and use intermittent chewing movements in a rhythmical fashion, add raisins and strips or pieces of dried fruit. These foods require a substantial amount of chewing. They provide a challenge to the mildly impaired child because they do not dissolve, and their natural sweetness usually increases saliva production. To handle them efficiently, the child must be able to chew and simultaneously swallow the excess saliva that is produced. This can be an excellent food to explore subtle minimal feeding problems.

◉ Develop tongue lateralization in chewing when transferring food from one side of the mouth to the other.
- ⓐ Set up a pattern and rhythm in food placement, alternating the placement to mimic the pattern used in transferring food across midline. For example, place a raisin on the right side. As soon as the child has finished the raisin, place a second one on the center of the tongue and ask the child to move it to the left. Repeat this side-center-side sequence with initial placement on the left side. As the rhythm becomes established, suggest that the child make the raisin placed on the right move to the left without stopping to swallow it right away.
  - ✧ It is appropriate to begin work on cross-midline transfers of food when a child is developmentally 18 to 24 months old and has developed chewing skill in moving the food from the side to the center and from the center to the side.
- ⓐ Expand the food transfer game. Suggest to the child that the food will move all the way from one side to the other. Use a piece of food and your finger on the teeth and tongue to demonstrate the movement across midline, ending up on the opposite side. Let the child explore this possibility independently. Introduce the activity as another way of moving and playing with food. Use tactile and visual cues to assist the child.
- ⓐ Have the child chew meat or other tough food that requires a grinding action and cross-midline transfer. As the child chews on one side, suggest that the other side would like a turn with the same piece of meat. If you have been playing turn-taking games, the idea that the two sides of the mouth need to take turns will delight a child.
  - ✧ Smooth transfers of chewy food from one side of the mouth to the other do not begin until the child is developmentally 2 years old. Look for a smooth, continuous movement, without pause in the center. It is appropriate to work on cross-midline transfers of food when a child is developmentally 2 years old and has developed chewing skill in moving the food from the side to the center and the center to the side.

◉ Increase the timing and coordination of the chewing pattern.

Possible Activities

🅰 Encourage rhythmical activities during chewing that build postural tone, provide proprioceptive input, and increase the rhythm and timing of chewing. Many children will stomp their feet spontaneously or kick rhythmically as they are chewing.

Food Transitions

◉ Reduce postural, sensory, and oral motor limits that interfere with the ability to handle more complex foods.

Possible Activities

🅰 Observe the relationship among the child's lip, cheek, jaw, and tongue movements and the limiting tone and movement patterns of the face and mouth.

🅰 Explore changes in positioning and body movement to discover ways of changing these oral-facial patterns. See Oral Control Issues: Limiting Areas on page 443 for suggestions for influencing tone and movement in the mouth.

🅰 When there are increases or decreases in tone and limiting movement patterns of the jaw, tongue, lips, and cheeks, work to reduce or eliminate them must precede any direct work to obtain a more advanced normal pattern. As these patterns diminish, the normal movements are facilitated. This can take place within the same therapy session and may seem to occur simultaneously if the child's system is easily changeable.

Sensory Transitions

◉ Organize and present new foods on a *taste* continuum that assures acceptance and success.

Possible Activities

🅰 Start with a familiar food. Vary the flavor slightly with a new, slightly different flavor.

🅰 To introduce a flavor that may not be readily accepted, try presenting the new drink using a straw in a glass with a lid. The lid decreases the smell of the food and may allow the child to taste it without immediate rejection due to the smell or sight of it.

🅰 Chilled foods seem to have less odor than warmed foods. Often, new flavors are tried more readily with chilled foods.

🅰 Ice cubes with a new flavor can melt slowly in a drink. The flavor enters the drink gradually as it is being consumed. Thus, the flavor change is subtle and more likely to be accepted.

🅰 Use the "around the bowl" method. In one bowl, offer a familiar food and a new food. First, present the familiar food. Then offer a spoonful that is mostly the familiar food with a tiny bit of the new food. If that flavor mix is accepted, offer several spoonfuls that way. Gradually work your way around the bowl as the child accepts more and more concentration of the new food flavor. When you get to any level of flavor concentration that seems to worry the child, go back to a familiar and safe flavor.

🅰 Reintroduce foods that the child has rejected in the past.

⊙ Organize and present new foods on a ***texture*** continuum that assures acceptance and success.

Possible Activities

🅐 Present new textures slowly with carefully selected changes added to familiar textures. Start with food the child can handle and work through the texture continuum as the child demonstrates the skills and the interest.

🅐 Start with a familiar food such as pudding or yogurt. Thicken it first. A gradual thickening of a familiar food enables the child to feel the thickness and pressure changes in the mouth, tongue, and pharynx while swallowing.

🅐 Take a food that the child enjoys, such as commercially pureed baby carrots, and prepare it differently. Try blending boiled carrots. The homemade blenderized carrots offer a familiar flavor with a similar, but slightly more textured sensation.

🅐 Vary the degree to which a homemade food is blenderized to provide slightly varied texture.

🅐 Grind a familiar food, such as carrots, apple, sweet potato, or pasta dish. Baby food grinders can make food a steady consistency without providing noticeable identifiable lumps to be spit out. Put foods through the grinder twice, if necessary. You can add liquids to keep the food moister.

🅐 Offer a familiar food with different variations. For example, baby cereal is quite smooth when mixed with formula or juice. Instant oatmeal is more textured. Quick-cooking oatmeal is more textured yet. Slow-cooked oatmeal is the most textured of all these types of oatmeal. Gradually changing the type of oatmeal can provide thicker and more textured sensations.

🅐 Gradually blend and grind foods less.

🅐 Mash soft foods such as bananas and soft cooked vegetables such as carrots, sweet and white potatoes, and squash. These foods can be mashed and smooth or include soft and easy-to-swallow lumps.

🅐 Add soft textured foods to thickened purees. Add well-cooked small pieces of pasta, such as alphabet-shaped pasta, to purees to add texture. You also can add crushed crackers or dried cereals, which will soften with the moisture.

🅐 Crush crumbs on top of foods to add texture variation.

🅐 Mash soft table foods to different degrees, allowing for bigger and bigger lumps.

🅐 Provide different textures within one mouthful. Soups and casseroles provide the opportunity to handle liquids and soft solids or multi-textured solids all within one mouthful.

🅐 Combine dry solids and wet or smooth foods. Sandwiches such as crackers and bologna or bread and cheese give texture variation. Crackers dipped in dips or spread with refried beans, cookies dipped in yogurt, or banana strips dipped in cream cheese and brown sugar and rolled in cracker crumbs can be flavorful texture combinations.

🅐 Use the "around the bowl" method. In one bowl, offer a familiar food texture, such as a puree, and a new texture, such as a thickened version of the puree. First, present the familiar texture. Then, offer a spoonful that is mostly the familiar texture with a tiny bit of the new texture. If the child accepts that, offer several spoonfuls of that mixture. Gradually work your way around the bowl as the child accepts more and more concentration of the new food texture. When you get to any level of texture concentration that seems to worry the child, go back to a familiar and safe texture.

⊙ Organize and present new foods on a ***temperature*** continuum that assures acceptance and success.

Possible Activities

🅐 Start with familiar and comfortable temperatures. Gradually offer foods that are slightly warmer or slightly colder.

🅐 Make ice cubes containing a familiar food flavor. Offer the child a familiar drink, such as a room temperature glass of chocolate milk. To increase acceptance of colder foods, add ice cubes made of chocolate milk to the drink. As the child drinks the milk, the ice cubes will melt, chilling the drink slightly. If you offer the drink more chilled to begin with, the child may reject it. However, if the temperature change is made gradually during the drinking of the milk, the child may accept it more readily.

Liquids to Smooth Solids

⊙ Build the child's acceptance of smooth, solid foods.

Possible Activities

🅐 Reduce postural, sensory, and oral motor limits that interfere with the ability to handle smooth solids.

🅐 Introduce tiny tastes of different, smooth pureed foods into the child's formula. When these same tastes are introduced on a finger or spoon, the taste aspect will be familiar.

🅐 Use the taste continuum for introducing new pureed foods as described in Food Transitions: Sensory Transitions in Foods on page 481.

🅐 Introduce stronger taste differences by offering a mixture of water and juice in a bottle or cup. Select juices such as apple, grape, apricot, cranberry, prune, and carrot. Initially, dilute the juices to reduce the sharpness of taste when they are presented. This approach is appropriate for infants 4 months and older who have not experienced different tastes. Change of taste in a liquid form prepares children for accepting a smooth solid that has taste and texture differences.

🅐 Dip your finger or the child's finger in different juices and let the child suck the finger to build familiarity and acceptance of taste.

🅐 Add commercial pureed fruits and vegetables to the child's milk or juice. Combine foods and liquids such as milk and rice cereal, apple juice and applesauce, apricot nectar and apricots, and carrot juice and carrots. By adding the solid form of a familiar juice, the child receives only a change in thickness or density of a taste that already is acceptable.

　　⊕ Introduce these thickened liquids from a cup with a wide lip, following the instructions for facilitating mature oral movements during cup drinking. See Sucking: Cup Drinking on page 466.

　　⊕ Encourage the child to slurp-suck, pulling the thick liquid into the mouth and regulating its flow.

🅐 Introduce the same thickened liquids from a spoon. Place the spoon at the front of the lips, using it as if it were the lip of a cup. Sometimes this is easier if a large tablespoon is placed so the child drinks from the side of the bowl instead of the front.

🅐 When feeding smooth solids that have not been diluted with liquid, use an appropriate size and shaped spoon for the child's mouth. Gradually increase the number of tastes that the child will accept. You can select tastes from commercial baby foods and table foods that have been processed in a blender and diluted to create a smooth texture.

🅐 Select foods from these categories to help the child move from liquids to smooth solids:
Thin liquids—water; broth; orange, apple, grape, and grapefruit juice
Heavy, "milky" liquids—melted ice cream, milkshakes, yogurt, pudding, custard
Heavy, "nectar" liquids—apricot, tomato, pineapple juice; blended fruit drinks
Pureed foods—commercial baby foods, homemade baby foods, table foods blended to a thin puree
Thickened foods—baby cereals, pureed foods thickened with wheat germ or rice cereal, table foods blended to a thick puree

🅐 Discuss family food preferences and styles with the child's parents. Offer suggestions of the type of food appropriate for the child from typical foods that are eaten in the home.

Smooth Solids to Lumpy Solids

◎ Build the child's acceptance of lumpy solid foods.

Possible Activities

🅐 Reduce postural, sensory, and oral motor limits that interfere with the ability to handle smooth solids.

🅐 Use the taste and texture continuums for introducing new lumpy solid foods as described in Food Transitions: Sensory Transitions in Foods on page 481.

🅐 Introduce smoothly blenderized table foods to the child's diet. This prepares the child for the taste characteristics of freshly prepared food. It is easier to adjust and regulate the amount of lumpiness in food when you prepare your own. The child must be familiar with the taste characteristics of food that will be introduced later in a ground or lumpy form. This taste change is an important step in the transition to solids for children whose main taste experience has been with commercial baby foods.

🅐 Prepare ground food using a baby-food grinder and homemade table foods. You can grind the food a second time and mix it with liquid if the child cannot handle the consistency created by the initial grinding. This step produces a combination of thickness and small lumps that are the same size and shape. Introduce this change in food consistency after the child has made the adjustment to thicker, smooth foods. The change can be made gradually, enabling the child to adjust to texture changes.

🅐 Thicken smooth solids with wheat germ, potato flakes, or dehydrated fruit and vegetable flakes. You also can introduce mashed foods such as ripe bananas, mashed potatoes, or scrambled eggs. Increase the thickness to a mild amount of generalized lumpiness as the mixture assumes a very solid form. This initial change in food consistency is appropriate as the child moves from smooth to lumpy solids. The change can be made gradually, enabling the child to adjust to texture changes.

🅐 Introduce foods with soft lumps that are not mixed evenly in another food. These include cottage cheese, mashed stew, and pasta with sauce. You can add mashed carrots, green beans, or beets to a thick base of mashed potatoes. Avoid vegetables that have an outer shell, such as peas, corn, and lima beans. You can add these when the child is more skilled in handling lumpy foods. Introduce this change in food consistency after the child has adjusted to ground solids with evenly distributed lumps. The change can be made gradually, enabling the child to adjust to texture changes.

🅐 Move directly into chewy solids that do not scatter in the mouth when chewed, bypassing the preliminary stage of lumpy solids. Return to this stage as chewing skills improve. See Food Transitions: Lumpy Solids to Chewy Solids on page 485 for options for introducing chewy solids. Children with oral sensory defensiveness may be extremely intolerant of food with small lumps. Often, the child handles larger pieces of food more effectively because he can be encouraged to chew them, while the smaller pieces presented independently do not immediately stimulate chewing. When the food becomes scattered in the mouth, the child may gag or spit it out.

🅐 Encourage the child to explore and accept textures in play with water, sand, cornmeal, and finger paints. Use foods for smearing and finger painting.

🅐 Encourage the child to put toys in the mouth for discriminative mouthing and oral exploration. Many of these toys have textures that can introduce the child to lumps and bumps not associated with food. Discriminative mouthing helps the child reduce the strength of the gag reflex and prepare the mouth for lumpy solid foods. See suggestions in the Combined Oral Sensorimotor Control: Mouthing section on page 441.

■ Reduce the child's tendency to gag when lumpy foods are placed in the mouth. Identify the cause of the child's gagging and follow the appropriate suggestions in the Gagging section on page 490.

■ Help the child develop the ability to organize a bolus and use a clearing swallow to clean the mouth. This includes activities for reducing limiting patterns of the jaw, tongue, lips, and cheeks, as well as those for facilitating a more normal sucking or chewing pattern. Particular attention is directed to the role of the cheeks in forming the bolus and preventing food particles from scattering.

■ If the child has major difficulty when you introduce dry foods or foods with discrete lumps, use a binder food. Alternate bites of hard, lumpy food with a clearing spoonful of a food that will bind together the loose pieces and form a more efficient bolus. Use foods such as applesauce, strained or blenderized fruits or vegetables, and cranberry sauce as binders. Teach the child to ask for spoonfuls of the binder food before eating food pieces that are uncomfortable or may cause gagging. As the child's skill in chewing and swallowing increases, she will have less need for the binder food.

■ Select foods from these categories to help the child move from smooth solids to lumpy solids:
Pureed foods—commercial baby foods, homemade baby foods, table foods blended to a thin puree
Thickened foods—baby cereals, pureed foods thickened with wheat germ or rice cereal, table foods blended to a thick puree
Mashed early solids—regular oatmeal; finely mashed bananas or other very ripe fruit; mashed avocado; mashed potatoes; mashed squash, carrots, or yams; soft scrambled eggs; mashed, soft-boiled eggs; mashed tofu
Textured early solids—tapioca pudding, applesauce, cookies crumbled and soaked in milk, some third stage food meats
Lumpy solids—cottage cheese, hamburger meat in a casserole, spaghetti, mashed macaroni and cheese, mashed rice and beans

■ Discuss family food preferences and styles with the parents. Offer suggestions of the type of food appropriate for the child from typical foods that are eaten in the home.

Lumpy Solids to Chewy Solids

◉ Build the child's acceptance of chewy solid foods.

Possible Activities

■ After the child accepts lumpy solids and is ready to expand chewing movements, add solid foods that require some chewing. Mince or cut table foods into fine chunks for easier handling. Raisins, dry cereal pieces, squares of soft cheese, canned green beans, and small chicken strips may be enjoyed as first finger-foods. Gradually move to foods that are harder to chew, such as beef, lamb, raw carrots, and raw celery, as chewing proficiency develops. Introduce foods that have a combination of two or more discrete consistencies, such as vegetable soup, dry cereal with milk, and gelatin with fruit chunks.

■ Work on chewing skills. See Chewing: Munching on page 477 and Chewing: Lateralization on page 478 for options for developing the ability to chew.

■ Select foods from these categories to help the child move from lumpy solids to chewy solids:
Easy chewy solids—raisins, cheese, canned green beans, chicken, tuna
Combination foods—noodle soup, vegetable soup, dry cereal with milk, gelatin with fruit chunks, many commercial toddler foods
Difficult chewy solids—roast beef, lamb chops, pork chops, raw carrots, raw celery

■ Discuss family food preferences and styles with the parents. Offer suggestions of the type of food appropriate for the child from typical foods that are eaten in the home.

Food Selection

Food and Oral Movement

⊙ Identify the sensory properties of individual foods and their relationship to the child's oral movement skills.

Possible Activities

🅰 Personally explore and examine the sensory properties of each food selected for a child. Put the food in your mouth and become aware of its sensory aspects. Is it heavy or light in the mouth? Is it grainy, smooth, or lumpy? Does it stick together in a solid mass or bolus when mouthed or chewed? Does it melt in the mouth? If so, how quickly? Does it break up into many pieces? How rapidly does it move to the back of the mouth and down the throat? Is it composed of a combination of several textures (such as an apple) or is there a single texture (such as a banana)? What is the taste? Tart? Bitter? Sweet? Sour? What is the temperature? Does the temperature vary during the meal? Self-discovered knowledge of food properties is remembered more easily and for a longer time than information obtained by reading or from another person.

🅰 Practice eating different foods while imitating the child's problems of the jaw, tongue, lips, cheeks, and head position. Vary the texture, temperature, taste, and smell while exploring different foods. Find out what changes make the food easier to eat. This will support the discovery of the specific movements required to handle the food effectively and which aspects of the child's sensory abilities and movement patterns interfere with the normal patterns. It also will contribute to an understanding of which foods are easier or more difficult for the child to handle. Select specific Participation Exercises from the *Mealtime Participation Guide* (Klein & Morris, 1999) that reflect the child's physical and sensory abilities and limitations.

Facilitating Normal Oral Movement

⊙ Identify and select foods whose sensory properties facilitate more normal oral movement for a child.

Possible Activities

🅰 Experientially identify the sensory properties of individual foods and their relationship to the child's oral movement skills. Use the general strategies below and described in Food Transitions: Sensory Transitions on page 481. Develop an in-depth understanding of the interplay between food and normal and limiting patterns of physical, sensory, and feeding development by completing the Participation Experiences in the *Mealtime Participation Guide* (Klein & Morris, 1999).

🅰 If the child has difficulty organizing the food into a bolus for swallowing or a tendency to aspirate before, during, or after the swallow, explore the differences between thicker and thinner foods and liquids.

⊕ Thicker, heavier food and liquid provides stronger tactile and proprioceptive cues. It moves more slowly through the oral and pharyngeal cavities and is less likely to bounce uncontrollably into the airway. A child who is learning to drink from a cup may have difficulty with the runny liquid moving rapidly over the mouth and face. The liquid may be moving so quickly that there is insufficient feedback for the tongue to adjust its configuration and collect the liquid more efficiently. Drinking abilities may improve with a heavier liquid such as a milkshake or a mixture of juice and applesauce. Many children who have difficulties with sucking and swallowing can use a more mature movement pattern when the food or liquid is thickened.

⊕ Thicker foods and liquids tend to get stuck in the mouth and throat if tongue and pharyngeal mobility is weak. In that case, the heavy consistency is a disadvantage for movement.

- ✛ Thin liquids in small quantities are handled in the same way as saliva. A child who handles secretions well may learn to swallow better if small drops of water or juice are used.
- ✛ Thicken pureed foods and liquids with cereal, wheat germ, dehydrated potato flakes, or a commercial thickener. Add less liquid when processing or grinding food. Substitute yogurt if the child cannot handle the thin consistency of milk.

▼ Explore the influence of thickness of food and liquid with any child who has difficulty organizing the food into a bolus for swallowing or a tendency to aspirate before, during, or after the swallow. More specific information on the effect of food consistency on a child's swallowing ability can be obtained through a videofluoroscopic swallowing study.

🄰 If the child has inefficient cheek and tongue action or difficulty with chewing, explore the differences between foods that stick together in the mouth and those that break apart.
- ✛ Foods that break apart into firm and diffuse pieces usually are more difficult to handle than those that maintain a more solid single mass as they are chewed. Once the food has broken apart, the child may find it impossible to create a bolus for chewing and may attempt to handle the pieces by sucking them. This causes coughing and choking as pieces escape and become stuck in the throat or are inhaled.
- ✛ Although ground meats such as hamburger often may be more difficult to chew than chicken or roast beef (which mat together when chewed), the particles of hamburger are gathered together when served as a sandwich. The bread becomes slightly gummy when wetted by saliva, serving as a binder to hold the pieces of meat together.

🄰 Crisp foods provide auditory as well as tactile and kinesthetic feedback for biting and chewing. They may help children develop greater precision of chewing than softer foods. It is important to observe the child's response to the small, firm pieces of food that are produced when biting a crisp food. If the pieces scatter in the mouth, they may cause problems and result in gagging or a reversion to sucking.
- ✛ Pieces of dry cereal, crackers, potato chips, and pretzels are some of the foods that can be used to help the child develop precision in biting and chewing.
- ✛ Crisp foods should be used in moderation. Many commercially available foods contain excessive amounts of salt, sugar, hydrogenated oils, or chemical preservatives. Foods that retain a small, firm shape should not be used if they cause the child to gag and choke.

🄰 The shape into which food is cut can increase its ability to facilitate more normal oral movements. Long strips of food that can be moved slowly into the side of the mouth as the child uses a rhythmical biting and chewing pattern are particularly effective in teaching chewing.
- ✛ Strips of chewy meat, sandwiches cut in 1-inch strips, and dried apple and apricot strips can help develop tongue lateralization in chewing. Carrot strips and other vegetables can be cooked until they are softened to the necessary consistency. Dried fruits and fresh fruits and vegetables also contribute to the child's nutritional needs.
- ✛ Thin strips of lunch meats such as skinned hot dogs, bologna, and pressed ham are excellent to use in the beginning stages of chewing because of their soft consistency. Some people may prefer not to use these foods extensively because they contain chemical preservatives. Some of these preservatives, such as sodium nitrite, may be dangerous if consumed in large quantities.

🄰 The size of the food pieces or amount given in a spoonful can facilitate more normal oral movements.
- ✛ A large mouthful of food facilitates mouth closure and lip activity in children who can produce these movements. The child who stuffs the mouth with food when self-feeding is increasing the sensory input of the food within the mouth cavity and improving the ability of the lips and cheeks to contain the food in the mouth.

- A small mouthful of smaller pieces of food facilitates more precise jaw, tongue, and cheek movement for chewing in children who can produce these movements.
- Vary the size of the mouthful given to the child. To observe the child's lip and cheek movements and ability to eat without losing food, give a relatively large spoonful of macaroni and cheese or other food that doesn't require a high level of chewing precision. To observe the precision of tongue movement in chewing, give small amounts of chewy foods such as meat or raisins.

A Explore the differences between foods of a single consistency and those with several consistencies. For example, an apple has a very chewy skin, moderately chewy pulp, and a thin, juicy liquid that is extracted by biting and chewing. The sweet taste of most apples triggers the production of extra saliva. To eat the fruit, an individual must be able to separate the juice from the pulp and swallow any excess liquid while chewing the firmer portions. The solid portion of the apple must be separated into pulp that is ready for swallowing and pulp and skin that requires additional chewing. In contrast, a banana or a piece of cheese creates a single consistency in the mouth. As the food is mixed with saliva, it holds together and becomes ready for swallowing at one time rather than several moments.

- Handling food with multiple consistencies requires a high level of coordination. Children who have mild feeding problems may have difficulty with foods such as gelatin with fruit chunks, orange segments, vegetable or meat soups, and dry cereal with milk. Include these combination foods when assessing mild coordination problems.
- Children who have difficulty with food with multiple consistencies may compensate by eating the different parts separately. For example, a child may drink the liquid part of the soup and then eat the solid pieces. Observing how a child handles a challenging food can tell you a great deal about areas of sensation and movement that may be less precise or skillful.
- Avoid combination foods until the child has developed chewing and swallowing abilities for less complex foods. Use these foods for evaluation and therapy when the child is ready to work on higher levels of oral sensorimotor coordination.

A Children with oral tactile defensiveness may be extremely intolerant of food with small lumps. Often, larger pieces of food are handled more efficiently because the child can be encouraged to chew them, while the smaller pieces presented independently do not immediately stimulate chewing. When the food becomes scattered in the mouth, the child may gag or spit it out. Differences in behavior should be noted in giving lumpy solids and chewy solids to the child with oral tactile hypersensitivity.

A Cold temperatures can alert the nervous system and prepare the mouth for a rapid swallow. Small bits of crushed ice or lemon sherbet can be used to improve a child's delayed swallow reflex. Cold may increase muscle tone when low tone and insufficient movement hamper feeding abilities.

▼ The use of cold in facilitating the swallow must be done with caution. Many children who have poor swallowing patterns also are hypersensitive to temperature extremes. Many have dental problems that cause discomfort when icy temperatures are used.

A Strong taste can alert the nervous system. This can increase muscle tone and improve the precision of oral movement. Sour and bitter tastes also tend to alert the system and facilitate more movement. Children who are poorly alerted to food, such as those who have a history of nasal congestion that limits their ability to smell food, are unmotivated to eat. They may respond and eat better when herbs or spices are added to their food.

- Children who have difficulty organizing and integrating sensory information may accept food more enthusiastically and use better feeding movements when alerting foods, such as those with sour or bitter tastes, are eliminated from the diet.
- Explore the role of taste. Observe patterns in each child's preference for different tastes. Observe the effect of taste on tone and movement in the body and mouth.

■ Small pieces of a hard, rough cereal, such as Grape-Nuts™ and granola, may increase tongue lateralization when they are placed on the lateral border of the tongue or between the teeth. When hidden in the cheek and lip pockets, they provide a stimulus for more active cheek and lip movement.

■ The use of small pieces of food to stimulate tongue, lip, and cheek movement is appropriate when the child is able to handle small pieces of food in the mouth without gagging and choking. It is particularly helpful for the child with low tone who experiences reduced skill and movement.

Limiting Normal Oral Movement

⊙ Identify and avoid foods with sensory properties that limit a child's normal oral movement.

Possible Activities

■ Experientially identify the sensory properties of individual foods and their relationship to the child's oral movement skills. Use the general strategies described in Food Selection: Food and Oral Movement on page 486. Develop an in-depth understanding of the interplay between food and normal and limiting patterns of physical, sensory, and feeding development by completing the Participation Experiences in the *Mealtime Participation Guide* (Klein & Morris, 1999).

■ Examine the child's preferences in food and liquid. When a child dislikes a food, often it is because of its sensory properties (e.g., texture, taste, temperature, smell). When these properties are perceived as unpleasant, noxious, or threatening, they may elicit greater changes in postural tone, more delayed or limiting mouth movements, gagging, spitting, or vomiting. When a child likes a food, usually its sensory properties support the child's needs and abilities.

⊕ It is possible for every feeding therapist and parent to approach a child's likes and dislikes with an attitude of discovery and learning. Patterns can emerge that enable adults to know more about the child's abilities and needs for feeding.

■ If the child creates a great deal of mucus or saliva and has difficulty handling secretions, explore the effect of specific foods on the amount, frequency, and thickness of the mucus.

⊕ Consider eliminating milk from the diet for a week to observe for differences. Milk increases mucus production for some children. Many children who have swallowing problems do not handle milk well. When dairy products are eliminated from the diet, other foods that are high in calcium should be increased.

⊕ Clear meat juices or homemade broth often cut through mucus and help the child to handle it.

⊕ Carbonated drinks sometimes are effective in clearing mucus from the throat. However, the sugar and chemical content of commercial sodas makes them inappropriate for frequent use. Sparkling mineral water can be given plain or mixed with a small amount of fruit juice for flavor.

⊕ Sweet foods and drinks tend to create more saliva. Consider reducing the intake of sweet foods if the child drools.

■ Children with oral defensiveness may reject very warm or very cold foods. Temperature extremes also may be uncomfortable for children with dental problems. Tooth decay, cavities, or metal fillings cause the teeth to be more sensitive to temperature. Refer the child for dental examination and care. If teeth must be filled, ask the dentist to consider using a substance that does not create discomfort with heat and cold. Explore every child's response to temperature differences in food.

Aspiration

◉ Identify and reduce the impact of gastroesophageal reflux and its role in the child's aspiration.

Possible Activities

🅰 Work with the child's physician to identify and reduce gastroesophageal reflux. Aspiration of refluxed stomach contents can occur long after a regular meal. This causes greater damage to the lungs than aspiration of food and liquid that is swallowed. See Chapter 22 for a discussion about gastroesophageal reflux and its treatment.

◉ Identify and reduce the impact of the aspiration of food and liquid into the airway.

Possible Activities

🅰 Prepare the child for a videofluoroscopic swallow study following the guidelines provided in Chapter 8.

🅰 Use diagnostic testing to identify the safest consistencies, amounts, and positions for feeding.

🅰 Limit the amount of food and liquid used in therapy. Develop greater oral motor coordination using nonfood strategies for improving oral function.

Gagging

◉ Identify the type of gag and reasons for the child's gagging.

Possible Activities

🅰 Carefully observe the child, environment, and situations in which gagging occurs.

🅰 Consider which of the following types of gagging are present.

✠ ***Coordination and Timing Gagging.*** Some children have difficulty organizing the food or liquid into a bolus for swallowing. The child may be unable to clear all of the food from the mouth. A portion remains on the back of the tongue in the area that triggers a normal gag reflex.

✠ ***Hypersensitivity Gagging.*** The normally protective gag reflex is overresponsive. It may seem to have "moved forward" as it is triggered by touch or food on the front of the tongue or lips. The hypersensitive gag reaction can come from an inconsistent or hyperreactive sensory system, reactions to certain medications, and a history of gastrointestinal disorders, such as gastroesophageal reflux. In all of these situations, the food passing across the lips, tongue, or pharynx causes the gagging reaction.

✠ ***Mucous Gagging.*** When a child produces thick mucus, it may become lodged in the nasopharynx or oropharynx, where it can trigger coughing or gagging. Many children discover that gagging actually dislodges the mucus and results in greater comfort. This type of gagging often occurs in the early morning or after a nap when the lack of movement results in more post-nasal drip and greater accumulation of mucus. It also is more frequent in children who do not receive adequate water in their diet.

✠ ***Structural Gagging.*** The structurally based gag usually looks different from a hypersensitivity gag initially. Often, the child can swallow the food texture, but gags or vomits after the food has gone partway down the esophagus. If a structural problem is suspected, an upper GI series will rule out the stricture.

- ✥ *Communication Gagging.* Sometimes children use gagging as a powerful communication tool. If children do not feel that their voice or body language is heard as they communicate a dislike for certain food types or textures, or if they feel ignored as they try to indicate fullness, they may clamp the mouth shut, push away the food, spit it out, or, finally gag or vomit to get the adult's attention.

- ✥ *Emotional Gagging.* Some children gag as a physiological response to the real or perceived emotional stress of mealtimes. Emotionally based gagging can occur from the stress of the mealtime interactions. It may develop from a history of negative oral experiences. Emotionally based gagging develops over time. Eventually, it can occur at the sight or smell of food.

- ✥ *Combination Gagging.* Frequently, gagging starts out with a specific cause such as sensory hypersensitivity, gastroesophageal reflux, or an early choking episode on a particular food texture. It easily can turn into an emotional response, which evolves out of fear of new or uncertain oral experiences. The child may see the parent's reaction and then learn to gag, or even vomit, to elicit parental attention or emphasize a refusal to eat. All children seem to go through a stage of trying to be independent and checking out the rules in attempts to be powerful and independent. Children who have a history that includes gagging or vomiting for physiological or sensory reasons have gagging in their repertoire of behavioral options.

A Rule out a structural basis for the gagging if there is any possibility of a stricture. The timing of the gagging will provide the clues for this referral. An upper GI, or barium swallow study, is used in ruling out these esophageal problems. If an esophageal stricture is discovered, a gastroenterologist or pediatric surgeon will treat it.

A Build a trusting relationship with the child. Support the child's knowledge that gagging does not have to be used to communicate. Incorporate ideas from the Trust section on page 423.

A Focus on the development of use of the mouth for pleasure and discovery without gagging. Incorporate the generalized and discriminative mouthing activities described in the Combined Oral Sensorimotor Control: Mouthing section page 441.

A Use the taste, texture, and temperature continuums for introducing new foods as described in Food Transitions: Sensory Transitions on page 481.

A Help the child develop the ability to organize a bolus and use a clearing swallow to clean the mouth. Use techniques that reduce the limiting patterns of the jaw, tongue, lips, and cheeks, as well as those that facilitate a more normal sucking or chewing pattern. Direct attention to the role of the cheeks in forming the bolus and preventing food particles.

A Use a binder food if the child has major difficulty with dry foods or those with discrete lumps. Alternate bites of hard, lumpy food with a clearing spoonful of a food that will bind together the loose pieces and form a more efficient bolus. Applesauce, strained or blenderized fruits or vegetables, and cranberry sauce are good binders. Teach the child to ask for spoonfuls of the binder food before eating food pieces that are uncomfortable or may cause gagging. As the child develops skill in chewing and swallowing, he will need the binder food less often.

A Reduce the gag reflex that is part of a hyperreaction to sensory input by following the guidelines in Hyperreaction: Bodily Sensory Input on page 419.

A A *gag distraction* approach can be effective. Select a distraction such as looking the other way, singing, or showing a toy or a book to the child. When the child gags, focus attention on the distraction rather than on the gag. In this way, the child learns to control the gag independently without undue adult attention directed toward it.

A Increase the amount of water in the child's diet in order to thin any mucus and reduce the amount of thicker mucus that becomes lodged in the child's throat.

A Watch the tilt. Give the child more control over the pace and presentation of food at mealtime. When the child feels some control and can give you permission to put the food in the mouth, the gag reaction can be reduced. The child who opens the mouth and moves forward toward the

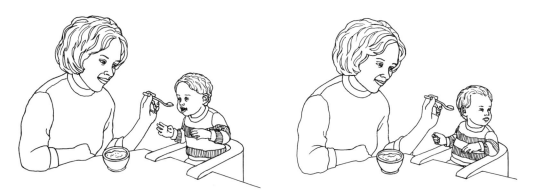

spoon generally is more relaxed and ready than the child who tilts away from the feeder. The child who pulls away as the food is being presented tends to have a stronger, more reactive gag.

A Observe how people in the child's environment react when gagging occurs. Does the gag occur in any predictable pattern that is related to the child's interaction with others? For many children, a gag reflex can serve a major communicative function. The child may be saying, "Get out of my mouth," "I don't like this food," "Please pay attention to me rather than the television," or "You can't make me do this." How does the child respond if you verbalize what you believe the child is trying to communicate? For example, say, "Johnny says, 'Yuck! I hate corn! Please Mommy, don't make me eat this'." Often, simply hearing a message that reflects the inner feelings will diminish the power of the gag. It also opens the lines of communication to negotiate whether it is necessary to eat the corn.

A Gagging and vomiting create discomfort for adults in the environment. Their continued attention to this behavior gives the child an arena for attention and control. If you suspect that the child is using gagging to get attention or engage others in a power struggle, explore some of the following ideas:

✤ Remove attention from the child when gagging begins. After determining that the child is physically safe, briefly leave the room. If it is inappropriate to leave the room, have a magazine or book available during the feeding session and focus on reading rather than on the child. Balance this procedure with touching the child's mouth when food is present, to give warmth and attention.

✤ When you feel yourself becoming angry or irritated from the gagging, say, "I must stop feeding you because it is hard to feed someone who is gagging. You can stay here and gag and vomit if you like. I am going into the living room to listen to music. I will be back in a while to continue the meal if you feel like eating more later." Give all of your messages as **_I messages_**. Let the child know what you want and how you are going to find what you want. This is very different from the **_you messages_** that tell the child what to do.

✤ Children who have a disability often feel very powerless. Gagging can become a way to assert a normal need to have some control over life. Find other ways in which the child can make choices and feel more in control. The child can choose which of two bowls or spoons to eat from or which food or drink to begin with.

✤ When the child vomits as part of the gag, this can be handled in a casual, matter-of-fact way. Clean it up without comment. Ask the child to help you clean up the mess if he is physically able to do so.

✤ Other ideas for dealing with attention and power behaviors are presented in *Children: The Challenge* by Dreikurs and Stoltz (1964).

✤ These ideas are helpful in reducing gagging and vomiting when you suspect that attention-getting or power are part of the picture. Your own reactions will let you know what purposes the behavior serves for the child. When attention is an issue, you usually feel irritated at the child. The child may stop gagging for a while and begin it again as soon as your attention is on something else. When a power contest is involved, you generally feel angry with the child for gagging. The child usually ignores requests to stop. Sometimes the child will stop briefly and then increase the amount of gagging.

🄰 Create an environment of warm acceptance for the child. Recognize that previous negative experiences associated with oral stimulation and feeding may have created strong emotional memories. Take time to help the child develop positive associations with the mouth. Initiate changes slowly. Allow the child to set the pace and create the timetable for moving on. Chapters 14 and 23 contain many suggestions for incorporating these concepts in the program.

Gastroesophageal Reflux

⊙ Reduce the impact of gastroesophageal reflux on the child's mealtime comfort and interest in eating.

Possible Activities

🄰 Work with the child's physician to identify and reduce gastroesophageal reflux.

🄰 See Chapter 22 for a discussion about gastroesophageal reflux, its treatment, and suggestions for management within the feeding program.

Retching

⊙ Reduce the impact of gastroesophageal reflux on the child's mealtime comfort and interest in eating.

Possible Activities

🄰 Work with the child's physician to identify and reduce retching.

🄰 See Chapter 22 for a discussion about retching, its treatment, and suggestions for management within the feeding program.

Mouth Stuffing

⊙ Identify why the child stuffs the mouth.

Possible Activities

🄰 Carefully observe the child, environment, and situations in which mouth stuffing occurs.

🄰 Consider which of the following types of mouth stuffing are present.

　✛ **Developmental.** As children approach the age of 24 months, they discover the amazing size of their mouth. A seemingly endless amount of food fits in the space, and their new ability to keep the lips tightly closed against pressure from the inside seems like a miracle. This leads parents to remind them to finish what is in the mouth before taking another bite. Once the sense of sensorimotor discovery and adventure has worn off, children return to more reasonably sized mouthfuls.

　✛ **Sensory.** When the mouth is fully stuffed with food, children obtain more sensory information about the boundaries of their mouths and the presence of food in the mouth. This often happens when oral sensation is reduced. The child may have a low level of awareness of the inside dimensions of the mouth and the feeling of food. The stuffing wakes up the mouth and helps the child know that there is still food in the mouth. Unpredictable movement of the food can be very uncomfortable when children experience oral sensory defensiveness. Many children with oral tactile defensiveness also stuff the mouth because it reduces the random tactile input to the cheeks when smaller pieces of food are moved around.

♦ **Oral Motor Control.** Mouth stuffing can occur when a child has difficulty using skillful tongue movements for chewing. Movements may be uncoordinated or limited in direction or strength. When there is a great deal of food in the mouth, a very small amount of tongue movement will push some food to the side for chewing. Smaller pieces require much more control of movement.

⊙ Increase the child's sensory awareness and comfort of smaller mouthfuls of food.

Possible Activities

🅰 Use foods that are spicy, crunchy, cold, or carbonated to wake up the mouth before the meal, intermittently during the meal, and after the meal. These four sensory inputs help a child become more aware of the mouth and organize oral movement more effectively. You can include foods such as pickles, raw carrots, and spicy dips, or add spices to other foods. The child can sip cold, carbonated mineral water between mouthfuls. Add lemon to the mineral water for extra sensory input if the child will accept it. Add ice to other liquids.

🅰 Have the child chew on ice before and during the meal. This alerts the mouth, but simultaneously reduces discomfort from oral sensory defensiveness.

🅰 Use a small table mirror, and occasionally have the child look at the mouth before taking another bite and at the end of the meal. Help the child learn what an empty mouth looks like and feels like.

🅰 Use a small vibrator massager before the meal to help build more awareness and movement in the tongue, lips, and cheeks.

🅰 Incorporate other appropriate activities from the Sensory Awareness: Face and Mouth section on page 411.

⊙ Increase the child's oral movement and chewing skills for handling of smaller mouthfuls of food.

Possible Activities

🅰 Use a small vibrator before the meal to build muscle tone in the cheeks and tongue if the child has low tone in these areas.

🅰 Brush the sides of the tongue when you brush the teeth. This can help improve tongue lateralization, which is needed for chewing. Use an electric toothbrush if the child will accept it.

🅰 Provide strong or frequent sensory stimulation to the insides of the cheeks. This can be done with a toothbrush or by pushing outward on the inside of the cheeks with your fingers. Chewing is a partnership between the tongue and the cheeks. Often, poor chewing coordination is caused by cheeks that are inactive.

🅰 Incorporate other appropriate activities from Chewing: Lateralization on page 478 and Lip and Cheek Control: Cheek Compression on page 435.

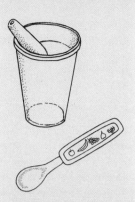

Chapter 18

Feeding Materials for Assessment and Treatment

▦ Choosing Feeding Materials

Selection

The appropriate selection of equipment to support and enhance a child's feeding abilities depends on an understanding of the purpose and selection criteria for each piece of equipment. Within a given equipment category, there are many commercially available and homemade choices for the typical population, as well as the special needs population. There are certain criteria that must be considered when choosing items for an effective feeding program. For example, a spoon that has a shallow bowl will allow the upper lip to remove food with greater ease. A deeper-bowled spoon will be more of a challenge in removing food with the lips, yet may be easier for a child who is learning self-feeding skills. The therapist must determine the appropriate bowl depth when picking a spoon for a child. Additionally, a child with oral hypersensitivity may need a spoon that does not transmit strong temperature sensations. A spoon size appropriate to a school-age child would be inappropriate for an infant because of differences in mouth size and shape. Looking at all the variables is important in choosing feeding equipment.

The challenge facing therapists working with feeding programs is to develop an internal set of criteria for different types of feeding equipment. This will enable them to be astute and informed consumers of available products. It helps to develop a feeding evaluation and therapy kit consisting of a variety of equipment. Therapists vary in their preferences for items to include, according to their experience, the population seen, and personal preferences. When developing the kit, remember that a feeding evaluation is part observation and utilization of utensils by the family, and part exploration of treatment options. To be able to explore several treatment options and make workable recommendations to the family, therapists must include a variety of pacifiers, bottles, cups, spoons, straws, and treatment materials. For example, a feeding kit might contain spoons of different sizes and shapes; bottles of different sizes, shapes, and types of construction; nipples of different shapes, sizes, lengths, and stiffness; pacifiers of different sizes, lengths, shapes, and shield construction; cups of different diameters, sizes, lip construction, and handles; and oral stimulation materials that vary in purpose, texture, shape, size, and stiffness.

Availability

Therapists should have a current purchasing source for each item in the box. Resources for Feeding Materials on page 502 provides a list of vendors and the types of products they carry. Therapists can add to the list or keep their own reference file. On page 505 is a helpful form for organizing feeding resource information. When therapists find equipment that meets the needs of children with feeding problems, it is important for them to give that feedback to the company from which they purchased the item. They can share their experience and enthusiasm for the product and suggest that this information be passed on to the manufacturer. There have been many excellent pieces of equipment that are no longer available. Perhaps if these companies had had extensive, ongoing, positive feedback from therapists and families who had benefited from the products, factors other than economic performance would have been considered and the products would still be available.

Manufacturing and marketing decisions frequently are determined by sales records and novelty. Culture and belief systems heavily determine the design and manufacturing process. Buyers for retail stores and individual customers have a mental image of cups, spoons, and pacifiers that are appropriate for infants and children. These often are related to the type of utensils that they used as children or as parents. For example, in the early 1990s, most of the first cups for young children had two handles, making it more difficult to hold for a child with poor grasp or the use of only one hand. Narrow or tapered cups without handles were rare. With a greater understanding of young children's needs and education of the consumer, a wide variety of narrow, handleless cups are now available. The manufacturing companies that initiated this trend took a risk, because the new products were different from those that buyers and consumers expected.

Marketing decisions play a large role in purchasing decisions. Toys that are designed for infants to put in the mouth when they are cutting teeth have been marketed for generations as **teether toys**. This term has stuck and has not been replaced or alternated with the more descriptive term **mouth toys** or **mouth learning toys**. Most parents of typically developing infants do not perceive the learning that takes place through the mouth with the toys that they purchase for their infants. A new term would create a much broader understanding of children's oral sensorimotor development, yet many companies do not want to promote or use a term that could jeopardize their sales.

Companies that manufacture and market products designed for the typical infant and child market make many key decisions based on total sales. If a product sells well over many years, it may continue to be available to many generations of families. More typically, a new product sells well for several years because it is novel or is associated with a current favorite television show or child's book. Toys, spoons, cups, and plates with Sesame Street®, Barney®, Batman™, Winnie the Pooh, Blue's Clues, and Teletubbies® have waxed and waned, depending on current child and family culture. When sales of a product begin to go down, the item usually is withdrawn from the market and a new one substituted. If the new item has the same underlying features, small changes in design will make very little difference. However, often the new item does not contain the design features that made it valuable to children with special feeding needs. Some companies continue to manufacture smaller quantities of a specialty item when they know of its value and sales potential to a specifically targeted market such as children with special feeding needs. Items that formerly were available on a more widespread basis with extensive marketing costs may be available to specialty catalogs or professional offices wishing to make bulk purchases. The manufacturer wins in this situation by saving money through reduced marketing. The special-needs consumer wins because the product continues to be available through specific distributors.

Professionals who recognize the needs of children with feeding difficulties also design specialty positioning, play, and feeding products. These products make valuable contributions to feeding therapists, parents, and the children who benefit from them. However, the therapists and other professionals who form small companies to carry their products often have a limited knowledge of business trends and marketing strategies. Financial capital may be available for designing and manufacturing the new product; however, poor business decisions or limited marketing resources may result in financial difficulties that cause a small company to go bankrupt or cease doing business.

Over the years, many items change. New concepts and products become available. Older product lines are discontinued as manufacturers follow trends in the marketplace and discontinue items that are not selling well. Other products disappear from the market as smaller companies go out of business or products imported from other countries are no longer available for a wide variety of reasons. The first edition of *Pre-Feeding Skills* (Klein & Morris, 1987) featured an expanded listing of both general and specific pre-feeding and feeding materials that the authors liked and were using. Many of these products or their manufacturers were unavailable by the end of the first year! In 1999, when the current edition was written, 40 of the 87 products (46%) were unavailable. Of the items that were still on the market, 18 of the 47 products (38%) were generic descriptions such as standard bottles, pre-emie nipples, or blowers and whistles. These are common items that usually are produced over the years by many different manufacturers. Another view of change is seen when looking at the 1999 *Mealtimes* catalog, a specialty resource for oral motor, feeding, and mealtime programs. Out of 40 feeding utensils (e.g., bottles, nipples, cups, spoons, straws), only 10 had been manufactured and were available to consumers in 1987! Seventy-five percent of the items had come onto the market in the intervening 12 years.

Selection Criteria

Choosing an Appropriate Pacifier

Guidelines for Use of a Pacifier

Babies are born with a strong suck and a physiological need to exercise the suck. Sucking provides pleasure as well as nourishment. It also represents the infant's first means of self-quieting. Babies suck their fists and fingers, and can benefit from a dry nipple or pacifier. Therapists should give careful consideration to the way in which a pacifier is used. Some mothers use the pacifier as a plug to keep the baby's mouth closed and quiet. Extensive use of pacifiers can lead to passive children who are happy only when their mouths are full. A pacifier should not be used to distract a child who needs adult attention and involvement. It is not a substitute for parent-child interaction.

A pacifier can be used with any infant who shows a tight suck, no tongue thrust, and enjoyment. If the baby spits it out, thrusts the tongue forward, or bites, use of a pacifier should be questioned because it usually is inappropriate when these behaviors occur. Many toddlers who experience sensory processing difficulties continue to benefit from pacifiers for self-calming and sensory organization.

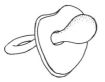 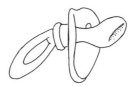 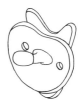

Criteria for an Effective Pacifier

■ The pacifier has an outer shield molded to the shape of the lips to provide sustained contact and stimulation for lip closure.

■ Pacifier shapes and sizes vary. A pacifier must fit the size and shape of the child's mouth.

■ The pacifier provides a thin or narrowed area between the gums for the child who has a jaw thrust or a bite reflex.

■ If the infant has difficulty making sensory transitions, the pacifier chosen should have the same or similar shape as the preferred nipple.

- Some infants are sensitive or allergic to latex. A non-latex pacifier should be selected if infants are in a high-risk group for latex allergies or have identified allergies.
- The pacifier is constructed so that it will not come apart when the baby sucks or chews on it.
- Some pacifiers are modified to allow medicine to flow as the infant sucks. These can be used prescriptively to provide liquid during sucking for infants who are transitioning from pacifier sucking to nipple sucking.

Choosing an Appropriate Nipple

Guidelines for Use of a Nipple

Nipples are chosen for a variety of reasons. Breast-feeding is generally a first choice, though commercially available nipples may be chosen or necessary. Nipples are chosen to provide appropriate and safe nutrition. In some instances, the mother's finger can become an initial "nipple" to stimulate a more active and coordinated sucking pattern.

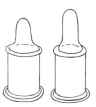   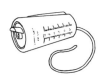

Criteria for an Effective Nipple

- The nipple fits the size and shape of the infant's mouth.
- The nipple flow rate is appropriate for the infant's abilities, the consistency of the liquid being presented, and the infant's feeding position. The holes in the nipple are not artificially enlarged, causing a rapid, uncontrolled flow of liquid. Some nipples feature an adjustable flow rate by turning the orientation of the nipple in the baby's mouth.
- The nipple provides an adequate stiffness or resistance to the individual infant's sucking pattern. A softer nipple may be more appropriate for the infant whose suck is weak or who tends to tire easily. The nipple should not collapse with the infant's sucking.
- The nipple provides a thin or narrowed area between the gums for the infant who has a jaw thrust or a bite reflex.
- Tubing that does not interfere with the nursing process and provides the infant with an additional regulated amount of liquid from a small container assists the liquid flow from the nipple of the breast-feeding mother.
- Thin tubing that attaches to the mother's finger, which is used to stimulate the infant's sucking, facilitates the liquid flow into the infant's mouth.

Choosing an Appropriate Bottle

Guidelines for Use of a Bottle

Though breast-feeding is highly regarded as optimum for babies, many parents make the decision to bottle-feed their own infant because of personal preference, the lifestyle of the parent, and the baby's sucking skills. Initially, parents hold the bottles, then gradually the infant holds them as skill and interest increase.

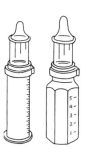 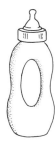 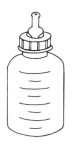 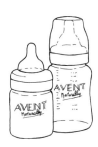 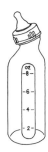

Criteria for an Effective Bottle

- The shape of the bottle supports the head-positioning needs of the infant.
- The bottle holds the appropriate amount of fluid. A bottle that is too small must be refilled during the feeding to provide the correct amount of fluid, disrupting the flow of the feeding process.
- The bottle is easy and pleasing for the infant to hold.
- The bottle fits the size and shape of the feeder's hand.
- The bottle is sturdy and unbreakable.
- The bottle can be colored or decorated to attract and maintain the infant's visual attention.

Choosing an Appropriate Cup

Guidelines for Use of a Cup

Infants indicate readiness for the cup with their eyes, reach, and interest in the cup drinking of others. Cup drinking provides different development challenges from breast-feeding and bottle-feeding. During cup drinking, the infant must move the liquids from the front of the mouth to the back for swallowing. This is in contrast with nursing or bottle usage in which the nipple places the liquid toward the back of the tongue in preparation for swallowing.

Children initially are dependent on adults to hold and guide the cup. Gradually, the child learns to drink from the cup independently. Most children learn to drink from a variety of cups. Some have lids, some are open, some have spouts, and some have a depressed lid and raised cup rim. Each cup style and shape offers different oral motor challenges. Cup drinking takes practice and is messy at first. Parents may prefer to choose cups that involve the least amount of spillage.

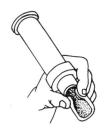 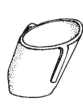 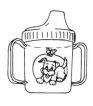 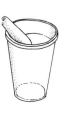 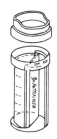 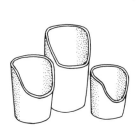

Criteria for an Effective Cup

- The cup can be tipped to get liquid at the bottom without tipping the child's head back.
- The cup does not shatter or break if the child bites the edge.
- The cup gives the feeder a clear view of the child's mouth.
- The cup provides a thick or rolled lip for extra stability if the child needs to hold the edge of the cup with the teeth.

- The cup provides a mechanism for graded control of the liquid flow for the child whose ability to handle a larger volume of liquid is poor.
- The cup is easy to hold and regulate liquid flow when held by an adult.
- The cup provides an appropriate physical shape and an appropriate means of holding for the child who is a self-feeder.
- The cup is colored or decorated when it is used specifically to attract and maintain the child's attention.
- The cup meets the need for success for both the child and parent. Many parents view a reduction in spilling as very important to the success of cup drinking.

Choosing an Appropriate Straw

Guidelines for Use of a Straw

Children must be developmentally ready to use a straw. Initially, children try to suck from the straw as they did the bottle. Straws provide different oral motor challenges from bottles and cups. Straw drinking can offer a greater level of independence in self-feeding for the physically challenged child.

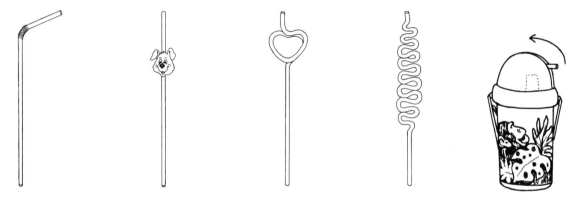

Criteria for an Effective Straw

- The straw can be tall, short, narrow, or wide, depending on the child's sucking skills.
- The straw can be cut, bent, or adjusted to teach a mature straw-drinking pattern.
- The straw does not shatter or break if the child chews or bites it.
- The straw can be used with other adaptive equipment to provide support or control for the lips.
- The straw provides a mechanism for graded control of the liquid flow for the child whose ability to handle a larger volume of liquid is poor.
- The straw can be used while sitting at the table or when the child is in the car seat or stroller. Travel straws included with cups that have lids reduce spillage and are important considerations for parents.

Choosing an Appropriate Spoon

Spoons provide the most important way to introduce children to pureed foods. However, these are not the only alternative. Fingers and mouthing toys also can provide an initial method of presentation of these foods.

Infants must be maturationally ready for pureed foods. Generally physicians recommend a developmental age of 4 to 6 months. Infants initially are fed by the feeder and gradually take over the process of feeding themselves with a spoon. Spoon feeding takes practice and can be messy at first.

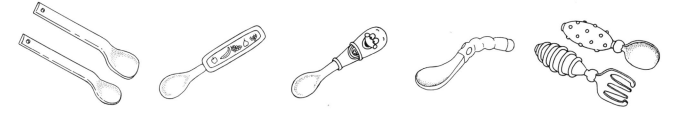

Criteria for an Effective Spoon

- The bowl is relatively flat so that food can be removed easily by the upper lip.
- The spoon does not shatter or break if the child bites it.
- The bowl fits the size of the child's mouth.
- Metal spoons are covered, coated, or have a plastic bowl for the child who is hypersensitive to temperature or taste or has a bite reflex.
- The length of the handle is appropriate for the feeder's hand for dependent feeding and appropriate for the child's hand for independent feeding.
- The spoon can fit into an adaptive handle for holding assistance when necessary.
- The spoon is interesting to the child who is learning independent spoon feeding. Color and design can attract and maintain the child's attention.
- The spoon is the appropriate weight for the child's independent feeding needs.
- The spoon has a pleasing texture for the child to hold.

Choosing Appropriate Oral-Facial Stimulation Materials

Guidelines for the Use of Oral-Facial Stimulation Materials

The oral-facial stimulation materials should satisfy one or more of the following purposes:
- stimulate a more active sucking pattern
- reduce hypersensitivity in the mouth
- reduce the strength of the tonic bite reflex
- increase acceptance of objects coming toward the face
- increase the amount of oral experience and exploration so the child will obtain better tongue, lip, and jaw movements for feeding and sound play
- increase oral organization

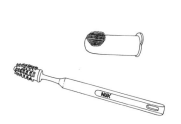 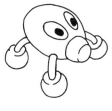 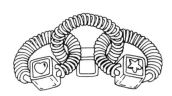 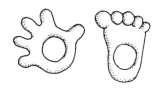

- The materials meet the general criteria for product safety. They are constructed of nontoxic materials and do not contain small parts that could come off in the mouth.
- The materials can withstand the physical stress of biting and mouthing.
- Any materials that are given to a child to explore without direct adult supervision must be constructed of materials that will not jab, poke, or injure the mouth or eyes.
- The materials can be easily cleaned and disinfected if used with more than one child.
- The materials are easy for the adult to use.
- The materials are constructed to withstand daily use.
- The materials promote oral-skill development appropriate to the child's needs and developmental level.

Resources for Feeding Materials

The following companies supply many of the feeding materials that the authors use in their programs. The sources and addresses for representative materials are correct as of May 2000. These are companies that have been in business for many years, and the authors anticipate that they still will be providing feeding and oral motor materials to consumers when you read this book. The majority of them market primarily through catalogs or the Internet. If a therapist is looking for a particular type of feeding material or specific product, he or she should contact one of these companies.

Ali-Med
297 High Street
Dedham, MA 02026
800-225-2610
http://www.alimed.com

Ali-Med has specialty catalogs for pediatrics and dysphagia. It carries a wide variety of books related to swallowing disorders and a selection of cups, spoons, and dishes from different manufacturers.

Children's Medical Ventures, Inc.
541 Main Street
South Weymouth, MA 02190
800-377-3449
http://www.childmed.com

Children's Medical Ventures specializes in designing and selling products for premature infants and babies. It carries a variety of simple positioning equipment for use in the NICU. Its unique pacifier line includes the Wee Thumbie,

Wee Soother, Soother, and Super Soother, which fit the mouths of prematures and other small infants. A variety of other catalogs also carry these products.

Equipment Shop
P.O. Box 33
Bedford, MA 01730
800-525-7681

The Equipment Shop manufactures the Flexi-Cut Cups and Maroon Spoons, which they sell directly to consumers as well as to stores and catalogs. They also carry therapy balls and a variety of toys and feeding equipment from other companies.

Kaplan
P.O. Box 609
Lewisville, NC 27023-0609
800-334-2014
http://catalog.kaplanco.com

Kaplan has a series of catalogs that provide equipment and materials for early childhood and special education needs. Kaplan's Concepts for Exceptional Children catalog carries a selection of general therapy materials for children with special needs, including a small selection of spoons, cups, and dishes.

Lact-Aid® International Inc.

P.O. Box 1066
Athens, TN 37371-1066
423-744-9090
http://www.lact-aid.com

Lact-Aid International manufacturers and sells the Lact-Aid Nursing Trainer System for breast-feeding mothers.

Maddak Inc.

P.O. Box 10894
Newark, NJ 07193
973-628-7600
http://www.maddak.com

Maddak's Ableware catalog provides an extensive source of aids for daily living. Although the majority of the products are geared toward adults, they have many feeding-related items (e.g., spoons, cups, dishes) that are appropriate for children.

Medela

1101 Corporate Dr.
McHenry, IL 60050
800-435-8316
http://www.medela.com

Medela is a leading manufacturer and supplier of equipment to support breast-feeding. Many of the products are highly supportive of infants and young children with sucking and swallowing difficulties. These include the Haberman Feeders, Hazelbaker™ FingerFeeder, Baby Cup, SoftFeeder, and Supplemental Nursing System.

New Visions—Mealtimes

1124 Roberts Mountain Road
Faber, VA 22938
800-606-3665, 804-361-2285
http://www.new-vis.com

New Visions' Mealtimes catalog is an exclusive provider of materials for oral motor, feeding, and mealtime programs. The current catalog lists most of the items mentioned in this book,

including mouth toys, toothbrushes, pacifiers, bottles, nipples, cups, straws, spoons, dishes, bibs, pillows, and other simple positioning equipment. In addition, the catalog carries books, videotapes, and a wide selection of music for mealtime programs.

One Step Ahead

P.O. Box 517
Lake Bluff, IL 60044
800-274-8440
http://www.onestepahead.com

The One Step Ahead catalog carries a variety of toys and daily living equipment for infants and toddlers. It has a continuously updated section of toys and feeding equipment to meet the needs of young children. The items include high chairs, booster seats, utensils, dishes, and food-preparation supplies.

Professional Development Programs

14398 N. 59th Street
Oak Park Heights, MN 55082
651-439-8865
http://www.pdppro.com

P.D.P. Products specializes in products that address the needs of children with sensory-integration disorders. It carries a series of infant and toddler toys, as well as toys for oral motor development. These include a large supply of blow toys and whistles.

Puppets That Swallow

9002 Stoneleigh Court
Fairfax, VA 22031
703-280-5070
http://www.playfulpuppets.com

Puppets That Swallow makes and sells a wide variety of hand puppets with a slit for swallowing in the back of the mouth.

The Right Start

5388 Sterling Center Drive, Unit C
Westlake Village, CA 91361
800-548-8531
http://www.rightstart.com

The Right Start catalog carries a wide selection of toys and daily living equipment for infants and toddlers. It has a continuously updated section of toys and feeding equipment to meet the needs of young children.

Sammons Preston

AbilityOne Corporation
4 Sammons Ct.
Bolingbrook, IL 60440
800-323-5547
http://www.sammonspreston.com

The Sammons Preston catalog carries general rehabilitation equipment and materials. It has a wide selection of specialty spoons, cups, and dishes for adults with feeding difficulties. Many items are appropriate for older children.

Therapro

225 Arlington Street
Framingham, MA 01702-8723
800-257-5376
http://www.theraproducts.com

Therapro offers an extensive catalog for therapists that features a large selection of daily living aids such as bowls, dishes, cups, and utensils.

Therapy Skill Builders®

555 Academic Court
San Antonio, TX 78283
800-211-8378
http://www.tpcweb.com

The Therapy Skill Builders' catalog carries many books that support the development of movement, sensory processing, and feeding. In addition, it has a small number of cups, spoons, and other materials to support feeding programs.

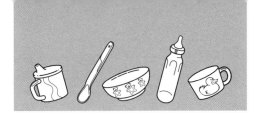

Feeding Equipment Resource Information

Date _____

Item _____

Source _____

Source address _____

_____

_____

_____

Source phone _____

Source fax _____

Source email/web site URL _____

Comments/Considerations _____

_____

_____

_____

_____

_____

_____

_____

_____

_____

_____

_____

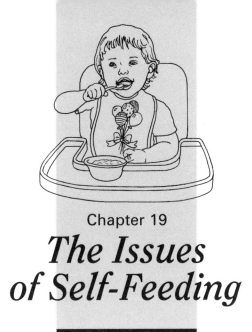

Chapter 19

The Issues of Self-Feeding

As infants and young children have positive experiences with foods and increasing opportunities to watch others eat, they begin to show signs of readiness for self-feeding that emerge as a process between infancy and toddlerhood (Gesell & Ilg, 1937). Older infants take more and more responsibility for the pace of the meal and the foods they eat. They demonstrate stronger preferences. Toddlers are psychologically and socially focusing on independence. The "do it myself" attitude often strongly dominates toddlers' mealtimes and gives the parents a strong indication of self-feeding readiness and a demand for independence.

Readiness for Self-Feeding

Children who are ready for self-feeding usually demonstrate a number of signs beginning in infancy. Developmentally they are

- **Anticipation.** The child shows anticipation of the next bite, opening his mouth, leaning forward, or otherwise letting the feeder know, "I want that food."
- **Eagerness and enjoyment.** The child is an eager participant in the mealtime process. The child paces the meal and communicates interest in the meal physically and socially. The child seems to enjoy the meal. Children who enjoy eating seem to show earlier interest in self-feeding.
- **Preferences.** The child shows food preferences, giving the parent clear messages about which foods he wants and does not want. These preferences can change from day to day.
- **Mouthing.** Children mouth their fingers and toys once they learn to bring their hands to their mouths and can grasp objects. They practice directing objects into the mouth and not into the nose or the ear! This is a helpful skill for self-feeding. They also practice putting their mouths around toys of different shapes and textures. They learn to work the hands with the lips, jaw, and tongue in these endeavors. Repetitive mouthing of objects helps refine the hand-to-mouth motion necessary for self-feeding with fingers and spoons.
- **Play with the food.** The child enjoys playing with the food. He or she may finger paint with it, touch and squish it, and smear it in his or her hair. This is how the child actively explores the food. Playing with food gives children opportunities to check it out as well as practice reaching, grasping, and releasing it.
- **Reach for the spoon.** The child reaches for the food, spoon, and cup, attempting to bring them to the mouth. This reaching is often the clearest sign that the children want to feed themselves.

This is often the time when parents give children their own spoons while they continue to feed them. The child's spoon gives her the opportunity to practice coordination for self-feeding while the parent provides a steady stream of nourishment.

■ **Do it myself.** The child initially reaches for the spoon and plays with it, sometimes getting the spoon and food in the mouth and sometimes in the ear! Sometimes the child becomes more interested in mouthing the spoon handle. It takes practice. The child's initial curiosity about the spoon can quickly turn into a demand to "do it myself." Children who are happy playing with their own spoons as their parents feed them may begin to refuse any food given by an adult as they express a preference for trying to do it themselves.

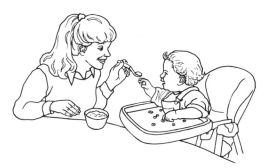

■ Learning Self-Feeding

Bottle-Feeding

Infants are born with the oral motor readiness to suck and swallow with the strength and coordination needed for survival. Their reflex development at birth serves as a foundation for mature skill acquisition. In contrast, the arms and hands are not developmentally ready at birth to actively participate in the feeding process. Children need to observe, imitate, and practice independent feeding skills as their motor skills mature.

Developmental Sequence

At 3 months, infants bring one or both hands to the mouth voluntarily while lying on the back. During the early months, they place their fingers in the mouth when lying on the tummy with the hand close to the turned head. The increased ability to bring their hands to the mouth in supine enables infants to use hand-to-mouth activities as a means of self-calming. By 3½ months, they not only recognize the bottle visually but also respond to it with active changes in movement. This anticipatory response is seen in facial expression, vocalization, sucking motions of the mouth, and the kicking or swinging of the legs and arms. By 4 months, babies can bring an object placed in the hand to the mouth with greater purposefulness and consistency.

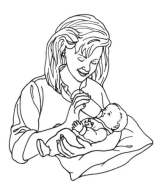

By 4 to 5 months, infants have begun to develop the shoulder control and stability they need for voluntary, direct, reaching movements. They begin to pat the bottle with one or both hands. The many hours spent in a prone position, lifting the head, turning it from side to side, and shifting their weight from elbow to elbow have contributed to the improvement in shoulder girdle stability. With this new steadiness, babies can place both hands on the bottle by the age of 4½ months.

Between 4 and 5 months of age, infants increase the amount of time they spend reaching in prone. Some infants are not given the opportunity to develop these prone-lying skills that contribute to shoulder girdle stability and weight shifting. As a result, some of their gross motor developmental skills lag behind those of other infants during the first year (Davis et al., 1998). The effect of this delay on hand skills and self-feeding has not been studied.

When infants spend time in prone, they explore varying degrees of elbow flexion and lift their bodies on extended arms. They spend a great deal of time rolling from prone to the side between 4 and 6 months of age. These weight changes help refine the reach-and-grasp control that results in the ability to independently hold a bottle by 5½ to 6 months. Although babies of this age can hold the bottle, their actual practice in holding the bottle varies. Some feeders continue to hold the bottle during the close togetherness time the parent and baby have established as their mealtime. Other feeders willingly allow the baby to hold the bottle while they hold the baby closely. Still other feeders give the baby the bottle for independent holding while the baby is in bed or in an infant seat. Many parents use a combination of these. Pediatricians, however, are increasingly discouraging babies from lying supine during bottle feeding because of the increased likelihood of ear infections. Therefore, the practice of handing the baby the bottle to hold independently in supine tends to be discouraged. Most babies are held by the feeder for bottle feedings, with the parent holding the bottle. This often reduces their opportunities to learn to hold the bottle.

When considering a baby's developmental skills, it is important to look at the overall picture. Does the baby have the opportunity to hold the bottle? Does the baby have the physical skills to bring the arms and hands to the midline? Does the baby have the ability to organize the hands on the bottle? Do not become too worried when infants do not hold the bottle if they can bring their hands to the bottle and hold it when the parent lets go of it.

Children vary in the age at which they are willing to discard the bottle. Some children give up the breast or bottle spontaneously as they gain skills with the cup. Others drink from a cup at mealtime and continue to want the bottle during naps, at bedtime, and during times of stress. Stressful situations such as illness, separation from parents, introduction to a new baby-sitter, or the birth of a baby brother or sister can become easier for the child with the organizing support of sucking from the bottle or breast. Remember that nonfeeding functions of the early sucking pattern can help organize behavior. Despite individual variations, most children give up the bottle by 18 to 24 months in favor of cup drinking.

Bottle Variations

Some children are not interested in holding the bottle independently. Others lack the physical skills to make the necessary forward arm movements. A number of commercial and homemade options are available to increase the child's independent ability to hold the bottle.

- **Diameter.** Commercially available bottles vary, with narrow and wide diameters. Wider bottles make it easy for the baby to rest both hands comfortably on the bottle. The infant does not need the added control required to bring the hands closer to the midline. The smaller diameter bottles hold less formula and are lighter in weight. They often work well for premature infants with tiny hands as well as for infants who hold the bottle with one hand.

- **Height.** There are tall and short bottles. The taller bottles often hold more liquid and are heavier when full. Many babies can hold the decreased weight of the filled shorter bottle before they have the strength to hold a taller, more filled bottle.

- **Shape.** There are a number of different angle-necked bottles, with different angles and angle designs. There are 2-, 4-, and 8-ounce bottles in various designs. Often, the angle neck is used to prevent the air intake that contributes to colic and to help the baby attain an easier chin-tuck position during sucking. These bottles tend to work best when the feeder holds the bottle. It is difficult for babies to put the nipple in the mouth with the correct orientation. They tend to rotate the bottle so that they either get no formula or must turn the head awkwardly to enhance the flow.

In addition to the angle necks on many bottles, there are other variations in shape that are more conducive to self-feeding. There are bottles with a cut-out middle, making the sides into handles. There are round-handled bottles that require less effort for the baby to bring his or her hands toward the midline. These handle variations sometimes give children extra help as they grasp the bottle with their little fingers. Novelty bottles shaped like cartoon characters, sport balls, and other creative shapes are designed for the parent's enjoyment. The infant will have the opportunity to hold and touch different shapes and angles while attempting self-feeding. Some of the shapes make bottle holding easier while others make it much more complicated.

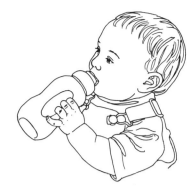

■ **Color and design.** This is the age of color and design in baby equipment. There are different solid-colored bottles and bottles with a multitude of colored designs and characters. The parents seem to enjoy the humor and bottle variety, and the infants seem to be attracted to the colors. Although babies have fed themselves for generations with clear bottles, the colorful designer bottles add interest to self-feeding.

■ **Bottle holders.** Some infants may benefit from a homemade bottle holder, which provides small, lateral handles that are easily grasped by little fingers. For many children, this is the amount of extra help they need for independent bottle holding. To make a bottle holder:

1. Cut an X in the middle of a plastic margarine container lid.

2. Mark four handhold spots.

3. Cut out the four handholds. Wind yarn through the holes to cover the outer portion of each handle.

4. Put the bottle through the X in the center of the holder. Now the child can hold the bottle by the handles.

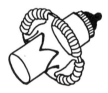

   Plastic margarine container lids come in different sizes. Large lids can be used initially if the child is having difficulty bringing the hands to the midline. Gradually move to smaller lids as the child's skills improve.

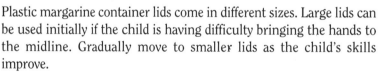

Facilitation of Bottle Holding

The way a baby is held can enhance or discourage bottle holding. Generally, the adult should bring both of the baby's arms forward during bottle-feeding. The baby's hands then can be placed on the bottle or on the feeder's fingers holding the bottle at the midline. This helps the baby feel that she is a more active part of the feeding. It gently encourages the baby positionally to hold the bottle and promotes a good head and neck position for swallowing. Babies who are held with one arm behind the feeder's back or with the arms spread out to the side do not have the opportunity to discover that they can bring their hands forward to help hold the bottle.

When babies have tighter muscles, it is more effective to gently push the elbows forward to place the hands on the bottle rather than pull the hands forward. When the therapist facilitates the movement from the shoulders and upper arms, he is working with the body's natural flow of movement. Most of the limiting tension and resistance to forward movement that prevents a child from bringing the arms forward independently originates in the shoulder girdle. Gently pushing the elbows and upper arms forward helps stop or break up this limiting pattern of tone and movement. When the therapist pulls the hands and lower arms, he must work against limiting pulls in the shoulder girdle.

This requires more effort and makes it difficult for the child to assist. It also is easier to reduce or fade assistance when it is given at the elbows.

Finger-Feeding

By 3½ months of age, infants visually recognize food or the bottle. This recognition, paired with the emergence of skilled hand-to-mouth activity, sets the foundation for finger-feeding. Babies begin to grasp objects placed in the hand and then discover that they don't have to wait for someone to give them what they want; they can reach for it and take it themselves. Parents often give their 5- to 6-month-old infants a teething toy to soothe swollen gums. Hard baby cookies also are introduced at this time. Babies quickly learn to mouth and gum these cookies, enjoying the sensation picked up by sensors in the emerging teeth. In the process, they also learn that certain textured, colored objects have taste and make a wonderful mess. With their new ability to bring hard cookies to the mouth, babies get ample practice in developing jaw control as well as tongue and lip mobility. This occurs long before they have the oral control to chew lumps of cookie or other foods.

By 6½ to 7 months of age, babies can feed themselves a cracker. An important developmental milestone has made self-feeding possible. When babies can sit independently, they no longer need to use their hands for support. Their arms and hands are free to tackle the job of learning to self-feed. They can concentrate on the excitement of stuffing the mouth with crackers and cookies.

By the age of 9 months, babies have developed more functional finger-feeding skills. The high chair provides security. Improved weight shift and balance abilities make it possible to wiggle and shift weight to find and explore food on the tray. Reach usually is unilateral and direct. The grasp is beginning to be more precise. Babies can use their thumb to rake food into the palm of the hand (a radial-palmar grasp). Gradually, this is refined into a raking or pinching movement of the extended thumb and index finger (an inferior pincer grasp). These children now have the grasp needed to tackle smaller pieces of food. Dry cereal pieces, peas, cheese squares, and macaroni are added to their self-fed diet. They also have improved their release skills, and they are able to use a straight or extended wrist when releasing larger food pieces. At this stage, smaller pieces of food provide a greater challenge, and release is clumsier. With practice and continued maturation of hand skills, finger-feeding abilities will improve (Erhardt, 1993).

Postural Support for Finger-Feeding

A child must have sufficient sitting balance to finger-feed. If the child is not well supported, her hands will not be free for the fine motor skill of self-feeding. If the child does not have adequate independent sitting balance, consider adapting the sitting situation to create a stable support. A high chair usually provides the front-back support to free up the arms and hands for the task of finger-feeding. Sometimes the child also needs side support. A couple of pillows, towel rolls, or favorite stuffed toys placed on the side can solve the problem. A different chair, extra cushions, or pads of rolled towels can provide the base of support that enables the child to develop a functional grasp with release of the food into a hungry mouth. Older, more physically challenged children may need further postural support with head supports, lateral trunk supports, or seat belts.

Finger Foods

At the finger-feeding stage, children are motivated to bring everything to the mouth. Feeders need to be sure that the finger foods presented provide pleasure and success so that the child wants to practice this important skill. The types of foods presented can help or hinder the success of finger-feeding. Along with interest in finger-feeding comes an emerging refinement in fine motor skills.

- **Handle foods.** Children will have success initially with large foods such as a bagel or hard baby cookie. The size allows for easier grasp, and no release is necessary. These foods are hard to break off and require sustained and varied hand-to-mouth skills. The hand, wrist, arm, and mouth must work together. Tinier pieces of food are difficult to grasp and place in the mouth. When a piece of cereal or a raisin becomes lost in the grasp, there is no tangible reward for bringing the hand and food to the mouth. Strips of food (e.g., a cookie, soft toast or bread, soft steamed vegetables such as cauliflower or broccoli flowerets) are large enough for the child to hold while providing a free end to stuff into the mouth.

- **Finger practice foods.** Dried cereals often are presented as first finger foods because they tend to melt when mixed with saliva. Often, parents place these directly into the child's mouth. Once parents know that the child can handle this texture and size of food orally, they let the child "chase" the food around the tray with the fingers. This offers the child opportunities to develop the use of isolated fingers and to refine oral movements. The child gradually learns to handle small pieces of other foods. Smaller cookie pieces, diced cooked fruits and vegetables, soft cheese, and bread give the child the chance to practice isolation of the thumb and fingers for a more refined grasp. These foods tend to be motivating enough for many children to stick with this task and move toward mastery. With time, the child is ready for different shapes and sizes, which provide many different reach, grasp, and release opportunities.

- **"Meltable" foods.** Foods such as dried and puffed cereals, cookies, crackers, and breads easily mix with saliva, therefore "melting" in the mouth. When mixed with saliva, they turn into an easily swallowed bolus.

- **"Squishable" foods.** Very ripe or canned fruits, cooked or canned vegetables, cooked pastas, and canned food-consistency foods are easily squished between the tongue and the palate. They provide flavor, nutritional variety, and the opportunity for tongue play without high risk for choking or gagging.

- **Safe foods.** Children should not be given foods that are round and similar in size to the airway because of possible choking and aspiration if the child loses oral control (Byard et al., 1996). Avoid whole grapes, nuts, popcorn, and hot dogs cut in circles. Grapes and hot dogs can be given to the young child if they are cut in smaller pieces or strips. Nuts and popcorn should not be given until well after the child's second birthday. This is an important time to keep a watchful eye as the child learns to coordinate arm and finger skills while refining oral motor skills.

Independent Spoon Feeding

As young children practice holding the bottle to drink and then learn to sit and finger-feed, they are preparing for the next step—spoon feeding. At first, children show interest in the spoon as another toy. They hold it, bang it, and mouth it at about 9 months of age. If food happens to be on the spoon and survives the shaking, banging, or tapping, the child may get a taste while mouthing the spoon. At this stage in development, children are learning to imitate sounds, movements, and games. If shown how to stir a spoon in the cup at the age of 9 months, they can imitate the action. They are interested in the process of taking the spoon to the mouth, and they grab at the spoon while being fed. They want to do everything themselves. Between 12 and 14 months of age, children bring filled spoons to the mouth. Because they don't yet have the coordination to rotate the wrist efficiently, they are apt to extend the wrist and turn the spoon over en route to the mouth. The ability to control lateral movements of the wrist comes several months later, making it possible to get most of the food into the mouth without spilling it.

During this stage, children are still learning to coordinate the combined action of the shoulder, elbow, and wrist needed for smoothly graded movement. To provide the needed stability, they lean or rest the arm or elbow against the body or chair. This proximal stability, provided externally by the environment, enables them to practice the more skilled distal movements of the forearm, wrist, and fingers. The importance of stability for mobility is primary. Most awkward maneuvers can be explained as lack of proximal control or as an early attempt to provide it through arm and body position. The arm may rest against the trunk as the forearm moves to the mouth. The arm may be abducted, with the upper arm held in an exaggerated position parallel to the floor. Children may even lock or "fix" the shoulder in this position to provide the stability they need to bring the grasped spoon and forearm toward the mouth.

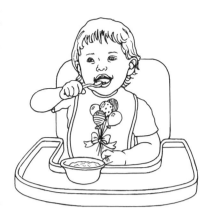

Practice improves these skills. Gradually, children develop more fluidity in movement. By the age of 15 to 18 months, usually they can scoop food and bring it to the mouth. When the spoon reaches the mouth, a child of this age generally turns it over to dump the food onto the tongue rather than clearing it off with the lips. There is still some spilling, but it is substantially less than it was at 12 months of age.

By 24 months of age, children can hold the spoon or fork for scooping and bring it to the mouth with the wrist supinated into a palm-up position. Before this, they tended to bring the spoon to the mouth with the palm down. This lack of supination was responsible for much of the food hitting the lap rather than the mouth. The child now has the control to use the top lip to remove food from the spoon as it enters the mouth.

At the age of 30 to 36 months, children show greater curiosity about utensils. They are adventurous with a fork and will use it to stab food. They try to serve themselves liquids and family-style portions of food. Independence continues to emerge as skills mature.

"Spoonable" Foods

Foods used for introduction to the spoon can influence the child's initial success and feeling of accomplishment. Foods that stick to the spoon help the child experience greater success while he or she develops and refines wrist control. Some foods are easy to use a spoon with and can provide early success. They include puddings, yogurt, oatmeal, creamed wheat or rice cereal, mashed white or sweet potatoes, refried beans, Spanish rice, and macaroni and cheese.

Soups and cereals with milk (common spoon foods) provide major challenges to the beginner. The child's inability to control lateral movements of the wrist while using the spoon causes liquids or foods such as corn or peas to fall off easily.

Children can be creative when faced with a reasonable feeding challenge. Often, they pick up food with their fingers and place it on the spoon. They may bring the spoon to the mouth with one hand while stabilizing the spoon with the other hand.

Bowl and Spoon Options in Spoon Feeding

A bowl or plate with a raised edge gives the beginning feeder something to scoop against. This helps the child focus on getting food onto the spoon and eliminates pushing food out of the bowl and onto the table.

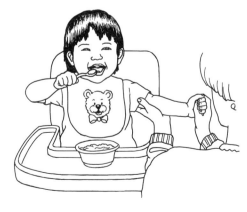

Children who are just learning eye-hand coordination and wrist control need short spoons. Spoon bowl shape, handle length, and handle shape should be considered when choosing a spoon.

The spoon bowl can be deep or flat. A flat shape makes it easier for the child to use the upper lip to remove food from the spoon. However, a slightly deeper spoon bowl may be more successful for the self-feeder. Food does not fall out of a deeper spoon bowl as easily as it does from a flat bowl. The spoon bowl can be round, laterally widened, or elongated like an adult teaspoon.

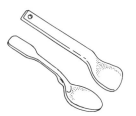 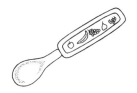 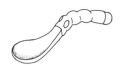 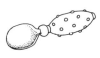

The child's degree of lateral wrist control should be considered when selecting a bowl. The beginner who has limited wrist stability may have an easier time with a laterally widened or round bowl. Some spoon bowls are bent at angles with the handle to provide a more direct approach to the mouth.

Handle length and shape can make a difference in early self-feeding success. The longer the handle, the more coordination required to bring the bowl of the spoon or fork into the mouth. In general, beginners need a short handle that makes the utensil a slight extension of their hand. Spoon handles come in various shapes and widths. Wider shapes may help the beginner or a child who has poor motor coordination. Little fingers often have an easier time holding a wider handle because it gives the child more physical contact with the spoon and provides a more stable grasp. Uneven shapes are available with cartoon character or other creative designs. These help some children and confuse others. Extra-wide shapes or shapes specially constructed for those with physical disabilities are available. Each is designed to facilitate success at a different skill level. An uneven shape may keep the spoon from tipping over. Specially constructed, prescriptive shapes may help the child move from a gross grasp to a more refined or mature palm-up grasp.

See Chapter 19 for a list of resources for specialty feeding equipment.

Teaching Self-Feeding With a Spoon

There are many ways to physically assist the beginner with spoon feeding. Sighted children learn about this process by watching others use a spoon and then imitating them. Most first attempts at spoon feeding are awkward as coordination to bring the grasped spoon to the mouth improves. Children usually have not yet developed the refined wrist control that they need to bring the filled spoon to the mouth smoothly, accurately, and consistently. Food may spill as the spoon is brought to the mouth. The spoon may miss the mouth, and the food may decorate the face. Feeders may need to look at the spoon, spoon bowl, and food consistency to be sure they provide optimum success. In addition, some physical support may be necessary.

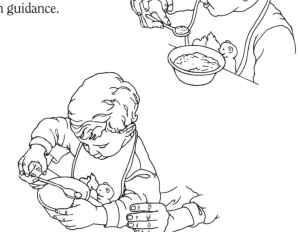

▪ The child can hold onto the feeder's hand as the spoon is brought to the mouth to provide minimum guidance.

▪ The child can hold the spoon as the feeder holds the end of the spoon.

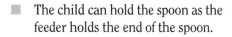

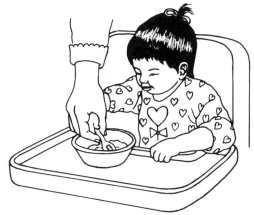

- The feeder can hold the child's hand on the spoon.

- A **utility handhold** can be used to help children who
are having difficulty because of physical and mental challenges. In this method, the feeder holds
the spoon in the child's palm by holding one finger on the spoon in the child's palm and the
thumb on the back of the child's wrist. This keeps the wrist in
hyperextension and assists the action of the child's fingers.
The feeder should not have his or her finger on the back of the
child's hand because this does not provide as much support
for wrist extension and suggests finger extension to the child.
Finger extension is not what is needed; finger flexion on the
spoon is the desired response! This utility handhold method is
preferable to holding the child's hand on the spoon because it
draws the child's sensory attention to the spoon in the palm
rather than feeling the feeder's hand over the back of the
child's hand. When the feeder holds his or her hand on the
child's hand, the child feels the feeder doing most of the work.
It is more difficult to fade assistance. The utility handhold
enables the child to assume more of the process more easily.

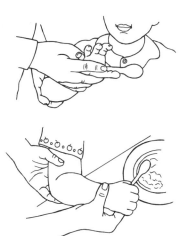

- When teaching tool or utensil use, the feeder can use ***backward chaining*** to help the child succeed. Backward or reverse chaining is a good step-by-step
learning tool based on Skinner's Law of Chaining. When using this type of instruction, the
adult provides assistance until the last step of the sequence is reached (Hagopian, Farrell, &
Amari, 1996; Wilson, Reid, Phillips, & Burgio, 1984). The child performs the last step independently, thereby successfully completing the task. The final behavior needed for the task is taught
first, and the initial behavior is taught last. This is how the name ***backward chaining*** is derived.
When teaching spoon use by this method, the adult helps the child scoop and bring the spoon
up toward the mouth. The child is responsible for bringing the spoon into the mouth and
removing the food. When the child is able to complete this step, a new one is added to the child's
responsibilities. The adult may continue to assist with the scooping process, but the child is
always allowed to bring the spoon to the mouth independently. Gradually, the feeder fades assistance as the child assumes more of the task. This concept and
process continues until the child is able to perform the entire
sequence independently.

- The child often experiences the best success when the feeder
helps him bring the elbow up to shoulder height after the food
has been scooped from the bowl. This exaggerated movement
of the elbow and shoulder (i.e., ***elbow exaggeration***) is similar
to movements seen in young children who are learning to use
a spoon. Children quickly discover that when they lift their
elbow to shoulder height, they spill less food from the spoon.
When they begin to use a spoon, they are still developing
refined control of the wrist. To manage the spoon, children
often lock the wrist in extension. If they hold their arm at the

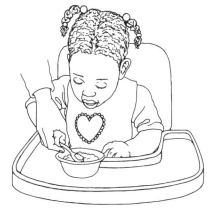

side of their trunk and lock the wrist in extension, the spoon tips over on the way to the mouth, spilling the contents. When they raise their elbow, the locked wrist directs the spoon right at the mouth, resulting in much more success. As children gain wrist control, they relax their arm at their side.

▓ A utility handhold with backward chaining and elbow exaggeration would proceed as follows:

1. The feeder helps the child scoop the food by moving the child's hand and spoon into the bowl. Many children benefit from using an exaggerated tap to the bottom of the bowl. This helps them reach the bottom of the bowl and get food on the spoon. Otherwise, many children scoop air instead of food! When the spoon is filled, the feeder helps the child direct the spoon all to the mouth, exaggerating the movement of the elbow to about shoulder height.

2. The feeder then helps the child scoop and bring the filled spoon halfway to the mouth, letting the child bring the filled spoon the rest of the way to the mouth. The feeder provides elbow support as needed as the child's hand independently brings the spoon to the mouth.

3. Next, the feeder helps the child scoop allowing the child to bring the filled spoon from the bowl to the mouth. The feeder may give gentle elbow support if the child needs it.

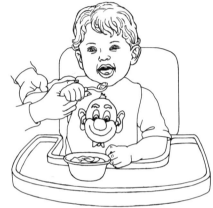

4. The feeder then gives a prompt toward the bowl for scooping because the child knows the process. The feeder may need to provide a little elbow support until the child gains the wrist control to accurately direct the spoon to the mouth.

   In this method, the feeder helps the child at the hand and elbow only as much as needed for success. The goal is for the child to take over independently, succeeding in the entire spoon feeding process.

Independent Cup Drinking

By the time infants can hold the bottle independently and bring everything possible into the mouth, they grab for an adult's cup or can of soda. Parents naturally take cues of interest from the child, and usually they playfully give the child a taste. The first taste is drooled or dribbled down the chin while the baby suckles the rim as if it were a bottle or approaches it with uncontrolled up-down jaw movements. The rapid flow of liquid from this new source may be poorly coordinated with breathing, resulting in a cough or splutter. By the age of 6 months, infants have a clearer interest in drinking from a cup that is held for them. They show beginning awareness that an object of this shape contains a liquid, and they reach toward it with the intent of getting a drink. Between 6 and 12 months of age, children play with cup drinking with much experimentation and spills.

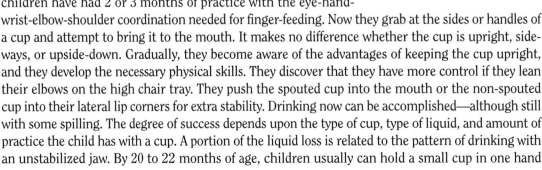

By the first birthday, sitting balance is well established and children have had 2 or 3 months of practice with the eye-hand-wrist-elbow-shoulder coordination needed for finger-feeding. Now they grab at the sides or handles of a cup and attempt to bring it to the mouth. It makes no difference whether the cup is upright, sideways, or upside-down. Gradually, they become aware of the advantages of keeping the cup upright, and they develop the necessary physical skills. They discover that they have more control if they lean their elbows on the high chair tray. They push the spouted cup into the mouth or the non-spouted cup into their lateral lip corners for extra stability. Drinking now can be accomplished—although still with some spilling. The degree of success depends upon the type of cup, type of liquid, and amount of practice the child has with a cup. A portion of the liquid loss is related to the pattern of drinking with an unstabilized jaw. By 20 to 22 months of age, children usually can hold a small cup in one hand while drinking with little liquid loss. The reduction in spills is a function of skills in self-feeding and the establishment of greater jaw stability that enables more precise lip control of the liquid. Skill in cup drinking continues to be refined, culminating in the emerging ability to pour liquids from a small container at 2½ years of age.

Teaching Cup Drinking

Picking the right liquid and cup and providing needed physical support are keys to success in cup drinking. Critical to success in this mealtime skill is jaw stability. The child must be able to hold the jaw open and quiet so that the lips can control the flow of liquid into the mouth. Many parents place a hand under the child's chin to provide extra jaw support. This helps beginning cup drinkers who lose considerable liquid as they chew on the cup with the wide jaw excursions of underdeveloped jaw stability. Some older, physically challenged children also need this support.

To succeed at cup drinking, children tend to push the cup into the lateral cheek corners. This gives them additional stability, allowing for more activity at the central lips in drawing in liquid and reducing spills from the lip corners. When helping coordination with cup drinking, be aware of the need for cup placement into the lateral lip corners. This provides external stability initially until the child has enough lateral lip control to provide that stability internally.

Types of Liquid

When teaching a child to use a cup, be sure the child likes the liquids used. Strained fruits or vegetables mixed with a little liquid can be offered to the infant at the age of 6 or 7 months. These represent enjoyable, familiar tastes. Thickened liquids in an open cup offer an excellent way to begin teaching cup-drinking skills as they flow slowly to the rim of the cup and are more easily controlled by the feeder. Because they move out of the cup more slowly, they are easier for the child to collect in the mouth. Using thickened liquids helps children learn to use an active suck to draw the liquid into the mouth. Thin liquids often are poured or dribbled into the infant's mouth from the spouted cup, offering babies limited opportunities to develop drinking skills. Babies who learn in this way often continue to tip the cup and slightly hyperextend the head to dump liquid into the mouth.

Older infants and children who have delays and physical disabilities also will benefit from the use of thickened liquids. More appropriate consistencies and tastes should be selected. These can include milk shakes, blended smoothies, applesauce diluted with other liquids, gazpacho, or fruits and vegetables that have been liquefied in a blender.

Cups should be filled with liquid to enable children to tip the cup slightly and drink without moving the head and neck into hyperextension. When very small amounts of liquid are placed in the cup, the child's tendency to tip the head back is increased, and liquid often is poured in without sucking.

Cup Variations

The most important criterion for cup size is that the cup fit the child's mouth. The size and shape of the cup rim needs to promote optimum lip closure, lateral lip and cheek control, and jaw stability. Cups with a small diameter often are easier to use than those with a large diameter. However, a wide diameter with a rolled rim often provides an optimum opportunity for jaw stabilization and subsequent improvements in lip and cheek control.

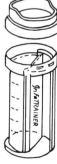

Many cup types are available for teaching cup-drinking skills. Parents and therapists can choose from among those with or without lids, with or without spouts, and a regular or a controlled flow. Cups come with no handles, one handle, or two handles. They also can be clear or opaque.

Parents often prefer lids that decrease some of the beginning cup drinker's mess. These lids also reduce mess when the child explores the art of throwing a cup. The feeder must decide whether to use a lid with or without a spout. The nonspout lid provides a learning situation that is closer to the lip and tongue control needed to drink from a regular cup. The child's mouth feels the edge of the cup and begins to learn the control that will be needed when the lid is removed.

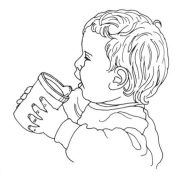

It is more efficient to move directly to the cup rim without using a spout. When a learning spout is provided, the child treats it as if it were a nipple, continuing the coordination patterns that are familiar from the bottle or breast. Many children become stuck at this stage and have greater difficulty moving on to the cup rim. Some children seem to need the familiarity provided by the spout. When spouted cups are selected, the feeder must evaluate the specific characteristics of the cup in relation to the child's current needs. Some cups have a wide spout that gives more support and fills the corners of the mouth, while others have a narrow spout that enables the child to develop more active lip control. Some spouts are angled diagonally from the top of the lid, while others are perpendicular to the lid. Some are long; others are short. Some are made of hard plastic; others are made of a soft silicone that is similar to the bottle nipple. A child who is having difficulty transitioning from the bottle to the cup may do well with a lid that has a soft spout. A child with low tone and exaggerated tongue protrusion may suck with the tongue inside the mouth when using a firm spout that places downward pressure on the tongue. Each type of cup must be considered in relation to the child's needs.

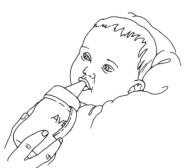

The decision to use a cup with handles depends on the child's physical abilities and needs at a particular stage in cup usage. For most children without handicaps, the presence or absence of handles makes little difference. Some children have more success using narrow, child-hand-sized cups without handles. Others rely on the handles to keep a firmer grasp on the cup. The handles can provide more security and a higher level of confidence that the grasp won't be lost. Children with a hemiplegia may find that they can assist more consistently if their involved hand is placed on the handle of a one-handled cup while their less involved hand holds the cup directly. Cups with two handles can be problematic for some children. The uneven lifting with double handles increases the difficulty instead of the independence of cup drinking. For others, the double handles used at snacktime inspire the weaker hand to help out in a motivating activity.

Some children are more successful with the improved proprioceptive feedback provided by weighted cups. Some commercial cups are weighted to allow the cup to right itself when put down. The creative feeder can use his or her imagination to provide weight for stabilization. For example, airplane-modeling clay can be put on the bottom of a specialty cup for added weight. Using modeling clay also helps keep a regular cup or glass from sliding.

Clear cups or those with cutout sides make it easier for the feeder to help the child regulate the amount of liquid flowing into the mouth. Brightly colored, opaque cups provide visual interest, but neither the feeder nor child can see the liquid flowing toward the rim of the glass. As a result, the child may suck and receive very little liquid or be flooded with liquid that moves rapidly into the spout and mouth when the cup is tipped.

All children should have guided experience drinking from non-spouted cups. Although intermittent opportunities are offered when the child reaches for the adult's glass, many parents and therapists avoid giving children cups without lids because of the risk of spilling. It is much easier for children to develop stabilized jaw control when they have extensive experience drinking from an open cup or glass.

Straw Drinking

It is difficult to determine specifically when children develop straw drinking skills. On many developmental checklists, the skill is included by age 2. In Morris' longitudinal study of six normal infants (1978), none had straw drinking experience at 15 months of age. Each child was given a straw, and they were shown how to get liquid through it. Within 5 minutes, all six children were drinking proficiently through a straw. During a small cross-sectional study (Morris, 1994), all the children between 8 and 28 months of age were able to drink from the straw. Thus, experience plays a major role. Parents vary when they introduce a straw. Some do not offer a straw until the child's second birthday. Many others give the baby a straw when they eat in a restaurant that provides straws for other members of the family. In addition, many infants move directly from cups with thin, narrow spouts to straws with juice boxes and sport bottles. These culturally based patterns tend to introduce children to this type of drinking at an earlier age.

Initially, straw drinking is accomplished by drawing several inches of straw into the mouth, curling the tongue around it, and using a suckling motion to create enough pressure to obtain the liquid. As the child matures, the tongue flattens, the jaw reduces its excursion, and the lips and cheeks play a major role in creating negative pressure that pulls the liquid up the straw. The child no longer bites the straw and is able to drink successfully with only a small portion of the straw between the lips.

Personal Exploration

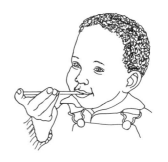

As always, it is helpful to remind yourself of the skills involved through personal experience. Get a straw and something to drink. Drink through the straw as you usually do. Put your fingers where your lips touch the straw. Remove the straw from your mouth. Notice from your finger placement how far forward the straw was in your mouth.

Put the straw in your mouth as if you were a young child with little straw-drinking experience. Take several inches of the straw into your mouth. Curl your tongue around it and suck the liquid. Explore different tongue motions. Slide your tongue backward and forward in the early suckle pattern. Hold your tongue steady, moving it up and down with the jaw in the later developing suck. Notice in both situations how much work your tongue and jaw must do, and how little work the lips contribute to the sucking.

Teaching Straw Drinking

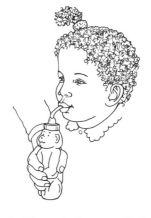

Many parents teach their child to drink from the straw by putting the straw into a glass of liquid and then putting a finger over the top of the straw. This creates a pressure that holds some of the liquid in the bottom of the straw. When the parent lifts the straw from the glass and puts the bottom end in the child's mouth, the liquid drips or flows in. As the child begins to get the idea that there is a desirable liquid in the straw, the angle of the straw can be lowered gradually. The child soon discovers how to close the lips and suck the liquid.

Another approach, usually a homemade option, involves a squeeze bottle made from a soft plastic doll bottle, squeezable mustard bottle, or honey bottle. A Mead Johnson Cleft Palate Nurser™ also can be used. The top of the squeeze bottle should be cut carefully so that a piece of clear plastic aquarium tubing or medical tubing or a flexible standard straw can be pulled through the hole. It is important to cut a small spout. The tubing must fit tightly in the spout so that suction is created. Some of the newer soft ketchup bottles have a cap with a hole the right size for tubing or a straw. Squeezing the bottle makes liquid come up the straw. The teacher can control how much liquid the child gets, how fast the flow arrives, and how often liquid is available for sucking. Some sports water bottles with a firm plastic spout operate on the same principle and work well in helping children learn to actively suck the liquid.

This method enables the feeder to do all the squeezing until the child gradually closes the lips and begins to suck independently. This is another example of the backward-chaining procedure in which the teacher guides the child to success.

Many children initially put their tongue around the straw and put the straw into the mouth and far back on the tongue before sucking. To help the child learn to suck from a straw using greater lip activity, the feeder gradually can place a shorter amount of the straw in the child's mouth. This can be done in a variety of ways.

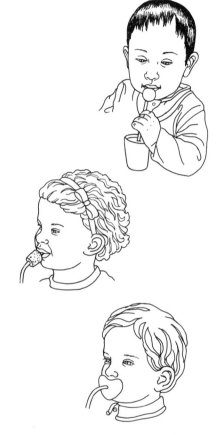

▨ Use a large bead at the end of the straw.

▨ Use a cork with a hole drilled in it. Fit the straw through the hole, allowing only as much straw as you wish to go in the child's mouth. This has the added benefit of providing a flattened surface to press against the lips for increased tactile and proprioceptive feedback.

▨ Mold and shape a piece of a moldable splinting plastic. Fit it over the straw and shape it to the child's lips. Make a hole in the center and regulate the amount of straw that passes through the hole into the child's mouth.

▨ Play and Self-Feeding

Self-feeding requires an extensive array of sensory and postural adjustments, as well as hand and mouth accommodations. Most of these are learned and practiced extensively by the typically developing infant during play (Erhardt, 1993, 1994). Children accommodate their fingers to the shapes of different objects as they reach, grasp, shake, and bang them. They bring them to their mouth for mouthing and teething. They develop sensory awareness in the hands and mouth, as well as interconnections between vision, hand, and mouth skills. These emerging abilities during nonfeeding play support the ability to locate the food the child wishes to pick up, grasp it, and bring it toward the mouth while opening the mouth an appropriate amount. The progression toward the skilled use of spoons, forks, and cups is supported by play activities such as pouring water into different containers in the bathtub, shoveling sand in the sandbox, cutting into pieces of play dough, and engaging in pretend food play with a favorite doll or stuffed animal.

Children with physical challenges often miss many spontaneous stages of play development because of their movement difficulties. They may need extensive assistance to hold toys or grasp and release them. Movements of the hand and toy toward the face for mouthing may be sudden and ungraded, causing the child to avoid this prerequisite for self-feeding. Movement patterns that are needed for self-feeding should be explored and incorporated initially into the child's play. This can become a very realistic self-feeding venture for the child when using the imagination to pretend. For example, the child might dip a gas tank hose (i.e., the finger) into a dish containing super gas (i.e., an empty dish that can be filled with anything in the child's imagination), and then bringing it to the car (i.e., the mouth). When the car is filled with the super gas, the car can fly above the trees! This scenario can be expanded or modified for the child to play with a variety of spoons, cups, dishes, and pretend foods. Learning the required movement patterns during play generally is more successful than in real feeding situations. When food and liquid are involved, the child has the additional challenges of dealing with the food and issues of hunger, spills, and oral manipulation of the food.

Sensory challenges pose a very different set of issues for play. Children who experience tactile defensiveness on the hands avoid touching many types of toys. They particularly may avoid touch to the palms or anything that feels wet or dirty on the hands. They often dislike playing with play dough or smearing finger paint. They may be very uncomfortable with sand play or pouring water. If children gag or experience oral defensiveness when toys are brought to the mouth, they may miss the early hand-to-mouth activities that are precursors of finger-feeding. These children benefit from an overall program to prepare them for better sensory modulation and integration before and during play activities.

Self-Feeding for the Child With Physical Challenges

Readiness

Readiness factors are easily considered with children who have normal muscle tone and motor development. What about the child who shows these readiness factors but lacks the physical skills to move easily into self-feeding? Many children have limits in motor control that make it physically impossible for independent feeding success or cause overflow throughout the body so that posture and oral motor control deteriorate. Therapists may have worked to help a child attain a level of quality in oral motor function only to watch this quality become lost when the child attempts to bring a spoon to the mouth. Following are some options for this common problem.

A child with multiple disabilities may demonstrate some readiness factors but not actually be indicating the need for self-feeding. The mouth opening in anticipation of the next bite may be the child's way of regulating the speed of the mealtime. The child may be saying, "I have swallowed this mouthful and now I am ready for another."

Eagerness to participate in the mealtime can be a demonstration of the child's enjoyment of the feeding process and communication with the feeder. It also may be the child's way of indicating food preferences. The physically involved child may not need to take a spoon in hand to indicate these preferences and participate actively.

Food play and attempts to reach for the food, spoon, or cup are clues that must be explored. Are the child's attempts to bring the cup to the mouth successful? Is sufficient liquid getting to the mouth? What degree of oral motor control does the child have while being fed? Does control deteriorate with self-feeding attempts? Does the child show an overflow of movement and tension that causes frustration during self-feeding attempts? Are you, as a therapist or parent, frustrated with the child's loss of oral motor control during self-feeding attempts? If you believe that the child's oral skills are not in jeopardy, you may encourage the next steps toward self-feeding. However, if you believe that oral skills for feeding and speech may be jeopardized, analyze the readiness factors more carefully.

Who is pushing for self-feeding right now? Is it the child? The parent? The teacher? The therapist? Is the child's interest in reaching for the spoon a way of saying, "I am interested and I want to help some?" Is it a demand to self-feed? Are the mother's questions about her child's mealtime independence a hope for the next developmental steps or a request to spend less time in the feeding process? Is the teacher's urging for independence an unspoken question about the appropriateness of the feeding program? All sides of these questions must be explored, and the pros and cons of all the answers must be weighed. Therapists must question whether the child's need to self-feed is so strong, because of family and peer pressure and his age, that they are willing to give-and-take with the quality of oral motor skills. Can this child's initial attempts at reaching for the cup or spoon be a way of saying, "I want to be a more active participant in this process?" Would it satisfy the child if more choices of cups, food order, and utensils were allowed? Could the child self-feed a cookie at snack time, but continue to be fed at meals in a way that promotes more quality of oral movements?

The goal is for optimum oral motor control in an environment of social acceptance. But as children grow older and become more self-conscious of their disability and their need for independence, it may be more important to let them feed themselves than to insist on precision in oral motor control.

Moving Toward Self-Feeding

As therapists make choices with children and their families that help move them toward independence in feeding, they can suggest strategies to increase children's physical accuracy and control.

1. **Stability.** Stability can increase control. Some children may need to rest their elbows on a wheelchair tray, or the tray height may need to be adjusted to optimize the control needed for drinking from a cup or using a spoon.

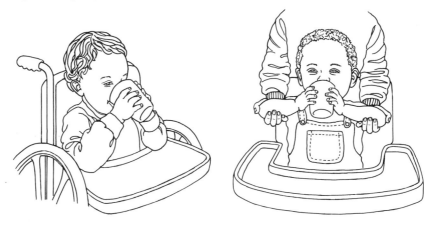

2. **Position.** A change in position can improve oral motor control during self-feeding. Many suggestions in Chapter 15 can improve self-feeding and oral-feeding skills.

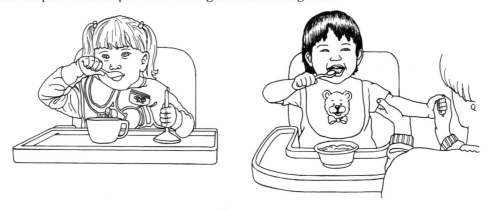

3. **Associated reactions.** Associated reactions usually interfere with self-feeding. Assistance with maintaining a stable non-leading hand can help the child be more accurate with the hand used for eating.

4. **Feeding Utensils.** Feeding utensils should support increased control and independence. Specialized modifications should be made in existing equipment when necessary, and should look the most normal and be age appropriate. Sometimes a lidded cup with a straw can allow independence when an open cup provides only frustration. Children often can be independent using a sports bottle or spouted water bottle while looking like all the other kids!

   A thicker, stickier textured food, a bowl or high-sided plate, and a spoon with an enlarged handle support independent spoon feeding. Some children need more help. Specially designed spoon handles or universal cuffs may make it easier for children to hold a spoon successfully.

5. **Timing.** Timing is important. As physically challenged children are learning to feed themselves, they may need short periods to practice eating favorite foods. The child may need to be fed the full nourishment of a meal by the parent, but can practice self-feeding with a dessert or snack. Sometimes, self-feeding the whole meal creates too much stress and is too fatiguing. The child may want to be independent in public but is quite messy with the spoon. Trying to eat with a spoon in the school cafeteria may be exhausting and extremely frustrating for everyone. The child's physical and social needs could be met by drinking a "power shake" meal from a straw in the cafeteria and eating independently from the spoon during meals at home.

Self-Feeding for the Child With Sensory Challenges

Readiness

Self-feeding is critically important for the child with sensory-based feeding issues. These children have great difficulty regulating the amount and type of input that is acceptable to their sensory system. There is a tremendous amount of variability from day to day and even from moment to moment. Because of the unpredictability of internal readiness to accept and process food in the mouth, many children develop a distrust of adults who feed them. In the early months, this can be reduced or alleviated when parents learn to read the child's readiness cues and allow the child to be the leader in the mealtime dance. However, when children learn to feed themselves, they have full control of what enters the mouth. Many children who are on feeding tubes do not venture into the area of oral feeding until they are able to feed themselves. Developing self-feeding skills often is the key to developing and refining eating and mealtime skills for this group of children.

Movement toward self-feeding may be delayed by tactile defensiveness in the hands. Children may avoid finger-feeding because they don't like the way food feels when they pick it up. They may move into spoon feeding slowly as they withdraw from the sensation of the spoon handle in their palm. Many compensate for this by using the more adult-like hold on the spoon with the thumb and fingers rather than the earlier child's grasp. This, however, offers less initial stability and makes it more difficult for the child to get the spoon to the mouth without spilling food.

Issues of spills and messiness are major deterrents for many children with sensory issues. They may handle a spoon or cup competently, but put it down and lose interest in eating if food gets on the spoon handle or their hands or if they spill liquid. This can become quite a challenge because self-feeding requires practice, and a certain amount of messiness will always be part of the initial stages.

Readiness for these children often is defined by their overall ability to handle sensory input during and after activities that improve sensory processing. Some readiness questions might include:

▓ Does the child use the hands to hold and manipulate a wide variety of toys?

▓ Does the child put fingers or toys to the lips or in the mouth?

▓ Does the child sit at the table and accept the presence of feeding utensils and food?

▓ Is the child interested in watching others eat?

- Is the child interested in spoons, forks, dishes, and cups as playthings?
- Does the child imitate physical actions of mealtime preparation or feeding (e.g., stirring, bringing a spoon to the mouth, feeding another person)?

Moving Toward Self-Feeding

Feeding and mealtimes often are emotionally laden battlefields for children with sensory-based feeding difficulties. They suspect anything involving food to be an ambush from adults to trick them into eating. Movement toward self-feeding must be gradual and come out of the child's comfort and readiness. Most of these children have the physical abilities and internal developmental timetable that support self-feeding. They may hold back because of their sensory discomfort. When steps are taken to reduce or eliminate the discomfort and opportunities are offered gradually, these children generally move easily toward feeding themselves. The following strategies make this journey easier.

- **Sensory preparation.** The guidelines presented in Chapter 14 should be introduced before self-feeding activities.

- **Sensory environment.** Self-feeding incorporates input from most of the senses. Children must attend to and integrate visual, auditory, tactile, proprioceptive, vestibular, olfactory, and gustatory information. Adults can simplify the sensory environment by selecting table mats, dishes, and utensils that are non-distracting. When possible, solid colors that are pleasing to the child should be selected, and dishes and utensils that contain visually complex patterns should be avoided. It is very difficult for some children to perceive pieces of food that are placed on the patterned surface of a dish or mat. Cups or spoons with complex shapes and patterns may be distracting or overwhelming to the child's sensory system.

- **Postural support.** Self-feeding requires stable postural support in the body. Many children with sensory-based feeding issues have marginally low postural tone and poor postural stability. They often hold or fix other parts of the body to obtain stability. The tension that is created as they do this may reduce their precision or accuracy in self-feeding. They may move a spoon too far into the mouth and gag themselves, or tip the cup too far and spill liquid down the chin. These sensory experiences can be upsetting and reduce their desire to feed themselves. In addition, the added tension or movement in the body creates additional sensory input that can contribute to sensory overload.

- **Proprioceptive and tactile input.** Activities providing deep tactile and proprioceptive input to the trunk, arms, and hands during the meal can be very helpful for some of these children. Some children are more aware of their own body when they wear a weighted vest during the meal or when an adult provides intermittent downward pressure to their shoulders. Firm grasp or clapping of the hands during the meal can increase awareness as well as reduce tactile defensiveness for many children.

- **Imitation and touch.** Many children with sensory issues learn to feed themselves more easily through visual guidance and imitation than manual guidance of the hand to the mouth. Often, the touch of an adult's hand is disorienting or disturbing if the child has sensory defensiveness. However, firm touch combined with verbal preparation may be acceptable (i.e., "I'm going to hold your hand and show you how it feels to get the spoon into your mouth easily"). Children who have additional difficulties with imitation and motor planning may need this type of guidance.

- **Utensils.** Children know what does and does not feel comfortable to their hands and mouth. Allow them to select the utensils they prefer by introducing them to play activities before using them to teach self-feeding. Observe the types of surface shapes and textures that the child accepts and avoids. Select two spoons or cups that have appealed to the child during play and ask the child which one she wants to use during the self-feeding session.

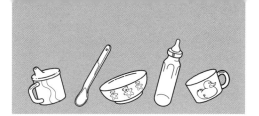

Table 19.1 Developmental Self-Feeding Summary

Developmental Age*	Skill
2 months	Infant brings the hands to the mouth in prone.
3 months	Infant brings the hands to the mouth in supine.
3½ months	Infant visually recognizes food and the bottle.
4 months	Infant pats the bottle with one or both hands. Infant can bring the hand to the mouth while holding an object.
4½ months	Infant holds the bottle with both hands.
5½ months	Infant holds the bottle independently with one or both hands.
5 or 6 months	Infant mouths and gums solid foods such as hard baby cookies.
6 months	Infant drinks from a cup held by an adult.
6½ or 7 months	Infant feeds self a cracker.
9 months	Infant is capable of independent finger-feeding. Infant holds and bangs the spoon.
9½ months	Infant stirs with the spoon in imitation.
12 months	Infant is capable of independent finger-feeding.
12 months	Child holds cup and drinks with some spilling. Child holds the handle of a cup while drinking.
12 to 14 months	Child brings a filled spoon to the mouth, turning the spoon over in the mouth.
15 to 18 months	Child scoops food and brings it to the mouth, spilling some.
18 to 24 months	Child gives up the bottle and drinks just from the cup.
20 to 22 months	Child can hold a small cup in one hand while drinking.
24 months	Child brings a spoon or fork to the mouth with the hand palm up.
30 months	Child can pour liquid from a small container.
31 or 32 months	Child feeds self with little spilling.
30 to 36 months	Child uses a fork to stab food.

*Developmental ages are approximate and may vary with individual children.

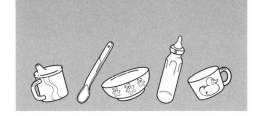

Table 19.2   Bottle-Feeding Summary

Developmental Age*	Skill
2 months	Infant brings the hands to the mouth in prone.
3 months	Infant brings the hands to the mouth in supine.
3½ months	Infant visually recognizes the bottle.
4 months	Infant pats the bottle with one or both hands. Infant can bring the hand to the mouth while holding an object.
4½ months	Infant can hold the bottle with both hands.
5½ months	Infant can hold the bottle independently with one or both hands.
18 to 24 months	Infant gives up the bottle.

*Developmental ages are approximate and may vary with individual children.

Table 19.3   Finger-Feeding Summary

Developmental Age*	Skill
2 months	Infant brings the hands to the mouth in prone.
3 months	Infant brings the hands to the mouth in supine.
3½ months	Infant visually recognizes food and the bottle.
4 months	Infant brings the hands to the mouth while holding an object.
5 or 6 months	Infant mouths and gums solid food such as hard baby cookies.
6½ to 7 months	Infant feeds self a cracker.
9 months	Infant is capable of independent finger-feeding.

*Developmental ages are approximate and may vary with individual children.

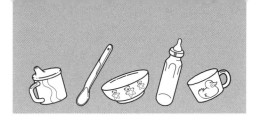

Table 19.4 Spoon and Fork Summary

Developmental Age*	Skill
2 months	Infant brings the hands to the mouth in prone.
3 months	Infant brings the hands to the mouth in supine.
4 months	Infant brings the hands to the mouth while holding an object.
9 months	Infant holds and bangs a spoon.
9½ months	Infant stirs with a spoon in imitation.
12 to 14 months	Child brings a filled spoon to the mouth, turning the spoon over en route to the mouth.
15 to 18 months	Child scoops food and brings the spoon to the mouth, spilling some.
24 months	Child brings a spoon or fork to the mouth with the hand palm up.
31 or 32 months	Child feeds self with little spilling.
30 to 36 months	Child uses a fork to stab food.

*Developmental ages are approximate and may vary with individual children.

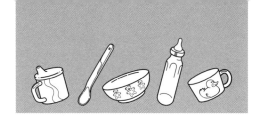

Table 19.5   **Cup Drinking Summary**

Developmental Age*	Skill
6 months	Infant drinks from a cup held by an adult. 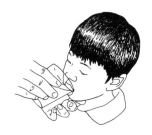
12 months	Child holds a cup and drinks with some spilling. 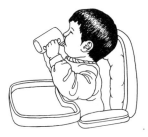
20 to 22 months	Child can hold a small cup in one hand while drinking. 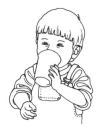
30 months	Child can pour liquid from a small container. 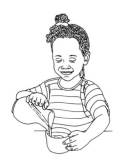

*Developmental ages are approximate and may vary with individual children.

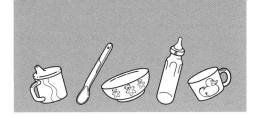

Table 19.6   Cup Drinking Oral Patterns Sequence

Developmental Age* and Oral Patterns

6 months	Child holds a cup and drinks with some spilling. 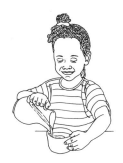
12 months	Sucking pattern Tongue may protrude under the cup. Holds the handle of a cup and drinks with some spilling. 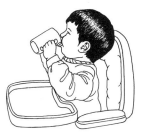
18 months	Sucking pattern External jaw stabilization achieved by biting the edge of the cup. Holds the handle of a cup and drinks with less spilling. 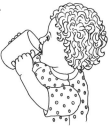
24 months	Sucking pattern Internal jaw stabilization achieved through balanced activity of jaw flexors and extensors Holds small glass with one or both hands; little spillage 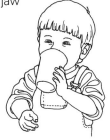

*Developmental ages are approximate and may vary with individual children.

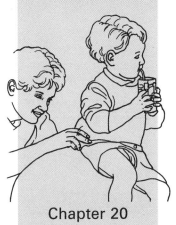

Chapter 20

Feeding and Speech: A Question of Relationships

▪ Parallel Versus Causal Relationships

Feeding and Early Speech Sounds

An ongoing question in the field of communicative disorders concerns whether there is a causal relationship between the motor control used for nonspeech-oral movements such as feeding and that used for speech production. Some scientists and academicians deny the relationship and propose that two control systems are responsible for a separate development of these skills. Their support comes from theoretical models and laboratory studies of neuromotor control that have compared specific muscle timing and coordination for sucking, chewing, and early speech production (Green et al., 1997; Moore & Ruark, 1996; Ruark & Moore, 1997). Their preliminary investigations have suggested that the coordinative organization for speech is distinct from the organization of sucking and chewing. They believe that speech motor control emerges in parallel with other oromotor activities but is not dependent upon feeding and nonspeech oral movements. Other scientists and clinicians believe that the two systems are closely related or operate in a causal fashion (Love, Hagerman, & Taimi, 1980; Marshalla, 1985). Their support comes from research, detailed clinical observations of children with typical and atypical development, and from their interpretation of theoretical models. Irrefutable data are nonexistent to support either view.

It is helpful to examine developmental similarities in the relationship of oral-movement patterns in feeding and speech. A parallel development occurs in the movements and processes considered necessary for speech production and those that occur in the development of feeding skills (Morris, 1985). For example, it is necessary to tighten the cheeks and pull them inward during sucking from the bottle or breast and while moving chewed food from the side to the center of the tongue for swallowing. This creates a central channel for food to pass to the back of the tongue for swallowing. A central grooving of the tongue also supports the oral stage of the swallow. This activation of the cheek muscles increases as the sucking pads diminish and the infant must rely on internal movements of control for stability and precise skills. A similar pattern is required in speech development. The contraction or inward tightening of the cheeks is necessary to direct the airstream forward and prevent lateral air leakage in the production of fricative consonants (/f/, /v/, /sh/, /zh/, /s/, /z/). A spreading and slight grooving of the tongue are needed to create an unobstructed channel for the air. Many other similar or parallel movement patterns exist between feeding and sound production. These include the sustained closure of the lips on the spoon during spoon feeding or on the cup in drinking, and the sustained closure of the lips used in making the bilabial consonant /m/. Tongue-tip elevation is observed during the mature swallow and for cleaning movements used during chewing. A similar elevation of the front of the tongue is predominant in speech development.

There are many similarities between the movements that infants experience during feeding and those that are combined with sound at a slightly later time. The six infants in Morris' longitudinal observation (1978) did not develop the speech movements of tongue-tip elevation (for /t/, /d/, or /n/) or teeth-lower lip (for /f/ or /v/) in their sound play before they appeared in feeding. Generally, the movements that occurred in feeding were refined for babbling and appeared several weeks or months later.

For example, elevation of the tongue tip emerges slowly during feeding as the infant shifts from the early suckle pattern to the up-down tongue action of the suck. This begins around 6 or 7 months of age. The elevated pattern also emerges in the swallow at this age, alternating with the earlier simple tongue protrusion. By the age of 9 months, babies show many instances in which tongue movement is separate from jaw movement, resulting in independent tongue-tip elevation.

Sound production follows a similar sequence, usually lagging behind the feeding patterns by several weeks or months. Most babies seem to increase vocal play and the variety of sounds just after they are introduced to lumpy and soft, mashed foods. The first consonants produced generally are those requiring sustained or intermittent contact of the lips. It is interesting that the sequence *ma-ma* occurs in almost every known language as the baby's symbol for the mother. This refinement of lip contact also is the first feeding movement that reaches a skilled level during nursing and early spoon feeding. By the time the infant is 6 to 9 months old, when babbling emerges and reaches its height, precise lip movements are used to eliminate the loss of liquid during bottle- or breast-feeding, to remove food from the spoon, and to prepare the lower lip for cleaning by the teeth. The same level of skill has not been developed for tongue movement. A backward-forward tongue movement predominates in feeding until the infant is 6 to 9 months of age. There is a gradual shift during this period toward tongue-tip elevation. The emergence of consonants produced by elevating the front of the tongue (/t/, /d/, and /n/) occurs for most babies after they have already produced lip sounds (/m/, /b/, and /p/). Initially, the jaw and tongue move together in saying *dada* or *nah-nah-nah*. Independent upward tongue movement will not occur for many months. Sounds produced with the back of the tongue elevated develop around the same time. It may be necessary for the infant to perceive separate movements of the front and back of the tongue during feeding for this distinction to occur in sound production. Sounds that require greater sophistication and a finer level of motor control (/f/, /v/, /s/, /z/, /sh/, /zh/, /ch/, /j/, /th/, /r/, and /l/) occur much later in the exploration of sound. These require movement patterns that are similar to those refined during the chewing process.

These similarities do not prove that feeding skills are prerequisite to talking. If this were the case, a child who is fed by tube would have no possibility of speaking. We know this is not true. Many children require tube feedings because of medical problems that are not associated with neurological disorders. Although some of these children show a delay in speech and language development, they do learn to talk. Other children with disorders of pharyngeal and esophageal control develop spontaneous speech. Does this imply that there is no relationship between the two skills? Do they indeed follow separate paths of development?

Children With Feeding Problems

These observations of children with normal oral motor control abilities must be balanced with observations of feeding and speech development in children with known oral-control problems. Clinical experience supports the view that when a child experiences difficulty with oral control in feeding, there will be similar oral-control problems in sound production and speech. For example, the child with lip retraction during feeding probably will show the same lip retraction pattern during speech. Moreover, improvements in jaw, tongue, and lip movements in feeding frequently lead to improved acquisition of speech sounds containing similar movements. Children who show dyspraxia of speech often show similar problems and have limited spontaneous experience with motor-planning skills in feeding. Their eating skills frequently are slightly delayed and may show poor refinement. Oral feeding patterns may show delayed development of tongue-tip elevation, poor sensory organization of the food into a bolus, and delayed ability to use the tongue in a refined fashion to clean the teeth or extract food that becomes caught in the cheek pouches.

How may one view these seemingly conflicting observations? The human central nervous system shows a high degree of efficiency and redundancy. The development of a common system to support the initial stages of feeding and early pre-speech development would fit this operational model. Infants move toward speech through an extended period of nonmeaningful sound play. They develop a predictable progression of vegetative noises, cooing, babbling, and jargonning sounds. (Oller, 1978; Stark, 1978a, 1978b; Stark, Bernstein, & Demorest, 1993). Many of the new sounds produced by the developing infant appear to begin with the combination of mouth movements explored during the handling of foods requiring more complex mouth movements (such as chewing) and simple sounds produced at the level of the larynx. Thus, feeding provides many of the motoric building blocks for babbling. Steeve, Moore, Green, and Engel (1999) found a similar pattern of specific muscle contractions and movement patterns of the jaw during chewing and babbling in 9-month-olds. The two patterns began to diverge by the age of 15 months, with babies at that age shifting to a jaw pattern for babbling that was more similar to that found in the speech of older children and adults. The most critical period of sound development for later speech development appears to be that of canonical babbling. This stage is most predominant between 6 and 10 months of age and is characterized by well-formed syllables that are often duplicated (e.g., **ba-ba-ba, di-di, muh-muh**). Oller found that late onset of canonical babbling beyond 10 months can be used as a predictor for identifying children who later will have speech and language delays (Oller, Eilers, Neal, & Cobo-Lewis, 1998; Oller, Eilers, Neal, & Schwartz, 1999).

As the infant develops a need for a set of repeatable movements to symbolize ideas, movements that are familiar and refined through feeding and babbling are selected. The infant has rehearsed the basic movement components of early speech for a year before needing similar articulatory speech movements. This preliminary learning could provide the basis for the speech motor-control system. Clearly, the patterns of coordination used in feeding are not adequate for sophisticated speech production. The requirements for speech motor control increase beyond those required for feeding. Two control systems may emerge sometime during the second year of life.

Feeding per se may not be the magical element that is required for preparation of the initial sensorimotor coordination. Children who have never eaten food orally, yet speak, support this statement. In most instances, these children have engaged in sensory play and exploration with the mouth. Because they have not experienced major motor difficulties, they are free to use the hands and mouth to discover the sensory variations in their world. The tongue, lips, cheeks, and jaw are engaged in the process of sensorimotor differentiation that sets the stage for speech. Thus, the key element may be the opportunity that the child has to develop sensorimotor control and differentiation within the mouth and to build a finely tuned awareness of oral movement. If this opportunity has been present and specific oral motor-control problems do not interfere with development and learning, the patterns needed for speech should be there. Essentially, this is what is observed in tube-fed children who have gastrointestinal, respiratory, or cardiac problems and those experiencing aspiration related to pharyngeal or esophageal mechanisms.

For the typically developing child, feeding provides an oft-repeated stage for learning sensorimotor control and differentiation. If the elements usually associated with feeding can be incorporated frequently into the child's learning, speech movements will be possible without the physical act of eating.

Observing some children who do not follow either of the patterns described has raised another interesting question. A number of children make major changes in their coordination during feeding without evidence of change in their sound production and sound play. A smaller group appears to develop changes in speech sounds without a similar advancement in feeding. Some children with severe sensory defensiveness avoid the more typical, organizing sensory input that comes from mouthing activities and textured foods. Some receive their nutrition through a feeding tube while others continue to eat a diet of liquids and pureed foods. Although babbling often is delayed in these children, they eventually talk despite their lack of external sensory input. Any theory must explain the exceptions as well as the underlying rule. A two-system control mechanism could be supported by these few clinical examples.

Learning is a function of the connections and interconnections made in the brain as new experiences are added. It is possible that the transference of movement patterns from feeding into speech production does not occur automatically but relies on the child's awareness of the potential connection. If feeding is worked on without any exploration or modeling of similar speech sounds, some children experience the *aha* phenomenon that enables them to use a potential pathway to speech. A child who experiences swallowing difficulties or sensory deviations in integrating the many sensations involved in eating solid foods may find it easier to develop higher-level coordinations during speech, which may bypass control areas that are difficult.

These conflicting views provide many implications for feeding programs. Because there is a strong possibility that feeding and speech control systems are related at least during the first year, it is important to include work on oral motor feeding patterns with any child who shows delays or deficits in feeding or nonfeeding oral movements. Yet it is not assured that simply working on feeding will resolve the child's difficulties with speech motor control for articulation. The connections and interconnections of learning must be built into the program.

It is also possible that feeding, sound play, and speech development are interconnected through the development of foundational sensorimotor skills. For example, oral-feeding patterns are highly stereotypic during the first 4 to 6 months of life. During this early period of growth, the primary focus of development is on the infant's postural stability in head and trunk control. Stability is a primary prerequisite for the development of separation of movement and greater mobility of the jaw, tongue, and lips. In their study of infants with Down syndrome, Cobo-Lewis, Oller, Lynch, and Levine (1996) found delayed development yet a similar age of acquisition of rhythmical hand-banging and rhythmical canonical babbling patterns. They suggested that common neuromuscular development and postural behaviors might internally link these rhythmical behaviors.

Work on oral movement patterns through movement, sensory exploration, and the facilitation of sound play is an essential part of the treatment program for any child who is not taking food orally. Sounds for babbling and speech often are possible for a tube-fed child long before the system can support the coordinations required for oral feeding. Because choking and aspiration usually are not a part of oral exploration and vocalization, the child can approach the learning of oral patterns with greater freedom. There also appears to be a reverse interconnection between feeding and sound production in the tube-fed child whose program includes an active exploration of movement for sound play. Although most infants develop the feeding patterns first and generalize their use to sound production, the tube-fed child is likely to learn the primary patterns through stimulation of sound production, and then generalize their use to the manipulation of food and liquids. All of these possibilities can be incorporated into a feeding program.

Asking the Right Questions

A definitive answer to the theoretical questions about the relationship between feeding and speech is not needed to take appropriate clinical action. As therapists work with children who are having difficulty developing the coordination patterns for speech sounds, they initially must observe whether the underlying sensorimotor and oral motor patterns are present.

■ Does the child have the underlying postural support and control for the oral movements used in feeding and speech?

■ Has the child experienced a wide variety of sensory inputs to the mouth through mouthing of the hands, toys, and objects?

■ What type of mouthing has the child engaged in? Has the child moved to the stage of discriminative mouthing? Does the child respond to discriminative sensory input with a wide variety of jaw, lip, and tongue movements?

- Has the child developed jaw stabilization patterns during eating and drinking that would support discrete, rapid movements of the tongue and lips for speech?
- Does the child have the essential movement patterns of the jaw, tongue, and lips during feeding that could be incorporated into speech (i.e., internal jaw stability in a semi-open position, precise lip closure, tongue flattening and grooving, tongue-tip elevation)?

Mealtime and Feeding Strategies

The following general strategies are helpful in providing children with feeding challenges with the underlying skills that lead toward speech.

- **Jaw Stability:** Work on the underlying sensorimotor strategies that support external and internal jaw stability.
- **Sensorimotor Exploration:** Engage the child in sensory exploration with the mouth to provide a wide variety of sensory information that can be used to organize movement. Encourage play and discovery with the lips and tongue to get many combinations of movements as possible.
- **Interconnection Bridges:** Assume that feeding and speech are related but not causal systems. Build bridges between the two. For example, if you are focusing on sustained upper and lower lip closure on the spoon during a snack, provide auditory models of the /m/ consonant that contains the same general movement. Offer comments such as "Mmmmmmm, that's good" or model words such as *more, milk*, or *yummy*.

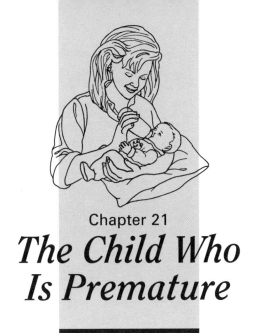

Chapter 21
The Child Who Is Premature

During the past three decades, technology has advanced sufficiently that tinier and tinier premature infants are being saved, with better and better outcomes. Significant advances in medical care have enabled neonatologists to support complicated respiratory and other system needs of these fragile infants. In addition to massive technological changes for these infants, there has been a growing transformation of care within neonatal nurseries. These nurseries are moving to more developmentally supportive, family-centered care—to a partnership with professionals and family that better supports the special relationship between the infant and the family as well as the neurobiological needs of the infant.

A major consideration in discharging a premature infant home to the family is usually the progression to full nipple feeds. Transitioning to nipple feedings is a challenge for the medically fragile and developmentally immature infant who was physiologically not ready to be born. These infants must learn to eat, and parents must learn to feed them before discharge can be considered. Because earlier release from the hospital promotes improved infant-family relationships and reduces the cost of care, early achievement of quality nipple feedings is an important goal. Supportive developmental-care changes in the nurseries have helped to promote and achieve this goal.

Developmentally Supportive Care

The concept of developmentally supportive care in the neonatal intensive care units (NICUs) is based on the Synactive Theory of Development created by Heidelise Als (1982, 1985, 1986, 1998). This approach is based on the premise that infants are active collaborators in their own care and that infant behavior provides the best base from which to design care. It focuses on the importance of the infant-parent relationship in the health and optimum development of the infant. This approach focuses on careful observation and understanding of the neurobehavioral and physiological organization of the infant. These observations form the basis of the Assessment of Preterm Infant Behavior (APIB; Als, 1982) and Neonatal Individualized Developmental Care and Assessment Program (NIDCAP; Als, 1985). They are created on the assumption that infants actively communicate their needs through their behavior. By understanding infant behaviors and responses, caregivers can understand their thresholds for stress and stability. Interventions focus on the preterm infant's self-regulation skills, coping skills, and development. Als' approach looks at how to make the life-saving intensive care nursery a supportive, nurturing environment that enhances the development of the infant and the family. This dramatically influences the early presentation of nutrients, understanding of infant readiness for oral feedings, the introduction of nippling, and parental involvement in feedings.

Feeding in the NICU

Nutrition Continuum for Premature Infants

Preterm infant feedings follow a number of different scenarios along a nutrition continuum from intravenous (IV) to orogastric (OG) to nasogastric (NG) to breast- or bottle-feedings, depending on the infant's medical and developmental needs. Initially, the preterm infant may require considerable medical support and receive initial nutrients intravenously through an umbilical catheter or other IV site. Once the baby's respiration, heart rate, and blood pressure are stabilized and the baby is on full enteral feedings, an orogastric tube may be used. Pumped breast milk or premature baby formula is provided slowly by an OG-tube. The feedings start small and build to full volume, with the IV feedings decreasing simultaneously as the OG feedings increase. The volumes are presented slowly to give the immature gastrointestinal system time to positively respond to the feedings. Immature guts lack the appropriate enzymes necessary for proper digestion. Slow introduction of the milk stimulates the production of these enzymes. Tolerance is monitored carefully so the infant does not develop necrotizing enterocolitis. Babies tolerate introduction of milk differently. Some move more rapidly toward full volume feeds and others take longer to tolerate the stimulation to their gut. The goal is for full feeds to be given through the OG-tube with no supplemental IV nutrients. Full-feed volumes are considered sufficient when the baby can take an average of about 120 kcal/kg per day or can demonstrate an appropriate weight gain. The OG-tube may be placed for each feeding or be indwelling. Some babies transition directly from OG to breast-feedings or bottle-feedings, while others who need more continuous small volume feedings may use the nasogastric tube. Breast-feedings and bottle-feedings are introduced as the baby demonstrates readiness.

Readiness Factors for Nippling

Nippling readiness is determined for each infant and parent based on infant maturation and stability rather than by a developmental sequence that says a baby should be ready to feed at a certain gestational age. Just because an infant is a certain age, such as 32 or 35 weeks, does not mean that he or she is stable enough for oral feedings. In an ideal, developmentally supportive approach, caregivers and parents observe the maturing infant for behavioral signs of stress and stability. Any interventions, including feeding, are contingent on readiness cues. They focus on helping the baby regain and maintain coordination throughout the activity.

Early feedings are introduced slowly. Parents and caregivers learn to observe signs of stability and stress in an infant before, during, and after nippling attempts. This gives them competence and confidence in feeding their infant. They also learn to make appropriate interventions to promote physiologic homeostasis and self-regulation. They are taught to interact with the baby in ways that prevent problems. Intervention is necessary if stability problems occur. By understanding the signs of stability and stress during feeding, the parents and infants will have more success. Sometimes these early feedings are met with success. At other times, infants need to grow and mature before they can be successful.

As defined in a developmentally supportive approach to care, the following self-regulatory behaviors reflect infant stability and readiness for feeding or indicate that an infant is nippling well or positively handling the feeding intervention:

- Stable physiologic systems including smooth and regular respiration, heart rate, and oxygen saturation. The infant's respiration should show no (or minimal) increase in respiratory effort from the baseline established before the feeding. Appropriate autonomic responses should be noted, and visceral indicators of stress should be considered.

- Good optimum color that shows no or minimal change from the baseline established before feeding.
- Good and consistent postural control throughout the body, as well as smooth movements and modulated muscle tone.
- Softly flexed posture.
- Hands that have nice tone and are held near the face or midline.
- Steady awake state.
- Good coordination of the suck-swallow-breathe triad.

The following are some of the behavioral signs of stress that occur during sucking and swallowing attempts. Caregivers need to become skilled at looking for color, state, autonomic function, and general signs of self-regulation. These must be observed regularly before presentation of any feeding or pre-feeding opportunity in order to minimize further stressing the infant. When stress signs are seen during the feeding, the baby is communicating stress and letting the feeder know modifications need to be made.

Color Changes

Often, synchrony in sucking, swallowing, and breathing is not achieved in early attempts to nipple. Or, once achieved, it can be disrupted in these early attempts at breast- or bottle-feeding. Being aware of the infant's color before beginning the feeding enables the feeder to notice subtle color changes during the feeding. An early sign of stress might be a subtle color change. This may occur slowly and be indicative of a steady decline in oxygen saturation. Some babies who feed too rapidly may depend on quick shallow breathing and may need to take deeper periodic breaths. Sudden color changes can occur with breath holding. Sometimes this is due to attempts to hold the breath when there is a fluid buildup around the airway. This can come from poorly organized sucking and swallowing from above the airway or from gastroesophageal reflux below. It is not uncommon for the fluid to trigger a vagal response if fluid is too close to the airway. A drop in heart rate then can be seen.

Change of State

Before initiating a feeding, the feeder must ensure that the baby is quiet, alert, and ready for the meal. This state enables the premature infant to focus on the feeding in a more organized fashion. Some infants will demonstrate rooting responses and more feeding enthusiasm while in this state. When this state changes, the feedings quickly can become disrupted. Though some babies will accelerate from fussiness to crying, more babies will fatigue or shut down. It is important to explore a multitude of reasons for the change in state because the intervention chosen must address the specific reason. For example, fussiness can be caused by anything from hunger to an uncomfortable position or a dirty diaper to desaturating oxygen to complaints about the complicated demands of nippling. Shutting down can be caused by too much exertion, respiratory or cardiac stress, feeding too rapidly, or decreased overall endurance.

Breathing Changes

Breathing effort needs to be observed before a feeding. As the baby engages in the workout called feeding, the rate and depth of breathing, the heart rate, and the shape of the airway change to accommodate the increased demands for oxygen. When there is respiratory compromise, the child's energy goes to support the cardiorespiratory needs and is not as available to support the demands of feeding. Coordination between sucking, swallowing, and breathing can become stressed. Signs of the respiratory compromise may be seen in fatigue, tachypnea, nasal flaring, changes in head position, shallow breathing, or inspiratory stridor.

Problems with swallowing control and timing can result in drooling, gulping, gurgling sounds in the pharynx, needing to swallow several times in succession, and coughing or choking. These problems often are seen in infants who are just learning to take the nipple.

Motor Changes

A common sign of stress in early nipplers may be loss of muscle tone, control, and endurance. This can be seen in the whole body as the arms go flaccid at the sides and the body loses central tone and control. Often it is seen as the mouth drops open in a flaccid gaping position.

Nonnutritive Sucking

Before presentation of the breast or bottle for feeding, premature babies can be offered a finger or pacifier to practice nonnutritive sucking. Clinical observation of nonnutritive sucking can give the caregiver information about the infant's readiness and organization for nipple-feeding. Strength of sucking, including the compression force and the suction or negative pressure, can be felt and observed. The negative-pressure suction will be felt as a resistance to the removal of the finger or pacifier. Autonomic responses and ability to self-regulate during this nonnutritive sucking should be noted. It is common practice to offer a finger or pacifier to an infant during tube feedings and to observe whether the infant attempts to suck. This can give caregivers many clues about readiness for introduction of the breast or bottle. Numerous studies have shown that sucking on the pacifier during tube feedings enhanced the readiness of many infants for oral feedings (Field et al., 1982; Measel & Anderson, 1979).

One commonly used approach is to offer the pacifier during tube feedings first in the comfort and isolation of the Isolette®. Gradually, as the infant can handle it, she may be held in the caregiver's arms. Caregivers should notice whether the infant can handle the tube feedings paired with the pacifier while being held. Gradually, the progression moves toward taking the bottle and breast while being held.

Some infants, however, have difficulty transitioning between the pacifier or finger and the breast or bottle. They, in turn, may have difficulty moving between the bottle and the breast or the breast and the bottle. Many infants have trouble when offered the breast or bottle after using the faster nonnutritive sucking pattern on the finger or pacifier. Many do not make the needed rate change and suck too quickly on the nipple, leading to gulping and then gagging or choking. Practice, however, does seem to help in transitioning between pacifier and breast or bottle.

Common Feeding Complications in Premature Infants

Premature infants may present with a number of complex issues in feeding despite attempts to carefully observe their stability and self-regulatory readiness for feeding interventions. The NIDCAP is used for assessment during feedings. The Neonatal Oral Motor Assessment Scale (NOMAS; Braun & Palmer, 1985; Palmer, 1993; Palmer, Crawley, & Blanco, 1993) also can be helpful in guiding observation of sucking, swallowing, and oral motor skills. The APIB can be helpful in assessing self-regulation, although it is not conducted during feeding. Following are some of the specific issues that complicate feeding in premature infants.

Medical Instability

Often preemies start out medically unstable. They need to be fully stabilized before feedings can be presented. The immature gastrointestinal system requires a very slow introduction to nutrients. Cardiopulmonary problems can contribute to poor coordination and timing of sucking, swallowing, and breathing. Irregularity in respiratory patterns can lead to poorly initiated, dysrhythmical, and inefficient sucking. Coughing, choking, and aspiration can occur with the poor synchrony of breathing.

Neurological Immaturity

The premature infant is neurologically immature. As with any developmental progression, infants vary. Most facilities now watch for the infant's early signs of readiness for introduction of the nipple and let that be their guide. Experience has shown that infants younger than 32 weeks gestation often can achieve the intraoral pressure necessary to influence the flow of milk, but they lose strength and coordination quickly. The 34-week-old not only will sustain longer sucking bursts but usually can swallow more fluid during each suck. This allows an increase in the volume of feeds. Most facilities wait until about 32 weeks, but report more nippling success at closer to 34 weeks gestation. However, babies as young as 32 weeks gestation have demonstrated the ability to coordinate sucking and swallowing in breast-feeding. When offered the bottle, these infants displayed difficulty with respiratory control and frequently demonstrated cyanotic episodes (Meier, 1988). Bu'Lock et al. (1990) reported that sucking, swallowing, and breathing are maturational skills that do not seem to be consistently achieved until 37 weeks post-conceptional age. The 37-week mark may well be when most infants are neurologically ready to fully support nutritional requirements orally. Most facilities introduce nippling before this time, based on a perception of readiness for the individual infant.

Problems With State Regulation

These problems already have been described in detail. They are central to the abilities of the infant to initiate and maintain good sucking.

Abnormal Muscle Tone

The infant may have very low or high muscle tone. There may be fluctuations in tone or combinations of hypertonicity and hypotonicity. Overall weakness can lead to lack of proximal stability of the neck, shoulders, and trunk. The full-term infant is born with physiological flexion because of the cramped intrauterine space in the weeks before birth. When a baby is born prematurely, there is more space to extend in the weeks and days before birth. Because of the lack of physiological flexion, the premature infant often has increased or exaggerated patterns of extensor movements. These bias the head position with cervical extension. The extended head and neck position, in turn, can influence the mechanics of sucking. Head extension patterns tend to bias the jaw toward a slightly more open posture, the cheeks into slight retraction, and the tongue slightly retracted. This extension pattern can work actively against the flexion pattern, which is optimal for sucking. Decreased muscle tone in the trunk can influence the mechanics of the internal organs of digestion. Decreased tone in the trunk, with thoracic flexion, can aggravate gastroesophageal reflux.

Immature or Altered Oral Mechanism

Premature infants often have very high and vaulted palates, influenced by extended ventilation. The soft and cartilaginous palate is easily molded to fit the shape of the endotracheal ventilation tube. This can influence tongue and nipple placement for sucking. These infants are born too early to have developed cheek (buccal) sucking pads, which provide some stability for sucking in full-term babies. They have weakened oral musculature, which influences jaw, cheek, and lip control. Often, oral reflexes are somewhat depressed, providing less initial support for the rooting, sucking, and swallowing processes.

Poor Oral Skills for Sucking and Swallowing

Sucking often is weak or poorly coordinated. Exaggerated jaw excursions decrease tongue mobility. Decreased lip seal can increase the work of sucking and reduce the efficiency of the suck. Poor sucking skills influence the coordination for bolus preparation in swallowing. Disorganization in the timing of sucking, swallowing, and breathing can be a common feeding challenge. It is important to distinguish between feeding patterns that simply are disorganized (i.e., a lack of overall sucking rhythm) and those in which jaw and tongue movements are dysfunctional (i.e., interruption of feeding by abnormal movements of the tongue and jaw) (Palmer, 1993).

Oral Hypersensitivity

Premature infants can become orally hypersensitive in response to the aversive oral stimulation they have experienced. Endotracheal tubes, extra corporeal membrane oxygenation (ECMO) treatments, and orogastric and nasogastric procedures can provide negative associations with the mouth. Pairing these negative interactions with delayed, positive oral-feeding experiences can lead to guarded and, ultimately, hypersensitive responses.

Oral Hyposensitivity

Some infants may become less sensitive, or hyposensitive, to oral input. They initially may have demonstrated rooting and early sucking responses only to have them ignored because of the multitude of tubes and procedures necessary for medical stability. Perhaps the repeated stimulation of these early responses with no positive reinforcement, such as food, decreases their level of responsiveness.

Slowed Growth

Premature infants who have problems with sucking and swallowing can have slowed-to-poor weight gain because they are consuming fewer calories and expending greater energy in feeding. The feeding may stop early because of poor state regulation. The infant may tire easily, taking in a smaller feeding and fewer calories, or may quit the feeding because of discomfort with suck-swallow-breathe synchrony or aspiration. While the baby is still in the hospital, this is prevented by orogastric or nasogastric feedings. In many hospitals, if the baby cannot establish weight gain secondary to oral feedings, he or she will receive supplemental tube feedings. These may not be continued once the baby has been discharged. At that point, weight gain and growth may begin to taper off.

Disruption in the Development of a Positive Feeding Relationship

Feeding has been described as a dance that depends on the abilities of the infant and the parent for success. The abilities of the infant are stressed and those of the parents are challenged in the environment of the NICU with multiple caregivers. The multitude of difficulties in feeding that a sick, premature baby can have can make the situation less than pleasant for infants and their parents, and can interfere with the development of a positive feeding relationship.

Parent Involvement in Feeding

Als describes parents as the primary nurturers, central to the survival and growth of the premature infant (Als, 1995). Ideally, in an environment of developmentally supportive care, the parents are involved early on with as much of the baby's daily care as possible. As they are educated about the signs of stress and stability, they develop the confidence to establish a partnership with the medical professionals and the baby in provision of care.

Before the trend for developmental care, parents often were bystanders in the care of their fragile, premature infant. The medical team provided the necessary pokes and probes in an environment of lights and bells, hustle and bustle. Parents felt helpless as they were unable to provide for their baby's needs, let alone hold him. This approach can lead to parent and baby depression, helplessness, and a disruption in the important bonding between parent and infant, both of whom need the comfort and security gained from mutual touch.

With the current focus on parent and infant attachment and more active, close, parental involvement in care of the preterm infant, parents are involved earlier in the feeding process. Comfort-touch is an early component of pre-feeding skills. In many hospitals, as soon as the baby is stabilized medically, parents are encouraged to participate in kangaroo-care holding of the baby (Anderson, 1991; Whitelaw, 1990). Both mothers and fathers are encouraged to hold their naked baby to their own skin. Many fathers describe this skin-to-skin holding as their first invitation to interact with their infant. The skin-to-skin contact is promoted as often as the baby can handle it. "Infants have been found to experience increased respiratory stability and more restful sleep when held by parents, while parents report that they experience a sense of calm and fulfillment" (Als & Gilkerson, 1995). It also has been shown to increase production of the mother's milk supply for breast-fed infants. This early, loving touch can provide a foundation of trust and closeness upon which to build a feeding relationship.

If the baby can handle it during kangaroo care, he or she can be put to the breast to nuzzle and experience the touches and smells of nursing. Initially, the infant may not be ready or have any idea how to nurse, but simply explores the nursing environment in a comfortable way. Babies let adults know when they are stable enough and interested in making beginning sucking attempts at the breast or the bottle. Their readiness may change from day-to-day and hour-to-hour as they are becoming neurologically and physiologically more stabilized.

Breast-Feeding

For most parents, the birth of a premature infant is an overwhelming time. The baby may be very sick and trying to survive. There may be tubes, machines, and medical staff surrounding the baby. Parents describe feelings of grief over the loss of the healthy baby they dreamed about bringing home. They may have fears about their child's future or may be trying to make it through the day or the hour! In the midst of all this stress, fear, and uncertainty may have been a dream about breast-feeding the baby. This dream used to be regularly shattered, as parents were not allowed even to hold their babies. Bottle-feeding was the norm. There have been many breakthroughs of understanding and supportive research about breast-feeding premature infants and the positive implications for baby and mother. Many hospitals are trying to create environments that promote early breast-feeding for these infants.

Breast milk has been shown to be important for premature infants, whether or not it is delivered by breast. Studies have shown that term ***breast milk*** (breast milk expressed by a mother of a term infant) has a different composition than ***preterm milk*** (Schanler & Oh, 1980). Preterm milk composition changes consistently with advancing gestation, but it has been reported to support adequate intrauterine rates of growth in preterm infants (Muhudhia & Musoke, 1989). There are differing opinions about whether fortification must be added to breast milk and whether specific nutrients such as calcium and phosphorus should be added. The composition of the milk given depends, in great part, on the baby and individual growth patterns. The fact that the composition of preterm milk changes over time and that it appears to be nutritionally appropriate gives further support to the importance of a mother's milk for her baby. The mother's body seems to know best what the infant needs. Whenever possible, hospitals use the milk expressed by the mother to feed the baby. Fresh milk is preferred because it provides the best immune-system support. Frozen milk is dated so it can be provided chronologically by orogastric feeding until the baby can take more feedings orally.

Even when hospital staff members are supportive of breast-feeding, it can be a challenge for the mother. Good sucking and swallowing often are not developed until 33 or 34 weeks of gestation. Before then, the mother must use a breast pump throughout the day. Frequent pumping is essential to establish and sustain lactation until breast-feeding occurs. Lactation experts suggest initiating breast pumping shortly after the delivery and then at least five times daily. Some even suggest rates up to 8 to 12 times daily. This takes quite a commitment. It is considerably less comfortable and relaxing to pump milk than to nurse an infant. Milk production can drop when influenced by stress.

In early efforts to breast-feed, the mother initially must receive support. Breast-feeding premature babies can provide significant challenges to even the most determined mother. Initial efforts vary for mothers and infants. Some healthy preemies do well from the beginning, while others take a long time to develop the coordination, discouraging the parent. Mothers need privacy to explore the breast-feeding relationship and yet need support. Some mothers find it hard to relax in the NICU with the noise and supportive inquiring staff wondering how things are going. Others do well. Many mothers in a retrospective look at their breast-feeding experience felt they expected too much in the beginning and wished they had been warned about how long it would take their baby to latch on and really nurse (Als & Gilkerson, 1995). They wished they had realized that it is a slow process for many mothers and that their slowness did not mean failure. It was helpful for them to realize that milk production increases over time and with nursing practice, and that initial slow milk production does not mean failure.

Experience has shown that there seem to be three turning points for the mother who is attempting to nurse her premature infant. If the mother gets too discouraged to continue the breast-feeding journey, it probably will be at one of these points. First is the overwhelming process of keeping up with the pumping of breast milk. The stress of "nursing" the pump, searching for the right handheld or electric pump, the frequency and time spent pumping, and the process of trying to keep up the supply of milk in light of NICU stresses, can discourage many mothers. Second, many mothers become discouraged when attempting to put the infant to the breast. They may not have been emotionally prepared for the slow process and time it takes for mother and baby to figure it out. Third, there can be discouragement when the mother attempts to discontinue all pumping and bottle supplementation. It may take a long time for the baby to make that transition and grow well. At these times, the mother who is breast-feeding her premature baby will need extra support and encouragement.

Babies bring their own challenges and stresses to the breast-feeding meal. By following the Als synactive model of supportive developmental care, the baby would be offered the breast only after careful observation determined that she was in a stable state of self-regulation. The baby would be held in a comfortable fashion that supports smooth respiration and an organized calm state. The infant's hands are allowed to be active and near the face or midline. The baby's self-regulation is monitored as the breast is offered in a slow and careful manner. The baby needs time to explore the breast and the nipple. Nuzzling at the breast may be all the infant can handle at first. Some babies can handle gentle stroking of the lips with the nipple, and they may open the mouth to try to take in the nipple. This can be complicated for the new mother. Trying to blend newly learned breast-feeding techniques with the baby's self-regulation needs can be tricky. A slow approach to learning these mutual skills is usually best for everyone.

Although the baby may show signs of good self-regulation at the beginning of a feeding attempt, it may be difficult at first to maintain this state, as the ongoing effort of nippling is required. NICU nurses, lactation specialists, or feeding therapists may have suggestions for optimizing success in breast-feeding while monitoring the baby's state regulation. Once the baby can self-regulate reasonably consistently, the mother may be able to more easily focus on the baby's breast-feeding skills.

Bottle-Feeding

Although breast-feeding has been shown to have advantages for baby and mother, it can be a formidable challenge within the NICU. Some settings are more supportive of the effort than others. Some mothers know from the beginning that they prefer to bottle-feed their infant. Some mothers who wanted to breast-feed know they are not up to the challenge in this setting and under these circumstances. For many babies, bottles are introduced as the first nippling experience or simultaneously with offerings of the breast. The same issues of stability and self-regulation apply here as with breast-feeding. Attempts must be made not to overwhelm the baby with this activity. As with the breast, first attempts can relate to nuzzling and touching the nipple. A rooting response may be an initial sign of readiness, as the lips and cheeks are stroked. Again, as with the breast, initial readiness on the part of the infant can change quickly as the nipple is actually presented. As in all feedings, it is up to the feeder to be an excellent observer of baby behavior, which tells the feeder when to move forward and make adjustments to best meet the baby's needs. Following are some interventions that can facilitate coordination in sucking and swallowing for the premature infant.

Milk Delivery Alternatives

A number of devices are available to help preterm infants develop early sucking and swallowing skills before they are fully ready to take the breast or bottle. Many of these alternatives were developed for infants whose mothers prefer the eventual alternative of breast-feeding. Some of these infants initially were given the bottle in the NICU, but they had difficulty shifting to breast-feeding when their suck was more mature. The use of a non-nipple milk delivery device appears to avoid this type of nipple confusion. Although nipple confusion is not an issue for most babies, some infants with more vulnerable sensory systems have trouble with this type of transition. By using a non-nipple milk delivery device, problems often are avoided while respecting the mother's preference for breast-feeding when the baby needs added help in stimulating the sucking response.

Supplemental Nursing Systems

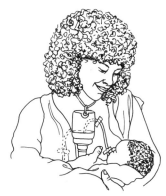

Both Medela and Lact-Aid make a feeding-tube device that assists mothers wishing to breast-feed an infant with sucking difficulties. It is used widely to give premature infants, failure-to-thrive infants, and infants with a weak suck long-term supplemental feedings at the breast. It is an excellent alternative to gavage feedings when the infant does not have a problem with aspiration. A container filled with breast milk is hung around the mother's neck and a thin tube is taped to the breast so that the end projects slightly past the nipple. The soft tube is very small and unnoticed by most babies. When babies take the nipple and areola into the mouth, they also take the tube. This can give babies an initial experience with breast-feeding even when the underlying strength of the infant's suck would make successful breast-feeding difficult without the device. There are different devices on the market, so it is important for parents and professionals to explore the alternatives with a lactation consultant.

Finger-Feeding

Finger-feeding offers many physiological and psychological benefits for the baby who is just learning to suck. The mother can tape a thin feeding tube to the end of her finger and use a small syringe to express breast milk or formula into the tube. Gentle stroking of the infant's tongue and palate with the finger stimulates sucking. As the suck is elicited, milk is gently released into the mouth. The intraoral stimulation promotes proper and sequential contraction of the tongue, jaw, and lips, and stimulates the mid-portion of the tongue where the nipple is drawn. Finger-feeding is the only

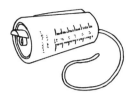

therapeutic method that provides the touch of human skin as in breast-feeding. This skin-to-mouth tissue contact enhances feedback between the caregiver and baby. Finger-feeding also allows the baby to pace the feed. The Hazelbaker FingerFeeder™ provides an easier and more efficient manner of delivering the milk to the oral tube than the older use of a syringe. This device provides a bulb feeder for the milk with the thin tubing attached. The milk bulb fits comfortably into the hand of the feeder, making it easier to handle the feeding device and the baby's oral needs.

Cup Feeding

Cup feeding also can be introduced as an early alternative to breast- or bottle-feeding. A small, flexible cup is placed on the infant's lips and tipped so that a small amount of milk enters the mouth when the baby begins to suck. This requires much less energy than sucking on the bottle or breast. Some cuplike devices such as Medela's SoftFeeder™ incorporate a valve and self-refilling reservoir, which makes it possible for the feeder to maintain a steady supply of milk.

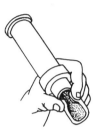

■ Development of Feeding Skills

Facilitating Coordination of Sucking and Swallowing

Parent Guidance

Early feedings are a team effort. Sometimes, the mother starts by introducing the breast. Sometimes, the nurses or feeding specialists offer the bottle. Sometimes, it is a combination of the two. In either case, parents can be centrally involved. They must be educated so that they feel competent in supporting state regulation and organization in the baby. The ability of premature infants to initiate feeding and coordinate sucking and swallowing depends greatly on their skills at self-regulation. Being able to assess stresses and stability will enable adults to choose the opportune time to present the breast or bottle. Initially, the nurse or feeding specialist can help monitor the infant's behavior. Parents initially learn these cues during nonfeeding situations and gradually move into the realm of feeding with greater confidence. As parents learn to recognize the cues, they can modify their behavior as the baby's behavior changes. Als describes this as co-regulation and a good interactive fit. Parents need to follow the baby's cues and let the baby lead the mealtime dance. This will help build the feeding relationship on a foundation of trust.

Position

Special consideration must be made for positioning premature infants during breast- and bottle-feeding. The baby's ability to assume and maintain a stable, coordinated, and organized position is one of the strong indicators of self-regulation in readiness to suck. Good support with the arms and legs close to the body seems to promote endurance. Premature infants nipple best when they come to the meal with calm bodily organization. Their hands often are at the midline and near the face with good and consistent postural control throughout the body. For some babies, swaddling provides the neutral warmth and containment that supports the organization they need for success. Breast-fed babies can be swaddled or held with their bodies slightly flexed and with one or both arms forward. A regular, horizontal baby position or a football hold (in which the baby is held to the mother's side with the infant's feet to her side) or a more upright position may be used. Most important in any position choice should be the baby's stability and ability to self-regulate. Feeder comfort also is an important consideration.

Preparatory Sensory Stimulation

The initiation of efficient sucking requires a rapid, organized response to the sensory input of the nipple. Touching or stroking the newborn's cheeks or lips elicits the rooting reaction—a highly organized opening of the mouth and turning of the head toward the stimulus. This presucking response helps the infant initially find the breast and open the mouth in preparation for latching on (Marmet & Shell, 1984). Some babies need time to organize a response. Others show a very disorganized response to the initial stimulation of the mouth. A number of studies have shown that applying sensory stimulation (e.g., stroking the lips and cheeks, gentle pressure to the base of the tongue, rubbing on the gums) before a scheduled bottle-feeding enhanced the infant's feeding skills as measured by increased weight gain, decreased hospital stays, and a reduction in the number of gavage feedings (Case-Smith, 1988; Gaebler & Hanzlik, 1996; Leonard, Trykowski, & Kirkpatrick, 1980). Individualized oral stimulation may help some healthy premature infants initiate a more organized sucking pattern.

Palmer (1993) makes the important distinction that babies who show a more disorganized sucking pattern need changes and adaptations only to the environment, such as decreasing the lighting and noise levels and minimizing the sensory input from handling. More specific sensory input and supportive manipulation of the oral mechanism may be more appropriate for infants who have a dysfunctional sucking pattern.

Imposed Breaks

Typically developing infants suck in a rhythmical pattern of sucking bursts and pauses. The burst periods include periods of 3 to 10 suck-swallow-breathe sequences, followed by a brief pause. Premature infants often have difficulty developing and coordinating their suck-swallow with respiration and developing a smooth sucking burst-pause pattern (VandenBerg, 1990). The feeder can impose breaks to allow the infant time to maintain or regain the self-regulation needed to nipple. Beginning nipplers can easily start a meal in an organized, self-regulated state and then become disorganized with the introduction of the nipple. They also may respond with increasing disorganization to other suck-swallow-breathe coordination stressors. Breaks can be used in anticipation of a stress signal or after one. They should be brief and used to reduce fatigue or reorganize breathing. To provide an imposed break, the feeder of a bottle-fed infant can tip the nipple down to reduce the flow of liquid in the nipple or remove the nipple from the baby's mouth. For some infants, the nipple becomes part of the organization of the feeding. Removing it can lead to further disorganization. It is important to break the suction by twisting the nipple or putting a finger in the corner of the mouth before removing the nipple to decrease the possibility of stress or choking when the nipple is removed. After a few seconds, the feeder can reassess the infant's readiness cues for continuing the feeding.

Imposed breaks also can be provided to breast-fed infants. The feeder's finger may need to gently enter the side of the mouth and break the seal to help the baby come off the breast. This works for some babies but is too disorganizing for others.

Bolus Size

The size of the bolus can affect the baby's ability to swallow with control. Loss of control of the bolus can lead to coughing and choking and completely disrupt the baby's state of organized calm. This can be controlled by regulating the number of sucks that are allowed before swallowing. The fewer the sucks, the smaller the bolus. The feeder can observe the baby's ability to handle the liquid and notice how many sucks he can handle before becoming stressed. This can provide the foundation for the number of sucks before providing a break. The feeder can build on the baby's coordination and skill level, then build a rhythmical progression of a specific number of sucks, followed by a break. Some babies may adaptively suck and then spit out saliva when they swallow. Often, this is the baby's way of reducing the bolus before swallowing until swallowing skills mature.

Flow Rate

The flow rate of the milk influences respiration, feeding abilities, and swallowing safety in infants (Als & Gilkerson, 1995; Mathew, 1991). There has been some interesting research recently on flow rates, which has an impact on swallowing control in these infants. Traditionally, red and blue preemie nipples have been used with premature infants. These nipples were designed by formula companies to reduce the stress on babies during sucking by providing a faster flow of liquid, thereby, presumably reducing effort. Meier (1988) concluded that the stress and fatigue seen in a number of premature infants during feedings was not caused by the efforts they expended in sucking, but by the effect of the fast flow rate on the breathing pattern. The infant sucking was disrupted in an effort to try to control the flow and regulate the breathing. Mathew (1988) did a functional comparison of nipple units for newborn babies and found that the Ross Laboratories yellow standard nipple had a slower flow rate than other commercially available nipples that he studied. It is vital to observe each premature infant individually to determine which nipple works best. It may be necessary to actually slow the flow rate for some premature infants to reduce the frequency of swallowing and provide them with greater time to organize their suck-swallow-breathe synergy.

Oral Support

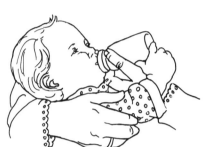

Premature babies are born before they have developed sucking pads. These pads develop at about 8 months in utero, well after most of these babies are born. Sucking pads consist of fatty tissue in the infant's cheeks that gradually is reabsorbed as the infant gets older. These are important for the baby's development because they create a firmness of the cheeks that provides the infant with additional stability in the oral system to support early sucking patterns. When this stability is combined with the small size of the oral cavity and the relatively large size of the tongue, the mouth is better able to achieve compression and suction in extracting liquid from the nipple. The lack of suck-

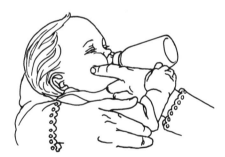

ing pads paired with the somewhat decreased oral tone and overall delayed rate of acquisition of head and neck control set a foundation of reduced stability for the premature infant. Additionally, there is a bias toward extension in the system of the premature baby. Sucking is a flexion skill. When the jaw is biased toward opening (i.e., extension), the jaw excursion is wider and the infant has to work harder just to get to the more flexed, closed-mouth starting position of sucking.

Although many infants need extra support, some do not. It is important to observe the infant's feeding attempts first and assess whether oral support is needed. Sometimes all the infant needs is a little bit of chin support to reduce the effort needed to maintain a closed-mouth position on the nipple and provide more stability. Other infants who need more support can get it by the feeder drawing their cheeks forward during sucking. These supports must be gentle and done with careful observation of the baby's regulatory state so as not to disrupt the feeding. Also, support must not disrupt the parent-infant feeding relationship. One

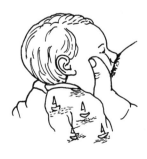

approach to providing oral support for the breast-feeding infant is known as the Dancer hand. The mother's breast and baby's jaw are cupped by the mother's hand, which tends to improve the seal of the baby's mouth around the breast in premature or neurologically impaired infants (Biancuzzo, 1999). The cheek support can be given to the top cheek, as the lower cheek receives positional stability from contact with the breast. A research study by Einarsson-Backes, Deitz, Price, Glass, and Hays (1994) compared the volume intake of formula in premature infants with an oral-support condition and without an oral-support condition. These infants showed a significant increase in volume when oral support was used, validating its use as an effective treatment technique to enhance sucking efficiency.

Demand Versus Scheduled Feedings

There are many unresolved questions about the best ways to approach feeding and growth in the premature infant. How do caloric density, feeding volume, weight, gestational age, and nippling skills influence the growth of these babies? Can these infants lead the feeding dance and grow sufficiently with self-regulation? The research is still inconclusive and more must be done.

Typically, NICU settings put newly nippling babies on a carefully designed schedule, offering feedings of a specified amount of breast milk or formula at a certain time. The baby is fed orally and given any unfinished feeding by orogastric tube. As the baby becomes a stronger nippler, the entire feeding is taken orally. This practice ensures regular nutrition and growth for the infant, but does not encourage the infant's individuality. The debate has continued about whether and when demand versus scheduled feedings are appropriate for this population.

Collinge, Bradley, Perks, Rezny, and Topping (1982) found that premature infants who were fed on demand took in as many calories as those fed on schedule. This was explained, in part, because the infant nipple feedings were completed by gavage feedings. Saunders, Friedman, and Stramoski (1991) found that partially nipple-fed premature infants who were fed on demand gained as much weight as infants fed on schedule. Again, however, if the infants did not take in the prescribed amount of formula orally, they were supplemented with tube feedings.

In an effort to look at the preterm infant's ability to regulate feedings and growth, Pridham et al. (1999) looked at the infant's ability to regulate volume and caloric intake rather than just the ability to time feedings in relation to each other. Healthy preterm infants were given the opportunity to initiate and terminate feedings as they desired (described as ad-lib feedings in this study). Caloric density, volume, and weight gain were all noted over a 5-day period. The researchers found overall that demand feedings had a negative effect on dietary intake assessed in calories and volume. They also found that weight gain was influenced by caloric intake, not the specific feeding regimen or just caloric density of the formula. As infants gained practice with full nipple feedings, the caloric intake of the demand feeders began to approach that of the infants on the scheduled feeding regimen. The research findings supported the concept that premature infants develop self-regulatory capacities with demand feedings. This study differed from previous studies in that Collinge's and Saunders' studies defined demand as the initiation of the feedings and researchers supplemented the feeding when the demand-fed babies did not take the predetermined amount. In the Pridham study, both initiation and termination of the feeding were infant controlled. This study, however, demonstrated that the demand-fed babies initially took in less than the 120 kcal/kg recommended by the American Academy of Pediatrics, but came closer to approaching this number as the study progressed. Study results, therefore, seemed to indicate that the experience of nipple feeding improves infant skill and ability to regulate dietary intake and, therefore, growth.

Research of this nature should continue. More hospitals need to investigate demand versus scheduled models and how to balance skill and maturation level, self-regulatory skills, appetite, and endurance with infant growth. In looking at the feeding relationship, the authors encourage the goal of infant-directed feedings with the parent in the support role as soon as the infant demonstrates readiness and ability to regulate growth.

Facilitating Growth and Development of Eating Skills in the Older Premature Infant at Home

Parental Guidance and Support

Parents must receive ongoing support in the feeding of their premature infant after discharge from the hospital. The baby's growth and progression to oral feedings are strong factors in the timing of discharge from the hospital. Often, the achievement of full oral feedings is established just before discharge. The parent and baby often still are working things out. Parents and babies must make the huge transition to the home environment. Parents describe feelings that vary from relief and joy to insecurity and panic. Many are overwhelmed. These emotions can and do strongly influence feedings.

Feeding guidance may take the form of daily phone calls, regular home visits, periodic consultation, or regular feeding treatment. The level of support needed will change as the baby matures and moves in and out of different developmental feeding stages. Feeding guidance should support a positive feeding relationship for the infant and parents.

Position

Posture and tone differences between premature and term babies may appear more pronounced as the infant matures. Older premature infants can develop stronger patterns of extension, especially in the neck and trunk, as they become more active in their movements against gravity. The patterns of extension can actively work against good sucking. A baby still needs a feeding position in which there is extension in the back, flexion at the hips, a forward and midline position of the arms, and a chin-tuck position of the head. The appearance of the chin tuck changes as the baby grows and develops a neck. The infant's earlier need to hyperextend the neck in attempts to maintain an open airway often is reduced as the respiratory system matures. The chin-tuck position, therefore, usually can be used more consistently to promote improved sucking strength and coordination.

As the baby grows, her size changes the dynamics of positioning, although the positioning concepts remain the same. The baby no longer is tiny enough to hold in one hand. Back extension cannot as easily be provided with the palm. Too much trunk flexion usually is not an issue in the tiny premature infant because of the size of the infant in relation to the feeder's hands. The feeder needs to be aware of the possibility of too much trunk flexion in older infants, as it can trigger more problems with gastroesophageal reflux (GER). For infants with reflux, the feeder must support the trunk with good extension to avoid unnecessary stress on the lower esophageal sphincter. The parent also may need to experiment with positions closer to upright to reduce the frequency of GER for some babies.

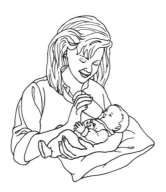
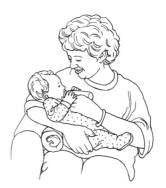

Parents may need help finding ways to coordinate the baby's postural alignment of the body with any oral support he or she needs. The parents and the infants must be comfortable if the feeding is going to work.

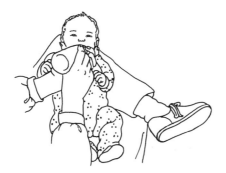
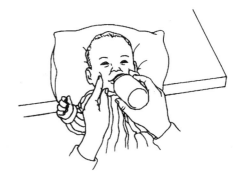

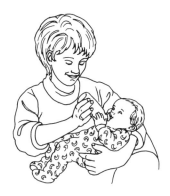

In addition, the angle between the nipple and the bottle can make feeding easier or more difficult for the adult and the baby. Some bottles are short and wide, controlling air flow into the nipple without a bend or angle. Others are angled to provide better liquid flow. Still other bottles are straight, but have an angle in an adapter between the bottle and nipple. Each of these alternatives works well, but some will be more successful for the individual baby and feeder, depending upon the specific positioning used and the size and shape of the adult's hands. Some angle-neck bottles help infants get a good chin-tuck position; others do not.

Prepare the Home Environment

Supportive developmental care in the hospital is provided with an understanding that everything in the environment has some impact on the baby. By structuring the NICU environment to minimize adverse reactions, the baby will be healthier and more available for learning. Parents may need help in preparing a calm and supportive environment for feeding in the home. Intense visual, auditory, and tactile stimuli can overstimulate the baby and interfere with an underlying ability to organize sucking and swallowing. Simple visual changes such as closing shutters or dimming the lights may make it much easier for the baby to nurse. Sound levels may need to be reduced or calming music used in a supportive fashion. Some babies do well with the neutral warmth of holding. Others need the organization provided by swaddling. Some babies and mothers prefer sitting in an overstuffed chair, while others need the gentle rocking of a rocker or glider chair. Each sensory channel should be considered when creating the optimum environment for feeding a baby who has specific sensory needs.

Oral Support

Infants who once needed cheek and jaw support may not need as much support when they get older, or they may need more support. Feeders need to follow the baby's lead, gradually removing supports as the baby takes over in an organized and efficient fashion. Changes can be made in the place and the amount of support. Sometimes, babies initially need cheek and jaw support. As they develop greater internal control, they may need assistive control only with the jaw or only with the cheeks. At times, the location of oral control remains the same but the amount of pressure is reduced as the baby takes over.

Flow rates of nipples may be changed as the baby matures. Faster or slower rates can facilitate improved sucking for different babies. Careful observation of the baby's sucking with different nipples can determine the rate needed. Some nipples offer a variable flow rate so that turning the nipple opens different combinations of holes. This makes it possible to begin with one flow rate and move to another during the meal, or to use different flow rates on different days, depending on the baby's coordination.

Generally, as babies mature, they need less assistance in coordinating sucking, swallowing, and breathing. The need for imposed breaks in feeding will decrease over time.

Transitions to Pureed Food

A number of factors must be considered when deciding to move a premature infant to pureed food. It can be a mistake to consider only the infant's chronological age. Healthy, term babies are offered purees between 4 and 6 months of age. How well they do depends on their neurological and developmental maturity. For example, a baby who was born at 28 weeks gestation and who chronologically is now 4 to 6 months of age is only 1 to 3 months of age when adjusted for prematurity. Even adjusting for prematurity, these infants may be quite different from term infants in their maturation and readiness because of postural and tone issues. The typical premature infant who is at a 4-month-old adjusted age does not look just like the typical 4-month-old term baby, largely because of differences in flexor tone and neurological maturation. Presenting purees to the 4-month-old term baby can be *very* different from presenting them to a 4-month-old preemie.

Each baby lets his feeders know the pace at which to move toward presentation of purees. As a rule of thumb, however, it is often better to present purees a bit later rather than earlier. Premature infants may try cereals or pureed baby foods at about 6 months adjusted age. This is when the infant is more apt to have the neurological organization and sensory experiences to enjoy them. In addition to the baby being neurodevelopmentally ready at the older age, many physicians prefer that the baby receive breast milk or formula until at least that age because there are more calories per ounce in these liquids than in most purees offered. The milk or formula provide greater opportunities for improved growth.

Babies with excessive extensor tone may react to pureed foods with excessive tongue extension or protrusion. Some babies who are introduced to purees too early show fussing and irritability, gagging, choking, or vomiting. Giving babies more opportunities for mouthing and playful oral exploration may better prepare them for this sensory change. These sensitive babies may need a variety of diluted tastes to be introduced during play with mouthing objects or on their own fingers. Once they demonstrate enjoyment and playful exploration of the tastes on these objects, they may more readily accept the spoon and larger quantities.

Transitions to Solids

Some premature children have difficulties with the transition to solids. There are many different factors that may contribute to this oversensitivity. For some, the early aversive oral experiences with ventilation, orogastric, and nasogastric tubes may carry over into the transition to textures in solid foods. For others, there may be neurological immaturity and disorganization—choking and gagging because of lack of oral control. What starts out as an oral disorganization can quickly become an emotional response to the texture change. Many premature children have gastroesophageal reflux throughout the first year of life. This can lead to increased gagginess in these children. Often, these children are treated for GER early in life but taken off all GER measures when blatant vomiting decreases. The more subtle characteristics of appetite suppression and gagginess may continue to influence these children, despite the obvious reduction in vomiting.

Transitions to solids must be done slowly, watching for the child's response and with the child in the lead. Often, these children have a difficult time moving from pureed baby food to third stage baby food containing random lumps and textures. Slowing down the texture transition and reducing the contrasts may be all these children need. Helping them handle thicker pureed foods, then blended and ground foods, and then lumpy mashed foods hidden in the thicker foods may be an easier transition for these children (see Chapters 14 and 17).

Monitor and Optimize Growth

In the NICU, every gram of weight gain is celebrated! Weight gain can mean things are going well, and every gram of weight moves the infant closer to the goal of going home. Parents bring their infants home and may expect the same rate of growth. They may feel a great deal of pressure to help their baby gain weight. Feeding problems can have a great impact on growth rates. Parents can become frustrated as they carefully watch intake and weight gain in their child. Parents need to find the delicate balance between supporting growth and pushing too hard for growth.

Premature infants have their own unique way of growing. Whereas term babies triple their birth weight in the first year of life, a healthy premature infant may have a ten-fold weight increase. The key word here is healthy. This rapid rate of weight gain is the baby's "catch-up" growth. The rapid growth requires considerable nutrition, more than is needed for the term baby. In addition, many of these babies have medical conditions, such as respiratory difficulties, that actually require increased calories. Providing these calories can be a major challenge for parents.

Standard growth charts are designed for healthy, term babies. In monitoring the growth of a premature child, physicians must adjust the baby's age for prematurity to provide a more reasonable comparison of weights. This adjustment for prematurity is usually done for 1 to 2 years. Some researchers have suggested that catch-up growth continues longer than that for very low birth-weight infants. Hack et al. (1996) concluded that in very low birth-weight infants (less than 1,500g), most catch-up weight occurred during infancy, but some continued until 8 years of age.

The baby's rate of growth and catch-up to above the 3rd percentile on standard growth charts is influenced by a number of factors. Catch-up growth appears more often in average-for-gestation-age babies (AGA) than in small-for-gestational-age babies (SGA). Intrauterine growth failure and neurological abnormalities can delay growth. The size of the baby at birth and gestational age will strongly influence growth rates. Raval (1998) found in her study at the University of Arizona Health Science Center that the tinier the baby, the smaller the chance of catching up to the 5th percentile by 1 year adjusted age. She found that by 1 year adjusted age:

- 85% of 24 weeks' gestation babies were less than the 5th percentile
- 64% of 25 weeks' gestation babies were less than the 5th percentile
- 31% of 26 weeks' gestation babies were less than the 5th percentile
- 36% of 27 weeks' gestation babies were less than the 5th percentile
- 20% of 28 weeks' gestation babies were less than the 5th percentile

Guo and associates (Guo et al., 1997; Guo et al., 1996; Roche, Guo, Wholihan, & Casey, 1997) found that growth parameters for premature infants of different birth weights and gestation ages differed enough from the traditional normative data that they warranted their own charting system. The proposed charts were based on revised height, weight-to-head circumference, and weight-for-length reference data for low birth weight (LBW; defined as equal to or less than 1,500 grams) and very low birth weight (VLBW; less than 1,500 grams) premature infants. The normative data was gathered on more than 4,500 preterm infants. This growth data is being distributed as a separate growth chart series for premature infants as IHDP growth percentiles for LBW for Premature Girls, LBW for Premature Boys, VLBW for Premature Girls, and VLBW for Premature Boys. Clinics following premature infants should consider using this type of adjusted growth chart when monitoring the growth velocities of premature infants.

This is important information for physicians as they monitor these babies. More and more investigators are researching growth patterns and nutritional needs for premature infants. In addition to the weight parameters for these infants, the height-to-weight ratio is significant. It compares the baby's weight to that of other babies of the same height. In many ways, this is a more significant relationship. A baby who weighs little compared to other babies her age may be absolutely proportionate when compared with babies of her height. Many settings, however, focus solely on the weight measurement, misinterpreting the baby's small size.

Without proper comparative data or growth-chart adjustments, these babies unfortunately can be misdiagnosed as having the condition known as failure-to-thrive. This can cause parents to worry unnecessarily and start pushing food and calories that the children are unable or unwilling to eat. This, in turn, can create a feeding problem—one of interaction—where one had not existed before. Parents never win in this type of food battle. The diagnosis of failure-to-thrive should be made with great caution in the very low birth-weight population.

All teams working with the feeding and nutritional needs of these infants and young children must be aware of these growth parameters because infant growth and growth rates often are considered in evaluations of treatment programs.

Table 21.1   A Comparison of Feeding Issues for Full-Term and Preterm Infants

Term Infant	Preterm Infant
Flexor baby	Extensor baby
Better neck, trunk, and shoulder stability	Poorer neck, trunk, and shoulder stability
Anatomically ready to suck	Anatomically at a sucking disadvantage
Strong suck	Weakened suck
Adequate lip seal	Inadequate lip seal
Sucking pads help cheek stability	Poor cheek stability
Sufficient jaw stability to maintain a good repetitive suck	Often insufficient jaw stability for maintaining a good suck
Adequate hunger and thirst signals	Inadequate hunger and thirst signals
Neurologically more organized	Often neurologically disorganized, irritable
More rhythmical suck-swallow-breathe coordination	Poorer rhythmical suck-swallow Less rhythmic in suck-swallow-breathing coordination
Intact oral motor reflexes	Incomplete oral motor reflexes

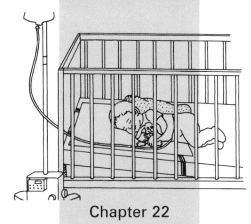

Chapter 22

The Child Who Has Gastrointestinal Discomfort

Gastrointestinal Discomfort and Feeding

The gastrointestinal (GI) system influences the desire to eat and the way children eat. It is designed to take in food, move it through a system of tubes and valves, absorb the fluids and nutrients necessary for nourishment and growth, and discard the unneeded byproducts of digestion in the form of urine or stool. It must have proper structure and physiology to work well. When all goes well, food and liquid are taken in, directed into the stomach and not into the lungs, and moved smoothly along the system. When all goes well, appetite is adequate to support good growth and nutrition. When all goes well, thirst and hunger cues are consistent and support good hydration and energy needs. When all goes well, appropriate nutrients are eaten and utilized. For many children with feeding problems, however, all is ***not*** well and the GI system may cause nausea, vomiting, retching, gagging, or even pain. These forms of GI discomfort can negatively influence the desire to eat as well as appetite and growth.

GI discomfort is caused when the structure, motility, or acid and hormone balance of the GI system are not functioning properly. Conditions that influence the direction and speed of nutrient flow through the system can cause GI discomfort. Sometimes, food and liquid move up instead of down the system, as seen in gastroesophageal reflux. Sometimes, food and partially digested material can get stuck while passing through the system, as seen in pyloric stenosis or constipation. Sometimes, food moves too slowly, as seen in stomach-emptying problems, or moves too rapidly, as in dumping syndrome or malabsorption problems. Sometimes, outside agents such as bacteria, viruses, or parasites interfere with proper functioning. Sometimes, the system is overzealous in its production of acid. Many acute and chronic illnesses take away appetite. Often the medications and treatments prescribed for these illnesses and conditions have an impact on the well-being of the GI system, and therefore, influence appetite. Overall stress and emotions also affect appetite and overall GI functioning.

It is very important for feeding therapists to understand the relationships between gastrointestinal symptoms and feeding, appetite, and growth in their assessment and treatment of children with feeding disorders. The most carefully planned feeding programs, oral motor techniques, and positioning changes will not be successful until the nausea, gagging, retching, vomiting, pain, and other GI symptoms are fully appreciated. A child's feeding issues can be made worse if gastrointestinal discomfort is not understood and treated properly. To better understand these issues and their relationship to a child's feeding issues, read Alicia's story.

Alicia

Alicia was a 2-month-old twin who was born at 35 weeks' gestation. Her sister was growing well, but Alicia was having a more difficult time. Her mother was beginning to feel stressed about feedings. Alicia had **good** meals and **bad** meals. During a good meal, she could take 4 ounces of formula happily and comfortably. During difficult meals, she would arch and push the bottle away as it was offered, or she would start the feeding, arch, and then become very fussy and almost inconsolable for an hour. The first therapist who saw Alicia focused strictly on the oral skills that influenced the stressed meal. She saw the baby arch, pull away, and not take the nipple into the mouth. She prescribed dimming the lights, swaddling the baby, and stimulating the lips with the mother's finger (i.e., moving the finger three times around the lips in one direction and then three times around the lips in the other direction). She suggested that Alicia might need ongoing therapy for underlying sensory problems. The mother went home to try the techniques, but after a week of implementing this approach, she felt there was no change. The recommendations did not make sense to her, based on what she knew about her baby.

Alicia's mother sought another opinion. The new therapist spent time with the mother, asking many questions in an effort to obtain the big picture. The therapist noted that the baby did have good, very organized, and happy meals. If the problem were predominantly due to sensory issues, why would some meals under identical sensory conditions look so organized? What might Alicia be trying to say to her mother with the arching and pushing of the bottle? As the therapist observed the baby, she saw the classic facial grimace of gastroesophageal reflux. Alicia spit up a little bit of formula into her mouth, even before the feeding started. She made a face indicating discomfort and displeasure. She tried to suck her pacifier and her finger in the classic effort to comfort herself and increase her swallowing (i.e., the saliva neutralizes the acid of reflux). Her mother described little coughs that Alicia made throughout the day. The therapist discussed these findings with the pediatrician. In partnership, they decided Alicia should be treated as if she had GER. Alicia was fed in a more upright position and was kept upright for longer periods after meals. She was not put in the moving swing immediately after meals. The doctor recommended a baby antacid. Then, medication to increase the motility of the gastrointestinal system was started. Alicia's mother noted immediate changes, with less stressful feedings. The little coughs stopped. The mother was thrilled and felt that someone had understood what her baby was going through. Alicia happily began taking full 4- to 6-ounce feedings every mealtime. Her mother described Alicia as a "new baby" whom she now enjoyed feeding. She was happy that Alicia, too, now enjoyed her meals.

There was a high probability that this baby and her mother would have developed an extremely stressful feeding relationship. All the signs were there. By a misreading of the feeding problem as purely a sensory one, the gastroesophageal influences were ignored. This baby would not have improved with the best sensory-based program if the gastrointestinal discomfort continued. If the discomfort continued for a significant period of time, mother and baby would have been extremely upset about mealtime. The feeding relationship would have been disrupted. The longer the stressful relationship continued, the more complicated the impact would have become on the total feeding pattern. In this case, once the GI discomfort was discovered and treated, the "sensory" problem magically disappeared and needed no further treatment. This is an important reminder that the big picture **must** be seen before precise oral motor techniques are recommended.

As seen in Alicia's case, the feeding therapist must understand the gastrointestinal symptoms that influence feeding. Therapists often are in a better position than physicians to interview parents in much greater detail about feeding issues. They may hear about and see the symptoms of GI discomfort before pediatricians become aware of them. In Alicia's case, her mother had seen the arching and grimacing but did not relate those to reflux or the feeding problem, so she had not reported them to the physician. She thought the grimacing was just "baby faces" and the arching was just Alicia's temper. When it was suggested that they might be related to reflux, the mother noticed the pattern all day long. The relationship with feeding became clear. The treatment chosen this time made sense to the mother and made a difference to Alicia.

Partnership With Physicians

The feeding therapist can play a significant role in partnership with pediatricians and gastroenterologists in management of GI discomfort as it relates to eating. Physicians are responsible for prescribing medical-management strategies including medications and surgeries. The feeding therapist can provide clinical data to the physician to help in the detective process of understanding the complete eating issues. Feeding therapists can provide mealtime management and interactive support for the family, and thereby have a great impact on the mealtime and the feeding relationship.

Often, feeding therapists are the extended eyes and ears of the physician. They know about mealtimes and what influences feeding. They get to see babies feed. Pediatricians usually do not. Therapists often are in a position to contact the physician to ask about possible GI conditions that may be influencing appetite, growth, and the feeding relationship. The partnership between feeding therapists and physicians is invaluable in defining the big picture of the mealtime for every child. When therapists refuse to become involved by making statements such as, "The physician will take care of that," "The doctor didn't suggest a GI problem, so there must not be one," or "The GI testing results said there was no problem, so there must not be one," they are missing the boat! Therapists know that physicians take care of as much as they can with the data they are given; however, sometimes physicians do not receive all the relevant information. Therapists must know that even when upper GI tests come back negative, there still can be a problem with GER. The clinical symptoms can indicate this. Feeding therapists need knowledge and a willingness to follow clinical intuition. Babies tell therapists what they need. Therapists need to listen and communicate that information to the rest of the team.

Common Gastrointestinal Symptoms That Influence Feeding

Common gastrointestinal symptoms of nausea, gagging, vomiting, constant fullness, retching, and pain influence children's appetite and mealtime interactions (Hyman, 1994; Nelson et al., 1998). However, these symptoms affect each child differently. The intensity of the child's response can depend on a number of factors. These include the severity and longevity of the GI symptom; the age of onset for the symptom; the type of medical and therapeutic treatment for the symptom; the parental reaction and sensitivity to the symptom; and the child's developmental stage, overall health, temperament, ability to provide cues about the symptom, and personal interpretation of the symptom.

For one child, a short-term intestinal flu may have no long-term effect on feeding. Another child may have an extended flu at the same time that lumpy food is being introduced. Nausea from the flu can contribute to gagging with texture changes. Some children with chronic, hourly vomiting may grow and thrive with no apparent effect on eating. Others who vomit once daily may arch, cry, and refuse all foods. Healthy children may react much differently to a short-term GI discomfort than chronically ill children. Some children can handle one or two GI discomforts but cannot deal collectively with several additional problems because the impact is too great. Some babies are described as easygoing. Nothing seems to bother them. They seem very resilient. Others seem set back by any discomfort. They are much less able to bounce back from stresses.

It is important that the feeding team members try to understand each child and his personal response to gastrointestinal discomfort. Each child and mealtime must be evaluated and treated according to the specific needs that are identified.

Now is a good time to look at some of the most common types of gastrointestinal discomfort to gain a more in-depth understanding of their causes and influences on feeding and appetite.

Nausea

Nausea is a general feeling of stomach distress with an urge to vomit. The nausea can be a subtle malaise or powerful urge to vomit. Anyone who has ever felt nauseous knows that it makes a person feel sick and unsociable, and it reduces appetite. Children do not want to eat when they feel nauseous, and if they do eat, they certainly do not eat as much as usual.

Nauseousness can be caused by a variety of conditions, including *acute illness*, such as gastrointestinal flu. The illness comes and then goes, causing a general malaise during its course. For some, severe headaches cause nausea. When the headache is gone, so is the nausea. Chronic disease processes, such as liver or kidney failure or some cancers, and their treatments also cause nausea.

Some *physiological processes* can cause nausea. Gastroesophageal reflux disease can cause a constant, low-grade nauseousness. This may lead to gagging, vomiting, and appetite suppression.

Treatment or *medications* for an acute or chronic illness sometimes have side effects that can cause nausea. For example, the antibiotics frequently prescribed for common ear infections can contribute to nauseous feelings. Often, children with feeding difficulties take more than one medication. Many medications can have vomiting, gagging, or nauseousness as side effects. The nausea caused by some medications is made worse when the medication is taken with food. For others, the side effect is worsened if taken without food.

Emotional influences such as stress, anger, or fear can be strong enough to elicit feelings of nausea in a child. Adults usually can identify when they have been so angry, stressed, or frightened that they felt nauseous. Children can move through similar emotions with similar GI results. Disruptions in the feeding relationship that influence bonding and attachment with the parent are said to affect GI comfort in infants. Stressed feedings can lead to stressed gastrointestinal tracts.

A classic symptom for many food *allergies* can be nausea, gastroesophageal reflux, and GI upset. The nauseousness can be caused immediately by a certain food or be the result of chronic low-grade allergic reactions to multiple foods.

Gagging

Children who gag while eating often do not want to eat or become much less enthusiastic about mealtime. Frequent gagging can be scary to children. In some situations, gagging can lead to vomiting. Gagging is influenced by many different situations, with a number of different types of gagging emerging.

Difficulty with timing and coordination of bolus formation and swallowing can cause *motor-based gagging*. The bolus is not well collected. A partially chewed bolus (or part of the bolus) can pass over the back or sides of the tongue before the child is ready to swallow it. The gagging is a motoric effort to keep a piece of food that is not the appropriate size for swallowing from reaching the airway. *Protective gagging* is seen regularly when inappropriate foods are swallowed. Hard food such as peanuts, chips, or other food requiring significant chewing (e.g., meat) can trigger gagging if given before a child has the oral motor maturation to handle it. Structural problems can cause *structural-based gagging*. An esophageal stricture or narrowing of the esophagus can cause a protective food-removal gagging response.

Some children have overly sensitive oral mechanisms that can lead to an overreactive gagging response. These children may gag with changes in food texture or taste. This *hypersensitivity gagging* often is triggered as the food touches the lips, tongue, or pharynx.

Some children produce and accumulate mucus that can trigger gagging. This *mucous gagging* is the child's attempt to clear the pharynx and airway. Mucous gagging often occurs when the child awakens in the morning or after a long nap when secretions are more likely to pool and remain unswallowed.

Some children use gagging as a way to communicate with the feeder. Perhaps the child wants to end the meal, and the feeder is not paying attention. *Communication gagging* is a way to let feeders know that the child wants them to listen and pay attention.

For some, gagging becomes an emotional reaction to the presentation of the meal. *Emotional gagging* is a response that is learned over time. The stress of the situation may cause GI discomfort. This type of gagging may occur as the parent is bringing food to the table or as the child smells a certain food. It may be the child's response to mealtimes that are too stressful.

Vomiting

Vomiting is a general descriptor for stomach contents that move up the esophagus and into the mouth or beyond. There are, however, different "looks" to vomiting. It can be frequent or infrequent, little spits or large projectile volumes. It can cause the baby distress or seem to go unnoticed. It can occur right after a meal or just before the next meal. It can be consistently evoked after eating certain foods or seem more random. It may seem to be provoked or unprovoked, stressed or unstressed. It can occur with movement or while sitting still. It can occur with an acute illness or be a chronic problem. Vomiting may be triggered by nauseousness or gagging. Some vomiting greatly influences appetite and growth while other instances seem to cause the baby little concern.

Fleisher (1994) uses the term *innocent vomiting* to refer to the common infant spitting up that does not involve nausea, pain, retching, or generalized fear or discomfort. It can happen as early as the newborn period and usually resolves itself between 6 and 18 months of age. Episodes range from a few times a week to a few times an hour. These infants grow well and generally seem unconcerned about the vomiting.

Some vomiting signals a *structural problem*. In pyloric stenosis, for example, the formula or food may be blocked as it tries to exit the stomach. Vomiting is the way the body chooses to rid itself of the food that will not pass. For some children, structural vomiting can occur with esophageal strictures as the esophagus rids itself of a bolus too large to pass through the esophagus and into the stomach.

Some vomiting is the body's way of *ridding itself of a substance* that it interprets as unhealthy. For some, it could be a swallowed poison. For others, it can be an allergic reaction to a formula or specific food. Vomiting, in this case, is the signal that something is wrong.

Many *acute or chronic illnesses* create GI disturbances sufficient to cause vomiting. If the episodes are brief and health is regained, there may be no effect. If the nausea and vomiting become chronic, appetite may be severely effected. An episode of food poisoning or a gastrointestinal flu can cause vomiting for a day or two. Most children recover from that type of illness with no long-term effects. However, vomiting as a result of chemotherapy for a cancer treatment may have a much more lasting effect on a child's appetite.

Cyclical vomiting is understood less well than other types of vomiting. It is defined by self-limited episodes of nausea and vomiting separated by symptom-free intervals (Fleisher & Matar, 1993). Each patient has a unique pattern of frequency and length of the vomiting cycles. It is diagnosed by its timing patterns and is treated symptomatically.

Some vomiting is related to a *chronic gastroesophageal reflux disease (GERD)*. These vomiting episodes may be episodic or frequent and seem to cause the infant moderate to severe discomfort. Sometimes, GERD symptoms develop over time and repetition of episodes. Nausea, pain, retching, arching, facial grimacing, and appetite suppression are common. The vomiting may be subtle little spit-ups or more forced, large projectile episodes. Sleep disturbances can occur. In more severe situations, GERD can lead to aspiration and mimic reactive airway disease.

Some children who have had sensitive GI systems learn to use vomiting as a way *to gain attention* or control the parent's behavior. The child may have had innocent vomiting or reflux that has mostly been resolved, but may have noticed how the parent responded when the vomiting occurred. Some children appear to enjoy the attention, positive or negative, that they receive following a vomiting episode. Others may have noticed that they did not need to eat the food that was presented when vomiting occurred. Perhaps the parent offered a favorite food or drink or special sympathy after a vomiting episode.

Some children resort to vomiting to *communicate* a powerful message. Perhaps the child tried to indicate he had finished eating. The feeder may have wanted the child to take just one more bite. The child first may have said no or shaken his head. If the feeder did not listen, the child may have pushed the food away. If the feeder still does not listen, the child may gag. If the feeder again does not listen, the child may resort to vomiting. Vomiting can be an escalation of the "No, *I* am in charge" message.

Vomiting has been described in the literature as a symptom of an ***impaired maternal infant relationship*** (Sanders et al., 1993).

Tube feeding–induced vomiting can occur when a bolus tube feeding is given too rapidly. When the feeder holds the syringe too high, the formula flows through the tube and into the stomach rapidly. The higher the syringe, the faster the flow. The lower the syringe, the slower the flow. When the stomach is filled too rapidly, the child may vomit. The concept of ***too rapidly*** varies by child. Some children can handle an 8-ounce bolus in 5 minutes. For others, 1 ounce in 15 minutes is too fast and will cause vomiting.

Constant Fullness

It is hard to be interested in eating if you have just eaten an entire Thanksgiving meal. Many children who eat poorly always act as if they have just finished a 12-course Thanksgiving meal! When children have a constant feeling of fullness, they are not interested in eating regular meals. This certainly deters them from trying new foods.

Constipation can be a classic reason that children feel full. Appetite is affected when the bowels fail to empty regularly and completely. The gastrointestinal system functions as a series of tubes. When the stomach is full, food needs to move through a tube to the small intestines and on to the large intestines and colon. When the large intestines and colon are full, there is nowhere for the contents of the small intestines to go and therefore, the contents of the stomach are slowed down. The fullness of the intestines gives a chronic feeling of fullness that deters appetite.

Poor stomach emptying can cause a feeling of fullness. Typically, the stomach completely empties between meals. This emptiness is part of the trigger for hunger signals for the next meal. For many children with feeding disorders, the stomach does not empty efficiently or at a usual pace. The stomach, therefore, may still be filled with one meal when the parent is offering the next. This is seen easily with tube-fed children. By checking for residuals before the meal, the parent knows if the last meal has left the stomach.

Timing of meals influences the feeling of constant fullness. Some children are fed by gastrostomy tube in a 24-hour-a-day drip method. These children may receive a small amount of food every minute of the day. The constant fullness they experience may diminish their interest and appetite for oral foods. Orally fed children also can have a constant feeling of fullness. Children who "graze" or munch on food all day may have a constant state of fullness with no real appetite for meals.

Food choice will influence the feeling of constant fullness. Some children commonly drink sugary drinks such as juice, sodas, and Kool-Aid™ throughout the day, between and during meals. The high sugar content suppresses appetite and can provide a false feeling of fullness before appropriate nutrients are taken in. High-fat foods are digested more slowly and, therefore, stay in the stomach longer than other foods. Many children who are growing poorly are placed on diets that include large quantities of high-fat, high-caloric formula shakes. It is common for these children to reject food at the next regularly scheduled snack-meal because of the slow rate at which the high-fat food leaves the stomach.

Retching

Retching is defined as making an effort to vomit. It looks like a vomiting, heaving effort without the emesis. Retching may or may not lead to vomiting. Either there is nothing in the stomach available to come up, or the child may have had a fundoplication and is not physically capable of bringing up stomach contents. Retching can be seen as an extreme gagging reaction. It can be seen after severe flu when the child already has vomited all available stomach contents. However, it is most often associated with a post-surgical course with a fundoplication (Borowitz & Borowitz, 1997). There is some evidence that retching is more common after a fundoplication in children who have gastric-emptying problems (Jolley et al., 1987). Some children who have had this surgery become very sensitive to changes in the expansion of the stomach as the food is offered. Retching may be a common response to each tube feeding.

Pain

Pain is suffering or distress associated with a warning that there is a problem in the body. In the gastrointestinal system, pain can be caused by gas bloat (Lundell, Myers, & Jamieson, 1994), colic (Dihigo, 1998; Iacono et al., 1991), gastroesophageal reflux, ulcers, or esophagitis. Pain can be severe or mild. How each child interprets it is personal. Some children have a very low tolerance for pain, while others seem to tolerate quite a bit of pain before it affects their functioning. The level of pain perception also is shaped by the child's relationship with the primary caregiver (Hamilton & Zeltzer, 1994). However, chronic pain usually negatively influences appetite.

Emotional Impact on the Gastrointestinal System

The relationship of emotions to the gastrointestinal system is easily understandable as each person looks at his or her own relationship to food. Many people eat more when they are nervous or stressed. Others stop eating or have no appetite during periods of stress. Reactions to stress and food are highly personal, as are the gastrointestinal responses. This also is the case with children. There is an intense personal bond between the child and the feeder. Disruptions in that bonding and attachment process have been documented to cause GI symptoms in infants. In early infancy, disrupted bonding is believed to be a contributor to colic (Dihigo, 1998). In later infancy, it can contribute to diarrhea, vomiting, and pain. Older children can develop pain and constipation. Because each of these symptoms can have other medical or physiological causes, it is extremely important to look at the whole picture. Therapists cannot look medically without looking psychologically. And they cannot blame the psychological relationship for issues that are medically based. However, remember that medically based feeding issues can lead to disruption in the feeding relationship and that disruption in the feeding relationship can lead to gastrointestinal symptoms. Often, what begins as a physiological or sensory problem can become an emotional reaction or aversion in a child. These complex interrelationships require that feeding therapists consider the total picture and become aware of the multiple influences on a child's mealtime behaviors in order to provide appropriate support for children and families.

Symptom Triggers

It is helpful to think of gastrointestinal symptoms as having underlying causes and a series of symptom triggers. The underlying cause may be physiological, such as GER (i.e., because of reduced resting pressure of the lower esophageal sphincter) or emotional (i.e., poor parent-child bonding). Yet the timing and frequency of the symptom is strongly influenced by environmental triggers that elicit or set off the symptom. Physical, sensory, and emotional triggers strongly influence gastrointestinal symptoms.

Physical discomfort such as the pain of an ulcer or esophagitis associated with GER can trigger GI responses of nausea, gagging, retching, or vomiting. Physical movement can change the relationship of the esophagus and the stomach and the resting pressure of the lower esophageal sphincter. This can cause upward movement of the gastric contents, followed by the GI responses associated with GER or vomiting. Increased abdominal tension and anxiety from the first sign of a cough or gag can trigger uncontrollable retching.

Sensory stimuli can set off a chain of events that cause GI discomfort. For an orally hypersensitive child, the stimulus of a finger in the mouth or the texture of a mouthful of food can cause a gag or a gagging reaction that turns into a vomiting episode. An unexpected taste or temperature change can lead to some GI reactions of gagging, retching, or vomiting. Mucus can trigger gagging and retching. A noisy environment or a radio playing loud music can trigger reflux in a sensitive infant.

Emotions can complicate the response of children. For some, the repeated pain or discomfort associated with eating can cause an emotional reaction of gagging or vomiting when the child sees or smells food. Other children may develop an emotional trigger that is stimulated each time the parent tries to help the child gain weight by offering "just one more bite." A specific therapist or care provider may serve as a stimulus to gagging triggered by emotional stress.

The distinction between an underlying causative agent for the gastrointestinal disorder and stimulus triggers is critical. Although medical management of the disorder is the physician's responsibility, feeding therapists can help children and families reduce the power of the triggers that elicit the symptoms. This may shift a gastrointestinal problem from causing severe interference with eating to a mild discomfort that the child can deal with.

■ Understanding and Treating Gastrointestinal Discomfort

Disorders of the gastrointestinal system can be structurally and motility based. Some of these disorders are described in Chapter 6. The feeding therapist must have a general knowledge of the most common gastrointestinal disorders and an understanding of treatment strategies that can be part of the overall feeding and mealtime program.

Understanding and Treating Esophageal Dysmotility

The bolus moves by peristaltic action through the esophagus to the stomach. Esophageal dysmotility occurs when the peristaltic movement is inadequate or a structural problem interferes with movement through the esophagus and into the stomach.

An *esophageal stricture* is a narrowing of the esophagus. Some children are born with this structural problem and others develop it, usually as a response to the chronic acid associated with gastroesophageal reflux. A stricture can be suspected from clinical observations. A very tight congenital stricture may be suspected at birth when there is a slowing of the flow of liquid through the esophagus combined with coughing episodes. Often, however, congenital strictures allow the passage of fluid, but become more obvious as the child transitions to pureed or solid foods that require a wider esophageal diameter for bolus passage. When the bolus cannot pass, the esophagus tries to rid itself of the bolus by inducing gagging or vomiting. Generally, just the problem bolus, not the entire meal, is vomited. The gagging usually is seen *after* the bolus has passed over the tongue. It appears to pass partway down the esophagus and then cause a delayed gag or vomiting episode.

Clinically, suspected strictures are definitively diagnosed most often with an upper GI barium study. The contrast material highlights the length and width of the stricture. Strictures must be treated medically. They may need surgical intervention or regular dilitations. Reflux-induced strictures may need a regimen of GER medications. Some children also have reduced esophageal motility below the stricture that has an impact on the movement of thicker and more solid foods to the stomach.

Surgical repairs of the esophagus also contribute to motility problems. Conditions such as tracheoesophageal fistula and esophageal atresia (which are discussed in detail in Chapter 6) can impair esophageal motility at or below the site of structural repair (Cavallaro, Pineschi, Freni, Cortese, & Bardini, 1992; Duranceau et al., 1977). Although these conditions generally have been repaired before infants work with a feeding therapist, the impact of the reduced esophageal motility can influence the child's desire and ability to move to oral feedings or add more solid foods to the diet.

Problems with *neurological control and coordination* also influence movement of food through the esophagus. A generalized esophageal motility disorder may influence the entire esophagus, or a more specific motility disorder may influence only the timing of the opening of the lower esophageal sphincter. *Achalasia* is a condition in which there is a high resting pressure of the LES that does not relax to allow the bolus to pass into the stomach. It often is associated with generalized esophageal dysmotility or occasionally can be the result of a tightly wrapped fundoplication. Esophageal dysmotility is diagnosed with a combination of clinical history, upper GI studies, and sometimes manometry.

Although there are differences in etiology for each of these conditions, each results in a dysmotility that interferes with the smooth passage of food into the stomach. All create similar issues for children and feeding therapists.

The challenges for the feeding therapist usually involve

- making clinical observations that may suggest a dysmotility problem. These must be reported to the physician as a part of the diagnostic effort.

- partnering with the physician and the family about the clinical impact of the dysmotility on the feeding process and the feeding relationship.

- supporting the infant in acquisition of the oral skills necessary for sucking and swallowing when they have been forgotten or disrupted.

- supporting the infant through a careful transition to thicker and more solid foods after medical treatment of the dysmotility. This includes being aware of the sensitivities and fear that may have developed and carefully listening to the child.

- guiding the parent in reading the infant's cues for timing variations as different food consistencies move through the esophagus. Liquids move more rapidly than solids. Some foods may need a liquid "chaser" to help them make it to the stomach.

Understanding and Treating Gastroesophageal Reflux

Gastroesophageal reflux is defined as the return of gastric contents into the esophagus. Most people reflux occasionally. Many babies spit up as a normal part of the maturation of their GI system. This is usually just innocent physiological vomiting and, although inconvenient, it often has minimal effects on feeding and will be outgrown with maturity of the GI system and increased postural control. However, when the chronic reflux symptoms cause changes in the child's health, appetite, and growth, then GERD or pathological gastroesophageal reflux is diagnosed. Some of the symptoms of reflux are overt, such as vomiting, and others are much subtler, making an accurate diagnosis more complicated. Because gastroesophageal reflux is such a common influence on children with feeding issues, it is important that feeding therapists fully understand its characteristics and diagnosis and their role in treatment. See tables 22.1 and 22.2 for common and unusual manifestations of GERD based on Tuchman (1994).

Table 22.1   Common Manifestations of Gastroesophageal Reflux Disease

Vomiting	Irritability
Nausea	Gagging
Sleep interruption	Esophagitis
Heartburn, chest pain	Frequent swallowing with facial grimaces
Frequent coughs, hiccups	Malnutrition
Aspiration	Reactive airway disease, wheezing, intractable asthma
Anemia	Hemetemesis (vomiting blood)
Stricture	Stridor, hoarseness
Waterbrash (the flow of salty saliva into the mouth)	

Table 22.2   More Unusual Manifestations of Gastroesophageal Reflux Disease

Sandifer Syndrome (arching and stiffening of the trunk, and torticollis-like posturing associated with GER pain)	Rumination
Apnea or cyanotic episodes	Acute life-threatening events
Infant "spells" (including seizure-like events)	Reflux and aspiration that mimics bronchopulmonary dysplasia

Symptoms of Gastroesophageal Reflux

It is important to note that the child does not need to have all the symptoms listed in tables 22.1 and 22.2 to have a diagnosis of GERD. It is a common misconception that an infant must have vomiting, for example, to have pathological GER. Some infants have appetite suppression, Sandifer syndrome, apnea episodes, or cyanosis with no vomiting at all. On the other hand, there can be a number of other causes for these symptoms. It is important to look at the whole picture to understand gastroesophageal reflux and its influences on feeding.

The upward movement of gastric contents into the esophagus may be influenced by the improper functioning of the lower esophageal sphincter or delayed emptying of the stomach contents. In the normal system, the LES resting pressure is usually high, maintaining gastric contents in the stomach. Inadequate resting LES pressure, inappropriate transient LES relaxation, or ineffective sphincter support (as in a hiatal hernia) can contribute to the upward movement of stomach contents. Meal size, gastric secretions, and gastric emptying affect gastric volume. Chronic obesity, tight clothing, and movements or position changes of the trunk can increase abdominal pressure. Coughing or forced expiration also can increase abdominal pressure and GER. Pressure changes within the chest or thorax can create reflux. Thoracic pressure changes associated with labored inspiration in bronchopulmonary dysplasia (BPD) and asthma can cause the upward movement of stomach contents. The supine position is noted to increase GER in reflux-prone infants.

Refluxed material in the esophagus is cleared by peristalsis of the esophagus paired with increased salivation and swallowing. The saliva neutralizes the acidity of the refluxed material (Helm et al., 1984). Acid allowed to stay in the esophagus can inflame the delicate esophageal tissues. This esophagitis can cause symptoms from mild nauseousness, gagging, irritability, and heartburn to severe pain or the development of strictures (Black, Haggitt, Orenstein, & Whitington, 1990; Fonkalsrud & Ament, 1996). Some children arch and stiffen seemingly in response to the discomfort of esophagitis. This arching is called Sandifer syndrome and can be associated with neck hyperextension, a torticollis-like posturing of the head and neck, or marked flexion to one side (Gorrotxategi et al., 1995b). This has been shown to improve esophageal clearance of refluxed material and usually resolves when the reflux is treated appropriately.

Respiratory symptoms due to GER may be difficult to differentiate from those due to primary respiratory disease. The refluxed material can irritate the larynx, causing a cough, hoarseness, or chronic aspiration. Reflux can be considered a possible contributor to respiratory problems when pneumonia is recurrent or chronic, when asthma is intractable, or when apnea in infants is obstructive (Balson, Kravitz, & McGeady, 1998; Blecker et al., 1995; Meyers & Herbst, 1982). GERD is a common factor in respiratory complications of neurologically disabled children who are chronically positioned on their backs. The acid in the esophagus also can lead to vagal nerve responses including apnea and cyanosis, which sometimes are life-threatening events (Gomes & Lallemand, 1992).

Gastrostomy tube feedings have been shown to increase the likelihood of GER symptoms (Berezin, Schwarz, Halata, & Newman, 1986; Grunow, Al-Hafidh, & Tunell, 1989; Heine, Reddihough, & Catto-Smith, 1995; Isch, Rescorla, Scherer, West, & Grosfeld, 1997). To better understand this, consider the following analogy: Imagine you are carrying a full cup of coffee as you are walking around the house or up and down stairs. To keep the coffee from splashing out of the cup as you move, notice how you move the cup slightly to compensate for the movements of your body. Now think about the anatomy of a gastrostomy tube. The tube is placed in the stomach. The inner balloon of the catheter or button tube pulls the stomach toward the abdominal wall, connecting the inside to the outside. Adhesions form over time to create a channel for the tube to pass through. This connecting channel essentially holds the stomach slightly tipped in one position, at the abdominal wall. The stomach, which used to be able to move slightly within the abdomen to compensate for body movements, now is secured at the abdominal wall. Remember that cup of coffee? What would have happened if you had held your hand rigidly still as you went up those stairs? It would have splashed out of the cup. The stomach seems similarly biased to "splash" stomach contents upward without the compensatory movements and with the tilt caused by the G-tube placement. For some children, the GER is significant enough to need treatment; for others, it is not.

Diagnosis of Gastroesophageal Reflux

Diagnosing GER and its contributing causes can be difficult (Catto-Smith, 1998). Many of its symptoms can be attributed to other disease processes. Diagnosis of GER is made in a number of ways. A good clinical history is extremely important. The Gastroesophageal Reflux Parent Questionnaire on page 581 can be helpful in obtaining information. Sometimes, physicians note clinical signs of GER and initiate a trial period of antireflux medications to see if the child improves. Sometimes, a more in-depth diagnostic workup is necessary.

Often, an upper GI series is chosen as a first study for several reasons. It is a noninvasive, outpatient study. If a child demonstrates GER episodes during the study, the duration and height of the refluxed material can be documented. There are, however, a number of drawbacks to the upper GI series for the diagnosis of gastroesophageal reflux. There can be high false positives and false negatives. A child who regularly refluxes may not show reflux during that particular study. The study does not indicate the frequency of reflux episodes or their effect on the child. Any information acquired from an upper GI study must be compared with the information in the child's clinical history. If GER is suspected from the history, further testing may be needed if no reflux is seen on this test.

A pH probe has been considered the gold standard for diagnosing reflux, but it is important to understand its strengths and limitations (Cucchiara et al., 1995; Ferreira et al., 1993; Gorrotxategi et al., 1995a; Hendrix, 1993). It quantifies the frequency and duration of acid reflux for a prolonged period of time, but it cannot detect nonacid reflux, as in the reflux associated with meals and postmeal (postprandial) reflux. Nonacid reflux can occur for up to 2 hours after a milk feeding. Although some clinicians have begun giving apple juice feedings at least once or even throughout the entire pH probe because of its pH of 4.0, there has been some concern about the likelihood that apple juice is handled differently in the GI tract than milk. This study can, however, document potentially dangerous conditions associated with reflux such as delayed clearance of refluxed acid, reflux during sleep, and reflux-induced coughing because the activities of the child are monitored along with the esophageal pH.

Additionally, scintigraphy or a technitium scan can be used to provide more information about GER (Orenstein, Klein, & Rosenthal, 1993; Tolia, Kuhns, & Kauffman, 1993a, 1993b). In contrast with the pH probe, the scan takes about an hour. The child ingests radioisotope-labeled food. This study can document any reflux episode, including postprandial reflux, regardless of the pH of the meal. This shorter study, however, also may miss refluxed episodes and make it difficult to extrapolate the frequency of the reflux.

Sometimes, an upper endoscopy is performed. This gives the physician a direct view of the esophageal tissue. Acute esophagitis inflammation can be documented. Biopsies can be taken to document esophageal changes. This cannot completely document how the inflammation affects a certain child (Black, Haggitt, Orenstein, & Whitington, 1990; Saraswat, Dhiman, Mishra, & Naik, 1994). Some children have been shown to have very mild esophagitis, but have significant GERD symptomatology. Others have had serious inflammation documented by endoscopy, with lesser symptoms.

Some children develop gastroesophageal reflux as a symptom of an allergy to cow's milk or other proteins in the diet. Iacono et al. (1991) studied 204 infants under a year of age who had been diagnosed with GER on the basis of 24-hour continuous pH monitoring and histologic examination of the esophageal mucosa. A diagnosis of cow's milk allergy was made in 85 infants (41%), suggesting that allergy testing should be done in infants with GERD (Cavataio, Iacono, Montalto, Soresi, Tumminello, Campagna et al., 1996, Cavataio, Iacono, Montalto, Soresi, Tumminello, & Carrocaio, 1996; Iacono et al., 1996). Other allergic infants may be identified clinically by changing their formula to an amino acid-based formula (Kelly et al., 1995).

Therefore, none of the diagnostic test procedures for gastroesophageal reflux are ideal or provide all the necessary information. The team must match the clinical and mealtime history, the parent report, and the child behaviors and growth patterns with the limited diagnostic information that can be obtained from different tests before determining management options. See Chapter 8 for a more detailed discussion of these evaluation tools for reflux.

Treatment of Gastroesophageal Reflux

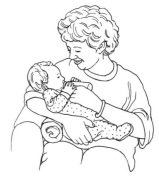

Treatment of gastroesophageal reflux can be as conservative as positioning and as invasive as surgery. It usually involves managing the problems occurring as a result of the reflux and treating the underlying causes. Although there is some disagreement as to the complete effectiveness of positioning for GER management, upright or prone positions have been noted to reduce episodes of reflux, in contrast with supine or reclined resting positions (Meyers & Herbst, 1982; Nordstrom, 1988; Orenstein & Whitington, 1983; Orenstein, Whitington, & Orenstein, 1983; Wolf & Glass, 1992). Some recommend an elevated prone position to further improve reflux episodes, although research support has been inconsistent. The prone and right-sidelying positions speed gastric emptying, as opposed to left side and supine positions (Yu, 1975). The prone position seems to decrease the likelihood of aspiration as compared with the supine position. Cloth slings can be used to position infants in an elevated prone position during sleep (Nordstrom, 1988). During waking hours, the infant should be in the upright position whenever possible. Orenstein et al. (1983) determined that there was an increased number of GER episodes when the infant was placed in a semireclined infant seat after a meal rather than in a prone position. This may be related to the slouched position of the chest in

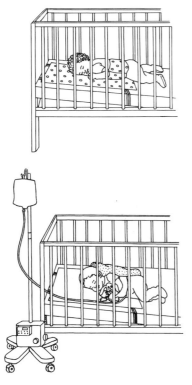

larger infants that creates a bend at the level of the LES. This bend was hypothesized to increase the intra-abdominal pressure and influence the retrograde movement of stomach contents. Smaller infants did not have increased reflux episodes in this position and did not experience the bend with the posterior tilt of the pelvis and a subsequent increase in abdominal pressure. These findings have led to the recommendation that infant seats be adapted when used to prevent reflux in infants. A foam insert can support the infant and give 90 degrees of flexion at the hips, flexion at the knees, and support at the lateral trunk. Some clinicians

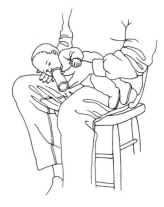

also provide a tiny towel roll at the lumbar spine to provide a more neutral or even a slight anterior tilt of the pelvis.

Thickening formula—with a ratio of 1 ounce of dry infant rice cereal to 2 ounces of formula—has been shown to increase caloric content of formula from approximately 20 calories per ounce to 30 calories per ounce and reduce regurgitation in infants. This provides extra nutritional support for infants with reflux who often are at high risk for malnutrition because of vomiting. This is needed, not only because good nutrition is important for good growth and development, but also because malnutrition impairs gastrointestinal motility (Tuchman & Walter, 1994). Although numbers of pH probe–documented GER episodes have not been shown to be significantly decreased with thickenings, the number and volume of actual regurgitation or vomiting episodes does decrease, sleep time is increased, irritability is decreased, and caloric value of intake is increased (Orenstein, 1992). Essentially, the baby retains more food.

Medications often are used to manage gastroesophageal reflux. These anti-reflux drugs work in a variety of ways. Antacids work in varying degrees to neutralize stomach acid and reduce the negative esophageal effects of acid exposure (Sutphen, Dillard, & Pipan, 1986). Antisecretory drugs called H2 blockers (e.g., ranitidine, cimetidine) reduce reflux by blocking the receptivity of the cells that produce hydrochloric acid in the stomach, thus reducing the amount of acid that is available (Lambert, Mobassaleh, & Grand, 1992; Thomson et al., 1994; Thomson, Kirdeikis, & Zuk, 1999). Some drugs block the production of gastric acid completely by acting as a proton pump inhibitor (e.g., omeprazole, lansoprazole) and are prescribed in cases of severe esophagitis (De Giacomo, Bawa, Franceschi, Luinetti, & Fiocca, 1997; Maton, Orlando, & Joelsson, 1999; Skoutakis, Joe, & Hara, 1995). Prokinetic drugs (e.g., cisapride) work in varying ways to increase upper gastrointestinal motility. They can improve peristalsis, increase LES resting pressure, reduce gastric-emptying time, and thus reduce the time the esophagus is exposed to acid (Brueton, Clarke, & Sandhu, 1990; Marcon, 1997; Schapira, Henrion, & Heller, 1990). These medications often are used in combinations in attempts to manage the symptoms of GER (McKenna, Mills, Goodwin, & Wood, 1995). Many children, however, experience little or no relief from these medications (Cucchiara et al., 1997; Kahrilas, Fennerty, & Joelsson, 1999; Lambert, Mobassaleh, & Grand, 1992). In addition, children and adults may experience a wide variety of side effects from medications, especially when they are given in combination (Farrington, 1996; Gray, 1998; Teare et al., 1995; Vandenplas et al., 1999).

Surgery usually is considered in situations where GER contributes to chronic aspiration problems or vomiting and cannot be managed with positioning or medications. A procedure called a fundoplication is performed in which a portion of the fundus of the stomach (i.e., **fundo**) is wrapped (i.e., **plication**) around the lower esophageal sphincter. This allows food and liquid to enter the stomach from the esophagus, but tightens the sphincter so that food, liquid, and air cannot move upward in the pattern of reflux. The most common fundoplication is the Nissen fundoplication, which uses a complete wrap around the sphincter (Luostarinen, 1993). In some instances, a Thal or a Toupet fundoplication is done as a partial wrap (Mayr, Sauer, Huber, Pilhatsch, & Ratschek, 1998; Ramachandran et al., 1996). These involve a looser wrap that can reduce some of the negative side effects of the Nissen procedure, especially when decreased esophageal motility is a concern.

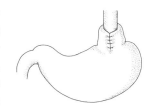

When successful, the fundoplication eliminates GER. It can, however, have side effects that influence feeding. In infants and toddlers with poor eating and early satiety, the fundoplication may worsen symptoms initially. Children may feel too full when they eat or develop a reduced tolerance to larger bolus feedings because of a reduction in the stomach's ability to relax and accommodate the volume of the meal (Vu et al., 1999). Many children are unable to burp or vomit. Some develop swallowing difficulties because the wrap is too tight for food to go down easily (Borowitz & Borowitz, 1997; Luostarinen, 1993; Wo et al., 1996). Gas may accumulate in the upper portion of the stomach and place pressure on the LES. Children experiencing this type of gas bloat often have a great deal of pain. This can be relieved by venting the feeding tube, but during the gassy periods the child can be very uncomfortable. Many children experience severe gagging and retching episodes.

Most of these problems appear to be experienced by children with neurological involvement who have pre-existing problems with gastrointestinal motility. These difficulties with delayed gastric emptying or dumping often increase after the fundoplication and contribute strongly to increased satiety, gas bloat (Lundell et al., 1994), gagging, and retching (Alexander, Wyllie, Jirousek, Secic, & Porvasnik, 1997; Jolley et al., 1987; Papaila et al., 1989). Borowitz and Borowitz (1997) described a child with mild neurological impairment who developed severe gagging, retching, and oral motor dysfunction following a Nissen fundoplication. The child stopped eating by mouth and resumed only after the Nissen was reversed. The reversal resulted in a cessation of the gagging and retching, as well as a return of oral motor function.

These observations have led to a diverse set of research findings and recommendations for the child with severe GERD who does not respond to medications. There is a fairly consistent view that children with neurological involvement should receive diagnostic tests for gastrointestinal motility (e.g., gastric emptying, intestinal manometry) to determine whether they are appropriate candidates for fundoplication surgery (Boix-Ochoa, Casasa, Gil-Vernet, & Marhuenda, 1990; Di Lorenzo, Flores, Hyman, 1991). Some physicians strongly recommend that a fundoplication be combined with a gastric-emptying procedure (e.g., pyloroplasty, pyloromyotomy, antroplasty), which surgically increases the opening of the pyloric sphincter from the stomach into the small intestine (Bustorff-Silva et al., 1999; Dunn, Lai, Webber, Ament, & Fonkalsrud, 1998; Fonkalsrud et al., 1995). Others recommend against this solution, finding more complications and a longer time for regaining feeding skills in children who have had a pyloroplasty (Maxson, Harp, et al, 1994). Still other physicians recommend against both the fundoplication and gastric-emptying procedures and deal with the problem of reflux by using a jejunostomy feeding tube that bypasses the stomach and deposits formula directly into the jejunum of the small intestine (Albanese, Towbin et al., 1993).

Many of the children seen with feeding difficulties associated with neurological disorders have an increase in the intensity of the GER symptoms because of their overall coordination difficulties. This may be influenced by poor peristalsis, poor swallowing control, and poor tone in the trunk. The symptoms may start out as physiological pain and discomfort, and may move to sensory and emotional aversion to eating. Treatment must be global, addressing all aspects of the problem. Medical diagnostic and treatment procedures must focus on identifying and remediating the underlying causes of GERD. Consideration must be given to the risks and benefits of each procedure in relation to the child's feeding and mealtime development. Therapy must work toward increasing positive oral motor and mealtime experiences and rebuilding a positive feeding relationship.

The challenges for the feeding therapist may include

- using the Gastroesophageal Reflux Parent Questionnaire to gather information about the impact of GER on a child's feeding.
- making clinical observations that may suggest gastroesophageal reflux. These must be reported to the physician as part of a team diagnostic effort.
- making ongoing clinical observations about stomach emptying and respiratory issues that might be influenced by GER. These must be reported to the physician as part of a team diagnostic effort.
- making ongoing clinical observations about the impact of GER on tube feedings. These must be reported to the physician as part of a team diagnostic effort.
- partnering with the physician and family about the clinical impact of gastroesophageal reflux on oral feeding and the feeding relationship.
- educating parents about the potential impact of various medical and surgical procedures to control reflux on the feeding process and feeding relationship.
- making suggestions regarding conservative measures for reflux control such as positioning and using thickened formulas.

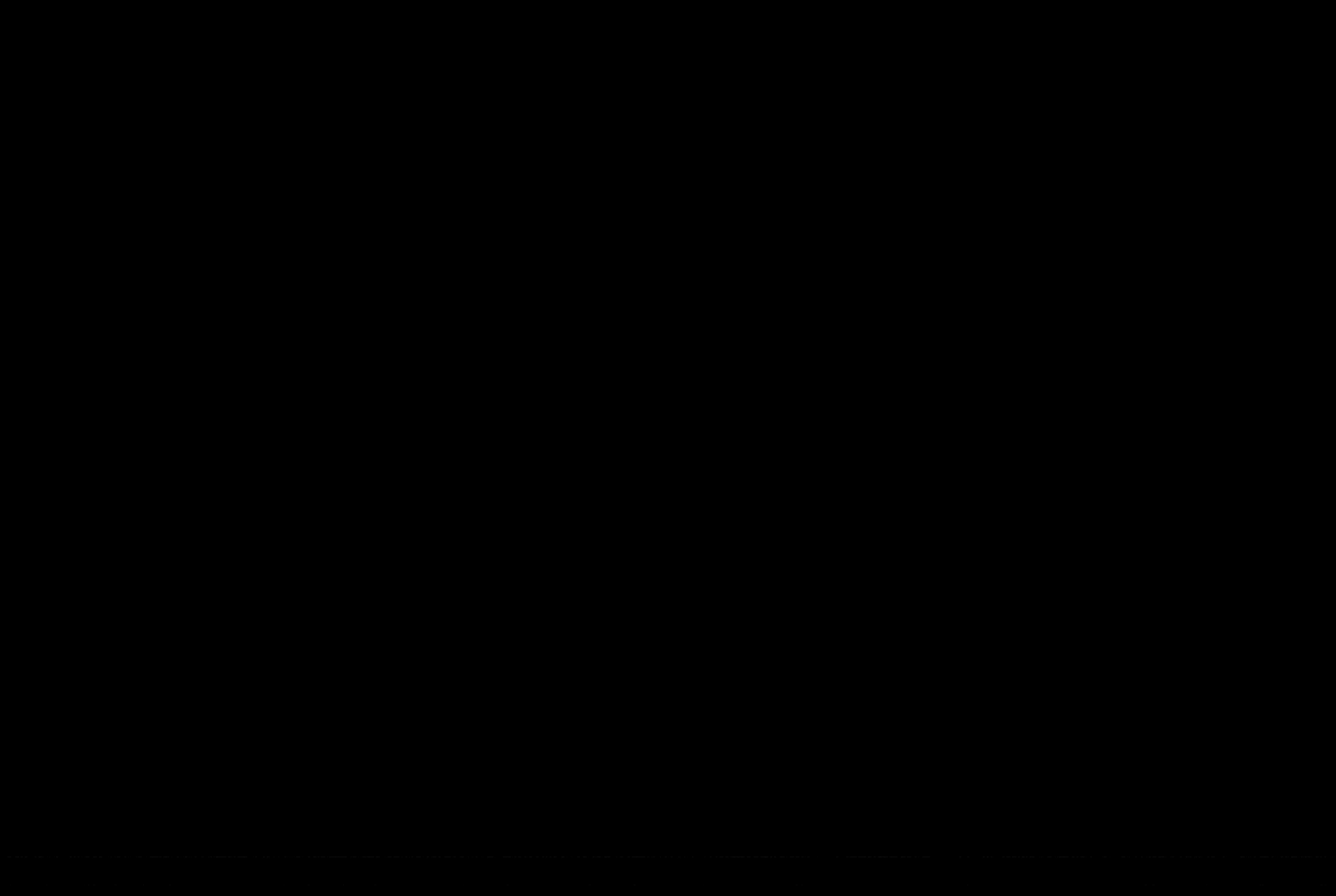

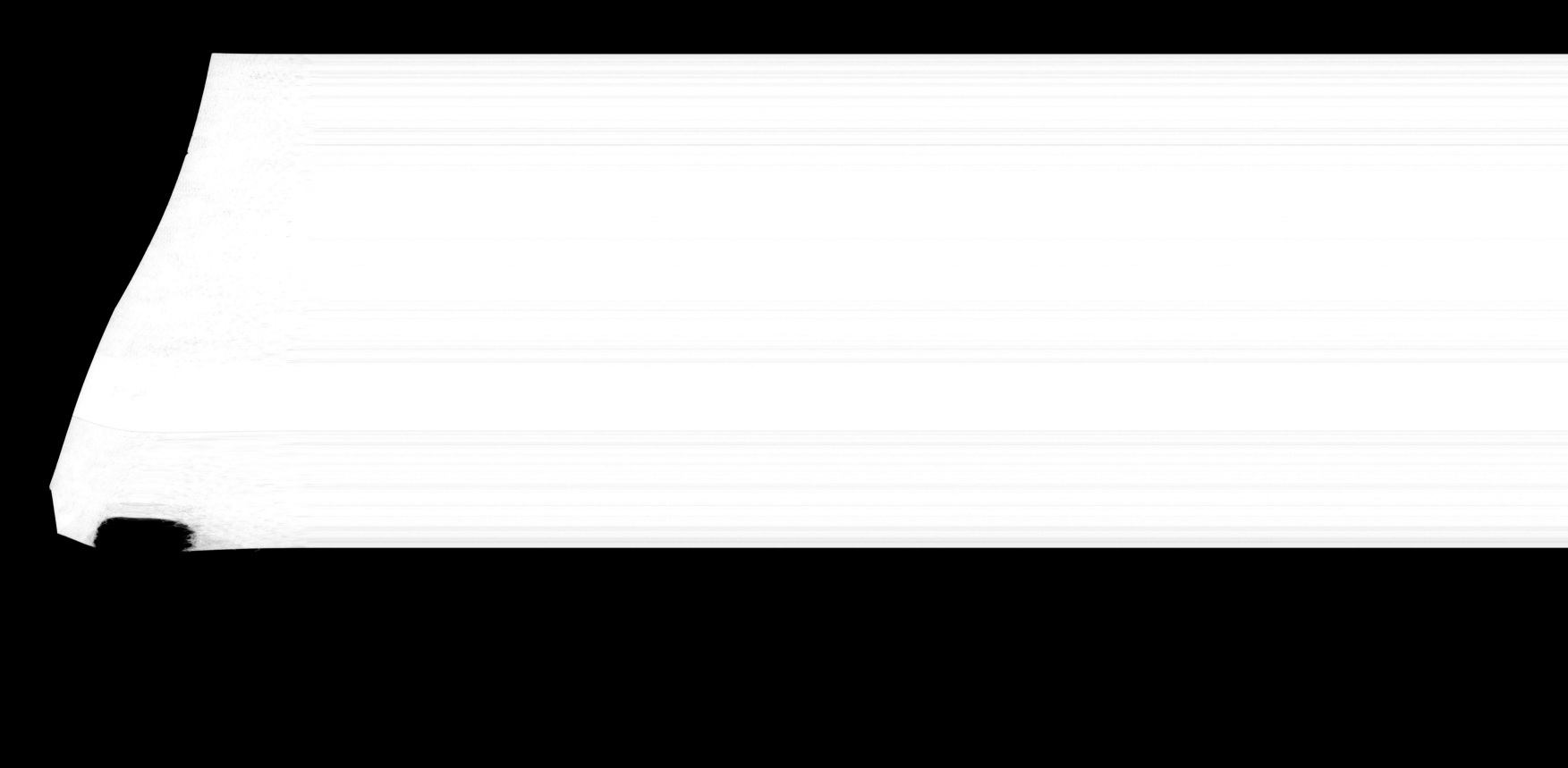

Understanding and Managing Retching

Retching is most commonly associated clinically with children who are being tube fed. The majority of these youngsters have received a Nissen fundoplication and are dealing with retching as a direct or indirect effect of their surgery. Some physicians tell parents that the vagus nerve (cranial nerve X) may have been damaged during surgery. Others feel that the problem is a functional effect of changes in gastric-emptying patterns. A series of medications or formula changes will be explored. Some children seem to get better and experience less retching over time, even without medical intervention. Others remain the same or get worse. Some physicians tell parents that nothing further can be done. Others work with the feeding team to search for answers and relief of these issues.

Clinical experience indicates that retching is composed of two distinct components. It clearly is a physiological event rooted in stimulation of the autonomic nervous system through the vagus nerve. However, like many other gastrointestinal dysfunctions, it also has a series of symptom triggers. Some of these triggers are stimulated by the child's response to the discomfort of retching. This is similar to the issues faced by women during childbirth and individuals who have chronic pain. Pain is increased through anticipation of pain and increased physical tension to fight the pain.

Reduction in pain and an improved quality of life are strongly influenced by approaches that teach the behavioral strategies (e.g., relaxation, self-empowerment, focusing, breathing skills, imagery) for working with the discomfort rather than fighting it (Arnstein, Caudill, Mandle, Norris, & Beasley, 1999; Caudill, 1994; Jones, 1988; Lieberman, Rosenberg, & Simkin, 1992). Caudill, Schnable, Zuttermeister, Benson, and Friedman (1991) found a 36% reduction in clinic visits among patients with chronic pain who participated in an outpatient behavioral medicine program in which they were taught nonpharmaceutical strategies for reducing their level of discomfort.

Reducing Retching

Many of the approaches used in pain management have been extremely effective in reducing the frequency and intensity of retching episodes in infants and children. The feeding therapist may try the following approaches.

Identify the subtle initial signals of gastrointestinal discomfort.

Carefully observe the child for body signals of initial discomfort during tube feedings. These may include facial expression, changes in the swallowing of saliva, increases in body tension, wiggling, shifts in attention, rumbling sounds in the stomach, coughing, and increases in hand-to-mouth patterns. Upon identifying the first signs of discomfort, initiate strategies to improve comfort. Responses to the final discomfort signals of gagging, coughing, retching, and vomiting are usually less effective in stopping the pattern.

Stop the flow of formula intermittently and at any early sign of discomfort.

Stopping the flow of formula allows the stomach to rest and adapt to a lesser level of discomfort. It prevents escalation of the autonomic nervous system into unstoppable gagging and retching.

Reduce physical, sensory, and emotional tension.

A diverse number of approaches can be used to reduce stress and increase physical and emotional relaxation. A well-supported position that encourages gastric emptying is important. Gentle movement, frequent venting of the gastrostomy tube, and music that calms and organizes the senses and emotions can be helpful. Children generally respond to their own combination of strategies that calm the nervous system and reduce emotional and sensory triggers.

Build the child's awareness and discovery of what helps.

Make the child a partner in finding out what makes a difference in the comfort level. These techniques may include softening the abdomen, putting gentle pressure on the abdomen, reminding the child to breathe more deeply, using a signal to the feeder to stop the flow of formula, sucking on a pacifier, or gently triggering a cough or gag that reduces pooling of mucus or saliva.

■ **Empower the child.**

Often, children who retch feel out of control. Their bodies seem to be taken over by an uncontrollable force that randomly makes them feel miserable. By working actively with strategies to reduce the final level of discomfort, children become more empowered. They feel less like victims of their bodies. This can help them shift their beliefs and establish new experiences in which they can move through the retching episodes with less distress. This in itself can reduce the power of pain or discomfort.

Understanding and Treating Poor Stomach Emptying

Movement of gastric contents from the fundus of the stomach to the pylorus requires muscular action. The stomach is not anatomically designed to allow gravity alone to move the food to the pyloric sphincter. Abnormal or inconsistent muscular activity in the stomach can lead to delays in emptying of the stomach. These delays can contribute to gastroesophageal reflux and projectile vomiting. Persistent vomiting with delayed emptying also can be caused by an ulcer or an irritation or growth in the stomach near the pylorus (Hayden, Swischuk, & Rytting, 1987). Medications used to treat GER often improve stomach emptying by increasing its motility. When more conservative measures have failed to achieve efficient stomach emptying, a pyloroplasty is performed to open up the distal stomach and accelerate gastric emptying. Issues relating to medications and surgical procedures are discussed in the previous section related to GER.

Delayed emptying of the stomach contributes to GER and gastrointestinal discomfort after a fundoplication. It also can reduce the child's interest in eating or the amount she eats because part of an earlier meal might still be in the stomach. Because of the stomach's shape and position in the abdomen, gastric emptying occurs more efficiently when the child is lying on the right side (Yu, 1975).

Some children experience too rapid an emptying of the stomach, often as a side effect of a Nissen fundoplication or pyloroplasty (Pittschieler, 1991; Samuk et al., 1996). Food passes rapidly through the stomach and into the small intestine, causing major difficulties with insulin and sugar regulation (Rivkees & Crawford, 1987). Strong autonomic symptoms such as increased salivation, nausea, sweating, lethargy, and pallor may be triggered (Veit et al., 1994). The sudden increase in saliva may cause severe physical and emotional distress for children who have swallowing difficulties. Treatment for dumping syndrome typically involves dietary changes that increase the amount of complex carbohydrates and fat in the diet (Khoshoo, Roberts, Loe, Golladay, & Pencharz, 1994).

The challenges for the feeding therapist may include

■ making clinical observations that may suggest stomach dysmotility problems. These must be reported to the physician as part of the diagnostic effort.

■ partnering with the physician about the clinical impact of stomach dysmotility on the feeding process and feeding relationship.

■ helping the family position the infant on the right side or prone after meals to help promote stomach emptying.

■ helping the child deal with increased saliva production during meals through a strategy such as sucking on a pacifier during tube feedings.

Understanding and Treating Constipation

Constipation, the passage of hard, dry stools, can negatively influence appetite. Children who are constipated often strain during the passage of stools or produce small pellet-sized stools. In an extreme state, constipation can cause fecal impaction or blockage of the intestines. Some of the causes include inadequate fluid intake, inadequate dietary fiber, allergy to cow's milk (Iacono et al., 1995), abnormal muscle tone affecting movement within the gastrointestinal tract, decreased physical activity, and malnutrition. It also can be a side effect of some medications. Improper positioning and lack of an established toileting routine can influence it. When constipation is a chronic problem, it decreases appetite and may have an impact on growth.

Many children with feeding difficulties are prime candidates for constipation. Sucking and swallowing problems may make it difficult, unpleasant, and time consuming to drink adequate liquid. Chewing problems influence dietary choices. Often, the diet does not include the high fiber fruits, vegetables, and grains that promote good movement of digested materials through the intestines. Common problems with muscle tone can reduce the amount and quality of movement needed to move waste materials through the digestive tract. Low muscle tone can make it difficult to recruit enough tone to push out an appropriate bowel movement. High tone can make it difficult to relax enough to release the bowel movement. Fluctuating tone can make a consistent pattern of sustained pushing difficult. Each of these tone issues can influence muscle tone in the abdominal-pelvic girdle and limit movement of the abdominal muscles that help support and stimulate the intestinal tract and help move the stool through the system. Decreased fluid, fiber, and movement can cause constipation in and of themselves. When all three factors affect a child at once, chronic constipation can occur. As a result, appetite can be suppressed and growth may be affected. It can easily become a vicious cycle.

Reducing Constipation

Because there are a number of influencing factors causing constipation, there are a number of treatment options that can be implemented. Although these measures can work individually, a combination usually is more effective.

■ **Increase the child's fluid intake.**

A general guideline is that a child needs 1.5 ounces of fluid per pound of body weight (100 cc/kg). A child weighing 20 pounds needs a minimum of 30 ounces of fluid per day. The amount of fluid needs to be increased in very warm weather and when there is severe constipation.

Whenever possible, children should be given water in addition to the fluid they receive in formulas and other drinks. Even when parents are advised to give drinks containing measurable calories, water should not be eliminated, as it is necessary for proper functioning of the cells (Batmanghelidj, 1995). Guidelines for adding water to the diet are provided in Chapter 16. Highly sweetened drinks (Klein & Delaney, 1994) and drinks containing caffeine (Batmanghelidj, 1995) such as sodas and KoolAid™ are best taken in moderation because they can slightly increase the child's fluid-intake needs.

When children have difficulty swallowing, taking in enough fluid can be a challenge. Strategies for improving sucking and swallowing skills may need to be a priority for therapy. Finding the bottle, cup, or straw that works best for that child and parent is imperative. While working on the oral skills to increase liquid intake, feeders can add fluid-based foods to the diet. Partially chilled gelatin desserts become thick and can be taken as a thick drink. When the child swallows the gelatin, the body uses it as fluid. Some children can take in slushies, popsicles, or frozen fruit bars more easily than regular liquids because these melt as a thin liquid. These options, though appealing to many children, do have high sugar content and must be considered as highly sweetened drinks. They do help increase the overall fluid amounts, but may increase the total fluid need slightly because of their sugary content.

■ **Increase the amount of fiber in the child's diet.**

We need to help parents "think fiber." Dietary fiber helps soften stools and can increase the movement of the intestines. It is imperative, however, that increases in dietary fiber be accompanied by increases in fluid. Without sufficient fluid intake, the fiber can actually slow down the movement in the intestines. Some children can chew and swallow many different dietary sources of fiber, including fresh fruits and vegetables, whole grain breads and cereals, nuts and seeds, and cooked beans and peas. For children with chewing and swallowing difficulties, however, the consumption of sufficient dietary fiber can be a creative challenge. Whenever possible, mash and grind instead of blending fiber foods to give the child larger pieces of fiber in the diet. Incorporate prunes and prune juices into the diet. Raisins, prunes, dried apricots, and apples can be blended and made into a spread for toast, or mixed in with oatmeal. Keep the skins on vegetables such as carrots and potatoes when making soups and vegetable dishes. Bran, seeds, and ground nutmeats can be sprinkled on casseroles, cereals, or soup dishes.

Increase the child's physical activity.

Physical activity can provide movement and physical stimulation for the abdomen, which helps keep the stool moving. Each child's physical skills are different. Some children can move in and out of many positions, walking, running, and keeping physically active. Others lead a more sedentary life because of their physical limitations and are dependent on adults for their movement experiences. Each family and therapist knows what physical activity is best for each child. There must be a conscious effort to incorporate physical activity into the day. This can be child or adult directed. Here are some physical exercises that can be incorporated into the day when the child is dependent on the adult for movement support.

Take a few moments to move the legs during diapering and dressing or after bathing.

1. Bring the child's knees up to the chest. Hold the position if this is comfortable for the child. Then move both knees to the right and hold. Then move both knees to the left and hold.

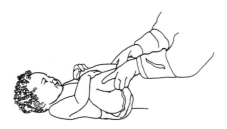
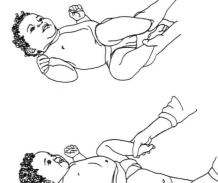

2. Move the legs slowly, as in pedaling a bicycle, pausing as each leg alternately is flexed with the other leg extended. When one leg is extended, the other is flexed.

Use specific massage strokes to enhance elimination and reduce constipation.

Specific massage techniques have been found useful as part of a total constipation-management plan, especially for infants and children who are dependent on adults for movement experiences. Using these techniques in combination with increased fluid and dietary fiber intake and increased general physical activity seems to be a winning combination. Drehobl and Fuhr (1991) suggest that the Water Wheel and Sun/Moon strokes can be effective in treating constipation.

Water Wheel

1. Get the child's permission to begin the massage.
2. Place one hand on the center of the child's abdomen.

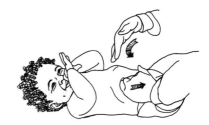

3. Slowly move that hand toward the groin area in a gliding motion.
4. Repeat the above motion with the other hand.
5. Alternate hands, performing this sequence slowly.

Sun/Moon Strokes

1. Get the child's permission to begin the massage.
2. Your left hand (the sun hand) moves clockwise around the abdomen in a circle.
3. Your right hand (the moon hand) follows after the left hand.
4. As you imagine the face of a clock, the left hand starts out at 9 o'clock. As it gets to 6 o'clock, the right hand begins moving in the same clockwise direction. The left hand stops at 5 o'clock and starts back at 9 o'clock. The right hand then finishes at 5 o'clock and goes back to 9 o'clock in the circular motion.

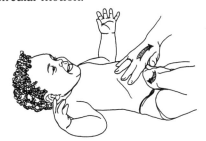 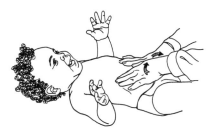

Drehobl and Fuhr recommend that the Water Wheel be done six times and the Sun/Moon be done six times in a sequence to help with constipation.

Review the medications that the child is taking.

Constipation can be a side effect of some medications. Read the labels and understand when GI side effects are possible. Physicians may be able to prescribe a different medication that does not have constipation as a side effect. At other times, just knowing the potential for constipation enables parents to offer extra fluid and fiber to try to avoid it.

Establish a toileting routine.

Parents sometimes need assistance in establishing a toileting routine for their child. Many begin by putting their child on the toilet after each meal, when there is a period of increased intestinal activity. Sitting in an upright position helps put the pressure on the abdomen that can aid in bowel movements. Some children use adaptive toilet seats. The occupational or physical therapist can help in ordering or designing an adaptive system if one is needed.

Developing a daily routine can be difficult for any family. We all lead very busy lives as we move from activity to activity. The schedule for a child with multiple disabilities can be extremely busy, with added doctor and therapy appointments. Finding a way to establish an orderly toileting routine may be a challenge, but it may be well worth the extra effort if it increases functional bowel movements and reduces constipation.

Reduce stress.

The gastrointestinal system is very personal. Stress for some people can cause diarrhea; for others it can cause constipation. As a general rule, less stress is helpful for the GI system. Slowing the pace, establishing routines, and developing stress-reducing strategies for the parent and the child can be an important component of any constipation program.

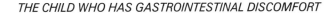

Understanding and Treating Gagging and Vomiting

Vomiting is a common symptom of childhood illnesses. In most instances of acute and chronic vomiting, feeding therapists are not involved in the management of the problem. However, when gagging or vomiting occur in a child who has feeding and growth difficulties, a feeding therapist may become involved. To understand and deal with vomiting, therapists must understand why it is occurring. They must understand the **_look_** of the gagging and vomiting. The following general questions will help adults understand a child's gagging or vomiting episodes.

- When did the vomiting start?
- Does the child gag before vomiting?
- Does the child gag without vomiting?
- How frequently does the child gag or vomit?
- Are the episodes little spit-ups or major projectile vomiting?
- Is the baby calm or upset during the gagging or vomiting?
- Does the gagging or vomiting happen before, during, or after a meal?
- Are there certain food textures that seem to influence the gagging or vomiting?
- Can you predict under what circumstances the child will gag or vomit?
- Does the child ever vomit during sleep?
- Does the child ever vomit small amounts and then swallow it?
- Do certain foods seem to cause vomiting?
- Does the gagging or vomiting occur when the child is stationary or moving?
- Does the gagging or vomiting seem to be provoked by certain triggers?
- Does the vomiting seem to be affecting the child's appetite?
- Are there any other health symptoms associated with the vomiting (e.g., headaches, fevers, other GI or neurological symptoms)?
- Does the vomiting episode bring up food, traces of blood, or just stomach juices?
- Does the child seem to be using the gagging or vomiting to communicate?
- Is the overall mealtime interaction between the parent and the child stressed?
- Could there once have been a sensory or physiological cause for the gagging or vomiting, but now it seems more emotional? What is the emotion?
- Do the gagging or vomiting episodes have a self-stimulatory quality to them?

Persistent vomiting always must be discussed with the child's primary care physician. Feeding therapists often are in situations where they hear parents talking about regular vomiting episodes with the children. They know vomiting can be a symptom of a number of conditions that influence feeding, so it must be taken seriously. Vomiting can be a symptom of structural and motility GI conditions. Oral hypersensitivity and gagging, difficulties with tube feeding, and allergies can lead to vomiting. In situations in which vomiting relates to feeding, feeding therapists often get involved. A disrupted feeding relationship can cause vomiting or be caused by vomiting.

Children who have had chronic discomfort or pain associated with meals may learn to gag or vomit in anticipation of future discomfort. Initially, the vomiting begins with a physiological basis. The child eats food and then vomits or hurts. Gradually, the child learns that food means discomfort and vomiting. The mere sight of food can trigger the vomiting response.

Gagging and vomiting also occur in children whose gastrointestinal structure and physiology is normal. They may have strong sensory and emotional triggers. Gagging that is stimulated by sensory changes in food, including texture, taste, and temperature, can trigger vomiting. The child who is hypersensitive orally may need to vomit to get rid of a worrisome mouthful of food or may vomit as a means of self-protection and avoidance of eating more of the food.

Sometimes, mealtimes become such emotional interactional challenges for children that they vomit at the sight of the meal. Stressed mealtime interactions or perceptions of mealtime stress can trigger it. Once a child starts a vomiting cycle, it can be difficult to stop. It seems to become easier to vomit as a result of a variety of triggers.

Medical Management

Whenever vomiting influences feeding and appetite, feeding therapists must involve the child's pediatrician or primary care physician. It is always important to help parents and physicians understand how the gagging and vomiting are influencing the child's interest in eating. Consultation by a wide variety of specialists (e.g., pediatric surgeon, gastroenterologist, neurologist, allergist) may be needed. Vomiting may be due to a structural problem that must be corrected surgically. Gastroesophageal reflux may cause the child's vomiting and require medical or surgical management. Vomiting may be a sign of neurological changes, as in Arnold Chiari Malformation. When the onset of vomiting is sudden, it may indicate neurological changes and a possible need for decompression surgery. Gagging and vomiting can be related to the food or environmental allergies that increase mucus production or trigger nausea or reflux.

Challenges for the Therapist

Challenges for the feeding therapist usually involve

- **rebuilding trust**

    Vomiting can have a structural or physiological basis that requires medical management. Feeding therapists do not provide the management, but may be in a position to recommend it or notice symptoms that need to be brought to the physician's attention. Vomiting, however, can continue after the medical management of the structural or physiological problem is completed. Children may need to relearn that eating is safe and will not hurt, or that food will no longer get stuck. The child must learn to trust.

    Johnny was 4. He still took in only pureed foods. He had been to traditional behavioral specialists to teach him to eat solids, but was making no progress. Whenever he ate food more textured than a puree, he continued to vomit. No matter what the reward or the punishment, there was no change. He finally was referred to a feeding specialist who noticed that Johnny did chew and swallow some foods that had limited texture. He actually seemed to like some of them. But 10–15 seconds after he swallowed the bolus, he would cough, gag, and eventually vomit that mouthful. The therapist suspected an esophageal stricture, which was confirmed by an upper GI series. No wonder he couldn't swallow solids, and no wonder the traditional behavioral approach did not work! The surgeon performed a series of esophageal dilatations and told his mother to go out and buy him a Big Mac™. Johnny would not eat the hamburger or other more solid foods for quite a while. He sometimes vomited with the introduction of new solid food. He needed to learn to trust his throat. He needed to rebuild confidence in his ability to chew food into a bolus and swallow it without choking. He did learn to eat that Big Mac, but it took time and a gradual thickening of the foods, a gradual increasing of texture, and a gradual introduction of chewable harder solids. Johnny slowly was taught to trust the adults who fed him and to trust himself through feeding therapy that followed his lead.

- **developing oral skills**

    Some children have had the introduction of oral foods delayed while waiting for appropriate surgical procedures. These children may never have had a chance to use the sucking and swallowing skills with which they were born. When skills are not used, they may be forgotten or disrupted. By the time surgical repairs are completed, an infant may not remember what his mouth is for. The feeding therapist can help the child redevelop these skills.

    Brian was born with an esophageal atresia. There was insufficient esophageal tissue available to reconnect the two parts of the esophagus. He needed to be tube fed for 5 months while waiting for esophageal growth. He needed constant suctioning by replogle tube to keep him from choking on the saliva that would collect in the upper esophageal pouch. At 5 months, the anastomosis (surgical reconnection of the esophagus) was completed, and Brian's mother was told she could feed him orally. Brian, however, had a different opinion. He had forgotten that his mouth was for feeding and had forgotten how to suck and swallow. He gagged or vomited when a nipple was offered. He seemed to believe that anything that came toward his face was a relative of the replogle tube and he wasn't going to have anything to do with it! The challenge for his mother and his feeding therapist was to teach him to trust and enjoy his face and mouth, and then teach him the oral skills of sucking and swallowing. Tube feedings were paired with playful oral activities and, gradually, tastes. Nonfeeding times included kisses and playful touches around the face and exposure to fun mouthing toys. Gradually, he began to bring the toys to his mouth and provide his own oral stimulation. Food was placed on some toys, and Brian gradually accepted small amounts of taste in this nonstressed play situation. As his enjoyment and skillful exploration of tastes increased, he showed interest in increased quantity of foods. He did not learn to drink from the nipple, but found cups, spoons, and mouthing toys acceptable ways to take in foods. He redeveloped his oral skills only after he could trust the adults in his environment to listen to him, follow his pace, and not to put scary things down his throat.

decreasing oral-pharyngeal hypersensitivities and hyperreactions

The procedures necessary to medically manage a number of gastrointestinal conditions can create overly sensitive gagging and vomiting responses. For example, children who have had nasogastric tubes repeatedly put in and taken out, extended periods on the ventilator, or constant replogle or trach tubes placed for suctioning can become fearful or overreactive to any change they feel in the mouth or pharynx. Likewise, children who have had constant nausea and gagging or vomiting because of gastroesophageal reflux can become overly sensitive to changes in the texture of foods.

Jayne had a history of severe gastroesophageal reflux. She gagged, arched, cried, vomited, and refused meals. Aggressive medical management with medications and general developmental maturation seemed to help. Eventually, the obvious symptoms of GER disappeared. She was taken off the reflux medications and introduced to more solid foods when she was a year old. She gagged and then vomited whenever a lump was presented. She could not get the lumps past her tongue. She ultimately was given a follow-up barium swallow study through which it was determined that she continued to have regular GER although she was not vomiting at any time other than mealtime. The GER could have caused chronic nausea and gagging, which easily can trigger vomiting. She was restarted on her medications and gradually reintroduced to textures. First, purees were thickened, then food was ground well, and gradually, soft lumps were mashed into the thickened foods. She explored crumbs on her lips and on toys in therapy. She slowly felt confident enough to try more solids and ultimately did well. In her situation, the feeding therapist's role included partnering with the physician on clinical symptoms that may have been influencing the repeated vomiting. It included oral mouthing and exploration, oral games, playful experiences around her mouth, and support for her mother in the gradual introduction of more textured foods.

reducing the emotion

Sometimes, there no longer is a physical reason for a child to gag or vomit. Sphincters are under control, and strictures are repaired. But the child still vomits. He gags and vomits when anything new is presented. He vomits whenever his mother feeds him, but with no one else. He vomits when he is angry or sad. When children are stressed or perceive stress, their gag and vomit response can be much more highly responsive.

Samuel is a child who easily vomits whenever he sits in a high chair. His mother offers him food and wants Samuel to take in one more bite because of her worries about his growth. Samuel leans backward, trying to get away from the food because he does not want it. Experience has shown that a child like Samuel is *much* more apt to vomit when he is stressed and pulling away from the feeder than when he is relaxed and leaning toward the feeder. The physical tilt between the feeder and the child can influence the child's stress level.

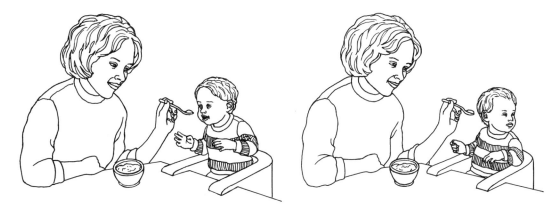

To reduce the emotion of the mealtime, this child may need some distractions. Appropriately chosen distractions can help the child think about something other than "Oh, my goodness, here comes the food. I need to spit up!" A well-chosen distraction can help him think about something else and divert the need to vomit. Caution must be taken when introducing distractions at mealtimes. For some children, distractions become such a vital part of the mealtime process that the child is only eating for the entertainment. The parent needs to add more and more distractions just to keep the meal going. Whenever possible, distractions should be related to the mealtime. The child can be given his own spoon to try to feed himself while the parent is offering spooned foods. Or she can have dried cereal on the tray so she can chase after it with her emerging pincer grasp while spooned food is offered. Sometimes, mealtime music or interesting mealtime conversation serves as a little distraction. An interesting spoon with a favorite character or special straw may provide enough entertainment to keep the child from thinking about gagging.

Some children may have strong emotional reactions to certain adults who feed them. A parent who has pushed the child to eat or has been involved in uncomfortable medical procedures may become associated with feeding and mealtime stress. The parent may need to take a vacation from feeding the child until the child begins to eat well for another person. This may be a therapist, grandparent, or the other parent. As the child begins to eat well for the other person, the parent can get back in the picture, first sitting in the same room, then sitting closer, then offering spoonfuls of a favorite food, and then offering the whole meal. The strength of the stressed emotion is diluted, and the child develops a new set of positive emotions surrounding mealtime.

As a general rule, the stressed emotions of the meal will decrease as the child feels more in control. As children feel that they are respected, being listened to, and have choices, they relax. They no longer feel threatened by anatomy that does not work, textures that are too scary, or interactions that are perceived as too aggressive.

Understanding and Treating Poor Appetite

Internal and External Regulators

Appetite is regulated by the hypothalamus in the brain and by a complex intermixture of neurotransmitters and hormones that provide the physiological messages to eat or stop eating. It also is guided by physical, sensory, emotional, and experiential cues and signals that direct the individual to specific foods. This chapter will not include a review of the neurochemical or psychological literature on appetite control, but will include a discussion of aspects of appetite regulation that relate to the mealtime partnership and gastrointestinal distress.

Satter's philosophy that there must be a division of responsibility at mealtimes has been repeated throughout this book (1983, 1987, 1990, 1999). It is the parent's responsibility to provide an appropriate diet of nutritious foods throughout the day, and it is the child's responsibility to decide which of those foods to eat and how much. Children must decide what goes into the mouth; forcing them to eat will backfire. How, then, can adults get children to eat, grow, and be healthy when they do not seem to have an appetite?

Appetite has internal and external regulators. Healthy children who have positive mealtime experiences from early infancy can internally regulate the amount of calories and nutrients that they take in. Numerous research studies have shown that the internal regulatory system makes spontaneous adjustments to guide children to eating the amount and type of food that they need. When children were given a food with a specific caloric density prior to a meal, their preference for that food was reduced at the next meal (Birch & Deysher, 1986). They also adjusted the number of calories eaten at the meal to compensate for the food they had eaten previously. When children's mealtime intake was examined over a 6-day period, a high degree of variability was noted from meal to meal (Birch et al., 1991). However, their daily energy intake remained relatively constant as the children adjusted their caloric intake at successive meals. Thus, if a child ate very little at lunch, he would eat larger amounts at dinner. This same ability to regulate the amount eaten through internal signals also has been observed in full-term and premature infants under the age of 12 weeks (Matheny et al., 1990; Pridham et al., 1999).

Although infants are born with a strong ability to internally self-regulate, this skill can become reduced when external factors that influence appetite awareness are present. Johnson and Birch (1994) found that the best predictor of children's ability to regulate energy intake was the amount of parental control in the feeding situation. They stated that "…mothers who were more controlling of their children's food intake had children who showed less ability to self-regulate energy intake. These findings suggest that the optimal environment for children's development of self-control of energy intake is that in which parents provide healthy food choices but allow children to assume control of how much they consume" (p. 653).

External regulators of food intake can consist of many different influences on appetite that interfere with the child's internal regulation system. In the typically developing child, the strongest interference is parental control (Johnson & Birch, 1994). Some external regulators, such as physical discomfort, pain, gagging, nausea, vomiting, retching, emotional discomfort, and stressed mealtime interactions have a negative impact on children's appetites. These external regulators can become more powerful than the internal regulators.

Most children start out with adequate internal regulation. Illness, discomfort, or stressed and unbalanced mealtime interactions can cause them to lose track of their inner regulation. Parents who take over the child's responsibility at mealtimes by deciding what, when, and how much the child is to eat can cause the child to lose the ability to determine the appropriate amounts to eat. This can cause undereating or overeating. Many of these children depend on the parent to determine when the meal should start and stop.

Children who are fed on strict schedules often lose their internal regulation skills very rapidly. Tube-fed meals usually are given on a strict schedule to maximize caloric intake. The child's hunger cues rarely are consulted. Children who eat orally have small meals and bigger meals, depending on appetite at the moment. They may skip some meals and then eat much larger amounts at a later meal. Tube-fed children tend to have the same size meals and the same caloric and nutritional content regardless of appetite cues. The tube-feeding schedule becomes an external regulator. Over time, the tube-fed child ignores the internal cues and can become dependent on the adult for caloric regulation. When calories in the tube-feedings are reduced to use hunger as an internal motivation for eating orally, the strategy may be ineffective. The child may ignore the physiological signals of hunger or misinterpret them because they have not been meaningful regulators of appetite.

Adults often describe the physiological signals for hunger and satiation as feelings of mild gastrointestinal discomfort. We eat or stop eating as a way of reducing the discomfort. When children have experienced the major signals of gastrointestinal distress, they often become confused by the more subtle signals of hunger or satiation. Some children are used to paying attention only when signals are very strong. They miss the weaker signals that tell them it is time to eat. Other children are very aware of hunger and satiation signals. However, their only experience with this type of physiological sensation tells them to expect discomfort. They may interpret a hunger signal as impending reflux or gas bloat. The signal then becomes a message to avoid eating rather than to eat. Even more commonly, the child may begin to recognize hunger and start to eat. The uncomfortable signals diminish, and the immediate hunger goes away. As the child eats or drinks more, the stomach begins to expand, and the muscles send sensory signals that eventually result in satiation and cessation of eating. However, some children seem to be alerted to the first signals that the stomach is filling and interpret the signals as gastrointestinal discomfort; thus, they stop eating.

As discussed earlier, delayed gastric emptying and constipation can give a child a constant feeling of fullness. Because the gastrointestinal system is still dealing with a previous meal, the child does not receive or respond to signals of hunger.

A low appetite also can result when children do not feel well. Although parents and physicians generally diagnose a clear-cut cold, ear infection, or flu, children also may have extended periods in which they simply are not feeling well. Their energy and appetite may be low. Their throat may be slightly sore and uncomfortable. They may be cutting teeth. They may have congestion in their ears or sinuses that is not obvious to adults. They may be experiencing mild nausea from an illness or as a side effect of medication. They are not overtly ill, but they are not well. As a result, they show a very low interest in eating or stop eating after the first edge of hunger is reduced. Because these children can show strong variability in their appetite levels, depending on their state of wellness, they create many frustrations for parents.

Why Is the Child's Appetite Poor?

Many questions can be asked to help the family, physician, and feeding therapist better understand why a child has a poor appetite.

- Does the child really have a poor appetite, or is the child just small and following his own growth curve?
- Is the child ill?
- Are the child's ears healthy? Is there an ear infection?
- Does the child have a sore throat?
- When did the family notice a change in the child's appetite?
- Does the poor appetite seem to be related to nausea, gagging, vomiting, retching, pain, diarrhea, or other GI symptoms?
- Does the child have gastroesophageal reflux?
- Does the child's stomach empty properly?
- Is the child chronically constipated?
- Are the child's teeth erupting? Is there tooth decay?
- Is the child offered food on a regular meal-snack schedule, or does the child graze all day?
- If the child is tube fed, what is the feeding schedule? Is the child bolus fed at mealtimes or drip fed all day and night?
- Is the child filling up on high-calorie formula, thereby having no interest in other foods orally?
- Is the child filling up on highly sweetened sugar drinks or foods throughout the day?
- Are the mealtime interactions stressful, thereby causing GI stress symptoms that suppress the appetite?

- Does the child have food allergies that may suppress appetite?
- Is the child's diet deficient in nutrients that impact on appetite, such as zinc?
- Is the child on medications that have appetite-suppressing side effects?

How poor appetites are treated depends greatly on the reason for them. Children need help to feel well enough to notice and trust their internal appetite regulators. Therapists need to look at the external regulators and determine what can be done to eliminate their influence on appetite. At times, the treatment may involve medical intervention or a change in mealtime schedules and food choices. Mealtime interactions can be altered so that they are more positive for the child and the parent. There must be a time of rebuilding of trust and making mealtimes more enjoyable.

Feeding therapists cannot afford to ignore the gastrointestinal aspects of a child's feeding and mealtime program. These gastrointestinal components must be addressed in every feeding program. Blending them with the more standard sensorimotor and oral motor strategies will increase the motor and sensory skills that support comfort and competence in eating.

Additional guidelines for supporting gastrointestinal comfort and increasing positive mealtime experiences are found in Chapters 16, 23, and 24.

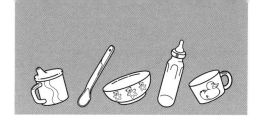

Gastroesophageal Reflux
Parent Questionnaire

Child's Name _____ Today's Date _____

Date of Birth _____ Child's Age _____

Parent Name(s) _____

Primary Care Doctor _____

Name of Parent Completing This Questionnaire _____

Medical and Feeding History

Medical history _____

Specialists your child sees _____

Feeding history _____

Are you or your child's physician worried about your child's growth pattern?   ☐ Yes ☐ No

    Current weight   _____

    Current height   _____

    Height-to-weight ratio   _____

    Head circumference   _____

Is an updated growth chart available?   ☐ Yes ☐ No
If yes, where?

Has your child had a hoarse voice?   ☐ Yes ☐ No

Does your child have a history of bronchitis?   ☐ Yes ☐ No

Does your child have a history of pneumonia?   ☐ Yes ☐ No

Does your child have a history of asthma?   ☐ Yes ☐ No

Does your child have a history of reactive upper airway disease?   ☐ Yes ☐ No

Does your child have a history of respiratory infections?   ☐ Yes ☐ No

Does your child wake up at night?   ☐ Yes ☐ No
If yes, how frequently?

Does your child drool?   ☐ Yes ☐ No
If yes, how frequently?

Does your child swallow with facial grimaces?   ☐ Yes ☐ No

Has your child ever had apnea spells?   ☐ Yes ☐ No
If yes, describe.

Does your child have ear infections?   ☐ Yes ☐ No
If yes, how frequently?

Does your child now have or ever had a gastrostomy tube?   ☐ Yes ☐ No
If yes, describe.

Does your child tend to be a happy or an irritable child?   ☐ Yes ☐ No
Describe.

Does your child ever seem to have eating-related pain?   ☐ Yes ☐ No
If yes, describe.

Has your child ever been treated for gastroesophageal reflux?   ☐ Yes ☐ No
If yes, what was the treatment?

Current medications

Is constipation a problem for your child?   ☐ Yes ☐ No
How often does he or she have a bowel movement?

Current Mealtime Routine

What is your child's current mealtime routine and schedule?

Current Formula   Quantity per feeding   per day
List other formulas your child has tried.

In what position do you feed your child?

Does your child spit up?   ☐ Yes ☐ No
If yes, describe.

How many times a day does your child spit up?

Are there episodes of forceful, projectile vomiting?   ☐ Yes ☐ No

---

Does your child spit up every week?   ☐ Yes ☐ No
Day?   ☐ Yes ☐ No

Does you child cough before spitting up?   ☐ Yes ☐ No
Describe the average quantity of vomiting.

When your child spits up:
    is it after meals?   ☐ Yes ☐ No
    is it during a meal?   ☐ Yes ☐ No
    is it between meals?   ☐ Yes ☐ No
    is it within an hour of the next meal?   ☐ Yes ☐ No

Is he or she more likely to spit up:
    ☐ liquids   ☐ solids   ☐ both liquids and solids

Does your child have a good appetite? ☐ Yes ☐ No
Describe.

List foods your child enjoys.

List foods your child does not enjoy.

Does your child gag when you offer some foods? ☐ Yes ☐ No
If yes, what foods?

Did or does your child have difficulty transitioning from liquids to purees? ☐ Yes ☐ No

Did or does your child have difficulty transitioning from purees to solid foods? ☐ Yes ☐ No

Comments

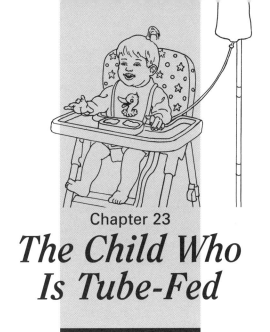

Chapter 23
The Child Who Is Tube-Fed

The use of supplemental feeding tubes to provide nutrition for children has undergone many changes through the years. These changes have required an expanding role for the feeding therapist. In the early 1970s, few children had feeding tubes. These generally were the sickest of children. There were no commercially available tube feeding formulas. Most feedings were homemade or infant formulas. School programs rarely saw tube-fed children. Now supplemental feeding tubes are used extensively to provide total or partial nutrition for many more children. The placement procedures have been streamlined, and even the look of the tubes has changed from bulky catheter tubes to feeding-buttons with insertable tubes. There are many commercially available formulas to replace the homemade varieties, and tubes are common in children attending public schools. Teams have expanded from a surgeon or gastroenterologist with an occasional feeding therapist to teams regularly including a surgeon, gastroenterologist, dietitian, nurse, speech-language pathologist, occupational therapist, physical therapist, and a multitude of other medical specialists. Always central to this team are the child and family. Feeding therapists no longer just support the transition from tube feeding to oral feeding. They frequently are involved when decisions for tube placement are made and as programs are established to optimize oral skills. They help educate families about tube feeding and troubleshoot problems with tube feeding as they relate to appetite, comfort, and oral feeding. They work closely with families and schools in the establishment of oral treatment programs that maximize children's oral skills. They support families as they struggle to incorporate tube feeding into the family mealtime.

■ The Decision to Tube Feed a Child

Tube Feedings and the Family

A tube is given to support life and make it easier for the child to grow without the risk of malnutrition, excessive fatigue, or aspiration. Though physicians may see the tube as an easy and safe way to supplement calories, parents often see it differently. They describe a multitude of emotions when faced with the recommendation of tube feeding their child.

Theoretically, the introduction of the tube could be a positive event—one that supports health, growth and learning. In practice, however, there are many mixed emotions in making the decision to tube feed a child. For some parents, the recommendation for supplemental tube feeding is a relief. The child may have been so sick or struggling so hard to eat and grow that the option to give extra calories by tube may be considered positively. The parents look forward to a sick child becoming much healthier and the undernourished child growing more easily. For other parents, the thought of the tube causes guilt and feelings of failure. In most cultures, there is considerable emotion surrounding feeding. In American culture, there is a strong emotional connection between feelings of adequacy as a woman and a mother and the ability and enthusiasm with which our children eat. Mothers often see their job as feeding their children and helping them grow. When children can't or won't eat in a way that meets their mothers' expectations, mothers wonder where they have failed. Often they have tried and re-tried every imaginable option before the tube was determined necessary. They may have tried changing feeding positions and techniques, changing formulas and mealtime schedules, or adding additional calories. The tube may represent a perceived inadequacy. Even when there is objective evidence that the child's feeding problems are unrelated to issues of mothering, often there is a nagging inner voice that says that if the mother were smart enough, creative enough, or persistent enough, her child would be able to eat. The tube can be perceived emotionally as the final symbol of failure even though logically the parent knows otherwise.

For some parents, there is fear of the unknown. What will the surgery be like? How will the tube be used? What if it comes out? How will I care for it? What will I tell my own mother and friends? Can my child ever go in the bathtub or swimming pool? Surgery is a scary thought for any parent. Some parents may have never seen a feeding tube and may imagine a horrible sight. Others may have seen a tube and were frightened by its appearance or permanency. If the child has neurological problems, there can be a strong, unspoken fear that once a child has been given a tube, it will be required forever. In a sense, the tube can represent the family's fear concerning the severity of the child's problem. Somehow if the tube would go away, it would mean that the child was less disabled and more like other kids.

Most parents grieve in some way for the loss of the dream for a perfectly healthy baby who grows well under the great care they can provide. After surgery, they may grieve over the scarred abdomen that will never again be perfect. Or they may grieve over their inability to lovingly prepare those homemade delicacies that they had dreamed about for their child.

Parents need information and support as they move forward in the decision for tube placement for their child. They may need help in seeing the tube as a nutritive support, as a friend and not an enemy. Although feeding tubes create a great deal of initial concern, parents usually end up experiencing the tube as providing the nutrition necessary for the child to gain needed weight while improving health. Tawfik, Dickson, Clarke, and Thomas (1997) surveyed 29 parents whose children had received a gastrostomy tube to find out whether they were happy with the outcome. These parents reported a reduction in their child's coughing, choking, and vomiting. The children gained weight, and the parents reduced the time spent feeding their child. Only one parent regretted the decision for the child to have a feeding tube.

Tube Feedings and the Child

How the tube feedings affect the child can vary with many factors. The site of tube placement makes a difference. Children receive supplemental tube feedings for different reasons at different times. Tiny, premature infants may receive their first supplemental feedings by orogastric tube (OG-tube) through the mouth because the nasal passages are so small. Later, they may need a nasogastric tube (NG-tube) that passes through the nose en route to the stomach. Still later, the child may need a gastrostomy tube (G-tube) directly into the stomach. Others receive the NG-tube as the first tube. It can be placed for each feeding or placed for a period of days or several weeks. Still other children receive the G-tube initially, bypassing the mouth completely.

Tubes that are inserted through the nose or mouth can create discomfort or distractions that may influence the child's overall perception of the mouth. In addition to different oral experiences created by different placement sites, the child will be influenced by the body's reaction to the food given through the tube. If the child handles the feedings well and grows easily, the tube will have a much more positive effect than if the child gags, retches, or vomits with tube feedings.

Some children are given the tube for total nutrition, while other children who can still eat orally may use a tube to supplement caloric intake. Children who continue to eat orally maintain the ability to receive the natural stimulation of the mouth with foods and liquids although swallowing sensations will vary with tube-site placement. The OG-tube or NG-tube will most directly and immediately affect swallowing.

When total tube feedings are initiated with no food orally, the mouth goes through many changes. The stimulation provided by touch to the mouth, feeding utensils (nipples, spoons, and cups), and food often disappears from the child's sensory experience. Small sucking and swallowing movements that may have been present but were inadequate to support nutrition are no longer stimulated and practiced. Over time, they appear to be forgotten and do not occur when a nipple or food is placed in the mouth. Negative and invasive stimulation to the face and mouth continues or increases as suctioning, intubation, tube insertion, and other life-enhancing procedures are carried out. Gradually, the mouth becomes unfamiliar with touch, taste, texture, and other stimuli that had pleasurable associations. The face and mouth can become physically hypersensitive to touch and taste. It is as if the nervous system increases its sensitivity to search for input that has been withdrawn with the addition of tube feedings. When sensory input is provided, it can be perceived as invasive, uncomfortable, sudden, and intense. The infant dislikes the way things feel and taste in the mouth. If there are problems with physical coordination, the baby may be unable to put fingers, fists, and toys in the mouth. The child is unable to participate in the exploration that is the primary path to learning. The infant becomes cautious about allowing anyone near the mouth. Much of the sensory input is uncomfortable and unpleasant. Suctioning and insertion of a nasogastric or orogastric tube occur frequently. With each invasion of the oral space, the child may strengthen a belief that sensations in the mouth are dangerous and unpleasant. A vicious circle begins as the infant erects barriers against anyone who would provide oral stimulation or offer food.

When tube feedings are initiated immediately after birth, the infant lacks the opportunity to build associations between positive sensations in the mouth and the reduction of hunger or the social interaction with another person that surrounds a meal. If oral feedings become possible later, the prime associations and motivations to take food by mouth are missing. The child may see no relationship between learning to handle food in the mouth and the satisfying feelings that come after a good meal. This can become a greater barrier to the establishment of oral feedings than the original sensorimotor problem.

Parents usually are given instruction in the physical management and mechanics of the tube feedings, but often are not given adequate guidance in adapting them to the parent-infant needs for physical contact and interaction. When tube feedings become mechanical without regard for the emotional aspects of feedings, the development of bonding and attachment can be delayed or altered. This can lead to stressed and unsatisfying parent-infant interactions.

Reasons for Tube Feeding

Babies should be fed by mouth whenever possible, but sometimes oral feedings alone are not enough. Essentially, supplemental feeding tubes are placed to help the child grow and receive adequate nutrition that otherwise was impossible. For some children, the tube becomes the sole source of nutrition, and for others, it becomes a way to add to inadequate oral nutrition. There are many reasons for lack of adequate growth and oral nutrition.

■ **Prematurity.** Premature infants under the gestational age of 33 weeks or who weigh 3 pounds have not reached the stage of development where strong sucking and swallowing patterns can support oral feedings. Orogastric or nasogastric tubes often are used until the infant's sucking skills can support growth.

■ **Anatomical Abnormalities.** Some children require total or partial tube feedings because of anatomical problems, such as esophageal atresia, a tracheoesophageal fistula, tumors, short bowel syndrome or strictures, until those problems are corrected.

- **Neurological Issues.** Some children lack the neurological coordination required to organize and move food in the mouth, and propel it to the back of the tongue and the pharynx for swallowing. Sucking and swallowing may be very slow or very uncoordinated, and the child might be unable to take in enough calories before becoming exhausted. These children may need supplementation for some or all of their nutrition while learning to take in food in a more organized and coordinated fashion.

- **Aspiration.** Because the respiratory system and the feeding system use the same passageway in the upper portion of the pharynx, difficulties with swallowing or breathing coordination can cause a child to aspirate, or draw food or liquid into the lungs rather than into the esophagus. These children often need to receive all nutrition by tube until their lungs heal and they no longer aspirate.

- **Fatigue.** Some children have such severe respiratory and cardiac difficulties or such low muscle tone that they do not have the energy to suck and swallow sufficiently for growth. They may need supplemental oral feedings.

- **Pending Surgeries.** Sometimes an infant has a complicated cardiac, liver, kidney, or other medical problem that will require surgery soon. Supplemental tube feedings may be used in this situation to improve growth and stamina with good nutrition before surgery. This often is the case with cardiac complications causing congestive heart failure.

- **Failure-to-Thrive.** Some children do not take in enough calories and nutrients orally to support their growth and ability to thrive. Tube feedings often are initiated to increase weight and nutritional status (Corwin et al., 1996; Gordon, 1996; Kovar, 1997).

- **Appetite.** Some children have insufficient appetite to support appropriate growth. These children may have ongoing disease processes or be on medications that grossly effect appetite. They may need some supplementation to their oral attempts at eating.

Feeding Tubes

Feeding tubes can be divided into a number of classification groups that have different risks and benefits to the child. The most common are *enteral tubes* that deliver a food formula by tube directly into the gastrointestinal system. A second group consists of *parenteral tubes* that bypass the gastrointestinal system and deliver a special formula intravenously by catheter into the bloodstream.

Enteral Tubes

Orogastric Tubes

The thin and flexible orogastric or orogavage tube (OG-tube) is passed from the mouth (oro-) to the stomach (-gastric). It is usually put in for a feeding and pulled after the feeding. It often is used short term with premature infants whose nasal passageways are too small to allow for the placement of a nasogastric tube (Greenspan, Wolfson, Holt, & Shaffer, 1990). Formula feedings can be given by bolus over 15 to 20 minutes, or can be used with a pump for continuous drip feedings.

Nasogastric Tubes

The thin and flexible nasogastric tube (NG-tube) is placed through the nose and extends to the stomach. This tube can be placed for a feeding and then removed, or it can be an indwelling NG-tube that is taped to the side of the face and left in for several days. Some of the smallest NG-tubes can be left in place for up to a month before changing. Placement of the NG-tube has the advantage of being temporary. Surgery is not required. Parents are taught to insert it appropriately with the help of a stethoscope. Often this tube is used when the infant needs supplementation for a short period of time, up to 2 to 3 months. This may be all some infants need to catch up on growth and become stronger feeders. The infant can eat by mouth with the NG-tube. Formula feedings can be given by bolus over 15 to 30 minutes or can be used with a pump for continuous drip feedings.

There are disadvantages to the NG-tube. Primarily, it may cause interference with the normal swallowing mechanism. In a radiographic study of 10 normal young adults, both wide-bore and fine-bore NG-tubes slowed swallowing by increasing the duration of movement of the bolus in oral and pharyngeal stages of swallowing as well as the duration of the opening of the upper esophageal sphincter (Huggins, Tuomi, & Young, 1999). Infants and young children have been observed clinically to stop swallowing their saliva, presumably from the discomfort created by the movement of the NG-tube. Constant placement and replacement of the tube can create nasal, pharyngeal, and esophageal irritation (Desmond, Raman, & Idikula, 1991). It can be uncomfortable and contribute to gagging or vomiting for some children. When the NG-tube is left in place during oral feeding, it can cause disorganization, swallowing delays, or oversensitivities for some children. Some families lose their sense of privacy because an indwelling NG-tube is constantly visible and advertises their child's medical and feeding difficulties to others.

Nasogastric tubes generally are used for short-term growth. Children with long-term growth and nutritional difficulties usually receive a gastrostomy tube. A small group of children seem to progress to oral feeding adequately despite long-term use of an NG-tube. Some have a high sensory threshold with lowered sensory awareness and seem less disturbed by sensations created by the feeding tube. Others adapt for no clear reason.

Nasojejunal Tubes

The nasojejunal tube (NJ-tube) is similar to the nasogastric tube. Like the NG-tube, it is inserted through the nose and threaded into the stomach. However, it passes through the stomach and ends in the jejunum of the small intestine. Because it follows a more complicated route, it is inserted by a physician, using endoscopic or radiographic guidance. The tube remains in place longer than the NG-tube.

It is uncommon for tubes to be placed lower than the stomach. It is only done when physicians feel the stomach is functioning poorly enough that it must be bypassed to prevent GER when medications have been ineffective and surgery is inappropriate. Because the NJ-tube bypasses the stomach, it may be recommended as a short-term treatment measure for children with severe GER, especially when this is exacerbated by delayed gastric emptying. Because food is delivered into the intestine below where it would be subject to digestion, a special predigested formula must be used. The intestines also require the slower delivery of a continuous drip feeding with a feeding pump rather than bolus feedings.

Gastrostomy Tubes

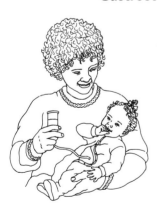

A gastrostomy tube (G-tube) bypasses the mouth completely and is placed directly into the stomach by a surgeon or gastroenterologist. It is inserted surgically under general anesthesia with a hospitalization required or is performed in an outpatient stay (with up to 1 day observation) by endoscopy. The latter is called a percutaneous endoscopic gastrostomy (PEG) (Gauderer, 1991). It is placed with pain medication and tranquilizers but without general anesthesia. Some surgeons prefer to use general anesthesia with younger children during the PEG procedure, but the surgery is relatively brief and the child receives much less anesthesia than in more standard surgical procedures. In either procedure, a catheter tube usually is used initially. After the pathway from the stomach through the abdominal tissue heals, sealing off the pathway to the stomach, a simpler feeding button with a removable tube can replace the catheter (Gauderer, Olsen, Stellato, & Dokler, 1988; Huth & O'Brien, 1987).

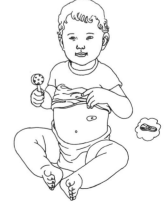

The catheter tube extends 12 to 15 inches from the tube site. It must be taped or carefully watched so it does not become pulled into the stomach. The extra length of tube usually is taped to the diaper or clothing to avoid unnecessary pulling on it. The button tube, on the other hand, lies flat against the abdominal skin. It does not have a length of tubing that comes from the stomach. Often, parents are pleased that it can be easily hidden with clothing and is less likely to be pulled out accidentally by the child's daily movements. The PEG procedure for inserting the gastrostomy tube and the use of a feeding button are the two most common feeding-tube situations encountered with children who have long-term tube feeding needs.

Jejunostomy, Duodenal, and Gastrojejunal Tubes

The jejunostomy, duodenal, and gastrojejunal tubes are variations on the gastrostomy tube in that they avoid the mouth and are placed in the abdomen for direct feedings. The duodenal tube (Duo-tube) is placed directly into the duodenum, the first part of the small intestine. The jejunostomy tube (J-tube) is placed into the jejunum, which is slightly farther down the intestines like the NJ-tube. The gastrojejunal tube (GJ-tube) is a two-branched tube that passes through the abdomen into the stomach. The second branch continues into the jejunum. Some children require medications that must go through the digestive process and are not assimilated well by the body when they are delivered directly to the jejunum. The GJ-tube allows medications to be given through the gastric port and food nutrients to be given through the jejunal port. Again, because the stomach is bypassed, a special predigested formula must be used.

Parenteral Tubes

Total Parenteral Nutrition

Total parenteral nutrition (TPN) is an intravenous procedure in which nourishment is delivered into a large central vein by a catheter. It is used predominantly for children who have major dysfunction of the gastrointestinal tract (Zlotkin, Stallings, & Pencharz, 1985). For example, in short bowel syndrome, the removal of an extensive portion of the intestines reduces the surface tissue that can absorb nutrients. Even though the diet might supply adequate nutrients, the body cannot take them in and use them. To prevent malnutrition from malabsorption, total parenteral nutrition sometimes is used. TPN formulas consist of highly concentrated nutrients that help children survive. However, the system has many negative consequences when used as a long-term feeding solution (Roy & Belli, 1985; Weber, Sears, Davies, & Grosfeld, 1981).

Impact on Oral Motor Treatment and Feeding

From a therapeutic perspective, feeding tubes can be divided into two general categories: those that are inserted through the oral-pharyngeal area (e.g., NG-tubes, OG-tubes, NJ-tubes) and those that are not (e.g., G-tubes, J-tubes, TPN tubes). This is an important distinction, therapeutically. The insertion and presence of a tube in the nose, mouth, or pharynx may compete with goals of a comprehensive oral motor treatment program. Because one of the program goals for feeding therapists is to develop a sense of pleasure and enjoyment with use of the mouth, this will be more difficult if tubes are constantly being inserted or must remain in the nasopharyngeal area. It is uncomfortable for some children to actively suck and swallow with the tube in place. Added breathing difficulties can arise when the tube occludes one small nostril. This also can compete with the development of good feeding skills.

If supplemental nourishment is necessary for an extended period of time, or if the mouth is already a stressed area, a gastrostomy tube generally would be the tube of choice. A G-tube enables nourishment to be supplied in a way that does not conflict with oral motor treatment goals. The area of tube insertion is separate from the oral-pharyngeal area. It may become much easier for the child to discover the pleasurable aspects of the mouth.

There is still a substantial controversy about the role of feeding tubes in the stimulation of gastroesophageal reflux. As discussed in Chapter 22, GER plays a substantial role in influencing many children's desire to eat by mouth. When a feeding tube increases reflux or triggers it when it previously has not been present, the addition of tube feedings may be solving one problem (i.e., aspiration or poor nutrition) while creating another (i.e., reflux with discomfort leading to rejection of oral feeding). Often, physicians and therapists have implied that nasogastric tubes do not create this problem while gastrostomy tubes have a high risk of causing reflux. The incidence of reflux with NG-tubes appears to be related, at least in part, to the size of the tube, with larger tubes creating more acid reflux and reducing the ability to clear refluxed acid from the esophagus (Noviski, Yehuda, Serour, Gorenstein, & Mandelberg, 1999).

Concern that gastrostomy procedures and tubes could cause reflux has strongly influenced medical procedures. Studies published in the early 1980s led to doing ***protective*** fundoplication surgery with each gastrostomy procedure (Jolley, Smith, & Tunell, 1985; Mollitt, Golladay, & Seibert, 1985; Wesley, Coran, Sarahan, Klein, & White, 1981). More recent studies have shown mixed results, especially when gastrostomy tubes have been inserted using the PEG procedure. Some have shown increased reflux in children who previously were diagnosed with GERD, as well as the onset of reflux in children who did not have it before surgery (Grunow et al., 1989; Langer et al., 1988). Others have shown that a PEG-tube does not increase or cause reflux (Borowitz, Sutphen., & Hutcheson, 1997; Launay et al., 1996). It is very important for feeding therapists to be aware of surgical and therapeutic complications related to feeding tubes so that they can be more effective in parent education and in dialogues with physicians.

Table 23.1   **Enteral Tube Comparisons**

	Orogastric Tube	**Nasogastric Tube**	**Nasojejunal Tube**	**Gastrostomy Tube**	**Jejunostomy Tube**
Placement	Mouth to stomach	Nose to stomach	Nose to jejunum	Directly in stomach	Directly in jejunum
Placement Method	Non-surgical	Non-surgical	Non-surgical	Surgical	Surgical
Who Puts the Tube in Initially?	Physician, nurse	Physician, nurse	Physician, nurse	Surgeon	Surgeon
Who Replaces the Tube?	Parent	Parent	Physician	Physician or parent	Physician
Nutrition	Commercial or homemade formula	Commercial or homemade formula	Pre-digested formula	Commercial or homemade formula	Pre-digested formula
Appearance	Shows	Shows	Shows	Does not show	Does not show
Influences Swallowing	Yes	Yes	Yes	No	No
Type of Feeding	Bolus or continuous	Bolus or continuous	Continuous	Bolus or continuous	Continuous

■ Management of Tube Feedings

Bolus or Continuous Drip Feedings

The type of feedings done with the tube will depend on the child and the reasons for tube placement. Some feedings are given by **bolus**. This type of feeding is intended to serve as a meal that fills the stomach, usually in 15 to 30 minutes. It usually is done by day, coinciding as closely as possible with the family meals. Other children are fed by **continuous drip**. For the drip feedings, the child's tube is connected to a special feeding pump. It is set for a certain number of ccs per hour for a certain number of hours (e.g., 40 ccs per hour for 10 hours). This method often is used for supplementation at night while the child is sleeping. Some children who receive bolus feedings also may use a feeding pump set at a high output rate so that the flow of formula is more even and predictable over a 30-minute period.

There are many variations on these methods. Under optimum circumstances, it is best to try to follow as normal a schedule as possible for children who are tube fed. Toddlers and older children who would be receiving three large meals and two small snacks per day can receive tube feedings with the same volume and timing. Some children receive bolus feedings by day and a continuous drip feeding at night. Their stomach capacity may not allow enough caloric intake in the daytime bolus feedings. Others receive boluses by day and night. This alternative is more difficult for parents who need their sleep, too! Some children receive four large bolus feedings for their complete daily nutrition, while others, whose stomach capacity is small, may receive many smaller bolus feedings. Some bolus feedings are given in 10 minutes; others take more than an hour. Some feedings are given following an oral feeding to provide the calories that the child has not taken by mouth. Others are given once before bed. Some children who need a very slow feeding rate may need a continuous feeding from the pump for almost 24 hours a day. This is usually done when the stomach does not tolerate more than a tiny amount at any given time.

The decisions regarding the way to use the tube for feeding depends on the health and capacity of the child's gastrointestinal system, the ability or inability to take food orally, and the family schedule. Often the schedule is rearranged when appetite is being stimulated to increase a child's interest in oral feedings.

Positioning for Tube Feeding

It is important to provide tube-fed children with the physical and emotional nourishment that independent oral feeders receive at the family mealtime. This goal will influence the positioning and place of the meals. If a baby is at an age when he typically would be held during a feeding, then it is appropriate to try to hold him during tube feedings. Physical and emotional closeness as well as time together remains important for parent-infant attachment and bonding. If a toddler would be sitting in the high chair at family meals, then she should be in the high chair at the family meal. An older child could be at the table or in a booster seat while being tube fed. When possible, the tube feedings should be incorporated into the family meal so that children are a part of the mealtime socialization. They will continue to learn a great deal from seeing others eat and share meals.

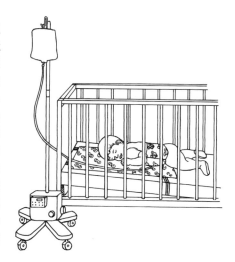

Some feeding schedules require the child to be fed when the family is not eating. The child still can be invited to join the family for mealtime socialization. Additional meals can take place as the schedule requires. These meals also can take place in a parent's arms, in the high chair, or at the family table.

Continuous drip feedings and night feedings require different considerations. A child who receives feedings by day and night through the feeding pump will have an extension tube on the pump that allows for movement. Some children who are walking will wear a child-sized backpack that carries a small, portable, feeding pump. This provides more freedom of mobility than being confined to a pump hanging from a wheeled IV stand. Children who are fed during sleep usually do best if positioned in prone with a slightly elevated bed or in a sidelying position on their right side. For the elevated prone position, a wedge can be positioned in the bed or a few books can be placed under the mattress to elevate the head of the bed. This prone position often works best with a special sling support (Nordstrom, 1988; Noviski et al., 1999). This cloth 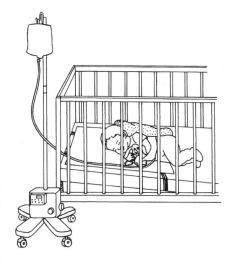 wrap helps position and keep the infant in prone while sleeping. A variety of positioning slings is available commercially. Some parents have made slings by sewing or taping a large pair of men's underpants to the bedsheet and slipping the child's legs through the holes. The sidelying position often is facilitated with a pillow or positioning roll at the child's back. Positioning on the right side facilitates more rapid stomach emptying because of the angle of the stomach and position of the pyloric outlet into the small intestine. Both positions seem to reduce the frequency of GER, which can be induced or aggravated during tube feedings.

Diet and Tube Feeding

Tube-fed children need to be monitored closely by the physician and dietitian. The tube is placed, and a formula and schedule are presented. All too often, the child remains on that same formula with the same schedule for months or even years. Just as the diet for orally fed children changes over time, maturity, and activity level, so must the diet of the tube-fed child. Healthy, orally fed children tend to eat more as they grow. They monitor their own growth needs and eat accordingly. Tube-fed children often are dependent on others for their feedings. The sense of hunger and appetite often is altered or confused. Parents and other team members must remember that the nutrient and caloric needs for these children change. Growth, nutrients, calories, and mealtime schedules need to be monitored. The goal is to do what is necessary to ensure a healthy pattern of growth for the child.

When the medical profession began using tube feeding to supplement feedings or provide total nutrition, most parents were blending their own formulas. As commercially prepared formulas became available, the trend shifted strongly away from homemade formulas. The commercially prepared formulas have been pasteurized to prevent food contamination. They are fast, easy, convenient, and readily available, and third-party payers often pay for them. This has eliminated the fuss and muss of formula preparation. The formula companies have done a highly effective job of marketing formulas as complete foods that provide everything the child needs. But do they? Now is a good time to look at the concept of dietary diversity and reconsider this approach (Morris, 1998a).

The human body was designed to receive a diversified diet. The breast-fed infant is exposed to dietary diversity at each meal because the taste of strong-tasting foods eaten by the mother passes into the breast milk. The fat content of the milk varies from the beginning to the end of the meal, again offering change and variety. By 6 months, the diet of the typical infant is expanded to include cereals, fruits, and vegetables. Anecdotal reports of bottle-fed infants suggest that there may be both a greater eagerness to transition to supplemental foods and a greater difficulty in making the transition to new tastes. Perhaps this occurs because of an inner drive and need for dietary diversity, as well as a lack of preparation for the shift to greater diversity because of the infant formula. Continued diversity in infant feeding is encouraged during the first year to provide a strong foundation for the variety that will support a nutritious diet for the child and adult.

The infant who is unable to take nutrients by mouth is limited in receiving dietary diversity. Like the bottle-fed infant, the baby who receives tube feedings generally is given a single formula during the first 6 months. However, the tube-fed child continues to receive this single dietary formula with none of the normal variation associated with typical growth and development. The formula will be changed as the child grows and requires a higher level of nutrients and calories; however, a formula similar to the infant formula generally is recommended. For example, if babies have been on a soy formula, a standard soy formula often is introduced when they are ready for a higher calorie formula.

The child's gut gains experience digesting only one formula if the same formula is provided day after day, year after year. After a while, the introduction of a new food or formula can cause a stooling reaction because the gut has lost some of its versatility and ability to deal with new foods. Is this optimal for the digestive system? When new foods or formulas are introduced slowly, in dilute form, the gastrointestinal system can re-establish efficiency for digesting a wider variety of foods.

In addition, we know we can taste foods that have been placed directly into the stomach by gastrostomy tube. These tastes come from wet burps that come up into the mouth and from dry burps which are air bubbles that come up into the nasopharynx. Even children who cannot create efficient burps because of a fundoplication appear to emit a formula odor from the mouth. Interpretation of taste comes from a combination of taste and smell. The olfactory system smells foods not just directly through the fragrance of the food in the air, but through the olfactory receptors in the nasopharynx that smell the burps from the stomach. Perhaps diets for tube-fed children should rotate formulas for diversity in the gut. Perhaps parents occasionally should feed children some pureed real foods through the tube or make homemade formulas to diversify the diet and provide tastes that may inspire totally tube-fed children to try new foods orally. These possibilities are discussed in the Treatment section of this chapter and in Chapter 16.

Tube Feeding Management Team

The child who is tube fed often acquires a very complex management team. In some situations, there are so many people that the family can easily become overwhelmed and confused. In other situations, there is not enough support for the family; the tube is placed and the parents are sent home with minimal understanding of tube feedings and the issues that they and their child will face. It is important for feeding therapists to learn as much as possible about tube feedings so that they can be a strong support for the family. Though there are a number of people who theoretically can be involved on the team, the nature of the tube-management support team will vary, depending on the experience of members and the setting in which support is provided. Some hospitals or clinic settings have primary care physicians, gastroenterologists, surgeons, nurses, dietitians, speech-language pathologists, occupational therapists, physical therapists, social workers, and psychologists under the same roof. Each may play an important role for the family in the management of tube feedings; likewise, the multitude of faces may overwhelm them. In isolated rural settings, a feeding therapist or dietitian may give the support. If the person has extensive tube feeding experience, this may be enough to manage many of the issues that arise. Team members working with tube feedings often are called upon to understand the mechanics of the tube feedings, dietary considerations, emotional aspects of feeding tubes, and the feeding relationship. It is important for feeding specialists to understand the full range of issues so that they can offer comprehensive support to families and serve as a link to other team members as they guide the family and child along the tube feeding process. Some communities have organized parent support groups for families whose children receive tube feedings. An electronic community also could provide worldwide support through parents and professionals who participate in listserv groups on the Internet.

■ Treatment

Referral for Treatment

When should a child be referred for treatment? Many infants and children are referred in infancy. Others are not referred until they are older. There are many advantages to beginning a treatment program as soon as tube feedings are recommended. It is important to *educate* parents about tube feedings, *prevent* problems from developing, and *optimize* oral motor control and oral enjoyment for exploration and feeding.

To develop appropriate referrals for treating these children, feeding therapists must clarify how they describe their work to themselves and other team members. The concepts that are usually associated with the terms *feeding therapy* and *traditional oral motor therapy* are not always the most appropriate for children who are on feeding tubes. The goals determined by feeding therapy versus traditional oral motor therapy versus comprehensive oral motor treatment can be very different. The therapists' goals and expectations in each of these treatments will determine the nature and timing of the therapeutic activities chosen. Although the differences between these therapy program names may seem semantic, it is important to look at their underlying differences in orientation.

Feeding Therapy

The primary goal of feeding therapy is oral feeding. The program may include many steps and components of an oral motor treatment program, but the context is different. Because the short-term goal is oral feeding, often there is a sense of haste and a diminished importance of each step along the way. The current step is only a way station toward a predetermined goal. If oral feeding is not achieved within a reasonable time, there is no sense of accomplishment—only a perception of failure. The primary emphasis within the program is placed on the mechanics of sucking and swallowing and increased food intake, and the child may become lost in the process. Activities to enhance positive interaction and communication may be missing. Feeding therapy always works toward the use of food and liquid in the program. Food may be introduced before the child has the requisite oral, pharyngeal, and respiratory skills.

Traditional Oral Motor Therapy

The primary goal in *traditional* oral motor therapy is to improve the function of the mouth, perhaps for feeding and perhaps for speech production and articulation. Therapists often use a *cookbook* of oral motor ideas to make therapy fun and to improve specific oral motor function. In this approach, there may be oral motor changes in children who have feeding tubes, but they may be limited. These programs frequently fail to look past the mouth into the other sensory, motor, emotional, and physiological systems that influence oral function.

Comprehensive Oral Motor Treatment

The primary goal of *comprehensive* oral motor treatment, as defined with tube-fed children, is to develop positive and enjoyable use of the mouth in all its functions. The treatment focus is to develop the appropriate use of the mouth in conjunction with respiratory and phonatory systems, in exploration, sound play, and as much oral feeding as possible. Food and liquid are not essential to the program (especially in the initial stages), and may not be included at all if the child has a severe swallowing disorder. Treatment strategies include opportunities for development of sensory awareness, perception, and discrimination within the mouth. Use of oral movement to explore and understand the world of toys, clothing, body parts, sounds, food, and liquid also is provided. Food and liquid may be introduced to provide smells, tastes, and temperatures, and to elicit specific oral movements when the child is medically able to handle them. Treatment always looks at the effects of the mouth on the feeding relationship and looks at the physiologic systems that have an impact on the mouth. It looks at the mouth as a part of a whole child, who is a part of a whole family! Oral feeding is the by-product of a total program, not the major goal. As a result, there is an ongoing sense of gain and accomplishment throughout the program that is not diminished by the slow attainment of oral-feeding abilities.

Comprehensive oral motor treatment provides support for the child and family, wherever they are on the journey between tube feeding and oral feeding. Guiding children from tube feeding to oral feeding is a process that involves many steps and considerations. It is not usually an either/or proposition. Most children develop skills from their own starting point on the continuum. They let us know if and how fast they can move along. Their medical status, growth, and development of oral skills determine the path taken along this continuum. Some children remain tube fed for extended periods, but need to continue to build the oral skills for oral exploration, swallowing, and oral hygiene. Some children become oral feeders for solids and continue to take liquids by tube. Oral skills for chewing and swallowing need to be developed or maintained. Other children become complete oral feeders by day with some nutrient supplementation at night. Still others move off the tube and onto complete oral feedings. By focusing only on feeding as the major goal and component in the program, the scope of the program is narrowed and many programming aspects that are essential to help the child progress are eliminated. The result may be frustration for the child, parent, and therapist. Comprehensive oral motor treatment supports the child anywhere on this continuum. Morris (1989) said: "The ultimate success of a (comprehensive) oral-motor treatment program is not measured by the child's progression to total oral feedings. It is measured by the emergence or enhancement of a child's ability to enjoy the mouth and use it for exploration with sensory awareness and discrimination. It is measured by the growth of a communicative child who uses vocalization, sound play, and gesture to interact with others" (page138).

These are important distinctions. An early referral for comprehensive oral motor treatment is always appropriate for a child who is receiving supplemental tube feedings. When therapists state that they are providing feeding therapy for children, referrals for early treatment may not be made if the physician feels that oral feeding would be dangerous or does not believe that the child will ever become an oral feeder. Comprehensive oral motor treatment programs focus strongly on parent-child interaction during mealtimes and on parent education. Even children who are medically unstable and cannot be physically handled by a therapist can benefit from early enrollment in this type of treatment program. By expanding thinking about comprehensive oral motor programs and educating physicians about them, more appropriate referrals will be made with greater consistency.

Role of the Feeding Therapist

Children who receive all or part of their nourishment through a tube create special challenges for parents and therapists. The level of involvement for the feeding therapist varies with the nature and intensity of the problems that led to initial tube placement. For some, the role is education and prevention; for others, it is ongoing consultation. Others need direct oral motor treatment, and still others need strong family support. Many families need a combination of these supports.

Education

Some families primarily need information. Feeding therapists can assume an important role by becoming a resource for educating the family about tube feeding. Parents want and need to learn all about the tube that their child is about to receive. How will it be put in? How does it work? Where do we get the supplies? What formula should we use? How should we hold our child during feedings? How can we prevent spitting up? What is the best timing for tube feeding so that our child will still be hungry for the oral feedings? When will our child be able to get rid of the tube? These and many other questions can overwhelm the family initially. A feeding therapist with experience in tube feeding can answer many of these questions or know where to get the answers from other team members.

The therapist needs to educate the family and the team to prevent problems. Many children start out simply needing the tube for supplemental nutrition and end up refusing all foods that they used to eat by mouth. This is devastating for parents and often can be avoided. Other children are put on tube feeding and not allowed to take anything orally. Parents need to be educated about what they can do to keep the child from neglecting the mouth, to optimize oral skills, and to continue to associate the mouth with feedings. Parents need to understand what to do in the beginning to prevent problems and what to do if they occur.

Ongoing Consultation

Some families and children need ongoing consultation to monitor progress. How is the family managing the tube feedings? How is the child growing? How is the child using his mouth? Is the child showing readiness factors to begin working toward more oral feeding? By monitoring the child and family's progress with tube feedings, feeding therapists can provide regular education, prevent future problems, or catch small problems before they become big ones. They can monitor oral skills and recommend more specific oral motor treatment as needed.

Family Support

It is important for families of tube-fed children to receive support, not only from the medical team, but also from other families who have children fed by tube. Many feeding therapists provide this support with other team members by offering opportunities for parents to come together and share their own experiences with tube feedings. Parents learn a great deal from each other, and therapists learn a great deal from parents.

Direct Oral Treatment

Many children have oral sensorimotor difficulties that influenced the decision to place the tube. These issues must be treated thoughtfully and comprehensively in partnership with the child, parents, and therapist. Direct oral motor treatment may involve food, depending on the nature of the child's medical issues. The goals of the program may range from improving the feeding relationship to optimizing feeding enjoyment to oral normalization and desensitization to experimentation with new foods tastes and textures to increasing the pleasure in increased quantities of food. (See Components of a Comprehensive Oral Motor Treatment Program later in this chapter).

Common Influences on Treatment

Children who are tube-fed demonstrate many different feeding issues and sensitivities depending on each child's oral experiences with and without foods, medical status, previous and current interactions around mealtimes, overall physical skills, and specific oral skills. The influences outlined in Chapter 24 that describe why children do not eat also impact the oral treatment program. Following is a discussion of the multiple influences on the child and family that affect the goals of the comprehensive oral motor treatment program.

Oral Experiences

Children's prior and current oral experiences strongly influence how they approach oral stimulation and feeding. Limiting or aversive responses to oral stimulation occur frequently when the infant has been deprived of positive sensory input to the mouth. Because many of these children require invasive procedures such as prolonged ventilation, suctioning, and tube insertion, they may develop a belief that the mouth is an unpleasant place. They avoid using it to explore and learn because it is uncomfortable. They become wary and watchful of anyone who approaches the mouth. Their attempts to protect or guard the area become deeply ingrained.

Some infants have tubes placed almost immediately if their medical status or poor sucking skills warrants it. These children then may have had no experiences with normal sucking and swallowing. They may "forget" how to use existing sucking and swallowing skills or may never have developed them. They may not have any experiences with tastes and textures and may end up missing the critical periods where the learning of oral skills is physiologically most easily achieved.

Medical Status

Many medical conditions make mealtime enjoyment difficult and healthy growth impossible. Children with cardiac difficulties may fatigue so quickly that mealtimes become exhausting. Respiratory difficulties are observed with high frequency. Respiratory issues contribute heavily to exhaustion and poor coordination of sucking and swallowing patterns with breathing. When given the choice of breathing or eating, these children choose breathing. Respiratory control problems contribute to fearfulness and caution as a general approach to new or unsuccessful experiences. They may become exaggerated when the child produces excessive mucus that collects in the pharyngeal airway. Children who aspirate may eat less because of their internal realization that the food or liquid is not good for them.

Many children have other disease processes, medications, or severe allergies that negatively influence appetite. Gastroesophageal reflux, for example, can strongly influence mealtime experiences. It is unpleasant for the child and caregivers. Constant acid irritation of the esophagus can reduce the infant's desire to take food by mouth because of the discomfort. Appetite is suppressed. Children quickly learn that eating means discomfort or pain, and therefore often avoid or reduce eating by mouth.

Children with many medical conditions have learned that mealtime is no fun! When supplemental feeding tubes are placed, many realize they feel so much better with a full tummy or have to work so much less at feeding that they voluntarily stop eating by mouth. They need to have their medical conditions treated and then may need to re-learn that eating can be enjoyed.

A review of 100 young infants fed by nasogastric tube showed a powerful relationship between medical factors and the length of time required for the baby to transition to complete oral feeding (Bazyk, 1990). The total number of medical complications showed a significant positive correlation with the length of the transition. Children who had 10 medical complications, for example, required a longer period for the transition than those who had fewer complications. Digestive, respiratory, and cardiac complications were strong predictors of a longer transition to oral feeding.

Mealtime Interactions

Children's personal-social interactions surrounding meals strongly influence their attitudes about meals and development of appropriate oral skills. Parents of tube-fed children often are guided in the mechanics of tube feeding, but not in the emotional aspects of feeding. If tube feedings become a mechanical process, children and parents can miss out on the nurturing, trust building, attachment, and bonding aspects of the mealtime relationship. Emotional responses to the feedings can express themselves as colic, irritability, gagging, retching and vomiting, and an unwillingness to try new things in the mouth.

Sometimes by the time the tube is placed, parents and therapists have tried everything. They have added calories, encouraged, prodded, and begged. They have bribed, coerced, and tricked. Sometimes the child has been forced to take in calories by well-meaning parents and relatives who are just trying to help the child grow. The overall effect may be a child who cringes when he sees food coming. Mealtime may have become a time of stress for all. The positive aspects of the mealtime relationship have been lost. Neither child nor parent enjoys the meal any longer. The positive mealtime relationship must be reestablished.

Physical Skills

Changes in muscle tone influence the effectiveness and coordination of skills for eating. Many tube-fed children have neurological issues that affect muscle tone, causing hypertonicity, hypotonicity, or fluctuations in tone. These tone changes affect the child's posture for eating and respiration. Poor trunk posture influences head and neck control. It also has an impact on the internal organization of the digestive process. Children who round their back in sitting often **bend** right at the level of the lower esophageal sphincter. This can promote or aggravate gastroesophageal reflux. Hyperextension of the neck, accompanied by scapular adduction and shoulder girdle elevation, is seen as the primary movement characteristic of many of these infants and young children. This position strongly influences oral and pharyngeal control, and affects the skills of bolus preparation and the safety of swallowing.

Oral Skills

Some children are born with poor oral skills that lead to the tube placement, while others develop them. Infants may have poor oral skills for many different reasons. Disorganized and arrhythmic sucking patterns are characteristic of many neurologically impaired tube-fed infants. Often a clear sucking rhythm is lacking. Movement may be further disorganized when touch or pressure is applied to the tongue with a nipple or spoon. Some children's oral skills at birth do not support good growth. When feeding tubes are given, the children may stop eating orally so that they do not have to work so hard. These are children who often seem to forget sucking and swallowing skills. When organizing input and experiences are not provided early, critical periods of development may be missed. Thus, when intervention finally is provided, these children may have bypassed the physiological stages at which learning is most easily achieved (Illingsworth & Lister, 1964).

Swallowing disorders preclude the development of successful oral feeding. Many children have difficulty using the tongue and lips to organize the bolus of food or liquid in the oral cavity and project it backward for the swallow. Small amounts of food may drip over the back of the tongue without eliciting a swallowing reflex. When the swallowing reflex fails to occur, the airway is open and unprotected, and the upper end of the esophagus does not open to allow food to pass. Aspiration of food into the lungs is the natural consequence. Some children have a delayed swallowing reflex. Instead of the pattern triggering from the backward movement of the tongue and the stimulation of the anterior pillars of fauces, swallowing is elicited after food or liquid has collected in the valleculae or pyriform sinuses. Although the swallow occurs, a portion of the bolus may be aspirated.

Some tube-fed children develop overreactive or underreactive responses to oral stimulation. These may occur with touch to the face and mouth, or as reactions to textures, tastes, smells, or temperatures. These will need to become more normalized as a part of an oral treatment program.

Components of a Comprehensive Oral Motor Treatment Program

A comprehensive oral motor treatment program is a holistic program, based on a global view of the needs of the child and the family. Many aspects of interaction, sensation, movement, learning, social skills, and communication are included. The focus of treatment is not strictly on the function of the mouth in feeding. The following components of the program must be considered in the development of a successful treatment program for children who are tube fed.

Establishing a Positive Mealtime and Treatment Relationship

A comprehensive program must begin with the reestablishment of a positive mealtime relationship for the parents and child at home and for the therapist and child during treatment. Just as the mealtime is a relationship between the parent and child, it also becomes a relationship between the child and therapist. The child's relationship with both is extremely important to the program's success. Parents and therapists come to the relationship with positive and negative experiences with feeding and oral treatment. The abilities of the therapist to convey the principles of the oral program and the abilities of the parent to understand and carry out recommendations at home also will strongly influence the program. Children come to the relationship with their own temperaments, experiences, attitudes about mealtimes, and skills. All of these influence where, when, and how to begin an oral treatment program with the goal that the child will enjoy oral exploration and have positive feelings about the mealtime.

Therapists can use many of the same strategies in establishing positive relationships with the child and parents. Parents need to be reminded about the importance of positive touch during tube feedings as well as throughout the day. Positions for tube feedings, when possible, should involve the same supportive, loving holding that a baby would receive during breast-feedings and bottle-feedings. In the same way that a parent would pause a feeding for burps or discomfort in bottle feeding, the parent of a tube-fed child can learn to be sensitive to signs of discomfort or fullness and create comfort pauses. Parents can be shown how to *listen* to the body language of widening eyes, changes in facial expression, signs of discomfort, and wiggling or arching. These may be cues to pause, slow down, or discontinue a tube-fed meal.

For children who have had negative experiences around the mouth, parents need to understand the importance of positive loving touch, not only orally, but also over the whole body. Positive and loving touch can be an important component in the reestablishment of trust in the feeding relationship. Touch and movement can be used in a highly communicative, interactive fashion during treatment and daily care. Pediatric massage techniques can be demonstrated so that loving touch is incorporated into the daily routine of the child (Drehobl & Fuhr, 1991). Parents can play interactive touch and oral stimulation games around the face and mouth. Kissing can become very powerful and rewarding therapy for both the parent and child. Favorite stuffed animals or dolls can help with the kissing and facial touches in a safe and familiar fashion. Combining songs with touch activities can provide a distracting, playful, and predictable rhythm.

Children must be given some control over the mouth to trust those around them. They must be allowed to let the parent and therapist know what feels good and what does not. They need to trust that they no longer will be forced to have unpleasant, frightening experiences around the mouth and at mealtimes. They must be allowed to give permission by actively participating in the presented activities or meals. Each child can learn to give permission by leaning forward into the experience or opening the mouth. Children will develop trust if the focus of treatment is to make the oral experiences enjoyable, with their active participation. Programs that try to desensitize the child by pushing unwanted stimulation into the mouth are incompatible with the goal of oral motor and mealtime fun.

In comprehensive oral motor treatment, the therapist and parents follow the child's lead. The child knows what she can handle, what feels good and what does not. The adult and the child establish a trusting mealtime relationship where the child gives permission for the activities presented. The therapist and child explore the aspects of oral treatment together. It is not a program where the therapist "does *to* the child." They dance *together*.

Establishing a Relationship Between the Mouth and Feeding

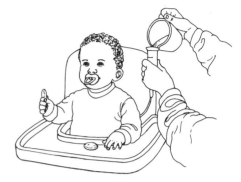

Children who are fed by tube from early infancy can forget that the mouth has anything to do with the feelings or the satiation that comes with a meal. Oral feeders are hungry, see the breast or bottle, eat, and then feel full. They easily learn to relate the feelings of fullness with the mouth and eating. Tube-fed babies receive a feeling of fullness through a tube that passes into the nose or stomach. In the child's experience, the mouth may have no relationship to the feeding. Some children who are on continuous drip feedings are fed all day. They never have an opportunity to experience hunger or satiation. This further complicates the relationship between the mouth and hunger. Early treatment can allow for associations to be made with smells and tastes during tube feeding by pairing oral-feeding stimuli with the tube feeding. Stimulating a nonnutritive suck with a pacifier or finger during tube feedings can result in reduced irritability, increased weight gain, and easier transition to oral feedings (Field, et al., 1982; McCain, 1995). Babies also can suck on the bottle or breast during a tube feeding if there are no swallowing difficulties. This can actively relate the feeling of fullness to the mouth and the smells and touches surrounding feedings. Whenever possible, the feeding schedule should include space between meals to allow for hunger to develop so that a hunger fullness cycle can be established.

Reducing the Impact of Medical Conditions That Influence Feeding

Ongoing medical management of the conditions and disease processes influencing feeding and appetite must be a priority. Though physicians usually control this treatment, feeding therapists can play an active role in communicating with the medical team. It is important to work in partnership with physicians to provide feedback about how different procedures and treatment options are influencing feeding, appetite, and overall goals in oral motor treatment. Although feeding therapists do not do medical procedures or prescribe medications, there are some ways they can support the medical management of these children. For example, the presence of gastroesophageal reflux is a pervasive factor in developing goals for an oral motor treatment program. The physician will treat the reflux medically, but the feeding therapist and other team members may need to help the family manage the daily reflux experiences.

Work in therapy can explore the child's acceptance of feedings, feeding sizes, and positioning during and after meals. Some children improve just by being fed smaller meals more often. Less volume can reduce the stress on the LES and stomach emptying. Thickening feedings with 1 tablespoon of baby cereal per 2 ounces of formula may reduce vomiting episodes. Some children have fewer reflux episodes when positioned prone or on their right side. This can be accomplished with prone positioning on the parent's lap or prone in bed. Elevating the crib mattress to a 30-degree angle or providing a pillow wedge with a 30-degree angle also helps reduce the number of reflux episodes. Some older children are helped by being fed in an upright prone position using a prone stander propped at a 45-degree angle. Studies by Orenstein (1988) and Widstrom et al. (1988) have suggested that nonnutritive sucking on a pacifier during tube feedings can reduce an infant's gastroesophageal reflux and enhance digestion.

Reflux has many trigger points that can complicate the feeding process. The therapist and the parent can explore these together. Some children with reflux have frequent vomiting episodes. Others gag frequently and have trouble differentiating between the need to burp and the need to vomit. Still others become overly sensitive to sensory changes in the mouth and pharynx and have difficulty transitioning from thin liquids to purees or from purees to textured solid foods. Some children induce gagging as they explore the mouth with fingers or toys. Children who have had an extensive history of reflux often end up having gagging and vomiting available to them in their repertoire of "things to do to get attention." This can lead to voluntary use of gagging in daily interactions. A hospitalized infant, for example, may discover that vomiting is a sure way to engage the one-to-one attention of the nursing staff or other adults. It can become a way in which a helpless child can show power over coercive adults. The communicative aspects of reflux and triggers for gagging must be explored carefully in the development of the comprehensive oral motor treatment programs.

Optimizing the Comfort and Enjoyment of Tube Feedings

It is difficult to begin or maintain a positive treatment program if the tube feedings themselves are aversive. Parents need to be educated in the optimum ways to provide the tube feeding and in reading the child's cues of feeding-related discomfort. The rate of formula delivery through the tube can be changed easily by raising or lowering the syringe or by reducing the feeding pump's delivery rate. Some children have a very small stomach capacity that must be expanded gradually. This often requires increasing the formula volume slowly. However, because the stomach volume is being increased, it is always being pushed to maximum capacity. This can cause gagging, retching, or vomiting if it is done too rapidly and without regard for the child's cues of discomfort.

Some children have increased sensitivity for bolus feedings after a Nissen fundoplication procedure. There can be excessive bloating, gagging, or retching. In extreme situations, the surgery can become undone with the intensity of the retching. This is very uncomfortable for the child and causes a reversion to the pre-fundoplication symptoms of GER. Therapists can help parents explore their children's tube feedings and find the combination of bolus size and method of delivery that causes the least stress. This may involve slowing the rate of the feeding. Over time, the feeding time gradually can be decreased. For some children, slowing the rate is not enough; there may need to be actual pauses or breaks. Other children need to be given smaller feedings more often to reduce the stress on the stomach. Still other children may need to return to continuous drip feedings to reduce the stomach stress and gradually work up to larger boluses.

Changes in bolus size and feeding rate need to be done very slowly. Children often remain on a smaller bolus size or slower feeding rate than their bodies can handle because changes are too sudden. Increasing bolus size by 5cc to10cc (⅙ to ⅓ ounce) at a time may take longer, but may allow the gastrointestinal system to gradually adjust without distress. It is also important to remain at the new rate for at least a week to allow the system to adjust and accept this as a comfortable level. Again, if increases are made too rapidly, some children's gastrointestinal systems will rebel, increasing symptoms of distress and discomfort.

Bolus size often can be increased more easily initially by using boluses of water. The stomach stretching provided by water boluses may be better accepted initially than calorically dense formula boluses because water moves through the stomach more rapidly. This gives the child an initial stimulus that stretches the stomach but does not continue to the point of discomfort. Digestion is not involved with clear water. This enables many children whose discomfort is associated with prolonged periods of stomach fullness to learn that they can feel "full" for short periods without feeling ill. This is an important concept for children who have learned to respond to the initial stretch of the stomach with tension and anticipation of gastric distress. Working with the medical team and family, the feeding therapist can help promote the optimum positive associations with the tube feedings.

In optimizing the comfort, enjoyment, and positive associations of tube feedings, therapists and team members can explore questions about dietary diversity and the possibility that the child's gastrointestinal distress may be related to an allergy or allergic sensitivity to the single formula. Different formulas can be used to provide diversified nutritional components and more varied experiences for the gut. The therapist may ask: Does the child need to be on this particular formula alone? Could there be some variation in the diet to provide some diversity for the gut? Would formula rotation be appropriate? Could three of four formulas with different nutritional components be rotated by giving a different formula every day?

An example for an older infant would be:

Day 1 = Similac™ (milk and corn based)

Day 2 = Nursoy™ Liquid (soy and no corn)

Day 3 = Compleat Pediatric™ (beef, fruits, and vegetables)

Day 4 = Peptamen Junior™ (predigested with hydrolyzed whey protein)

Could a serving of a blended food be given by tube at least once a day to alter the diet and give different taste and smell experiences? Would a homemade blended diet be possible? The therapist would ask these questions of the medical team and have the family work closely with a dietitian to develop the diverse diet that best meets the needs of that child and family. A more in-depth discussion of rotary, diversified diets in relationship to allergy and food sensitivities is found in Chapter 16.

Improving Postural Control of the Head, Neck, and Trunk

Any oral motor treatment program should begin with a look at the child's whole body. If the team starts with the mouth alone, it might ignore the basis for some of the oral difficulties. Work that builds or normalizes postural tone in the trunk and develops postural stability enables the child to release any holding tension in the neck, shoulders, arms, and legs. As tone is built up and stabilized with handling and sensory input, new automatic movements are facilitated. These include patterns that involve capital flexion (chin tuck with a straight neck) and activation of the lateral and diagonal control of the abdominal muscles. Greater neck flexion and a balance of flexion and extension for upright head control bring the tongue and lips into a more forward position and reduce inefficient posturing of the mouth and pharynx. As control is developed in the neck flexors and in the oblique abdominal muscles, greater stability is provided for the rib cage. This, in turn, allows for increased chest expansion during inspiration. Activation of the entire abdominal-pelvic muscle girdle allows for better support of the stomach and abdominal contents, and a reduction of colic, excessive burping, and gastroesophageal reflux. Contraction of the abdominals is also necessary for regulating vocalization for sound play and speech.

Initial work frequently is carried out in supine, sidelying, and prone to enable the infant to develop a clear sensory feedback of the movement without having to deal with the added control required in antigravity positions of sitting and standing.

Improving Control of the Pharyngeal Airway

At birth, infants can make the postural adjustments of the pharyngeal wall, which maintain the airway tube at a constant diameter regardless of head and neck position. If this did not occur, there would be constant changes in diameter as the tube bent with neck flexion and extension, and the tongue would tend to move into the airway when the infant was in supine. This pharyngeal airway maintenance assures the body of a constant amount of air inflow through a stable intake tube.

It is important to determine the extent to which the infant or child depends on compensations such as neck hyperextension or tongue protrusion to enhance the diameter of the airway. These compensations must not be taken away without dealing with the underlying difficulties.

The increased production and poor handling of mucus constitutes a major difficulty in airway clearance for many children. The reason for the mucus should carefully be investigated. Mucus is produced by the body as a secretion to lubricate tissue or as an excretion to rid the body of something that is inimical to the system. Thus, when a person has a cold, he produces additional mucus as a binder to flush toxins out of the system. Increased mucus occurs when the body is not producing adequate elimination through the bowels or skin, when food has been aspirated, and when there is an allergy or sensitivity to foods, chemicals, or inhalants.

Using the Mouth to Explore the Environment

Often, tube-fed infants have missed the richness of sensory information that occurs in typical babies as they mouth everything they can. Babies mouth their own fingers, toes, bibs, and rattles. They experience the sensory variation in mouthing provided by the breast or bottle, their own skin, fabric textures, and hard and soft plastic toys. The mouth feels surfaces that are smooth and rough, and sizes that are big and small. The jaw, lips, cheeks, and tongue all respond to the shape and texture of the mouthed object. Holding these objects in the mouth provides one of a baby's first opportunities to move the tongue separately from the jaw. The child learns to move the tongue to the side, forward, up, and down, exploring the sensory wonderland of mouthing toys. A discriminative type of exploration gradually replaces the earlier random, generalized mouthing pattern. Oral skills expand, and interpretation of information becomes more sensitive. Infants begin to find similarities in mouthed objects and experience contrasts of sensations. Clothing offers many sensory contrasts for the mouth. Young children find zippers, buttons, and shoelaces with the tongue, and contrast the sensations with those produced by the surrounding fabric. The development of greater discriminative skills and stereognosis in the mouth improves sensorimotor organization and articulatory skills in children who do not have neurological impairment.

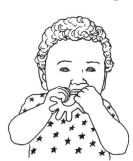

Helping children mouth their own fingers or toys can be a part of everyday life as well as a central part of an oral treatment program. The child's own body is the first toy. It can be used very effectively for mouthing. Fingers and toes provide a wealth of sensory information for the mouth. The child can experience the feeling of one finger versus the entire hand and use the tongue to explore a group of fingers versus the thumb. The fingers can be laced together and both thumbs inserted into the mouth to explore a new sensation. There are many varied and wonderful mouthing toys available that can be explored. When children are active participants in bringing toys to the mouth, they will integrate more sensory information from the toy. Children who gag easily typically accept fingers or toys that they direct to their own mouth more easily than toys put in their mouth by another person. Oral exploration can be paired with games and songs for further variation in activities.

When it is medically appropriate, children can take tastes off toys. Once a child has played with the mouthing toy and seems to enjoy it, it can be dipped in regular or diluted juice or broth to slowly introduce flavors. Thus, taste and texture variations can be introduced slowly, always following the child's lead. Food tastes can be placed on the child's fingers or toes. As the fingers and toes find the mouth in play, the child, instead of the therapist, introduces tastes. Finger painting with pureed fruit or vegetables can be encouraged on the high-chair tray or on a mirror. Gradually, the tastes can be painted on the lips. With the introduction of foods, the child is exposed to smells, temperatures, and visual impressions with the finger painting. Crumb textures can be introduced with the finger painting or on the mouthed objects. This new texture may not be as scary in a play activity or as a byproduct of mouthing a familiar toy. Feeding therapists must be very aware of their internal agendas as well as the child's response to the introduction of taste. A strong sense of trust must be built before bringing food-related stimuli into the child's play. When adults introduce tastes with the ulterior motive of tricking the child into eating, the strategy often fails. When it is done as part of a program to expand the child's overall enjoyment of sensations, the child initially may reject the input, but accept it on another occasion.

Normalizing the Response to Stimulation

Many tube-fed children develop overly sensitive or undersensitive reactions to sensory experiences involving the mouth. Another goal of a comprehensive oral motor treatment program is to help normalize the child's responses to stimulation.

Whether the child's responses to stimulation are from negative oral experiences, fear of new experiences, or sensory or emotionally based, treatment must progress slowly. Attention must be placed on building the child's trust in oral play and increasing the child's ability to get hands to the mouth and use the lips and tongue to explore the environment. The positive interaction between adult and child needs to be built gradually, allowing the child to gain confidence that the therapist is a partner in exploring the body and mouth—not another invader.

It is important to begin with sensory experiences that the child ***does*** enjoy. Find them. They ***do*** exist. They may be deep pressure touch, soft touch, warm touch, or vibration. Children may be drawn to their own fingers, a favorite toy, the bathtub, or their mother's hand. When touch is introduced, it always should be presented so that children can see it coming. This avoids sensory surprises. The therapist should let the child reach out and be a part of the touch and play. The exploration should begin at the part of the body where the child is most comfortable. In many cases, this is ***not*** the mouth or even the head. Initial touch may involve the child's foot or abdomen. The games then can move the touch to the chest, head, cheeks, and mouth, as the child allows. It is vitally important to listen carefully. If the last touch came too close and began to cause discomfort, the observant feeding therapist can shift the touch to a safer and more comfortable area.

Rhythm and music make these activities more fun and predictable for the child. If the touching is paired with a song, the child can anticipate a touch playfully. A song rhythm can be tapped along the child's body from the foot to the knee to the tummy to the chest and up to the face. When presented in this fashion, children often are more comfortable by the time the touch nears the face than if the face were approached directly. Touch paired with movement also can help the child anticipate what is next. When the child sits on a swing or therapy ball, movement can provide a rhythmical base for touching as the child moves nearer and farther from the therapist.

Variety, intensity, and duration of stimulation are increased until the child's threshold for comfort and easy acceptance is reached. The therapist watches for any limiting patterns of tone or movement that have occurred in the past. The stimulation is increased gradually as the therapist helps the child control or stop the undesired response. Focus is placed on finding ways to make the sensory input interesting, communicative, comforting, and acceptable while gradually pushing back the limiting threshold and building a more appropriate response and reaction.

Identifying and Facilitating a Swallowing Reflex

It is critical to determine whether a swallowing reflex is present before food and liquid are used in the program. The feeding therapist can check for a swallowing reflex by observing the child's control of saliva and spontaneous swallowing or by using a straw or other pipette to place small drops of water on the back of the tongue. A history that suggests chronic aspiration may preclude presentation of liquid. In either case, the therapist should feel for the elevation of the larynx-hyoid complex in the neck and elevation of the root or base of the tongue. She should observe whether the child chokes or coughs after small amounts of food or liquid are given. If there is no sign of a swallowing reflex, the therapist can proceed cautiously, working to enhance sensory and motor skills in the front of the mouth without using food or liquid. Initial work to achieve an appropriate swallow pattern can begin by using toys, pacifiers, or fingers that help the child increase oral motor control. An effective swallow often can be triggered by work to increase the strength, duration, and timing of the suckle pattern. As respiratory problems become less threatening, swallowing function is likely to return. Stimulation of the faucial arches with cold temperatures also can make it easier to obtain a swallowing reflex (Kaatzke-McDonald, Post, & Davis, 1996).

Once a consistent swallowing reflex is achieved, it is difficult to be certain clinically that swallowing of liquids or foods other than saliva will be safe. Although the timing and components of the swallowing response can be analyzed through videofluoroscopy, the child must be able to swallow at least a third of a teaspoon of liquid mixed with saliva for several swallows to get any reasonable information from the study. At this stage, the therapist may need to work in collaboration with the medical management team to introduce tiny amounts of liquid or puree for increased swallow and taste practice before a videofluoroscopy just to ensure more useable information from the study. This decision depends on many factors, including the intactness of the swallow reflex, the child's medical history and current medical status, and the therapist's experience.

Tube-fed children pose a challenge to the parent and therapist that is potentially frightening. In the back of each mind is the fear that the child might choke, aspirate, or die in the process of learning to swallow. Caution is appropriate; fear is not. It is much easier to prevent these problems than it is to deal with them. Postural drainage, suctioning, facilitation of a cough, and careful selection of the type and amount of liquid or food will sharply reduce the amount of conflicting mucus in the mouth and pharynx during attempts to swallow. The possibility of aspiration will be reduced by paying careful attention to positioning so that the head is not in hyperextension, by developing the prerequisite oral movements before adding food for oral stimulation, and by thoroughly preparing the child physically and sensorially for swallowing.

Many children will experience mild aspiration on the path to oral feedings. Therefore, foods must be selected carefully to reduce the danger of aspiration pneumonia and lung damage. A small amount of diluted, water-based liquid is the least harmful. Food and liquid containing fat are less easily assimilated by the lungs and should be avoided until there is no indication of aspiration. This includes dairy products, meat broths, and other animal foods. Foods that tend to produce an increase in mucus for the specific child also should be avoided. These may include milk-based products, grains, and some sweets. Fresh pureed vegetables and fruits are appropriate when semisolids are added to the diet. Vegetables (if the child will accept them) are preferable to fruits because they do not rely on sweet taste for acceptance.

If there is a history of extensive aspiration, it is wise to introduce oral feedings where suctioning equipment is available. However, with good preparation and introduction of food only when the infant can handle it, this precaution is not critical. Work on feeding should be done only when the child is conscious and awake. Gentle oral stimulation may be done when the child is asleep or comatose, but food and liquid should not be placed in the mouth unless the child is alert and aware of what is happening.

Facilitating a Rhythmical Suckle-Swallow

Rhythmicity is the underlying component of all coordinated behaviors. When it is absent or distorted in sucking and swallowing, the resulting incoordination precludes successful oral feeding. The extension-retraction pattern of the suckle-swallow assists in moving a liquid or food bolus to the back of the mouth for the swallow. Because the suckle facilitates the swallow, often the swallowing response can be improved by concentrating on developing a strong, rhythmical, sustained suckle. This pattern occurs at a rate of about one suckle-swallow per second. This is the underlying rhythm-tempo seen in other systems, such as the walking gait and heartbeat.

Initially, the tongue is stroked in a downward and forward direction by the therapist's finger or by the infant's finger under the therapist's guidance. If there is any type of rhythm present in the suckle, it should be followed and gradually altered to fit the one-per-second rate. The use of music with a 4/4 rhythm and a tempo of 60 beats per minute (e.g., largo and adagio movements of baroque music) can be extremely helpful in augmenting this underlying body tempo. Rocking at the same rhythm and tempo also can enhance the pattern.

As the suckling rhythm emerges, water, juice, or small amounts of pureed fruits and vegetables can be placed on the stroking finger. Eventually the stroking can be done with a plastic medicine dropper, syringe, modified pacifier, or moistened cotton swab. This allows larger amounts of liquid or food to be added gradually to the rhythmical tongue movements of the suckle. When the child can take small amounts from a spoon, the rhythm can be sustained by using a downward tip to the spoon with rhythmical contact on the tip of the tongue. It is extremely important that this progression proceed slowly and within the child's physical and emotional tolerance. If too much liquid is presented, the child may automatically stop the rhythmical suck to defend a vulnerable swallowing or respiratory system.

Improving Tone and Movement in the Jaw

Because of the anatomical attachment of the other structures of the face and mouth with the jaw, problems such as jaw thrust, jaw retraction, or exaggerated downward excursions reduce the efficiency of other parts of the oral mechanism. Opening and closing movements of the jaw are strongly influenced by the position of the head and neck. Treatment approaches that create a more normal balance between extensor and flexor patterns throughout the body will favorably influence the control of the jaw. Activities to normalize the child's response to oral-sensory stimulation can reduce a tonic bite reflex when combined with handling and positioning to normalize postural tone.

Improving Tone and Movement in the Lips and Cheeks

It is important to work for active use of the lips and cheeks in drawing food and liquid into the mouth and retaining it within the cavity in preparation for swallowing. If the suckling pattern can be elicited from stimulation at the lips, the infant will be better able to control the intake. At first, the therapist can build tone in the face through playing patty-cake on the cheeks, vocalizing, patting the lips to make interesting sounds, and firmly applying face lotion to the cheeks. Stroking firmly with a circular motion around the lips can encourage greater lip activity and a forward posturing for the suck. These activities should be presented in a communicative, interactive fashion, playing around the mouth while smacking the lips, making funny sounds, or blowing raspberries.

The stimulation from an electric toothbrush can stimulate tone and movement in the lips and cheeks. The stretch of the cheek as the toothbrush is cleaning the cheek-side of the teeth can promote a drawing in of the cheek and lip corners. Sometimes, finger toothbrushes or a variety of infant tooth-cleaning options can be used.

Improving Tone and Movement in the Tongue

The tongue is often hypotonic, thick, and bunchy. Increased force and tone may occur during protrusion. The configuration often deviates from the normal flattened tongue with central grooving. This normal configuration provides a channel for passage of the bolus from the front to the back of the mouth for the swallow. Treatment approaches to improve tongue tone and develop a more appropriate configuration often include downward bouncing or patting on the tongue with the finger, a toy, a teething biscuit, or the NUK™ toothbrush trainer set. This is done in a context of sound play or with the rhythm of folk music. As tone increases, greater flattening and movement occurs. The tongue can be stroked to obtain a central grooving or a lateral or upward movement. A rhythmical suckle-swallow then can be facilitated from the lips or tip of the tongue.

Toothbrushing also stimulates tone and movement in the tongue. Brushing the center of the tongue can facilitate flattening and a more central groove while brushing the sides can stimulate tongue lateralization. As the child becomes more comfortable with a range of sensations in the mouth, the adult can vary the input by using sponge brushes, finger toothbrushes, and electric toothbrushes.

Facilitating Voicing and Sound Play

Vocalization and sound play are actively encouraged in all phases of the program. When the emphasis during oral motor activities is shifted to play and vocalization, there is less association with unsuccessful or unpleasant past experiences with feeding. Emphasis is placed on combining respiration with vocalization and interesting sounds produced by the therapist, paired with easy movement of the child. Jiggling the chin, tapping the lips or tongue, and other physical maneuvers will encourage the child to produce sound. Older children may enjoy blowing bubbles while making noises.

With infants and children developmentally younger than the age of 5 months and children unable to produce voice because of a tracheostomy or severe neuromotor damage, the therapist may produce sounds to get attention without requiring vocal interaction. With older infants and children who are able to vocalize, therapists may expect some direct vocal contagion and imitation.

It is important to work for the sensorimotor experiences that provide speech production possibilities. This includes awareness of many ways of valving the vocal tract, the auditory feedback from different valving maneuvers, and the type and extent of contact of the lips, tongue, and jaw. The therapist can manually help the child experience these contrasts. Vegetative noises, vowels, and consonants produced by the child should be imitated, reinforcing the production and creating a dialogue. The therapist can develop pleasure and joy in sound play, the infant may be able to explore sound contrasts independently.

Various combinations of tongue, lip, and jaw movement can be practiced with sound and without food. Improved sensory discrimination and sensorimotor control for sound play can improve the similar coordinations involved in oral feeding. Vocalization provides greater action of the pharynx, larynx, and mouth. It also may indirectly facilitate some swallowing and reduce mucus lodged in the mouth and pharynx. It helps a therapist define the status of the larynx and any vocal fold closure difficulties. When the child has difficulty with vocal fold closure and airway protection during swallowing, work to improve vocal fold control during vocalization can be invaluable.

Programming Total Communication

The tube-fed child who has neurological problems is at high risk for not developing oral communication. There are parallels between the movements and coordinations that develop in feeding and those that emerge in early sound production (Morris, 1985). Whether there is a causal relationship between feeding and the normal acquisition of speech motor control is debatable. It is clear, however, that infants and children who have severe disorders of oral control for feeding will have similar difficulties with the finer coordinations needed for intelligible speech production. Deprivation of oral-sensory experiences that organize movement for speech can have a profound effect on speech and language development of the tube-fed child, even when there is no neurological impairment.

Programming for infants older than the developmental age of 8 months should include a strong emphasis on total communication. By that age, infants have a sense of causality and are capable of communicative intent. The development of turn-taking behaviors, expansion of means-ends abilities, and eye-gaze rules should be included. Emphasis should be placed on using simple gestures (e.g., waving, reaching to be picked up, pointing with vocalization) by the age of 12 months. Formal gestures or signs and pointing to pictures to indicate needs, wants, and simple ideas can be encouraged by 18 months. Ideally, the program would include all aspects of communication—gestures, pictures, vocalization, and some word approximations. The goal is to enable the child to use the most complete communication system available for expression.

Creating a Learning Environment

Tube-fed children often experience invasive procedures critical to physical survival. They may have felt pushed or forced to eat. As a result, they may erect a series of internal barriers to protect themselves from further invasion. They may discover how important the act of eating by mouth is perceived by others. They learn quickly that adults really want them to eat. Thus, eating becomes a tool in the battle for autonomy, and refusal to eat may become an effective weapon against powerful adults in their environment. The mealtime environment, therefore, must undergo changes to make it more fun. In behavioral terms, if we want to change the behaviors, we must change the stimulus. Following is a look at how to create a more positive learning environment to support positive eating behaviors.

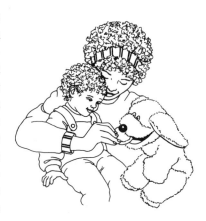

Pressure is reduced when spoons or cups are introduced playfully and games are used to make mealtime fun. Puppets or dolls create a sense of shared adventure. The therapist can explore having the child feed him, another child, a stuffed bear, or a doll. The child can play with food, watch the family prepare food, plant a vegetable garden, participate in family meals, and even play with pretend food.

The most important challenge that a therapist faces is creating an environment that enables these children to develop trust and an inner knowledge of their own capabilities. This often involves the willingness to acknowledge each child's inner wisdom and respect the need to progress slowly. The therapist should let the child be in charge of the movement when food enters the mouth. The therapist also should avoid invading the child's mouth by stopping the movement of the spoon about an inch away from the mouth and letting the child move forward and remove the food from the spoon.

The direct or indirect communication of expectations for oral feeding should be monitored by the therapist and discussed openly with the family. One needs both a belief in the infant's ability to develop and learn oral motor skills that will result in oral feeding, and a true acceptance of the current status as a nonoral feeder. Infants and children sense adults' expectations and demands for success or failure. When parents and therapists are able to accept the child, even if tube feeding continues indefinitely (or forever), any demands that inhibit progress will not interfere with the treatment program. Occasionally, the parent or therapist may firmly believe that little can be done for the infant but there is an obligation to try. This may occur after several months into the program if expectations have been unrealistically high. The child will perceive these underlying feelings of pessimism and discouragement and may attempt to fulfill them. The belief system, then, can result in failure and a confirmation of the underlying negative belief.

The fear of permanent tube feeding may be accompanied by unspoken feelings that the infant is not acceptable as a nonoral feeder and that the child must change rapidly in the treatment program to win basic love and acceptance. In this case, the child may become discouraged and may not make progress because of the conditionality involved in being accepted. When demands are made, counterdemands often emerge. A power struggle may develop in which the infant refuses to eat by mouth as a way of controlling the parent and defying the unspoken demand.

The therapist must be willing to release an attachment to results. When the child's progress is linked to feelings of professional and personal worth, creativity becomes lost. Progress appears to be enhanced by an ability to trust an intuitive sense of what the child needs or is ready for at each session. There also must be a trust in the child's inner wisdom, which accepts change and progress as appropriate for each moment. The greatest overall progress in treatment is made when the parent and therapist are able to accept the child, have a preference and a belief that the child eventually will become an oral feeder, and trust the child's timetable. Gains are made when faith in the child's underlying abilities is high, when demands are reduced, and a program that allows for growth is initiated.

Music can be used in the learning environment to provide the mutual playfulness and pleasure found in moving and interacting to the rhythm and flow of the melody. Folk music with a clear, regular rhythm and a simple, repeated melody is highly effective with children with severe feeding disorders. Calming background music and music with a tempo of one beat per second enables both the feeder and the child to become entrained to the rhythmical, slow tempo that enhances sensorimotor organization. Music containing the special sound combinations known as Hemi-Sync™ creates a more equal balance of activity in both the right and left hemispheres of the brain and is effective in focusing attention and enhancing learning. Stress is reduced, and the feeder and child can become open to new possibilities when music is used. The protective barriers, which the child has needed to feel safe, gradually are eliminated, and the child discovers the potential that lies within.

Timing

Although the specific elements of a program are important, the most critical aspect is the timing in which each component is introduced and emphasized. Each child and family is unique, and generalizations may be dangerous. However, the following observations apply to many different children.

The underlying medical problem influencing feeding must be treated. It is difficult, for example, to convince children that eating is fun when they feel pain or discomfort during or after a meal. The feeding therapist can be a link in the medical management of the feeding difficulties. The most basic underlying elements of function or dysfunction should receive the greatest emphasis in the program. For example, if the child has a severe cardiac condition, it must be remediated before the child will have enough energy to eat. If there are severe difficulties with pharyngeal airway maintenance, these must be dealt with before one can expect there to be a functional suckle-swallow response. If there is gastroesophageal reflux, it must be treated to optimize physical comfort before the child can develop an increased interest in feeding. If there are problems with hypersensitivity or hyposensitivity, therapists can help normalize the child's response to sensory information. If the child is fearful of feeding, adults must try to make the mealtime and feeding experience safe and pleasant or learning will be compromised. If this underlying prerequisite is not given an initial priority, the child will be unable to use and integrate sensory information and develop new motor responses.

The therapist must have a clear sense of the components of sensory and motor development and must skillfully analyze the child's abilities and deficits. All treatment must be done within the framework of a whole child within a whole family. Initial goals will be directed toward building the skills and abilities that form the foundation for higher-level feeding skills.

Specific activities should be built on the child and family's interests and abilities. Children and adults learn most efficiently when they are allowed to use their strengths and individual learning styles. There are no techniques for improving respiratory and oral motor skills that can be applied to all children or used by all families. The technique becomes an idea for obtaining improved function in a specific area. In the hands of a creative therapist, the technique becomes a theme with infinite variations. These variations emerge from the uniqueness of each child, family, and therapist. An observation that the child enjoys the bathtub or water play in a basin may lead to introducing a spoon or syringe to stir the water, using a sponge for water play around the face, and letting drops of water enter the mouth on bathtub toys. The child may incorporate the oral stimulation and early swallowing of water in this environment because it is familiar, fun, and nonthreatening. The same procedures presented in a mealtime context might be rejected immediately because of previous associations with fear and failure.

■ Transition to Oral Feeding

The Continuum From Tube Feeding to Oral Feeding

There is a continuum from non-oral feeding to oral feeding. Rarely an either/or situation, it is a *process*. There is a great deal of variation in how children and families respond to tube feeding and the transition journey toward oral feeding. Some children require total tube feedings with no oral feedings. Some progress to taking small snacks orally. Some children can eat solids but receive all liquids by tube because of the risk of aspiration. Some children eat by mouth but need extra calories by tube to grow. Other children move to oral feeding, demonstrating the ability to grow and thrive without the tube. Where children begin and how they move on this continuum depends on many factors. Long-term difficulties in moving to oral feeding rarely are caused by a single factor, but rather by a complex mixture of factors. In a comprehensive oral-treatment program, the child directs the approach. Therapy can provide experiences and opportunities, but the child tells adults how fast to travel and what direction to go on this journey.

For children who are tube-fed and taking some foods by mouth, there is always the temptation to push them rapidly toward total oral feeding. Many children who have remained at the tasting stage for long periods have been described as having a feeding aversion or feeding resistance (Archer & Szatmari, 1990; Handen et al., 1986). Some of these children are directed into intensive programs that use a behavior-modification model to get them to eat (Blackman & Nelson, 1987). Although there are similarities in breaking down the components of eating, building on a child's successes, and modifying aspects of the feeding environment, the philosophical base for behaviorally based programs is in sharp contrast to the concepts described here (Kedesdy & Budd, 1998). Children with feeding tubes who show ongoing resistance to learning to eat may benefit from some of the concepts and strategies that are discussed in Chapter 24.

Many questions arise regarding how and when to help a child take larger amounts and a greater variety of foods orally. Readiness factors must be considered, and multiple team players may be involved.

Readiness Factors

There are a number of factors that must be considered when any transition toward oral feeding is contemplated.

Resolution of the Original Problems

The therapist must know whether the medical conditions that led to tube feeding in the first place have been resolved. For example, if the child had the tube placed because of aspiration, is aspiration still present? If fatigue required supplemental feedings due to a cardiac condition, has the cardiac condition been resolved? Did the necessary surgeries occur? Are more surgeries scheduled? If the child had an esophageal fistula or atresia, have the necessary surgical procedures been successfully completed, allowing the food to move easily from the mouth to the stomach? If these original conditions continue to be a problem for the child, an active focus on transitioning to oral feeding usually is inappropriate.

Overall Health of the Child

The transition to oral feeding typically involves some reduction in tube feedings. The assumption is that the child will begin to feel hunger and make up the difference in calories by eating more orally. However, this may not happen immediately. Even when children are ready for this step, it may take time for them to understand what is happening and increase oral intake. If children are unwell, they may respond by getting ill or by losing too much weight. When they are not feeling well, they may lack the internal drive and motivation to move to oral feeding. Thus, before moving to a tube-weaning program the therapist must ask many health-related questions. Is the child in good health? Has the child generally been healthy over an extended period of time or is good health only a recent phenomenon? Has a consistent pattern of growth been shown over time? Are the child's height, weight, and head circumference in appropriate proportion?

Swallowing Safety

Many children initially are given feeding tubes because they cannot swallow safely. They aspirate food or liquid or are at high risk for aspiration. As their prerequisite skills for oral feeding improve, their ability to swallow safely often improves. They begin to eat small amounts with good coordination and without external indicators that they are aspirating. This, however, is quite different from taking full meals orally. Some children can handle small amounts of food and liquid, even with some aspiration, safely. These same children may be silent aspirators or may become more uncoordinated and lose their margin of swallowing safety when they must take larger amounts or eat for a longer time. If there has been any history of aspiration or a videofluoroscopic swallow study that showed risk of aspiration, the VFSS should be repeated before encouraging larger amounts and varieties of food or liquid. Even without a history of swallowing difficulties, therapists may need to ask questions in this area. Do we know that the child currently has a safe and efficient swallowing mechanism? Is a video-fluoroscopic swallow study necessary to document the swallowing skills?

Status of Oral Skills

Clearly, the child's oral skills play a major role in determining readiness to transition to oral feeding. When they are limited or cannot be sustained over a period of 30 to 45 minutes, children often resist moving into prolonged periods of oral feeding. What oral skills does the child have available? How does the child handle liquids? Purees? Solids? Can the child successfully handle changes in texture? Does the child have competence in using bottles, cups, straws, spoons, or forks? Could the child eat the volume of food needed to support nutrition within 30 minutes?

Hunger

Hunger provides the internal regulation for eating orally. Many tube-fed children have missed the gastrointestinal experiences that create contrasting sensations of hunger and satiation. Does the child have a sense of hunger? Does the child understand that the mouth and food eaten orally play a major role in reducing hunger? Can the child's stomach comfortably accept bolus feedings? Is the child fed on a schedule that resembles a family eating schedule?

Child Readiness

Children progress toward oral feeding when they are interested in this way of taking in food and when they are ready. Readiness is an internal phenomenon. Adults can provide the encouragement and introduce children to the experiences that seem to promote readiness. However, readiness itself is perceived and directed by children, not by adults. Does the child show signs of interest in eating? Interaction with foods and liquids stimulates enjoyment and involvement. Children usually reach for food or the spoon and try to put it in the mouth. Does the child feel well enough to eat? Does he have an appetite or let an adult know when he would like to eat (orally or by tube)? Does the **child** really want to eat orally or is this the goal of the parents or therapist?

Parent Readiness

Helping a child make the transition from tube feeding to oral feeding takes time and commitment from parents. It is important to know whether the parents really are ready for their child to move to oral feeding. Parents become the team leaders in this process. Much of the effort will rest on their shoulders. Is this what they want? Do they understand all the issues involved in transitioning the child to oral feedings? Do they feel they have the patience to let the child lead the pace? These issues need to be explored and discussed together from the beginning.

The team will work together in the decision-making process of transitioning to oral feeding. Physicians must determine if the child's medical condition is stabilized and whether the child is healthy enough to move to oral feeding. Videofluoroscopic swallow studies can be done, as needed, to determine the safety of the swallowing mechanism. The dietitian may work closely with the family to follow growth patterns and caloric needs. Feeding therapists can provide oral motor treatment to help the child use oral skills in the most efficient and positive manner. They can look for signs of feeding readiness. The team members can work with the family to understand the family's readiness for this process. Following are ways in which the feeding therapist can provide comprehensive oral motor treatment to support the transition to oral feeding.

The Continuum of Oral Preparation

From Nonfoods to Foods

Moving from nonfood to food situations must be done slowly and with respect for the child's needs and abilities. At first, a taste may be presented on the finger or in drops of water. Then the intensity of the taste or the quantity of liquid is increased gradually, the child's response is observed carefully, and additional challenges are provided only when the child shows readiness. A wide exploration of taste and texture should continue to be combined with extensive oral play. Small drops of liquid are similar in taste and amount to the saliva that a child already may be able to swallow successfully. When liquid is introduced gradually with mouth play to develop tongue and lip movement, it may be swallowed with relative ease. The therapist can increase the amount by working progressively with cotton swabs, a medicine dropper, small syringe, infant spoon, and cup. Liquid, however, may pose a major problem for those who have substantial difficulties in coordinating breathing and swallowing. Some children need to start with a pureed consistency.

Pureed foods appear to be easier for some children who need stronger sensory cues of weight, texture, and taste to organize the sensorimotor response in moving the food to the back of the mouth. The slightly thicker, heavier consistency doesn't flow out of control as rapidly as liquid. Because of the slightly greater time and control allowed by the thicker food or a thickened liquid, the suckle-swallow is improved. Other children appear to need the consistency of the semisolid foods, followed by drops of liquid, to clear the back of the tongue and pharynx.

The child should continue to enjoy the taste and texture transition to purees if they are presented carefully. There is a tendency for infants to stop the rhythmical tongue movements and revert to old patterns when food initially is introduced by spoon. Panic, disorganized mouth movements, and protective tongue retraction may occur. In some situations, the child has had negative experiences with the spoon that can trigger fear and protective responses. The therapist should consider introducing the purees on the child's finger, a familiar mouth toy, or pacifier. It is critical that the emphasis be placed on sustaining a rhythmical suckle movement of the tongue. If this is lost, the amount of food presented on the tongue should be reduced or the food thinned until the rhythmical movement returns. When the child becomes fearful, old patterns of head extension, body arching, and overall incoordination may appear, increasing the risk of choking and aspiration.

Children will show their preferences in how they make taste and texture transitions. Some prefer strong flavors, while others prefer diluted ones. Some prefer to move from tiny amounts of thin liquids to larger amounts of the liquid. They then may move to nectar consistencies and then expand their skills with different feeding utensils such as a bottle, cup, or straw. Others move from liquid tastes to purees and gradually on to solid foods. Still others quickly leap from liquid tastes to crumbs and meltable foods, then on to more challenging solids, refusing any offerings of wet foods.

Feeding Utensils

Often therapists are asked whether an infant should be placed on the bottle or breast if initial feeding difficulties required that tube feedings be given. Much depends on the strengths, specific problems, and age of the infant. If a rhythmical sucking pattern is present and tongue retraction does not increase when the nipple is inserted, feeding from the bottle or breast may be a realistic goal. A rhythmical suckle on a finger or thin cloth or sponge dipped in water, breast milk, or formula can prepare the infant for bottle-feeding or breast-feeding. The Hazelbaker™ FingerFeeder can be used to feed the baby off the adult finger. A soft, preemie nipple may be used to obtain an easier suck. If the infant can continue a rhythmical suck-swallow without excessive liquid loss or choking, a juice nipple with a slightly larger hole, a Haberman™ feeder, or a supplemental nursing system for breast-feeding may be used.

Many babies move directly to cup drinking, bypassing the nursing or bottle-feeding stage. The age of the child and the severity of the oral motor difficulties will influence the decision. Some babies have severe sensitivities to the touch of the nipple in the mouth. Some become disorganized with the presentation of the nipple, resulting in tongue retraction or disorganized movement. Some infants cannot maintain the energy level and organization needed for nipple feeding. For these children, cup drinking can be more appropriate.

Still other babies and young children show their greatest eating skills with the spoon. They seem able to control the amount and movement of food or liquid more efficiently, especially when they learn to use an active movement of the lips to draw food into the mouth from the spoon. These children may bypass the bottle, breast, and cup stages initially and take all solid foods and a small amount of liquids from the spoon. They may continue to receive larger amounts of liquid by tube until they have developed the ability to coordinate their sucking-swallowing-breathing pattern for a larger volume of thin or thick liquids.

Guidelines for feeding equipment to support weaning from feeding tubes are discussed in Chapter 18.

Mealtime Modeling

When there are strong signs that a child may be developing greater interest in eating and moving to oral feeding, the child must move from the lap, floor, or bed to the family table for tube feeding during regular mealtimes. This step can be built into the initial stages of the program for most children. It builds an association between the satiation of hunger provided by the tube feedings and the sights and smells of a regular meal within the social context of a family mealtime. The child may be given spoons, bowls, or food on the tray to encourage feeding play. Children who show interest in tastes can be given food and liquid to taste. The emphasis is on the positive mealtime experience and mealtime imitation rather than on the quantity of food.

Dietary Preparations for Oral Feedings

Dietary support should parallel efforts to prepare the mouth for oral feeding. Increasing nutritional variation in the tube diet may help prepare the child's mouth, nose and gut for new foods. Problems can develop when only formula is given by tube and cereal, fruit, vegetables, and juices are only offered orally. Children with a genetic predisposition toward allergy may develop allergic triggers from repeated challenges of the food sources in a formula that is given at every meal. These children may develop allergic or hypersensitive reactions to new foods that are offered by mouth. These reactions can trigger increased mucus, abdominal discomfort, pain, headache, or feelings of irritability and unwellness. The child may associate the oral feedings with discomfort and refuse to eat. If individual foods are pureed, diluted with water, and given occasionally by tube, allergic or hypersensitive responses can be identified before the child has experienced them orally.

If the child has high caloric needs and can take only tube feedings, it may be difficult to provide adequate non-formula calories in a volume that can be tolerated by tube. In that case, non-formula meals via the tube may be deferred until stomach capacity is greater and a larger diameter tube can be inserted, which would require less dilution of the food. However, mini-meals of different foods can be given by tube, and the child's reaction can be observed. Because of the immature digestive system, pureed foods should not be given before an infant is 4 months old. When they are added by tube, new foods should be added at 3- or 4-day intervals in the same way new foods are introduced to the typically developing infant. Consult the child's physician or a dietitian to determine the best diet when the child is ready to begin the transition to oral foods.

Learning to enjoy new foods and a healthy diet is extremely important in helping children move from tube feedings to oral feedings. It is very easy to get into the trap of giving children only sweet tastes and junk foods because they may be more interested in these foods. This can become a big trap. Children continue to be drawn to the types of food that they are given as they are learning to eat. If adults really want children to be capable of supporting their body's nutritional needs orally, they need to think in terms of healthy foods and dietary diversity from the very beginning. The focus in therapy should be on helping children learn to accept and enjoy small tastes of a wide variety of foods. Therapy should not emphasize increasing the amount of one or two foods. Therapists can begin with the types of taste that are easiest for the child, but they must help the child move to new foods and new tastes from the beginning. For some children, this may be simply changing the brand of food so that the change is very small. However, the overall goal is to develop a wide variety of tastes that the child will like and accept. It often is hard for families to develop a long-range view when they want their child to eat now. But it really is worth it in the end. Parents and therapists can start with the small steps in the beginning that take them to what they really want—children who are happy, comfortable, and well-nourished as oral feeders.

Hunger as an Ally

A successful transition to oral feeding depends on the child's association of oral feeding with hunger and its reduction, and on the child's physical ability to take some food orally. In preparation for the transition to oral feedings, the tube feeding schedule can be modified to promote both hunger and a more normal mealtime routine. Hunger can and should be used as an ally in encouraging the child to take more by mouth. Tube feedings can be adjusted so that their volume and timing is similar to an oral-feeding pattern of three large meals and two smaller snack meals per day. When smaller, more frequent tube feedings are given or a continuous drip-feeding pattern is used, children never feel the sensations of hunger or satiation. Their system is unprepared for the internal cues that create the motivation needed to accept oral feedings. Some children have been fed all of their calories by continuous drip feedings at night. Parents and professionals hope that they will be hungrier during the day. This works for some children but not for others. Some children have been tube fed for so long on such a schedule that they do not identify hunger at all. A daytime bolus-feeding schedule may more readily provide the child with the contrasting sensations of satiation and hunger that can be more easily associated with food and eating.

As a hunger-satiation pattern is established, the parent should identify the time of day when the child's energy level is the highest and mood is the best. Most parents notice that some meals are consistently better for their child. They can identify when the child seems hungry **and** most willing to take on the challenge of an oral meal.

Once the child shows interest and skill in eating foods and the parents can identify optimum times for mealtime challenges, hunger can be used creatively to enhance the child's motivation in eating. There are many ways to rearrange the feeding schedule and the calories. The decision depends on the child's hunger, interest in foods, and stomach capacity. It also depends on the family routine. The child's growth, nutrition, and fluid needs must be watched closely. The physician or dietitian usually works with the family and feeding therapist during this transition. Here are some of the options often used by the team to optimize hunger with oral feedings. Several of these options may be tried before the best alternative is found for a specific child.

- When the child is on a daytime meal-snack-meal-snack-meal bolus schedule, feed the child orally at the time the tube feeding takes place.
- When the child is on a daytime meal-snack-meal-snack-meal bolus schedule, postpone one of the feedings for half an hour or more to maximize hunger. Then offer food by mouth before the tube feeding.
- When the child is on a daytime meal-snack-meal-snack-meal bolus schedule, reduce the calories of a tube feeding before the oral meal. Make up the calories later as needed.
- When the child is on a daytime meal-snack-meal-snack-meal bolus schedule, skip a snack entirely and provide the oral foods at the beginning of the next meal or a half-hour before the bolus feeding begins. Make up the snack calorie by tube during or after the last feeding of the day.

- When the child is on a daytime meal-snack-meal-snack-meal bolus schedule, skip a snack entirely and provide the oral foods at the beginning of the next meal or a half-hour before the bolus feeding begins. Do not make up the calories by tube, thus reducing the overall daily caloric count.

- Move the tube feedings to a nighttime continuous drip schedule to promote daytime hunger. The optimum oral feedings may take place after 1 PM or 2 PM.

- Dilute the tube feedings with water by a determined percentage to give fewer calories overall and maximize hunger. Some dietitians reduce the caloric content by 25% and add water to maintain the optimum fluid level.

- Feed the child orally by day and supplement necessary calories by night or at naptime. This is important when the child's self-perception is that of an oral feeder and the option of supplementary tube feedings is not as obvious.

A time limit of 15 to 30 minutes should be set for oral feedings. During this period, the child is allowed to eat as much as desired. The remainder of the meal then is given by tube. The child should enjoy the social interactions, mealtime conversations, and mealtime atmosphere. There should be encouragement and support without coercion, force, or pressure to eat. The parents need to know that the tube is still there as a nutritional support. Whatever the child does not take by mouth can easily be given by tube.

Too many transitions to oral feeding bog down at this point as prematurely enthusiastic parents and therapists put direct or indirect pressure on the child to eat more. If calories are decreased too drastically early in the weaning process, stress will increase and the program can fail. Parents want their children to remain healthy and not lose weight. A rapid reduction in calories can put too much pressure on the parents to help the child take in enough food. This, in turn, can put pressure on the child to eat more than is comfortable. Weaning a child from a feeding tube is a process, not an end destination. It often can be a slow process. The tube is there to help until the child is very capable and willing to take in sufficient food by mouth. Parents and therapist *must* listen to the child and let the child set the pace. Health, good growth, and positive mealtime experiences are the most important goals.

Removing the Feeding Tube

An indwelling feeding tube (e.g., gastrostomy tube) should remain in place following a complete transition to oral feedings. Oral feedings should become fully stabilized and the child's needs for liquids and solids should be satisfied orally even in time of illness before the tube is removed and the insertion closed. The premature removal of the tube may create excessively long meals for the child and feeder, and may introduce the possibility of malnutrition or failure to thrive, especially during times of illness.

Maturation and Change

Time and maturation can be important allies for many infants in developing better feeding patterns. This is primarily related to changes in anatomical structures and reduction of primary respiratory problems that occur during the first year of life. When feeding difficulties are increased by a disproportionately small jaw or by difficulty in maintaining the size of the pharyngeal airway (as in micrognathia or Pierre Robin sequence), anatomical changes will occur over time. The downward and forward growth of the mandible and the elongation of the pharynx, which begin at 4 to 6 months, can play a positive role. These anatomical changes increase the pharyngeal airspace for breathing and provide a larger area for tongue movement, thus reducing stress on the respiratory and feeding systems. Poor health related to respiratory or cardiac difficulties may be reduced as the infant matures. With greater ease of breathing and greater energy, progress in oral feeding may become easier.

The contribution of time and maturation to the process does not mean that referral for treatment and an intervention program should not begin during the first year. Emphasis during the initial stage of treatment should be placed on the development of postural control, communication and interaction during nonoral feedings, normalization of oral sensitivity, and oral exploration.

The role of change in human behavior is important to recall when working with young children. As the infant matures, the sensory feedback from the restrictive, nonfeeding patterns becomes familiar and is incorporated into the developing body image and self-concept. When change becomes possible through therapeutic handling and stimulation, it is unfamiliar and may be frightening. There is a tendency to cling to the old pattern. This is particularly true when the habitual pattern included compensations that enhanced survival. Thus, a child who choked during swallowing may find it difficult to use a suckling response to draw liquid into the pharynx. Another child may resist swallowing semisolid foods, knowing that swallowing produced a sense of suffocation when respiratory abilities were stressed by oral feeding. These old habits and perceptions must be acknowledged, and the therapist must resist pushing the child into new behaviors. The therapist is a guide who introduces new possibilities. The child is encouraged to explore these new ways of being. If the changes are presented as something new and interesting, they may be accepted when the child is ready because there is no battle and no image to be preserved. Therapists frequently strive for repeated gains and changes without pause. This often pushes the infant or child to the point where there may be a functional retreat into less mature but familiar behaviors. Natural plateaus must be allowed and encouraged. The child needs these pauses to stabilize a newly learned behavior before moving on.

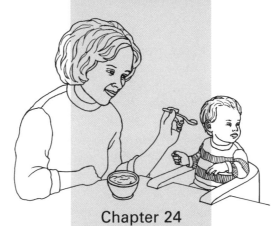

Chapter 24

The Child Who Refuses to Eat Enough

Many children do not eat enough to grow properly because of obvious feeding issues. They may lack the proper muscle tone or oral structure. They may be tube fed and just learning to eat by mouth. They may have been chronically ill and have no appetite. They may have cardiac problems that have an impact on their endurance.

For these children, the reasons for poor appetite and slowed growth are relatively understandable. However, there is a group of children with feeding problems that cannot be explained so simply. At first glance, these children may seem to be reasonably capable eaters, but they just do not eat enough to grow properly. Their parents and pediatricians have significant concerns: Why won't this child eat enough? Why does he refuse to eat a good meal? These children can be a challenge for parents and feeding specialists.

It is helpful to look at who these children are and play detective to explore possible explanations. In most cases, there is not a single explanation, but rather a series of reasons why a child refuses to eat enough food to grow well.

Andy, who is 2½ years old, came to the assessment with his mother. She was asked to bring food that showed the therapist what brought out Andy's best and worst eating skills. She also was asked to bring his favorite utensils so that he would feel comfortable eating in an office situation. Andy's mother walked in the door with 14 kinds of food. She brought lots of things to try because she is never sure of what he will like at a meal. She also indicated that she needed to offer many foods at each meal at home. She brought a cassette tape player, Andy's favorite tape, a stuffed toy, and a couple of books. She also brought his favorite cup and spoon—the only spoon he will use at a meal. By the amount of material the mother brought, the therapist could see that mealtime had become a struggle. But how, when, and why did that struggle start?

Tommy, 18 months old, always has had a poor appetite. He prefers smooth foods such as yogurt, pudding, and ice cream. He can eat spaghetti and macaroni and cheese. He still gags on meats and more dense foods. His parents, concerned about his weight, give him the foods he enjoys. Upon further questioning of the parents, the therapist learned that Tommy spit up frequently. He had been on gastroesophageal reflux medication. He stopped his regular vomiting when he was a year old, so the medication was discontinued. Why isn't Tommy eating more? Why is he stuck on smooth foods? What interferes with his appetite?

Julia is Mrs. Jones' first child. Mrs. Jones prepares highly nutritious meals for her family and is very concerned that Julia is not eating enough. She indicates that she tries and tries to get Julia to eat more at each meal so that she has a well-balanced and nutritious diet. Julia pushes her away, wants to do it herself, and fusses every time she is in the high chair. No one enjoys meals. How did this well-meaning mother and perfectly healthy child end up with mealtimes being such a struggle?

Frankie, a 3-year-old, has a poor appetite. He picks and pokes at his food. He will eat whatever is offered, but only in small quantities. He cannot be convinced to eat larger amounts. He has constant allergies to airborne allergens. He has recurrent ear infections and constant phlegm and gastrointestinal discomfort. When and why did his poor appetite begin?

Darria is 3½ years old and has been on a feeding tube since birth because of initial respiratory and gastrointestinal difficulties. For the past 18 months, she has eaten small amounts of food by mouth but seems interested only in eating a tiny amount of a limited number of foods. A psychologist told Darria's mother that the child had a strong feeding resistance because of feeding aversion related to her early medical history. Why is Darria having such difficulties making the transition to oral feeding?

These children have many differences in history and mealtime experiences. What they have in common is a history of poor growth or a very high risk of future undernutrition. Their personal mealtime experiences are such that they do not take in enough calories or variety of foods orally. They seem to have the foundational oral skills necessary to eat sufficient food. For some reason, they don't have the appetite and motivation to eat more. It is helpful to take an in-depth look at these children and their complicated mealtime issues. For most of these picky eaters who take in insufficient calories, there is a layering of issues that fit together and result in a negative impact on mealtimes for the child and the parent.

The Personal Nature of Eating

Most healthy children are born wanting to eat. When their system works, they seek out food and monitor their own intake so that they eat enough for good growth. How much a child needs for growth is an individual matter that depends on genetics, muscle tone, and energy expenditure. Are the child's parents short or tall, thin or obese? Is the child active or sedentary? Does the child tend to have a high metabolism or a slow one? Children's appetite changes from day to day and from week to week, depending on the demands on their bodies. Caloric intake can vary widely during the day; but, overall, when everything works, most children grow adequately.

Layered on top of the child's unique caloric and energy needs is a personal relationship to food and personal interpretations of mealtime experiences and reactions. The personal nature of eating patterns complicates the understanding of appetite. Some factors that strongly influence feeding for some children may have a minimal impact on others. Chapters 6 and 22 contain an in-depth discussion of the factors that limit feeding skills and the specific impact of gastrointestinal discomfort. For example, gastroesophageal reflux has a very different impact on different children. Why can some children spit up 25 to 30 times a day and still maintain the desire to eat and thrive? How are these children different from other children who may not actually spit up but may arch, gag, and have no appetite? Why would some children with a wheat or gluten allergy eat anything placed in front of them and seem oblivious to their chronic gastrointestinal upset and general allergic symptoms, while others lose all interest in food because of the symptoms? Why do some children demand to do it themselves and have nothing to do with adult help at the meal, while others happily eat whatever is offered, any time it is offered, by anyone who offers it? Why can some children deal with mealtime situations with a highly controlling parent who carefully regulates how much food is put in the mouth, what is eaten, and how messy the meal becomes, while others rebel against this type of parental control? Why do some children with mild sensory integrative issues thrive, eating only the smooth foods or crunchy foods that they eat best, while others with similar sensory problems lose their appetite? The answer is personal. It is individual.

There is never just one explanation for these children's problems, but a series of explanations. What starts out as one issue easily spirals into another and then turns into a tornado of mealtime difficulties that affects the whole family. Once again, therapists need to look at the entire situation to identify the initial influences on feeding, the trigger events, and the layers of influence that seem to worsen the mealtime situation. These features must be placed in perspective with the current situation in order to understand how a parent's well-meaning struggle to provide good nutrition for a child has led to conflict and choices to stop eating enough to thrive.

Feeding therapists need to understand the nature of growth and the variables that should create concern for parents and professionals. They must understand the complex mixture of physical, sensory, communication, mealtime, and learning variables that influence children and their families.

Parents often are frustrated by frequent comments from family, friends, and professionals that imply that eating is a simple skill. Everyone eats, and if a child does not have a severe, visible handicapping condition (such as cerebral palsy), it is hard to understand why the child would choose not to eat or to eat a very limited diet. Multiple diagnostic tests may rule out the more obvious reasons for noneating or show a nonsignificant degree of the problem. In the end, parents frequently are told that the child has a behavioral feeding problem. Their child's problem is described with terms such as feeding resistance, feeding refusal, feeding aversion, and infantile anorexia.

Growth Issues: To Be Concerned or Not Concerned?

Before looking in depth at children who are not eating enough to grow, it is helpful to look at the parameters used to differentiate good growth from poor growth.

Growth Charts

Standardized growth charts have been developed to guide physicians and dietitians in following a child's growth over time. The charts provide normative data on the rate of growth, measuring height, weight, and head circumference. They also offer height-to-weight comparisons to aid understanding of how a child's weight relates to that of other children of the same height. Often, many important decisions about feeding and nutrition strategies are made based on these charts, so it is important to understand them, interpret them, and understand what information these charts can and cannot provide.

When looking at the growth record for a child to determine good or poor growth, it is important to consider several factors.

- **Look at the trend.** One isolated point in time usually will not provide sufficient information about a child's growth from which to make decisions. Both of the following children have a plot on the weight growth curve at the 5th percentile. Taken in isolation as one point below the 5th percentile, each child's case might be misinterpreted. Melissa has followed a consistent growth trend along the 5th percentile since early infancy. She seems to be a smaller child who is following her own petite growth pattern with no problems eating. Becoming worried about her diet and pushing her to eat more each day could cause a feeding problem. Susan, however, has followed a growth curve along the 75th percentile for most of her life and recently fell to the 5th percentile This trend should be a red flag, requiring a feeding assessment and a more in-depth look at this child and her mealtime interactions.

- **Look at all of the growth parameters.** Growth can be measured in a variety of ways, including height, weight, head circumference, and height-to-weight ratio. When a child receives inadequate nutrition, the weight curve usually is the first parameter to slow down, then the length. The body naturally shunts nutrients to the head first for protection, so head circumference tends to be the last parameter to be influenced by malnutrition. Head circumference is an important factor in the overall picture of growth. If a child's head is not following an appropriate growth trend, this can indicate severe malnutrition or possible neurological difficulties.

The height and weight trends, the head circumference, and weight-to-height ratio provide much more information about the child's growth trends.

Although he is 5 years old, Billy's height and weight are both similar to those of a 3-year-old. His height and weight curves indicate he is small. But his height-to-weight ratio indicates that he is well proportioned and at an appropriate weight for children of his height.

On the other hand, Ryan has the height of a 5-year-old and the weight of a 3-year-old. He is tall while his weight is low. The height-to-weight ratio provides more information for interpretation. Compared to other children of his height, Ryan is very thin. A look at family growth patterns, feeding routines, and strategies may be appropriate for Ryan, whereas Billy may not elicit such worry.

▦ **Measure accurately.** Children are weighed on different scales in different offices. Sometimes children have their clothes on, including bulky shoes (or even leg braces), and sometimes they are naked. Sometimes they have a dry diaper, sometimes a wet one, and sometimes none. There can be great variation in weight among children when such inconsistencies exist. Height measurements can vary even more. Dietitians usually measure children on a length board, which provides the most accurate linear measurement. Many medical personnel have a child lie on the paper-covered examining table and draw lines at the head and feet. Because the child often wiggles and the measurements are quick, the lines can vary considerably in accuracy. This can result in growth charts on which the child actually appears to have shrunk in height.

When parents are concerned about their child's growth, this measurement roller coaster of inconsistencies and different scales can be very upsetting. When parents are upset and worried about their child's growth, the child *is* affected.

▦ **Use the correct chart.** Many children seen by feeding specialists have issues other than feeding. The growth of children with certain genetic syndromes can be measured according to a set of growth charts that have been adjusted for children with the specific syndrome. This is true for such conditions as Down syndrome, Turner's syndrome, and Williams syndrome. It can be misleading to look at these children on a regular growth chart. The data may lead to incorrect results and unnecessary pressure on the family.

Tony has Down syndrome. On a regular chart, his age of 27 months and weight of 23 pounds indicates that he is below the 5th percentile for weight. This might be worrisome when looked at in isolation. However, when he is compared with other children of his age who have Down syndrome, he is between the 25th and 50th percentile for weight.

▦ **Adjust for prematurity.** Premature babies need to have their age adjusted for prematurity. Although dietitians and physicians vary on how long to make adjustments, most correct for prematurity at least through the first year of life. Many correct the age for prematurity through the second year, and some even adjust into elementary school.

Increasing amounts of data now are available on low birth weight (LBW) and very low birth weight (VLBW) premature infants and their growth outcomes after the first year of life. Hack et al. (1996) found that catch-up growth to above the 3rd percentile occurs for very low birth weight infants who have experienced earlier growth failures. Although most catch-up growth (defined as increased growth velocity after a temporary growth arrest) occurs during infancy, it continues until the child is 8 years old. Results of the study showed catch-up growth occurred more often in average-for-gestational-age babies (AGA) than in small-for-gestational-age babies (SGA) after intrauterine growth failure. Children with major neurosensory abnormalities did not show catch-up growth after 20 months of corrected age.

Studies have included proposals for revised height, weight-to-head circumference, and weight-for-length reference data for low and very low birth weight premature infants based on a collection of normative data for more than 4,500 preterm infants (Guo et al., 1996, 1997; Roche et al., 1997). The weight-for-length growth velocities for these children varied enough from the current normative data for the researchers to propose new charts. This growth data is being distributed in Infant Health and Development Program (IHDP) growth percentiles for LBW (weight equal to or less than 1,500 gms) and VLBW (weight less than 1,500 gms), with each calculated for premature girls and premature boys.

Raval (1998) found that the size of the baby at birth and gestational age strongly influence growth rates. She found that the tinier the baby, the less chance of its catching up to the 5th percentile by 1 year adjusted age (see Chapter 21).

A significant number of small premature babies, even after age is adjusted for prematurity, may still be below the 5th percentile at 1 year. This may be a natural progression for that baby. If this smaller growth trend, interpreted in isolation of other factors, is seen as a serious problem in an infant who is otherwise developing well, the physician may encourage the family to push the child to eat more. Although the team should support optimum nutrition for optimum growth for every baby, increasing parental stress with the diagnosis of poor growth and pushing the baby to eat more may create feeding relationship problems. Monitoring the infant's weight must be done within the context of the big picture.

Growth trends in premature infants are important information for physicians to know as they monitor these babies. Not only must they adjust their expectations based on corrections for prematurity, but they also must be realistic about growth expectations based on the child's birth and growth history. Whether the child was premature (and by how many weeks), average for gestational age, small for gestational age, or intrauterine growth retarded (IUGR) seems to influence early growth patterns. Being aware of these trends and looking at each baby's unique trends, height-weight relationships, head circumference, and developmental skills helps the team understand the big picture of growth for the child.

Look at the big picture. It is important to look at the big picture of growth and keep individual pieces of data in perspective. The growth chart describes points in time and trends in growth. It provides preliminary information that may require a look into the history and feeding issues for that child. The information that growth charts provide is part of the picture, but it is not the whole picture and certainly not the *only* picture. Remember that growth charts can *describe* growth but should not *dictate* growth (Satter, 1987).

It is important to be sure that growth really is a problem for a child before turning it into a problem. If growth charts have been evaluated carefully and the child's nutritional status is a concern, the feeding team can take the next step in the discovery process. The team can begin to uncover the layers of issues that have an impact on the child and family and may create problems in growth and nutrition.

Pediatric Undernutrition or Failure to Thrive?

Poor growth and pediatric undernutrition are important problems for children. Kessler and Dawson (1999) indicate that chronic pediatric undernutrition can contribute to decreased immunological resistance; decreased physical activity; and long-term impairments in cognitive development, school performance, and social-affective competence. Children need to receive proper nutrition, but making sure they get it should be done carefully. Poorly growing children and their families need sensitive support.

How a child's growth patterns are described can affect mealtime interactions. Kessler and Dawson (1999) recommend using more descriptive terms such as *pediatric undernutrition, growth deficiency,* and *growth failure* instead of a more emotionally laden term such as *failure to thrive.* They suggest looking beyond the traditional labels of organic and nonorganic failure to thrive and using a multifaceted approach to diagnose and treat these children.

Many children with pediatric undernutrition are labeled as failure to thrive. Smith and Berenberg (1970) warned the medical profession to be cautious about confusing a description of poor growth with a diagnosis of failure to thrive. However, many children still receive that label when a growth parameter is below the 5th percentile despite a look at trends, weight-for-height ratios, history, or diagnosis (see Table 24.1). In these situations, does the diagnosis help the child or enhance treatment? Parents are very aware of the negative connotations of the diagnosis of failure to thrive. They often describe a sense of failure and blame that can interfere with the success of otherwise appropriate therapeutic interventions. Their feelings of failure and discouragement can make an undernutrition problem worse.

Table 24.1	**Classic Failure to Thrive Diagnosis**

- Attained growth is less than the 3rd percentile on NCHS Growth Chart.*
- Weight for height is less than the 5th percentile on the NCHS Growth Chart.
- Rate of growth has fallen off a previously established growth curve.
- The downward crossing of equal to or greater than two major percentiles on the NCHS Growth Chart.

*National Center for Health Statistics

Pediatric undernutrition can be caused by problems ranging from inappropriate feeding practices to serious underlying illnesses (Frank, Needlman, & Silva, 1994). Historically, children with poor growth were classified as having nonorganic or organic reasons for their growth failures (Homer & Ludwig, 1981). Even the term *mixed category* does not seem to adequately answer the question of why a child is not growing. In organic failure to thrive, traditionally there is a specific major organ-system illness or dysfunction, a physical reason that explains why the child is not growing. Inorganic failure to thrive seems to be a diagnosis of exclusion. If medical personnel cannot identify an organic problem easily, they tend to label it as inorganic failure to thrive. Unfortunately, traditionally this diagnosis is interpreted as meaning the problem is the parent's fault. The mixed category or multidimensional classification system is being used more often to recognize an organic etiology that is complicated with a psychological component (Kedesdy & Budd, 1998). There are children who are failing to grow secondary to clear-cut medical problems such as metabolic disorders, liver dysfunction, and cystic fibrosis. Other children are failing to grow because the family is homeless and does not have enough money to buy the amount and types of food that support adequate nutrition. Many situations, however, are not as easy to diagnose. Many children have physiological influences on their feeding that are complicated by a layering of events, emotions, and situations.

Feeding teams need to look at all parameters—growth patterns, medical history, individual child and family situations, and mealtime interactions—in order to understand undernutrition. Once the team has concluded that the child has a growth issue and that pediatric undernutrition is a concern, then the growth and feeding assessment can move forward.

A Continuum of Concern

Although this chapter primarily focuses on children who cannot maintain an appropriate rate of growth through oral intake alone, many other children share these same problems. Noneating represents a continuum of concern, not a single point on the dietary map. This continuum begins with children who are described as *picky eaters*. Their diets may be limited to a set of favorite foods, and they continue the normal stage of neophobia for food beyond the typical 2- to 3-year-old age period. They typically get enough to eat and a diet that is diversified enough to support their nutritional and growth needs. The majority of these children will move through this period if their parents are creative and patient while setting limits around mealtime and allow their children to eat or not eat what is served. If parents cater to their children's picky whims, these children will continue to be picky eaters for long periods of time, even into adulthood.

Some children move from being picky eaters to being ***extremely selective eaters***. These youngsters have severely limited diets and strong aversions to food tastes, textures, and colors. Their food choices often are guided by a private logic that determines which foods are safe or comfortable to eat. With some children, these choices are easy to understand. For example, a child who has a history of poor chewing may avoid foods that require resistive chewing, even when her physical abilities are adequate for chewing more complex foods. A child with oral sensory defensiveness may reject any food that has a texture. Other children make their selections in ways that are unclear to adults. For example, one child went through a phase where he would eat only pureed foods that were purple. No one could identify any logical connection between the color purple and his feeding history.

Many children act as if specific foods or groups of food are dangerous and need to be avoided at all costs. Children in this group usually get enough to eat of the foods that they will eat. Some fail to grow well because of limited dietary diversity. For example, one 2-year-old lived on ice cream, cheese, and white bread. She ate an abundance of these foods but was below the 5th percentile in weight and was extremely thin. She consumed an appropriate number of calories, but limitations in the types of nutrients in her diet did not support her overall growth. Other children inexplicably grow well and remain healthy while eating diets that are limited in variety and calories. Although some children in this group of extremely selective eaters show appropriate growth, many remain in a marginal area of undernutrition. They constantly are at risk for growth and nutrition problems. Because of this, their extreme dietary selectivity causes major concerns for their parents.

At the far end of the continuum are children described as ***noneaters***. These children refuse to eat both the amount and the types of food that would support their growth and nutrition. They have growth problems as determined by standard measures and are in the group that has failure to thrive or pediatric undernutrition. Many of these children have strongly aversive reactions to eating and mealtimes. At the extreme are children who receive their nourishment through a feeding tube. Although Chapter 23 includes a discussion about these children, many of the concepts in this chapter are applicable when the child is ready to make the transition from tube feedings to oral feedings.

Children in each of these groups may have physical, sensory, structural, or experiential reasons that triggered their refusal to eat certain foods or to eat enough food to thrive as oral feeders. When children do not eat, parents become frightened. They also may feel that their children are defying them or rejecting them and the food. Food is strongly equated with love and acceptance in most cultures. When children reject food that is prepared and offered by a caring parent, many parents feel personally rejected. When parents are afraid or feel rejected or challenged, they frequently respond by trying to get their children to eat more food. This often sets into motion a process that leads toward greater food refusal and a greater risk of undernutrition.

■ Layers of Influence

The *Now* of Mealtime

By the time a feeding assessment is requested for children with poor eating patterns or poor growth, parents and professionals have tried a multitude of partial solutions. Time has passed, and both the children and their parents have developed habits and responses to mealtime behaviors. It is important for the feeding therapist to look at what is happening ***now*** as she reviews the sequence of events that led to the child's current mealtime choices. How did the child and parent arrive at the current situation? What physiological factors, parent and child belief systems, and interactions with the environment led this child to develop undernutrition problems?

The past plays a role in understanding the current situation. However, no matter what has happened in the past and whatever the reasons for the mealtime issues, the starting point for assessment and treatment is "what is happening ***now***" at each mealtime.

- Are there current difficulties in physical, sensory, or structural areas that influence the ease and comfort with which the child is able to eat?
- What does the family do to help this child grow?
- How does the child feel about mealtimes?
- How do the parents feel about mealtimes?
- Who is stressed and why?
- To what lengths has the family gone to try to help the child grow? Is there tricking, bribing, coercing, or forcing?
- Are there distractions or mealtime entertainment?
- Is the child punished for not eating?
- Have either the child or parents given up on making mealtime changes?
- Are the parents and child engaged in a power struggle?

In the *now*, many families are adding all the calories they possibly can at each meal. They have food available at all times. The child nibbles and grazes all day. Parents often describe feeling like short-order cooks, preparing special meals for their child. They play the child's favorite tape or video, read her favorite book, and surround her with her favorite toys. They may be tricking, bribing, coercing, begging, or forcing the child to eat. When the feeding therapist knows to what lengths the family has gone to get this child to grow, she begins to understand parental concerns and the stress that surrounds mealtimes. Understanding the *now*, the therapist can begin to peel away some of the layers of factors that influence the child's growth and mealtime skills and habits. What lies beneath the extravagant mealtime efforts to get the child to eat? What factors have influenced the child's mealtimes? When did the feeding problems begin? With this basis of understanding, the feeding therapist can begin to look below the surface and try to understand how the child feels about eating and how today's mealtime responses have developed from a complex layering of influences.

Initial Influences: The First Layer

After hearing and seeing the *now* of mealtime, the feeding therapist must review the child's history with the parents to identify possible initial influences on feeding. Children with growth and eating difficulties today started with problems in infancy. Parents often look back and describe a number of issues in the infant's early feeding history that gives clues to the beginning of these feeding difficulties.

Medical

Feeding issues often begin with medical events that influence children's physical endurance, gastrointestinal comfort, breathing, and overall wellness. These structural and physiological problems may remove the child from a typical mealtime setting. The child may receive nutrition intravenously or through a feeding tube while ill or unable to handle food or liquid orally. The child may experience rampant gastroesophageal reflux that creates pain at each meal and throughout the day. Respiratory problems associated with bronchopulmonary dysplasia (BPD) may make it difficult to coordinate sucking, swallowing, and breathing, as well as increase feelings of anxiety and fear. Cardiac difficulties may create such severe endurance problems that eating becomes too much work. Serious breathing and feeding difficulties may require ventilation and the regular placement and replacement of nasogastric tubes. The infant may experience formula intolerance and chronic gastrointestinal discomfort, resulting in a trial of multiple formulas before finding one that works. The child may have eaten well until hospitalized for a severe viral disease or uncontrolled seizures. Following the illness, he may refuse to eat, often because he does not feel well enough or lacks the necessary energy.

Sensorimotor

Many children's journeys toward eating competence are delayed or made tougher by difficulties with movement coordination or sensory processing. The histories of these infants may include early regulatory problems, including difficulties with sensory modulation. Extreme sensitivities to sound, light, touch, or movement may have made early infant care and feeding a major challenge for both infant and parents. The infant's sensory interpretation of feeding stimuli and motor responses can influence early experiences with eating. Some infants experience difficulties with postural tone and movement coordination that make it difficult to latch on properly for breast-feeding or to coordinate the flow of liquid during swallowing. Other infants may succeed with bottle- or breast-feeding but experience random periods of choking and coughing due to inconsistent or poorly organized sucking coordination. Problems initially may have been noticed when the baby became upset unless the formula was at a very specific temperature. The transition to cereals and pureed foods often creates challenges for children with sensorimotor difficulties. The changes required in sensory processing or motor organization skills become too great, and expansion of eating into this more challenging area comes to a halt. The introduction of textured foods also creates major difficulties for children who have problems with sensory hyperreaction or sensory defensiveness.

Recent research has identified mild sensorimotor disabilities and immature and abnormal oral-motor functioning in a significant proportion of a group of socioeconomically deprived, inner-city infants diagnosed with nonorganic failure to thrive (Mathisen, Skuse, Wolke, & Reilly, 1989; Reilly, Skuse, Wolke, & Stevenson, 1999; Skuse, 1985).

Mealtime Interaction

Some parents have difficulty reading infant cues of readiness to eat or cues of satiety to stop the meal. Cues may be ignored or misread, leading to mealtime interaction difficulties. Some infants do not give clear or consistent mealtime cues because of their sensorimotor difficulties (Mathisen et al., 1989). Parents who might do well with typical baby cues can be lost when trying to understand their infant's unique message system. Poor giving of or reading of cues and a multitude of other communication issues can cause disruptions in the mealtime relationship.

Environment

The environment in which children eat and grow affects their abilities and attitudes about eating. An environment that is calm, nurturing, and predictable provides a very different type of mealtime support than one that is chaotic, busy, and inconsistent. Environments that are filled with distractions may be very disorienting for infants who experience difficulties with sensory regulation. Families that experience poverty may have difficulty keeping enough food in the house to provide for their children's nutritional needs. Parents who are dealing with depression or eating disorders such as anorexia may forget to feed the child or offer amounts or types of food that are inappropriate for the child's needs.

Interpretation and Action: The Second Layer

Trigger Events

Although some children begin their journey toward feeding with major medical, physical, or sensory difficulties, these problems usually are dealt with by giving the child nonoral feedings or initiating a therapy program. When children move toward the second layer of refusing to eat, typically there are ***trigger events*** or situations that stimulate the development of the feeding problem.

Some acute illnesses trigger feeding problems by reducing appetite and the energy needed for eating. If a child has mild gastroesophageal reflux, an upper respiratory infection can make the reflux worse. If this caused increased gagging and nausea when the child was introduced to lumpy foods, the child may associate increased gagging with lumps and textures. He might interpret lumps with discomfort and refuse new foods. Some medications reduce appetite or cause mild nausea. If a child begins a medication that reduces appetite at a time when the parent has started to become concerned about growth, the child may perceive a push to eat just when she feels least like eating. A mealtime struggle can ensue. A choking episode may cause increased tension and vigilance in the parent when the child is offered foods with lumps. The child also may become concerned and respond with increased caution and a regression in acceptance and exploration of food textures.

Trigger events also can be traced to social interactions that created pressure on the child to eat. Parents do not always agree on the best way to handle developmental feeding issues in children. Conflicts emerge as a result of different viewpoints or parental actions. These can intensify when dealing with the extended family. For example, a grandmother may disagree with her daughter's low-key handling of her grandchild's tendency to dawdle and eat small amounts of food. During her infrequent visits, the grandmother forces the child to eat and provokes loud arguments with her daughter about the child's eating style. Sometimes the child's strong need for independence is in direct conflict with the parent's need for neatness and control. A trigger event does not have to be a major conflict. It can be as simple as the parent refusing to let the child reach for the spoon and interact with the food in a messy way. This may cause the child to react by refusing to open the mouth and then throwing the bowl on the floor.

Beliefs and Interpretation

Interpretation is the key to action. Similar events occur in the lives of many different children and parents. Each event is filtered through a nervous system that is more or less sensitive and through a variety of different personal temperaments. This colors the event with a degree of intensity and importance that differs for each individual. Most important, specific events are interpreted in relation to each individual's personal belief system (Kaufman, 1991).

Beliefs about mealtimes and eating guide the initial action that parents and children take. When the beliefs of the child and parent are incompatible, conflict can arise. For example, the child may believe that "I don't eat green or yellow foods. They taste yucky!" The mother may believe that "Children must eat vegetables every day in order to grow well." When the child acts in harmony with his belief about vegetables and refuses to eat them, his action confronts his mother's belief. This creates a level of discomfort for the mother, stimulating her to take action. The mother also holds other beliefs that influence the action she takes. She may believe that she can reason with her 2-year-old and convince him that vegetables are good for him. She may believe that she can get him to eat the vegetables by taking away a privilege or making him sit at the table until the vegetables are gone. She may believe that adults make the rules and children must be forced to comply with them; he will eat his vegetables! Each of these beliefs about parenting, learning, and the underlying relationship between parents and children will guide her actions.

Both children and parents act to defend their personal beliefs and views of reality. If an overt action to defend an important belief does not take place (due to other beliefs), the individual's discomfort level may increase. For example, the mother may decide to ignore her child's refusal of vegetables because she intellectually thinks that this is a phase of development that he will outgrow. However, she may be uncomfortable about this decision and unconsciously look for the negative effects of not eating vegetables on her child's health and growth. She may intermittently coax or bribe her child to eat just a couple of bites in order to reduce her own growing anxiety. Her son may pick up her nonverbal worries and concerns and interpret them in his own way to decide whether to comply with her request or to extend his noneating of vegetables to fruits as well.

When parents find themselves in this type of a quandary, they try to increase their own comfort level by assuming responsibility for their child's eating. They find ways to get involved with what and how much the child eats at each meal. When this happens, the feeding issues move to a whole new level.

In order to meet the needs of both the child and family, the feeding therapist needs to identify and consider the relative importance of events that create the special layers for this specific child. The therapist can explore the following questions.

- What events and early experiences began the progression toward the current feeding problem?
- When did these problems begin? How did the child react?
- How severe were the events that led toward the child's initial refusal to eat?
- Does the initial problem or event that triggered the child's eating difficulties still exist? If the problem is not resolved, how severe is it now? If the difficulty is no longer present, how long did the child experience the problem before it was resolved?
- How did the parents feel about the child's initial refusal to eat?
- How did the parents initially react when the child showed difficulties or differences in feeding behaviors? What actions did they take to get the child to eat more or eat different foods?
- What is the child's basic emotional style and temperament? How does this interact with actions taken to increase eating?
- Did the child feel safe during this period?
- Did the child feel pressure to eat from the parents or others in the environment?
- How did the child react to the parents' actions to increase food intake?
- How did the parents respond to the counterpressure from the child?
- How would you describe the child's personal interpretation of the feeding events that have been experienced?
- What did the child do to defend his personal position or belief about eating and mealtimes?

Children choose behaviors to take care of themselves and their perceived needs. One child may confront pressures to eat with a strong refusal to open the mouth. A second child may passively open the mouth and eat. A third child may protest mildly and then vomit the food after it has reached the stomach. Still another child may accept the pressure and eat the minimal amount to reduce immediate parental concern.

In order to understand a child's choices, the therapist needs to understand why the child might have chosen one set of behaviors over another. The therapist needs to look at the child's unique, underlying constellation of experiences. Then, and only then, can the therapist begin to put together a picture of the elements that started and perpetuated the feeding problem.

For most children, a complicated mixture of feeding interactions and growth difficulties develops as a result of many smaller events. Each of the small events adds to the total mixture that becomes a major event in the child's world view. Feeding difficulties for these children are created from a mixture of physiology, sensorimotor influences, mealtime interactions, and environmental factors that become paired with the child's beliefs and interpretations of these events.

For example, a child may have very mild gastroesophageal reflux, which by itself does not create a discomfort level that would interfere with eating. If the same child also has a mild-to-moderate difficulty with sensory modulation or sensory defensiveness, the sensory input from mild reflux may be interpreted as more intense or uncomfortable at mealtimes. This may reduce the child's ability to enjoy mealtimes and reduce her enthusiasm for eating. Because both reflux and sensory processing difficulties vary in frequency and intensity, the child may be more uncomfortable and reduce eating on some days but not on others. If a chaotic family environment is added to the mixture, with parental pressure to eat more, these multilayered issues can turn into a full-fledged feeding problem.

Common Beliefs and Their Roots

Although each child's experiences and belief systems are unique, a number of common ones seem interrelated. These beliefs emerge from children's experiences and perceptions of food and its impact on their bodies and emotions.

The child who has experienced **gastroesophageal reflux** may act on beliefs that say:

- "Food hurts my tummy."
- "If I eat your food, I feel sick."
- "When my tummy feels full, I need to stop before I throw up."

The child who has experienced **oral motor coordination problems** may act on beliefs that say:

- "Eating is scary."
- "I could choke if I ate that."
- "This is just too much work!"

The child who has experienced **oral sensory defensiveness** may act on beliefs that say:

- "Eating is dangerous."
- "If I move this food around in my mouth, it will attack me! If I hold it for a long time, maybe it will go away."
- "This is just too much work!"
- "I don't feel safe."
- "Eating hurts my mouth."

The child who has experienced **respiratory difficulties** may act on beliefs that say:

- "I can't breathe when I have food in my mouth."
- "Swallowing is scary and dangerous because I have to stop breathing."
- "Eating makes me feel too tired. I just don't have the energy to eat and breathe too."

The child who has experienced **conflicts around eating** may act on beliefs that say:

- "No one can make me eat!"
- "You can put it in my mouth but you can't make me swallow."

Is It a Behavior Problem?

The word **behavior** is descriptive and neutral. The *New Oxford Dictionary of English* (1989) defines **behavior** as "the way in which one acts or conducts oneself, especially towards others; or the way in which an animal or person behaves in response to a particular situation or stimulus." Adults and children choose behaviors that they feel are in their best interest—behaviors that are in line with their beliefs and that support what they most want at any given moment. Some therapists choose to spend a beautiful weekend sitting in a windowless conference room learning about feeding problems because, at that moment, their desire to expand their knowledge in this area is stronger than their desire to play tennis or go to the beach. Others choose to attend the workshop because an employer requires it, and they want to keep their job. A 2-year-old may choose to eat a new food because it has been presented in a way that stimulates her curiosity and this satisfies a driving curiosity about the environment. Another may choose to reject the new food because he is afraid that it is dangerous and could kill him. Both children make their choices based on a perception or belief (based on their knowledge and experience) that they are acting in their best interests at the moment.

However, in our society, the words **behavior** and **behavioral** have developed a negative connotation. When professionals and parents can't explain why a child doesn't eat, they often say the child has a behavioral feeding problem. They try to decide whether the child has a **real** reason not to eat or whether "it's just behavioral." Everything that a child or adult does reflects an automatic or conscious behavioral choice. When we judge behaviors as good or bad, our decisions reflect the bias of our belief system. When we learn to think in a broader and more accepting way, we can simply ask why a child or parent chooses one behavior over another. Because we are not judging the behavior or using the term to describe something negative, we are in a better position to understand the dynamics of the child's mealtime.

A Look at the Layers

It is helpful to review the children whose feeding examples were introduced in this chapter and visualize a conceptual layering of feeding influences.

Andy

Andy, who is 2½ years old, came to the assessment with his mother. She was asked to bring food that showed the therapist what brought out Andy's best and worst eating skills. She also was asked to bring his favorite utensils so that he would feel comfortable eating in an office situation. Andy's mother walked in the door with 14 kinds of food. She brought lots of things to try because she is never sure of what he will like at a meal. She also indicated that she needed to offer many foods at each meal at home. She brought a cassette tape player, Andy's favorite tape, a stuffed toy, and a couple of books. She also brought his favorite cup and spoon—the only spoon he will use at a meal. By the amount of material the mother brought, the therapist could see that mealtime had become a struggle. But how, when, and why did that struggle start?

A further look at Andy's history showed that he was small at birth and grew slowly during infancy. He had a severe respiratory illness when he was 8 months old and was sick for about a month. After that, he did not seem to regain his pre-illness interest in foods. As he continued to grow slowly, his pediatrician became concerned and encouraged his mother to "get him to take more foods." She started by offering a few more bites. Andy turned away and refused them. In a desperate effort to "get in those extra calories," she held his chin and forced him to take the food.

Andy had an illness and resultant poor appetite at the same time that his mother was worried about his weight. Her desperation led her to disregard his mealtime communications of fullness. His refusals became more common. Andy began to realize how important eating was to his mother at the same time he began to strive for a 2-year-old's typical need for independence and beginning autonomy. Refusing became part of the mealtime game for Andy. He began to realize he could hold out for favorite foods and that his mother, concerned about his weight gain, would give him anything he wanted. She became an expert at mealtime entertainment. At first, she noticed he ate better when she read a book. Gradually, he wanted more—a book *and* a videotape. The entertainment necessary to keep him at the meal continued to increase until all the paraphernalia that was brought to the office visit was a part of each meal (see Figure 24.1).

Tommy

Tommy, 18 months old, always has had a poor appetite. He prefers smooth foods such as yogurt, pudding, and ice cream. He can eat spaghetti and macaroni and cheese. He still gags on meats and more dense foods. His parents, concerned about his weight, give him the foods he enjoys. Upon further questioning of the parents, the therapist learned that Tommy was a baby who spit up frequently. He had been on gastroesophageal reflux medication. He stopped his regular vomiting at about 1 year of age so the medication was discontinued.

Tommy, according to his mother, was a very "spitty baby." Although her older son also had spit up while being burped, her experience with Tommy was quite different. At times, Tommy's spitty burps resulted in vomiting of the whole meal. Tommy wanted to eat very small amounts. He would cry for his bottle, suck 1 to 2 ounces, and then push the bottle away. An hour later, he would cry again and

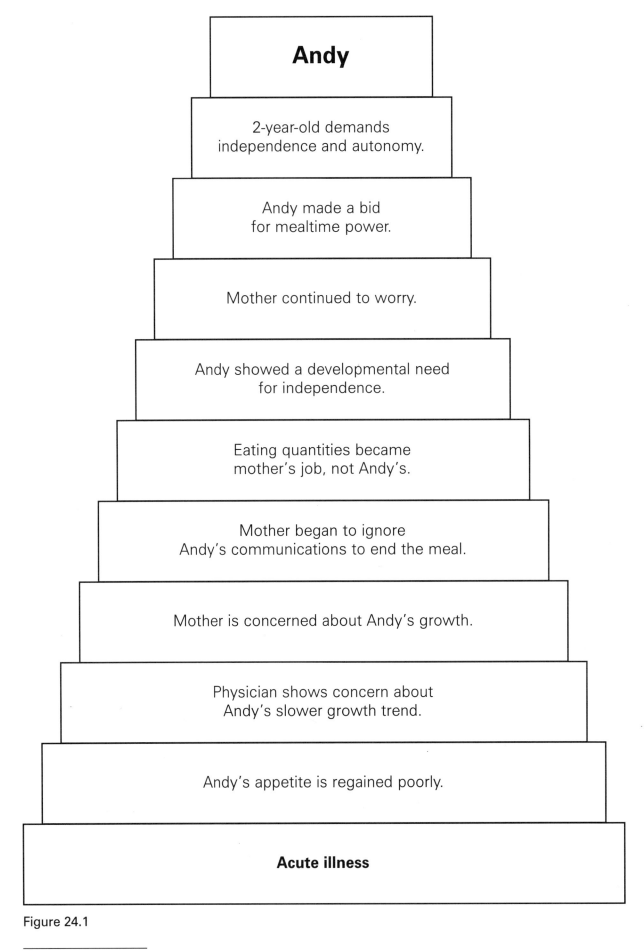

Figure 24.1

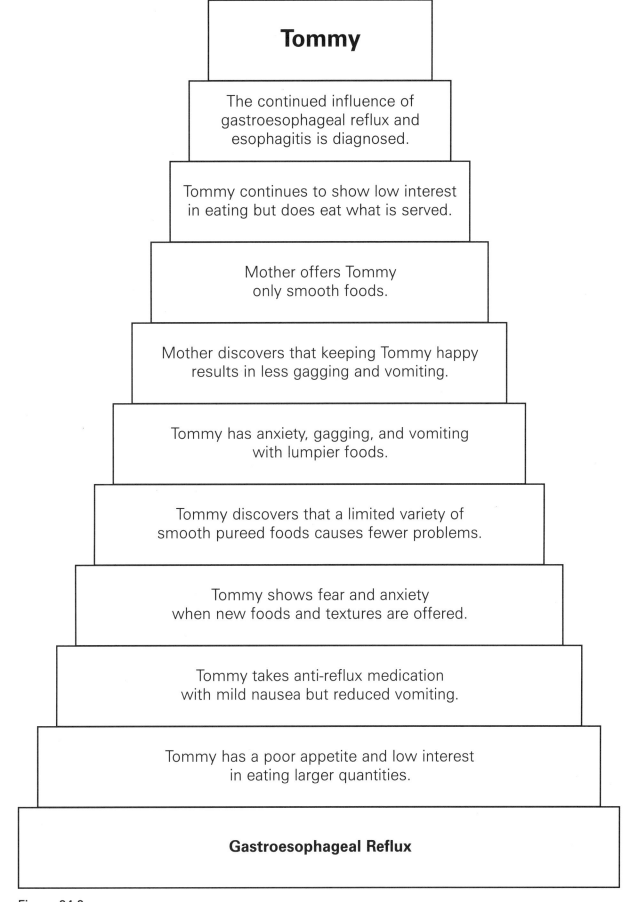

Tommy

The continued influence of gastroesophageal reflux and esophagitis is diagnosed.

Tommy continues to show low interest in eating but does eat what is served.

Mother offers Tommy only smooth foods.

Mother discovers that keeping Tommy happy results in less gagging and vomiting.

Tommy has anxiety, gagging, and vomiting with lumpier foods.

Tommy discovers that a limited variety of smooth pureed foods causes fewer problems.

Tommy shows fear and anxiety when new foods and textures are offered.

Tommy takes anti-reflux medication with mild nausea but reduced vomiting.

Tommy has a poor appetite and low interest in eating larger quantities.

Gastroesophageal Reflux

Figure 24.2

take another ounce or two. His total intake during the day was slightly low, and his mother was worried that he wasn't getting enough to eat. The pediatrician told her that his weight gain was low but still adequate and suggested that Tommy might have problems with gastroesophageal reflux. He prescribed a trial period of an anti-reflux medication when Tommy was 4 months old. Tommy continued to take small amounts of formula at each mini-meal, but spit up less. He now vomited only when he cried and was upset. His periods of upset seemed to be triggered by the medication, which often made him gag and act as if he had an upset stomach. Because the overall reflux seemed to be reduced, Tommy continued to take the medication until he was 1 year old. Tommy was very uninterested in eating new foods.

When his mother introduced pureed consistency foods, he gagged and cried. The crying often resulted in vomiting. His mother persisted by thinning the food with milk and making it smooth enough for Tommy to accept it. Yogurt, pudding, and ice cream became his favorites. Tommy no longer gagged until his mother introduced lumpier foods. Once again, she thinned them down until he could accept a few very soft foods with fairly uniform lumps such as macaroni and cheese and spaghetti. If she offered him other foods that had larger lumps or a thicker, heavier consistency, Tommy became anxious and would gag as soon as the food entered his mouth. If he became too upset, he would vomit. Because his mother did not want to upset him, she would give him the smooth foods that he liked. Gradually, Tommy reverted to eating a diet that consisted primarily of very soft, smooth foods. He continued to show a low interest in eating and wiggled and squirmed after eating only 1 to 2 ounces of food. He seemed physically uncomfortable during and after meals if he ate larger amounts.

A 24-hour pH probe for gastroesophageal reflux was done when Tommy was 18 months old. He had active gastroesophageal reflux with mild esophagitis. Because he no longer spit up or vomited, his parents and physician had assumed that this problem had been resolved. Because he was hungry, he was able to eat small amounts of food. He became more uncomfortable and anxious when the volume of food increased in his tummy. When he was anxious, his tummy became more upset and he felt like vomiting. He taught his mother not to upset him with more difficult foods and to give him only foods that he knew didn't cause him problems (see Figure 24.2).

Julia

Julia is Mrs. Jones' first child. Mrs. Jones prepares highly nutritious meals for her family and is very concerned that Julia is not eating enough. She indicates that she tries and tries to get Julia to eat more at each meal so that she has a well-balanced and nutritious diet. Julia pushes her mother away, wants to do it herself, and fusses every time she is in the high chair. No one enjoys meals. How did this well-meaning mother and a perfectly healthy child end up with mealtimes being such a struggle?

For 5 years, Julia's mother wanted to have a child. When she discovered that she was pregnant, she was overjoyed. She spent the last months of her pregnancy reading every book on child development that she could find. She was particularly interested in the relationship between nutrition and children's intelligence. She decided to breast-feed Julia to give her a strong nutritional advantage. Julia ate well for the first 6 months. She was a strong and aggressive breast-feeder who liked to eat and gave her mother clear signals of hunger and fullness. Her mother felt emotionally nourished by her daughter's avid desire to eat and acceptance of her breast milk. Julia continued to eat well until her mother added supplemental foods to her diet at 6 months. She sat on her mother's lap and tried to reach for the spoon as her mother fed her cereal, fruit, and vegetables. Her mother knew that children couldn't use a spoon to feed themselves until they were older. She pushed Julia's hand away each time Julia wanted to be physically involved with the meal. Julia learned to swipe at the spoon with her hand and knock it from her mother's hand. This made a mess, which upset her mother. Her mother learned to hold Julia down and restrain her hands so that she couldn't reach out. Julia fussed and seemed less interested in eating, but continued to do so because she was hungry. The restraint

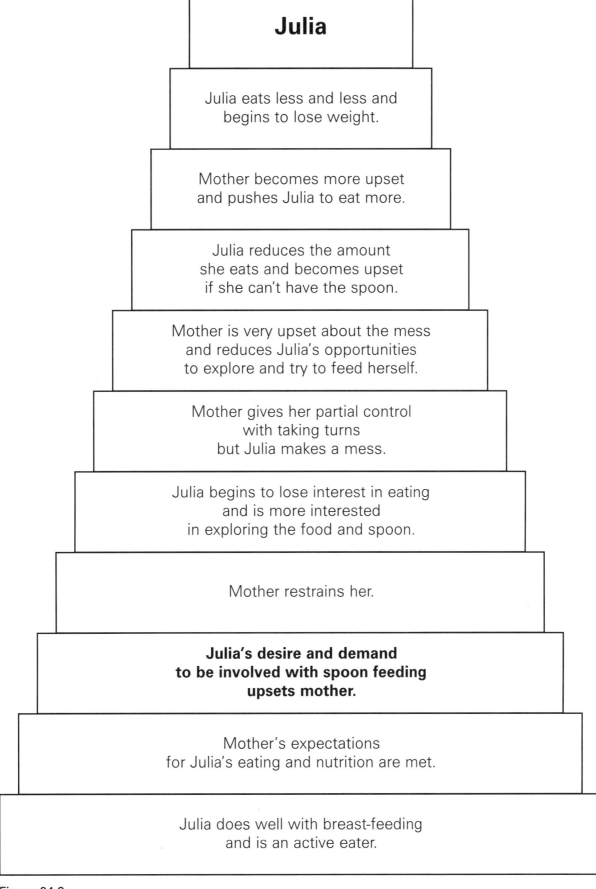

Julia

Julia eats less and less and begins to lose weight.

Mother becomes more upset and pushes Julia to eat more.

Julia reduces the amount she eats and becomes upset if she can't have the spoon.

Mother is very upset about the mess and reduces Julia's opportunities to explore and try to feed herself.

Mother gives her partial control with taking turns but Julia makes a mess.

Julia begins to lose interest in eating and is more interested in exploring the food and spoon.

Mother restrains her.

Julia's desire and demand to be involved with spoon feeding upsets mother.

Mother's expectations for Julia's eating and nutrition are met.

Julia does well with breast-feeding and is an active eater.

Figure 24.3

solution worked until Julia was 9 months old and began to sit in a high chair. She wanted to put her hands in the food and put the food into her mouth by herself. Her mother was horrified! Her beautiful baby daughter was a mess, and food flew everywhere. Her mother pulled Julia's hands out of the food and cleaned her up. She couldn't stand the messiness and didn't have time for the extra work that it created. As her emotions escalated, Julia's mother forgot that babies at Julia's age want and need to be involved in the first stages of finger feeding. All she could think about was getting her child fed without the mess and getting her to eat a balanced diet.

Julia became fussy every time her mother put her in the high chair. Although she was hungry, Julia tried to get down or push away the bowl of food. She usually ate just enough to make the hunger go away and then shifted to confronting her mother about who would put the food into her mouth. When her mother gave her a turn, she loved to play with the food and bang the spoon on the tray. This upset her mother who could see only that Julia was playing and not eating enough. When her mother grabbed the spoon and tried to get her to take another bite, Julia clamped her mouth closed. She coaxed Julia to take more, and Julia angrily tried to grab for the spoon (see Figure 24.3).

Frankie

Frankie, a 3-year-old, has a poor appetite. He picks and pokes at his food. He will eat whatever is offered, but only in small quantities. He cannot be convinced to eat larger amounts. He has constant allergies to airborne allergens. He has recurrent ear infections and constant phlegm and gastrointestinal discomfort. When and why did his poor appetite begin?

Frankie was a sickly baby. He had frequent periods of diarrhea and colic. His parents and pediatrician tried different formulas, but nothing seemed to make a difference. Frankie accepted new foods without a problem during infancy and early childhood. He did not complain or seem to have strong food preferences or dislikes. He ate what was served but usually picked and poked at his food as if he were trying to decide how much to eat. During the summer and fall, Frankie's nose ran and he sneezed. During the winter, he often had chronic ear infections. As a toddler, he complained that he didn't feel good and that his tummy hurt. Frankie continued to eat but had to be coaxed to eat enough to maintain his weight. His parents and pediatrician were concerned that he wasn't growing as fast as other 3-year-olds. His mother continued to remind him to eat, and Frankie usually took several more bites without complaint before pushing his plate away. If his mother continued to coax or bribe him to eat, Frankie became angry and said his tummy hurt. His mother took him to the pediatrician, who said that Frankie wasn't sick. He felt that although Frankie had periods of poor health, Frankie had learned not to eat in order to get his mother's attention. He stated that Frankie had a behavioral feeding problem and that his parents should be stricter about getting him to eat all the food that was served. His mother did not agree and changed pediatricians. The second doctor believed that Frankie might be allergic to foods and pollens, and referred him to an allergist. Frankie was diagnosed with a chronic allergy to cow's milk and wheat, as well as multiple allergies to pollens and environmental chemicals. When the underlying problem was dealt with, Frankie's interest in eating increased and he began to grow (see Figure 24.4).

Darria

Darria is 3½ years old and has been on a feeding tube since birth because of initial respiratory and gastrointestinal difficulties. For the past 18 months, she has eaten small amounts of food by mouth but seems interested in eating only a tiny amount of a limited number of foods. A psychologist told her mother that Darria had a strong feeding resistance because of feeding aversion related to her early medical history. Why is Darria having such difficulties making the transition to oral feeding?

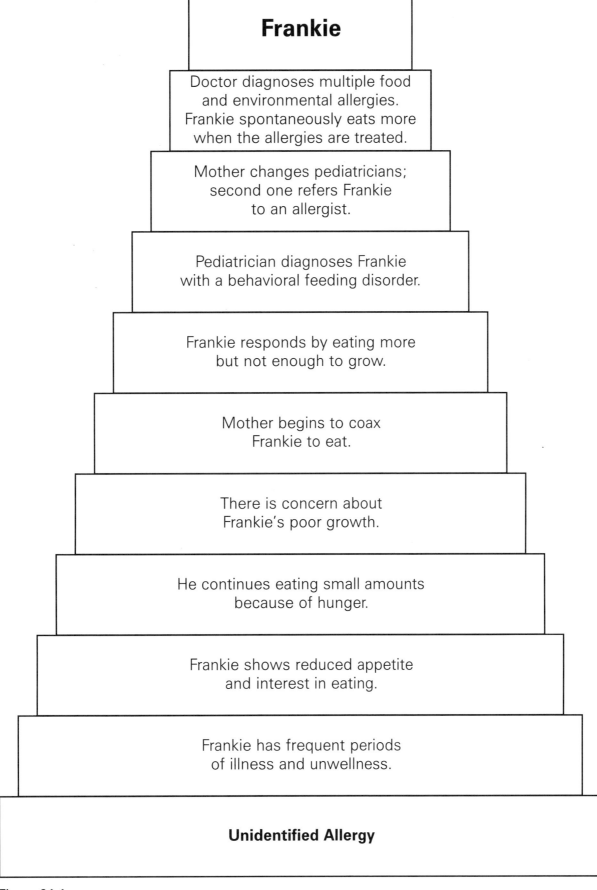

Figure 24.4

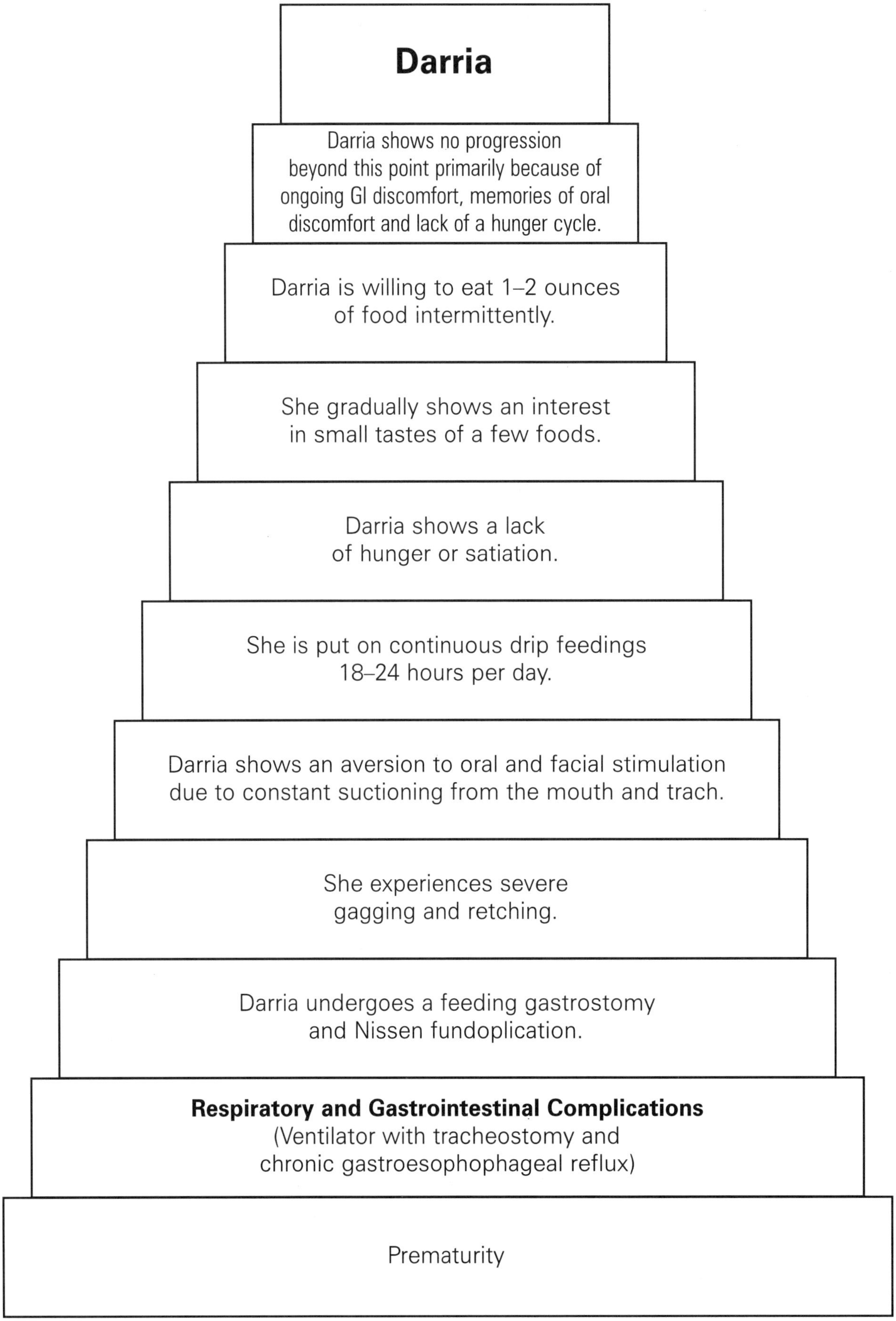

Darria

Darria shows no progression beyond this point primarily because of ongoing GI discomfort, memories of oral discomfort and lack of a hunger cycle.

Darria is willing to eat 1–2 ounces of food intermittently.

She gradually shows an interest in small tastes of a few foods.

Darria shows a lack of hunger or satiation.

She is put on continuous drip feedings 18–24 hours per day.

Darria shows an aversion to oral and facial stimulation due to constant suctioning from the mouth and trach.

She experiences severe gagging and retching.

Darria undergoes a feeding gastrostomy and Nissen fundoplication.

Respiratory and Gastrointestinal Complications
(Ventilator with tracheostomy and chronic gastroesophophageal reflux)

Prematurity

Figure 24.5

Darria was born prematurely at 26 weeks and had multiple medical complications during her first year of life. She remained hospitalized and on a ventilator until she was 7 months old, and she continued to receive oxygen through a tracheostomy until she was 2 years old. She had severe gastroesophageal reflux with vomiting, which did not respond to medication. Attempts to wean Darria from the nasogastric tube to oral feedings were unsuccessful because of her respiratory and gastrointestinal problems. At 7 months, she received a gastrostomy tube and a Nissen fundoplication. After the gastrointestinal surgery, Darria began to gag and retch. She continued to receive frequent suctioning of the secretions in her tracheostomy and thick mucus that accumulated in the back of her throat when she retched. She was weaned from her tracheostomy and oxygen when she was 2 years old and began to see a feeding therapist. Because of her gastrointestinal difficulties, Darria was fed by continuous drip for 18 hours a day. Her retching stopped when bolus feedings were discontinued and she was given no more than 2 to 3 ounces of formula each hour. She was off the pump between 10 a.m. and 4 p.m. each day. Her feeding therapist and parents focused strongly on developing Darria's feeding skills during this period. Gradually, Darria began to accept touch to her face and mouth and show brief interest and acceptance of small tastes. Her pattern of interest in food and small tastes continued but did not increase. A clinical psychologist recently recommended that Darria enter an 8-week inpatient program at the local hospital for treatment of her feeding aversion (see Figure 24.5).

Treatment Strategies

Addressing the Layers

Physiology, beliefs, and environmental responses contribute in multiple ways to noneating choices. This is a multilayered phenomenon that cannot be addressed solely on one level. Therapists who deal only with the physiology without looking at the beliefs and environmental interactions miss vital information and opportunities. Those who deal only with the mealtime behaviors without correcting the physiology or understanding the beliefs create partial solutions that are apt to fail.

Many treatment programs address only one aspect of the mealtime situation. Some professionals encourage families to add more calories to the diet. But this will not work if the child has no appetite or believes that food causes discomfort. Some set up elaborate behavior modification strategies to reward the child for taking a certain number of bites. But if the mealtime environment is chaotic or the child has continued gastrointestinal discomfort or oral defensiveness, the child will not show progress. Some programs focus on enhancing parenting behaviors and develop guidelines for offering the child food. But effective presentation skills cannot convince a frightened child to eat a food he perceives as threatening. His beliefs need to be understood. His emotional needs must be met first.

If professionals look only at the surface choices made by the child or parent and do not address the underlying issues, they may eliminate a specific behavior. They later may notice that the child has adopted a new behavior to support the same underlying belief or relieve a contingent discomfort. For example, a child may have a low appetite and a belief that eating the food will cause discomfort. He throws the food and gets up from his chair in an attempt to end the meal and stop adult pressures to continue eating. His therapist develops a behavior modification program to stop the child's throwing of food and increase the amount of time the child stays at the table. With contingencies to reinforce staying at the table and extinguish food throwing, the child may stop throwing food and sit at the table for longer periods in order to watch a favorite video used as a reinforcer. However, this may have no impact on the child's caloric intake. The child will continue to find other ways to refuse to eat because the underlying problem has not been addressed. Some children in this situation clamp their mouths shut to avoid the spoon. Other children will press the tongue against the palate to limit the amount of food entering the mouth; still others learn to vomit to get rid of the food. Professionals and parents *must* look at the reasons for the underlying behavior. If the complex layers of issues remain, the problem simply will pop up again or occur with other variations.

Although 4-year-old **Robin** has been in a feeding program since she was 1 year old, she has made very little progress. She remains on a gastrostomy tube and has strongly aversive responses to adults who approach her face and mouth. As an infant, she had severe respiratory and gastrointestinal problems related to her prematurity. She was weaned from the ventilator but remained on supplemental oxygen via a nasal cannula until she was 2 years old. She was an irritable baby and toddler, and constantly sucked on her fist in an attempt to calm herself. When she became upset, she would stick her fingers down her throat and gag. During one of her frequent periods of hospitalization, she was referred to a behavioral psychologist who developed a program to stop her from putting her hands in her mouth and gagging. Within 3 months, the gagging stopped and the program was considered a success. However, Robin seemed more irritable and unhappy. She had difficulty sleeping and was particularly jumpy and upset by specific sounds in her environment. She hated her bath and cried when she went outside on a windy day. Two months after the gagging stopped, Robin began to grind her teeth. The intense tooth grinding increased whenever she was upset. The psychologist again hospitalized Robin to extinguish her tooth grinding. During the hospitalization, she was seen by an occupational therapist who believed that Robin had severe problems with sensory overload and auditory and tactile sensory defensiveness. She felt that even if the behavioral program stopped the tooth grinding, Robin would find another sensory-based behavior to take its place. She recommended that the staff discontinue the behavioral program until the sensory issues were resolved. With a strong sensory integration program, Robin's ability to process sensory information increased, and her need for the strong proprioceptive input of gagging and tooth grinding disappeared. She became more interested in food and began to eat.

Every program will be unique because each child has a different history, set of beliefs and perspectives, and parents. However, a common series of guidelines can be used when approaching the mealtime problems and developing an effective program.

Identifying the Layers

The first step in any program is to gain a perspective on both the history of the problem and the current mealtime situation. Through logical and intuitive analyses, the feeding therapist can begin to identify the layers that have influenced mealtime interactions for the child and the parents.

Making Changes

The underlying goal of all therapy (e.g., feeding therapy, psychotherapy, educational therapy) is to help people make changes in their lives. Feeding therapists must be familiar with concepts of human learning and change, and they should incorporate these concepts into the therapy program (see Chapter 13). A successful mealtime program can address ways of helping children release their fears, change their beliefs, and adopt a new set of behaviors. An effective program can help children move toward eating a more varied diet or taking in more food by building the child's desire to eat rather than simply to please others.

A substantial portion of an effective program will be directed toward helping parents understand mealtime dynamics and know how they can support their children in making changes. They can get in touch with their own beliefs and the role that they play in the choices that they make. This may help them to accept and honor the natural division of responsibility at mealtimes.

Treating Underlying Physiological Influences on Feeding

Feeding therapists should consider the possibility that mild physiological problems continue to play a role in the child's poor appetite or refusal to eat. Often the role of mild problems is discounted because by themselves they cannot account for the child's feeding refusal. Feeding therapists often need to take the initiative in making referrals to diagnose and treat any medical or physiological influences on the child's appetite and mealtime.

Understanding and Respecting the Child's Beliefs

When therapists and parents mentally and emotionally put themselves in the child's shoes, they begin to understand more about the situation. They can imagine how they would feel in the child's mealtime situation. They can pretend that they are children and imagine their responses to the underlying problem and the current mealtime. Once adults understand the child's experiences and perspective, they can begin to understand the underlying beliefs that triggered and perpetuated the total mealtime pattern. With understanding, they can move forward more sensitively to create an environment in which the child feels comfortable enough to gradually release old perceptions of the mealtime and adopt new behaviors.

Exploration and the Child's Relationship to Food

Many children who refuse to eat consider food to be an enemy. They associate food with mealtimes and with efforts of adults to make them eat it. Yet young children can learn to make friends with new foods by playing with them. When they stir, pat, smear, pour, and make designs with an unfamiliar food, they experience that food's sensory qualities. What color is it? What does it smell like? What does it feel like on the hands? Is it smooth or does it have some texture? Is it wet or dry? Children add other sensations to their play as they lick a finger or take a small taste from the spoon used for stirring. Gradually, they develop the comfort to explore food with the mouth as they begin to eat small amounts.

When food play is separate from the child's meal, children know that they are not expected to taste or eat the food. This gives them confidence and greater willingness to experience the food in other ways. Food play can begin with pretend foods such as a soft plastic apple or plastic slices of bread and cheese. The child can explore these foods with the lips and tongue or pretend to feed them to a doll or stuffed animal. A real apple, bread, or cheese can be introduced into the play as the child becomes more comfortable and accepting of real food. Strips or small cubes of cheese can become the eyes, nose, mouth, and hair on an apple face or piece of bread. For an older child, a boat could be hollowed out of a cucumber or zucchini. The emphasis should be on the familiarization that comes through play. If adults try to convince children to take a bite of the food, the children may become suspicious that the adult has an ulterior motive. They begin to perceive the situation as another trick to get them to eat rather than enjoyable food exploration.

Helping the Feeding Relationship

When children are not growing, their feeding relationships usually change. Adults respond to children's eating choices in a wide variety of ways, but the basic relationship and interaction during the meal must be examined. Satter (1987) said, "If distortions in feeding are not the cause of the poor growth, they are almost certain to be the effect." Whether the relationship is the cause or the result of the feeding issues, it must be dealt with as a part of the total picture. It must be addressed in an understanding and nonjudgmental manner that supports family members' ability to change their roles in the current feeding relationship. Although all parents want their children to thrive and be healthy, they must learn to accept them unconditionally. Children's lovability and acceptance should not depend upon the amount of food they eat. Therapists can help parents learn to shift their desire for the child to eat differently from a demand for eating to a preference that the child will be comfortable eating enough to grow and be healthy. When children are supported with love and acceptance, they are more likely to learn and shift their eating patterns.

Mealtime Environments That Maximize Success

Many mealtime habits and behaviors for parents and children develop when children have poor growth patterns and parents become concerned. Often, these mealtime patterns have had a long time to grow and have become established because children's feeding patterns usually do not change rapidly. Establishing an environment that optimizes success is a necessary foundation from which to build positive mealtime behaviors.

Division of Responsibility

The division of mealtime responsibility is a critically important starting place (Satter, 1987, 1999). In this model, parents are responsible for selecting food that is developmentally and nutritionally appropriate for the child. Parents decide what foods are offered, how they are presented, and when and where the meal is held. Children are responsible for how much they eat and even whether they eat at all.

When parents get overly involved in how much their children eat, children lose track of their role in the mealtime. Some children rely too heavily on the parent to tell them what to eat and learn to ignore their own internal cues of hunger and fullness. Satter (1987) suggests that understanding the division of responsibility enables parents to know that they have done all they can. This frees them up to respect the child and maintain the relationship rather that getting caught up in the struggles and anxiety about eating.

Researchers have discussed the use of natural and logical consequences to guide the child's eating and mealtime behaviors (Dinkmeyer, McKay, & Dinkmeyer, 1997; Dreikurs, Cassel, & Kehoe, 1992; Dreikurs & Grey, 1993; Dreikurs & Stoltz, 1964). They also agree that eating is the child's responsibility. When children choose not to eat (for whatever reason), they are subject to the law of natural consequences. Their inner hunger drive is engaged if parents do not interfere with the process, and they soon learn that it is in their best interest to eat. Logical consequences link the child's behavioral choice to a consequence that makes sense to both child and parent. For example, when children throw food or disrupt the meal, parents can let them know that this is not a socially acceptable way to deal with their problems. Children who throw food may be required to clean up what they have thrown. This may include washing walls or vacuuming carpets. If they continue to throw food, they might be required to eat away from other people so that their behavioral choice does not interfere with the others' meal.

Meal-Snack Schedule

Most children seem to grow best when they are offered meals and planned snacks at regularly scheduled times. Pragmatically the typical meal-snack-meal-snack-meal schedule supports growth for young children. It enables the child to develop hunger because no additional foods are offered between meals. It supports the caloric needs of children by not making them wait too long between opportunities to eat. Snacks are planned as mini-meals. As adults, we often think of snacks as the spontaneous eating of cookies, chips, or a candy bar. We even call these ***snack foods***. For children, snacks should be planned and have high nutritional value. Snacks may consist of cheese, crackers, and a glass of milk; refried beans and a tortilla with a few grapes; or raw vegetables dipped into guacamole or salad dressing.

Grazing

Many children who have poor growth often are allowed to munch and nibble throughout the day in an effort to get them to eat. Eating is encouraged in whatever manner and timeframe that the child will accept. However, when food or liquid is available constantly, the child never is quite hungry enough to take a substantial meal. The nibbling takes the edge off hunger and seems to interfere with mealtime caloric intake. Children usually eat less and grow poorly when they are allowed to graze. Grazing should be discouraged in the mealtime program. Some children need smaller, more frequent meals because of gastrointestinal problems or coordination difficulties that result in long mealtimes. Small meals can be planned every 2 to 3 hours for these children; however, the key is to plan them and incorporate them as a routine part of the child's day.

Food Choices

Adults should offer children foods with a wide variety of nutrients. Daily meals should include protein sources, fruits, vegetables, grains, and fats. Ideally, a child should be comfortable with 4 to 5 different food choices in each category. Thus, in therapy, the targeted goal for dietary diversity might be four different vegetables, four different fruits, etc. This does not mean that children will eat every food group at every meal. Children's appetite and interest vary from meal to meal. However, children usually seem to manage to create a balance in their nutritional intake over time.

Rejected Foods

Children reject foods. At certain developmental ages, they are highly suspicious of new foods (i.e., neophobia) and find it very easy to say *no*, preferring to eat more familiar foods. When children refuse a specific food, it is important to introduce it again at another time. Children who love green beans this week may reject them the next. This does not necessarily mean they dislike the food. It simply means that on this day, at this time, the child is not interested in this particular food. Adults experience this type of shifting preference as well. They are not always in the mood for Mexican food, Italian food, or Chinese food. They are not always in the mood for a sandwich or a dessert. So too, children are not always in the mood for a food that the parents have served. If the parents, however, believe that the child dislikes the food because it was rejected before, and take the food off the list of options, inevitably the list of food choices will become smaller and smaller. Soon, the parents complain that the child eats only four foods. It is important to reintroduce rejected foods and encourage children to take small tastes. Research supports the concepts that up to 10 taste exposures may be needed before a child actively chooses and eats a new food (Birch & Marlin, 1982; Birch, McPhee, et al., 1987).

Liquid Intake

Because children are drawn to sweet tastes, parents and therapists frequently offer them juices and other sweet drinks. Given too liberally, these drinks may suppress appetite and replace milk and water that are needed for ideal growth. Skinner and her colleagues studied a group of typically developing children between 24 and 36 months of age (Skinner, Carruth, Moran, Houck, & Coletta, 1999). They found that there were no statistically significant differences in children's height or body mass index related to fruit juice intake. They did find, however, that the amount of soda pop that the children drank was negatively related to intake of milk and fruit juice. Smith and Lifshitz (1994) looked at the amount of fruit juice consumed by children diagnosed with nonorganic failure to thrive. They found a clear-cut relationship between children's deterioration of weight and linear growth and the excess consumption of fruit juices. In some instances, apple juice contributed to 25% to 60% of the child's daily caloric intake, replacing other more calorie and nutrient-dense foods. Children with feeding refusal issues often decide quickly which foods and liquids are safe and which are not. Because they frequently do not feel safe around food, the liquids they initially select may become the only liquids they will drink. Adults should offer children a variety of liquids and keep juices and sweet drinks in balance.

Caloric Intake

Caloric intake varies from meal to meal and from day to day. Children and adults do not eat completely well-balanced meals at every mealtime. Some meals are big meals, while others are lighter. Children are hungrier at some meals than others. Even when adults offer children all the food groups, there is no guarantee that the child will eat them. Children must decide for themselves when they have had enough. Adults must learn to listen to them. If adults decide how much is enough for children, children learn to ignore their internal appetite cues and become dependent on others for eating decisions. This can lead to weight problems later.

Mealtime Location

Children need to have a specific place to eat. This provides some of the structure and routine that children need to become comfortable with a new approach to mealtimes. A high chair, booster seat, picnic table, or TV-tray can provide an environment from which the child can focus on the meal. When a specific mealtime location has become associated with mealtime pressures, the physical locale or the type of seating arrangement will need to be changed. Mealtimes will be more successful if the physical setup for meals is different from the one that the child associates with pressure and failure. Some children with sensory-based feeding difficulties are more adventurous and interested in food when they are sitting in their car seat during a trip in the car. The vestibular movement provided by the car may enhance their ability to focus and process the sensory information in food. In addition, they seem to know that the parent is busy driving the car and cannot be as directly involved in whether the child eats.

Feeling Safe

Children who refuse to eat often feel vulnerable around food and mealtimes. They have private reasons for not eating that are not acknowledged by adults. They may be concerned that the food will make them feel ill or uncomfortable. They may refuse to eat as a way of feeling valued or powerful. In each instance, the child does not feel safe. Feelings of safety are vital to making changes and exploring new experiences that have caused distress. Adults help children feel safe by giving them legitimate choices and being trustworthy. Children can count on what the adult says or does without having to expend energy being on the lookout for deceit and trickery. Children also feel safe when they feel less stress in themselves and in those around them.

Children must know that they can get food out of the mouth safely. Many children refuse to taste or let any food into the mouth because they believe that this commits them to eating it. When children know that they can get the food out of the mouth when they need to, they are much more likely to put it into the mouth. If they feel threatened or unsafe, they will fight any attempt to put the spoon or food in the mouth. Children with sensorimotor difficulties may become very frightened when they have food in their mouth. When children are scared or uncomfortable, they generally stop moving the mouth. Food sits on the tongue and frequently reaches the area that stimulates a gag reflex or falls over the back of the tongue, causing coughing and choking. Teaching children many ways of removing food from the mouth is a critically important part of every program. They can use their fingers, wipe it off the tongue with a napkin, push it out with the tongue, or spit it out. Each of these strategies helps children organize the sensorimotor skills in the mouth that also support forming an efficient bolus for swallowing. Many children can learn to bite off a piece of food and spit it out immediately. As this becomes comfortable, they may progress to holding the food in the mouth or moving it around the mouth before spitting it out. Gradually, they learn to chew it briefly without swallowing and then to swallow small amounts of food as they chew. Guidelines for food removal are also an important part of the program. Children can learn that there is a special "all done bowl" or a plate for food that comes out of the mouth. When children taste food with permission to chew it and spit it out, they gain more positive experience with food. They learn that they do not have to like everything that goes into the mouth. They also learn that some foods or tastes are acceptable. As they gain more positive experience in a safe and supported environment, they begin to swallow foods easily and independently.

Exploration

Children must be allowed to explore new foods that are part of the meal. They need to touch, smell, and taste new foods. They might not eat any of the food the first few times it is offered. With greater familiarity the child may stir, touch, poke, smear, or pat the foods. Food may go into and come out of the mouth repeatedly. Gradually, the child may think that the food is safe enough to chew and swallow. The mealtime exploration is a very important part of mealtime comfort and safety.

Parents may wish to separate major periods of food exploration from the mealtime itself when children are older and eating with the family. A food-play period can be set aside for major types of exploration of new foods. Once the child is familiar with the food, parents can introduce it as part of the regular mealtime.

Small Steps

Children who have developed an aversion to eating or to specific aspects of the mealtime environment must develop the courage to address their fears and move through the aversive situation in a new and more comfortable way. This becomes possible when children are supported emotionally and can approach the challenging situation in very small steps. For example, a child who gags or vomits when he sees food on the table may learn to help set the mats, plates, and utensils on the table and be in the same room with feeding-related objects while controlling the urge to gag. Weeks later, the same child may put serving bowls of food on the table. Gradually, in very small successful steps, the child is comfortably able to sit at the table and enjoy the smell and small tastes of food.

Focus of Attention

Therapists and parents should look carefully at the mealtime environment. In most instances, children need as few distractions as possible in order to focus on the mealtime. At times, however, children may need a distraction in order to eat more. Parents and therapists must be sure that the mealtime distraction is a part of the meal and not an outside distraction. Nonmealtime distractions such as videos, books, and toys take the child's attention away from the meal and focus it on entertainment. Whenever possible, adults can offer distractions that keep attention on the meal. Giving children dried cereal while they are offered spooned foods can keep them interested as they chase the cereal around the tray with their emerging fine motor skills. Offering children their own spoon can keep them from grabbing the feeder's spoon. This may be another way to give children their own mealtime distraction while enabling the feeder to present the spoon foods without using an outside distraction.

Distractions enable children to reduce their focus on situations or sensations that are uncomfortable or distressful. Television and videotapes offer a type of distraction that has many hypnotic features. Children may immerse themselves in the action of the videotape and eat in a very automatic, unconscious manner. When this type of distraction becomes part of the child's routine, it is difficult to stop. This is another area where the concept of small steps leads to success. The child's videotape gradually can be shifted to one that has a music background, preferably a tape that has real children interacting rather than cartoon characters. At a later point, the TV can be turned so that the child may have the auditory distraction but not the combined visual and auditory distraction. Singing some of the songs on the tape with a parent during the meal gradually can lead the child into a shared mealtime interaction. Other types of calming or focusing music can be used in the background helping the child make the shift toward music as an auditory distraction to music as an auditory support.

Background music during the meal can contribute to a relaxed focus of attention. Metamusic™ containing Hemi-Sync™ sound frequencies has been particularly helpful in reducing stress and creating a more open and attentive focus for learning to eat in new ways (Morris, 1996). Chapter 13 includes strategies for using music during mealtimes.

Novelty

Children are attracted to new things. Some children eat best when all food choices are presented at once, while others maintain their interest in the meal longer when the foods are presented one at a time. To provide novelty, parents might introduce string cheese when the child is almost finished with the spaghetti. When she seems done with the string cheese, they could offer cooked veggies and dip. After the veggies, apple slices appear. When the apple slices are eaten, a pudding ends the meal. In addition to providing novelty, this approach enables the child to experience the completion of small steps rather than the overwhelming confrontation with a large plate of food.

Another way to incorporate novelty into the meal is to offer familiar foods in a different way. Parents and the therapist might try using a cookie cutter to provide special shapes for sandwiches or cheese. They can make sandwiches out of waffles instead of bread or put brightly colored juice ice cubes into the drink.

Rules

Children look to parents to establish a mealtime routine with predictable rules. Meals happen at a relatively predictable time of day, in a particular place. Food is to be eaten, not thrown or fed to the dogs. Milk is to be drunk and not made into a lake on the high chair tray. Mealtime guidelines are established gradually as the child has the developmental and cognitive skills to understand and comply with them. Children seem to thrive on the adult-created structure that provides a safety in knowing what to expect. Within the umbrella of adult mealtime structure, children make their own creative decisions. Of the foods offered, they decide what to eat, how much to eat, what foods to eat first, and what foods to eat last. They decide when to pause and when to eat, when to fill the tummy and when to socialize.

Family Mealtimes

Children learn an incredible amount of information about mealtime from sitting at the table with the family. They observe how to use spoons, forks, and cups, and how to hold a sandwich. They learn that a banana is peeled before eating, and that the orange peels are the handles while eating an orange slice. They learn the communication and social aspects of the meal. When children are fed in isolation of the family mealtime, they miss out on excellent learning opportunities.

Team Support

Some children do not grow well. The complexity of the issues that influence mealtime may necessitate a number of diagnostic and support services to help a child and family improve their mealtimes.

Alternative Approaches

A variety of approaches to dealing with children who refuse to eat are available to therapists and parents. This book presents a child- and family-centered approach. The most common approaches, however, are based on psychological and behavioral models. These include treatment models that reflect the belief that failure to thrive is rooted primarily in dysfunction in the underlying parent-child relationship (Chatoor, 1989; Chatoor, Ganiban, Colin, Plummer, & Harmon, 1998) and in models that view it as a learned maladaptive response to the sensory stimuli surrounding food and mealtimes (Johnson & Babbitt, 1993; Stark et al., 1994; Thompson et al., 1977). Kedesdy's and Budd's (1998) more recent attempt to integrate behavioral and biological approaches to children's feeding disorders reflects a growing trend among practitioners to view the multiple layering of difficulties experienced by these children.

The philosophy and strategies used in behavior modification programs for feeding are widely implemented for children who refuse to eat. These reflect views on human learning and change and are discussed in detail in Chapter 13.

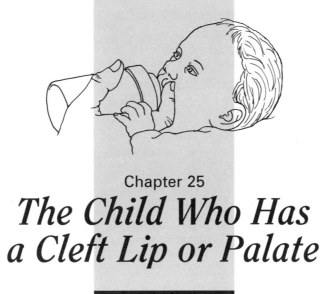

Chapter 25

The Child Who Has a Cleft Lip or Palate

Clefting is one of the most common birth defects. Feeding specialists must have a clear understanding of the physical impact of clefting on the processes of sucking, swallowing, and chewing to help the family discover the most successful ways for the baby to eat. However, the team must be able to look past the anatomy of clefts to see the multitude of factors that can have an impact on this very specific feeding relationship. The physical appearance of clefting, the grieving over the imperfect baby, the mechanics of feeding, the worries over proper growth, and the promise of surgeries and extensive medical follow-up can have a powerful influence on the family.

■ Clefts

Types of Clefts

A basic understanding of the concept of clefting is important to appreciating the issues facing children with clefts, their families, and their health-care team.

Clefting, as with most disorders, includes a large spectrum of severity, ranging from the simplest type of cleft lip or mild clefting of the soft palate to the most severe bilateral complete cleft lip and palate. A cleft is a separation of parts of the mouth that are usually joined together during the early weeks of fetal development.

A cleft lip is the separation of one or both sides of the upper lip and often of the upper alveolar or dental ridge. The cleft of the lip can be incomplete, affecting primarily the lip and not extending into the nasal cavity, or it can be complete, including separation of the dental ridge and lip and extending through the nasal cavity. When the cleft occurs on one side of the nose, it is unilateral, and when it occurs on both sides, it is bilateral.

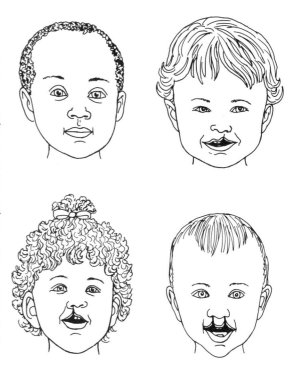

Clefts of the palate may occur in the bony hard palate or the soft palate at the back of the mouth. A cleft palate may occur with or without a cleft lip. It can occur as a unilateral, complete cleft through the soft and hard palates on one side or as a bilateral, complete cleft through the soft and hard palates on both sides. A submucous cleft occurs when the tissue connecting the two sides of the hard or soft palate is incomplete even though the surface tissue is present. A submucous cleft is invisible to the eye at birth but often can be found when the palate is checked carefully with a finger. In the submucous cleft, muscles are not joined even though the lining of the roof of the mouth is intact. Cleft palates can be left-sided or right-sided, except for the cleft of the soft palate or the submucous cleft, which are always in the middle.

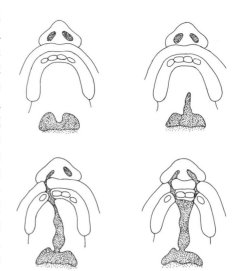

Incidence of Clefting

There are some notable racial, geographic, and sexual differences in the incidence of clefting. Clefts of the lip, palate, or both are more common in Asian or Native Americans than in Caucasian babies, and they are more common in Caucasian babies than in African-Americans (Kaufman, 1991; Melnick, 1986). Unilateral clefts are more common on the left side than the right, and they are more common than bilateral clefts. When they are bilateral, the left side is usually the more affected side. More males have cleft lips and palates than females, but more females than males have isolated cleft palates (Hagberg, Larson, Milerad, 1998).

Etiology of Clefting

There does not seem to be a consensus in the literature as to the cause and pathogenesis of clefting. It is known that genetic and environmental causes are involved (Kaufman, 1991). Sometimes clefting is seen in isolation of other physical or neurological conditions, and other times, it is seen as a part of a collection of characteristics such as in Pierre-Robin malformation, Treacher-Collins syndrome, or Crouzon disease.

According to current theory, clefts of the lip result from failure of the facial process to fuse. The face begins to develop embryologically between the 7th and 9th weeks. The maxillary processes fuse to form the upper lip and primary palate by the 7th week in utero. The lateral palatal processes of the maxilla grow in an upward and oblique direction until they arch over the tongue and fuse at the midline of the oral cavity. Fusion begins as the right and left anterior portions of the hard palate connect in midline by about 9 weeks. By the 12th week, the palatal processes fuse to form the secondary palate or soft palate (Kaufman, 1991). In general, development moves from the front to the back during the 9th to 12th weeks of prenatal development. Thus, the midline closure of the lips occurs before closure of the hard palate. The hard palate closes before midline closure occurs in the soft palate. This gradual meeting of the separate lateral structures and the forming of a midline connection explains the variability seen in the development that produces a cleft of one or more structures. The amount of clefting depends partially upon which weeks of prenatal development (and the closure occurring at that time) were involved in the causative aspects of the child's cleft. Therefore, it is possible to have either a cleft of the lip, of the palate, or of both.

Numerous studies have made the associations between clefting and environmental teratogens. Connections between anticonvulsants, maternal smoking (Kaufman, 1991; Khoury, Gomez-Farias, Mulinare, 1989) and steroids (Melnick, 1986) have been drawn. There may be a predisposition for certain individuals to be biologically susceptible to clefting when influenced by these factors.

Team Support

The family with a baby who has a cleft lip, palate, or both needs support. Team members must find ways to nourish the whole child and the whole family, which will need information and emotional and medical support. The baby will need help in finding his own way of feeding, adjusting to the cleft, and adjusting to future surgeries. The degree of clefting and the multitude of issues that influence the feeding relationship will influence the amount of help the family and the baby need.

Team members must be sensitive to the issues that go beyond the cleft and feeding techniques. Parents who have given birth to a baby with a cleft of the lip or palate often need to adjust to the fact that their dreams of a perfect baby are shattered. Many describe an initial process of grieving and distress. Emotional support can come through family members, physicians, psychologists, feeding specialists, and friends. Feeding usually is the next most immediate issue that parents must face. Some babies with clefts of the lip or palate have few feeding problems, but others experience more difficulty. It is important to pair the family with a specialist trained in the baby's complicated feeding issues. This specialist must be aware of the importance of the feeding relationship as well as the specifics of feeding techniques and adaptations that support good growth in these babies. Medical support will be needed in the form of ongoing follow-up treatment as well as surgical management. Nutritional management may be needed through a dietitian or the pediatrician. Later, the baby may need speech therapy, otolaryngology and audiological support, and dental and orthodontic management. The family may leave the hospital not just with their newborn, but with a whole team. For some, this is comforting and for others it may be overwhelming!

The cleft palate team ultimately may include a pediatrician, surgeon, feeding specialist, nutritionist, social worker, psychologist, speech-language pathologist, otolaryngologist, dentist, and orthodontist.

Surgical Management

Clefts of the lip and palate are closed through surgery. Timing depends on the type of surgery necessary, the child's condition, and the surgeon's preference. Surgical procedures often are initiated during the first months after birth. The lip is repaired first. Some bilateral clefts of the lips require more than one surgery for closure and possibly an additional procedure for cosmetic purposes. Because more extensive surgery is required to repair the palate, the surgeon usually waits until the infant has reached a predetermined weight. Several operations and grafts may be required to obtain maximum closure. Most plastic surgeons seem to delay the initial palatal repair until the baby is at least 1 year old. A temporary dental splint or plate may be used to assist in feeding and to maintain the upper jaw in alignment between surgeries. Orthodontia may be required later to correct for misalignment of the teeth caused by defects in the dental arches.

▨ Feeding the Child With a Cleft

Nutrition and Growth Patterns

Children with clefts frequently have a slower weight gain during the first 2 to 3 months than other infants. This often is caused by difficulties with feeding, which can add to the stress of having a baby with a cleft. The pressure for the baby to grow increases with the knowledge that the baby must achieve a certain weight before the lip and palatal repairs can be made. Good nutrition is also very important for healing after surgery. As the baby and mother discover a successful feeding technique and ultimately the lips are repaired, babies usually begin to improve in the feeding and show some catch-up growth. As babies do better, mothers relax and the feeding experience becomes more positive and fulfilling for all. Feeding methods should be chosen that ensure the best feeding relationship and optimum growth for the baby.

The Mechanics of Sucking and Swallowing With Clefts

Healthy babies search for the nipple with a rooting reaction and begin a sucking movement as soon as the nipple touches the lips and enters the mouth. Babies with clefts have these same reactions. Complications in feeding arise for them because their sucking and swallowing reflexes are present but do not function efficiently because of their differences in anatomy.

Both lips and palate are important in the feeding process. The lips help hold on to the nipple. They close together to keep liquid in the mouth. They work with the gums to compress the areola to help with milk "let down." They create a strong sensory connection between the mother and baby. The palate separates the mouth from the nasal cavity. It provides the upper boundaries of the mouth needed in creation of negative-pressure suction. It provides a place against which the tongue can push in placement and control of the nipple. Its shape helps the tongue find an organized resting place in the mouth.

Clefting can influence the mechanics of sucking, to varying degrees, depending on its location and severity. Remember that good sucking requires positive and negative pressure. The positive pressure is achieved by the compression of the lips and the gums on the nipple. The negative pressure is achieved by the vacuum and negative-pressure suction created by drawing liquid from the breast or bottle into the mouth. The effectiveness of the negative-pressure suction achieved by a baby depends on the location and the severity of the cleft. Babies with a cleft may still be able to use a good positive compression of the gum ridge on the nipple as well as the necessary negative-pressure suction. The tongue fills the mouth and can adapt to many types of clefts of the lip. Lips also can be supported externally in a more closed position to assist in suction.

Babies with clefts of the palate, however, cannot achieve and maintain the optimum vacuum for negative pressure because there is no closed intraoral environment. The mouth is open to the nasal cavity, which is open for intake of air. Regular breast-feeding, therefore, is unlikely when there is severe palatal clefting. With some small clefting, there is a reduction in the negative pressure, but the breast-feeding process may still work. For babies with small posterior clefts, the tongue may take up the space of the cleft, causing less reduction in the negative pressure. When infants cannot make this type of compensatory movement, a small cleft can have a significant negative impact on sucking (Glass & Wolf, 1999). Large clefts, however, simply do not allow for the negative-pressure suction that is needed in the breast- and bottle-feeding processes. Depending on the cleft size and location and the baby's skills, there are some adaptations in breast-feeding that may work for some mothers and babies. For others, adapted bottle-feeding is a much more successful alternative.

Feeding Babies Who Have Clefts

Generally, infants with a cleft of the lip alone or an isolated cleft of the soft palate have less trouble with breast- and bottle-feeding. Assuming there are no associated neurological difficulties or syndromes, the degree of difficulty in feeding seems strongly correlated with the degree and location of the clefting (Clarren, Anderson, & Wolf, 1987). More complex clefts of the palate provide special challenges to the mother and the baby. It may take some time to discover comfortable methods of feeding.

Feeding specialists must carefully look beyond the mechanical issues of the clefting. The feeding interactions can be influenced by multiple factors, all of which can improve or worsen the feeding process. Some parents adjust quickly to the arrival of a ***different*** baby. Other parents spend more time with their grief, anger, and sadness. Some parents have the time and patience to work at breast-feeding with a baby who may or may not be successful. Others need to move on immediately to adapted bottle systems with pumped breast milk to provide the nourishment of breast-feeding with a simpler method of feeding. Some parents feel quite coordinated and can handle any type of bottle system. Others feel awkward and need the simplest system described in simpler terms. Some parents and babies figure it out right away and go home enjoying their mealtimes together. Other parents and babies need and want support for a longer time. The process of feeding these babies is one of discovery. Following are some methods that help babies and parents move beyond feeding success to mealtime enjoyment.

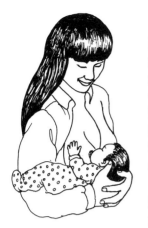

Breast-Feeding

Each family is unique, and the possibility of breast-feeding should be discussed with the mother and her physician if there is a desire to nurse the baby. The decision to breast-feed may prove to be a challenge or may need to be altered completely with the birth of a baby with a cleft, but it should be explored if the mother desires (Danner & Cerutti, 1984; Hagberg et al., 1998). Often, babies with a cleft of only the lip can breast-feed. Obviously, the more involved the lip, whether it is unilateral or bilateral, complete or incomplete, the greater influence it will have on the nursing success. Clefts of the palate must be considered individually in breast-feeding.

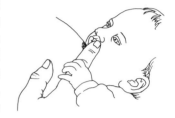

Sometimes it is helpful for the infant to be held with the cleft lip side next to the breast. The mother's soft breast may help create a lip seal not achievable with a regular nipple. With a good lip seal, the non-cleft side can function more normally. The seal can be created with the mother's thumb taking up space at the site of the cleft or by gently pressing the parts of the upper lip toward each other. Because the baby must empty both breasts, the mother will need to use a different position for each breast. For example, if the infant has a cleft of the right side of the lip, the regular left-arm baby hold is effective for nursing at the mother's left breast. To maintain the same head position and relationship of the cleft lip to the breast, the mother can use a football hold to enable the infant to nurse at her right breast. In this position, the infant is held along the mother's side, facing her, rather than across her lap. It is essentially the same position as with the left breast but the baby is now at the right breast.

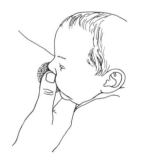

Some babies with severe clefts of the lips need more support than the soft breast tissue to achieve more closure during nursing. These babies may need to have the lip segments gently moved together with the mother's fingers. In this situation, the side with the cleft lip would be up toward the mother in the feeding position rather than down being supported by breast

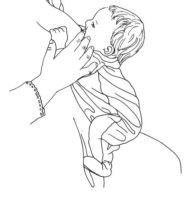

tissue. The goal of this support is to close the cleft as much as possible and in a comfortable way that does not interfere with the nursing process. This closed lip support may give the baby a more secure grasp of the breast and better closure during sucking and swallowing. The baby frequently will need more support when nursing on one side than on the other. Babies who have a bilateral cleft of the lip may need even more lip support and different positioning during nursing. Sometimes, what works well is a more upright position in which the baby straddles the mother's leg or lies on the mother's chest with the mother leaning slightly back in the chair. The baby's ability to adapt to the cleft lip and the feeder's ability to coordinate the lip support will vary. It may take some time for the mother-baby team to find out what works best.

Nursing a baby who has a cleft of the palate provides increased challenges for mother and baby. Most attempts to nurse these infants using regular techniques fail because babies with a palatal cleft cannot achieve the same degree of negative-pressure suction as babies with an intact palate. This can frustrate the baby and the mother, leading to stress that can challenge the bonding process and the feeding relationship. From the beginning, parents need to fully understand the mechanics of sucking and the limitations created by the open cleft. There needs to be an understanding that the more involved the cleft, the more complications there will be for successful breast-feeding.

For some babies, adapted breast-feeding aids can be used. Medela provides a number of lactation support systems for breast-feeding mothers. (See the discussion of milk delivery alternatives in Chapter 21.) Some mothers enjoy the closeness of the baby rooting and sucking at the breast while using pumped breast milk in a lactation pouch or supplemental nursing device (e.g., Supplemental Nursing System or Lact-Aid) for an even milk flow.

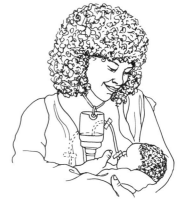

Some mothers feed the baby from a bottle using pumped breast milk while letting the baby "nurse" at the breast for comfort and closeness. Still other mothers use a specially molded palatal obturator or plate (see the description later in this chapter) while using modified breast-feeding holds and cheek support. Supplemental breast milk is then pumped and given by a supplemental nursing system or bottle until it is determined whether the baby can take in enough breast milk through breast-feeding to grow. Some mothers try breast-feeding while initially dripping breast milk into the baby's mouth to encourage more patience as the baby waits for the let-down response. A syringe or supplemental nursing device can be used for this.

Breast-feeding specialists can provide a very important support for mothers determined to make breast-feeding work for their babies. The patience of the mother and the baby, the frustration tolerance, and the degree of the clefting will have a significant impact on the baby's ability to get better at breast-feeding attempts and grow appropriately.

Bottle-Feeding

For some mothers, bottle-feeding is a first choice, whether it is with pumped breast milk or formula. For others, it is disappointing not to be able to successfully breast-feed. Feeding specialists should be aware of the impact these emotions can have on the feeding process. Whatever choice the family makes or must make, the focus of support should be on nurturing the loving and positive feeding relationship.

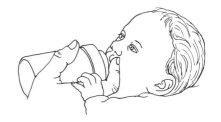

There are commercially available nipples and bottles for infants with cleft lips and palates. Although it may be necessary to purchase special equipment, it is important to explore normal adaptations first. These can include adjusting the way in which the baby is held, and exploring different sizes and types of nipples and bottles. Each infant with a cleft is different. Each parent has different skills and needs. The feeding method created should be personally designed for the individual mother and baby.

Babies who have clefts of the lips may be able to use any commercially available nipple and bottle, with the feeder adapting only the feeding position and the amount of lip support.

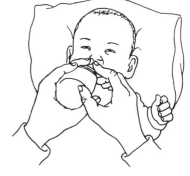

Cleft palates, however, will require more specific considerations. A baby with a cleft palate will find the regular bottle system difficult because it works predominantly on the principle of suction or negative intraoral pressure. This baby's positive-pressure compression action on a regular nipple will only lead to frustration as tiny drops of liquid slowly drip from the bottle. Without the negative-pressure suction, feedings may be long, fatiguing, and frustrating. The baby will need a bottle system that assists with the easier flow of liquid. Some babies may need nipples with enlarged holes to maximize the flow of liquid. Others need bottle systems with entirely different designs that do not require negative-pressure suction for success.

The feeding system chosen should offer another option for movement of liquid into the baby's mouth. The nipples that work best will enable the baby or parent to control the flow of liquid. The Haberman feeder is an excellent option. It has been created to function on the principle of positive pressure. The Haberman is uniquely designed to respond to the baby's ability to compress the nipple with the lips and gums. A one-way valve prevents backflow, allowing the liquid to flow only in the direction of the mouth when the nipple is compressed. The slit opening can be turned to modulate liquid flow from slow to fast. The baby's natural compression response allows liquid to flow when the baby gives a chewing pressure on the nipple. The liquid stops flowing when the baby pauses. This enables the baby to control the rate of the feeding. If the baby is having difficulty, the mother also can influence the flow by rotating the nipple in the mouth. This changes the angle of the slit, allowing for a faster or slower flow rate as the baby compresses the nipple. If necessary, the feeder can apply pressure to the nipple to create a flow if the baby is unable or too fatigued to do so. The feeder should do this carefully, being very attentive to the baby's cues for rate of liquid flow and pauses.

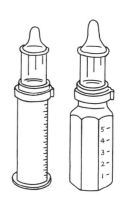

Another common bottle system used for babies who have clefts of the palate is the Mead Johnson Cleft Palate Nurser. This nipple is slightly longer than a regular nipple and has a crosscut for easier flow. It has a soft, plastic, flexible bottle that the feeder can easily squeeze to move liquid into the baby's mouth as the baby compresses the nipple and indicates readiness. The baby gets some of the liquid by the compression action on the crosscut nipple and some by the feeder's action. It is important to remember, however, that the parent is in charge of most of the flow rate. The feeder must be very sensitive to the baby's cues about how fast or slow to squeeze the liquid and when to pause. A feeder who is very sensitive to these cues and a baby who gives clear cues are the variables that work best for this system. When these factors go well, the feeding is pleasant and safe, and provides an opportunity for important bonding to take place. If the adult frequently misreads the infant's cues, the mealtime can become tense and unsatisfying for both. Most often, it just takes time for the mother and the baby to fine-tune their communication during this mealtime dance.

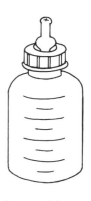

Other bottle systems are developed regularly. The most important factors to consider are:

- Does the feeding technique provide as normal a mother-infant interaction as possible?
- Does the system give the baby control of liquid flow rate?
- Does it work on a positive-pressure compression system?
- Does the nipple compress easily?
- Is the flow rate rapid enough without being too fast?
- Is the nipple soft to reduce unnecessary fatigue?
- Is it readily available?
- Is it affordable?
- Is it safe?
- Can it be easily cleaned?

With any of these bottle systems, a more upright feeding position is recommended. A semi-sitting position allows gravity to move the liquid into the pharynx while directing it away from the nasal cavity, ears, and cleft. Feeding should be slow enough to prevent choking, coughing, and loss of liquid into the nasal cavity. It should be fast enough to prevent fatigue. The baby should be burped frequently, as there seems to be a much higher incidence of air swallowing during feeding with clefts. Parents may be encouraged to feed the infant smaller amounts of liquid at each feeding and to increase the number of feedings per day.

Palatal Obturator

Most babies learn to feed well with adapted breast- and bottle-feeding techniques. Others may need extra help. A palatal obturator is one option considered for some babies with a cleft of the palate (Clarren, et al., 1987; Goldberg, Ferguson, & Miles, 1988; Kogo, et al., 1997; Osuji, 1995; Trenouth & Campbell, 1996). The obturator, also called a plate, is a plastic insert that forms an artificial palate that not only separates the nasal cavity from the mouth, but also helps bring the tongue forward. The forward part of the tongue side of the obturator usually has grooves, which can help position the tongue. This artificial palate provides a surface against which the baby can support the nipple with the tongue during sucking. It does not, however, change the intraoral pressure needed to create the vacuum for the negative-pressure part of sucking. When an obturator is determined to be necessary, an impression is made of the baby's upper jaw. The obturator can be made of hard or soft plastic or a combination. It can be taken in and out as needed for cleaning. Many babies adapt to the obturator reasonably quickly; others do not. Sometimes, several fittings and adaptations are needed to eliminate pressure sores. Adjustments will need to be made as the baby grows.

A number of factors should be considered when making the decision to use an obturator. The baby and the mother ideally should be allowed a short time to establish feeding without an obturator because most baby-mother teams with good mealtime support establish very positive and yet individual ways of feeding. Obturators can be considered in instances where the cleft is particularly large, there are significant neurological problems, or the probability of failure to establish adequate feeding and growth is high. This option should be explored before a full cycle of failure and despair is established and the feeding relationship and bonding are disrupted. Community resources and support also should be factors. Many communities do not have professionals with extensive experience in fitting and adjusting obturators. Adapted feeding techniques, extensive family support, and, in extreme circumstances, nasogastric feedings may be used. In other communities, obturators are common and regularly fitted before nasogastric feedings are considered. As with all issues concerning the management of clefts, the decisions are individual and depend on many medical and personal factors.

Spoon Feeding

Cleft lip repair usually has been completed by the time the infant weighs 10 to 12 pounds. This weight usually is attained before pureed baby foods or cereals are introduced. However, the palate usually is left open until the child is 12 to 18 months old.

Babies who have cleft lips and palates can and do transition to pureed foods. Adults must be aware initially of whether the infant is developmentally ready for more solid foods and spoon feeding. Often, it is better to wait a bit longer to introduce these foods to babies who have clefts to ensure optimum oral control of the food. As food is introduced, the feeder must go slowly enough that the baby has success and enjoys the food. It is important that the feeder use the same sequence and guidelines that would be used with any baby, letting the infant indicate when it's time to move to the next developmental challenge of food taste, quantity, and texture. The feeder must take care to present the mouthfuls slowly while observing the baby's reaction. Rapid feeding or mouthfuls that are too large can cause excess choking or nasal loss of food. The baby needs to feel in control of each bite while gradually learning how to direct the food around the cleft. The feeder should let the baby lean forward or open the mouth to indicate desire and give permission for presentation of the next mouthful. The spoon should remain in the mouth long enough for the baby to remove food with the lips. This also helps the baby develop lip mobility after surgery.

Textured Foods and Chewing

The transitions to textured or lumpy foods and finally to bite-size table foods generally occur in the same sequence as for other children, although sometimes a bit more slowly. Because these transitions usually occur before surgery to close the cleft palate, the child needs to control lumps that arrive at the palatal openings.

The feeder should present these foods slowly and at the child's pace. The child can practice with finger-foods such as soft or hard baby cookies. This is identical to the way solids are introduced to children who are unimpaired. The small pieces that break off as the baby gums or munches the cookie usually are not frightening as they are mashed with the tongue and swallowed. The child gradually becomes proficient at guiding mashed or finely cut foods past the cleft. Periodic choking may occur as the infant learns new motor skills. This is seen in all children who are learning to handle more challenging foods. If the food falls from the nose or becomes stuck in the palate, the feeder should remove it with a finger or a cotton swab without alarming the child. The food will not interfere with breathing. Foods such as peas or rice tend to scatter and become lost in the mouth. Gravy or other sauces help these foods stick together in a bolus that can be swallowed more easily. Some parents avoid more acidic foods such as citrus juices and spicy sauces until after the palate has been repaired.

Older Children With a Cleft Palate

The child usually has discovered a very functional way to eat even before the cleft is completely closed. As the mouth grows, problems with the teeth and dental arches may become more prominent, and the child may receive periodontal or orthodontic care. Attention to alignment of the teeth is important for the development of mature chewing patterns. Speech difficulties are common as the child learns to use the surgically repaired palate. A speech-language pathologist should be consulted about questions regarding the quality of speech for these children.

Babies Who Continue to Have Feeding Problems

Most infants who have a cleft lip or palate learn to eat proficiently with modifications in positioning, equipment, and timing. Clefting is a structural or anatomical problem. Infants who have a normally-functioning central nervous system are able to develop muscle movements that compensate for difficulties caused by the cleft. Occasionally, infants continue to have feeding difficulties despite the usual modifications. They may adapt poorly to surgery to close the palate and have increased feeding difficulties after closure because of difficulty adapting to new sensations and movements. Often, these difficulties are signals that the infant may have other problems. Even mild incoordination with problems of sensation and movement can reduce an infant's ability to compensate for the cleft. An infant with a cleft who continues to have significant feeding problems should be observed carefully for indications of other neurological issues or syndromes that involve clefts. In some situations, continued problems may be an indicator of other issues in the feeding relationship. These factors should be investigated.

General Strategies for Feeding Children With a Cleft Lip or Palate

The following general strategies are helpful when guiding the feeding program of children with cleft lips and palates.

Focus on the Feeding Interaction

Parents need time and support to adjust to the anatomical and feeding differences in their infants. The baby's structural problems create emotional and physical challenges. The primary focus in a feeding program should be placed on strategies that support the mealtime interaction between the baby and the parent. This will include the use of positioning and equipment adaptations to improve the physical support for eating.

Seek Simplicity

Begin with the simplest adaptations in positioning and equipment. Move to more specialized or complex equipment if the simpler adjustments are not effective. The easier the adaptation or compensation, the easier it will be for parents to focus on the baby and their relationship with him or her rather than on the adaptation.

Identify and Incorporate Effective Compensations

Infants with structural problems such as cleft lips and palates have trouble eating because their structure interferes with the ability to develop sucking pressures and keep food out of the nasal area. Therapy is directed toward finding ways of compensating for these structural difficulties. Compensations may include

- positioning the child in a more upright posture for eating
- using the fingers or mother's breast to provide closure or support for an open lip cleft
- using bottles and nipples that do not require negative-sucking pressure
- using palatal obturators to seal a portion of the palatal cleft

Move Slowly to Feeding Success

Remember that these infants need time to adjust or adapt their movements to an anatomical structure that is not designed for efficient eating. Offer food slowly and provide physical, sensory, and emotional support for learning.

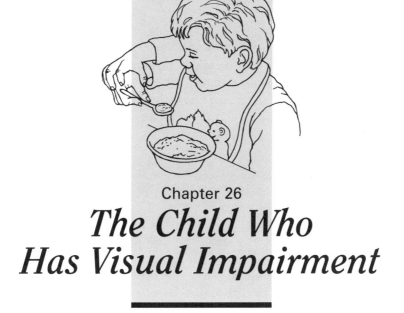

Chapter 26
The Child Who Has Visual Impairment

Visual impairment and blindness affect the development of independent eating skills and play a major role in the way in which the feeder and the child interact.

◼ The Infant

Feeding a blind baby is very much like feeding a sighted baby. The same threads of trust, nurturing, and bonding are being developed. The finely tuned communication and reciprocal reading of cues guide the mealtime dance. The baby needs to feel safe and build trust in the feeder, who needs to feel secure in the knowledge that the baby is feeding well and growing. Sighted infants use their vision integrally as part of this mealtime bonding process. They recognize their parents and begin to expect certain touches and care from them. They visually learn the routine of feeding and how to recognize the breast or bottle and associate them with the pleasant feelings of sucking and hunger satiation. Blind children, on the other hand, do not have the benefit of sight in making these associations. They learn to recognize parents and the approaching mealtime by touch, smell, and sound. Parents need to understand the baby's nonsighted way of learning and figure out sensitive ways of communicating, "It is mealtime" or "Do you want to eat now?"

Personal Exploration

One excellent way for you, as parents and support team members, to understand what a blind baby might experience in the feeding process is to close your eyes and either have a friend feed you or imagine that you are being fed. Notice what works and does not work as the bottle or spoon is presented. You may discover important lessons and sensitivities for feeding a child who has a visual impairment.

Preparation

Visually impaired babies must be active participants and partners in the mealtime process. Adults need to account for the visual limitations as they prepare them for a meal. Their baby's hands become the eyes in exploration and learning about the environment. Guiding the baby's hands to the breast or bottle enables him to *see* the environment of the meal, from early infancy. Helping the visually impaired infant hold the feeder's fingers as the bottle is held, or guiding the baby to touch the breast or bottle, will give him an image of where the milk comes from. The tactile exploration of the bottle or breast enables the baby to make the image associations that sighted babies make.

Having the baby *see* by following the adult's hands to the bottle and breast becomes even more important as the baby moves from breast- and bottle-feeding to the sensory challenges of pureed and then solid foods and into the world of cups and straws. Repeatedly seeing through the guide of the adult hands provides the baby with information of how the eating process really works. This incidental learning provides the foundation that the infant needs for more active involvement in the feeding process.

Breast-fed babies learn to understand the positioning, touches, and smells that accompany the presentation of the breast. They need to be guided to the breast, and to touch, massage, and explore the skin-to-skin contact of breast-feeding. The baby can put his hands on the breast and find the nipple with the hands and mouth. This begins to provide the infant with spatial information about the important triad of breast, hands, and mouth. This early information supports the infant's developing ability to bring the hands and toys to the mouth for sucking and mouthing. The way the baby is positioned in the feeder's arms or swaddled in a certain blanket, or the movement of the rocking chair may be enough to alert the baby that the feeding is being offered. Some feeders play specific music at mealtime or talk about the meal with certain words or a tone of voice. Over time, these sensory cues can help the visually impaired baby prepare for the meal.

Bottle-fed babies rely on different cues, but the concept is the same. Blind babies need to feel adult hands moving through the process of bottle-feeding. From the beginning, feeders can place the baby's hands on their hands or on the bottle as it is presented. They can guide the baby to feel the whole bottle from its base to the nipple. This enables the baby to see the process of feeding and be prepared for it. With her hands on the bottle, the baby knows it is mealtime and can be prepared for presentation of the nipple. Some feeders put a sock or a cloth sleeve over the bottle to draw the baby's tactile attention to it.

Control

Babies eat and grow best when they are in charge of the initiation, pace, and timing of the meal. They need to be in control of what they let in their mouths. Before the feeder places a nipple in a baby's mouth, she should have the baby's permission. By granting permission, the baby is saying, "I am relaxed and ready for the feeding. No surprises!" Sighted babies can use vision to control the situation from a distance. For example, they can see the bottle coming and make decisions about whether they want it before it even touches them. They can turn away or even bat at the bottle if they are not ready for it. A blind baby does not have the benefit of seeing the bottle coming. If it is merely placed in the baby's mouth, it can be a surprise and an unpleasant experience. A number of these unpleasant experiences can lead to a dislike of the mealtime or aversions to touch around the mouth. Blind infants who are allowed to touch the bottle before it touches the mouth can make the decision about whether they are ready for a feeding. If they are not ready for a feeding, they can push the bottle away or close the mouth. If they want to eat, they can bring the bottle to the mouth, or the feeder can gently stroke the baby's lips or cheek with it and let the baby turn the head and open the mouth to the nipple to further indicate readiness. A baby fed in this type of sensitive environment is more likely to have positive, more fulfilling mealtime experiences. The baby can trust that when she is offered the bottle, she will be respected whether she wants it or not. If the baby is fed in an environment of surprises where someone else is in control, she may fear what is coming next. Mealtimes can become a time of tension, fear, sensory surprises, and discomfort rather than experiences of complete nourishment, relaxation, and bonding.

It takes awhile for babies to give consistent cues about their feeding desires, and it sometimes takes a parent awhile to understand these cues. Fraiberg (1974) describes the difficulties experienced by parents of blind infants. The typical communication signals of smiling and eye contact that are familiar triggers of interaction and mealtime communication for most adults are elicited by vision. Blind infants do not communicate through eye gaze and facial expression. Parents must learn to look for hand signals and other body signs that may be unique to their infant's emerging communication system.

The baby's visual impairment and the parents' worries may further complicate this situation. Sometimes, a visually impaired baby may cry at the presentation of the bottle. He may not be saying, "I am not hungry," but rather, "I did not like that unexpected touch." It takes time to sort out the messages and respond appropriately. Physically involving the baby and consistently pausing with the nipple at the lips or cheeks seems to give the baby the information that there will be no surprises. When babies reject a bottle after this type of presentation, they are less likely to be saying, "I did not like the unexpected touch." Cues may be easier to read.

Mouthing! Mouthing! Mouthing!

Mouthing toys helps prepare the mouth for the challenges of new textures. Sighted babies engage in many hours of this preparation. Babies put their fingers and toes in their mouths. They also put rattles, bibs, toys, and whatever they can reach in their mouths. To reach for a toy, they need to see what they are reaching for before they can pick it up and put it in the mouth. Visually impaired babies also learn to reach, but they are more cautious and need more help in doing so. They tend to be more stationary babies, staying where they are placed. They are not as easily enticed out of their very safe, immediate environment because they are not sure what lurks beyond. They do not see the toys surrounding them. They need to learn to explore or search with their fingers and hands. This will influence the kinds and numbers of mouthing experiences they have. By the time they are at an age where other babies are being introduced to pureed foods, they may not have the same sitting or mobility skills or have had anywhere near the number of mouthing experiences that prepare other babies for the challenge of new foods. Some visually impaired babies do not like to mouth at all at this stage. It is important to help parents of visually impaired babies learn to help their babies explore with their mouths and hands. This tactile exploration will be important for their hands as well as their mouths, and can better prepare them for foods, textures, and transitions.

Change Sensory Variables Slowly

All babies need to guide adults as to when they are ready to make changes in their mealtime diet. Feeders look for developmental, growth, interaction, and appetite cues to know when a baby is prepared to handle pureed foods or when finger foods should be introduced. It may not be as easy to determine readiness in visually impaired babies. They may be a bit older when they learn to sit up. They cannot watch others eat, so they are less likely to reach for food or drink taken by others. They may be more cautious in their exploration of different textures. Therefore, the decision to try a new food or texture often rests on the shoulders of parents and pediatricians. By default, the decision often is determined by chronological age rather than developmental readiness. To ensure the most pleasant experiences with new tastes and textures, it is important to go slowly and watch the baby's feedback at each step of the way.

Once again, imagine yourself as a visually impaired baby. Imagine that you have been happily eating from the breast or bottle. You are very secure with the flavor and texture of breast milk or formula. What would it be like if someone suddenly put a mouthful of sweet potatoes in your mouth? You may like it and indicate that you want more. It is also just as possible, and maybe even more likely, that you would make a face, push away, or spit it out. It may even have been enough of a sensory surprise to cause you to gag or vomit. If you had a more extreme reaction, it is possible that the next time sweet potatoes are presented, you would be less than thrilled. If you are a very cautious individual, you may become extremely concerned at the next mealtime, wondering if another sensory surprise awaited you. If you had several of these experiences, you might be worried about any pureed texture or spooned food, or even the sound of a baby food jar being opened!

Just as it was important to get the visually impaired baby's permission to put the bottle in her mouth, it is also important to get her permission and active involvement when introducing new tastes and textures. The feeder should watch for signs of mouthing or help the baby mouth a variety of textured toys. Often, babies put particular toys or fingers that they crave in their mouths. These toys or fingers can become an excellent spoon substitute for introducing tastes. Pureed foods and crumbs can be put on the mouthing toys as an introduction to new tastes and textures.

The feeder must be careful not to overwhelm the baby with the introduction of a new sensation. The feeder should change sensory variables slowly and start with small amounts. Many babies will take *tiny* tastes quite nicely off of their own finger or favorite mouthing toy. When a baby puts a familiar textured toy in the mouth and then happens to get a small taste of some new food, it is usually much different from encountering a spoonful of something new, such as sweet potatoes, in the mouth. The baby is more relaxed with finding food on the finger or toy because it is his finger or toy, and he is in charge. Visually impaired babies are much more likely to be stressed by a new flavor on a new spoon when someone else is in charge and they have no control. Again, giving the baby some control can make a big difference. Watch for cues and continue to listen to the baby. If the baby acts as if it is an interesting flavor (e.g., smacking the lips, playing with the food with his tongue or fingers), the adult may offer another small taste.

These first pureed food experiences should be tastes only. The taste should be so small initially that there is minimal texture. As amounts are increased, the feeder should move from liquid to runny purees to thicker purees slowly, always watching for the child's reaction. The child should guide the decisions the adult makes regarding changes in taste, texture, and temperature.

Just as the visually impaired baby needed to feel the bottle to see the process, so must she also see spoon feeding through touch. She must see the parent eating from his spoon by putting her hands on her father's hands as he feeds himself. She can feel the feeder's mouth as he chews and the throat as he swallows. She can see the process of spoon feeding as she feels the feeder fill the spoon and bring it to her mouth and feel her own swallow. She may even have an easier time with initial attempts at spoon feeding if the first pureed food presented is one she has tried and enjoyed when taking tastes off of mouthing toys. This way, she is familiar with the taste while she is learning to see the spoon-feeding process. It is critically important that there be no surprises.

As babies get used to a new food taste, they learn to use their sense of smell as an introduction or a warning that the food is there. The older baby quickly learns how foods smell and makes decisions accordingly. Smell can tell a baby if it is a familiar food but may not be of much help in preparing for texture differences. Giving tastes on the lips is another nice way of preparing the baby for a new texture. After the feeder has helped the baby put a new taste on his lips, he has the option of bringing that food into his mouth. He has control over how much of it to try.

It is difficult to prepare a child for temperature changes. When the child is older, she can feel the cup or bottle and understand temperature differences. The baby, however, will not be able to understand the significance of these differences. Feeling the bottle is one way to prepare for the liquid temperature. Changes in spooned food temperature can be more challenging. Many visually impaired babies have a narrow range of tolerance for temperature differences. This may be their way of controlling the safety of their meals. Again, gradual changes may be best. For some babies who will drink only warmed formula, feeders may try making a tiny ice cube of formula. When it is put into the warmed bottle at the beginning of the feeding, it melts gradually. As the baby drinks, the temperature gradually changes. Babies often learn to expand their temperature tolerance in this way.

Prevention

The visually impaired baby is at high risk for oral and tactile sensitivities. This is understandable if you imagine yourself blind and going through life at the mercy of the sensory surprises around you! A baby may not initially be overly sensitive to touch, taste, or temperature, but may easily develop these hypersensitivities due to lack of experiences or negative experiences. For self-preservation, these babies learn to avoid many touches. Efforts must be made to provide visually impaired babies with loving massage and different safe touches from their earliest months. They can be helped in learning to explore with their mouths and hands. Their mealtime experiences can be safe and sensitive, with the baby having control. People should listen carefully to what these babies are saying about their mealtime and touch needs. By helping parents and therapists communicate sensitively with visually impaired babies, many hypersensitivities can be avoided. Prevention is key. Once the oversensitivities have been developed, they are much harder to overcome because of the strong emotional component.

Mealtimes for the Older, Visually Impaired Child

Older visually impaired children need the same sensitive approach as visually impaired babies. They need to be prepared for the meal, follow a routine, actively participate in the mealtime process, and be helped to try new things slowly. They also need to be taught mealtime independence and manners.

Preparation

The visually impaired child needs to be prepared for the self-feeding process, which begins in infancy as the baby is guided to hold the bottle. This not only prepared her as the bottle approached, but it also gave her the image of what happens at a meal. By repeatedly experiencing the process of bottle-feeding, the baby has the information needed to imitate that process and try to feed herself. Mouthing and tasting helped her refine the hand-to-mouth and oral skills to move to new foods and bring them to the mouth. As the baby becomes older and is presented pureed foods and gradually solids, she learns a great deal about mealtimes. If the experiences have been positive and she has been an active participant, she will have the information and courage to try to feed herself. To help the blind child see the meal with her hands, it is important to guide her hands through all aspects of the meal as well as offer a regular opportunity to feel the adult finding the spoon, scooping, biting, and crunching foods.

Routine

Older, visually impaired children usually benefit from a predictable mealtime routine. They may be acutely aware that mealtime is approaching from the smells of the cooking, the sounds of the meal preparation and the sensation of feeling hungry. Some children prepare themselves for the meal by actually assisting in some of the preparation. Meals happen around the same time each day. They occur at a specific table with a specific chair. The plate is placed in front of the child, with the utensils and the cup always in the same place.

Exploration

Visually impaired babies are encouraged to do lots of mouthing. Older children who have had mouthing experience are encouraged to explore new foods, as their flavors and textures still need to be introduced slowly. Visually impaired children use their senses of smell and touch to check out the food before it gets near the mouth. Willingness to try new foods is personal and depends on individual experiences and preferences. Some children try anything! Other children are much more cautious and need encouragement.

It is important that feeders talk to these children about the foods they are eating and being offered. They should talk about the properties of the food and make exploration of it fun and safe. These children need to be encouraged to smell, feel, and lick foods. Many families, therapists, and education facilities enjoy involving these children in the preparation of food. This is an excellent way to safely explore new food tastes, textures, and smells.

Continue to Go Slowly With Sensory Changes

Familiarity

Remember that each food is a combination of unique tastes, textures, and temperatures. The visually impaired child may be willing to explore one aspect of that combination, but not all at the same time. This requires creative approaches on the part of the feeder, who may need to start with what the child already knows and accepts. Sometimes it helps to try a new flavor in a familiar texture, such as giving the child a new flavor of the pudding after she already likes vanilla. Sometimes foods can be mixed. Vanilla pudding can be swirled with the new butterscotch flavor. Cautious children may need a tiny amount of butterscotch swirled in their pudding. More courageous children may try the new flavor enthusiastically. Sometimes the flavor needs to remain the same with the texture changing gradually. In the sweet potato example, the baby may feel safe with baby-food pureed sweet potatoes and gradually may enjoy a combination of blended, real sweet potatoes with the pureed. Eventually, she may eat plain, mashed sweet potatoes enthusiastically.

Separate Tastes

The feeder initially should keep tastes separate as much as possible so that the child learns the taste and smell of different foods. Mixing foods together decreases the child's awareness of taste preferences and the sensitivity to subtle differences in taste.

Reintroduce Rejected Foods

Many children spit out a new food when it is presented, and mothers often present the food several times before deciding whether the child likes or dislikes it. The confusion with visually impaired children is that they may not like a food for different reasons. Perhaps it is the taste. Maybe it is the texture. It could be the temperature. Rejected foods need to be reintroduced, but it may be necessary to try again with a different texture or temperature, or a diluted taste. Sometimes, the new food can be tried in a different combination of foods. Children usually don't eat foods they don't like, so reintroduction of foods must be done sensitively while keeping the visual impairment in mind. Power contests can result if children suspect that they are being tricked into eating an undesired food that is mixed with foods they like. They also are triggered if children feel forced to eat foods they do not like. Unfortunately, too many sensory surprises for visually impaired children can lead to oral hypersensitivities and stronger food rejections.

Incidental Learning and Imitation

Sighted people learn so much through incidental learning and imitation. Visually impaired children miss out on this important aspect of learning. Sighted children watch people feeding themselves. They reach for their mother's cup or their father's plate. They want to try what parents are doing. They need repeated exposure to seeing mealtime activities before they try them.

Because of the limitations in vision, blind children generally are more passive learners. They tend to do less traditional imitation. They frequently rely on others to move them through an activity. Although this is one way for them to learn, there are many other ways of mastering feeding skills. They need to be supported in feeling their world and the activity around them. In feeding, this can be feeling how the feeder eats a meal or feeds himself. They can feel the spoon being held, the feeder scooping the food, the spoon being filled, and the spoon moving to the mouth. They can feel lips closing around the spoon, the mouth chewing the food, the feeder swallowing, and then the spoon returning to the bowl. They can feel the differences in mouth movements of chewing a pretzel or an apple, or sucking from a straw. Without feeling another perform this task, how can the visually impaired child be expected to know what others do and what is expected of them?

The strategy of **hand-under-hand** teaching is used actively in deaf-blind education (Miles, 1998). Geraldine Larrington, occupational therapist with the Arizona State School for the Deaf and Blind, discusses this method of exploration and support as critical in the incidental learning and imitation process of visually impaired infants and children (1999, personal communication). The hand-under-hand method enables the child to feel the movements of others as the activity is being performed. Feeling activities in this way can be a precursor to imitation for the visually impaired child. In feeding, the feeder's hand is **under** the child's hand. The child's hand rests on the feeder's hand, and she feels the motions the feeder goes through while eating. This provides information that will enable the visually impaired child to imitate these movements later. It provides the spatial overview of the meal. The child receives information about how much force to use in scooping food, the timing of the meal, the direction of forces, and spatial patterns between hands and mouth. This approach provides the kinesthetic information about feeding that can prepare the child and help her learn new skills faster with more security and fewer sensory and motor surprises.

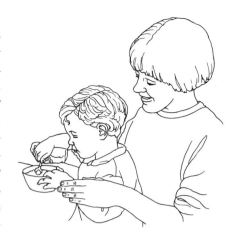

Parents need not have their hands under the child's hands for every meal and every mealtime activity. It should be done daily for at least part of a meal to continue to give information. Sighted children, after all, do not watch their parents eat **every** meal. They get distracted by other things. They do, however, have regular opportunities to see others eat. Visually impaired children need these same opportunities.

Teaching Independent Feeding

Sighted children generally acquire independent eating skills through visual imitation accompanied by verbal instructions from feeders. Verbal directions alone are not effective in teaching blind children to eat independently. Adults need to help them feel others eating and guide them to experience it themselves. When the child enjoys the meal and succeeds as an active participant, the meal is successful. Strategies, therefore, include:

- involving the child in feeding from an early age
- using regular hand-under-hand activity exploration
- pausing in the mealtime process to provide the opportunity for the child to try the activity independently
- giving physical guidance throughout the components of the meal
- providing experiences that allow the child to relate to verbal guidance, feedback, and support

Personal Frame of Reference

To begin, the child needs to establish a personal frame of reference at the table. Boundaries are critical to children who have visual impairments. They need to explore the mealtime setting by locating mealtime boundaries. A place mat or a rimmed cookie sheet can define the parameters of the eating space. The child can scan the mealtime space with his fingers to become aware of objects located there. The child learns to keep his hands in contact with the table and make scanning or trailing motions with the fingers, moving slowly across the table to identify the location and height of upright objects that are within reach. Is there a bowl? A plate? A cup? Which utensils are on the place mat? Those who are setting the table and serving the food should help by putting dishes, utensils, and napkins in the same place until the visually impaired child develops the skill to identify differences in routine.

Physical Success in Self-Feeding

What is most important is that the visually impaired child have enjoyable meals and success in eating! The child needs to feel control over the food and comfortable with the process. The feeder must determine the optimum methods for teaching success by following the child's lead. This will vary with the child and the activity. Often, it is helpful for feeders to try these different methods to feel the subtle differences and understand which aspects of the techniques to emphasize. The following strategies are helpful.

Check Out the Supports

Feeders need to consider the same supports that they would for a sighted child. Check out the spoon. Is it short enough for success? Is the food being used sticky enough to stay on the spoon en route to the mouth? Does the child need help lifting the elbow to shoulder height while guiding the spoon to the mouth? Some feeders grasp the end of the spoon and give it a little help to ensure added success as the child approaches the mouth.

Provide Hand-Under-Hand Opportunities

Provide hand-under-hand opportunities for all aspects of self-feeding. Give the child the experience of *seeing* the feeder scoop food and bring a filled spoon to the mouth, stab foods with a fork, drink from a cup, chew a crunchy apple, or even wipe the face with a napkin. The family can continue to give these imitation opportunities as the child is being physically helped in other ways.

Provide Opportunities for Trial-And-Error Learning

Often, blind children who have had extensive incidental-learning experiences with hand-under-hand exploration of feeding have sufficient *vision* of the activity that they can try to imitate it—just as sighted children do. They still will misguide the spoon to the mouth and make a mess—just as sighted children do. They still will need practice to get the correct end of the spoon to the mouth—just as sighted children do. Often, just the process of trial and error paired with the desire for the food is enough to set a good foundation for independence with the spoon. Some blind children, however, need extra physical help.

Provide Guidance With the Spoon Handle

Some children who have the idea of how to feed themselves may just need a parent to hold the end of the spoon handle and give a small amount of guidance as the child brings the spoon to the mouth.

Provide Extra Elbow Support

Some children just need slight assistance lifting the elbow as they guide the filled spoon to the mouth.

Provide Hand-Over-Hand Help

Many feeders try to guide new spoon users using a hand-*over*-hand method. This method calls for the feeder's hand over or around the child's hand while the feeder physically guides the child through the whole motion. This method works for many children. Although this method helps the child accurately get the food into the mouth, it may not be the best way to help the blind child understand the process and be independent. The child cannot see what is happening and can only feel the adult hand. The touch draws attention to the back of the hand in the adult-dominated activity. This does not give the child the opportunity to initiate and plan the movement; it leads to passive rather than active learning.

Use the Utility Handhold

Another approach to the physical guidance of the spoon is the utility handhold described in Chapter 19. In this technique, the spoon is held in the hand by pressing the spoon handle into the palm with pressure that puts the wrist into a slight extension, causing the fingers to close more naturally around the spoon. The child feels the spoon in the hand but may be less overwhelmed by the tactile input of the hand-over-hand approach commonly used. With the utility handhold and support at the elbow, the feeder can guide the child while remaining very sensitive to the child's attempt to do this with greater independence.

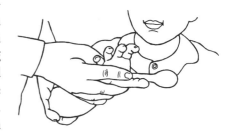

Use Backward Chaining to Build Success

The backward-chaining process of fading support as the child takes over is described in Chapter 19. In this process, the adult does as much as necessary for the child to succeed, but not too much to take over. Essentially, the child is supported into success.

Fine-Tuning the Mealtime

Experience with eating provides the information needed to help visually impaired children and their parents fine-tune the mealtime routine. Children learn to stabilize the plate with one hand while stabbing or cutting with the other. The assisting hand on one side of the plate also helps the visually impaired child determine the size of the plate. This makes it easier to scoop, stab, or cut the food appropriately. One hand can be used to hold a piece of bread, roll, or tortilla as a *pusher* for difficult foods on the plate. Bowls or plates with higher sides are helpful in collecting difficult foods without the need for a pusher. Children learn to return the utensil to the same place so that they can find it again during the meal.

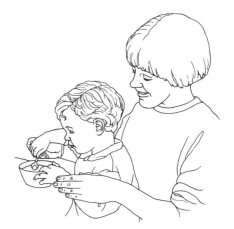

A blind child needs to learn to bend the trunk forward so that the face is directly above the plate. This can be taught verbally but will be more meaningful if taught incidentally by experience. It often is easier for the child to learn this while sitting on the adult's lap. As the adult is giving food from a spoon, the child can be guided to feel the bowl of food with one hand while feeling the adult hand scooping and offering the food. The adult can lean forward while guiding the spoon to the mouth. This gives the child the perspective of the bowl, spoon, and table in relation to his body, and it gives subtle cues about successfully guiding a filled spoon to

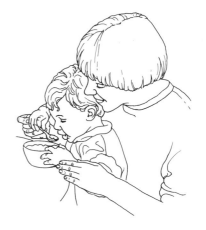

the mouth. The hand on the bowl helps the spoon hand find the food. Later, as the child sits next to the adult, the adult can use one hand to guide the spoon hand. This is accompanied by placing the child's other hand on the bowl and having a hand on the back of the child's neck to move the child forward to the spoon as the spoon approaches the mouth. This helps avoid major spills in case food falls from the fork or spoon. This subtle learning comes most quickly from incidental hand-under-hand learning opportunities. This is a subtle component of eating that sighted children learn through vision and feedback. The blind child needs this type of incidental learning opportunity to allow the verbal feedback to make sense.

Blind children learn to find the last food in the bowl or on the plate by feel. If the sighted adult scoops right to the last morsel of food, the child will not have had the opportunity to search for it. Adults need to help the child search by feel. The back of the spoon or fork can tap along the plate to find remaining food.

Many people establish the pattern of presenting specific food groups at a specific place on the plate. For example, the meat may be at 6 o'clock, the vegetables at 3 o'clock, the bread at 9 o'clock, and the fruit at 12 o'clock. This routine can add to a sense of security and safety about mealtime and can help the child feel calmer about the new tastes and textures that might be presented. Then changes can occur from a place of calm predictability rather than chaos and unpredictability.

With experience, children learn to identify foods by smelling them, sensing their temperature, and learning their tactile characteristics that can be sensed through the utensils. For example, how much pressure is required on the fork to stab or pick up a particular food successfully? Children discover that the need for different-sized bites can be identified by their weight on the utensil. Different amounts of liquid in a cup can be sensed by cup weight and by feeling the level of liquid at the top of the cup.

Vision Loss and Severe Feeding Challenges

A typically developing blind child and his family encounter challenges in the acquisition of everyday skills. Some of the potential difficulties with feeding can be avoided by good prevention techniques. However, the sensory challenges for feeding are greatly increased when visually impaired children have other medical and sensory diagnoses and neurological complications. Suggestions in this chapter can be modified and integrated with other information in this book that addresses feeding issues with children who have other physical, sensory, structural, and experiential difficulties.

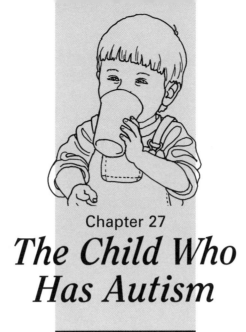

Chapter 27

The Child Who Has Autism

Children with Autism Spectrum Disorders tend to be very picky eaters. Just how picky depends on many factors.

A variety of different but related disorders are included in this spectrum. There is not yet full agreement on a classification system that is reliable and valid in describing and defining an intervention plan for each of the subgroupings (Siegel, 1999). The umbrella diagnostic category under the DSM-IV system (American Psychiatric Association, 1994) is Pervasive Developmental Disorder (PDD). It includes Asperger's syndrome, Pervasive Developmental Disorder-Autism Disorder, and Pervasive Developmental Disorder-Not Otherwise Specified (PDD-NOS). Children in these categories have difficulty with imitation, communication, language, social interactions, repetitive routines, and processing of sensory information (Rogers, 1999). Many show a reduction in eye contact. Both verbal and nonverbal language skills are impaired. Many parents describe a limited range of interests and activities, repetitive, and stereotypic behaviors. Among these disorders, characteristic symptoms can be from mild to severe.

All of the characteristics influencing these disorders can affect eating and mealtime behaviors. Restricted intake, reduced variety of foods, difficulty accepting any new foods, and trouble with change in the mealtime environment or routine are common complications for these children and their families. Mayes and Calhoun (1999) administered their Checklist for Autism to 143 young children with autism. Seventy-four percent of these children had feeding disorders, which included behaviors such as limited food preferences, hypersensitivity to textures, retaining food in the mouth, inconsistency in eating over time, and pica.

This can cause great concern for parents and care providers. Although there are many similarities among these children, it is difficult to generalize with this group because of the great variability in their behaviors. In order to simplify communication, in this chapter the term *autism* will be used to refer to all children who have an Autistic Spectrum Disorder.

Sensory Variables and Mealtimes

Many children with autism have significant sensory challenges (Ayres & Tickle, 1980; Baranek, Foster, & Berdson, 1997; Kientz & Dunn, 1997; Mayes & Calhoun, 1999). Mealtime challenges seem to be strongly related to how the child's sensory system processes information. We know that these children have difficulty organizing and responding to the large amounts of sensory information that surround and bombard them daily. Their neurological circuits do not seem to process information clearly and understandably. Some sensory responses seem to be hyperreactive, while others seem hyporeactive. Sensory receptivity appears to vary in sensitivity from time to time. Sensory overload occurs.

Heightened Sensitivities

Frequently, heightened sensitivities to sound, smell, taste, touch, temperature, and movement are noted (Baranek et al., 1997; Dunn & Fisher 1983; Kientz & Dunn 1997; Kootz, Marinelli, & Cohen, 1982). Hearing may be hyperacute, and the child may perceive certain soft sounds as loud and overpowering. Children with autism often appear to be overwhelmed and overloaded by the confusing, strongly stimulating sensory information surrounding the meal.

It is very helpful for therapists to think about and internally recreate the strong sensory aspects of a meal. A heightened sense of smell is common among children with autism (Mayes & Calhoun, 1999). Before food is seen, the smells permeate the room. These smells can contribute to a very positive meal or a rejection of the food before it is even presented. Parents describe these children as sniffing everything, seemingly as a screening method before interaction. This increased olfactory awareness can make the introduction of new foods very difficult. Many children can sense a *slight* change in a food even before the food is presented. One child could smell a difference between two brands of toasted O cereals. The cereal looked the same, but the smell (although the same to the feeders) was markedly different for the child who had autism. One toasted O cereal was rejected in favor of the other.

Often, parents are frustrated when the tiniest change in food preparation can take a usually enjoyed food and place it on the rejection list. A child may eat a favorite homemade stew with enthusiasm most of the time, but then unexpectedly reject it. The child's mother wonders what she did differently that caused her child's atypical reaction. It may have been the preparation or one of a number of other factors. The child may have experienced an increased hypersensitivity to a taste in the food because of fatigue. Slight nasal congestion may have distorted the taste, causing the child to assume that it was a new food that could not be trusted. Some children will eat only one food for an extended period of time and then reject that food altogether. This causes parents and therapists to wonder what caused the change. They wonder whether to offer the food again or find another food that is acceptable.

Many children with autism respond with heightened sensitivity to changes in food texture. Often, this first is seen as the child moves from liquid to pureed foods and then from pureed to lumpy foods. Some children prefer crunchy, dry foods once they have learned to chew and will reject all smooth or wet foods. There often are very particular and personal preferences along the sensory continuum of foods (see Chapter 14). These hypersensitivities to sensory change make it difficult for parents to introduce new flavors or foods. They make it almost impossible to give the child medications or introduce new diets.

Sometimes heightened sensitivities cause children to gag or vomit when tasting, smelling, or touching a food, or even when watching someone else eat a food. One parent said her son gagged whenever he saw someone else eat spaghetti. Another child vomited when he saw lipstick on a woman, and another child gagged when he saw balloons. These children overgeneralize uncomfortable sensory-based feeding reactions to other aspects of the mouth. Helping them handle touch in more comfortable ways often has important carryover into the realm of the meal.

Sensory Overload

Mealtimes provide rich sensory experiences. These experiences make mealtimes delightful when all is going well with sensory processing. However, all is not going well with the sensory systems of many children who have autism. It is this multisensory aspect of the mealtime that can make meals so stressful for these children. Sensory modulation difficulties and sensory overload are common (Dunn & Fisher, 1983; Kientz & Dunn, 1997; Kootz et al., 1982; Neisworth, Bagnato, & Salvia, 1995). Most people can focus on the most important sensory variables in their environment and ignore the rest. However, a child who has autism may experience sensory overload as a result of the barrage of incoming sensory information that is undifferentiated and out of balance.

Often, these children seem to be in a state of sensory bombardment. Some children report that hearing sounds feels like they are being touched from a distance. They perceive that they are engulfed by sound. The sounds of traffic outside, the noise of the air conditioner unit, chairs scraping on the floor, the dog barking, and regular conversation can be overwhelming for the sound-sensitive child. The onslaught of sensory information is cumulative.

The feeding therapist can get a sense of the child's dilemma by imagining being in a noisy restaurant and feeling overwhelmed by the high sound level. To the overpowering input of sound, add in the feeling of the touch of clothing on the body, other children bumping the chair as they run by, and the feeling of the carpet on the feet. Now add the sight of moving people and objects, and the busy array of colors and shapes. Add movement experiences and smells. Through creating this inner experience, a therapist can begin to understand what these children may be experiencing, even before the food arrives and they are expected to eat. When children face the dilemma of sensory overload, they must create complex strategies for coping. Some have temper tantrums. Some cover their ears. Some close their eyes and move into their own world, while others find stereotypic behaviors to organize this chaos. It is easy to understand why many of these children have poor appetites and eat a very limited diet.

Motor Planning Deficits

Many children with autism experience problems imitating the movement patterns of others (DeMeyer et al., 1972; Smith & Bryson, 1994). Stone, Ousley, and Littleford (1997) found that deficits were more pronounced in the autistic child's imitation of body movements than they were in the imitation of action on objects. Jones and Prior (1985) suggest that the combination of severe difficulties with motor imitation and a wide variety of soft signs of neurological dysfunction indicates that dyspraxia underlies these children's failure to learn to use gestures. Young children learn many meal time skills and behaviors, including self-feeding, from watching and imitating others. The addition of a motor-planning deficit seems to increase mealtime frustrations for children who can't seem to figure out how to make their mouths work for chewing or their hands work for scooping food and feeding themselves.

◾ Communication Variables and Mealtimes

Communication is one of the primary functions of mealtime. Infants and children who are learning eating and drinking skills rely heavily on nonverbal communication signals to guide the meal. Parents learn to understand their child's likes and dislikes, preferred pace for eating, and choices among the foods and liquids that are available at the meal. From this nonverbal dialogue, a mealtime dance emerges in which the child and adult share responsibility and provide ongoing feedback to each other. As discussed in Chapter 13, children communicate through eye gaze, body movement, facial movement, and vocalization. They look at the food or spoon. They reach for the bowl. They look at a glass across the table and grab the adult's hand to guide it toward the glass while intermittently looking toward the adult to ask for help in reaching the liquid. They open their mouths while using their eyes to visually invite the feeder to move the spoon more rapidly into the mouth. They smile and show delight in the food or frown and spit it out. They squeal or make pleasurable sounds as they let the person feeding them know that they are happy about the food.

Many of the characteristics of children with autism interfere with this mealtime dance and the partnership that it represents. Researchers have videotaped a series of free-play sessions with parents and their children with autism (Loveland, Landry, Hughes, Hall, & McEnvoy, 1988; Mundy, Sigman, Ungerer, & Sherman, 1986). When compared with mental-age matched groups of normal 2-year-olds and children with developmental language delays, the children with autism had more instances of nonresponsiveness to the parent. They produced fewer affirming responses, less turn-taking vocalization, and fewer gestures. They also were less likely to initiate communication than other children. Their parents were more likely to initiate the communication and to use commands. Deficits in nonverbal-indicating behaviors best discriminated the children diagnosed as having autism from the other groups. In a similar study, Landry and Loveland (1988) found that children with autism were less able than other children to respond correctly to language or gestures used to direct their attention. They also found these children used attention-directed pointing and showing less frequently.

Many of these children show major difficulties with focus of attention (Courchesne et al., 1994; Harris, Courchesne, Townsend, Carper, & Lord, 1999), the use of eye gaze (Mirenda, Donnellan, & Yoder, 1983; Tiegerman & Primavera, 1984), the ability to initiate and respond to joint attention (Lewy & Dawson, 1992; Loveland & Landry, 1986), communicative intent (Prizant & Wetherby, 1987), and use of facial expression and shared affect with others (Kasari, Sigman, Mundy, & Yirmiya, 1990; Yirmiya, Kasari, Sigman, & Mundy, 1989).

In a study of parents' perception of their children's emotional expressiveness, Capps, Kasari, Yirmiya, and Sigman (1993) found that children with autism were perceived as showing more negative emotion and less positive emotion than comparable groups of mentally retarded or normal children. Even when children smiled when praised after completing puzzles correctly, many did not look up to share their pleasure with the parent or experimenter or look at the puzzle to associate their pleasure with mastery of the task. Some children pulled away and tried to avoid the adult when praise was given (Kasari, Sigman, Baumgartner, & Stipek, 1993).

These studies support what clinicians and parents frequently experience when sharing a meal with children who have autism. Many of these youngsters act as if they are in an internal world into which adults are not invited. Many are easily distracted during the meal or shift from an interest in eating into stereotypic behaviors (e.g., flipping the fingers, spinning bowls and plates) that are incompatible with eating. They do not look at the feeder during the meal and give fewer positive responses to the food than other children. Their facial expressions often fail to predict their physical and emotional responses to the meal. For example, Jasmine consistently showed a very bland facial expression or smiled at the food. Once the spoon reached her mouth, she clamped the mouth closed and refused to open it for the food. This pattern of smiling and opening the mouth, followed by clamping it closed continued with each spoonful. Adam whined, pushed back, and acted highly distressed as the spoon approached. However, he opened his mouth willingly and smacked his lips, inviting his mother to place the spoon in his mouth. These mixed messages can be extremely confusing for a feeder. One mother commented, "Jason screams when he's full, and he screams when he's hungry. I never know whether to keep feeding him or to take the food away!"

Children with autism often fail to guide their feeders during the meal. While typically developing children will reach for or look at the glass when they are thirsty, children with autism may simply fuss or refuse to take the spoon when it is offered. The feeder may not know whether the child dislikes the food, needs a pause, wants a different food, has finished the meal, or simply needs a sip of liquid. They have difficulty engaging their feeder interactively and initiating the messages that guide the feeder through the meal.

When children are not communicating in ways that are clear to those feeding them, adults may overcompensate and become more directive. They often take over roles and decisions that belong to the child. Stress increases when children are less responsive and show fewer clear social interactions with parents (Kasari & Sigman, 1997). Some children with autism seem to be very sensitive to this shift in adult behavior and respond by demanding more control in the few areas in which they are comfortable.

Coping Strategies

Picky Eaters

In an effort to cope with the sensory and communication stresses at mealtimes, children with autism often compensate by limiting sensory input and withdrawing further from the social and communicative aspects of the meal. Both food and sensory engagement increase the amount and complexity of the sensory input of a meal. It is easier to avoid the sensory surprises of mealtimes by eating only familiar foods and simplifying communicative signals. As babies, many of these children completely reject breast-feeding in favor of bottle-feeding. This may be related to the reduced touch to the face that is experienced with the bottle. Other infants, however, may adopt breast-feeding readily and nurse continuously in short bursts of nutritive and nonnutritive sucking. The constant rhythm from sucking may be calming and organizing to these infants, enabling them to cope more effectively. They stick to their mothers like glue and want to use them as a pacifier 24 hours a day. Many of these babies, however, continue to demand the comfort and rhythmicity of sucking at the breast or bottle and will reject any transition to supplemental foods. These infants may significantly limit the flavors and textures of foods they will eat. They avoid anything new or unknown. The child will retreat into familiar routines and refuse to move beyond them if the food has a new visual appearance, smell, or flavor, or is offered in a new way. When a new food is tried and determined to be unacceptable, it (and any similar foods) may be placed in the child's rejection category.

This pickiness goes above and beyond the ordinary picky eating behaviors with which parents are familiar. Typical strategies for expanding foods in children's diets often do not work. Some parents indicate that their child will eat no more than 4 to 6 different foods. At times, the child is inconsistent and picky even with this limited diet. Some of the most common foods that these children include in their diets are pancakes, waffles, yogurt, milk, pretzels, chips, or other wheat- and milk-based meals. Unfortunately, vegetables and fruits are all too often avoided, though some children complicate this generalization by eating only fruits or only vegetables. The child's intake of meat or other high protein sources can be random or nonexistent. This mealtime inflexibility causes great concern for parents who are trying their best to provide well-balanced, nutritional foods.

Control

Children with autism can become very inflexible at mealtimes. When the environment is a confusing place, children attempt to simplify it by controlling it. Many children with autism control the mealtime environment to protect themselves from overload and make the meal more predictable and less frightening. Others may control it because their parents become highly directive and verbal in pushing them to eat. To control their mealtime world, these children may insist on sitting only in a certain seat, using a specific place mat, sitting next to one familiar person, using the same spoon at every meal, and eating very specific foods. Any change in the routine that the child has defined as safe can trigger tantrums or a refusal to eat. Parents often feel as if they are willing to do anything to reduce the mealtime stress and accommodate their child's demands. They understand intuitively that these demands represent real needs for their child and seem to be driven by a desperation that equates them with the child's survival. For this reason, they are more likely to give in to the child's demands than they would if they perceived them as an unreasonable bid for attention or power.

Limiting Transitions

Children with autism often have difficulty moving from one activity to the next. Transitions into or out of the mealtime environment can cause tantrums. The tantrum may have nothing to do with whether the child is hungry or dislikes the food. Difficulty with transitions permeates mealtimes for most of these children. Mealtimes are full of transitions, including transitions from the previous activity to the meal, from one food to another, from one texture to the other, from food to liquid, and from one mouthful to the next. For a child who is sensitive to transitions, the meal may be a roller coaster of transitions and worries. Some children refuse to eat or eat limited amounts to reduce the number of transitions with which they must cope.

Feedback From Older Children and Adults

Many parents are frustrated when their child selectively eliminates one food after the other from the diet. Rather than increasing dietary variety, many children with autism reduce it as they become older. Some parents have described the process "as if these foods all of a sudden became aversive." The child's reactions to many foods have the quality of a fight-or-flight survival reaction. Adults with Asperger's syndrome who have sensory-based feeding issues have indicated that the foods they refuse **simply cannot** be eaten. The food offered may seem foreign and not even within the category of food. Adults with typical sensory processing abilities have difficulty understanding these aversions. Imagine how you would feel and respond if someone offered you a glass of kerosene to drink or a piece of carpet to eat. You **know** that these are **not** foods and should not be eaten! Many children on this sensory aversion continuum appear to have intense reactions. They **know** that for them, a particular food is **not** to be eaten. Just as coercion, bribing, and force would not persuade you to drink the kerosene or eat the carpet, these techniques do not work well with these picky eaters.

Adults who can describe food-related sensory experiences in their youth say they hated the battles that evolved around the family meal. They indicate they would rather not eat or would prefer to eat alone than to feel pressured to eat foods whose smell, texture, or taste is unacceptable to them. Many feel that the stress of mealtimes worsened their physical reactions to the food and created long-term problems. Many become adults with picky eating habits that influence their lives, but they learn to live with these habits. Forcing children does not help them learn to eat and enjoy meals. Forcing creates added stress on the mealtime relationship and on family dynamics.

Nutrition and Growth

Growth Worries

Parents often worry that their children will not grow properly and will be malnourished because of their dietary limitations. Although, ideally, mealtimes are a time of nourishing the whole child, they can become a time of parental stress. Parents frequently feel rejected when their children constantly refuse the foods that they prepare and offer. Adding a new food to the diet may be a very slow and drawn-out process.

In spite of the fact that children with autism typically eat a very limited selection of foods, they may grow appropriately. Quinn (1995) says that "adequate growth in terms of weight and height for age, as well as weight for height, does not appear to be a concern." Many of these children are average or large for their age. In a sample taken by Quinn, 90% of the children had a weight-for-height ratio greater than or equal to the 50th percentile. Of that group, 76% had weight-for-height greater than the 75th percentile. Raiten and Massaro (1986) also report nutritional adequacy in the 7-day dietary records of 40 children with autism.

Some parents report growth issues beginning when their child transitions from pureed foods to table foods. Often, this is the time, before a diagnosis of autism has been given, when parents begin to notice subtle differences between their child and other children. A retrospective look at a child's growth records may show this trend. As the child matures, there may be other periods of slowed growth that center around times of change and transition (e.g., entering a new school, adjusting to new teachers or new residential situations).

Despite the fact that these children are eating few foods and their nutritional variety is limited, the majority seem to grow quite well. Some, however, clearly do not grow appropriately and are malnourished. In some cases, this is related to the specific foods that the child will eat. Clark, Rhoden, and Turner (1993) described an 8-year-old boy with autism who developed rickets and visual impairment because of severe deficiencies of vitamins A and D in his diet. The child's dietary history showed that for several years he had eaten nothing but french fried potatoes and water.

Longitudinal studies of growth and dietary status of children with autism have not been done, nor have any studies focused on the specific relationship between dietary intake and the severity of feeding difficulties for the child with autism. Children may grow in height and weight but have marked or subtle deficiencies in vital nutrients that can influence their overall state of wellness. Because feeding dysfunction frequently accompanies autism, careful attention should be paid to potential nutritional deficiencies. In his article on dietary influences on neurotransmitters in the brain, Zeisel (1986) points out that "Even when gross malnutrition is not present, subtle changes in diet may modulate brain function."

Dietary Challenges

Ongoing research studies and a variety of less structured clinical trials suggest that some children with autism have special dietary issues that influence their overall ability to function competently. Some of these issues may directly worsen their autistic behaviors. Many of these issues have additional implications for the child's relationship to food and mealtimes.

Gastrointestinal Abnormalities

Horvath, Papadimitriou, Rabsztyn, Drachenberg, and Tildon (1999) studied 36 children with autism who underwent upper gastrointestinal endoscopy with biopsies, intestinal and pancreatic enzyme analyses, and bacterial and fungal cultures. Gastrointestinal symptoms included chronic diarrhea, gaseousness, and abdominal discomfort and distension. On histological examination, 25 of the 36 children had reflux esophagitis, 15 had chronic gastritis, and 24 had chronic duodenitis. Twenty-one children had low intestinal carbohydrate digestive enzyme activity despite normal pancreatic function. The researchers concluded that "Unrecognized gastrointestinal disorders, especially reflux esophagitis and disaccharide malabsorption, may contribute to the behavioral problems of the nonverbal autistic patients."

In another study, Horvath and colleagues (Horvath, et al., 1998) described an increased pancreaticobiliary secretory response in children with autism as compared with nonautistic patients when some of these children with autism were given an intravenous administration of the pancreatic peptide hormone secretin. All three children with autism showed a significant amelioration of their gastrointestinal symptoms as well as a marked improvement in their behavior 5 weeks after receiving secretin. Behavioral changes included improved eye contact, greater alertness, and an expansion of expressive language.

Because this initial study suggested that treatment with secretin might influence more than gastrointestinal symptoms, other studies are in progress. A recently published study of 60 children (Sandler et al., 1999) looked only at the effect of a single dose of secretin on standardized behavioral measures on the Autism Behavior Checklist (Krug, Arick, Almond, 1980) using a double-blind trial. There was no significant difference at the end of 4 weeks between the children who received secretin and those who received a placebo. The researchers did not look at concomitant measures of gastrointestinal function in these children.

Although the greatest public interest has been in the non-gastrointestinal effects of secretin, the work of Horvath and colleagues suggests that more research is needed in understanding the overall contribution of the GI system to autism. Children who do not have autism but have gastrointestinal discomfort are less interested in eating and show more negative affect than other children (see Chapter 22). The added sensory processing and communication difficulties seen in autism would severely complicate children's experiences with pain or discomfort in the gastrointestinal system.

Gastrointestinal discomfort may guide food selection choices for some children and increase their beliefs that food is dangerous to their well-being.

Food Allergy

Many parents of children with autism have noted that their children were adversely affected by eating certain foods. When these foods were eliminated from the diet, the children's behavior improved and they appeared to be less autistic. Research is beginning to support these observations for many children.

A number of studies have shown an increased risk for food allergy in children with autism. Luccarelli and his colleagues (Lucarelli et al., 1995) evaluated 36 patients who had autism for food allergies. These patients were placed on a diet that eliminated cow's milk and any other foods that gave a positive allergic response after a skin test. Researchers noted a marked improvement in the patients' behavioral symptoms after 8 weeks on the diet. They also looked for immunological signs of food allergy in children with autism who were on a free choice diet. They found these children had significantly higher levels of antigen-specific antibodies for casein, a protein component of milk, as compared with a healthy control group. They suggest that allergy may play a role in the central nervous system disturbance of infantile autism.

O'Banion, Armstrong, Cummings, and Stange (1978) studied an 8-year-old boy with autism who had disruptive behaviors (including biting, scratching, and object throwing), uncontrolled laughter, and hyperactivity. They measured the frequency of his behaviors when he was fed a typical diet, during a fasting period, with the presentation of individual foods, and during a period when he was fed only foods that had not provoked a negative reaction. Their results documented that foods such as wheat, corn, tomatoes, sugar, mushrooms, and dairy products triggered his behavioral disorders.

Increased intestinal permeability has been described as a diagnostic symptom of allergy and as a way in which peptides derived from foods can pass through the gut mucosa, triggering an allergic response (Ahmed & Fuchs, 1997; Laudat, Arnaud, Napoly, & Brion, 1994). Researchers in another study used an intestinal permeability test with 21 children who had no known intestinal disorders. Altered intestinal permeability was found in 9 of the 21 patients (43%) with autism but in none of the 40 control patients (D'Eufemia et al., 1996).

Central Nervous System Toxicity

Incomplete digestion of foods containing gluten and casein can produce a toxic opioid substance that negatively affects brain function. Gluten is a protein contained in wheat and many other cereal grains (e.g., barley, rye, oats). Casein is the protein derived from cow's milk and other dairy products. During the digestion of protein, the body produces amino acids. Some of these amino acids combine to form peptides. Some peptides mimic the effects of neurotransmitters known as endorphins, which have a morphine-like or opioid effect on the brain. The digestion of both gluten and casein produces peptides with opioid activity. However, most people's digestive system breaks these peptides down further or the peptides are excreted so that they are not absorbed into the bloodstream. If these toxic peptides pass into the circulatory system in large numbers, they can pass through the blood-brain barrier and affect brain function.

Although there are many reasons why opioid peptides enter the brain, one theory is that this is related to the increased permeability of the intestinal wall, a condition often referred to as "leaky gut." This condition, which is discussed in greater detail in Chapter 16, may be more prevalent in children who have autism than those who don't (D'Eufemia et al., 1996). A number of researchers have hypothesized that the poor digestive breakdown of gluten and casein causes a toxic opioid response in the brains of children with autism, contributing to the behavioral symptoms of the disorder (Gillberg, 1995; Reichelt et al., 1981; Sahley & Panksepp, 1987; Sher, 1997). They describe positive effects when gluten and casein are removed from the diets of individuals with autism.

This theory has received support from the research of J. Robert Cade and his colleagues, who studied the effect of beta-casomorphine-7, a peptide derived from the breakdown of casein in milk on the brains of rats (Sun & Cade, 1999; Sun, Cade, Fregly, & Privette, 1999). They found support for the concept that the peptide crosses the blood-brain barrier and activates opioid receptors, affecting brain regions similar to those that are involved in schizophrenia and autism (Sun et al., 1999). A second study observed the behavioral responses of rats that received intravenous administration of beta-casomorphine-7. The animals responded with restlessness, inactivity, avoidance of other animals, and reductions in sound recognition and social interaction (Sun & Cade, 1999). The researchers noted that these same behaviors are characteristic of autism in humans.

Edelson and Cantor (1998) describe the growing evidence that chronic exposure of the developing nervous system to environmental toxins contributes heavily to the neurodevelopmental problems seen in autism. One study of 20 children with autism showed that all the children had abnormal liver detoxification profiles. Blood analyses of 18 of these children found that 16 had levels of toxic chemicals that exceeded the adult maximum tolerance. They concluded that these toxins interact with immune system dysfunction to increase the development of behaviors found in Autistic Spectrum Disorders.

Supplements

There is poor agreement in the literature on the importance of dietary supplements for children with autism. Over the years, a variety of nutritional supplements have been suggested and used by parents, physicians, and dietitians. Some have targeted increasing the overall nutritional level of those children whose dietary intake is limited (Clark et al., 1993). Others have focused on specific nutrients in food supplements that provide high-level nutrition for the body and enhance the immune system (Nisinzweig, 1999). Still others have been specifically directed at potential deficits that could be related to underlying contributing factors for autism. These have included high quality, balanced vitamin and mineral supplements, with an emphasis on calcium, magnesium, and zinc. The amino acid L-glutamine that is used to increase the growth of the villi in the small intestine may be used to address gastrointestinal issues and improve absorption of nutrients from the intestine. The use of digestive enzymes, especially those involved in the breakdown of protein (e.g., bromelain from pineapples and papaya), also may be helpful in breaking down the peptides in the gut more completely.

Research has included specific studies of the effect of high doses of vitamin B6 (balanced with magnesium) on the behavior of children with autism (Kleijnen & Knipschild, 1991). Rimland, Callaway, and Dreyfus (1978) conducted a double blind study of the use of vitamin B6 with 16 children with autism who had previously improved when given the supplement. Their behavior deteriorated significantly when the B6 was withdrawn. A later questionnaire asked 4,000 parents of children with autism to rate a variety of treatment interventions (Rimland, 1988). Parents gave the highest rating for their child's improvement to the use of high-dose vitamin B6 and magnesium. Rimland's original findings on the effect of vitamin B6 were supported by additional research that showed it was more effective when combined with magnesium (Lelord, Callaway, & Muh, 1982; Martineau et al., 1985).

Dietary Implications for Feeding Programs

The awareness of the potential role of diet for children with autism continues to grow. Many parents are involved in exploring dietary interventions with their children. Although research can describe the effect of various treatments in groups of children, it cannot define whether a specific intervention is appropriate for a specific child. Children with Autistic Spectrum Disorders are a heterogeneous group, and causal and contributing factors are undoubtedly different for different children. Therefore, parental observations and well-designed trials of different dietary strategies can be effective and appropriate for individual children.

Many families have observed positive changes in their children with dietary changes, the addition of supplements, or both. Physicians and dietitians should be consulted when any major dietary change is considered. Chapter 16 contains more specific information on the role of dietary management for children with feeding difficulties. Changing the diet or adding new supplements can be extremely difficult for many children with autism. Many already eat such a limited diet that eliminating one or more foods from that diet becomes an almost impossible challenge for parents. Dairy and wheat products are two of the most frequent foods that are recommended for elimination because of their high allergy potential and their role in opioid toxicity from casein and gluten. A child's diet frequently consists primarily of milk and wheat products. Parents working to make this type of dietary change will need support in helping the child take in enough new foods to make up for the calorie and nutrient loss caused by elimination of preferred foods. Dietary supplements can be added gradually, using the same guidelines as those for adding new foods. The principles of slow change and sensory support ultimately lead toward greater acceptance and greater success for the child and family.

Research and clinical investigations continue to provide new insights as well as new questions for therapists and parents of children with autism. At present, much of the research is conflicting and contradictory. Children with Autistic Spectrum Disorders are linked diagnostically by a set of similar characteristics; however, they represent a highly diverse group. As a result, contradictory results in research studies and findings that conflict with clinical practice will continue. Many of these differences are related to the small size of the groups studied and the current lack of ability to define the most important variables in the children studied. Parents of children with an Autistic Spectrum Disorder need to explore alternatives with informed professionals and discover what strategies work best for their own youngsters.

Sensory-Based Treatment

Although autism creates a wide range of challenges for children and their families, sensory processing difficulties have the strongest impact on the child's mealtime behaviors. Many of the nonverbal communication deficits and inconsistencies are rooted in problems with the sensory system. Treatment must address the child's overall sensory processing and integration as a foundation for changing specific feeding related difficulties (Ayres & Tickle, 1980). A review of Chapter 14 provides a strong overview of the sensory system and the difficulties experienced by children with sensory-based feeding difficulties.

A number of research studies support the validity of using a sensory-based approach with children who have autism. Preliminary research indicates that touch-pressure has a calming effect for children with autism and can reduce high levels of arousal that interfere with learning (Edelson, Edelson, Kerr, & Grandin, 1999; Field, et al., 1997). Case-Smith and Bryan (1999) examined the social responses of children with autism who participated in a 10-week program of occupational therapy that emphasized sensory integration. Four of the five children showed decreases in nonengaged behavior during free play sessions in the child's preschool. Studies have demonstrated increases in eye contact (Slavik, Kitsuwa-Lowe, Danner, Green, & Ayres, 1984) and vocalization (Ray, King, & Grandin, 1988) when children with autism participated in activities that provided vestibular stimulation.

Making a Positive Difference at Mealtimes

Each child is unique. Each child communicates as functionally as possible. Each nervous system has its own creative way of organizing and coping with sensory information. What works for one child and family may not work for another. What works one week may not work the next. A favorite food today may be completely rejected tomorrow. Some suggestions will make a difference immediately; others may take months to affect change. This is, by definition, the nature of the sensory and communicative systems of children with autism. However, some general suggestions based on extensive clinical experience with children with autism can be helpful.

Handling the Sensory Challenges of Mealtimes

- **Start early.** Although a diagnosis of autism rarely is made in early infancy, many of these children experience early regulatory disorders including sensory-based feeding difficulties (Baranek, 1999). Whenever possible, begin supportive mealtime strategies as early in infancy as possible. Feeding therapists can guide parents through difficult feeding transition periods as the child moves from liquids to pureed foods and from pureed to lumpy foods. Work toward dietary diversity in all food groups. Offer a wide variety of pureed foods. The larger the dietary repertoire, the greater the possibility that the child will assume that foods are safe and comfortable to eat. Explore alternating between commercially prepared purees and homemade purees. The textures and tastes are slightly different. Acceptance of these slight taste and texture variations can help children through more pronounced sensory changes as they move toward lumpy foods. Provide opportunities for children to develop positive oral experiences. Encourage mouthing of a variety of different toys and feeding utensils with different textures and shapes. Pair positive mouthing experiences with food. Feeding the child from different spoons or dipping favorite mouthing toys in interesting tastes can prepare children for increased acceptance of textured foods.

- **Treat the whole child.** These children usually need highly specialized treatment to help them learn to handle environmental sensory input. Children with overall difficulties with sensory processing can benefit from sensory integration strategies that help them learn to use tactile and vestibular information more comfortably and effectively. Experience has shown that it is very difficult to address the mouth and mealtime needs in isolation. Children with autism show the greatest improvement when oral sensorimotor and mealtime issues are addressed within a prescriptive sensory treatment program.

- **Reduce stress and increase the child's focus of attention at the meal.** Provide sensory activities before and during the meal that help reduce the child's anxiety and increase focus of attention. These include engaging the child in activities that provide deep touch-pressure and vestibular stimulation before the meal. Many children with autism have responded extremely well to music containing the binaural beat sounds of Hemi-Sync (Morris, 1996). These strategies for learning are discussed in detail in Chapters 13 and 14. When children are calm and focused, they are able to process the communication and sensory challenges of mealtime more effectively.

- **Know that the child's sensory reaction is real.** Even though adults have difficulty understanding why a certain food is being rejected, it is vital for them to understand that the child's reaction is *real*. It is serious for that child. The child wants parents and therapists to listen. Something in the child says, "Do not eat that!" The challenge for adults is to discover what aspects of the food are being rejected so that they can offer the same food again in a different way. Was the food offered on a different spoon? Was the food warmer this time than last? What aspects of the texture are being rejected?

- **Create a balance between routine and variation.** Children with the sensory processing difficulties of autism need a predictable structure to help organize their experiences. It is very helpful to schedule mealtimes at specific times and in specific locations. Use a specific chair, spoon, and place mat. Develop routines for offering the foods that are familiar and predictable. It is important, however, to balance this need for familiarity with the need for flexibility and acceptance of small variations. For example, a different spoon could be used on some days to offer food that the child likes. A different place mat could be introduced on another day. Applesauce could come from a spoon on some days and from a cup on other days. These small changes can broaden the child's experience and perspective, and widen the circumstances under which the child will eat. When new foods are offered, however, the familiar spoon and place mat become very comforting and very important. When the child is eating at a restaurant where the sensory input is more challenging, a familiar cup or spoon can make the difference between eating and not eating.

When small changes in routine are not introduced during the early stages of learning to eat, the child may become pickier, and change can disrupt all aspects of eating.

- **Maintain a familiar and predictable mealtime environment when making changes in food.** When offering a new food, adults always should validate the child's need for control and routine. Use the child's familiar spoon, plate, cup, and place mat. Have the child sit in the favorite seat at the table. Offer the new food from an environment that is routine, familiar, and nonstressful for the child.

- **Offer new foods at snack time or during therapy.** Because children who have autism depend upon a routine at mealtimes, they may reject new foods. The introduction of a new food may end a meal. Some children are so worried about change that they cannot finish a meal that includes a sensory surprise. Many parents and therapists find that children are more likely to accept new food tastes, textures, and temperatures when they are introduced at times other than mealtimes. Snack times or food-play times in therapy are potentially safer times to try new flavors or textures. Many children are more receptive to trying new foods with a therapist than they are with a parent. Often, this is because the child attributes safety and comfort to the parent at mealtimes, and new eating experiences are more likely to trigger uncertainty. Sometimes therapy can be a place for new experience that then can be transferred to snack time and then mealtime at home.

- **Make changes slowly.** It is vitally important to avoid dramatic sensory surprises with children who have the type of sensory aversions seen in autism. The difficulty comes with anticipating what will be a ***dramatic sensory surprise*** for individual children. The heightened senses of smell and touch may make the slightest flavor or texture change an aversive one for some children yet have a relatively small effect on others. Some children can handle larger increments of change than others. Parents know their children best and can provide excellent collaboration with therapists in developing a plan for sensory change. A general rule, however, is to start with a familiar food and make tiny changes only in one sensory arena. For example, keep the texture the same but change the flavor slightly, or keep the flavor the same and change the texture slightly. Know that some children have a much stronger aversion to even the slightest change, so go slowly. A child who eats pancakes may not notice the difference when an extra egg is included in the batter to increase the protein content. However, if two eggs are added, the child may refuse to eat any pancakes and may look at them suspiciously even when the number of eggs is reduced. In the same fashion, a few grains of cinnamon can change the flavor slightly but in an acceptable fashion, while a larger amount would be rejected. Some parents add pureed carrots, squash, or applesauce very gradually to increase their child's vegetable or fruit intake. Pancakes and waffles are easy to modify because the strong syrup smell can camouflage small amounts of other foods that have been added. Although these changes work well for some children, others show an intense awareness of the slightest change even before the food is placed in front of them.

- **Begin with a familiar flavor.** Many parents have succeeded in introducing new flavors by very gradually changing the flavor of a familiar food or drink. Tiny increments of change work for some children who ordinarily reject larger changes in taste. For example, the flavor of a drink can be modified by adding a flavored ice cube to a familiar drink. As the ice cube melts, the new flavor will blend into the drink. The flavor change is gradual. Because the drink begins with a very familiar taste, the child is more likely to accept the change. A child who prefers to drink soda can have the soda gradually mixed with ice cubes of juice. Gradually, more and more juice can be added. The ice cube method seems to work well when straw cups with a lid are used. This reduces changes in the smell and color of the drink. Many children who drink sodas prefer the sensory stimulation of the carbonation. Club soda or sparkling mineral water gradually can be substituted for commercial sodas after the child makes the initial shift in accepting fruit juices mixed with soda. This type of change should be done slowly but it has the benefit of increasing the child's intake of calories and nutrients through fruit juice and decreasing the empty calories and chemical additives found in commercial soda.

- **Mask the smell of the new food.** The heightened sense of smell seen in many children with autism complicates the presentation of new foods. Foods can be rejected because they smell different. Food molecules that stimulate smell and taste are more volatile and active when they are warm. To reduce the smell of new flavors, use chilled foods. Many parents have had success when they provide liquids in a cup with a lid. The lid masks the smell and the appearance of the liquid, and prevents many children from rejecting it simply on the basis of sight or smell. Some children are more open to trying the liquid again once they have experienced the first taste. If a change, however, is made too dramatically, the child may reject all future tastes from cups with lids. Remember to make the changes slowly.

- **Offer foods and supplements that provide a high level of nutrition.** Parents must evaluate the nutritional content of all foods that they offer their child. Because many children with autism are extremely picky eaters, they may eat smaller quantities of food and a more limited variety of foods. Thus, every mouthful offered should contribute to the child's nutritional well being. Dietitians often recommend vitamin and mineral supplementation for children who have very picky eating behaviors. The strong taste of liquid vitamins and the texture of chewable vitamins may provide a challenge for parents. Some parents add a crushed chewable vitamin very gradually to a favorite food. Others introduce Ovaltine™, Instant Breakfast™, or similar drink enhancers to provide a higher concentration of vitamins and minerals. Many parents have succeeded with these supplements by mixing them with a favorite drink, freezing the drinks into ice cubes, and melting them gradually into familiar drinks. Chapter 16 contains suggestions for increasing nutrition through food and food supplements.

Handling the Communication Challenges of Mealtimes

- **Assume that everything the child does has a communicative function.** Adults often forget that children with autism are communicating at all times. Every self-stimulatory, refusal, withdrawal, or acting-out behavior is the child's way of letting others know what they are experiencing and what they need.

- **Observe the child's patterns of communication.** Adults must observe the child carefully and notice how the child communicates likes; dislikes; and levels of sensory awareness, overload, or discomfort. It is helpful to compare the child's communicative responses in different environments and with different types and levels of sensory input.

- **Create a positive learning and communication environment.** Children with autism continually deal with sensory, communicative, and cognitive challenges that reduce their availability for learning at mealtimes. It is particularly important to consciously consider and choreograph a learning environment that meets their needs and provides them with ample opportunities to guide the meal through communication. See Chapter 13 for additional strategies for enhancing the learning and communication environments at mealtime.

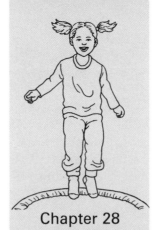

Chapter 28

The Child Who Has Minimal Involvement

When people think about feeding problems, they usually imagine children who have major difficulties with sucking, swallowing, biting, and chewing. They maintain a mental checklist of landmarks. If a child eats table foods, chews meat, and drinks from a straw, it is assumed that all is well. Children who pass through the major stages of feeding development usually are not referred for a feeding evaluation. However, children with mild or minimal sensorimotor involvement may experience difficulties that influence their feeding and speech development.

These children often are misdiagnosed or slip through developmental screenings and evaluations. Parents and professionals may believe that the child is just messy during meals and doesn't really have a feeding problem. Parents of preschoolers with persistently unclear articulation are told that speech automatically will improve as their children mature. When children accept new foods slowly or engage in precise rituals around mealtime, they are described as picky eaters. Even if the mild feeding issues are identified correctly, the child may not be enrolled in a treatment program. When therapy services and funding are limited, professionals may reserve treatment for children with more severe impairment.

Children with minimal feeding issues have many individual sensorimotor, oral motor, and pre-speech characteristics. These features cluster into several clearly observable traits that can be used to refer a child for services. Any child who drools, engages in persistent mouth stuffing, or shows significant delays in articulatory or expressive language development should receive a detailed evaluation of oral motor skills in feeding.

The Issues

Drooling

All children lose control of saliva and drool as they are developing control of gross motor and fine motor movements. As infants progress to more challenging motor skills such as sitting, standing, walking, and running, drooling occurs. Control of drooling is automatic. It requires a high level of sensorimotor organization to swallow automatically while focusing attention on a new skill. In normal development, children often revert to earlier, more familiar patterns during the acquisition stage of learning. The development of stability is a major component of normal development, and stability of the head, neck, and shoulder girdle is prerequisite to fine motor control of the mouth. When this control is lacking, drooling is likely to occur. It is seen as infants move toward stability in an upright and mobile position such as walking or running. Babies may achieve some of their initial control or stability by tensing the jaw or tongue. This results in a loss of swallowing control and drooling. Gradually, as skill and control increase, extra tension in the body drops out and drooling stops.

These same issues may be seen in youngsters who have mild difficulties with postural tone and movement. Because proximal stability is not well developed, the child continues to tighten muscles for extra steadiness. The shoulders will elevate, the jaw will tense, and the tongue will press against the palate. As a result, the oral structures are not free to move fluidly. The child drools. If the child has not had the opportunity to explore movement during feeding or play with nonfeeding mouth movements, the quality of feeding movements—including aspects of speed, precision, and overall coordination—may be deficient.

In some children, drooling may indicate that mild problems exist in sensory awareness or organization. The child may be unaware of wetness on the face and be unable to monitor the pressure cues within the mouth that trigger an automatic swallow. Still other children may have mild problems with oral motor coordination that become exaggerated when upper respiratory problems are present. If the child cannot breathe through the nose, an open-mouth posture may invite drooling in situations that involve effort.

Mouth Stuffing

Most young children will stuff food into the mouth as they are learning to refine their eating skills (Morris, 1978). They appear to love the sensory input and the challenge of filling the mouth and closing the lips around the food so nothing falls out. They swish soft food such as applesauce around inside the closed mouth and relish the way it feels. They fill their mouths with water and pat their cheeks, causing the water to spray out. Although young children delight in these mouth-stuffing activities, they readily pass through this stage. By the time they are 3 years old, they cooperate with cultural conventions that discourage such stuffing.

Some children engage in mouth stuffing for a very different set of reasons (Morris, 1997a). Mouth stuffing can signal sensory or motor difficulties in oral motor control. When the mouth is fully stuffed with food, children obtain more sensory information about the boundaries of their mouths and the presence of food in the mouth. This often happens when oral sensation is reduced. Imagine eating a meal after you have received a shot of Novocain at the dentist's office. Your sense of touch is deadened, and small pieces of food are lost in the mouth cavity. When children face a similar challenge, they stuff as much food as possible into the mouth. The pressure from the food wakes up the mouth and tells them they need to keep chewing and swallowing. Imagine filling your mouth with a quarter of a peanut butter and jelly sandwich. Your mouth is stuffed, and you definitely know where that sandwich is! Now imagine a kernel of corn in your mouth. Imagine the greater awareness you need to find the kernel of corn and the more refined oral skills to move it precisely.

Many children with low oral awareness may stuff the mouth and not clear the food when the meal is finished. They may not be aware that there is still food in the mouth. Other children who stuff deal with a condition called oral defensiveness. These youngsters experience highly distressful sensations from food taste or texture. Unpredictable movement of the food can be very uncomfortable. Many children with oral tactile defensiveness stuff the mouth because it reduces the random tactile input to the cheeks when smaller pieces of food are moved around.

Many of these children stuff their mouths because they are in a hurry. Their attention flits from one area to another. They are disorganized and have trouble focusing on the meal. They get up from the table, run around, and forget that they have chunks of food in the mouth. They may cough and choke when the combination of low awareness and poor focus of attention interact.

Mouth stuffing also is present when a child has difficulty using skillful tongue movements for chewing. Movements may be uncoordinated or limited in direction or strength. When there is a great deal of food in the mouth, a very small amount of tongue movement will push some food to the side for chewing. Smaller pieces require much more control of movement.

It is important to distinguish between mouth stuffing that is a normal developmental behavior and that which is a compensation for sensorimotor difficulties. Typically developing children have the sensory awareness and the motor skill to remove all food from the mouth at the end of the meal. Children with poor awareness or movement limitations often leave pieces of food in the mouth after eating. Some children are sure that their mouths are empty when there is still food on the tongue or in the cheek pockets. Often, parents find pieces of food pocketed between the gums and the cheeks when they brush their child's teeth at night. Many children with difficulties in sensory awareness love foods with strong flavors. Salsa, lemon juice, pickles, and barbecue sauce often are favorites. Other children seem to prefer strong sensory textures such as crunchy foods. There may be less mouth stuffing with these high-awareness flavors or textures. This could be a clue that the child's mouth stuffing is related to a sensory difficulty. The child with motor difficulties may push food up into the roof of the mouth where it becomes stuck. When the food later falls down, the child may be surprised and gag or choke on the unexpected mouthful.

Delays in Expressive Speech and Language

Children can show delays in speaking for many reasons. One possibility is the lack of motor control and organization needed for producing speech sounds. This aspect should be ruled out for every child who is not speaking single words by the age of 2 years. A mild problem with oral motor control can make intelligible speech difficult. Some children do their best to talk even though others fail to understand; others give up and prefer silence to overt frustration.

When the history and nonspeech patterns of oral movement in these children are examined, several patterns emerge. Many children have a history of limited sound play as infants (Morris, 1997a). They did not go through the babbling stage of combining sounds. If they did babble, it was stereotyped and lacking in the richness of different sound combinations. They may not have enjoyed or spent much time mouthing a variety of textured toys. These children may be unusually picky eaters with strong dislikes and preferences for a few foods. As infants, they may have had difficulty making the transition to solid foods, especially those with lumps. Observations of feeding patterns show difficulties with chewing, problems with foods of varied consistencies, and a lack of playfulness and exploitation of the sensory properties of food. Transfers of food across midline may be slow or done only with a pause in the center of the tongue. Drooling or choking may occur when the child has to swallow a liquid portion of the food while chewing or retaining a solid portion in the mouth. New food consistencies often are refused rather than explored.

Some children lack variations in the way in which more challenging movements can be performed. For example, if they are invited to explore different ways in which a raisin can be moved in the mouth, they may become confused or repeat the same movements. These difficulties with fine adjustments of movement and motor planning may reflect a central programming difficulty known as dyspraxia. Later, these children may be diagnosed as having a developmental dyspraxia of speech.

The Underlying Sensorimotor Issues

Children with minimal feeding involvement commonly experience difficulties with movement and sensory processing. The following sensorimotor challenges contribute strongly to the specific characteristics observed in their feeding and prespeech patterns (Morris, 1997a).

Low Tone in the Trunk With Poor Postural Stability for Movement

Children who experience primary difficulties with low postural tone often compensate for their instability with movements that can reduce the skilled functioning of the oral, respiratory, and phonatory systems. Often, elevation of the shoulder girdle with increased tension, clenching tension in the jaw, and firm pressing of the tongue against the hard palate are seen in attempts to provide greater stability for movement. These patterns contribute to tension and poor coordination in the parts of the body that are required for skilled feeding and speech movements.

Low tone in the muscles of the jaw, lips, and cheeks can lead to a chronic open position of the mouth. This contributes to weaker, less precise oral movements during feeding and loss of food and saliva during eating.

Poor Differentiation of Movement

Skilled movement requires a balance between stability and mobility. This balance leads to the ability to refine movement so that only those muscle patterns needed in the skill are used. Patterns of stability in the jaw provide the foundation for greater separation and differentiation of lip and tongue movements. Initially, the tongue and jaw work together. With greater stability of the jaw, the child learns to move the tongue independently. The combined movements, however, may be retained in cup drinking or speech for some children. Because jaw movement is much slower and less precise than tongue or lip movement, the speech of children who have not developed the separation may be slower or less skillful than normal.

Poor Sensory Awareness and Discrimination

The quality of eating and drinking patterns is compromised when children have poor sensory awareness and discrimination. Mouth stuffing frequently indicates difficulties with oral sensory awareness. This stuffing may increase children's awareness of food and make it easier for them to organize and swallow solid foods. Some children swallow foods before chewing them adequately because they lack the sensory organization and discrimination to determine the size and resistance of the food. Poor attention to sensory details during eating can lead to greater loss of food and liquid from the mouth during eating or to drooling after the meal. These same difficulties in oral sensory discrimination can influence the accuracy of articulation in speech development (Speirs & Dean, 1989; Speirs & Maktabi, 1990).

Poor Attention

Some children with hyperactivity or attention deficit disorders have difficulty focusing attention on the refined aspects of any activity. This may interfere with the attention needed to chew a mouthful completely. Many of these children swallow foods whole or poorly chewed. Intermittent choking or gagging may occur. For these children, the awareness of the sensory aspects of the food may be available to them, but the fact that the body is *on the go* may not allow enough focus to sufficiently chew a meal. Activities to help the child calm and focus attention before and during the meal may be needed to enable the child to focus on the details of eating. For some of these children, there is decreased sensory awareness in the oral area that affects attention to the oral management of food.

Sensory-Processing Difficulties

Children who experience difficulties processing and integrating sensory information often show mild sensorimotor difficulties in feeding and speech. Sensory integrative disorders strongly influence the development of skilled movements of the body and mouth, and make it more difficult for the child to learn new skills through sensory avenues that are affected. Motor-planning or apraxic difficulties, if present, make the learning of speech very difficult.

Motor-Planning Difficulties

The child with motor-planning problems may have difficulty imitating movements such as elevation, depression, or lateralization of the tongue; smacking, rounding, or spreading movements of the lips; and varying degrees of opening and closing movements of the jaw. Some children experience motor-planning issues when they are given new foods. If these foods require complex sensory decisions or the child cannot identify the salient sensory features, eating may require cognitive processing. The child has to figure out where the food is and how to move it or retrieve pieces that are stuck between the teeth. This poses an overwhelming challenge for some children. Many children who are diagnosed later as having developmental apraxia of speech don't play with their food like typically developing youngsters. They don't explore the sensory features of the food or discover creative ways to roll peas across the plate or blow bubbles in the milk. When these feeding characteristics are accompanied by other sensory-processing difficulties, they may reflect a motor-planning problem.

Children whose speech delays are related to developmental dyspraxia usually have normal or slightly delayed feeding skills. However, movements of the mouth that are observed during feeding cannot be reproduced at a voluntary level for speech. These youngsters often have an early history of delayed onset of babbling and difficulty transitioning to solid foods. They may remain picky eaters with limited food preferences.

An Approach to Therapy

Treatment of minimally involved children can be a major challenge. The differences and difficulties they experience with eating and drinking often seem unimportant when they are infants and toddlers. As they grow up, their continued drooling, messy eating, and challenges with speech cause more concern to their parents and teachers. Those who make decisions about granting services are aware that these children are different, but still will deny them services because they are not considered severe enough. Others will receive therapy that does not address their underlying needs.

The approaches used for children with mild feeding and oral motor problems will depend upon the specific characteristics and needs of the child. Therapy should be directed predominantly at the underlying sensorimotor issues that influence the child.

Asking the Right Questions

As therapists work with children who have minimal feeding difficulties, they initially must observe whether the underlying sensorimotor and oral motor patterns are present.

- Does the child have the underlying postural support and control for refined oral-feeding movements?
- Can the child maintain control in the oral area while engaged in balancing stressing movements and position transitions?
- Does the child have the underlying sensory-processing skills for skilled oral feeding? Is there good sensory awareness and discrimination?
- Has the child developed jaw stabilization patterns to support skilled, differentiated movements of the tongue and lips during eating and drinking?
- Can the child imitate movements of the jaw, lips, and tongue that are used automatically during eating or drinking?
- Does the child have the ability to keep attention focused throughout an activity?

Mealtime and Feeding Strategies

Specific work to improve the child's oral feeding skills can be incorporated into individual therapy sessions and the child's classroom as the underlying sensorimotor issues are addressed. Many minimally involved children need individual therapy rather than simply group experience in the classroom. Feeding skills also are sensorimotor skills, and like other sensorimotor skills such as sitting, walking, and hopping, children may require special therapy to learn a new or unfamiliar movement. Often, new patterns of chewing or swallowing will be taught initially by a therapist or teacher with special skill or training in feeding skills. The following general strategies and activities are helpful in working with children with mild feeding challenges.

Postural Stability and Control

Many of these children have low tone and poor postural stability for movement. It is important in therapy to focus on developing the underlying postural stability and control that support refined oral-feeding movements. Activities to develop greater stability in the trunk and shoulder girdle are appropriate when the child shows shoulder girdle elevation, protrusion of the shoulder blades, and other indications of central unsteadiness. These may include bouncing and jumping, which often are favorite activities of children who have the physical control to engage spontaneously in these activities. Many of these activities stimulate the righting and equilibrium reactions that enable the child to reach a higher level of sensorimotor integration and coordination. Supervised jumping on a small mini-trampoline or rebounder can provide many opportunities for building stability, exploring movement variations, and building aerobic support for improved breathing and voicing patterns.

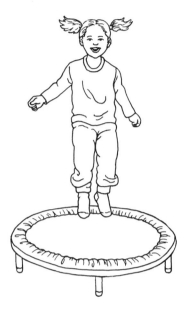

When children have marginally low postural stability, they often use a compensatory tension in the shoulder girdle, rib cage, jaw, or tongue to help them become more stable. Often, the child is not consciously aware of these patterns. As they become part of the child's sensory feedback of movement, they may continue in situations where the underlying postural stability issues have been resolved. It can be very helpful to incorporate activities or games that involve conscious contrasts in movement and tension of different parts of the body. For example, the child could feed himself with the right arm while consciously tightening the left arm or the jaw. This could be contrasted with self-feeding while the jaw and arm remain relaxed or *soft*.

Sensory Processing

Assistance with sensory processing may take many different forms. Some children have clear-cut difficulties with sensory modulation and integration. Many of them already are receiving therapy from an occupational therapist with experience in sensory integration. Others may not, either because their difficulties are subtler or this type of service is unavailable in their school system or community. Where overall problems in sensory processing are suspected, the child should be referred for consultation to an occupational therapist who is qualified to evaluate children with sensory integration dysfunction.

Within the feeding and mealtime program, however, the feeding therapist can apply many general principles. These are discussed in detail in Chapter 14.

Treatment sessions can engage the child in sensory exploration with the mouth to provide a variety of sensory information that can be used to organize movement as well as sensory processing. Many activities can be incorporated into the program that help the child build sensory awareness and discrimination. These would include the use of foods with high sensory information to wake up the mouth and visual feedback with mirrors to provide information on whether there is residual food in the mouth.

Increasing Attention

It is extremely important to help children develop their focus of attention before and during the meal. Some children will need to become more alert, while others will benefit from a calmer focus or a quiet area in which they can have their meal. Activities that provide vestibular, proprioceptive, and deep touch-pressure input can help many children become more organized and ready before they come to the table. Specific music that provides sensory organization and focus of attention can be incorporated into the mealtime (see Chapter 13). As food textures become more complex, the child must be able to focus attention on the grinding of complex foods until they are prepared into an appropriate bolus for swallowing. Children who have difficulty maintaining focus on a mouthful of food often swallow it whole or only partially chewed. Weighted vests or collars can provide proprioceptive information through the upper body that assists postural stability and increases a child's focus of attention. A variety of oral activities also helps focus of attention (Oetter et al., 1988). This may include increasing the thickness or resistance of liquids (e.g., thick milk shakes), using a long straw, and incorporating foods that provide a great deal of sensory information (e.g., strong tastes, crunchy textures).

Differentiation of Oral Movement

Children whose feeding issues fall in the mild or minimal range frequently have poor differentiation of oral movement. Their feeding is quite functional, but often feeding movements are imprecise. This may result in drooling, messiness during the meal, mouth stuffing, or avoidance of specific foods because of the subtle sensorimotor challenges that they pose.

Specific feeding activities should emphasize the prerequisite movements and sensory awareness required for fine motor control and motor planning. This can include activities to build awareness of two-point discrimination, to explore and discover movement options, and to follow the higher level sequences of oral-feeding development. Many specific treatment activities or techniques can be built around the normal developmental sequences described in Chapter 5. These could include work for more precise transfer of food from one side of the mouth to the other, graded opening of the jaw for foods of different thickness, and holding the cup gently with the teeth to develop external stability of the jaw during drinking.

Activities that provide the opportunity for the child to separate jaw, lip, and tongue movements from movements of the head, neck, and shoulder girdle are helpful. In the oral area, work on the underlying sensorimotor strategies that support external and internal jaw stability is essential.

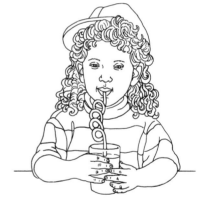

When there is low tone in the jaw or lips and cheeks, activities that incorporate specific muscle stimulation (e.g., tapping, vibration) or resistance can assist the development of saliva control and prevent drooling. Activities might include drinking a thick liquid through a long straw in a variety of shapes. In general, straw drinking can be very helpful in improving muscle tone in the lips and cheeks.

Activities that emphasize jaw movement against resistance, such as eating a snack while wearing a bathing cap or a cap with a chinstrap, can focus increased attention on jaw awareness. The child then can move from conscious awareness of jaw and lip movement to automatic responses by working with many distractions. Initially, keeping distractions to a minimum enables the child to focus awareness on the area of primary activity. As singing and fine motor or gross motor activities are added, the focus of attention is shifted to these events. The control of oral movements becomes integrated into the total activity at an automatic level. Vocalization and generalized exploration of sound should be incorporated during movement activities to enable the child to experience tongue, lips, and jaw that are free to move.

Children learn initial motor planning with the mouth when they have the opportunity to play with their food. They explore different quantities of food in the mouth, different locations, and different combinations of food. Because of their oral-sensorimotor delays or difficulties or early family preferences for neatness and serious eating at the table, many children miss this important stage of development. This makes little difference for children who can engage in oral motor-planning skills in other ways. Children who have difficulty organizing and planning movement sequences, however, can benefit from returning to this stage during therapy. Play and exploration with food can help them move from a more automatic use of oral movement with eating to a more conscious activity that involves movement planning.

Choosing Snack Foods

As new skills develop, children need many opportunities to practice the new patterns at home or school (Morris, 1997b). The classroom provides many occasions for continued learning and change. Snack time occurs in every classroom and home. Often, it is considered a time to physically refresh the children with food or an opportunity to work on language and social skills. When food is carefully selected, snack time can provide major opportunities to develop sensorimotor skills for feeding.

Food can be selected for snacks that meet specific goals for individual children and to provide opportunities for all children in the group to increase their experience with different kinds of food. Several types of food provide excellent opportunities for children with sensorimotor difficulties:

- **Foods with multiple textures.** Foods that consist of more than one texture are very challenging for children. Some foods have two or more textures that can be visibly observed; others tend to produce extra juice or saliva when they are chewed. The child must swallow the liquid and extra saliva produced by the food while continuing to chew the more solid parts. Often, children who have mild difficulties with oral control drool or lose liquid when they eat combination foods. Foods that could be given at snack time include unpeeled apple wedges; orange wedges; raisins; Jell-O with fruit chunks; firm, dry cereal with milk; or salad with pieces of different raw vegetables.

- **Foods that require extended chewing.** Children with mild feeding problems often resist foods that require extended chewing. Foods that could be given at snack time to increase chewing skill include raw carrots, raw celery, beef jerky, or strips of rare roast beef, steak, or other firm meat. Although candy and other sweet foods should be discouraged as a regular snack, licorice twists and sugar-free bubble gum are wonderful for encouraging extended chewing and chewing without drooling.

- **Foods that can be served in many sensory variations.** Foods that can be served in many different taste and texture combinations lend themselves beautifully to work on sensory discrimination and language. They also provide ways of making smaller, more gradual changes for children who are resistant to eating new foods. Foods that could be given at snack time to focus on sensory changes in taste and texture include crackers with toppings such as peanut butter, Swiss cheese, cheddar cheese, cream cheese, or cream cheese and jelly. Alternatively, one could take a theme of cheese and vary the type of cracker.

- **Foods that encourage playful exploration.** Young children typically love to explore and make discoveries with food. They enjoy hiding pieces of food in different parts of the mouth, feeling the mouth stuffed with food, and playing with different amounts of food in the mouth. Foods that encourage exploration include raisins or other dried fruits and firm cereal pieces. Chewing sugar-free bubble gum also develops playful exploration. Dipping hard foods in smooth foods can provide many opportunities for tongue exploration. For example, three-ring pretzels can be dipped in onion dip. The dip then can be licked off each part of the pretzel with the tongue accommodating to the varying shape challenges of the pretzel.

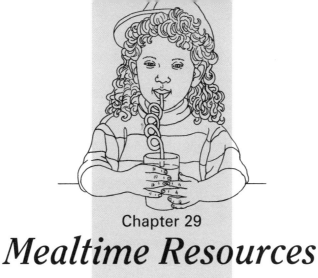

Chapter 29

Mealtime Resources

We really like the following resources. These have become part of our own libraries that we go back to regularly to remind ourselves of foundational skills for feeding and mealtime development.

Books on Mealtime and Feeding Development

Normal Development of Functional Motor Skills: The First Year of Life by Rona Alexander, Regi Boehme, and Barbara Cupps. Therapy Skill Builders, 1993.

> This wonderful book makes normal development come alive! As it takes you through the first 12 months of a baby's life, you will develop a strong appreciation for the interaction and interplay of all aspects of development. Each developmental stage includes an overview of the anatomical, postural, gross motor, fine motor, oral motor, feeding, respiratory, and phonatory development. The book is well-researched, providing current references and a convenient summary chart for quick referral at the end of each developmental stage. Use this resource for planning treatment for infants and preschool children with neurological involvement and developmental disabilities.

Pediatric Videofluoroscopic Swallow Studies: A Professional Manual with Caregiver Guidelines by Joan C. Arvedson and Maureen A. Lefton-Greif. Communication Skill Builders, 1998.

> This book will become an important reference for health-care professionals who are working with infants and children who have swallowing and feeding difficulties. The authors provide a detailed discussion of the anatomy and physiology of feeding and swallowing, and explore the differences between adult and infant anatomy. The unique differences between pediatric and adult swallowing studies are described along with the rationale for using different procedures to evaluate and interpret videofluoroscopic swallowing studies in children.

Out of the Mouths of Babes: Discovering the Developmental Significance of the Mouth by Sheila Frick, Ron Frick, Patricia Oetter, and Eileen Richter. PDP Press, 1996.

> This booklet is packed full of information for parents and therapists about the importance of the mouth in all areas of life. The authors of *M.O.R.E.* describe the timing and integration of the suck/swallow/breath synchrony in feeding, postural development, speech development, health, alertness, and the organization of behavior. Suggestions and strategies for home and school are included.

Feeding and Nutrition for the Child with Special Needs: Handouts for Parents by Marsha Dunn Klein and Tracy Delaney. Therapy Skill Builders, 1994.

> This practical collection of 195 handouts on feeding and nutrition has been developed for the busy therapist. The reproducible pages provide thousands of practical techniques and organized information for parents and caregivers. This library of diverse handouts gives you information on the ***how's*** and ***what's*** of feeding and nutrition for infants and children with special needs. All handouts are cross-referenced and space is provided to individualize the instructions for each child.

Neurodevelopmental Strategies for Managing Communication Disorders in Children with Severe Motor Dysfunction, edited by M. Beth Langley and J. Lombardino. Pro-Ed, 1991.

> Many feeding and communication programs are established on the foundation of the Neuro-Developmental Treatment approach (NDT). This approach to treatment was developed more than 30 years ago by Berta and Karel Bobath. Chapters in this clinical handbook were contributed by a special group of experienced clinicians whose work in the feeding and pre-speech areas is based on the NDT approach.

Evaluation and Treatment of Swallowing Disorders, 2nd Edition by Jeri A. Logemann. College Hill Press, 1997.

> Jeri Logemann is a pioneer and prolific researcher in the area of swallowing disorders. This book gives the reader in-depth information on normal and limiting areas of swallowing and dysphagia.

Manual for the Videofluorographic Study of Swallowing, 2nd Edition, by Jeri A. Logemann, Pro-Ed, 1993.

> An important resource for videofluoroscopic swallowing studies, this manual provides therapists with specific procedures for bedside and radiographic assessment of the oropharyngeal swallow as well as the treatment for swallowing disorders. Treatment techniques are described for application and evaluation in the radiographic study, and sample protocols are provided for patients with particular swallowing disorders.

Mealtime Participation Guide by Marsha Dunn Klein and Suzanne Evans Morris. Therapy Skill Builders, 1999.

> This is the most valuable book available for guided learning about feeding and mealtimes. The authors have created a guidebook that supports both individual and group learning. Each of more than 130 participatory experiences provides a list of goals, materials needed, a script for leading the activity, and discussion questions. A detailed summary of typical and variable responses to each activity is provided. This extensive guide includes both physical and imagination mealtime experiences. This is the ultimate tool for training students, staff, and parents.

Child of Mine: Feeding With Love and Good Sense, Second Edition by Ellyn Satter. Bull Publishing, 2000.

> This wonderful resource looks at feeding from pregnancy through the toddler period, special issues of feeding, and the feeding relationship. It covers all the basics of child nutrition, including nutrition for pregnancy, breast-feeding versus bottle feeding, calories and normal growth, introduction of solid foods to the infant diet, feeding and the toddler, overweight children, and childhood eating disorders. This and all of Ellyn Satter's works are excellent resources for parents and feeding therapists alike.

How to Get Your Kid to Eat—But Not too Much by Ellyn Satter. Bull Publishing, 1987.

> Ellyn Satter provides the reader with great basic principles of feeding and developmental stages of eating and addresses special feeding problems. Her concept of the Division of Responsibility is central to feeding and treating children with feeding difficulties. This is a ***must*** for parents and feeding therapists!

Secrets of Feeding a Healthy Family by Ellyn Satter. Kelcy Press, 1999.

> This book offers a practical guide for sorting through conflicting demands, sifting through health hysteria, planning wisely, and delightfully managing family meals. It empowers and inspires the reader to love and cook favorite foods and teach children to do the same. It provides chapters on eating management, the feeding relationship, food selection, you and your own eating, recipes, cooking, preparing and planning meals, shopping, and nutrition education. This is another ***must*** from Ellyn Satter.

Feeding and Swallowing Disorders in Infancy: Assessment and Management by Lynn Wolf and Robin Glass. Therapy Skill Builders, 1992.

> This book is essential if you work with infants with feeding and swallowing disorders! This practical resource integrates information in the areas of sucking, swallowing, and breathing to aid in evaluation and treatment of infants between birth and 12 months. The research-based text addresses diagnosis, evaluation, treatment, and follow-up for infants with varying types and degrees of feeding dysfunction.

Videotapes

Breastfeeding Your Baby: Positioning by Chele Marmet. Medela, 1991.

> Breast-feeding is a learned art. Although breast-feeding is the most natural thing to do, and breastmilk is the best food for a baby, the act of breast-feeding is a skill that must be learned. *Breastfeeding Your Baby: Positioning* teaches that skill. This video is essential for therapists working in the NICU or with any mother who wishes to breast-feed. When an infant has special needs, positioning becomes especially important in assisting the mother-infant partnership during feeding. Lactation consultant Chele Marmet demonstrates techniques for proper positioning of the baby and mother, presentation of the breast, and assisting the baby in latching on to the breast.

Series: Feeding with Love and Good Sense by Ellyn Satter. Ellyn Satter Associates, 1997. Contains *Feeding with Love and Good Sense: The Infant, Feeding with Love and Good Sense: The Older Baby, Feeding with Love and Good Sense: The Toddler, Feeding with Love and Good Sense: The Preschooler.*

> Every feeding clinic should have this videotape! Ellyn Satter does a fabulous job of teaching parents about communication/interaction at mealtimes in this videotape, formerly issued as a series of four 15-minute tapes and now updated. She is respectful of children and parents and teaches about mealtime development and interactions in clear, concise ways. These tapes help adults to understand feeding from the child's perspective and to be sensitive to their own behaviors and the impact of those behaviors on the child and the child's eating. Each tape focuses on reading the child's cues, helping to promote mastery skills in feeding, and understanding the division of responsibility in feeding.

Catalog

Mealtimes. New Visions, 1124 Roberts Mountain Rd., Faber, VA 22938, 800-606-3665; http://www.new-vis.com

> This unique catalog brings together in one place a diverse collection of materials to teach and stimulate oral-motor, feeding, and mealtime behaviors. Included are mouth toys, feeding equipment, books, videotapes, and music to support learning.

■ Internet

Feed Your Mind, http://www.new-vis.com

The Feed Your Mind section of the New Visions Web site is full of Information Papers related to feeding, oral motor treatment, and mealtime programs. Written by Suzanne Evans Morris, Ph.D., these papers reflect current thinking and treatment exploration. New materials are added monthly.

Appendix A
Pre-Feeding Global and Sequential Charts

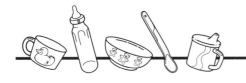

Developmental Pre-Feeding Checklist:
A Global Approach

Name _____ C.A. _____ Assessment date _____

		Present—Spontaneous	Present With Facilitation	Not Present
1 Month				
Feeding position	Supine with the head slightly elevated; or prone; or reclining at an angle of less than 45 degrees; or sidelying			
Food types	Is fed only liquids from the bottle or breast			
Food quantity	Takes 2 to 6 ounces of liquid per feeding, at 6 or more feedings per day			
Sucking liquids	Uses a suckling or sucking pattern with the bottle or breast. Loses some liquid during sucking			
Swallowing liquids	Swallows thin liquids with a suckle-swallow pattern. Tongue may protrude slightly through the lips with an extension-retraction movement			
Coordination of sucking, swallowing, and breathing	Sequences two or more sucks from the breast or bottle before pausing to breathe or swallow			
Control of drooling	Rarely drools because of minimal saliva production			
3 Months				
Feeding position	Is fed in a supported semi-sitting position, reclining at an angle of 45 to 90 degrees			

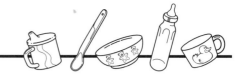

Pre-Feeding Checklist: A Global Approach (continued)

		Present—Spontaneous	Present With Facilitation	Not Present
	3 Months (continued)			
Food quantity	Takes 7 or 8 ounces of liquid per feeding, at 4 to 6 feedings per day			
Sucking semi-solids from a spoon	If soft or pureed foods are presented, uses a suckling or sucking pattern as food approaches or touches the lips. Upper lip does not assist in food removal.			
Swallowing semi-solids	If soft or pureed foods are presented, uses a primitive suckle-swallow response to move food into the pharynx. Some food is pushed out of the mouth. Periodic choking, gagging, or vomiting can occur.			
Coordination of sucking, swallowing, and breathing	Sequences 20 or more sucks from the breast or bottle. Swallowing follows sucking with no discernable pauses when hungry. Pauses for breathing are infrequent. Occasional coughing or choking indicates poor coordination of sucking, swallowing, and breathing.			
Jaw, lip, and tongue movements	Uses only suckling and sucking patterns			
	4 to 6 Months			
Food transitions	Usually cereals and pureed foods are introduced. Usually the cup is introduced for liquids.			
	5 Months			
Food quantity	Takes 9 or 10 ounces of food or liquid per feeding, at 4 to 6 feedings per day			

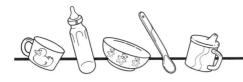

Pre-Feeding Checklist: A Global Approach (continued)

		Present— Spontaneous	Present With Facilitation	Not Present
5 or 6 Months				
Jaw movements in biting	Uses a primitive phasic bite-and-release pattern on a soft cookie. Biting rhythm is regular, and there is no controlled, sustained bite. May revert to sucking the cookie instead of biting it			
Jaw movements in chewing	Jaw movement is predominantly the primitive phasic bite-and-release pattern with a regular, stereotypic rhythm. May use diagonal rotary movements if food is placed on the side of the mouth for chewing or transfer to the middle of the mouth. May use intermittent nonstereotypic vertical movements with greater variability in up-down movement and speed			
Tongue and lip movements in chewing	Uses suckling or sucking patterns			
6 Months				
Food type	Is fed thin liquids and pureed foods			
Sucking liquids from breast or bottle	Uses a suckling or sucking pattern with the bottle or breast. No longer loses liquid during sucking, although may lose some when initiating or terminating the suck or as the nipple is removed			
Sucking liquids from a cup	Uses a suckling or sucking pattern or a mixture of sucking and suckling for cup drinking. Uses extension-retraction tongue motions during drinking or as the cup is offered or removed. Wide jaw excursions are common. Loses liquid			

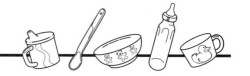

Pre-Feeding Checklist: A Global Approach (continued)

		Present— Spontaneous	Present With Facilitation	Not Present
	6 Months (continued)			
Sucking soft solids from a spoon	At 6 or 7 months, visually or tactilely recognizes the spoon. The jaw quiets and remains in a stable, open position until the spoon enters the mouth. The tongue quiets to accept the spoon.			
Swallowing liquids	At 6 to 8 months, swallows liquid from the cup with no observable elevated tongue-tip position. Tongue may move forward with extension-retraction during the swallow. This may alternate with a pattern of simple protrusion between the teeth. Lips may be open during the swallow. May lose liquid			
Swallowing semi-solids	Swallows some thicker pureed foods and tiny, soft, slightly noticeable lumps. May use simple tongue protrusion or extension-retraction movements. Food is not pushed out by the tongue, although minor losses of food occur.			
Coordination of sucking, swallowing, and breathing	Uses long sequences of sucking, swallowing, and breathing with breast or bottle. When taking liquids from a cup may have continuous sucks followed by uncoordinated swallowing. Much liquid is lost. Larger mouthfuls may result in coughing or choking.			
Jaw movements in chewing	Uses nonstereotypic vertical movements. Up-down pattern is more variable and less automatic than the phasic bite-and-release pattern. Uses diagonal rotary movement when moving the tongue to the side to assist with chewing food placed between the biting surface of the gums. Also may use the phasic bite-and-release pattern			

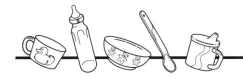

Pre-Feeding Checklist: A Global Approach (continued)

		Present—Spontaneous	Present With Facilitation	Not Present
6 Months (continued)				
Tongue movements in chewing	Tongue moves up and down in a munching pattern, with no lateralization when solid foods are placed in the center of the mouth. Some lateralization may occur when food is placed on the side, between the biting surfaces of the gums. Sucking movements may alternate with the munching and chewing patterns.			
Lip movements in chewing	Upper or lower lip draws slightly inward when food is left on it. When food is placed between the lateral biting surfaces of the gums, the cheek and lip on that side tighten asymmetrically to keep it in place for chewing. Does not yet use teeth and gums to clean food from the lips			
Control of drooling	Rarely drools in supine, prone, or sitting. May drool in these positions if babbling or when using hands for reaching, pointing, or manipulating objects; or when teething; or during or immediately after feeding or when given particular foods			
7 Months				
Feeding position	Is fed sitting, with the seat back at 90 degrees. External support is required for sitting (a restrainer, pillows, a tray, or a person).			
Food quantity	Takes 11 or more ounces of food and liquid per feeding, at four to six feedings per day			

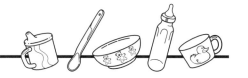

Pre-Feeding Checklist: A Global Approach (continued)

		Present—Spontaneous	Present With Facilitation	Not Present
	7 Months (continued)			
Tongue movements in chewing	Tongue begins to show more lateralization, with a gross rolling movement or simple horizontal shift when food is placed on the side, between the biting surfaces in the molar area.			
	8 Months			
Food types	Is given liquids, pureed foods, ground or junior foods, and mashed table foods			
Sucking soft solid food from a spoon	Upper lip moves downward and forward to posture or rest on the spoon and assist in food removal.			
	9 Months			
Feeding position	Is fed sitting, with the seat back at 90 degrees. No external support is needed. Security continues to be provided by the high chair, but the seat belt is used for safety, not support.			
Sucking liquids	Uses both the suckling and sucking patterns while drinking from the bottle or breast. No longer loses any liquid during sucking initiation or when the nipple is removed from the mouth			
Swallowing semi-solids	Uses an up-down sucking pattern. Simple tongue protrusion between the teeth or gums. Some extension-retraction of the tongue may continue intermittently.			

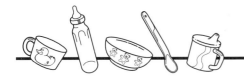

Pre-Feeding Checklist: A Global Approach (continued)

		Present—Spontaneous	Present With Facilitation	Not Present
	9 Months (continued)			
Coordination of sucking, swallowing, and breathing	Uses long sequences of continuous sucks during cup drinking. Still has difficulty coordinating sucks with swallowing and breathing. Although longer, coordinated sucks are possible, usually takes up to three sucks before stopping or pulling away from the cup to breathe			
Control of drooling	No longer drools when attempting newly acquired gross-motor skills, such as rolling and belly crawling. Drooling occurs during but not immediately before or after teething.			
Jaw movements in biting	Holds a soft cookie between the gums or teeth without biting all the way through. Maintains a quiet jaw and a holding posture as the feeder assists in breaking off a piece. With firmer cookies, may alternate this holding pattern with a phasic bite pattern			
Jaw movements in chewing	Primarily uses a nonstereotypic vertical movement with variations in the amount of up-down movement and speed. Uses diagonal rotary movements as the tongue moves from the center of the mouth to the side for chewing. Occasionally may use the phasic bite-and-release pattern when chewing food between the upper and lower central incisors			

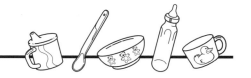

Pre-Feeding Checklist: A Global Approach (continued)

		Present— Spontaneous	Present With Facilitation	Not Present
	9 Months (continued)			
Tongue movements in chewing	Continues to use lateral tongue movements with ease when food is placed on the side of the mouth. Begins to transfer food from the center of the tongue to the side. May use intermittent extension-retraction movements with a difficult food transfer			
Lip movements in chewing	Lips are active with the jaw and make contact at the sides or in the center as the jaw moves up and down. Upper lip comes forward and down actively during chewing. Upper or lower lip draws inward when food is on it.			
	10 Months			
Sucking soft solids	Lower lip draws inward as the spoon is removed or if food remains on the lower lip. Upper lip actively moves forward, downward, and inward to remove food from the spoon.			
	12 Months			
Food types	Is given liquids and coarsely chopped table foods, including easily chewed meats			
Sucking liquids	May continue with the bottle or breast at bedtime, but takes liquid primarily from the cup. Uses a sucking pattern. Extension-retraction motion of the tongue is rare. Jaw excursions may be up-down or backward-forward. Tongue may protrude slightly beneath the cup to provide some additional stability. May lose liquid during sucking			

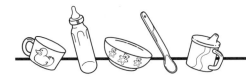

Pre-Feeding Checklist: A Global Approach (continued)

		Present—Spontaneous	Present With Facilitation	Not Present
	12 Months (continued)			
Food types	Is given liquids and coarsely chopped table foods, including easily chewed meats			
Sucking liquids	May continue with the bottle or breast at bedtime, but takes liquid primarily from the cup. Uses a sucking pattern. Extension-retraction motion of the tongue is rare. Jaw excursions may be up-down or backward-forward. Tongue may protrude slightly beneath the cup to provide some additional stability. May lose liquid during sucking			
Swallowing liquids	Swallows liquid from the cup with tongue tip elevated intermittently. May alternate this position with an extension-retraction pattern or simple tongue protrusion. Lips may be open during the swallow.			
Swallowing semi-solids	Swallows semi-solid foods with an intermittently elevated tongue-tip position. This tongue pattern may alternate with a pattern of simple tongue protrusion. Swallows with easy lip closure. No loss of food or saliva			
Swallowing solids	Swallows ground, mashed, or chopped table foods with noticeable lumps. Uses an intermittently elevated tongue tip, but may have simple tongue protrusion. No extension-retraction movements during swallowing			

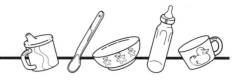

Pre-Feeding Checklist: A Global Approach (continued)

		Present— Spontaneous	Present With Facilitation	Not Present
	12 Months (continued)			
Coordination of sucking, swallowing, and breathing	When taking liquids from a cup, swallowing follows sucking with no pause. Sequences of at least three suck-swallows occur when thirsty. Intake during each suck-swallow is less than one ounce. Some coughing and choking may occur if the liquid flows too fast.			
Jaw movements in biting	Uses a controlled, sustained bite on a soft cookie. With a hard cookie, may not be able to sustain the bite (because of lack of teeth or weak biting power) and may revert to a phasic bite or sucking			
Tongue movements in chewing	Can transfer food from the center of the tongue to both sides of the mouth. Intermittent extension-retraction movements may occur with a difficult food transfer.			
Lip movements in chewing	Lips are active during chewing. Uses upper incisors or gums to clean food from the lower lip as it is drawn inward. May lose food or saliva while chewing			
	15 Months			
Sucking semi-solids from a spoon	Upper incisors are used to clean the lower lip as it draws inward. Uses a sucking pattern or a mixture of sucking and suckling. May playfully bite on the spoon, but the phasic bite reflex has been integrated and is no longer present			

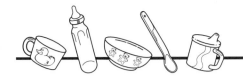

Pre-Feeding Checklist: A Global Approach (continued)

		Present— Spontaneous	Present With Facilitation	Not Present
	15 Months (continued)			
Coordination of sucking, swallowing, and breathing	When taking liquids from a cup, swallowing follows sucking with no pause. Pattern is well coordinated, and coughing and choking rarely occur. Sequences at least three suck-swallows while drinking one ounce or more without a major pause.			
Control of drooling	No longer drools when attempting newly acquired advanced gross-motor skills, such as walking and running. If cutting teeth, some drooling may occur			
Jaw movements in chewing	Diagonal rotary movements are smooth and well coordinated.			
Lip movements in chewing	Upper and lower lips are active during chewing and cleaning. Corner of the lip and the cheek draw inward to assist in controlling food placement and movement. This occurs more frequently, with a wide variety of food transfers in chewing.			
	18 Months			
Feeding position	Is fed sitting unsupported at the family table or at a small child's chair and table. The high chair is no longer needed for safety and security.			
Food types	Is given liquids and coarsely chopped table foods, including most meats and many raw vegetables			

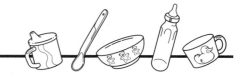

Pre-Feeding Checklist: A Global Approach (continued)

		Present—Spontaneous	Present With Facilitation	Not Present
	18 Months (continued)			
Sucking liquids from a cup	Uses a sucking pattern. External jaw stabilization is obtained by biting down on the edge of the cup. Upper lip is closed on the edge of the cup, providing a better seal for drinking. Tongue does not protrude from the mouth or rest beneath the cup. Minimal wide jaw excursions up-down or backward-forward if stabilization is not used			
Swallowing semi-solids	Tongue-tip elevation is used intermittently or consistently for swallowing. Simple tongue protrusion may occur during swallowing. No extension-retraction movements of the tongue			
Swallowing solids	Swallows solid foods with easy lip closure and no loss of food or saliva. Tongue-tip elevation used for swallowing. Some simple tongue protrusion may continue during swallowing.			
Control of drooling	No longer drools when attempting early fine-motor tasks, such as self-feeding, undressing, or random play. Drooling may occur if teething			
Jaw movements in biting	Uses a controlled, sustained bite on a hard cookie. May use overflow or associated arm or leg movements during biting. May pull the head backward into slight extension to assist with the bite			
Lip movements in chewing	Can chew with the lips closed, and does so intermittently. Lips are closed for chewing primarily when needed to prevent food from falling out. May lose food or saliva while chewing			

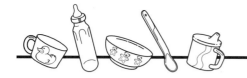

Pre-Feeding Checklist: A Global Approach (continued)

		Present—Spontaneous	Present With Facilitation	Not Present
	21 Months			
Jaw movements in biting	Uses a controlled, sustained bite on a hard cookie with no overflow or associated arm or leg movements. No longer extends the head to assist with biting. Opens the mouth wider than necessary to bite foods of various thicknesses			
	24 Months			
Sucking liquids from a cup	Uses an up-down sucking pattern, with the cup held between the lips. Internal jaw stabilization is emerging.			
Swallowing liquids	Swallows liquid from the cup with easy lip closure. No liquid loss during drinking or when the cup is removed from the lips. Elevated tongue position is used more consistently for swallowing.			
Swallowing solids	Swallows solid foods, including those with a combination of textures, with easy lip closure as needed. No loss of food or saliva. Tongue-tip elevation used for swallowing. No simple tongue protrusion during swallowing			
Control of drooling	No longer drools when attempting more advanced fine-motor tasks, such as drawing, fine finger movements, or two- or three-word speech combinations			
Tongue movements in chewing	Can transfer food from either side of the mouth to the other side without pausing in the center. Occasionally may use extension-retraction movements with a difficult food transfer			

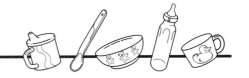

Pre-Feeding Checklist: A Global Approach (continued)

		Present— Spontaneous	Present With Facilitation	Not Present
24 Months (continued)				
Lip movements in chewing	Adequate lip movement during chewing. Can keep the lips closed during chewing, but does so only when needed to retain the food. No longer loses food or saliva			
Sucking liquids from a cup	Uses a sucking pattern and active internal jaw stabilization without biting the edge of the cup. Internal stabilization occurs most of the time during drinking sequences of more than two sucks. May use slight up-down jaw motions or hold the edge of the cup with the teeth			
Sucking semi-solids from a spoon	Tongue is used in a free, sweeping motion to clean food from the upper or lower lips. Tongue elevation and depression are independent of jaw movement. May be able to use skillful tongue-tip action. Slight lateral movements of the jaw may occur.			
Swallowing liquids	Tongue-tip elevation is used consistently for swallow. Swallowing occurs with no observable extension-retraction pattern and no tongue protrusion. Easy lip closure, with no loss of liquid during drinking or when the cup is removed from the lips			
Swallowing semi-solids	Swallows with no loss of food or saliva. Uses tongue-tip elevation for swallowing. No tongue protrusion			
Jaw movements in biting	Uses a controlled, sustained bite while keeping the head in midline when food is presented for biting on both sides of the mouth. Is able to grade the opening of the jaw when biting foods of various thicknesses			

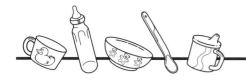

Pre-Feeding Checklist: A Global Approach (continued)

		Present—Spontaneous	Present With Facilitation	Not Present
	24 Months (continued)			
Jaw movements in chewing	Jaw movement continues to be a mixture of nonstereotypic and diagonal rotar movements. Uses circular rotary movements when transferring food across the midline from one side of the mouth to the other			
Tongue movements in chewing	Can transfer food rapidly and skill-fully from the center to the side, from the side to the center, and from side to side across midline. Uses precise tongue-tip elevation. No extension-retraction movements occur, even with difficult food transfers.			

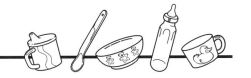

Developmental Pre-Feeding Checklist:
A Sequential Approach

Name _____ C.A. _____ Assessment date _____

Approximate Age	Skill	Present—Spontaneous	Present With Facilitation	Not Present
	Feeding Positions			
1 month	Supine with the head slightly elevated			
	OR			
	Prone			
	OR			
	Reclining at an angle of less than 45 degrees			
	OR			
	Sidelying			
3 months	Supported semi-sitting position, reclining at an angle of 45 to 90 degrees			
7 months	Sitting, with the seat back at 90 degrees. External support is required for sitting (a restrainer, pillows, a tray, or a person).			
9 months	Sitting, with the seat back at 90 degrees. No external support is needed. Security continues to be provided by the high chair, but the seat belt is used for safety, not support.			
18 months	Sitting unsupported at the family table or at a small child's table and chair. The high chair is no longer needed for safety and security.			

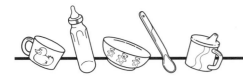

Pre-Feeding Checklist: A Sequential Approach (continued)

Approximate Age	Skill	Present— Spontaneous	Present With Facilitation	Not Present
	Food Quantity			
Birth to 1 month	Takes 2 to 6 ounces of liquid per feeding (six or more feedings per day)			
3 months	Takes 7 or 8 ounces of liquid per feeding (four to six feedings per day)			
5 months	Takes 9 or 10 ounces of food or liquid per feeding (four to six feedings per day)			
7 months	Takes 11 or more ounces of food and liquid per feeding (four to six feedings per day)			
	Food Types Eaten			
1 month	Is fed only liquids from the bottle or breast			
4 to 6 months	Is usually introduced to cereals and pureed foods			
8 months	Is given liquids, pureed foods, ground or junior foods, and mashed table foods			
12 months	Is given liquids and coarsely chopped table foods, including easily chewed meats			
18 months	Is given liquids and coarsely chopped table foods, including most meats and many raw vegetables			
	Sucking Liquids From the Bottle or Breast			
1 month	Suckling or sucking pattern with the bottle or breast. Loses some liquid during sucking.			

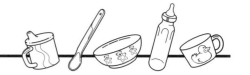

Pre-Feeding Checklist: A Sequential Approach (continued)

Approximate Age	Skill	Present—Spontaneous	Present With Facilitation	Not Present
	Sucking Liquids From the Bottle or Breast (continued)			
6 months	Suckling or sucking pattern with the bottle or breast. Does not lose liquid during sucking, although may lose some when initiating or terminating the suck or as the nipple is removed			
9 months	Uses both the suckling and sucking patterns while drinking from the bottle or breast. No longer loses any liquid during sucking initiation or when the nipple is removed from the mouth			
12 months	Takes liquid primarily from the cup. May continue with the bottle or breast at bedtime			
	Sucking Liquids From the Cup			
4 to 6 months	Is introduced to liquids from the cup			
6 to 8 months	Suckling pattern, or a mixture of sucking and suckling for cup drinking. Extension-retraction motions of the tongue during drinking or as the cup is offered or removed. Wide jaw excursions are common. Loses liquid			
12 months	Sucking pattern. Extension-retraction motion of the tongue is rare. Jaw excursions may be up-down or backward-forward. Tongue may protrude slightly beneath the cup to provide some additional stability. May lose liquid during sucking			

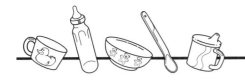

Pre-Feeding Checklist: A Sequential Approach (continued)

Approximate Age	Skill	Present—Spontaneous	Present With Facilitation	Not Present
	Sucking Liquids From the Cup (continued)			
18 months	Sucking pattern. External jaw stabilization is obtained by biting down on the edge of the cup. Upper lip is closed on the edge of the cup, providing a better seal for drinking. Tongue does not protrude from the mouth or rest beneath the cup. Minimal wide jaw excursions up-down or backward-forward if stabilization is not used			
24 months	Uses an up-down sucking pattern, with the cup held between the lips. Internal jaw stabilization is emerging.			
24 months +	Uses a sucking pattern and active internal jaw stabilization without biting the edge of the cup. Internal stabilization occurs most of the time during drinking sequences of more than two sucks. Slight up-down jaw motions or holding the edge of the cup with the teeth also may occur.			
	Sucking Soft Solid or Pureed Foods From the Spoon			
Under 3 months	Does not take food from a spoon.			
3 months	If soft or pureed foods are presented, uses a suckling or sucking pattern as food approaches or touches the lips. Lip does not assist in food removal.			

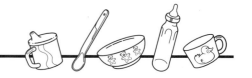

Pre-Feeding Checklist: A Sequential Approach (continued)

Approximate Age	Skill	Present— Spontaneous	Present With Facilitation	Not Present
	Sucking Soft Solid or Pureed Foods From the Spoon (continued)			
6 or 7 months	Visual or tactile recognition of the spoon. The jaw becomes quiet and remains in a stable, open position until the spoon enters the mouth. The tongue rests quietly to accept the spoon.			
8 months	Upper lip moves downward and forward to posture or rest on the spoon and assist in food removal.			
10 months	Lower lip draws inward as the spoon is removed or if food remains on the lower lip. Upper lip actively moves forward, downward, and inward to remove food from the spoon.			
15 months	Upper incisors are used to clean the lower lip as it draws inward. Uses a sucking pattern or a mixture of sucking and suckling. Playful biting on the spoon may occur, but the phasic bite reflex has been integrated and is not present.			
24 months +	Tongue is used in a free, sweeping motion to clean food from the upper or lower lips. Tongue elevation and depression are independent of jaw movement. Skillful tongue tip action may be present. Slight lateral movement of the jaw may occur.			
	Swallowing Liquids			
1 month	Swallows thin liquid with a suckle-swallow pattern. Tongue may protrude slightly through the lips with an extension-retraction movement.			

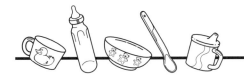

Pre-Feeding Checklist: A Sequential Approach (continued)

Approximate Age	Skill	Present— Spontaneous	Present With Facilitation	Not Present
	Swallowing Liquids (continued)			
6 to 8 months	Swallows liquid from the cup with no observable elevated tongue tip position. Tongue may move forward with an extension-retraction movement pattern during the swallow. This may alternate with a pattern of simple protrusion between the teeth. Lips may be open during the swallow. May lose liquid			
12 months	Swallows liquid from the cup with a tongue tip that is intermittently elevated. This position may alternate with an extension-retraction pattern or simple tongue protrusion. Lips may be open during the swallow			
24 months	Swallows liquid from the cup with easy lip closure. No liquid loss during drinking or when the cup is removed from the lips. Elevated tongue position is used more consistently for swallowing.			
24 months +	Tongue tip elevation is used consistently for swallow. Swallowing occurs with no observable extension-retraction pattern and no tongue protrusion. Easy lip closure, with no loss of liquid during drinking or when the cup is removed from the lips			

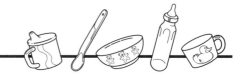

Pre-Feeding Checklist: A Sequential Approach (continued)

Approximate Age	Skill	Present— Spontaneous	Present With Facilitation	Not Present
	Swallowing Semi-Solids			
Under 3 months	Does not take semi-solids.			
3 months	If soft or pureed foods (semi-solids) are presented, uses a primitive suckle-swallow response to move food into the pharynx. Some food is pushed out of the mouth. Periodic choking, gagging, or vomiting can occur.			
6 or 7 months	Tongue shows an extension-retraction pattern or simple protrusion between the teeth or gums. Food is not pushed out by the tongue, although minor losses of food occur.			
9 months	Uses an up-down sucking pattern. Simple tongue protrusion between the teeth or gums. Some extension-retraction of the tongue may continue intermittently.			
12 months	Swallows semi-solid foods with an intermittently elevated tongue-tip position. This tongue pattern may alternate with a pattern of simple tongue protrusion. Swallows with easy lip closure. No loss of food or saliva			
18 months	Uses tongue tip elevation intermittently or consistently for swallowing. Simple tongue protrusion may occur during swallowing. No extension-retraction movements of the tongue			
24 months +	Swallows with no loss of food or saliva. Uses tongue tip elevation for swallowing. No tongue protrusion during swallowing			

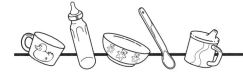

Pre-Feeding Checklist: A Sequential Approach (continued)

Approximate Age	Skill	Present— Spontaneous	Present With Facilitation	Not Present
	Swallowing Solids			
6 to 8 months	Swallows some thicker pureed foods and tiny, soft, slightly noticeable lumps. May use simple tongue protrusion or extension-retraction movements			
12 months	Swallows ground, mashed, or chopped table foods with noticeable lumps. Uses an intermittently elevated tongue tip, but may have simple tongue protrusion. No extension-retraction movements during swallowing			
18 months	Swallows solid foods with easy lip closure as needed. No loss of food or saliva. Tongue tip elevation used for swallowing. Some simple tongue protrusion may continue during swallowing.			
24 months +	Swallows solid foods, including those with a combination of textures, with easy lip closure as needed. No loss of food or saliva. Skillfully swallows foods that have a combination of textures. Tongue tip elevation used for swallowing. No simple tongue protrusion during swallowing			

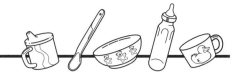

Pre-Feeding Checklist: A Sequential Approach (continued)

Approximate Age	Skill	Present— Spontaneous	Present With Facilitation	Not Present
	Jaw Movements in Chewing			
Under 5 months	Uses only suckling and sucking			
5 months	Jaw movement is predominantly the primitive phasic bite-and-release pattern with a regular, stereotypic rhythm. Diagonal rotary movements may occur if food is placed on the side of the mouth for chewing or transfer to the middle of the mouth. Nonstereotypic vertical movements with greater variability in up-down movement and speed may occur intermittently.			
6 months	Jaw movement consists primarily of nonstereotypic vertical movements. Up-down pattern is more variable and less automatic than the phasic bite-and-release pattern. Diagonal rotary movement of the jaw occurs when the tongue moves to the side to assist with chewing food placed between the biting surface of the gums. The phasic bite-and-release pattern also may occur.			
9 months	Jaw movement is primarily a nonstereotypic vertical movement with variations in the amount of up-down movement and speed. Diagonal rotary movements occur as the tongue moves from the center of the mouth to the side for chewing. Phasic bite-and-release pattern may occur occasionally when chewing food between the upper and lower central incisors.			
15 months	Diagonal rotary movements are smooth and well-coordinated.			

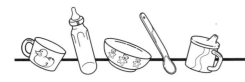

Pre-Feeding Checklist: A Sequential Approach (continued)

Approximate Age	Skill	Present— Spontaneous	Present With Facilitation	Not Present
	Jaw Movements in Chewing (continued)			
24 months +	Jaw movement in chewing continues to be a mixture of nonstereotypic and diagonal rotary movements. Circular rotary movements occur when transferring food across the midline from one side of the mouth to the other.			
	Tongue Movements in Chewing			
Under 6 months	Uses sucking or suckling patterns.			
6 months	Tongue moves up and down in a munching pattern, with no lateralization when solid foods are placed in the center of the mouth. Some lateralization may occur when food is placed on the side, between the biting surfaces of the gums. Sucking movements may alternate with the munching/chewing patterns.			
7 months	Tongue begins to show more lateralization, with a gross rolling movement or simple horizontal shift when food is placed on the side, between the biting surfaces in the molar area.			
9 months	Lateral tongue movements continue to occur with ease when food is placed on the side of the mouth. Begins to transfer food from the center of the tongue to the side. Intermittent extension-retraction movements may occur occasionally with a difficult food transfer.			

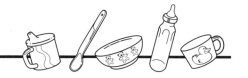

Pre-Feeding Checklist: A Sequential Approach (continued)

Approximate Age	Skill	Present—Spontaneous	Present With Facilitation	Not Present
	Tongue Movements in Chewing (continued)			
12 months	Can transfer food from the center of the tongue to both sides of the mouth. Intermittent extension-retraction movements may occur with a difficult food transfer.			
24 months	Can transfer food from either side of the mouth to the other side without pausing in the center. Extension-retraction movements may occur occasionally with a difficult food transfer.			
24 months +	Can transfer food rapidly and skillfully from the center to the side, from the side to the center, and from side to side across midline. Uses precise tongue tip elevation movements. No extension-retraction movements occur, even with difficult food transfers.			
	Lip Movements in Chewing			
Under 6 months	Uses sucking or suckling motions.			
6 months	Upper or lower lip draws slightly inward when food is left on it. When food is placed between the lateral biting surfaces of the gums, the cheek and lip on that side tighten asymmetrically to keep it in place for chewing. Does not yet use teeth and gums to clean food from the lips			
9 months	Lips are active with the jaw during chewing, and make contact at the sides or in the center as the jaw moves up and down. Upper lipcomes forward and down actively during chewing. Upper or lower lip draws inward when food is on the lip.			

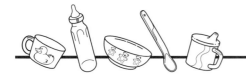

Pre-Feeding Checklist: A Sequential Approach (continued)

Approximate Age	Skill	Present— Spontaneous	Present With Facilitation	Not Present
	Lip Movements in Chewing (continued)			
12 months	Lips are active during chewing. Uses upper incisors or gums to clean food from the lower lip as it is drawn inward. May lose food or saliva while chewing			
15 months	Upper and lower lips are active during chewing and cleaning. Corner of the lip and the cheek draw inward to assist in controlling food placement and movement. This occurs more frequently, with a wide variety of food transfers in chewing.			
18 months	Can chew with the lips closed, and does so intermittently. Lips are closed for chewing primarily when needed to prevent food from falling out. May lose food or saliva while chewing			
24 months	Adequate lip movement during chewing. Can keep the lips closed during chewing, but does so only when needed to retain the food. No longer loses food or saliva			
	Coordination of Sucking, Swallowing, and Breathing			
1 month	Sequences two or more sucks from the breast or bottle before pausing to breathe or swallow.			
3 months	Sequences twenty or more sucks from the breast or bottle. Swallowing follows sucking with no discernible pauses when hungry. Pauses for breathing are infrequent. Occasional coughing or choking indicates poor coordination of sucking, swallowing, and breathing.			

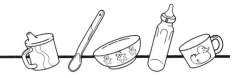
Pre-Feeding Checklist: A Sequential Approach (continued)

Approximate Age	Skill	Present— Spontaneous	Present With Facilitation	Not Present
	Coordination of Sucking, Swallowing, and Breathing (continued)			
6 months	Uses long sequences of sucking, swallowing, and breathing, with breast or bottle. When taking liquids from a cup, may have continuous sucks followed by uncoordinated swallowing. Much liquid is lost. Larger mouthfuls may result in choking or coughing.			
9 months	Uses long sequences of continuous sucks during cup drinking. Still has difficulty coordinating sucks with swallowing and breathing. Although longer, coordinated sucks are possible, usually takes up to three sucks before stopping or pulling away from the cup to breathe.			
12 months	When taking liquids from a cup, swallowing follows sucking with no pause. Sequences of at least three suck-swallows occur when thirsty. Intake during each suck-swallow is less than one ounce. Some coughing and choking may occur if the liquid flows too fast.			
15 months	When taking liquids from a cup, swallowing follows sucking with no pause. Pattern is well coordinated, and coughing and choking rarely occur. Sequences at least three suck-swallows while drinking one ounce or more without a major pause			

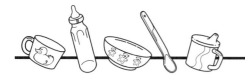

Pre-Feeding Checklist: A Sequential Approach (continued)

Approximate Age	Skill	Present— Spontaneous	Present With Facilitation	Not Present
	Control of Drooling			
1 month	Rarely drools because of minimal saliva production.			
6 months	Rarely drools in supine, prone, or sitting. May drool in these positions if babbling or when using hands for reaching, pointing, or manipulating objects			
	OR			
	May drool due to teething			
	OR			
	Drools only or primarily during or immediately after feeding or when given particular foods			
9 months	No longer drools when attempting newly acquired gross motor skills, such as rolling and belly crawling. Drooling occurs during but not immediately before or after teething.			
15 months	No longer drools when attempting newly acquired gross motor skills, such as walking and running. If cutting teeth, some drooling may occur.			
18 months	No longer drools when attempting early fine motor tasks, such as self-feeding, undressing, or random play. Drooling may occur if teething.			
24 months	No longer drools when attempting more advanced fine motor tasks, such as drawing, fine finger movements, or two- or three-word speech combinations.			

Reproducible Forms

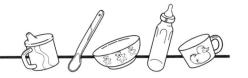

Pre-Feeding Checklist: A Sequential Approach (continued)

Approximate Age	Skill	Present— Spontaneous	Present With Facilitation	Not Present
	Jaw Movements in Biting			
5 or 6 months	Uses a primitive phasic bite-and-release pattern on a soft cookie. Biting rhythm is regular, and there is no controlled, sustained bite. May revert to sucking the cookie instead of biting it.			
9 months	Holds a soft cookie between the gums or teeth without biting all the way through. Maintains a quiet jaw and holding posture as the feeder assists in breaking off a piece. With firmer cookies, may alternate this holding pattern with a phasic bite pattern.			
18 months	Uses a controlled, sustained bite on a hard cookie. May use overflow or associated arm or leg movements during biting. May pull the head backward into slight extension to assist with the bite			
21 months	Uses a controlled, sustained bite on a hard cookie with no overflow or associated arm or leg movements. No longer extends the head to assist with biting. Opens the mouth wider than necessary to bite foods of various thicknesses			
24 months +	Uses a controlled, sustained bite while keeping the head in midline when food is presented for biting on both sides of the mouth. Is able to grade the opening of the jaw when biting foods of various thicknesses			

Appendix B
Spanish Translations
of Parent Questionnaires

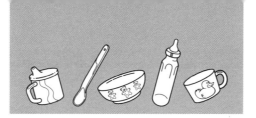

Cuestionario Alimenticio Para Padres
Habilidades de Comer y Beber

Nombre del niño   Fecha dia de hoy

Fecha de nacimiento   Edad del niño

Nombre de padre(s)

Médico principal

Nombre de padre llenando el cuestionario

Historia Clínica e Inquietudes con Respecto al Comer y Beber

¿Tiene algunas inquietudes con respecto a la alimentación de su hijo? Descríbalas.

¿De cuáles enfermedades ha sufrido su hijo? ¿Le han hecho cirugías?

¿Le da medicaciones a su hijo? ¿Cuáles?

¿Cuáles evaluaciones o estudios de alimentación le han hecho a su hijo?

¿Han consultado con un dietista? Si lo han hecho, favor de anotar el nombre y la frecuencia de las consultas.

¿Está recibiendo terapia su hijo? Si contestó sí, ¿de qué tipo y con cuál terapeuta?

¿Asiste su hijo a un programa preescolar o de escuela? Si contestó sí, favor de anotar el sitio.

(continuado)

Describa las primeras etapas de la alimentación de su hijo:

☐ ¿Fue amamantado?   ¿Por cuanto tiempo?   ¿Hubo problemas?

☐ ¿Usó biberón?   ¿Hubo problemas?

¿Cuál tipo de formula le dió/da de comer a su bebé?

¿Cómo toleró la formula su bebé?

¿Cuándo introdució los purés (e.j., First Foods o hechos en casa)?

¿Cómo reaccióno su hijo al probar el puré?

¿Cómo se acomodó al avanzár de puré a comidas grumosas y sólidos?

¿Cuándo empezaron los problemas de alimentación?

Rutina Actual de Alimentación

¿Con qué frecuencia come y bebe su hijo? ¿Cuáles son sus horas normales para comer y tomar bocados?

¿Cuáles comidas/bebidas le da normalmente a su hijo para:

¿el desayuno?

¿la comida ("lonche")?

¿la cena?

¿bocaditos entre comidas?

(continuado)

¿Cómo está preparada la comida? (Indique todos los que se apliquen.)

☐ Líquido regular

☐ Líquido espeso

☐ Comida comercial para bebé de First o Second Foods

☐ Preparada en la licuadora

☐ Comida molida o comercial de Third Foods

☐ Comida de mesa blandita

☐ Comida regular de mesa (fácil)

☐ Comida regular de mesa (difícil)

☐ Otra (por favor sea específico)

¿Cuáles de estas comidas maneja su hijo con facilidad?

¿Cuáles de estas comidas maneja su hijo con dificultad?

¿Qué usa normalmente para alimentar a su hijo? (Indique todos los que sean aplicables.)

☐ Pecho	☐ Tenedor	☐ Biberón
☐ Dedos	☐ Taza	☐ Popote
☐ Cuchara		

¿Cuáles de los siguientes puede usar su hijo él solo?

☐ Tenedor	☐ Cuchara	☐ Biberón
☐ Dedos	☐ Taza	☐ Popote

¿Prefiere su hijo ciertos sabores? ¿Cuáles?

¿Prefiere su hijo ciertas texturas de comida? ¿Cuáles?

¿Prefiere su hijo la comida a ciertas temperaturas (e.j., fría, tibia, caliente, al tiempo)?

(continuado)

¿Quién normalmente le da de comer a su hijo?

¿Quién más puede darle de comer a su hijo?

¿Dónde le da de comer a su hijo (e.j., en una silla, sentado en sus piernas)?

¿Cuánto tiempo toma para darle de comer a su hijo?

¿Qué cantidad, de promedio, de comida y líquido ingiere su hijo dentro de ese tiempo?

¿Sufre su hijo de alergias a ciertas comidas?

¿Sufre de alergias algún familiar (e.j., a comidas, sustancias químicas, polen o mohos)?

¿Tiene problemas su hijo con:
    ¿Ahogo, nauseas? (Favor de describir)

    ¿Reflujo gastroesofágico? (Favor de describir)

    ¿Vómitos? (Favor de describir)

    ¿Estreñimiento? (Favor de describir)

Otros comentarios:

_____

Firma de padre

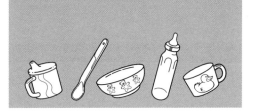

Cuestionario Alimenticio Para Padres
Nutrición Enteral con Tubo y Alimentación Oral de Primeras Etapas

Nombre del niño   Fecha dia de hoy

Fecha de nacimiento   Edad del niño

Nombre de padre(s)

Médico principal

Nombre de padre llenando el cuestionario

Historia Clínica e Inquietudes con Respecto a la Nutrición por Tubo

¿Tiene algunas inquietudes con respecto a la alimentación de su hijo? Descríbalas.

¿De cuáles enfermedades ha sufrido su hijo? ¿Le han hecho cirugías?

¿Le da medicaciónes a su hijo? ¿Cuáles?

¿Cuáles evaluaciones o estudios de alimentación le han hecho a su hijo?

¿Han consultando con un dietista? Si lo han hecho, favor de anotar el nombre y la frecuencia de las consultas.

¿Esta recibiendo terapia su hijo? Si contestó sí, ¿de qué tipo y con cuál terapeuta?

¿Asiste su hijo a un programa preescolar o de escuela? Si contestó sí, favor de anotar el sitio.

Describa las primeras etapas de la alimentación de su hijo:
- ☐ ¿Fue amamantado?   ¿Por cuanto tiempo?   ¿Hubo problemas?
- ☐ ¿Usó biberón?   ¿Por cuanto tiempo?   ¿Hubo problemas?

¿Cuál tipo de formula le dió/da de comer a su bebé?

(continuado)

¿Cómo toleró la formula su bebé?

¿Cuándo introdució los pures (e.j., First Foods o hechos en casa)?

¿Cómo reaccióno su hijo al probar el puré?

¿Cómo se acomodó al avanzár de puré a comidas grumosas y sólidos?

¿Cuando empezaron los problemas de alimentación?

Describa la historia de alimentación por tubo de su hijo.

¿Cuáles exámenes diagnosticos se han hecho? ¿Cuando?

¿Qué tipo de tubo usa su hijo?
- ☐ ¿Nasogástrico?
- ☐ ¿Gastrostomia?   ¿De qué tipo?   ☐ ¿Botón?   ☐ ¿Yeyunostomia?
- ☐ ¿Catéter?
- ☐ ¿Otro?

¿Porqué usa tubo de alimentación su hijo?

¿Cuándo le colocaron el tubo a su hijo?

¿Quién colocó el tubo? ¿Dónde?

(continuado)

¿Tuvo su hijo una funduplicatura?

¿Cómo reaccionó su hijo a la funduplicatura?

¿Cuál médico supervisa a su hijo mientras se le alimenta por tubo?

¿Cómo se ha acostumbrado su hijo al tubo?

Rutina Actual de Alimentación

¿Cuál formula usa para alimentar a su hijo por tubo?

¿Quién le da de comer a su hijo normalmente?

¿Quién más le puede dar de comer a su hijo?

¿Dónde le da de comer por tubo a su hijo (e.j., en una silla, sentado en sus piernas, en la cama)?

¿Cuál horario siguen las alimentaciones por tubo de su hijo?

    ¿De día?

    ¿De noche?

¿Si usa bolo alimenticio, cuanto dura cada alimentación?

¿Experimentan usted o su hijo dificultades con la alimentación por tubo? Si existen problemas (e.j., cantidad, regulación, náusea, ahogo, vómito), por favor descríbalos. ¿Cuando ocurren, y como los maneja?

(continuado)

Llene lo siguiente si su hijo ingiere comida o líquido por la boca.

¿Quién le da de comer a su hijo normalmente?

¿Dónde le da de comer a su hijo normalmente (e.j., en una silla, sentado en sus piernas, en la cama)?

¿Cuáles comidas o líquidos le ofrece a su hijo?

¿Prefiere su hijo ciertos sabores? ¿Cuáles?

¿Prefiere su hijo ciertas texturas de comida? ¿Cuáles?

¿Prefiere su hijo la comida a ciertas temperaturas (e.j., fría, tibia, caliente, al tiempo)?

¿Cuanto dura cáda alimentación oral?

¿Experimentan usted o su hijo dificultades al comienzo de alimentaciones orales? Si hay problemas (e.j., interés, tos, movimientos de boca), por favor descríbalos. ¿Cuando ocurren y como los maneja?

¿Sufre su hijo de alergias a la comida o otras cosas?

¿Sufre algún familiar de alergias (e.j., comida, sustancias químicas, polen, moho)?

(continuado)

¿Tiene su hijo problemas con:

¿Ahogo, nauseas? (favor de describir.)

¿Reflujo gastroesofágico? (favor de describir)

¿Vómito? (favor de describir)

¿Estreñimiento? (favor de describir)

Otros comentarios:

_____

Firma de padre

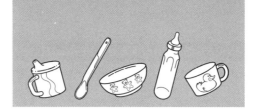

Cuestionario Para Padres
con Respecto a Reflujo Gastroesofágico

Nombre del niño   Fecha dia de hoy

Fecha de nacimiento   Edad del niño

Nombre de padre(s)

Médico principal

Nombre de padre llenando el cuestionario

Historia Clínica y de Alimentación

Historia clínica

Especialistas que consulta su hijo

Historia de alimentación

¿Está usted o su médico preocupado sobre el crecimiento de su hijo?	☐ Sí	☐ No
Peso actual _____		
Estatura actual _____		
Proporción de peso a estatura _____		
Circunferencia de cabeza _____		
¿Está disponible una tabla de crecimiento actualizada? Si contestó sí, ¿donde?	☐ Sí	☐ No
¿Ha estado ronco su hijo?	☐ Sí	☐ No
¿Tiene historia de bronquitis su hijo?	☐ Sí	☐ No
¿Tiene historia de neumonía su hijo?	☐ Sí	☐ No
¿Tiene historia de asma su hijo?	☐ Sí	☐ No
¿Tiene historia su hijo de enfermedades reactivas de la vía aérea superior?	☐ Sí	☐ No
¿Tiene historia su hijo de infecciones del sistema respiratorio?	☐ Sí	☐ No
¿Despierta su hijo durante la noche? Si contestó sí, ¿con qué frecuencia?	☐ Sí	☐ No
¿Babea su hijo? Si contestó sí, ¿con qué frecuencia?	☐ Sí	☐ No
¿Hace muecas su hijo cuando traga?	☐ Sí	☐ No
¿Ha sufrido su hijo de apnea? Si contestó sí, descríbalo.	☐ Sí	☐ No

(continuado)

¿Tiene su hijo infecciones del oído Si contestó sí, ¿con qué frecuencia?	☐ Sí	☐ No

¿Tiene o ha tenido su hijo un tubo de gastrostomia? Si contestó sí, descríbalo.	☐ Sí	☐ No

¿Es su hijo alegre o irritable? Descríbalo	☐ Sí	☐ No

¿Sufre dolor su hijo cuando come? Si contestó sí, descríbalo.	☐ Sí	☐ No

¿Ha recibido su hijo tratamiento para reflujo gastroesofágico? ¿Si contestó sí, cuál fue el tratamiento?	☐ Sí	☐ No

Medicaciones actuales

¿Sufre su hijo de estreñimiento? ¿Con qué frecuencia evacúa su hijo?	☐ Sí	☐ No

Rutina Actual de Hora de Comer

¿Cuál rutina y horario sigue para darle de comer a su hijo?

Formula actual	Cantidad de formula	Por día

Indique otras formulas qué su hijo ha probado.

¿En qué posición alimenta a su hijo?

¿Escupe su hijo la comida? Si contestó sí, describalo.	☐ Sí	☐ No

¿Cuantas veces al dia arroja su hijo?		
¿Son episodios de vómito fuerte?	☐ Sí	☐ No
¿Escupe su hijo cada semana? ¿Día?	☐ Sí ☐ Sí	☐ No ☐ No
¿Toce su hijo antes de arrojar?	☐ Sí	☐ No

Describa la cantidad actual de vómito.

Cuando su hijo arroja:		
¿Es despues de comer?	☐ Sí	☐ No
¿Es durante la comida?	☐ Sí	☐ No
¿Es entre comidas?	☐ Sí	☐ No
¿Es dentro de una hora de la proxima comida?	☐ Sí	☐ No

Es más probable qué arroje:
   ☐ Líquidos   ☐ Sólidos   ☐ Líquidos y sólidos

(continuado)

¿Tiene buen apetito su hijo?   ☐ Sí   ☐ No
Descríbalo.

_____

Apunte comidas que su hijo disfruta.

_____

Apunte comidas que su hijo no disfruta.

_____

¿Hay comidas que le causan náusea a su hijo?   ☐ Sí   ☐ No
Si contestó sí, ¿cuáles comidas?

_____

¿Le costó dificultad a su hijo cambiar de líquidos a pures?   ☐ Sí   ☐ No
¿Le costó dificultad a su hijo cambiar de pures a sólidos?   ☐ Sí   ☐ No
Comentarios

Mealtime Participation Experiences

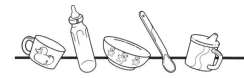

5. Retraction Patterns

Purpose

To simulate retraction patterns of movement and explore their influences on eating and drinking

Materials

Thin liquid (e.g., water or juice)

Soft, smooth food (e.g., yogurt, pudding, or applesauce)

Cracker

Raisins

Teaspoon

Cup

Guide

In this exercise you will think "pull back," and retract each part of your body. Exaggerate the retraction to better experience this limiting factor on function. As you retract each part, play with degrees of retraction and degrees of tightness. Be very retracted or just a little bit retracted. Try to focus on each individual body part and isolate it—noticing how the retraction feels in contrast with your usual muscle tone and movement patterns. As you try to retract each part in isolation from the rest of your body, notice which other body parts are affected by the retraction pattern. Notice when it affects function.

Retract your shoulders

...your neck

...your arm

...your jaw

...your lips and cheeks

...your tongue

Take several small sips of liquid from your cup in the way you normally would, appreciating the whole process. Notice the involvement of your body, mouth, sense of taste, and your general impressions of drinking this liquid. Do not analyze the parts. Just get the big picture. Slow things down so that you can pay attention to exactly what is happening. This will be your contrast experience as you explore what happens when you drink with retraction patterns.

With your shoulder girdle retracted, pick up your cup again and take a drink. Gradually add jaw retraction as you drink. Add lip and cheek retraction. Finally, add tongue retraction.

Notice how the retraction pattern in your body and mouth influences your ability to drink. Play with different combinations of retraction in the mouth. Discover the feeling of tongue retraction by itself and tongue retraction combined with lip retraction. As you drink, explore differing amounts of retraction. Try extreme retraction. Now try a milder degree of retraction. Notice the amount of body and mouth retraction that affects your ability to drink easily and skillfully.

Be aware of the challenges you experience as you drink with retraction patterns. Be aware of any changes or compensations you make to succeed in drinking the liquid.

When you have finished your exploration of drinking from the cup, **repeat this activity with each of the following foods.**

Notice what happens to your body and mouth as you try each food with a retraction pattern. Be aware of differences in your skill with each food and the compensations you use to succeed.

- Take a smooth food from a spoon.
- Bite through and chew a cracker.
- Chew several raisins.

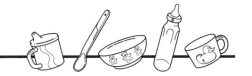

If You Have Time

Think of a person you know who has retraction patterns of movement. Pretend you are this individual. Use your body to sit and eat in the same way as this individual. Discover the eating challenges this person might encounter.

Discussion

How did retraction patterns in one part of your body affect other parts of your body?

What happened in your mouth when you tried to eat or drink each food when you were imitating a retraction pattern?

How did the intensity of the pattern influence your ability to eat and drink? How much retraction was too much?

How did the retraction pattern affect your ability to drink and eat the different foods?

Which food or liquid was easiest? Which the most difficult? Why?

Which retraction patterns in your mouth most affected your ability to eat and drink?

What did you do differently to succeed despite this limitation? What compensations did you use?

Did you enjoy your meal?

Do you think you would have responded differently if someone else had been feeding you?

Summary Theme

Body. Simulating retraction patterns is one way to build understanding of their influence on the mealtime skills of individuals with feeding issues. As we attempt to isolate the retraction in one part of the body, we are aware that it influences tone and function of other body parts. In general, the more proximal the retraction, the more global the effect. Retraction in the shoulders strongly influences overall posture and provides a poor base for the more distal movements of the head, neck, and oral area. As we look at compensations in each challenge, we notice that we can adjust for retraction in the body. We usually do this by shrugging our shoulders tightly and extending our head. This puts stress and tension on the entire oral-motor structures for eating.

Drinking. The neck and jaw are the most proximal parts of the oral-motor system. The more distal parts such as the lips, cheeks, and tongue rely on the stability and tone of the neck and jaw to provide the foundation for more controlled movement. When the neck is extended and the jaw is retracted, all skills in eating become more difficult. The lips, cheeks, and tongue usually are less controlled when trying to function on the foundation of retraction.

There can be considerable spillage in taking a sip of water. The jaw may have difficulty closing sufficiently and providing the forward, controlled stability necessary for supporting the cup. The lateral lips can lose much of the liquid because of their pulled-back, retracted, position. Many people will develop compensation strategies to prevent this loss of liquid.

Spoon. The lower lip provides a stable place for the spoon to rest. Without the controlled jaw as a foundation, the lips cannot function efficiently. The retracted jaw interferes with smooth functioning of the lips and cheeks. The upper lip may have difficulty connecting smoothly with the lower lip to take food from the spoon because of the retracted pull. The central portion of the upper lip may have trouble moving separately from the lateral lips to take food from spoons with deep bowls. Most people develop some type of compensatory strategy to prevent food loss.

Biting and chewing. The jaw provides the power to bite through foods. When the lower jaw is retracted, the teeth are no longer in proper alignment, and both the control and force of biting are reduced. Biting involves holding the food and controlling jaw movement in a graded fashion so that the teeth move through the food. A cracker usually is held momentarily between the teeth and then bitten with just the right amount of downward pressure. When the jaw is tense and pulled back, biting and chewing become almost impossible! Most people develop some type of compensatory

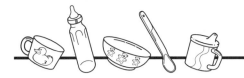

strategy to bite the food and manipulate it in the mouth for chewing.

Chewing a cracker requires both the upper and lower jaws to work together to break up the food. A retracted jaw, cheeks, lips, and tongue make it difficult to chew more complicated foods. Chewing requires the food to be over the teeth. The tongue, influenced by retraction patterns, usually cannot move freely enough to place food over the teeth. Many foods may be swallowed whole.

Summary Variations

Body. Many individuals compensate for retraction in the shoulders and jaw by tipping their head back into extension while eating and drinking. The amount of head-position compensation depends on the degree and intensity of the retraction. This pattern also is used as a strategy to prevent food or liquid from falling out of the mouth.

Drinking. People can use a wide variety of compensations while drinking with retraction patterns. Some tip their heads back and pour the liquid in. Others push the rim of the cup firmly into the lip corners to provide control not offered by the restricted freedom of movement often seen in a retraction pattern. They may have neck and swallowing tightness as they shrug and retract their shoulders tightly. Preparing the bolus for swallowing and the swallow itself may be difficult. Tipping the head back also is the most common compensation to prevent liquid from falling out of the mouth.

Spoon. Retraction in the lips and cheeks may result in difficulty removing food from a spoon. People can use a wide variety of compensations while taking food from the spoon. Some people tip their heads back and dump the food in the mouth. Others scrape the food off the spoon with their upper teeth so as not to use the lips in food removal. The type of compensation will depend upon the amount of retraction in the face and the type of food and utensil. Tipping the head back is the most common compensation to prevent food from falling out of the mouth.

Biting and chewing. People can use a wide variety of strategies to compensate for retraction of the jaw, lips, cheeks, and tongue in biting and chewing. Some people cannot bite through foods at all because of the retraction and tension in the jaw. Some break off pieces of cracker and place them over the teeth with their fingers. Others break the food using the teeth without any help or stability from the retracted lips.

Chewing is extremely difficult when the jaw, cheeks, and lips are retracted. When the tongue is retracted, movements are quite limited. The tongue moves most frequently toward an inward and backward direction, compatible with the overall pattern of retraction. Some limited backward-forward movements also may be present. The lateral movements needed for placement of food over the teeth usually are absent, or occur with difficulty. It is easy to choke and difficult to eat a wide variety of foods. Tipping the head back is the most common compensation to prevent food from falling out of the mouth.

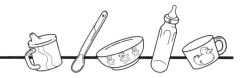

1. Smooth Food From a Spoon

Purpose

To experience the body and mouth patterns used when feeding yourself a smooth food from a spoon

Materials

Smooth food (e.g., applesauce, pureed baby fruit, yogurt, or pudding)

Teaspoon

Guide

Take several small spoonfuls of the smooth food in the way you normally would, appreciating the whole process. Notice the involvement of your body, mouth, sense of taste, and your general impressions of eating this food. Do not analyze the parts yet. Just get the big picture.

Now, try another mouthful—this time in slow motion. Slow things down so that you can pay attention to exactly what is happening.

Notice how you get food from the container.

Notice what happens to your body and mouth as you bring the spoon toward your mouth.

Notice what happens as you put the spoon in your mouth.

Notice your jaw, your cheeks and lips, and your tongue.

Notice how you move the food to the back of your mouth to swallow.

Discussion

What happened to your body in anticipation of each bite?

What did your mouth do as the spoon approached?

How and where did the spoon and food come into the mouth?

How did you get food off the spoon?

What did you do with the food when it was in your mouth?

How did you get it to the back of your mouth?

What happened when you swallowed?

Summary Theme

As we feed ourselves, we prepare our body and mouth ahead of time for the presentation of the spoon and food. We may bring our upper body slightly forward to meet our arm and hand as the spoon approaches the mouth. The mouth usually opens slightly before the spoon reaches the mouth. The jaw is stable, and the tongue is quiet. As the jaw begins to move upward, the upper lip moves downward to help remove food from the spoon. The lower lip may draw inward for cleaning after the spoon is removed from the mouth. Once the food is in the mouth, the tongue and cheeks work together to gather it into a bolus that can be moved backward for the swallow. The tongue elevates and propels the bolus of food backward for a swallow. When we swallow, we hold our breath briefly to protect our airway. The larynx elevates, which provides airway protection and opens the cricopharyngeus muscle at the top of the esophagus.

Summary Variations

Preparation. Some people bring the upper body and mouth forward to meet the spoon. Others simply bring the arm, hand, and spoon to the mouth.

Mouth opening. The amount of mouth opening will vary depending on the size of the spoon and the amount of food. A wider opening may be used if you like the food, and a smaller opening may be used if

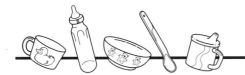

the taste is unclear or the food is less preferred. The tongue may be forward in the mouth, or even slightly protruding. The degree of flattening and cupping of the tongue will vary among participants.

Spoon entry. The spoon may enter the mouth in the center or slightly to the right or left. It may be placed directly on the tongue or have very little direct contact with the tongue.

Food removal. The upper lip usually is involved in removing food from the spoon. However, the degree of involvement may vary. Some people use their upper teeth to scrape food from the spoon.

Moving the food in the mouth. You may move food rapidly in the mouth, using the tongue and cheeks to keep it in the middle. The amount and type of cheek and tongue action varies with the size of the mouthful, the speed of eating, and the amount of pleasurable tasting.

Swallowing. The actual swallow is similar in all adults. However, there will be variations in the number of swallows used to clear the mouth.

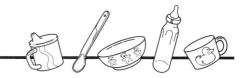

15. Lip Variations in Spoon Feeding

Purpose

To experience lip and cheek movement variations while eating from a spoon

Materials

Smooth food (e.g., applesauce, pureed baby fruit, yogurt, or pudding)

Teaspoon

Partners

Guide

Take several small spoonfuls of the smooth food in the way you normally would, appreciating the whole process. Notice the involvement of your body, mouth, sense of taste, and your general impressions of eating this food. Do not analyze the parts yet. Just get the big picture. This will be your contrast experience of your normal lip usage.

Now take more mouthfuls, each time trying a different variation in lip and cheek control, including:

- Very relaxed or low-toned lips and cheeks
- Pulled-back or retracted lips and cheeks
- Pursed lips with tense cheeks

Slow things down so that you can pay attention to exactly what is happening with the lips as you compare these variations with each other and with your contrast experience.

Notice what happens to your body and mouth as you bring the spoon toward your mouth.

Notice what happens as you put the spoon in your mouth.

Notice your jaw, cheeks and lips, and tongue.

Notice specifically what your lips and cheeks do as the food approaches.

Notice the activity of each lip and the parts of each lip as food is removed from the spoon.

Notice how your lips and cheeks help as you manipulate the food in your mouth.

Notice your lip and cheek involvement as you move the food to the back of your mouth to swallow.

Discussion

What did your trunk, head, and neck do as the spoon approached?

What happened to your lips as the spoon approached?

How did your cheeks and jaw help as the lips moved? What happened with each lip variation?

What did your lower lip do in food removal from the spoon? What happened with each lip variation?

How did your upper lip help remove food from the spoon?

What happened with each lip variation?

What did the corners of your lips and cheeks do as the food was removed from the spoon? What happened with each lip variation?

Did the center of your lips work separately from the lateral lips? What happened with each lip variation?

What parts of your lips are in contact with the spoon and when? What happened with each lip variation?

How and where did you get the stability needed for the movement of the lips? What happened with each lip variation?

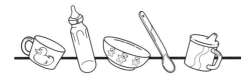

What happened to the lips as the food was being manipulated in the mouth and prepared for swallowing? What happened with each lip variation?

Which lip and cheek variation created the greatest overall challenge for you? Which variation was the most uncomfortable? Why?

Summary Theme

Typical lip activity. The lips, cheeks, and jaw work together during eating. The jaw provides the stability from which the lips and cheeks work when removing food from the spoon. The cheeks and lips automatically work together. It is difficult for one to work without the other because muscle fibers from the cheeks help form the obicularis oris muscle of the lips.

The lips open in anticipation of the spoon. The amount of mouth opening will vary, depending on the size of the spoon and the amount of food. A wider opening may be used for preferred foods, and a smaller opening may be used if the taste is unclear or the food is less desired. The spoon often rests on the lower lip, which provides the stability to support it. The upper lip removes the food from the spoon. In order for the upper lip to remove the food, the lateral lip corners must tighten and the central upper lip must become more active. As the food is manipulated in the mouth, the lips serve as a gate, helping to keep the food and liquid in the mouth. During swallowing, the lips close to help create the intraoral pressure necessary for an efficient swallow response.

Very relaxed or low-toned lips. Lowered muscle tone usually causes a slightly open, resting posture of the mouth. The amount and variation in lip activity are reduced because there is not enough gradation of tension to create variations. More food spillage and drooling is seen because of the difficulty controlling food inside the mouth.

Pulled-back or retracted lips. Lip retraction makes food removal difficult. The process for food removal requires a forward and downward action of the lips, which is the opposite movement of lip retraction. People with lip retraction will use a wide variety of compensations to take food into the mouth. Lip retraction functions in combination with cheek retraction. The tightness at the lips and cheeks makes the activity of sucking the food and bolus formation difficult. Food is lost with increased drooling and spillage unless the person uses a compensatory pattern to keep it from falling out.

Pursed lips. This tight forward pucker of the lips can be likened to the action that we see in a cloth laundry bag as it is closed with a drawstring. This action is never seen in typical lip action. When the person with this variation attempts to open in response to the spoon, the pursing usually interferes with basic opening control. Food removal is very difficult when the lips are pursed. Pursed lips are inefficient in serving as a gate to keep food in the mouth during sucking, bolus preparation, and swallowing.

Summary Variations

Typical lip variations. Some people open their lips in anticipation of the mouthful. Others wait until the lips are touched before opening. Some prefer to use their upper teeth to scrape the food from the spoon, or may retract slightly, to avoid the sensory contact with the food. The amount and type of lip and cheek action needed to take the food from the spoon vary with the size and texture of the mouthful, the size and shape of the spoon, the speed of eating, and the amount of pleasurable tasting. Some people may swallow with the lips parted slightly, especially it there is some nasal congestion requiring separated lips for more efficient breathing.

Very relaxed or low-toned lips. There may be only minor differences between the central and the lateral lips. The upper lip may rely more on gravity to place it on the spoon. Decreased muscle tone may reduce the efficiency of the lips in keeping the food in the mouth during bolus preparation.

The lips may remain slightly or grossly opened during the swallow. This will change the efficiency of the swallow and often causes a reversed tongue movement during the swallow. The wave action of the tongue may be from back to front with the stability at the back of the tongue. Tongue protrusion may be used during swallowing.

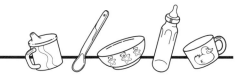

Pulled-back or retracted lips. Some people with lip retraction compensate for their inability to use the lips to remove food by biting on the spoon or trying to scrape the spoon with their teeth. When they have difficulty keeping the food in their mouth, they often tip the head back into extension to let gravity move the food back for a swallow.

Pursed lips. Lip pursing often is combined with a slight retraction pattern of the lips. Some people who have difficulty opening their mouth may compensate by biting on the spoon. Others may tilt the head back and drop the food into a slightly open, pursed mouth. They often tip the head back into extension to let gravity move the food back for a swallow and to keep the food from falling out.

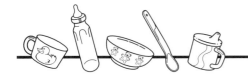

12. Sensory Defensiveness to Touch in the Mouth

Storyboard

Characters   A typical adult

A child with sensory defensiveness in the mouth

Setting   Mealtime

Story   Scene 1: Remember an unpleasant food texture in the mouth.

Scene 2: Imagine you are a child with sensory defensiveness in the mouth. Pretend you are given a texture that elicits a negative reaction.

Purpose   To provide a frame of reference for sensory defensiveness with touch/texture in the mouth

To begin to understand oral sensory defensive reactions

Brief Guide

Scene 1

Think about a food texture that is uncomfortable to you. Imagine that food in your mouth.

Scene 2

Now imagine you are a child who has sensory defensive reactions to touch/texture in the mouth. You are given a food whose texture makes you feel extremes of discomfort, pain, or rage. Notice how it affects your mealtime.

Expanded Guide

Remember a food texture that is not agreeable to you. Perhaps it is the rubberiness of octopus, the slipperiness of custard, or the sliminess of mushroom in your mouth. Perhaps for you it is something else… What is that food for you?… Imagine that food in your mouth. (Pause)… Feel its texture on your tongue… against your palate… between your teeth as you chew slowly… Try to swallow it… Notice how it feels… Notice your physical and emotional reaction.

Allow this scene and memory to fade… Take a deep, full breath, and be aware of the air moving in and out of your chest. (Pause)… Take a sip of water to cleanse your palate.

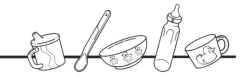

Now pretend you are a child who has sensory defensive reactions to various texture touches in your mouth… You are given a tiny morsel of cake and it feels like a rock on your tongue… Feel that rock… What do you do with the rock??? **or**… Imagine this one… You take a bite into a graham cracker… The broken pieces in your mouth feel to you like broken glass… The points are sharp… the edges hurt your mouth… Feel the glass… What do you do with the glass? Notice your physical and emotional responses to these imagined food textures.

Allow this scene and memory to fade… Take a deep, full breath, and be aware of the air moving in and out of your chest. (Pause).

Discussion

Did you remember a food that is not an agreeable texture? If you could not think of any, you are lucky! If you did think of one, what was it?

How did that food make you feel in your mouth?

Did you notice an emotional reaction to that food?

Do you think you could "learn" to like that food?

How did you feel as a child who has sensory defensive reactions to texture in the mouth?

What was it like seeing a crumb of cake but interpreting it as a rock? **or** biting a graham cracker and interpreting it as broken glass?

What did you feel in your mouth for each?

Did you have an emotional response to either?

What did you do when the uncomfortable food was in your mouth?

Do you know a child who seems to interpret some food textures in this type of extreme fashion?

Imagine how you would approach new food textures if you regularly had this type of defensive response to foods.

Have you asked an older child to describe reactions to certain disagreeable food textures? What insight did you glean?

Summary Theme
Scene 1

Many participants have had disagreeable responses to a particular food or foods. These foods usually elicit wrinkled faces as they are being discussed. Some focus on the texture with exaggerated words such as "disgusting, slimy, slippery, gross… ." Most participants indicate they could never and would never learn to like this food… End of discussion!!

Most adults can easily identify textured foods that they do not like and can avoid those foods. They do not cook them at home, and they certainly do not choose to order them at restaurants. If, by chance, they are caught by surprise with that food in a dish served in public, most participants have discovered polite, sometimes subtle ways to avoid eating, or avoid swallowing that food. The old "quietly spit it out in the napkin" trick seems to work quite well.

Scene 2

It is difficult for us to fully feel or understand the sensory defensiveness of children. We can observe reactions or ask older children about their responses. But mostly, we can notice the contribution of the sensory defensiveness to texture on their approach to mealtime.

Many participants try hard to imagine the "rock" or the "broken glass" in their mouth. Though these are definitely foreign concepts, they may spit out the food, wipe it off their tongue, gag, or imagine vomiting. They, first and foremost, seem to do anything within their power to rid themselves of that texture. Some describe extreme caution as they continue the meal, being fearful that another texture may be interpreted in such a negative fashion.

Summary Variations

Some participants can eat any texture, any flavor, and any kind of food. They may have never known a food they did not like. For these few, experiencing a disagreeable food can only be done in the imagination. Others have many food preferences that are guided by food texture. These participants will

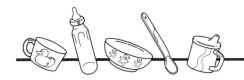

think of many examples of disagreeable food textures. It seems helpful to the group discussion when these participants can share their personal reactions to foods.

Children with sensory defensiveness to food texture in the mouth respond in a variety of ways. Some become very fearful of all foods and may limit their food intake to a very few familiar foods. Others check foods out carefully before trying them, looking them over, smelling them, or perhaps touching them cautiously to the lips or tongue before putting them in the mouth. Response to food for these children will be, however, extreme fight or flight. Their bodies give them strong messages to get away from the situation at all costs. Types of emotional responses and duration of the effects of the emotional responses will vary. These can include screaming, hitting, gagging, vomiting, and throwing the food.

As in all sensory responses, participants who are physically tense may have stronger sensory and emotional reactions to the imagined stories.

References

A

Abrams, C. K., Siram, S. M., Galsim, C., Johnson-Hamilton, H., Munford, F. L., & Mezghebe, H. (1992). Selenium deficiency in long-term total parenteral nutrition. *Nutrition in Clinical Practice, 7*(4), 175–178.

Achterberg, J. (1985). *Imagery in healing: Shamanism and modern medicine*. Boston: Shambhala Press.

Ackerman, D. (1991). *A natural history of the senses.* New York: Vintage Books.

Ahmed, T., & Fuchs, G. J. (1997). Gastrointestinal allergy to food: A review. *Journal of Diarrhoeal Diseases Research, 15*(4), 211–223.

Ainsworth, M. D. S., & Bell, S. M. (1969). Some contemporary patterns of mother-infant interactions in the feeding situation. In A. Ambrose (Ed.), *Stimulation in early infancy.* New York: Academic Press.

Akinbami, F. O., Brown, G. A., & McNeish, A. S. (1989). Intestinal permeability as a measure of small intestinal mucosal integrity: Correlation with jejunal biopsy. *African Journal of Medicine and Medical Sciences, 18*(3), 187–192.

Alexander, F., Wyllie, R., Jirousek, K., Secic, M., & Porvasnik, S. (1997). Delayed gastric emptying affects outcome of Nissen fundoplication in neurologically impaired children. *Surgery, 122*(4), 690–697; discussion 697–698.

Alexander, R., Boehme, R., & Cupps, B. (1993). *Normal development of functional motor skills: The first year of life.* San Antonio, TX: Therapy Skill Builders.

Alpers, D. H. (1994). Zinc and deficiencies of taste and smell. *Journal of the American Medical Association, 272*(16), 1233–1234.

Als, H. (1982). Manual for the assessment of preterm infants' behavior (APIB). In H. E. Fitzgerald (Ed.), *Theory and research in behavioral pediatrics* (pp. 65–132). New York: Plenum Press.

Als, H. (1985). *Observation of newborn behavior (NIDCAP).* Boston: Brigham and Women's Hospital.

Als, H. (1986). A synactive model of neonatal behavioral organization: Framework for the assessment of neurobehavioral development in the premature infant and for support of infants and parents in the neonatal intensive care environment. *Physical and Occupational Therapy in Pediatrics, 6*(3–4), 3–53.

Als, H. (1998). Developmental care in the newborn intensive care unit. *Current Opinion in Pediatrics, 10*(2), 138–142.

Als, H., & Gilkerson, L. (1995). Developmentally supportive care in the neonatal intensive care unit. *Zero to Three, 15*(6), 2–10.

Alton, G., Kjaergaard, S., Etchison, J. R., Skovby, F., & Freeze, H. H. (1997). Oral ingestion of mannose elevates blood mannose levels: A first step toward a potential therapy for carbohydrate-deficient glycoprotein syndrome type I. *Biochemical and Molecular Medicine, 60*(2), 127–133.

Amabile, T. M. (1998). How to kill creativity. *Harvard Business Review, 76*(5), 76–87, 186.

Amabile, T. M., Hennessey, B. A., & Grossman, B. S. (1986). Social influences on creativity: The effects of contracted-for reward. *Journal of Personality and Social Psychology, 50*(1), 14–23.

Aman, M. G., Mitchell, E. A., & Turbott, S. H. (1987). The effects of essential fatty acid supplementation by Efamol in hyperactive children. *Journal of Abnormal Child Psychology, 15*(1), 75–90.

American Academy of Pediatrics: Committee on Nutrition. On the feeding of supplemental foods to infants. (1980). *Pediatrics, 65*(6), 1178–1181.

American Academy of Pediatrics Committee on Nutrition. (1992). American Academy of Pediatrics Committee on Nutrition: The use of whole cow's milk in infancy. *Pediatrics, 89*(6 Pt 1), 1105–1109.

American Dietetic Association. (1995). Position of The American Dietetic Association: Phytochemicals and functional foods. *Journal of American Dietetic Association, 95*(5), 493.

American Psychiatric Association. (1994). *Diagnostic and statistical manual of mental disorders—Fourth edition* (DSM-IV). Washington, D.C.: Author.

Anderson, G. C. (1991). Current knowledge about skin-to-skin (kangaroo) care for preterm infants. *Journal of Perinatology, 11*(3), 216–226.

Archer, L. A., & Szatmari, P. (1990). Assessment and treatment of food aversion in a four year old boy: A multidimensional approach. *Canadian Journal of Psychiatry, 35*(6), 501–505.

Ardran, G. M., Kemp, F. H., & Lind, J. (1958a). A cineradiographic study of bottle feeding. *British Journal of Radiology, 31*(361), 11–22.

Ardran, G. M., Kemp, F. H., & Lind, J. (1958b). A cineradiographic study of breast-feeding. *British Journal of Radiology, 31*(363), 156–162.

Arnstein, P., Caudill, M., Mandle, C. L., Norris, A., & Beasley, R. (1999). Self efficacy as a mediator of the relationship between pain intensity, disability and depression in chronic pain patients. *Pain, 80*(3), 483-491.

Arvedson, J. C., & Lefton-Greif, M. (1998). *Pediatric videofluoroscopic swallow studies: A professional manual with caregiver guidelines.* San Antonio, TX: Communication Skill Builders.

Astor, F. C., Hanft, K. L., & Ciocon, J. O. (1999). Xerostomia: A prevalent condition in the elderly. *Ear, Nose and Throat Journal, 78*(7), 476–479.

Augustin, P., & Hains, A. A. (1996). Effect of music on ambulatory surgery patients' preoperative anxiety. *AORN Journal, 63*(4), 750, 753–758.

Ayres, A. J. (1972). *Sensory integration and learning disorders.* Los Angeles: Western Psychological Services.

Ayres, A. J., & Tickle, L. S. (1980). Hyper-responsivity to touch and vestibular stimuli as a predictor of positive response to sensory integration procedures by autistic children. *American Journal of Occupational Therapy, 34*(6), 375–381.

Ayres, B. R. (1987). The effects of a music stimulus environment versus regular cafeteria environment during therapeutic feeding. *Journal of Music Therapy, 24*(1), 14–26.

B

Babbitt, R. L., Hoch, T. A., Coe, D. A., Cataldo, M. F., Kelly, K. J., Stackhouse, C., & Perman, J. A. (1994). Behavioral assessment and treatment of pediatric feeding disorders. *Journal of Developmental and Behavioral Pediatrics, 15*(4), 278–291.

Baer, M. T., & Harris, A. B. (1997). Pediatric nutrition assessment: Identifying children at risk. *Journal of American Dietetic Association, 97*(10 Suppl. 2), S107–S115.

Bagley, M. T. (1984). *200 ways of using imagery in the classroom.* Monroe, NY: Trillium Press.

Bailey, D. J., Andres, J. M., Danek, G. D., & Pineiro-Carrero, V. M. (1987). Lack of efficacy of thickened feeding as treatment for gastroesophageal reflux. *The Journal of Pediatrics, 110*(2), 187–189.

Ballentine, R. (1978). *Diet and nutrition: A holistic approach.* Honesdale, PA: Himalayan Institute Press.

Balson, B. M., Kravitz, E. K., & McGeady, S. J. (1998). Diagnosis and treatment of gastroesophageal reflux in children and adolescents with severe asthma. *Annals of Allergy, Asthma, and Immunology, 81*(2), 159–164.

Bamford, O., Taciak, V., & Gewolb, I. H. (1992). The relationship between rhythmic swallowing and breathing during suckle feeding in term neonates. *Pediatric Research, 31*(6), 619–624.

Bandla, H. P., Davis, S. H., & Hopkins, N. E. (1999). Lipoid pneumonia: A silent complication of mineral oil aspiration. *Pediatrics, 103*(2), E19.

Baranek, G. T. (1999). Autism during infancy: A retrospective video analysis of sensory-motor and social behaviors at 9–12 months of age. *Journal of Autism and Developmental Disorders, 29*(3), 213.

Baranek, G. T., Foster, L. G., & Berdson, G. (1997). Tactile defensiveness and stereotyped behaviors. *The American Journal of Occupational Therapy, 51*(2), 91–95.

Bartz, A. H., & Deubler, D. C. (1990). Identification of feeding and nutrition problems in young children with neuromotor involvement: A self-assessment. *Journal of Pediatric Perinatal Nutrition, 2*(2), 1–15.

Bassette, R., Fung, D. Y., & Mantha, V. R. (1986). Off-flavors in milk. *Critical Review in Food Science and Nutrition, 24*(1), 1–52.

Batmanghelidj, F. (1995). *Your body's many cries for water: You are not sick, you are thirsty!* (2nd ed.). Falls Church, VA: Global Health Solutions.

Baxter, M. R. (1994). Congenital laryngomalacia. *Canadian Journal of Anaesthesia, 41*(4), 332–339.

Bazyk, S. (1990). Factors associated with the transition to oral feeding in infants fed by nasogastric tubes. *American Journal of Occupational Therapy, 44*(12), 1070–1078.

Beauchamp, G. K., & Cowart, B. J. (1985). Congenital and experiential factors in the development of human flavor preferences. *Appetite, 6*(4), 357–372.

Beauchamp, G. K., & Moran, M. (1984). Acceptance of sweet and salty tastes in 2-year-old children. *Appetite, 5*(4), 291–305.

Beck, M. A. (1999). Selenium and host defence towards viruses. *Proceedings of the Nutrition Society, 58*(3), 707–711.

Bekaroglu, M., Aslan, Y., Gedik, Y., Deger, O., Mocan, H., Erduran, E., & Karahan, C. (1996). Relationships between serum free fatty acids and zinc, and attention deficit hyperactivity disorder: A research note. *Journal of Child Psychology and Psychiatry and Allied Disciplines, 37*(2), 225–227.

Bell, D., & Hale, A. (1963). Observations of tongue-thrust swallow in preschool children. *Journal of Speech and Hearing Disorders, 28*(2), 195–198.

Belmont, J. R., & Grundfast, K. (1984). Congenital laryngeal stridor (laryngomalacia): Etiologic factors and associated disorders. *Annals of Otology, Rhinology and Laryngology, 93*(5 Pt 1), 430–437.

Bendich, A., & Langseth, L. (1995). The health effects of vitamin C supplementation: A review. *Journal of American College of Nutrition, 14*(2), 124–136.

Benton, D., & Cook, R. (1991). The impact of selenium supplementation on mood. *Biological Psychiatry, 29*(11), 1092–1098.

Berezin, S., Schwarz, S. M., Halata, M. S., & Newman, L. J. (1986). Gastroesophageal reflux secondary to gastrostomy tube placement. *American Journal of Disease in Childhood, 140*(July), 699–701.

Biancuzzo, M. (1999). *Breastfeeding the newborn: Clinical strategies for nurses*. St. Louis, MO: Mosby.

Billeaud, C., Guillet, J., & Sandler, B. (1990). Gastric emptying in infants with or without gastro-esophageal reflux according to the type of milk. *European Journal of Clinical Nutrition, 44*(8), 577–583.

Birch, L. L. (1987). The role of experience in children's food acceptance patterns. *Journal of the American Dietetic Association, 87*(Suppl. 9), S36–S40.

Birch, L. L. (1989). Effects of experience on the modification of food acceptance patterns. *Annals of the New York Academy of Sciences, 561,* 209–216.

Birch, L. L. (1998a). Development of food acceptance patterns in the first years of life. *Proceedings of the Nutrition Society, 57*(4), 617–624.

Birch, L. L. (1998b). Psychological influences on the childhood diet. *Journal of Nutrition, 128*(Suppl. 2), 407S–410S.

Birch, L. L., & Deysher, M. (1986). Caloric compensation and sensory specific satiety: Evidence for self regulation of food intake by young children. *Appetite, 7*(4), 323–331.

Birch, L. L., & Fisher, J. A. (1995). Appetite and eating behavior in children. *Pediatric Clinics of North America, 42*(4), 931–953.

Birch, L. L., & Fisher, J. O. (1997). Food intake regulation in children: Fat and sugar substitutes and intake. *Annals of the New York Academy of Sciences, 819,* 194–220.

Birch, L. L., Johnson, S. L., Andresen, G., Peters, J. C., & Schulte, M. C. (1991). The variability of young children's energy intake. *New England Journal of Medicine, 324*(4), 232–235.

Birch, L. L., Johnson, S. L., & Fisher, J. A. (1995). Children's eating: The development of food-acceptance patterns. *Young Children, 50*(2), 71–78.

Birch, L. L., & Marlin, D. W. (1982). I don't like it: I never tried it: Effects of exposure on two-year-old children's food preferences. *Appetite: Journal for Intake Research, 3*(4), 353–360.

Birch, L. L., Marlin, D. W., & Rotter, J. (1984). Eating as the "means" activity in a contingency: Effects on young children's food preference. *Child Development, 55,* 431–439.

Birch, L. L., McPhee, L. S., Bryant, J. L., & Johnson, S. L. (1993). Children's lunch intake: Effects of midmorning snacks varying in energy density and fat content. *Appetite, 20*(2), 83–94.

Birch, L. L., McPhee, L., Shoba, B. C., Pirok, E., & Steinberg, L. (1987). What kind of exposure reduces children's food neophobia? Looking vs. tasting. *Appetite, 9*(3), 171–178.

Black, D. D., Haggitt, R. C., Orenstein, S. R., & Whitington, P. F. (1990). Esophagitis in infants: Morphometric histological diagnosis and correlation with measures of gastroesophageal reflux. *Gastroenterology, 98*(6), 1408–1414.

Black, M. M., & Nitz, K. (1996). Grandmother co-residence, parenting, and child development among low income, urban teen mothers. *Journal of Adolescent Health, 18*(3), 218–226.

Blackman, J. A., & Nelson, C. L. A. (1985). Reinstituting oral feedings in children fed by gastrostomy tube. *Clinical Pediatrics, 24*(8), 434–438.

Blackman, J. A., & Nelson, C. L. A. (1987). Rapid introduction of oral feedings to tube-fed patients. *Developmental and Behavioral Pediatrics, 8*(2), 63–67.

Blecker, U., de Pont, S. M., Hauser, B., Chouraqui, J. P., Gottrand, F., & Vandenplas, Y. (1995). The role of 'occult' gastroesophageal reflux in chronic pulmonary disease in children. *Acta Gastroenterologica Belgica, 58*(5-6), 348–352.

Bly, L. (1999). *Baby treatment based on NDT principles*. San Antonio, TX: Therapy Skill Builders.

Bly, L., & Whiteside, A. (1997). *Facilitation techniques based on NDT principles*. San Antonio, TX: Therapy Skill Builders.

Bock, S. A., & Atkins, F. M. (1989). The natural history of peanut allergy. *Journal of Allergy and Clinical Immunology, 83*(5), 900–904.

Boehme, R. (1988). *Improving upper body control: An approach to assessment and treatment of tonal dysfunction*. San Antonio, TX: Therapy Skill Builders.

Boix-Ochoa, J., Casasa, J. M., Gil-Vernet, J. M., & Marhuenda, C. (1990). Surgical considerations: upper gastrointestinal motility disorders (chapter 26). P. E. Hyman (Editor), *Pediatric Gastrointestinal Motility Disorders* (pp. 387–402). Atlanta, Georgia: Children's Motility Disorder Foundation.

Bonn, M. (1994). The effects of hospitalisation on children: A review. *Curationis, 17*(2), 20–24.

Bonny, H. L., & Savary, L. M. (1983). *Music and your mind*. Port Townsend, WA: ICM Press.

Boris, M., & Mandel, F. S. (1994). Foods and additives are common causes of the attention deficit hyperactive disorder in children. *Annals of Allergy, 72*(5), 462–468.

Borowitz, S. M. & Borowitz, K. C. (1997). Oral dysfunction following Nissen fundoplication. *Dysphagia, 7,* 234–237.

Borowitz, S. M., & Borowitz, K. C. (1997). Gastroesophageal reflux in babies: Impact on growth and development. *Infants and Young Children, 10*(2), 14–26.

Borowitz, S. M., & Rocco, M. (1986). Acute water intoxication in healthy infants. *Southern Medical Journal, 79*(9), 1156–1158.

Borowitz, S. M., Sutphen, J. L., & Hutcheson, R. L. (1997). Percutaneous endoscopic gastrostomy without an antireflux procedure in neurologically disabled children. *Clinical Pediatrics (Phila), 36*(1), 25–29.

Bosma, J. F. (1963a). Maturation of function of the oral and pharyngeal region. *American Journal of Orthodontics, 49*(2), 94–104.

Bosma, J. F. (1963b). Oral and pharyngeal development and function. *Journal of Dental Research, 42*(1), 375–380.

Bosma, J. F. (1967). Human infant oral function. In J. F. Bosma (Ed.), *Symposium on oral sensation and perception* (pp. 98–110). Springfield, IL: Charles C. Thomas.

Bosma, J. F., Hepburn, L. G., Josell, S. D., & Baker, K. (1990). Ultrasound demonstration of tongue motions during suckle feeding. *Developmental Medicine and Child Neurology, 32*(3), 223–229.

Bosma, J. F., Vice, F. L., Heinz, J. M., Giuriati, G., & Hood, M. (1990). Cervical auscultation of suckle feeding in newborn infants. *Developmental Medicine and Child Neurology, 32*(9), 760–768.

Boudraa, G., Touhami, M., Pochart, P., Soltana, R., Mary, J. Y., & Desjeux, J. F. (1990). Effect of feeding yogurt versus milk in children with persistent diarrhea. *Journal of Pediatric Gastroenterology and Nutrition, 11*(4), 509–512.

Boyd, L. D., Palmer, C., & Dwyer, J. T. (1998). Managing oral health related nutrition issues of high risk infants and children. *Journal of Clinical Pediatric Dentistry, 23*(1), 31–36.

Boyle, C. L., & Render, G. F. (1982). The relationships between the use of fantasy journeys and creativity. *Journal of the Society for Accelerative Learning and Teaching, 7*(3), 269–281.

Brady, D. B. (1997). *Binaural-Beat Induced Theta EEG Activity and Hypnotic Susceptibility* [Web Page]. URL http://www.monroeinstitute.org/research/hypnotic.html.

Braun, M. A., & Palmer, M. M. (1985). A pilot study of oral-motor dysfunction in "at risk" infants. *Physical and Occupational Therapy in Pediatrics, 5*(4), 13–25.

Brazelton, T. B. (1993). Why children and parents must play while they eat: An interview with T. Berry Brazelton, MD. *Journal of the American Dietetics Association, 93*(12), 1385–1387.

Bruce, E. J., Schultz, C. L., & Smyrnios, K. X. (1996). A longitudinal study of the grief of mothers and fathers of children with intellectual disability. *British Journal of Medical Psychology, 69*(Pt 1), 33–45.

Brueton, M. J., Clarke, G. S., & Sandhu, B. K. (1990). The effects of cisapride on gastro-oesopageal reflux in children with and without neurological disorders. *Developmental Medicine and Child Neurology, 32*, 629–632.

Brug, J., Glanz, K., & Kok, G. (1997). The relationship between self-efficacy, attitudes, intake compared to others, consumption, and stages of change related to fruit and vegetables. *American Journal of Health Promotion, 12*(1), 25–30.

Bryant, C. A. (1982). The impact of kin, friend and neighbor networks on infant feeding practices: Cuban, Puerto Rican and Anglo families in Florida. *Social Science and Medicine, 16*(20), 1757–1765.

Bui, H. D., Dang, C. V., Chaney, R. H., & Vergara, L. M. (1989). Does gastrostomy and fundoplication prevent aspiration pneumonia in mentally retarded persons? *American Journal on Mental Retardation, 94*(1), 16–19.

Bu'Lock, F., Woolridge M. W., & Baum, J. D. (1990). Development of co-ordination of sucking, swallowing and breathing: Ultrasound study of term and preterm infants. *Developmental Medicine and Child Neurology, 32*(8), 669–678.

Burgess, J. R., Stevens, L., Zhang, W., & Peck, L. (2000). Long-chain polyunsaturated fatty acids in children with attention-deficit hyperactivity disorder. *American Journal of Clinical Nutrition, 71*(Suppl. 1), 327–330.

Burks, W., Bannon, G. A., Sicherer, S., & Sampson, H. A. (1999). Peanut-induced anaphylactic reactions. *International Archives of Allergy and Immunology, 119*(3), 165–172.

Burns, K., Chethik, L., Burns, W. J., & Clark, R. (1991). Dyadic disturbances in cocaine-abusing mothers and their infants. *Journal of Clinical Psychology, 47*(2), 316–319.

Bustorff-Silva, J., Fonkalsrud, E. W., Perez, C. A., Quintero, R., Martin, L., Villasenor, E., & Atkinson, J. B. (1999). Gastric emptying procedures decrease the risk of postoperative recurrent reflux in children with delayed gastric emptying. *Journal of Pediatric Surgery, 34*(1), 79–82; discussion 82–83.

Byard, R. W., Gallard, V., Johnson, A., Barbour, J., Bonython-Wright, B., & Bonython-Wright, D. (1996). Safe feeding practices for infants and young children. *Journal of Paediatrics and Child Health, 32*(4), 327–329.

C

Caine, J. (1991). The effects of music on the selected stress behaviors, weight, caloric and formula intake, and length of hospital stay of premature and low birth weight neonates in a newborn intensive care unit. *Journal of Music Therapy, 28*(4), 180–192.

Campbell, D. (1992). *One hundred ways to improve teaching using your voice & music: Pathways to accelerate learning.* Tucson, AZ: Zephyr Press.

Campbell, D. (1997). *The Mozart effect: Tapping the power of music to heal the body, strengthen the mind, and unlock the creative spirit.* New York: Avon Books.

Cannon R. A., & Stadalnik R. C. (1993). Postprandial gastric motility in infants with gastroesophageal reflux and delayed gastric emptying. *Journal of Nuclear Medicine, 34*(12), 2120–2123.

Cantekin, E. I., McGuire, T. W., & Griffith, T. L. (1991). Antimicrobial therapy for otitis media with effusion ('secretory' otitis media). *Journal of American Medical Association, 266*(23), 3309–3317.

Capdevila, F., Vizmanos, B., & Marti-Henneberg, C. (1998). Implications of the weaning pattern on macronutrient intake, food volume and energy density in non-breastfed infants during the first year of life. *Journal of the American College of Nutrition, 17*(3), 256–262.

Capps, L., Kasari, C., Yirmiya, N., & Sigman, M. (1993). Parental perception of emotional expressiveness in children with autism. *Journal of Consulting and Clinical Psychology, 61*(3), 475–484.

Carruth, B. R., Skinner, J., Morris, S., Houck, K., Coletta, F., & Cotter, R. (1994). Infant age and readiness feeding cues in healthy infants. Unpublished study.

Carter, C. M., Urbanowicz, M., Hemsley, R., Mantilla, L., Strobel, S., Graham, P. J., & Taylor, E. (1993). Effects of a few food diet in attention deficit disorder. *Archives of Disease in Childhood, 69*(5), 564–568.

Casas, M. J., Kenny, D. J., & McPherson, K. A. (1994). Swallowing/ventilation interactions during oral swallow in normal children and children with cerebral palsy. *Dysphagia, 9*(1), 40–46.

Casas, M. J., McPherson, K. A., & Kenny, D. J. (1995). Durational aspects of oral swallow in neurologically normal children and children with cerebral palsy: An ultrasound investigation. *Dysphagia, 10*(3), 155–159.

Case-Smith, J. (1988). An efficacy study of occupational therapy with high-risk neonates. *American Journal of Occupational Therapy, 42*(8), 499–506.

Case-Smith, J., & Bryan, T. (1999). The effects of occupational therapy with sensory integration emphasis on preschool-age children with autism. *Amercian Journal of Occupational Therapy, 53*(5), 489–497.

Caskey, O. (1896). Accelerating concept formation. *Journal of the Society for Accelerative Learning and Teaching, 11*(3), 137–147.

Catto-Smith, A. G. (1998). Gastroesophageal reflux in children. *Australian Family Physician, 27*(6), 465–469, 472–473.

Caudill, M. (1994). *Managing pain before it manages you.* New York: Guilford Press.

Caudill, M., Schnable, R., Zuttermeister, P., Benson, H., & Friedman, R. (1991). Decreased clinic use by chronic pain patients: response to behavioral medicine intervention. *Clinical Journal of Pain, 7*(4), 305–310.

Cavallaro, S., Pineschi, A., Freni, G., Cortese, M. G., & Bardini, T. (1992). Feeding troubles following delayed primary repair of esophageal atresia. *European Journal of Pediatric Surgery, 2*(2), 73–77.

Cavataio, F., Iacono, G., Montalto, G., Soresi, M., Tumminello, M., Campagna, P., Notarbartolo, A., & Carroccio, A. (1996). Gastroesophageal reflux associated with cow's milk allergy in infants: Which diagnostic examinations are useful? *American Journal of Gastroenterology, 91*(6), 1215–1220.

Cavataio, F., Iacono, G., Montalto, G., Soresi, M., Tumminello, M., & Carroccio, A. (1996). Clinical and pH-metric characteristics of gastro-esophageal reflux secondary to cows' milk protein allergy. *Archives of Disease in Childhood, 75*(1), 51–56.

Chad, K., Jobling, A., & Frail, H. (1990). Metabolic rate: A factor in developing obesity in children with Down syndrome? *American Journal of Mental Retardation, 95*(2), 228–235.

Chaitow, L., & Trenev, N. (1990). *Probiotics.* London: Thorsons.

Chandra, R. K. (1997a). Food hypersensitivity and allergic disease: A selective review. *American Journal of Clinical Nutrition, 66*(2), 526S–529S.

Chandra, R. K. (1997b). Nutrition and the immune system: An introduction. *American Journal of Clinical Nutrition, 66*(2), 460S–463S.

Chatoor, I. (1989). Infantile anorexia nervosa: A developmental disorder or separation and individuation. *Journal of the American Academy of Psychoanalysis, 17*(1), 43–64.

Chatoor, I., Ganiban, J., Colin, V., Plummer, N., & Harmon, R. J. (1998). Attachment and feeding problems: A reexamination of nonorganic failure to thrive and attachment insecurity. *Journal of American Academy of Child and Adolescent Psychiatry, 37*(11), 1217–1224.

Chatoor, I., Menvielle, P., & O'Donnell, R. (1989). *Observation scale for mother-infant-toddler interaction during feeding.* Washington, DC: Children's Hospital Medical Center.

Chlan, L. L. (1995). Psychophysiologic responses of mechanically ventilated patients to music: A pilot study. *American Journal of Critical Care, 4*(3), 233–238.

Clark, J. H., Rhoden, D. K., & Turner, D. S. (1993). Symptomatic vitamin A and D deficiencies in an eight-year-old with autism. *Journal Parenteral Enteral Nutrition, 17*(3), 284–286.

Clarren, S., Anderson, B., & Wolf, L. S. (1987). Feeding infants with cleft lip, cleft palate, or cleft lip and palate. *Cleft Palate Journal, 24*(3), 244–249.

Cobo-Lewis, A. B., Oller, D. K., Lynch, M. P., & Levine, S. L. (1996). Relations of motor and vocal milestones in typically developing infants and infants with Down syndrome. *American Journal of Mental Retardation, 100*(5), 456–467.

Cogbill, T. H., Moore, F. A., Accurso, F. J., & Lilly, J. R. (1983). Primary tracheomalacia. *Annals of Thoracic Surgery, 35*(5), 538–541.

Colley, J. R. T., & Creamer, B. (1958). Sucking and swallowing in infants. *British Medical Journal, 16*(2), 422–423.

Collinge, J. M., Bradley, K., Perks, C., Rezny, A., & Topping, P. (1982). Demand vs. scheduled feedings for premature infants. *Journal of Obstetric, Gynecologic, and Neonatal Nursing, 11*(6), 362–367.

Condon, W. S. (1975). Multiple response to sound in dysfunctional children. *Journal of Autism and Childhood Schizophrenia, 5*(1), 37–56.

Condon, W. S., & Sander, L. W. (1974). Synchrony demonstrated between movements of the neonate and adult speech. *Child Development, 45*(2), 456–462.

Conley, S. F., Werlin, S. L., & Beste, D. J. (1995). Proximal pH-metry for diagnosis of upper airway complications of gastro-esophageal reflux. *Journal of Otolaryngology, 24*(5), 295–298.

Contento, I. R., Basch, C., Shea, S., Gutin, B., Zybert, P., Michela, J. L., & Rips, J. (1993). Relationship of mothers' food choice criteria to food intake of preschool children: Identification of family subgroups. *Health Education Quarterly, 20*(2), 243–259.

Contento, I. R., Michela, J. L., & Williams, S. S. (1995). Adolescent food choice criteria: Role of weight and dieting status. *Appetite, 25*(1), 51–76.

Corwin, D. S., Isaacs, J. S., Georgeson, K. E., Bartolucci, A. A., Cloud, H. H., & Craig, C. B. (1996). Weight and length increases in children after gastrostomy placement. *Journal of American Dietetic Association, 96*(9), 874–879.

Courchesne, E., Townsend, J., Akshoomoff, N. A., Saitoh, O., Yeung-Courchesne, R., Lincoln, A. J., James, H. E., Haas, R. H., Schreibman, L., & Lau, L. (1994). Impairment in shifting attention in autistic and cerebellar patients. *Behavioral Neuroscience, 108*(5), 848–865.

Cowart, B. J., & Beauchamp, G. K. (1986). The importance of sensory context in young children's acceptance of salty tastes. *Child Development, 57*(4), 1034–1039.

Cox, D. R., Skinner, J. D., Carruth, B. R., Moran, J., & Houck, K. S. (1997). A Food Variety Index for Toddlers (VIT): Development and application. *Journal of American Dietetic Association, 97*(12), 1382–1388.

Cozzi, F., Steiner, M., Rosati, D., Madonna, L., & Colarossi, G. (1988). Clinical manifestations of choanal atresia in infancy. *Journal of Pediatric Surgery, 23*(3), 203–206.

Crook, W. G. (1980). *Tracking down hidden food allergy.* Jackson, TN: Professional Books.

Cucchiara, S., Minella, R., Campanozzi, A., Salvia, G., Borrelli, O., Ciccimarra, E., & Emiliano, M. (1997). Effects of omeprazole on mechanisms of gastroesophageal reflux in childhood. *Digestive Diseases and Sciences, 42*(2), 293–299.

Cucchiara, S., Santamaria, F., Minella, R., Alfieri, E., Scoppa, A., Calabrese, F., Franco, M. T., Rea, B., & Salvia, G. (1995). Simultaneous prolonged recordings of proximal and distal intraesophageal pH in children with gastroesophageal reflux disease and respiratory symptoms. *American Journal of Gastroenterology, 90*(10), 1791–1796.

Cunningham, K. F., & McLaughlin, M. (1999). Nutrition. In D. B. Kessler & P. Dawson (Eds.), *Failure to thrive and pediatric undernutrition: A transdisciplinary approach* (pp. 99-119). Baltimore: Paul H. Brookes Publishing.

Curtis, D. M. (1990). Infant nutrient supplementation. *Journal of Pediatrics, 117*(2 Pt 2), S110–S118.

Cusatis, D. C., & Shannon, B. M. (1996). Influences on adolescent eating behavior. *Journal of Adolescent Health, 18*(1), 27–34.

D

Daly, J. M., & Fritsch, S. L. (1995). Case study: Maternal residual attention deficit disorder associated with failure to thrive in a two-month-old infant. *Journal of the American Academy of Child and Adolescent Psychiatry, 34*(1), 55–57.

Danner, S. C., & Cerutti, E. R. (1984). *Nursing your baby with a cleft palate or cleft lip.* Rochester, NY: Childbirth Graphics.

Davidson, P. W., Myers, G. J., Cox, C., Axtell, C., Shamlaye, C., Sloane-Reeves, J., Cernichiari, E., Needham, L., Choi, A., Wang, Y., Berlin, M., & Clarkson, T. W. (1998). Effects of prenatal and postnatal methylmercury exposure from fish consumption on neurodevelopment: Outcomes at 66 months of age in the Seychelles Child Development Study. *Journal of American Medical Association, 280*(8), 701–707.

Davis, B. E., Moon, R. Y., Sachs, H. C., & Ottolini, M. C. (1998). Effects of sleep position on infant motor development. *Pediatrics, 102*(5), 1135–1140.

de Boissieu, D., Matarazzo, P., Rocchiccioli, F., & Dupont, C. (1997). Multiple food allergy: A possible diagnosis in breast-fed infants. *Acta Paediatrica, 86*(10), 1042–1046.

Decsi, T., & Koletzko, B. (1995). Do trans fatty acids impair linoleic acid metabolism in children? *Annals of Nutrition and Metabolism, 39*(1), 36-41.

De Giacomo, C., Bawa, P., Franceschi, M., Luinetti, O., & Fiocca, R. (1997). Omeprazole for severe reflux esophagitis in children. *Journal of Pediatric Gastroenterology and Nutrition, 24*(5), 528–532.

Delany, H. M. (1993). Nutritional support by tube jejunostomy. *Journal of the Association for Academic Minority Physicians, 4*(1), 26–29.

Dellert, S. F., Hyams, J. S., Treem, W. R., & Geertsma M. A. (1993). Feeding resistance and gastroesophageal reflux in infancy. *Journal of Pediatric Gastroenterology and Nutrition, 17*(1), 66–71.

DeMeyer, M. K., Alp, ern, G. D., Barton, S., DeMyer, W., Churchill, D. W., Hingtgen, J. N., Bryson, C. Q., Pontius, W., & Kimberlin, C. (1972). Imitation in autistic, early schizophrenic, and nonpsychotic subnormal children. *Journal of Autism and Childhood Schizophrenia, 2*(3), 254–287.

Demmelmair, H., Festl, B., Wolfram, G., & Koletzko, B. (1996). Trans fatty acid contents in spreads and cold cuts usually consumed by children. *Zeitschrift fur Ernahrung-swissenschaft, 35*(3), 235–240.

DeNardi, F. G., & Riddel, R. H. (1991). The normal esophagus. *The American Journal of Surgical Pathology, 15*(3), 296–309.

Denney, A. (1997). Quiet music: An intervention for mealtime agitation? *Journal of Gerontological Nursing, 23*(7), 16–23.

Desmond, P., Raman, R., & Idikula, J. (1991). Effect of nasogastric tubes on the nose and maxillary sinus. *Critical Care Medicine, 19*(4), 509–511.

Dettwyler, K. A. (1986). Infant feeding in Mali, West Africa: Variations in belief and practice. *Social Science and Medicine, 23*(7), 651–664.

D'Eufemia, P., Celli, M., Finocchiaro, R., Pacifico, L., Viozzi, L., Zaccagnini, M., Cardi, E., & Giardini, O. (1996). Abnormal intestinal permeability in children with autism. *Acta Paediatrica, 85*(9), 1076–1079.

Dhur, A., Galan, P., & Hercberg, S. (1990). Relationship between selenium, immunity and resistance against infection. *Comparative Biochemistry and Physiology C, 96*(2), 271–80.

Dick, T. E., Oku, Y., Romaniuk, J. R., & Cherniack, N. S. (1993). Interaction between central pattern generators for breathing and swallowing in the cat. *Journal of Physiology, 465*, 715–730.

Dietz, W. H., & Stern, L. (1999). *American Academy of Pediatrics guide to your child's nutrition: Making peace at the table and building healthy eating habits for life.* New York: Villard.

Dihigo, S. K. (1998). New strategies for the treatment of colic: Modifying the parent/infant interaction. *Journal of Pediatric Health Care, 12*(5), 256–262.

Di Lorenzo, C., Flores, A., & Hyman, P. E. (1991). Intestinal motility in symptomatic children with fundoplication. *Journal of Pediatric Gastroenterology and Nutrition, 12*(2), 169–173.

Dinkmeyer, D. Sr., McKay, G., & Dinkmeyer, D. Jr. (1997). *The parents handbook: Systematic training for effective parenting.* Circle Pines, MN: American Guidance Services.

DiPietro, J. A., Cusson, R. M., Caughy, M. O., & Fox, N. A. (1994). Behavioral and physiologic effects of nonnutritive sucking during gavage feeding in preterm infants. *Pediatric Research, 36*(2), 207–214.

DiPietro, J. A., Hodgson, D. M., Costigan, K. A., & Johnson, T. R. (1996). Fetal antecedents of infant temperament. *Child Development, 67*(5), 2568–2583.

Di Scipio, W., & Kaslon, K. (1982). Conditioned dysphagia in cleft palate children after pharyngeal flap surgery. *Psychosomatic Medicine, 44*(3), 247–257.

Dodds, W. J. (1989). The physiology of swallowing. *Dysphagia, 3*(4), 171–178.

Dodds, W. J., Stewart, E. T., & Logemann, J. A. (1990). Physiology and radiology of the normal oral and pharyngeal phases of swallowing. *American Journal of Roentgenology, 154*(5), 953–963.

Donnellan, A. M., Mirenda, P. L., Fassbender, M., & Fassbender, L. (1984). Analyzing the communicative functions of aberrant behavior. *Journal of the Association for Persons With Severe Handicaps, 9*(3), 201–212.

Donner, M. W., Bosma, J. F., & Robertson, D. L. (1985). Anatomy and physiology of the pharynx. *Gastrointestinal Radiology, 10*(3), 196–212.

Dowling, S. (1977). Seven infants with esophageal atresia: A developmental study. *Psychoanalytic Study of the Child, 32,* 215–256.

Drehobl, K. F., & Fuhr, M. G. (1991). *Pediatric massage for the child with special needs.* [Videotape]. San Antonio, TX: Therapy Skill Builders.

Drehobl, K. F., & Fuhr, M. G. (2000). *Pediatric massage for the child with special needs—Revised.* San Antonio, TX: Therapy Skill Builders.

Dreikurs, R., Cassel, P., & Kehoe, D. (1992). *Discipline without tears* (2nd Ed.). New York: Dutton/Plume.

Dreikurs, R., & Grey, L. (1993). *The new approach to discipline: Logical consequences.* New York: Dutton/Plume.

Dreikurs, R., & Stoltz, V. (1964). *Children: The challenge.* New York: NAL/Dutton.

Drotar, D. (1991). The family context of nonorganic failure to thrive. *American Journal of Orthopsychiatry, 61*(1), 23–34.

Dua, K. S., Ren, J., Bardan, E., Xie, P., & Shaker, R. (1997). Coordination of deglutitive glottal function and pharyngeal bolus transit during normal eating. *Gastroenterology, 112*(1), 73–83.

Duniz, M., Scheer, P. J., Trojovsky, A., Kaschnitz, W., Kvas, E., & Macari, S. (1996). Changes in psychopathology of parents of NOFT (non-organic failure to thrive) infants during treatment. *European Child and Adolescent Psychiatry, 5*(2), 93–100.

Dunn, J. C., Lai, E. C., Webber, M. M., Ament, M. E., & Fonkalsrud, E. W. (1998). Long-term quantitative results following fundoplication and antroplasty for gastroesophageal reflux and delayed gastric emptying in children. *The American Journal of Surgery, 175*(1), 27–29.

Dunn, W., & Fisher, A. G. (1983). II. Sensory registration, autism and tactile defensiveness. *SI Newsletter of AOTA, 6*(2), 3–4.

Duranceau, A., Fisher, S. R., Flye, M., Jones, R. S., Postlethwait, R. W., & Sealy, W. C. (1977). Motor function of the esophagus after repair of esophageal atresia and tracheoesophageal fistula. *Surgery, 82*(1), 116–123.

Dykman, K. D., Tone, C., Ford, C., & Dykman, R. A. (1998). The effects of nutritional supplements on the symptoms of fibromyalgia and chronic fatigue syndrome. *Integrative Physiological and Behavioral Science, 33*(1), 61–71.

Dykman, K. D., & Dykman, R. A. (1998). Effect of nutritional supplements on attention-deficit hyperactivity disorder. *Integrative Physiological and Behavioral Science, 33*(1), 49–60.

E

Edelson, S. B., & Cantor, D. S. (1998). Autism: Xenobiotic influences. *Toxicology and Industrial Health, 14*(4), 553–563.

Edelson, S. M., Edelson, M. G., Kerr, D. C., & Grandin, T. (1999). Behavioral and physiological effects of deep pressure on children with autism: A pilot study evaluating the efficacy of Grandin's Hug Machine. *American Journal of Occupational Therapy, 53*(2), 145–152.

Edwards, M., Ashwood, R. A., Littlewood, S. J., Brocklebank, L. M., & Fung, D. E. (1998). A videofluoroscopic comparison of straw and cup drinking: The potential influence on dental erosion. *British Dental Journal, 185*(5), 244–249.

Efron, D., Jarman, F., & Barker, M. (1997). Side effects of methylphenidate and dexamphetamine in children with attention deficit hyperactivity disorder: A double-blind, crossover trial. *Pediatrics, 100*(4), 662–666.

Ein, S. H., & Friedberg, J. (1981). Esophageal atresia and tracheoesophageal fistula: Review and update. *Otolaryngologic Clinic of North America, 14*(1), 219–249.

Einarsson-Backes, L. M., Deitz, J., Price, R., Glass, R., & Hays, R. (1994). The effect of oral support on sucking efficiency in preterm infants. *The American Journal of Occupational Therapy, 48*(6), 490–498.

Eisenberger, R., & Cameron, J. (1996). Detrimental effects of reward: Reality or myth? *The American Psychologist, 51*(11), 1153–1166.

Elinoff, V. (1993). Remission of dysphagia in a 9-year-old treated in a family practice office setting. *American Journal of Clinical Hypnosis, 35*(3), 205–208.

Ellison, S. L., Vidyasagar, D., & Anderson, G. C. (1979). Sucking in the newborn infant during the first hour of life. *Journal of Nurse-Midwifery, 24*(6), 18–25.

Engle, P. L., & Nieves, I. (1993). Intra-household food distribution among Guatemalan families and a supplementary feeding program: Behavior patterns. *Social Science Medicine, 36*(12), 1605–1612.

Epstein, G. (1989). *Healing visualizations: creating health through imagery.* New York: Bantam Books.

Epstein, S., Pronsky, Z. M., Crowe, J. P., & Young, V. (2000). *Powers and Moore's food medication interactions* (11th ed). Birchrunville, PA: Food-Medication Interactions.

Erhardt, R. P. (1993). Finger feeding: A comprehensive developmental perspective. *Pediatric Basics, 66*(Fall), 2–6.

Erhardt, R. P. (1994). Utensil feeding: A comprehensive developmental perspective. *Pediatric Basics, 70*(Fall), 2–9.

Ernst, J. A., Rickard, K. A., Neal, P. R., Yu, P. L., Oei, T. O., & Lemons, J. A. (1989). Lack of improved growth outcome related to nonnutritive sucking in very low birth weight premature infants fed a controlled nutrient intake: A randomized prospective study. *Pediatrics, 83*(5), 706–716.

F

Fagerli, R. A., & Wandel, M. (1999). Gender differences in opinions and practices with regard to a "healthy diet." *Appetite, 32*(2), 171–190.

Falconer, J. A., Roth, E. J., Sutin, J. A., Strasser, D. C., & Chang, R. W. (1993). The critical path method in stroke rehabilitation: Lessons from an experiment in cost containment and outcome improvement. *Qualitative Review Bulletin, 19*(1), 8–16.

Farquharson, J., Cockburn, F., Patrick, W. A., Jamieson, E. C., & Logan, R. W. (1992). Infant cerebral cortex phospholipid fatty-acid composition and diet. *Lancet, 340*(8823), 810–813.

Farrington, E. (1996). Cardiac toxicity with cisapride. *Pediatric Nursing, 22*(3), 256.

Fashakin, J. B., & Oladimeji, S. (1986). Effect of ascorbic acid on the availability of iron in weaning foods. *Annals of Nutrition and Metabolism, 30*(5), 324–330.

Ferreira, C., Lohoues, M. J., Bensoussan, A., Yazbeck, S., Brochu, P., & Roy, C. C. (1993). Prolonged pH monitoring is of limited usefulness for gastroesophageal reflux. *American Journal of Diseases in Childhood, 147*(6), 662–664.

Field, T. (1986). Models for reactive and chronic depression in infancy. *New Directions for Child Adolescent Development, 34*(1), 47–60.

Field, T. (1998). Maternal depression effects on infants and early interventions. *Preventive Medicine, 27*(2), 200–203.

Field, T., & Goldson, E. (1984). Pacifying effects of nonnutritive sucking on term and preterm neonates during heelstick procedures. *Pediatrics, 74*(6), 1012–1015.

Field, T., Ignatoff, E., Stringer, S., Brennan, J., Greenberg, R., Widmayer, S., & Anderson, G. C. (1982). Nonnutritive sucking during tube feedings: Effects on preterm neonates in an intensive care unit. *Pediatrics, 70*(3), 381–384.

Field, T., Lasko, D., Mundy, P., Henteleff, T., Kabat, S., Talpins, S., & Dowling, M. (1997). Brief report: Autistic children's attentiveness and responsivity improve after touch therapy. *Journal of Autism and Developmental Disorders, 27*(3), 333–338.

Finnie, N., Bavin, J., Bax, M., Browne, M., & Gardiner, M. (1997). *Handling the young child with cerebral palsy at home* (3rd ed.). Boston: Butterworth-Heinemann Medical.

Fireman, P. (1988). Otitis media and its relationship to allergy. *Pediatric Clinics of North America, 35*(5), 1075–1090.

Fisher, J. O., & Birch, L. L. (1995). Fat preferences and fat consumption of 3- to 5-year-old children are related to parental adiposity. *Journal of the American Dietetic Association, 95*(7), 759–764.

Fleisher, D. R. (1994). Functional vomiting disorders in infancy: Innocent vomiting, nervous vomiting, and infant rumination syndrome. *Journal of Pediatrics, 125*(6 Pt 2), S84–S94.

Fleisher, D. R., & Matar, M. (1993). The cyclic vomiting syndrome: A report of 71 cases and literature review. *Journal of Pediatric Gastroenterology and Nutrition, 17*(4), 361–369.

Fletcher, S. G., Casteel, R. L., & Bradley, D. P. (1961). Tongue-thrust swallow, speech articulation and age. *Journal of Speech and Hearing Disorders, 26*(3), 201–208.

Fonkalsrud, E. W., & Ament, M. E. (1996). Gastroesophageal reflux in childhood. *Current Problems in Surgery, 33*(1), 1–70.

Fonkalsrud, E. W., Ashcraft, K. W., Coran, A. G., Ellis, D. G., Grosfeld, J. L., Tunell, W. P., & Weber, T. R. (1998). Surgical treatment of gastroesophageal reflux in children: A combined hospital study of 7467 patients [see comments]. *Pediatrics, 101*(3 Pt 1), 419–422.

Fonkalsrud, E. W., Bustorff-Silva, J., Perez, C. A. Q. R., Martin, L. & Atkinson, J. B. (1999). Anireflux surgery in children under 3 months of age. *Journal of Pediatric Surgery, 34*(4), 527–531.

Fonkalsrud, E. W., Ellis, D. G., Shaw, A., Mann, C. M. Jr., Black, T. L., Miller, J. P., & Snyder, C. L. (1995). A combined hospital experience with fundoplication and gastric emptying procedure for gastroesophageal reflux in children [see comments]. *Journal of the American College of Surgeons, 180*(4), 449–455.

Fox, C. A. (1990). Implementing the modified barium swallow evaluation in children who have multiple disabilities. *Infants and Young Children, 3*(2), 67–77.

Fraiberg, S. (1974). Blind infants and their mothers: An examination of the sign system. In M. Lewis and L. Rosenblum (Eds.). *The effect of the infant on its caregiver.* New York: Wiley & Sons.

Frank, D. A., Needlman, R., & Silva, M. (1994). What to do when a child won't grow. *Patient Care,* March 15, 107–128.

Frank, L., Marian, A., Visser, M., Weinberg, E., & Potter, P. C. (1999). Exposure to peanuts in utero and in infancy and the development of sensitization to peanut allergens in young children. *Pediatric Allergy and Immunology, 10*(1), 27–32.

Freeman, J. M., Kelly, M. T., & Freeman, J. B. (1996). *The epilepsy diet treatment: An introduction to the ketogenic diet.* New York: Demos Publications.

Frick, S., Frick, R., Oetter, P., & Richter, E. (1996). *Out of the mouths of babes: Discovering the developmental significance of the mouth.* Hugo, MN: PDP Press.

Friel, J. K., Gibson, R. S., Kawash, G. F., & Watts, J. (1985). Dietary zinc intake and growth during infancy. *Journal of Pediatric Gastroenterology and Nutrition, 4*(5), 746–751.

Fung, K. P., Rubin, S., & Scott, R. B. (1990). Gastric vovulus complication Nissen fundoplication. *Journal of Pediatric Surgery, 25*(12), 1242–1243.

G

Gaebler, C. P., & Hanzlik, J. R. (1996). The effects of a prefeeding stimulation program on preterm infants. *The American Journal of Occupational Therapy, 50*(3), 184–192.

Galland, L. (1987). Biochemical abnormalities in patients with multiple chemical sensitivities. *Occupational Medicine, 2*(4), 713–720.

Gardiner, T. (2000a). Absorption, distribution, metabolism, and excretion (ADME) of eight known dietary monosaccharides required for glycoprotein synthesis and cullular recognition processes: Summary. *GlycoScience, 1*(12), 1–7

Gardiner, T. (2000b). Biological activity of eight known dietary monosaccharides required for glycoprotein synthesis and cellular recognition processes: Summary. *GlycoScience, 1*(13), 1–7.

Garfield, C. A., & Bennett, H. Z. (1984). *Peak performance: Mental training techniques of the world's greatest athletes.* Los Angeles: J. P. Tarcher.

Gauderer, M. W. L. (1991). Percutaneous endoscopic gastrostomy: A 10-year experience with 220 children. *Journal of Pediatric Surgery, 26*(3), 288–294.

Gauderer, M. W. L., Olsen, M. M., Stellato, T. A., & Dokler, M. L. (1988). Feeding gastrostomy button: Experience and recommendations. *Journal of Pediatric Surgery, 23*(1), 24–28.

Geertsma, M. A., Hyams, J. S., Pelletier, J. M., & Reiter S. (1985). Feeding resistance after parenteral hyperalimentation. *American Journal of Diseases in Children, 139*(3), 255–256.

Gershon, M. D. (1998). *The second brain.* New York: HarperCollins.

Gesell, A., & Ilg, F. L. (1937). *Feeding behavior of infants: A pediatric approach to the mental hygiene of early life.* Philadelphia: J. B. Lippincott.

Gibbs, C. H., Wickwire, N. A., Jacobson, A. P., Lundeen, H. C., Mahan, P. E., & Lupkiewicz, S. M. (1982). Comparison of typical chewing patterns in normal children and adults. *Journal of the American Dental Association, 105*(1), 33–42

Gibson, E. L., Wardle, J., & Watts, C. J. (1998). Fruit and vegetable consumption, nutritional knowledge and beliefs in mothers and children. *Appetite, 31*(2), 205–228.

Gibson, J. J. (1967). The mouth as an organ for laying hold on the environment. In James F. Bosma (Ed.), *Symposium on Oral Sensation and Perception* (pp. 111–136). Springfield, IL: Charles C. Thomas.

Gibson, R. S., Vanderkooy, P. D., MacDonald, A. C., Goldman, A., Ryan, B. A., & Berry, M. (1989). A growth-limiting, mild zinc-deficiency syndrome in some southern Ontario boys with low height percentiles. *American Journal of Clinical Nutrition, 49*(6), 1266–1273.

Gilger, M. A., Boyle, J. T., Sondheimer, J. M., & Colletti, R. B. (1997). A medical position statement of the North American Society for pediatric gastroenterology and nutrition: Indications for pediatric esophageal manometry. *Journal of Pediatric Gastroenterology and Nutrition, 24*(5), 616–618.

Gillberg, C. (1995). Endogenous opioids and opiate antagonist in autism: Brief review of empirical findings and implications for clinicians. *Developmental Medicine and Child Neurology, 37*(3), 239–245.

Giordano, B. P. (1992). The impact of genetic syndromes on children's growth. *Journal of Pediatric Health Care, 6*(5 Pt 2), 309–315.

Giovannini, M., Biasucci, G., Luotti, D., Fiori, L., & Riva, E. (1995). Nutrition in children affected by inherited metabolic diseases. *Annali dell'Istituto Superiore di Sanita, 31*(4), 489–502.

Gisel, E. G. (1988a). Chewing cycles in 2 to 8 year old normal children: A development profile. *American Journal of Occupational Therapy, 42*(1), 40–46.

Gisel, E. G. (1988b). Development of oral side preference during chewing and its relation to hand preference in normal 2- to 8-year-old children. *American Journal of Occupational Therapy, 42*(6), 378–381.

Gisel, E. G. (1988c). Tongue movements in normal 2- to 8-year-old children: Extended profile of an eating assessment. *American Journal of Occupational Therapy, 42*(6), 384–389.

Gisel, E. G. (1991). Effect of food texture on the development of chewing of children between six months and two years of age. *Developmental Medicine and Child Neurology, 33*(1), 69–79.

Gisel, E. G., & Patrick, J. (1988). Identification of children with cerebral palsy unable to maintain a normal nutritional state. *Lancet, 1*(8580), 283–286.

Gisel, E. G., Applegate-Ferrante, T., Benson, J. E., & Bosma, J. F. (1995). Effect of oral sensorimotor treatment on measures of growth, eating efficency and aspiration in the dysphagic child with cerebral palsy. *Developmental Medicine and Child Neurology, 37*, 528–543.

Gisel, E. G., Schwaab, L. M., Lange-Stemmler, L., Niman, C. W., & Schwartz, J. L. (1986). Lateralization of tongue movements during eating in children 2 to 5 years old. *American Journal of Occupational Therapy, 40*(4), 265–270.

Gisel, E. G., & Schwob, H. (1998). Oral form discrimination in normal 5- to 8-year-old children: An adjunct to an eating assessment. *Occupational Therapy Journal of Research, 8*(4), 195–209.

Glass, R. P., & Wolf, L. S. (1999). Feeding management of infants with cleft lip and palate and micrognathia. *Infants and Young Children, 12*(1), 70–81.

Godfrey, S., Avital, A., Maayan, C., Rotschild, M., & Springer, C. (1997). Yield from flexible bronchoscopy in children. *Pediatric Pulmonology, 23*(4), 261–269.

Goldberg, W. B., Ferguson, F. S., & Miles, R. J. (1988). Successful use of a feeding obturator for an infant with a cleft palate. *Special Care in Dentistry, 8*(2), 86–89.

Gomes, H., & Lallemand, P. (1992). Infant apnea and gastroesophageal reflux. *Pediatric Radiology, 22*(1), 8–11.

Goodall, R., Earis, J. E., Cooper, D. N., Bernstein, A., & Temple, J. G. (1981). Relationship between asthma and gastroesophageal reflux. *Thorax, 36*(2), 116–121.

Gordon, N. (1996). Nutritional management of the disabled child: The role of percutaneous endoscopic gastrostomy. *Developmental Medicine & Child Neurology, 39,* 66–68.

Gorrotxategi, P., Eizaguirre, I., Saenz de Ugarte, A., Reguilon, M. J., Emparanza, J., Mintegui, J., Garay, J., & Ruiz Benito, A. M. (1995a). Characteristics of continuous esophageal pH-metering in infants with gastroesophageal reflux and apparent life-threatening events. *European Journal of Pediatric Surgery, 5*(3), 136–138.

Gorrotxategi, P., Reguilon, M. J., Arana, J., Gaztanaga, R., Elorza, C., de la Iglesia, E., & Barriola, M. (1995b). Gastroesophageal reflux in association with the Sandifer syndrome. *European Journal of Pediatric Surgery, 5*(4), 203–205.

Graedon, J., & Graedon, T. (1995). *The people's guide to deadly drug interactions*. New York: St. Martin's Press.

Gramm, H. J., Kopf, A., & Bratter, P. (1995). The necessity of selenium substitution in total parenteral nutrition and artificial alimentation. *Journal of Trace Elements in Medicine and Biology, 9*(1), 1–12.

Gray, V. S. (1998). Syncopal episodes associated with cisapride and concurrent drugs. *The Annals of Pharmacotherapy, 32*(6), 648–651.

Green, J. R., Moore, C. A., Ruark, J. L., Rodda, P. R., Morvee, W. T., & Van Witzenburg, M. J. (1997). Development of chewing in children from 12 to 48 months: Longitudinal study of EMG patterns. *Journal of Neurophysiology, 77*(5), 2704–2716.

Greenspan, J. S., Wolfson, M. R., Holt, W. J., & Shaffer, T. H. (1990). Neonatal gastric intubation: Differential respiratory effects between nasogastric and orogastric tubes. *Pediatric Pulmonology, 8*(4), 254–258.

Greenspan, S. I. (1985). *First feelings*. New York: Penguin Books.

Greenspan, S. I. (1995). *The challenging child*. Reading, MA: Addison-Wesley.

Greenspan, S. I., & Lourie, R. S. (1981). Developmental structuralist approach to classification of adaptive and pathologic personality organizations: Infancy and early childhood. *American Journal of Psychiatry, 138*(6), 725–735.

Greger, J. L. (1999). Nondigestible carbohydrates and mineral bioavailability. *The Journal of Nutrition, 129*(Suppl. 7), 1434S–1435S.

Grunow, J. E., Al-Hafidh, A. S., & Tunell, W. P. (1989). Gastroesophageal reflux following percutaneous endoscopic gastrostomy in children. *Journal of Pediatric Surgery, 24*(1), 42–45.

Guilfoyle, G., & Carbone, D. (1996) *The facilitation of attention utilizing therapeutic sounds* [Web Page]. URL http://www.monroeinstitute.org/research/hsj-1997-spring-attention-guilfoyle-carbone.html.

Guinard, J. X., & Brun, P. (1998). Sensory-specific satiety: Comparison of taste and texture effects. *Appetite, 31*(2), 141–157.

Guo, S. S., Roche, A. F., Chumlea, W. C., Casey, P. H., & Moore, W. M. (1997). Growth in weight, recumbent length, and head circumference for preterm low-birthweight infants during the first three years of life using gestation-adjusted ages. *Early Human Development, 47*(3), 305–325.

Guo, S. S., Wholihan, K., Roche, A. F., Chumlea, W. C., & Casey, P. H. (1996). Weight-for-length reference data for preterm, low-birth-weight infants. *Archives of Pediatric and Adolescent Medicine, 150*(9), 964–970.

H

Hack, M., Weissman, B., & Borawski-Clark, E. (1996). Catch-up growth during childhood among very low-birth-weight children. *Archives of Pediatric and Adolescent Medicine, 150*(11), 1122–1129.

Hagberg, C., Larson, O., & Milerad, J. (1998). Incidence of cleft lip and palate and risks of additional malformations. *The Cleft Palate-Craniofacial Journal, 35*(1), 40–45.

Hagopian, L. P., Farrell, D. A., & Amari, A. (1996). Treating total liquid refusal with backward chaining and fading. *Journal of Applied Behavioral Analysis, 29*(4), 573–575.

Halstead, L. A. (1999). Role of gastroesophageal reflux in pediatric upper airway disorders. *Otolaryngology—Head and Neck Surgery, 120*(2), 208–214.

Hamilton, A. B., & Zeltzer, L. K. (1994). Visceral pain in infants. *The Journal of Pediatrics, 125*(6 Pt 2), S95–S102.

Hammer, L. D. (1992). The development of eating behavior in childhood. *Pediatric Clinics of North America, 39*(3), 379–394.

Hampl, J. S., Taylor, C. A., & Johnston, C. S. (1999). Intakes of vitamin C, vegetables and fruits: Which schoolchildren are at risk? *Journal of American College of Nutrition , 18*(6), 582–590.

Handen, B. L., Mandell, F., & Russo, D. C. (1986). Feeding induction in children who refuse to eat. *Archives of Diseases in Children, 140*(Jan), 52–54.

Hanson, M. (1976). Tongue thrust: A point of view. *Journal of Speech and Hearing Disorders, XLI,* 172–184.

Hanson, M. L., & Cohen, M. S. (1973). Effects of form and function on swallowing and the developing dentition. *American Journal of Orthodontics, 64*(1), 63–82.

Harris, C. S., Baker, S. P., Smith, G. A., & Harris, R. P. (1984). Childhood asphyxiation by food. *Journal of the American Medical Association, 251*(17), 2231–2235.

Harris, N. S., Courchesne, E., Townsend, J., Carper R. A., & Lord, C. (1999). Neuroanatomic contributions to slowed orienting of attention in children with autism. *Cognitive Brain Research, 8*(1), 61–71.

Hayden, C. K. Jr, Swischuk, L. E., & Rytting, J. E. (1987). Gastric ulcer disease in infants: US findings. *Radiology, 164*(1), 131–134.

Healy, J. M. (1990). *Endangered minds: Why children don't think and what we can do about it*. New York: Simon & Schuster Trade.

Hegardt, P., Lindberg, T., Borjesson, J., & Skude, G. (1984). Amylase in human milk from mothers of preterm and term infants. *Journal of Pediatric Gastroenterology and Nutrition, 3*(4), 563–566.

Heine, R. G., Reddihough, D. S., & Catto-Smith, A. G. (1995). Gastro-oesophageal reflux and feeding problems after gastrostomy in children with severe neurological impairment. *Developmental Medicine and Child Neurology, 37,* 320–329.

Heitlinger, L. A. (1983). Enzymes in mother's milk and their possible role in digestion. *Journal of Pediatric Gastroenterology and Nutrition, 2*(Suppl. 1), S113–S119.

Helm, J. F., Dodds, W. J., Pelc, L. R., Palmer, D. W., Hogan, W. J., & Teeter, B. C. (1984). Effect of esophageal emptying and saliva on clearance of acid from the esophagus. *New England Journal of Medicine, 310*(5), 284–248.

Hendrix T. R. (1993). pH monitoring: Is it the gold standard for the detection of gastroesophageal reflux disease? *Dysphagia, 8*(2), 122–124.

Hennequin, M., Faulks, D., Veyrune, J. L., & Bourdiol, P. (1999). Significance of oral health in persons with Down syndrome: A literature review. *Developmental Medicine and Child Neurology, 41*(4), 275–283.

Herrmann, N. (1988). *The creative brain.* Lake Lure, NC: Brain Books.

Herzog, D. B., & Rathbun, J. M. (1982). Childhood depression: Developmental considerations. *American Journal of Diseases in Children, 136*(2), 115–120.

Hillemeier, A. C., Lange, R., McCallum, R., Seashore, J., & Gryboski, J. (1981). Delayed gastric emptying in infants with gastroesophageal reflux. *Journal of Pediatrics, 98*(2), 190–193.

Hirama, H. (1989). *Self-injurious behavior: A somatosensory treatment approach.* Baltimore: CHESS Publications.

Hirtz, D. G., & Nelson, K. (1998). Magnesium sulfate and cerebral palsy in premature infants. *Current Opinions in Pediatrics, 10*(2), 131–137.

Hjern, A., Kocturk-Runefors, T., & Jeppson, O. (1990). Food habits and infant feeding in newly resettled refugee families from Chile and the Middle East. *Scandinavian Journal of Primary Health Care, 8*(3), 145–150.

Hoch, T. A., Babbitt, R. L., Coe, D. A., Ducan, A., & Trusty, E. M. (1995). A swallow induction avoidance procedure to establish eating. *Journal of Behavior Therapy and Experimental Psychiatry, 26*(1), 41–50.

Hodge, C., Lebenthal, E., Lee, P. C., & Topper, W. (1983). Amylase in the saliva and in the gastric aspirates of premature infants: Its potential role in glucose polymer hydrolysis. *Pediatric Research, 17*(12), 998–1001.

Hofmann, P. A. (1993). Critical path method: An important tool for coordinating clinical care. *The Joint Commission Journal on Quality Improvement, 19*(7), 235–246.

Hogan, R. W. (1999). *The PDR pocket guide to prescription drugs.* New York: Pocket Books.

Holman, R. T. (1998). The slow discovery of the importance of omega 3 essential fatty acids in human health. *The Journal of Nutrition, 128*(Suppl. 2), 427S–433S.

Homer, C., & Ludwig, S. (1981). Categorization of etiology of failure to thrive. *American Journal of Diseases in Childhood, 135*(9), 848–851.

Honjo, S. (1996). A mother's complaints of overeating by her 25-month-old daughter: A proposal of anorexia nervosa by proxy. *International Journal of Eating Disorders, 20*(4), 433–437.

Horvath, K., Papadimitriou, J. C., Rabsztyn, A., Drachenberg, C., & Tildon, J. T. (1999). Gastrointestinal abnormalities in children with autistic disorder. *Journal of Pediatrics, 135*(5), 559–563.

Horvath, K., Stefanatos, G., Sokolski, K. N., Wachtel, R., Nabors, L., & Tildon, J. T. (1998). Improved social and language skills after secretin administration in patients with autistic spectrum disorders. *Journal of Association of Academic Minority Physicians, 9*(1), 9–15.

Host, A., Jacobsen, H. P., Halken, S., & Holmenlund, D. (1995). The natural history of cow's milk protein allergy/intolerance. *European Journal of Clinical Nutrition, 49* (Suppl. 1), S13–S18.

Howell, E. (1985). *Enzyme nutrition: The food enzyme concept.* Wayne, NJ: Avery Publishing Group.

Hudson, R., & Distel H. (1999 Feb 6). The flavor of life: Perinatal development of odor and taste preferences. *Schweizerische Medizinishe Wochenschrift, 129*(5), 176–181.

Huggins, P. S., Tuomi, S. K., & Young, C. (1999). Effects of nasogastric tubes on the young, normal swallowing mechanism. *Dysphagia, 14*(3), 157–161.

Humphry, R. (1991). Impact of feeding problems on the parent-infant relationship. *Infants and Young Children, 3*(3), 30–38.

Huth, M. M., & O'Brien, M. E. (1987). The gastrostomy feeding button. *Pediatric Nursing, 13*(4), 241–245.

Hyman, P. E. (1994). Gastroesophageal reflux: One reason why baby won't eat. *Journal of Pediatrics, 125*(6), S103–S109.

I

Iacono, G., Carroccio, A., Cavataio, F., Montalto, G., Cantarero, M. D., & Notarbartolo, A. (1995). Chronic constipation as a symptom of cow milk allergy. *Journal of Pediatrics, 126*(1), 34–39.

Iacono, G., Carroccio, A., Cavataio, F., Montalto, G., Kazmierska, I., Lorello, D., Soresi, M., & Notarbartolo, A. (1996). Gastroesophageal reflux and cow's milk allergy in infants: A prospective study. *The Journal of Allergy and Clinical Immunology, 97*(3), 822–827.

Iacono, G., Carroccio, A., Montalto, G., Cavataio, F., Bragion, E., Lorello, D., Balsamo, V., & Notarbartolo, A. (1991). Severe infantile colic and food intolerance: A long-term prospective study. *Journal of Pediatric Gastroenterology and Nutrition, 12*(3), 332–335.

Illingsworth, R. S., & Lister, J. (1964). The critical or sensitive period, with special reference to certain feeding problems in infants and children. *Journal of Pediatrics, 65*(6), 839–848.

Irwin, R. S., French C. L., Curley F. J., Zawacki, J. K., & Bennett, F. M. (1993). Chronic cough due to gastroesophageal reflux. Clinical, diagnostic, and pathogenetic aspects. *Chest, 104*(5), 1511–1517.

Isaacs, J. S., Georgeson, K. E., Cloud, H. H., & Woodall, N. (1994). Weight gain and triceps skinfolds fat mass after gastrostomy placement in children with developmental disabilities. *Journal of American Dietetic Association, 94*(8), 849–854.

Isch, J. A., Rescorla, F. J., Scherer, III, L. R., West, K. W., & Grosfeld, J. L. (1997). The development of gastroesophageal reflux after percutaneous endoscopic gastrostomy. *Journal of Pediatric Surgery, 32*(2), 321–324.

J

Jacobson, M. F., & Schardt, D. (1999). *Diet, ADHD and Behavior.* Washington, D.C.: Center for Science in the Public Interest.

Jantz, J. W., Blosser, C. D., & Fruechting, L. A. (1997). A motor milestone change noted with a change in sleep position. *Archives of Pediatrics and Adolescent Medicine, 151*(6), 565–568.

Jarvinen, V., Meurman, J. H., Hyvarinen, H., Rytomaa, I., & Murtomaa, H. (1988). Dental erosion and upper gastrointestinal disorders. *Oral Surgery, Oral Medicine, and Oral Pathology, 65*(3), 298–303.

Jenkins, N. H. (1994). Whatever happened to family dinner? *Vegetarian Times,* (December), 53–57.

Johnson C. R., & Babbitt, R. L. (1993). Antecedent manipulation in the treatment of primary solid food refusal. *Behavior Modification, 17*(4), 510–521.

Johnson, R. K., Goran, M. I., Ferrara, M. S., & Poehlman, E. T. (1996). Athetosis increases resting metabolic rate in adults with cerebral palsy. *Journal of the American Dietetic Association, 96*(2), 145–148.

Johnson, S. L., & Birch, L. L. (1994). Parents' and children's adiposity and eating style. *Pediatrics, 94*(5), 653–661.

Jolley, S. G., Smith, E. I., & Tunell, W. P. (1985). Protective antireflux operation with feeding gastrostomy. Experience with children. *Annals of Surgery, 201*(6), 736–740.

Jolley, S. G., Tunell, W. P., Leonard, J. C., Hoelzer, D. J., & Smith, E. I. (1987). Gastric emptying in children with gastroesophageal reflux. II: The relationship to retching symptoms following antireflux surgery. *Journal of Pediatric Surgery, 22*(10), 927–930.

Jones, B., & Donner, M. W. (Eds.) (1991). Anatomical and physiological overview. In *Normal and abnormal swallowing: Imaging in diagnosis and therapy.* New York: Springer-Verlag.

Jones, C. (1988). *Mind over labor.* New York: Viking Press

Jones, L. C., & Heermann, J. A. (1992). Parental division of infant care: Contextual influences and infant characteristics. *Nursing Research, 41*(4), 228–234.

Jones, V., & Prior, M. (1985). Motor imitation abilities and neurological signs in autistic children. *Journal of Autism and Developmental Disorders, 15*(1), 37–46.

Joshipura, K. J., Ascherio, A., Manson, J. E., Stampfer, M. J., Rimm, E. B., Speizer, F. E., Hennekens, C. H., Spiegelman, D., & Willett, W. C. (1999). Fruit and vegetable intake in relation to risk of ischemic stroke. *Journal of American Medical Association, 282*(13), 1233–1239.

Judd, P. L., & Kenny, D. J. (1990). Anatomic and physiologic aspects of disordered feeding: A dental perspective. *Journal of Neurologic Rehabilitation, 4,* 85–96.

Jun Tze, W., Dunn, H. G., & Rothstein, R. L. (1981). Endocrine profiles and metabolic aspects of Prader-Willi syndrome. In *The Prader-Willi syndrome* Holm, Vanja A.//Sulzbacher, Stephen//Pipes, Peggy ed., (pp. 281–291). Baltimore: University Park Press.

Justice, B. (1987). *Who gets sick: Thinking and health.* Houston, TX: Peak Press.

K

Kaatzke-McDonald, M. N., Post, E., & Davis, P. J. (1996). The effects of cold, touch and chemical stimulation of the anterior faucial pillar on human swallowing. *Dysphagia, 11,* 198–206.

Kadrabova, J., Mad'aric, A., Kovacikova, Z., Podivinsky, F., Ginter, E., & Gazdik, F. (1996). Selenium status is decreased in patients with intrinsic asthma. *Biological Trace Element Research, 52*(3), 241–248.

Kahn, A., Montauk, L., & Blum, D. (1987). Diagnostic categories in infants referred for an acute event suggesting near-miss SIDS. *European Journal of Pediatrics, 146*(5), 458–460.

Kahrilas, P. J. (1997). Anatomy and physiology of the gastroesophageal junction. *Gastroenterology Clinics of North America, 26*(3), 467–486.

Kahrilas, P. J., Dodds, W. J., Dent, J., Logemann, J. A., & Shaker, R. (1988). Upper esophageal sphincter function during deglutition. *Gastroenterology, 95*(1), 52–62.

Kahrilas, P. J., & Ergun, G. A. (1994). Esophageal dysphagia. *Acta Oto-Rhino-Laryngolica Belgica, 48*(2), 171–190.

Kahrilas, P. J., Fennerty, M. B., & Joelsson, B. (1999). High- versus standard-dose ranitidine for control of heartburn in poorly responsive acid reflux disease: A prospective, controlled trial. *American Journal of Gastroenterology, 94*(1), 92–97.

Kaminski, J., & Hall, W. (1996). The effect of soothing music on neonatal behavioral states in the hospital newborn nursery. *Neonatal Network, 15*(1), 45–54.

Kannan, S., Carruth, B. R., & Skinner, J. (1999). Cultural influences on infant feeding beliefs of mothers. *Journal of the American Dietetic Association, 99*(1), 88–90.

Kant, A. K., Schatzkin, A., Block, G., Ziegler, R. G., & Nestle, M. (1991). Food group intake patterns and associated nutrient profiles of the US population. *Journal of American Dietetic Association, 91*(12), 1532–1537.

Kaplan, B. J., McNicol, J., Conte, R. A., & Moghadam, H. K. (1989). Dietary replacement in preschool-aged hyperactive boys. *Pediatrics, 83*(1), 7–17.

Kaplan, M. D., & Baum, B. J. (1993). The functions of saliva. *Dysphagia, 8*(3), 225–229.

Kasari, C., & Sigman, M. (1997). Linking parental perceptions to interactions in young children with autism. *Journal of Autism and Developmental Disorders, 27*(1), 39–57.

Kasari, C., Sigman, M., Mundy, P., & Yirmiya, N. (1990). Affective sharing in the context of joint attention interactions of normal, autistic, and mentally retarded children. *Journal of Autism and Developmental Disorders, 20*(1), 87–100.

Kasari, C., Sigman, M. D., Baumgartner, P., & Stipek, D. J. (1993). Pride and mastery in children with autism. *Journal of Child Psychology and Psychiatry and Allied Disciplines, 34*(3), 353–362.

Kaufman, B. N. (1975). *Son rise: The miracle continues.* New York: H.J. Kramer.

Kaufman, B. N. (1991). *Happiness is a choice.* New York: Fawcett Columbine.

Kaufman, F. L. (1991). Managing the cleft lip and palate patient. *The Pediatric Clinics of North America, 38*(5), 1127–1147.

Kaufman, S. L., & Kaufman, B. N. (1987). The joy of "special" parenting. *Mothering,* (Spring), 90–96.

Kaul, A., & Rudolph, C. D. (1998). Gastrointestinal manometry studies in children. *Journal of Clinical Gastroenterology, 27*(3), 187–191.

Kedesdy, J. H., & Budd, K. S. (1998). *Childhood feeding disorders—Biobehavioral assessment and intervention.* Baltimore: Paul H. Brookes Publishing.

Kelly, G. S. (1999). Nutritional and botanical interventions to assist with the adaptation to stress. *Alternative Medicine Review, 4*(4), 249–265.

Kelly, K. J., Lazenby, A. J., Rowe, P. C., Yardley, J. H., Perman, J. A., & Sampson, H. A. (1995). Eosinophilic esophagitis attributed to gastroesophageal reflux: Improvement with an amino acid-based formula. *Gastroenterology, 109*(5), 1503–1512.

Kennedy, C. M. (1996). Are children's early emotions antecedents to risk taking? *Pediatric Nursing, 22*(6), 553–557, 567.

Kennedy, C. M., & Lipsitt, L. P. (1998). Risk-taking in preschool children. *Journal of Pediatric Nursing, 13*(2), 77–84.

Kennerly, R. C. (1994) *An empirical investigation into the effect of beta frequency binaural beat audio signals on four measures of human memory.* [Web Page]. URL http://www.monroeinstitute.org/research/human-memory-kennerly.html.

Kessler, D. B., & Dawson, P. (1999). *Failure to thrive and pediatric undernutrition—A transdisciplinary approach.* Baltimore: Paul H. Brookes Publishing.

Khoshoo, V., Roberts, P. L., Loe, W. A., Golladay, E. S., & Pencharz, P. B. (1994). Nutritional management of dumping syndrome associated with antireflux surgery. *Journal of Pediatric Surgery, 29*(11), 1452–1454.

Khoury, M. J., Gomez-Farias, M., & Mulinare, J. (1989). Does maternal cigarette smoking during pregnancy cause cleft lip and palate in offspring? *American Journal of Disease in Childhood, 143*(3), 333–337.

Kientz, M. A., & Dunn, W. (1997). A comparison of the performance of children with and without autism on the Sensory Profile. *American Journal of Occupational Therapy, 51*(7), 530–537.

Kishnani, P. S., Boney, A., & Chen, Y. T. (1999). Nutritional deficiencies in a patient with glycogen storage disease type Ib. *Journal of Inherited Metabolic Disease, 22*(7), 795–801.

Kitzinger, S., & Kitzinger, C. (1991). Food as metaphor. *Mothering,* (Fall), 43–47.

Kleijnen, J., & Knipschild, P. (1991). Niacin and vitamin B6 in mental functioning: A review of controlled trials in humans. *Biological Psychiatry, 29*(9), 931–941.

Klein, J. O. (1999). Management of acute otitis media in an era of increasing antibiotic resistance. *International Journal of Pediatric Otorhinolaryngology, 49*(Suppl. 1), S15–S17.

Klein, M. D. (1999). Parents have learning styles, too! How to help your therapist help your child. In R. Erhardt (Ed.), *Parent articles about NDT.* San Antonio, TX: Therapy Skill Builders.

Klein, M. D., & Delaney, T. A. (1994). *Feeding and nutrition for the child with special needs: Handouts for parents.* San Antonio, TX: Therapy Skill Builders.

Klein, M. D., & Morris, S. E. (1999). *Mealtime participation guide.* San Antonio, TX: Therapy Skill Builders.

Kleiner, S. M. (1999). Water: An essential but overlooked nutrient. *Journal of American Dietetic Association, 99*(2), 200–206.

Kliempt, P., Ruta, D., Ogston, S., Landeck, A., & Martay, K. (1999). Hemispheric-synchronisation during anaesthesia: A double-blind randomised trial using audiotapes for intraoperative nociception control. *Anaesthesia, 54*(8), 769–773.

Knill, C. (1983). Body awareness, communication and development: A programme employing music with profoundly handicapped. *International Journal of Rehabilitation Research, 6*(4), 489–492.

Knobeloch, L. M., Ziarnik, M., Anderson, H. A., & Dodson, V. N. (1995). Imported seabass as a source of mercury exposure: A Wisconsin case study. *Environmental Health Perspectives, 103*(6), 604–606.

Koenig, J. S., Davies, A. M., & Thach, B. T. (1990). Coordination of breathing, sucking, and swallowing during bottle feedings in human infants. *Journal of Applied Physiology, 69*(5), 1623–1629.

Kogo, M., Okada, G., Ishii, S., Shikata, M., Iida, S., & Matsuya, T. (1997). Breast feeding for cleft lip and palate patients, using the Hotz-type plate. *Cleft Palate-Craniofacial Journal, 34*(4), 351–353.

Kohn, A. (1993). *Punished by rewards: The trouble with gold stars, incentive plans, A's, praise, and other bribes.* Boston: Houghton Mifflin.

Koivisto U. K. (1999). Factors influencing children's food choice. *Annals of Medicine, 31*(Suppl. 1), 26–32.

Koivisto, U. K., & Sjoden, P. O. (1996). Reasons for rejection of food items in Swedish families with children aged 2-17. *Appetite, 26*(1), 89–103.

Kong, C. K., Tse, P. W., & Lee, W. Y. (1999). Bone age and linear skeletal growth of children with cerebral palsy. *Developmental Medicine and Child Neurology, 41*(11), 758–765.

Koo, W. W., & Tsang, R. (1984). Bone mineralization in infants. *Progress in Food and Nutrition Science, 8*(3-4), 229–302.

Kootz, J. P., Marinelli, B., & Cohen, D. J. (1982). Modulation of response to environmental stimulation in autistic children. *Journal of Autism and Developmental Disorders, 12*(2), 185–193.

Kovar, A. J. (1997). Nutrition assessment and management in pediatric dysphagia. *Seminars in Speech and Language, 18*(1), 39–49.

Kozielec, T., & Starobrat-Hermelin, B. (1997). Assessment of magnesium levels in children with attention deficit hyperactivity disorder (ADHD). *Magnesium Research, 10*(2), 143–148.

Kramer, S. S. (1989). Complications following esophageal atresia repair. *Dysphagia, 3*(3), 155–156.

Krasnewich, D., & Gahl, W. A. (1997). Carbohydrate-deficient glycoprotein syndrome. *Advances in Pediatrics, 44,* 109–140.

Krebs, N. F., Hambidge, K. M., & Walravens, P. A. (1984). Increased food intake of young children receiving a zinc supplement. *American Journal of Diseases in Childhood, 138*(3), 270–273.

Krick, J., Murphy, P. E., Markham, J. F. B., & Shapiro, B. K. (1992). A proposed formula for calculating energy needs of children with cerebral palsy. *Developmental Medicine and Child Neurology, 34*(6), 481–487.

Krick, J., Murphy-Miller, P., Zeger, S., & Wright, E. (1996). Pattern of growth in children with cerebral palsy. *Journal of American Dietetic Association, 96*(7), 680–685.

Krick, J., & Van Duyn, M. A. (1984). The relationship between oral-motor involvement and growth: A pilot study in a pediatric population with cerebral palsy. *Journal of American Dietetic Association, 84*(5), 555–559.

Krug, D. A., Arick, J., Almond, P. (1980). Behavior checklist for identifying severely handicapped individuals with high levels of autistic behavior. *Journal of Child Psychology and Psychiatry, 21*(3), 221–229.

L

Lambert, J., Mobassaleh, M., & Grand, R. J. (1992). Efficacy of cimetidine for gastric acid suppression in pediatric patients. *Journal of Pediatrics, 120*(3), 474–478.

Lambert, S. A. (1996). The effects of hypnosis/guided imagery on the postoperative course of children. *Journal of Developmental and Behavioral Pediatrics, 17*(5), 307–310.

Lambrenos, K., Weindling, A. M., Calam, R., & Cox, A. D. (1996). The effect of a child's disability on mother's mental health. *Archives of Disease in Childhood, 74*(2), 115–120.

Lancon, J. A., Haines, D. E., & Parent, A. D. (1998). Anatomy of the shaken baby syndrome. *The Anatomical Record, 253*(1), 13–18.

Landry, S. H., & Loveland, K. A. (1988). Communication behaviors in autism and developmental language delay. *Journal of Child Psychology and Psychiatry and Allied Disciplines, 29*(5), 621–634.

Lane, J. D., Kasian, S. J., Owens, J. E., & Marsh, G. R. (1998). Binaural auditory beats affect vigilance performance and mood. *Physiology and Behavior, 63*(2), 249–252.

Langer, J. C., Wesson, D. E., Ein, S. H., Filler, R. M., Shandling, B., Superina, R. A., & Papa, M. (1988). Feeding gastrostomy in neurologically impaired children: Is an antireflux procedure necessary? *Journal of Pediatric Gastroenterology and Nutrition, 7*(6), 837–841.

Langley, M. B., & Lombardino, J. (Eds.). (1991). Neurodevelopmental strategies for managing communication disorders in children with severe motor dysfunction. Austin, TX: Pro-Ed.

Langley, W. F., & Mann, D. (1991). Central nervous system magnesium deficiency. *Archives of Internal Medicine, 151*(3), 593–596.

Langmore, S. E., Schatz, K., & Olson, N. (1991). Endoscopic and videofluoroscopic evaluations of swallowing and aspiration. *Annals of Otology, Rhinology and Laryngology, 100*(8), 678–681.

Lanphear, B. P., Byrd, R. S., Auinger, P., & Hall, C. B. (1997). Increasing prevalence of recurrent otitis media among children in the United States. *Pediatrics, 99*(3), E1.

Larson, C. (1985). Neurophysiology of speech and swallowing. *Seminars in Speech and Language, 6*(4), 275–291.

Laudat, A., Arnaud, P., Napoly, A., & Brion, F. (1994). The intestinal permeability test applied to the diagnosis of food allergy in paediatrics. *West Indian Medical Journal, 43*(3), 87–88.

Launay, V., Gottrand, F., Turck, D., Michaud, L., Ategbo, S., & Farriaux, J. P. (1996). Percutaneous endoscopic gastrostomy in children: Influence on gastroesophageal reflux. *Pediatrics, 97*(5), 726–728.

Lawless, H. (1985). Sensory development in children: Research in taste and olfaction. *Journal of the American Dietetic Association, 85*(5), 577–582, 585.

Lawlor, M., Handley, P., & Lawlor, M. (1997). *The creative trainer: Holistic facilitation skills for accelerated learning.* New York: McGraw Hill.

Lawrence, R. A., & Lawrence, R. M. (1999). *Breastfeeding: A guide for the medical profession.* St. Louis, MO: Mosby.

Learman, L. A., Avorn, J., Everitt, D. E., & Rosenthal, R. (1990). Pygmalion in the nursing home: The effects of caregiver expectations on patient outcomes. *Journal of American Geriatric Society, 38*(7), 797–803.

Leder, S. B. (1998). Serial fiberoptic endoscopic swallowing evaluations in the management of patients with dysphagia. *Archives of Physical Medicine and Rehabilitation, 79*(10), 1264–1269.

Leder, S. B., Sasaki, C. T., & Burrell, M. I. (1998). Fiberoptic endoscopic evaluation of dysphagia to identify silent aspiration. *Dysphagia, 13*(1), 19–21.

Lelord, G., Callaway, E., & Muh, J. P. (1982). Clinical and biological effects of high doses of vitamin B6 and magnesium on autistic children. *Acta Vitaminologica et Enzymologica, 4*(1–2), 27–44.

Leonard, E. L., Trykowski, L. E., & Kirkpatrick, B. V. (1980). Nutritive sucking in high-risk neonates after perioral stimulation. *Physical Therapy, 60*(3), 299–302.

Lewis, J. A., & Counihan, R. F. (1965, August). Tongue-thrust in infancy. *Journal of Speech and Hearing Disorders, 30,* 280–282.

Lewy, A. L., & Dawson, G. (1992). Social stimulation and joint attention in young autistic children. *Journal of Abnormal Child Psychology, 20*(6), 555–566.

Lieberman, A. B., Rosenberg, D., & Simkin, P. (1992). *Easing labor pain: the complete guide to a more comfortable and rewarding birth.* Cambridge MA: Harvard Common Press.

Little, J. P., Matthews, B. L., Glock, M. S., Koufman, J. A., Reboussin, D. M., Loughlin, C. J., & McGuirt, W. F. Jr. (1997). Extraesophageal pediatric reflux: 24-hour double-probe pH monitoring of 222 children. *The Annals of Otology, Rhinology and Laryngology, 169*(Suppl), 1–16.

Lockridge, T. (1997). Now I lay me down to sleep: SIDS and infant sleep positions. *Neonatal Network, 16*(7), 25–31.

Logemann, J. A. (1993). *Manual for the Videofluorographic Study of Swallowing* (2nd ed.). Austin, TX: Pro-Ed.

Logemann, J. A. (1997). *Evaluation and treatment of swallowing disorders.* (2nd ed.) San Diego, CA: College-Hill Press.

Logemann, J. A. (1997). Role of the modified barium swallow in management of patients with dysphagia. *Otolaryngology— Head and Neck Surgery, 116*(3), 335–338.

Lonnerdal, B. (1985). Dietary factors affecting trace element bioavailability from human milk, cow's milk and infant formulas. *Progress in Food and Nutrition Science, 9*(1-2), 35–62.

Love, R. J., Hagerman, E. L., & Taimi, E. G. (1980). Speech performance, dysphagia and oral reflexes in cerebral palsy. *Journal of Speech and Hearing Disorders, 451,* 59–75.

Loveland, K. A., & Landry, S. H. (1986). Joint attention and language in autism and developmental language delay. *Journal of Autism and Developmental Disorders, 16*(3), 335–349.

Loveland, K. A., Landry, S. H., Hughes, S. O., Hall, S. K., & McEnvoy, R. E. (1988). Speech acts and the pragmatic deficits of autism. *Journal of Speech and Hearing Research, 31*(4), 593–604.

Lozanov, G. (1978). *Suggestology and outlines of Suggestopedy.* New York: Gordon and Breach.

Lozoff, B., & Brittenham, G. M. (1987). Behavioral alterations in iron deficiency. *Hematology/Oncology Clinics of North America, 1*(3), 449–464.

Lucarelli, S., Frediani, T., Zingoni, A. M., Ferruzzi, F., Giardini, O., Quintieri, F., Barbato, M., D'Eufemia, P., & Cardi, E. (1995). Food allergy and infantile autism. *Panminerva Medicine, 37*(3), 137–141.

Lundell, L. R., Myers, J. C., & Jamieson, G. G. (1994). Delayed gastric emptying and itl relationship to symptoms of 'gas float' after antireflux surgery. *European Journal of Surgery, 160* (3), 161–166.

Luostarinen M. (1993). Nissen fundoplication for reflux esophagitis. Long-term clinical and endoscopic results in 109 of 127 consecutive patients. *Annals of Surgery, 217*(4), 329–337.

Lynch, B. J., & Rust, R. S. (1994). Natural history and outcome of neonatal hypocalcemic and hypomagnesemic seizures. *Pediatric Neurology, 11*(1), 23–27.

Lynch, E. W., & Hanson, M. J. (1992). *Developing cross-cultural competence: A guide for working with young children and their families.* Baltimore: Paul H. Brookes Publishing.

Lyon, A. J., Preece, M. A., & Grant, D. B. (1985). Growth curve for girls with Turner syndrome. *Archives of Disease in Childhood, 60*(10), 932–935.

M

Machtinger, S., & Moss, R. (1986). Cow's milk allergy in breast-fed infants: the role of allergen and maternal secretory IgA antibody. *Journal of Allergy and Clinical Immunology, 77*(2), 341–347.

Macknin, M. L., VanderBrug Medendorp, S., & Maier, M. C. (1989). Infant sleep and bedtime cereal. *American Journal of Diseases of Children, 143* (September), 1066–1068.

Maggioni, A., & Lifshitz, F. (1995). Nutritional management of failure to thrive. *Pediatric Clinics of North America, 42*(4), 791-810.

Mahler, M. S., Pine, F., & Bergman A. (1975). *The psychological birth of the human infant.* New York: Basic Books.

Mandel, I. D. (1987). The functions of saliva. [Special issue]. *Journal of Dental Research, 66,* 623–627.

Mandell, M. (1976). Factors contributing to a state of increased suseptibility. In Dickey, Lawrence, D. (Eds.), *Clinical Ecology* (pp. 570–576). Springfield, IL: Charles C. Thomas.

Mandell, M. (1979). Physical and mental allergies in children. In M. Mandell, & L. W. Scanion, *Dr. Mandell's 5-day allergy relief system* (pp. 148–208). New York, NY: Pocket Books.

Mandell, M. (1982). Allergy a factor in cerebral palsy? *Prevention, 34*(2), 67.

Mangione-Smith, R., McGlynn, E. A., Elliott, M. N., Krogstad, P., & Brook, R. H. (1999). The relationship between perceived parental expectations and pediatrician antimicrobial prescribing behavior. *Pediatrics, 103*(4 Pt 1), 711–718.

Manolson, A. (1992). *It takes two to talk: A parent's guide to helping children communicate.* Toronto: Hanen Centre.

Marcon, M. A. (1997). Advances in the diagnosis and treatment of gastroesophageal reflux disease. *Current Opinions in Pediatrics, 9*(5), 490–493.

Margetts, B. M., Martinez, J. A., Saba, A., Holm, L., Kearney, M., & Moles, A. (1997). Definitions of "healthy" eating: A pan-EU survey of consumer attitudes to food, nutrition and health. *European Journal of Clinical Nutrition, 51*(Suppl. 2), S23–S29.

Marley, L. S. (1984). The use of music with hospitalized infants and toddlers: A descriptive study. *Journal of Music Therapy, 21*(3), 126–132.

Marlier, L., Schaal, B., & Soussignan, R. (1998). Bottle-fed neonates prefer an odor experienced in utero to an odor experienced postnatally in the feeding context. *Developmental Psychobiology, 33*(2), 133–145.

Marmet, C., (1991). *Breastfeeding your baby: Positioning.* [Videotape]. McHenry, IL: Medela.

Marmet, C., & Shell, E. (1984). Training neonates to suck correctly. *Maternal Child Nursing, 9*(November/December), 401–407.

Marshalla, P. R. (1985). The role of reflexes in oral-motor learning: Techniques for improved articulation. *Seminars in Speech and Language, 6*(4), 317–335.

Martineau, J., Barthelemy, C., Garreau, B., & Lelord, G. (1985). Vitamin B6, magnesium, and combined B6-Mg: Therapeutic effects in childhood autism. *Biological Psychiatry, 20*(5), 467–478.

Matheny, R. J., Birch, L. L., & Picciano, M. F. (1990). Control of intake by human-milk-fed infants: Relationships between feeding size and interval. *Developmental Psychobiology, 23*(6), 511–518.

Mathew, O. P. (1988). Nipple units for newborn infants: A functional comparison. *Pediatrics, 81*(5), 688–691.

Mathew, O. P. (1991). Breathing patterns of preterm infants during bottle feeding: Role of milk flow. *The Journal of Pediatrics, 119*(6), 960–965.

Mathew, O. P., & Bhatia, J. (1989). Sucking and breathing patterns during breast- and bottle-feeding in term neonates: Effects of nutrient delivery and composition. *American Journal of Diseases in Children, 143*(May), 588–592.

Mathew, O. P., Clark, M. L., & Pronske, M. H. (1985). Breathing pattern of neonates during nonnutritive sucking. *Pediatric Pulmonology, 1*(4), 204–206.

Mathew, O. P., Clark, M. L., Pronske, M. L., Luna-Solarzano, H. G., & Peterson, M. D. (1985). Breathing pattern and ventilation during oral feeding in term newborn infants. *Journal of Pediatrics, 106*(5), 810–813.

Mathiesen, K. S., Tambs, K., & Dalgard, O. S. (1999). The influence of social class, strain and social support on symptoms of anxiety and depression in mothers of toddlers. *Social Psychiatry and Psychiatric Epidemiology, 34*(2), 61–72.

Mathisen, B., Skuse, D., Wolke, D., & Reilly, S. (1989). Oral-motor dysfunction and failure to thrive among inner-city infants. *Developmental Medicine and Child Neurology, 31,* 293-302.

Mathisen, B., Worrall, L., Masel, J., Wall, C., & Shepherd, R. (1999). Feeding problems in infants with gastro-esophageal reflux disease: A controlled study. *Journal of Paediatrics and Child Health, 35*(2), 163–169.

Maton, P. N., Orlando, R., & Joelsson, B. (1999). Efficacy of omeprazole versus ranitidine for symptomatic treatment of poorly responsive acid reflux disease—a prospective, controlled trial. *Alimentary Pharmacology and Therapeutics, 13*(6), 819–826.

Matthews, B. L., Little, J. P., McGuirt, W. F., Jr., & Koufman, J. A. (1999). Reflux in infants with laryngomalacia: Results of 24-hour double-probe pH monitoring. *Otolaryngology—Head and Neck Surgery, 120*(6), 860–864.

Mayes, S. D., & Calhoun, S. L. (1999). Symptoms of autism in young children and correspondence with the DSM. *Infants and Young Children, 12*(2), 90–97.

Mayr, J., Sauer, H., Huber, A., Pilhatsch, A., & Ratschek, M. (1998). Modified Toupet wrap for gastroesophageal reflux in childhood. *European Journal of Pediatric Surgery, 8*(2), 75–80.

McCain, G. C. (1995). Promotion of preterm infant nipple feeding with nonnutritive sucking. *Journal of Pediatric Nursing, 10*(1), 3–8.

McCann, J. B., Stein, A., Fairburn, C. G., & Dunger, D. B. (1994). Eating habits and attitudes of mothers of children with non-organic failure to thrive. *Archives of Disease in Childhood, 70*(3), 234–236.

McCraty, R., Barrios-Choplin, B., Atkinson, M., & Tomasino, D. (1998). The effects of different types of music on mood, tension, and mental clarity. *Alternative Therapies in Health and Medicine, 4*(1), 75–84.

McGraw, M. B. (1966). *The neuromuscular maturation of the human infant.* New York: Hafner.

McGuire, J. K., Kulkarni, M. S., & Baden, H. P. (2000). Fatal hypermagnesemia in a child treated with megavitamin/megamineral therapy. *Pediatrics, 105*(2), 18.

McKenna, C. J., Mills, J. G., Goodwin, C., & Wood, J. R. (1995). Combination of ranitidine and cisapride in the treatment of reflux oesophagitis. *European Journal of Gastroenterology and Hepatology, 7*(9), 817–822.

McKenzie, R. C., Rafferty, T. S., & Beckett, G. J. (1998). Selenium: An essential element for immune function. *Immunology Today, 19*(8), 342–345.

Measel, C. P., & Anderson, G. C. (1979). Nonnutritive sucking during tube feedings: Effect on clinical course in premature infants. *Journal of Obstetric, Gynecologic, and Neonatal Nursing, 8*(5), 265–272.

Medoff-Cooper, B. (1995). Infant temperament: Implications for parenting from birth through 1 year. *Journal of Pediatric Nursing, 10*(3), 141–145.

Meier, P. (1988). Bottle- and breast-feeding: Effects on transcutaneous oxygen pressure and temperature in preterm infants. *Nursing Research, 37*(1), 36–41.

Melnick, M. (1986). Cleft lip with or without cleft palate: Etiology and pathogenesis. *California Dental Association Journal, 14*(12), 92–96.

Mennella, J. A. (1995). Mother's milk: A medium for early flavor experiences. *Journal of Human Lactation, 11*(1), 39–45.

Mennella, J. A. (1996). The flavor world of infants: A cross-cultural perspective. *Pediatric Basics, 77*(Summer), 2–8.

Mennella, J. A., & Beauchamp, G. K. (1991). Maternal diet alters the sensory qualities of human milk and the nursling's behavior. *Pediatrics, 88*(4), 737–744.

Mennella, J. A., & Beauchamp, G. K. (1993a). Early flavor experiences: When do they start? *Zero to Three, 14*(2), 1–7.

Mennella, J. A., & Beauchamp, G. K. (1993b). The effects of repeated exposure to garlic-flavored milk on the nursling's behavior. *Pediatric Research, 34*(6), 805–808.

Mennella, J. A., & Beauchamp, G. K. (1997). Mothers' milk enhances the acceptance of cereal during weaning. *Pediatric Research, 41*(2), 188–192.

Mennella, J. A., & Beauchamp, G. K. (1998a). Early flavor experiences: Research update. *Nutrition Reviews, 56*(7), 205–211.

Mennella, J. A., & Beauchamp, G. K. (1998b). Infants' exploration of scented toys: Effects of prior experiences. *Chemical Senses, 23*(1), 11–17.

Mennella, J. A., Johnson, A., & Beauchamp, G. K. (1995). Garlic ingestion by pregnant women alters the odor of amniotic fluid. *Chemical Senses, 20*(2), 207–209.

Merritt, S. (1990). *Mind, music and imagery: Unlocking your creative potential.* New York: Plume.

Meyers, W. F., & Herbst, J. J. (1982). Effectiveness of positioning therapy for gastroesophageal reflux. *Pediatrics, 69*(6), 768–772.

Michel, D. E., & May, N. H. (1984). The development of music therapy procedures with speech and language disorders. *Journal of Music Therapy, 9*(Summer), 74–80.

Miles, B. (1998). The importance of hands for the person who is deaf-blind. *D-B Link: National Information Clearinghouse on Children Who Are Deaf-Blind, 5,* 1–12.

Miller, A. J. (1986). Neurophysiological basis of swallowing. *Dysphagia, 1,* 91–100.

Miller, A. J. (1993). The search for the central swallowing pathway: The quest for clarity. *Dysphagia, 8* (3), 185–194.

Miller, M. J., Martin, R. J., Carlo, W. A., & Fanaroff, A. A. (1987). Oral breathing in response to nasal trauma in term infants. *Journal of Pediatrics, 111*(6 Pt 1), 899–901.

Miller, M. J., Martin, R. J., Carlo, W. A., Fouke, J. M., Strohl, K. P., & Fanaroff, A. A. (1985). Oral breathing in newborn infants. *Journal of Pediatrics, 107*(3), 465–469.

Miller, S. B., & Toca, J. M. (1979). Adapted melodic intonation therapy: A case study of an experimental language program for an autistic child. *Journal of Clinical Psychiatry, 40*(4), 201–203.

Mirenda, P. L., Donnellan, A. M., & Yoder, D. E. (1983). Gaze behavior: A new look at an old problem. *Journal of Autism and Developmental Disorders, 13*(4), 397–409.

Mollitt, D. L., Golladay, S., & Seibert, J. (1985). Symptomatic gastroesophageal reflux following gastrostomy in neurologically impaired patients. *Pediatrics, 75*(6), 1124–1126.

Moore, C. A., & Ruark, J. L. (1996). Does speech emerge from earlier appearing oral motor behaviors? *Journal of Speech and Hearing Research, 39*(5), 1034–1047.

Morgan, J. (1987). What nurses learn from structured observations of mother-infant interactions. *Issues in Comprehensive Pediatric Nursing, 10,* 67–73.

Morris, S. E. (1978). A longitudinal study of feeding and pre-speech skills from birth to three years. Unpublished study.

Morris, S. E. (1981). Communication/interaction development at mealtimes for the multiply handicapped child: Implications for the use of augmentative communication systems. *Language, Speech, and Hearing Services in Schools, XII*(October), 216–232.

Morris, S. E. (1982). *Pre-Speech Assessment Scale: A rating scale for the measurement of pre-speech behaviors from birth through two years.* Clifton, NJ: J. A. Preston.

Morris, S. E. (1985). Developmental implications for the management of feeding problems in neurologically impaired infants. *Seminars in Speech and Language, 6*(4), 293–315.

Morris, S. E. (1989). Development of oral-motor skills in the neurologically impaired child receiving non-oral feedings. *Dysphagia, 3,* 135–154.

Morris, S. E. (1991). Facilitation of learning. In M. B. Langley & L. J. Lombardino (Eds.), *Neurodeveloopmental strategies for managing communication disorders in children with severe motor dysfunction* (pp. 251–296). Austin, TX: Pro-Ed.

Morris, S. E. (1992). Eating readiness cues: Introducing supplemental foods. *Pediatric Basics, 61*(Summer), 2–5.

Morris, S. E. (1994). A cross-sectional study of eating readiness skills from four to twenty-eight months. Unpublished study.

Morris, S. E. (1996). Music and Hemi-Sync in the treatment of children with developmental disabilities. *Open Ear,* (2), 14–18.

Morris, S. E. (1997a). *Feeding and pre-speech characteristics: Children with mild sensorimotor impairment* [Web Page]. URL http://www.new-vis.com/fym/papers/p-feed5.htm.

Morris, S. E. (1997b). *Why evaluate and treat mild feeding delays and limitations* [Web Page]. URL http://www.newvis.com/fym/papers/p-feed6.htm.

Morris, S. E. (1997c). Opening the door with Metamusic. In D. J. Schneck & J. K. Schneck (Eds.), *Music in human adaptation.* Blacksburg, VA: Virginia Polytechnic Institute and State University.

Morris, S. E. (1998a). *Formula rotation for children who receive tube feedings* [Web Page]. URL http://www.new-vis.com/fym/papers/p-feed7.htm.

Morris, S. E. (1998b). *Mouth stuffing* [Web Page]. URL http://www.new-vis.com/fym/papers/p-feed11.htm.

Morris, S. E. (1999a). Component charts for feeding development. In S. Morris (Ed.), *Feeding and pre-speech issues: The mild and moderately impaired child* (10th ed.). Faber, VA: New Visions.

Morris, S. E. (1999b). Components of efficient oral feeding. In S. Morris (Ed.), *From tube to table: A new vision for children who receive non-oral feedings* (1st ed.). Faber VA: New Visions.

Muhudhia, S. O., & Musoke, R. N. (1989). Postnatal weight gain of exclusively breast-fed preterm African infants. *Journal of Tropical Pediatrics, 35*(5), 241–244.

Mundy, P., Sigman, M., Ungerer, J., & Sherman, T. (1986). Defining the social deficits of autism: The contribution of non-verbal communication measures. *Journal of Child Psychology and Psychiatry and Allied Disciplines, 27*(5), 657–669.

Muñoz, K. A., Krebs-Smith, S. M., Ballard-Barbash, R., & Cleveland, L. E. (1997). Food intakes of US children and adolescents compared with recommendations. *Pediatrics, 100*(3 Pt 1), 323–329.

Murdock, M. (1987). *Spinning inward.* Shambhala Publications.

Murray, L., Fiori-Cowley, A., Hooper, R., & Cooper, P. (1996). The impact of postnatal depression and associated adversity on early mother-infant interactions and later infant outcome. *Child Development, 67*(5), 2512–2526.

Murray, M. T. (1996). *Encyclopedia of nutritional supplements: The essential guide for improving your health naturally*. Rocklin, CA: Prima Publishing.

Murray, R. (1996). Glycoproteins. In R. Murray, D. Granner, P. Mayes, & V. Rodwell (Eds.), *Harpers Biochemistry* (pp. 648–666). Stamford, CT: Appleton and Lange.

Murray, R., Eddy, D. E., Bartoli, W. P., & Paul, G. L. (1994). Gastric emptying of water and isocaloric carbohydrate solutions consumed at rest. *Medicine and Science in Sports and Exercise, 26*(6), 725–732.

Mutanen, M., & Mykkanen, H. M. (1985). Effect of ascorbic acid supplementation on selenium bioavailability in humans. *Human Nutrition, Clinical Nutrition, 39*(3), 221–226.

Myers, G. J., Davidson, P. W., Shamlaye, C. F., Axtell, C. D., Cernichiari, E., Choisy, O., Choi, A., Cox, C., & Clarkson, T. W. (1997). Effects of prenatal methylmercury exposure from a high fish diet on developmental milestones in the Seychelles Child Development Study. *Neurotoxicology, 18*(3), 819–829.

N

National Academy of Sciences. (1995). *Recommended dietary allowances* (10th edition). Washington, DC: National Research Council, Food and Nutrition Board.

Neidig, J. R., Megel, M. E., & Koehler, K. M. (1992). The critical path: An evaluation of the applicability of nursing case management in the NICU. *Neonatal Network, 11*(5), 45–52.

Neisworth, J. T., Bagnato, S. J., & Salvia, J. (1995). Neurobehavioral markers for early regulatory disorders. *Infants and Young Children, 88*(1), 8–17.

Nelson, S. P., Chen, E. H., Syniar, G. M., & Christoffel, K. K. (1998). One-year follow-up of symptoms of gastroesophageal reflux during infancy. *Pediatrics, 102*(6), E67.

Newman, J., & Taylor, A. (1992). Effect of a means-end contingency on young children's food preferences. *Journal of Experimental Child Psychology, 53*(2), 200–216.

Nisinzweig, S. (1999). Phytochemicals and glyconutrients in autistic children. *Proceedings of the Fisher Institute,1*(3), 12–14.

Nolte, D. L., Provenza, F. D., & Balph, D. F. (1990). The establishment and persistence of food preferences in lambs exposed to selected foods. *Journal of Animal Science, 68*(4), 998–1002.

Nordstrom, D. G. (1988). Cloth sling for treatment of infant gastroesophageal reflux. *The American Journal of Occupational Therapy, 42*(7), 465–468.

Notestine, G. E. (1990). The importance of the identification of ankyloglossia (short lingual frenulum) as a cause of breastfeeding problems. *Journal of Human Lactation, 6*(3), 113–115.

Noviski, N., Yehuda, Y. B., Serour, F., Gorenstein, A., & Mandelberg, A. (1999). Does the size of nasogastric tubes affect gastroesophageal reflux in children? *Journal of Pediatric Gastroenterology and Nutrition, 29*(4), 448–451.

Nowak, A. J. (1993). What pediatricians can do to promote oral health. *Contemporary Pediatrics, 10*(April), 90–106.

Nsouli, T. M., Nsouli, S. M., Linde, R. E., O'Mara, F., Scanlon, R. T., & Bellanti, J. A. (1994). Role of food allergy in serous otitis media. *Annals of Allergy, 73*(3), 215–219.

O

O'Banion, D., Armstrong, B., Cummings, R. A., & Stange, J. (1978). Disruptive behavior: A dietary approach. *Journal of Autism and Childhood Schizophrenia, 8*(3), 325–337.

Oetter, P., Richter, E., & Frick, S. M. (1988). *M.O.R.E.: Integrating the mouth with sensory and postural functions*. Hugo, MN: PDP Press.

Oller, D. K. (1978). Infant vocalization and the development of speech. *Allied Health and Behavioral Sciences, 1*(4), 523–549.

Oller, D. K., Eilers, R. E., Neal, A. R., & Cobo-Lewis, A. B. (1998). Late onset canonical babbling: a possible early marker of abnormal development. *American Journal of Mental Retardation, 103*(3), 249–263.

Oller, D. K., Eilers, R. E., Neal, A. R., & Schwartz, H. K. (1999). Precursors to speech in infancy: the prediction of speech and language disorders. *Journal of Communication Disorders, 32*(4), 223–245.

Oller, D. K., Wieman, L. A., Doyle, W. J., & Ross, C. Infant babbling and speech. *Journal of Child Language, 3*, 1–11.

Olson, J. R., & Morris, S. E. (1978). Problem solving with parents of children with cerebral palsy. In R. E. Hartbauer (Ed.), *Counseling in communication disorders* (pp. 227–269). Springfield, IL: Charles C. Thomas.

Orenstein, S. R. (1988). Effect of nonnutritive sucking on infant gastroesophageal reflux. *Pediatric Research, 24*(1), 38–40.

Orenstein, S. R. (1992). Gastroesophageal reflux. *Pediatrics in Review, 13*(5), 174–182.

Orenstein, S. R., Klein, H. A., & Rosenthal, M. S. (1993). Scintigraphy versus pH probe for quantification of pediatric gastroesophageal reflux: A study using concurrent multiplexed data and acid feedings. *Journal of Nuclear Medicine, 34*(8), 1228–1234.

Orenstein, S. R., Magill, H. L., & Brooks, P. (1987). Thickening of infant feedings for therapy of gastroesophageal reflux. *The Journal of Pediatrics, 110*(2), 181–186.

Orenstein, S. R., & Whitington, P. F. (1983). Positioning for prevention of infant gastroesophageal reflux. *The Journal of Pediatrics, 103*(4), 534–537.

Orenstein, S. R., Whitington, P. F., & Orenstein, D. M. (1983). The infant seat as treatment for gastroesophageal reflux. *The New England Journal of Medicine, 309*(13), 760–763.

Ornstein, R. (1998). *The right mind: Making sense of the hemispheres*. Northglenn, CO: Harvest Books.

Ostrander, S., & Schroeder, L. (1979). *Superlearning*. New York: Delta Press.

Osuji, O. O. (1995). Preparation of feeding obturators for infants with cleft lip and palate. *Journal of Clinical Pediatric Dentistry, 19*(3), 211–214.

O'Sullivan, E. A., Curzon, M. E., Roberts, G. J., Milla, P. J., & Stringer, M. D. (1998). Gastroesophageal reflux in children and its relationship to erosion of primary and permanent teeth. *European Journal of Oral Sciences, 106*(3), 765–769.

Oue, T., & Puri, P. (1999). Smooth muscle cell hypertrophy versus hyperplasia in infantile hypertrophic pyloric stenosis. *Pediatric Research, 45*(6), 853–857.

The Oxford Dictionary of English. (1989). Oxford, England: Oxford University Press.

P

Palmer, M. M. (1993). Identification and management of the transitional suck pattern in premature infants. *Journal of Perinatal and Neonatal Nursing, 7*(1), 66–75.

Palmer, M. M., Crawley, K., & Blanco, I. A. (1993). Neonatal oral-motor assessment scale: A reliability study. *Journal of Perinatology, 13*(1), 28–35.

Papaila, J. G., Wilmot, D., Grosfeld, J. L., Rescorla, F. J., West, K. W., & Vane, D. W. (1989). Increased incidence of delayed gastric emptying in children with gastroesophageal reflux: A prospective evaluation. *Archives of Surgery, 124*(8), 933–936

Parraga, I. M., Weber, M. A., Engel, A., Reeb, K. G., & Lerner, E. (1988). Feeding patterns of urban black infants. *Journal of the American Dietetic Association, 88*(7), 796–800.

Patrick, J., & Gisel, E. (1990). Nutrition for the feeding impaired child. *Journal of Neurological Rehabilitation, 4,* 115–119.

Patterson, B. H., Block, G., Rosenberger, W. F., Pee, D., & Kahle, L. L. (1990). Fruit and vegetables in the American diet: Data from the NHANES II survey. *American Journal of Public Health, 80*(12), 1443–1449.

Pearcey, S. M., & De Castro, J. M. (1997). Food intake and meal patterns of one year old infants. *Appetite, 29*(2), 201–212.

Pearlman, C. (1984). The effects of level of effectance motivation, IQ, and a penalty/reward contingency on the choice of problem difficulty. *Child Development, 55*(4), 537–542.

Pearson, F. G., Cooper, J. D., & Nelems, J. M. (1978). Gastroplasty and fundoplication in the management of complex reflux problems. *The Journal of Thoracic and Cardiovascular Surgery, 76*(5), 665–672.

Perusse, L., & Bouchard, C. (1999). Role of genetic factors in childhood obesity and in susceptibility to dietary variations. *Annals of Medicine, 31*(Suppl. 1), 19–25.

Phillips, S. F., & Wingate, D. L. (Eds.). (1998). *Functional disorders of the gut.* New York: Churchill Livingstone.

The physician's desk reference. (1998). Montvale, NJ: Medical Economics.

Pickler, R. H., Frankel, H. B., Walsh, K. M., & Thompson, N. M. (1996). Effects of nonnutritive sucking on behavioral organization and feeding performance in preterm infants. *Nursing Research, 45*(3), 132–135.

Pickler, R. H., Higgins, K. E., & Crummette, B. D. (1993). The effect of nonnutritive sucking on bottle-feeding stress in preterm infants. *Journal of Obstetric, Gynecologic, and Neonatal Nursing, 22*(3), 230–234.

Pitchford, P. (1993). *Healing with whole foods—Oriental traditions and modern nutrition.* Berkeley, CA: North Atlantic Books.

Pittschieler, K. (1991). Dumping syndrome after combined pyloroplasty and fundoplication. *European Journal of Pediatrics, 150*(6), 410–412.

Plaxico, D. T., & Loughlin, G. M. (1981). Nasopharyngeal reflux and neonatal apnea. *American Journal of Diseases in Children, 135*(9), 793–794.

Pliner, P., & Loewen, E. R. (1997). Temperament and food neophobia in children and their mothers. *Appetite, 28*(3), 239–254.

Ploysangam, A., Falciglia, G. A., & Brehm, B. J. (1997). Effect of marginal zinc deficiency on human growth and development. *Journal of Tropical Pediatrics, 43*(4), 192–198.

Porter, G., & Norris, P. (1985). *Why me?* Walpole, NH: Stillpoint Publishing.

Pouderoux, P., & Kahrilas, P. J. (1997). Function of upper esophageal sphincter during swallowing: The grabbing effect. *American Journal of Physiology, 272*(5 Pt 1), G1057–G1063.

Pouderoux, P., Shi, G., Tatum, R. P., & Kahrilas, P. J. (1999). Esophageal solid bolus transit: Studies using concurrent videofluoroscopy and manometry. *American Journal of Gastroenterology, 94*(6), 1457–1463.

Powell, G. F., & Bettes, B. A. (1992). Infantile depression, nonorganic failure to thrive, and DSM-III-R: A different perspective. *Child Psychiatry and Human Development, 22*(3), 185–198.

Price, G. M. (1983). Sensitivity in mother-infant interactions: The AMIS Scale. *Infant Behavioral Development, 6*(3), 352–360.

Prichard, A., & Taylor, J. (1980). *Accelerating learning: The use of suggestion in the classroom.* Novato, CA: Academic Therapy.

Pridham, K. F. (1987). Meaning of infant feeding issues and others' use of help. *Journal of Reproductive and Infant Psychology, 5*(3), 145–152.

Pridham, K., Kosorok, M. R., Greer, F., Carey, P., Kayata, S., & Sondel, S. (1999). The effects of prescribed versus ad libitum feedings and formula caloric density on premature infant dietary intake and weight gain. *Nursing Research, 48*(2), 86–93.

Prizant, B. M., & Wetherby, A. M. (1987). Communicative intent: A framework for understanding social-communicative behavior in autism. *Journal of American Academy of Child Adolescent Psychiatry, 26*(4), 472–479.

Prochaska, L. J., & Piekutowski, W. V. (1994). On the synergistic effects of enzymes in food with enzymes in the human body: A literature survey and analytical report. *Medical Hypotheses, 42*(6), 355–362.

Putnam, P. E. (1997). Gastroesophageal reflux disease and dysphagia in children. *Seminars in Speech and Language, 18*(1), 25?37.

Putnam, P. E., & Orenstein, S. R. (1992). Hoarseness in a child with gastroesophageal reflux. *Acta Paediatrica, 81*(8), 635?636.

Q

Quinn, H. P. (1995). Nutrition concerns for children with pervasive developmental disorder/autism. *Nutrition Focus, 10*(5), 1–4.

R

Ragneskog, H., Brane, G., Karlsson, I., & Kihlgren, M. (1996). Influence of dinner music on food intake and symptoms common in dementia. *Scandinavian Journal of Caring Sciences, 10*(1), 11–17.

Ragneskog, H., Kihlgren, M., Karlsson, I., & Norberg, A. (1996). Dinner music for demented patients: Analysis of video-recorded observations. *Clinical Nursing Research, 5*(3), 262–277; discussion 278–282.

Raiten, D. J., & Massaro, T. (1986). Perspectives on the nutritional ecology of autistic children. *Journal of Autism and Developmental Disorders, 16*(2), 133–143.

Ramachandran, V., Ashcraft K. W., Sharp R. J., Murphy P. J., Snyder C. L., Gittes G. K., & Bickler S. W. (1996). Thal fundoplication in neurologically impaired children. *Journal of Pediatric Surgery, 31*(6), 819–822.

Rance, F., & Dutau, G. (1999). Peanut hypersensitivity in children. *Pediatric Pulmonology, 18*(Suppl.), 165–167.

Randolph, T., & Moss, R. (1990). *An alternative approach to allergies: The new field of clinical ecology unravels the environmental causes of mental and physical ills.* New York: HarperCollins.

Rapp, D. J. (1991). *Is this your child?: Discovering and treating unrecognized allergies.* New York: William Morrow and Company.

Rapp, D. J. (1996). *Is this your child's world?* New York: Bantam Books.

Raval, D. (1998). Unpublished research data. Tucson, AZ: University of Arizona Health Science Center.

Ray, T. C., King, L. J., & Grandin, T. (1988). The effectiveness of self-initiated vestibular stimulation in producing speech sounds in an autistic child. *The Occupational Therapy Journal of Research, 8*(3), 187–191.

Reichelt, K. L., Hole, K., Hamberger, A., Saelid, G., Edminson, P. D., Braestrup C. B., Lingjaerde, O., Ledaal, P., & Orbeck, H. (1981). Biologically active peptide-containing fractions in schizophrenia and childhood autism. In J. B. Martin, S. Reichlin, & K. L. Bick (Eds.), *Neurosecretion and Brain Peptides* (pp. 627–643). New York: Raven.

Reilly, S. M., Skuse, D. H., Wolke, D., & Stevenson, J. (1999). Oral-motor dysfunction in children who fail to thrive: Organic or non-organic. *Developmental Medicine & Child Neurology, 41*(2), 115–122.

Reitman, D. (1998). The real and imagined harmful effects of rewards: Implications for clinical practice. *Journal of Behavior Therapy and Experimental Psychiatry, 29*(2), 101–113.

Rempel, G. R., Colwell, S. O., & Nelson, R. P. (1988). Growth in children with cerebral palsy fed via gastrostomy. *Pediatrics, 82*(6), 857–862.

Revol, O., Rochet, T., Maillet, J., Gerard, D., & de Villard, R. (1994). Depression in children: Etiological, clinical and therapeutical aspects. *Archives of Pediatrics, 1*(6), 602–610.

Riese, M. L. (1990). Neonatal temperament in monozygotic and dizygotic twin pairs. *Child Development, 61*(4), 1230–1237.

Rimland, B. (1988). Controversies in the treatment of autistic children: Vitamin and drug therapy. *Journal of Child Neurology, 3*(Suppl. S), 68–72.

Rimland, B., Callaway, E., & Dreyfus, P. (1978). The effect of high doses of vitamin B6 on autistic children: A double-blind crossover study. *American Journal of Psychiatry, 135*(4), 472–475.

Rings, E. H., Grand, R. J., & Buller, H. A. (1994). Lactose intolerance and lactase deficiency in children. *Current Opinions in Pediatrics, 6*(5), 562–567.

Rivkees, S. A., & Crawford, J. D. (1987). Hypoglycemia pathogenesis in children with dumping syndrome. *Pediatrics, 80*(6), 937–942.

Roberts, S. B., Heyman, M. B., & Tracy, L. (1999). *Feeding your child for lifelong health.* New York: Bantam Books.

Roche, A. F., Guo, S. S., Wholihan, K., & Casey, P. H. (1997). Reference data for head circumference-for-length in preterm low-birth-weight infants. *Archive of Pediatric and Adolescent Medicine, 151*(1), 50–57.

Rodman, D. P., Stevenson, T. L., & Ray, T. R. (1995). Phenytoin malabsorption after jejunostomy tube delivery. *Pharmacotherapy, 15*(6), 801–805.

Rogers, S. J. (1999). Intervention for young children with autism: From research to practice. *Infants and Young Children, 12*(2), 1–16.

Rolls, B. J. (1986). Sensory-specific satiety. *Nutrition Reviews, 44*(3), 93–101.

Rosenthal, R. (1974). The Pygmalion effect lives. *Psychology Today, 7*(4), 54–63.

Rosenthal, R., & Jacobson, L. (1968). *Pygmalion in the classroom.* New York: Holt, Rhinehart & Winston.

Rowe, K. S., & Rowe, K. J. (1994). Synthetic food coloring and behavior: A dose response effect in a double-blind, placebo-controlled, repeated-measures study. *Journal of Pediatrics, 125*(5 Pt 1), 691–698.

Roy, C. C., & Belli, D. C. (1985). Hepatobiliary complications associated with TPN: An enigma. *Journal of the American College of Nutrition, 4*(6), 651–660.

Rozlog, L. A., Kiecolt-Glaser, J. K., Marucha, P. T., Sheridan, J. F., & Glaser, R. (1999). Stress and immunity: Implications for viral disease and wound healing. *Journal of Periodontology, 70*(7), 786–792.

Rozin, P., & Millman, L. (1987). Family environment, not heredity, accounts for family resemblances in food preferences and attitudes: A twin study. *Appetite, 8*(2), 125–134.

Ruark, J. L., & Moore, C. A. (1997). Coordination of lip muscle activity by 2-year-old children during speech and nonspeech tasks. *Journal of Speech-Language-Hearing Research, 40*(6), 1373–1385.

Russell, G. F., Treasure, J., & Eisler, I. (1998). Mothers with anorexia nervosa who underfeed their children: Their recognition and management. *Psychological Medicine, 28*(1), 93–108.

Russell, R. (1993). *Using the whole brain: Integrating the right and left brain with Hemi-Sync sound patterns*. Norfolk, VA: Hampton Roads.

Russell, R. M., Cox, M. E., & Solomons, N. (1983). Zinc and the special senses. *Annals of Internal Medicine, 99*(2), 227–239.

Rywerant, Y., & Feldenkrais, M. (1991). *The Feldenkrais Method: Teaching by handling*. New Canaan, CT: Keats.

S

Sabourin, M. E., Cutcomb, S. D., Crawford, H. J., & Pribram, K. (1990). EEG correlates of hypnotic susceptibility and hypnotic trance: Spectral analysis and coherence. *International Journal of Psychophysiology, 10*(2), 125–142.

Safranek, M. G., Koshland, G. F., & Raymond, G. (1982). Effect of auditory rhythm on muscle activity. *Physical Therapy, 62*(2), 161–168.

Sahley, T. L., & Panksepp, J. (1987). Brain opioids and autism: An updated analysis of possible linkages. *Journal of Autism and Developmental Disorders, 17*(2), 201–216.

Saito, Y., Hashimoto, T., Sasaki, M., Hanaoka, S., & Sugai, K. (1998). Effect of selenium deficiency on cardiac function of individuals with severe disabilities under long-term tube feeding. *Developmental Medicine and Child Neurology, 40*(11), 743–748.

Sampson, H. A. (1999). Food allergy. Part 1: Immunopathogenesis and clinical disorders. *Journal of Allergy and Clinical Immunology, 103*(5 Pt 1), 717–728.

Sampson, L. K., Georgeson, K. E., & Royal, S. A. (1998). Laparoscopic gastric antroplasty in children with delayed gastric emptying and gastroesophageal reflux. *Journal of Pediatric Surgery, 33*(2), 282–285.

Samuk, I., Afriat, R., Horne, T., Bistritzer, T., Barr, J., & Vinograd, I. (1996). Dumping syndrome following Nissen fundoplication, diagnosis, and treatment. *Journal of Pediatric Gastroenterology and Nutrition, 23*(3), 235–240.

Sanders, K. D., Cox, K., Cannon, R., Blanchard, D., Pitcher, J., Papathakis, P., Varella, L., & Maughan, R. (1990). Growth response to enteral feeding by children with cerebral palsy. *Journal of Parenteral Enteral Nutrition, 14*(1), 23–26.

Sanders, M. R., Patel, R. K., Le Grice, B., & Shepherd, R. W. (1993). Children with persistent feeding difficulties: An observational analysis of the feeding interactions of problem and non-problem eaters. *Health Psychology, 12*(1), 64–73.

Sandler, A. D., Sutton, K. A., DeWeese, J., Girardi, M. A., Sheppard, V., & Bodfish, J. W. (1999). Lack of benefit of a single dose of synthetic human secretin in the treatment of autism and pervasive developmental disorder. *New England Journal of Medicine, 341*(24), 1801–1806.

Sandstead, H. H. (1994). Understanding zinc: Recent observations and interpretations. *Journal of Laboratory and Clinical Medicine, 124*(3), 322–327.

Sandstead, H. H. (1995a). Is zinc deficiency a public health problem? *Nutrition, 11*(Suppl. 1), 87–92.

Sandstead, H. H. (1995b). Requirements and toxicity of essential trace elements, illustrated by zinc and copper. *American Journal of Clinical Nutrition, 61*(Suppl. 3), 621S–624S.

Saraswat V. A., Dhiman R. K., Mishra A., & Naik S. R. (1994). Correlation of 24-hr esophageal pH patterns with clinical features and endoscopy in gastroesophageal reflux disease. *Digestive Diseases and Sciences, 39*(1), 199–205.

Satter, E. (1986). The feeding relationship. *Journal of the American Dietetic Association, 86*(3), 352–356.

Satter, E. (1987). *How to get your kid to eat. . .but not too much.* Palo Alto, CA: Bull.

Satter, E. (1990). The feeding relationship: Problems and interventions. *Journal of Pediatrics, 117* (2 Pt 2), S181–S189.

Satter, E. (1991). Children obesity demands new approaches. *Obesity & Health,* (May/June), 42–43.

Satter, E. (1995). Feeding dynamics: Helping children to eat well. *Journal of Pediatric Health Care, 9*(4), 178–184.

Satter, E. (1997). *Feeding with love and good sense.* [Videotape]. Madison, WI: Ellyn Satter Associates.

Satter, E. (1999). *Secrets of feeding a healthy family.* Madison, WI: Kelcy Press.

Satter, E. (2000). *Child of mine: Feeding with love and good sense.* (2nd ed.). Palo Alto, CA: Bull Publishing.

Saunders, R. B., Friedman, C. B., & Stramoski, P. R. (1991). Feeding preterm infants: Schedule or demand? *Journal of Obstetric, Gynecologic, and Neonatal Nursing, 20*(3), 212–218.

Scariati, P. D., Grummer-Strawn, L. M., & Fein, S. B. (1997). Water supplementation of infants in the first month of life. *Archive of Pediatric and Adolescent Medicine, 151*(8), 830–832.

Scartelli, J. P. (1982). The effect of sedative music on electromyographic biofeedback assisted relaxation training of spastic cerebral palsied adults. *Journal of Music Therapy, 19*(4), 210–218.

Schanler, R. J., & Oh, W. (1980). Composition of breast milk obtained from mothers of premature infants as compared to breast milk obtained from donors. *Journal of Pediatrics, 96*(4), 679–681.

Schapira, M., Henrion, J., & Heller, F. R. (1990). The current status of gastric prokinetic drugs. *Acta Gastroenterologica Belgica, 53*(4), 446–457.

Scheinberg, I. H., & Sternlieb, I. (1996). Wilson disease and idiopathic copper toxicosis. *American Journal of Clinical Nutrition, 63*(5), 842S–845S.

Schmidt, M. (1990). *Childhood ear infections: What every parent and physician should know about prevention, home care, and alternative treatment*. Berkeley, CA: North Atlantic Books.

Schmidt, M. A., Smith, L. H., & Sehnert, K. (1994). *Beyond antibiotics: 50 (or so) ways to boost immunity and avoid antibiotics*. Berkeley, CA: North Atlantic Books.

Schmidt, T., Pfeiffer, A., Hackelsberger, N., Widmer, R., Pehl, C., & Kaess, H. (1999). Dysmotility of the small intestine in achalasia. *Neurogastroenterology Motility, 11*(1), 11–17.

Schwaab, L. M., Niman, C. W., & Gisel, E. G. (1986). Comparison of chewing cycles in 2-, 3-, 4-, and 5-year-old normal children. *American Journal of Occupational Therapy, 40*(1), 40–43.

Schwartz, J. L., Niman, C. W., & Gisel, E. G. (1984). Chewing cycles in 4- and 5-year-old normal children: An index of eating efficacy. *American Journal of Occupational Therapy, 38*(3), 171–175.

Scott, T. J. (1980). The use of music to reduce hyperactivity in children. *American Journal of Orthopsychiatry, 40*(4), 677–680.

Scrimshaw, N. S., & Murray, E. B. (1988). The acceptability of milk and milk products in populations with a high prevalence of lactose intolerance. *American Journal of Clinical Nutrition, 48*(Suppl. 4), 1079–1159.

Sears, C. J. (1994). Recognizing and coping with tactile defensiveness in young children. *Infants and Young Children, 6*(4), 46–53.

Sears, W. (1989). *The fussy baby: How to bring out the best in your high-need child.* New York: Signet.

Sears, W. (1996). *Parenting the fussy baby and high-need child.* Boston: Little, Brown and Company.

Sears, W., & Sears, M. (1999). *The family nutrition book: Everything you need to know about feeding your children–from birth through adolesence.* Boston: Little, Brown and Company.

See, D. M., Cimoch, P., Chou, S., Chang, J., & Tilles, J. (1998). The in vitro immunomodulatory effects of glyconutrients on peripheral blood mononuclear cells of patients with chronic fatigue syndrome. *Integrative Physiological and Behavioral Science, 33*(3), 280–287.

Seibert, J. J., Byrne, W. J., & Euler, A. R. (1983). Gastric emptying in children: Unusual patterns detected by scintigraphy. *American Journal of Roentgenology, 141*(1), 49–51.

Seligman, M. E. P. (1991). *Learned optimism.* New York: Knopf.

Serfaty-Lacrosniere, C., Wood, R. J., Voytko, D., Saltzman, J. R., Pedrosa, M., Sepe, T. E., Russell, R. R. (1995) Hypochlorhydria from short-term omeprazole treatment does not inhibit intestinal absorption of calcium, phosphorus, magnesium or zinc from food in humans. *Journal of American College of Nutrition, 14*(4), 364–368.

Seth, R., & Heyman, M. B. (1994). Management of constipation and encopresis in infants and children. *Gastroenterology Clinics of North America, 23*(4), 621–636.

Shafarman, S. (1997). *Awareness heals: The Feldenkrais Method for dynamic health.* Reading, MA: Perseus Press.

Shaker, R., Kern, M., Bardan, E., Taylor, A., Stewart, E. T., Hoffmann, R. G., Arndorfer, R. C., Hofmann, C., & Bonnevier, J. (1997). Augmentation of deglutitive upper esophageal sphincter opening in the elderly by exercise. *American Journal of Physiology, 272*(6 Pt 1), G1518–G1522.

Shankar, A. H., & Prasad, A. S. (1998). Zinc and immune function: The biological basis of altered resistance to infection. *American Journal of Clinical Nutrition, 68*(Suppl. 2), 447S-463S.

Shaw, L., Weatherill, S., & Smith, A. (1998). Tooth wear in children: An investigation of etiological factors in children with cerebral palsy and gastroesophageal reflux. *Journal of Dentistry for Children, 65*(6), 484–486, 439.

Shawker, T. H., Sonies, B. C., Hall, T. E., & Baum, B. F. (1984). Ultrasound analysis of tongue, hyoid, and larynx activity during swallowing. *Investigative Radiology, 19*(2), 82–86.

Shawker, T. H., Sonies, B. C. & Stone, M. (1984). Sonography of speech and swallowing. In R. C. Saunders & M. Hill (Eds.), *Ultrasound Annual* (pp. 237–260). New York: Ravens Press.

Sher, L. (1997). Autistic disorder and the endogenous opioid system. *Medical Hypotheses, 48*(5), 413–414.

Shiao, S. Y., Chang, Y. J., Lannon, H., & Yarandi, H. (1997). Meta-analysis of the effects of nonnutritive sucking on heart rate and peripheral oxygenation: Research from the past 30 years. *Issues in Comprehensive Pediatric Nursing, 20*(1), 11–24.

Ship, J. A., Fox, P. C., & Baum, B. J. (1991). How much saliva is enough? *Journal of the American Dental Association, 122*(3), 63-69.

Sicherer, S. H. (1999). Manifestations of food allergy: Evaluation and management. *American Family Physician, 59*(2), 415–424, 429–430.

Sicherer, S. H., Burks, A. W., & Sampson, H. A. (1998). Clinical features of acute allergic reactions to peanut and tree nuts in children. *Pediatrics, 102*(1), e6.

Siegel, B. (1999). Autistic learning disabilities and individualizing treatment for autistic spectrum disorders. *Infants and Young Children, 12*(2), 27–36.

Sinden, A. A., & Sutphen, J. L. (1991). Dietary treatment of lactose intolerance in infants and children. *Journal of American Dietetic Association, 91*(12), 1567–1571.

Singer, L. T., Davillier, M., Preuss, L., Szekely, L., Hawkins, S., Yamashita, T., & Baley, J. (1996). Feeding interactions in infants with very low birth weight and bronchopulmonary dysplasia. *Journal of Developmental and Behavioral Pediatrics, 17*(2), 69–76.

Singer, L. T., Salvator, A., Guo, S., Collin, M., Lilien, L., & Baley, J. (1999). Maternal psychological distress and parenting stress after the birth of a very-low-birth-weight infant. *Journal of the American Medical Association, 281*(9), 799–805.

Skikne, B. S., Lynch, S. R., & Cook, J. D. (1981). Role of gastric acid in food iron absorption. *Gastroenterology, 81*(6), 1068–1071.

Skinner, J. D., Carruth, B. R., Houck, K. S., Bounds, W., Morris, M., Cox, D. R., Moran, J., III, & Coletta, F. (1999). Longitudinal study of nutrient and food intakes of white preschool children aged 24 to 60 months. *Journal of the American Dietetic Association, 99*(12), 1514–1521.

Skinner, J. D., Carruth, B. R., Houck, K., Coletta, F., Cotter, R., Ott, D., & McLeod, M. (1997). Longitudinal study of nutrient and food intakes of infants aged 2 to 24 months. *Journal of the American Dietetic Association, 97*(5), 496–504.

Skinner, J. D., Carruth, B. R., Houck, K., Moran, J., III, Coletta, F., Cotter, R., Ott, D., & McLeod, M. (1997). Transitions in infant feeding during the first year of life. *Journal of the American College of Nutrition, 16*(3), 209–215.

Skinner, J. D., Carruth, B. R., Houck, K., Moran, J., III, Reed, A., Coletta, F., & Ott, D. (1998). Mealtime communication patterns of infants from 2 to 24 months of age. *Journal of Nutrition Education, 30*(1), 8–16.

Skinner, J. D., Carruth, B. R., Moran, J., III, Houck, K., & Coletta, F. (1999). Fruit juice intake is not related to children's growth. *Pediatrics, 103*(1), 58–64.

Skinner, J. D., Carruth, B. R., Moran, J., III, Houck, K., Schmidhammer, J., Reed, A., Coletta, F., Cotter, R., Ott, D. (1998). Toddlers' food preferences: Concordance with family members' preferences. *Journal of Nutrition Education, 30*(1), 17–22.

Skoutakis, V. A., Joe, R. H., & Hara, D. S. (1995). Comparative role of omeprazole in the treatment of gastroesophageal reflux disease. *Annals of Pharmacotherapy, 29*(12), 1252–1262.

Skuse, D. H. (1985). Non-organic failure to thrive: A reappraisal. *Archives of Disease in Childhood, 60*(2), 173–178.

Slavik, B. A., Kitsuwa-Lowe, J., Danner, P. T., Green, J., & Ayres, A. J. (1984). Vestibular stimulation and eye contact in autistic children. *Neuropediatrics, 15*(1), 33–36.

Smith, C. A., & Berenberg, W. (1970). The concept of failure to thrive. *Pediatrics, 46*(5), 661–663.

Smith, I. M., & Bryson, S. E. (1994). Imitation and action in autism: A critical review. *Psychological Bulletin, 116*(2), 259–273.

Smith, M. M., & Lifshitz, F. (1994). Excess fruit juice consumption as a contributing factor in nonorganic failure to thrive. *Pediatrics, 93*(3), 438–443.

Smith, W. L., Erenberg, A., Nowak, A., & Franken, E. (1985). Physiology of sucking in the normal term infant using real-time US. *Radiology, 156*(2), 379–381.

Solomons, N. W. (1982). Factors affecting the bioavailability of zinc. *Journal of the American Dietetic Association, 80*(2), 115–121.

Solomons, N. W. (1985). Biochemical, metabolic, and clinical role of copper in human nutrition. *Journal of the American College of Nutrition, 4*(1), 83–105.

Solomons, N. W., Rosenfield, R. L., Jacob, R. A., & Sandstead, H. H. (1976). Growth retardation and zinc nutrition. *Pediatric Research, 10*(11), 923–927.

Sonies, B. C. (1997). *Dysphagia: A continuum of care.* Gaithersburg, MD: Aspen.

Sonies, B. C., Wang, C., & Sapper, D. J. (1996). Evaluation of normal and abnormal hyoid bone movement during swallowing by use of ultrasound duplex-Doppler imaging. *Ultrasound in Medical Biology, 22*(9), 1169–1175.

Speirs, R. L., & Dean, P. M. (1989). Toffee clearance and lingual sensory and motor activities in normal children and in children with articulation problems of speech. *Archives of Oral Biology, 34*(8), 637–644.

Speirs, R. L., & Maktabi, M. A. (1990). Tongue skills and clearance of toffee in two age-groups and in children with problems of speech articulation. *Journal of Dentistry for Children, 57*(5), 356–360.

Springer, S. P., & Deutsch, G. (1997). *Left brain, right brain: Perspective from cognitive neuroscience.* San Francisco: W. H. Freeman.

Stallings, V. A. (1997). Calcium and bone health in children: A review. *American Journal of Therapeutics, 4*(7–8), 259–273.

Stallings, V. A., Zemel, B. S., Davies, J. C., Cronk, C. E., & Charney, E. B. (1996). Energy expenditure of children and adolescents with severe disabilities: A cerebral palsy model. *American Journal of Clinical Nutrition, 64*(4), 627–634.

Stark, L. J., Mulvihill, M. M., Powers, S. W., Jelalian, E., Keating, K., Creveling, S., Byrnes-Collins, B., Harwood, I., Passero, M. A., Light, M., Miller, D. L., & Melbourne, F. (1996). Behavioral intervention to improve calorie intake of children with cystic fibrosis: Treatment versus wait list control. *Journal of Pediatric Gastoeroenterology and Nutrition, 22*(3), 240–253.

Stark, L. J., Powers, S. W., Jelalian, E., Rape, R. N., & Miller, D. L. (1994). Modifying problematic mealtime interactions of children with cystic fibrosis and their parents via behavioral parent training. *Journal of Pediatric Psychology, 19*(6), 751–768.

Stark, R. E. (1978a). Features of infant sounds: the emergence of cooing. *Journal of Child Language, 1*(5), 1–12.

Stark, R. E. (1978b). Infant speech production and communication skills. *Allied Health and Behavioral Sciences, 1*(2), 131–151.

Stark, R. E., Bernstein, L. E., & Demorest, M. E. (1993). Vocal communication in the first 18 months of life. *Journal of Speech and Language Research, 36*(3), 548–558.

Start, K. (1998). Treating phenylketonuria by a phenylalanine-free diet. *Professional Care of Mother and Child, 8*(4), 109–110.

Staum, M. J. (1983). Music and rhythmic stimuli in the rehabilitation of gait disorders. *Journal of Music Therapy, 20*(2), 69–87.

Steeve, R. W., Moore, C. A., Green, J. R., & Engel, N. M. (1999) Physiologic development of mandibular coordination in 9-month-old children [Web Page]. URL http://faculty.washington.edu/spchphys/moore.ppt.

Stevens, L. J., Zentall, S. S., Deck, J. L., Abate, M. L., Watkins, B. A., Lipp, S. R., & Burgess, J. R. (1995). Essential fatty acid metabolism in boys with attention-deficit hyperactivity disorder. *American Journal of Clinical Nutrition, 62*(4), 761–768.

Stevenson, R. D. (1995). Use of segmental measures to estimate stature in children with cerebral palsy. *Archive of Pediatric and Adolescent Medicine, 149*(6), 658–662.

Stevenson, R. D., Hayes, R. P., Cater, L. V., & Blackman, J. A. (1994). Clinical correlates of linear growth in children with cerebral palsy. *Developmental Medicine and Child Neurology, 36*(2), 135–142.

Stevenson, R. D., Roberts, C. D., & Vogtle, L. (1995). The effects of non-nutritional factors on growth in cerebral palsy. *Developmental Medicine and Child Neurology, 37*(2), 124–130.

Stigson, L., & Kjellmer, I. (1997). Serum levels of magnesium at birth related to complications of immaturity. *Acta Paediatrica, 86*(9), 991–994.

Stone, W. L., Ousley, O. Y., & Littleford, C. D. (1997). Motor imitation in young children with autism: What's the object? *Journal of Abnormal Child Psychology, 25*(6), 475–485.

Stordy, B. J. (2000). Dark adaptation, motor skills, docosahexaenoic acid, and dyslexia. *American Journal of Clinical Nutrition, 71*(1 Part 2), 323–326.

Sturniolo, G. C., Montino, M. C., Rossetto, L., Martin, A., D'Inca, R., D'Odorico, A., & Naccarato, R. (1991). Inhibition of gastric acid secretion reduces zinc absorption in man. *Journal of American College of Nutrition, 10*(4), 372–375.

Suarez, F. L., Savaiano, D. A., & Levitt, M. D. (1995). Review article: The treatment of lactose intolerance. *Alimentary Pharmacology and Therapeudics, 9*(6), 589–597.

Sullivan, S. A., & Birch, L. L. (1994). Infant dietary experience and acceptance of solid foods. *Pediatrics, 93*(2), 271–277.

Sun, Z., & Cade, J. R. (1999). A peptide found in schizophrenia and autism causes behavioral changes in rats. *Autism, 3*(1), 85–95.

Sun, Z., Cade, J. R., Fregly, M. J., & Privette, R. M. (1999). B-Casomorphin induces Fos-like immunoreactivity in discrete brain regions relevant to schizophrenia and autism. *Autism, 3*(1), 67–83.

Sutphen, J. L., Dillard, V. L., & Pipan, M. E. (1986). Antacid and formula effects on gastric acidity in infants with gastroesophageal reflux. *Pediatrics, 78*(1), 55–57.

T

Tamborlane, W. V. Ed. (1997). *The Yale guide to children's nutrition.* New Haven: Yale University Press.

Taylor, L. J., & Faria, S. H. (1997). Caring for the patient with a gastrostomy/jejunostomy tube. *Home Care Provider, 2*(5), 221–224.

Tawfik, R., Dickson, A., Clarke, M., & Thomas, A. G. (1997). Caregivers' perceptions following gastrostomy in severely disabled children with feeding problems. *Developmental Medicine and Child Neurology, 39*(11), 746–751.

Teare, J. P., Spedding, C., Whitehead, M. W., Greenfield, S. M., Challacombe, S. J., & Thompson, R. P. (1995). Omeprazole and dry mouth. *Scandinavian Journal of Gastroenterology, 30*(3), 216–218.

Thach, B. T. (1997). Reflux associated apnea in infants: Evidence for a laryngeal chemoreflex. *American Journal of Medicine, 103*(5A), 120S–124S.

Thach, B. T., & Weiffenbach, J. (1973). The lateral tongue reflex in low birth weight infants. In J. F. Bosma (Ed.), *Fourth Symposium on Oral Sensation and Perception.* Springfield, IL: Charles C. Thomas.

Thaut, M. H., McIntosh, G. C., & Rice, R. R. (1997). Rhythmic facilitation of gait training in hemiparetic stroke rehabilitation. *Journal of Neurological Sciences, 151*(2), 207–212.

Thaut, M. H., Miltner, R., Lange, H. W., Hurt, C. P., & Hoemberg, V. (1999). Velocity modulation and rhythmic synchronization of gait in Huntington's disease. *Movement Disorders, 14*(5), 808–819.

Thommessen, M., Kase, B. F., Riis, G., & Heiberg, A. (1991). The impact of feeding problems on growth and energy intake in children with cerebral palsy. *European Journal of Clinical Nutrition, 45*(10), 479–487.

Thommessen, M., Riis, G., Kase, B. F., Larsen, S., & Heiberg, A. (1991). Energy and nutrient intakes of disabled children: Do feeding problems make a difference? *Journal of American Dietetic Association, 91*(12), 1522–1525.

Thompson, C. K., Hall, H. R., & Sison, C. E. (1986). Effects of hypnosis and imagery training on naming behavior in aphasia. *Brain and Language, 28*(1), 141–153.

Thompson, J. M. (1998). *Nutritional requirements of infants and young children–practical guidelines.* Oxford: Blackwell Science.

Thompson, R. J., Jr., Palmer, S., & Linscheid, T. R. (1977). Single-subject design and interaction analysis in the behavioral treatment of a child with a feeding problem. *Child Psychiatry and Human Development, 8*(1), 43–53.

Thomson, A. B., Babiuk, L., Kirdeikis, P., Zuk, L., Marriage, B., & Bowes, K. (1994). A dose-ranging study of ranitidine and its effect on intragastric and intra-oesophageal acidity in subjects with gastro-esophageal reflux disease. *Alimentary Pharmacology and Therapeutics, 8*(4), 443–451.

Thomson, A. B., Kirdeikis, P., & Zuk, L. (1999). Comparison of 200 mg cimetidine with multiple doses of antacid on extent and duration of rise in gastric pH in volunteers. *Digestive Diseases and Sciences, 44*(10), 2051–2055 [MEDLINE record in process].

Tiegerman, E., & Primavera, L. H. (1984). Imitating the autistic child: Facilitating communicative gaze behavior. *Journal of Autism and Developmental Disorders, 14*(1), 27–39.

Toledo, C., Alembik, Y., Aguirre Jaime, A., & Stoll, C. (1999). Growth curves of children with Down syndrome. *Annales de Genetique, 42*(2), 81–90.

Tolia, V., Kuhns L., & Kauffman, R. (1993a). Correlation of gastric emptying at one and two hours following formula feeding. *Pediatric Radiology, 23*(1), 26–28.

Tolia, V., Kuhns, L., & Kauffman, R. E. (1993b). Comparison of simultaneous esophageal pH monitoring and scintigraphy in infants with gastroesophageal reflux. *American Journal of Gastroenterology, 88*(5), 661–664.

Tomaski, S. M., Zalzal, G. H., & Saal, H. M. (1995). Airway obstruction in the Pierre Robin sequence. *Laryngoscope, 105*(2), 111–114.

Torem, M. S. (1992). Therapeutic imagery enhanced by hypnosis. *Psychiatric Medicine, 10*(4), 1–12.

Towne, B., Guo, S., Roche, A. F., & Siervogel, R. M. (1993). Genetic analysis of patterns of growth in infant recumbent length. *Human Biology, 65*(6), 977–989.

Trahms, C. M., & Pipes, P. L. (1997). *Nutrition in infancy and childhood* (6th ed.). New York: Brown and Benchmark.

Trefler, E. (1993). *Seating and mobility for persons with physical disabilities.* Tucson, AZ: Therapy Skill Builders.

Treloar, D. M. (1994). The effect of nonnutritive sucking on oxygenation in healthy, crying full-term infants. *Applied Nursing Research, 7*(2), 52–58.

Trenouth, M. J., & Campbell, A. N. (1996). Questionnaire evaluation of feeding methods for cleft lip and palate neonates. *International Journal of Paediatric Dentistry, 6*(4), 241–244.

Trowbridge, J., & Walker, M. (1986). *The yeast syndrome.* New York: Bantam Books.

Tuchman, D. N., & Walter, R. S. (1994). *Disorders of feeding and swallowing in infants and children: Pathophysiology, diagnosis and treatment.* San Diego, CA: Singular Publishing Group.

Tunkel, D. E., & Zalzal, G. H. (1992). Stridor in infants and children: Ambulatory evaluation and operative diagnosis. *Clinical Pediatrics, 31*(1), 48–55.

Tunnessen, W. W. Jr, & Oski, F. A. (1987). Consequences of starting whole cow milk at 6 months of age. *Journal of Pediatrics, 111*(6 Pt 1), 813–816.

U

U.S. Department of Agriculture & U.S. Department of Health and Human Services. (1995). *Nutrition and your health: Dietary guidelines for Americans.* Washington DC: United States Government.

Uauy, R., Mena, P., & Valenzuela, A. (1999). Essential fatty acids as determinants of lipid requirements in infants, children and adults. *European Journal of Clinical Nutrition, 53*(Suppl. 1), S66–S77.

Uauy, R., Peirano, P., Hoffman, D., Mena, P., Birch, D., & Birch, E. (1996). Role of essential fatty acids in the function of the developing nervous system. *Lipids, 31*(Suppl.), S167–S176.

Udall, J. N. Jr, & Suskind, R. M. (1999). Cow's milk versus formula in older infants: Consequences for human nutrition. *Acta Paediatrica, 88*(Suppl. 430), 61–67.

V

Valdez, I. H., & Fox, P. C. (1991). Interactions of the salivary and gastrointestinal systems. I. The role of saliva in digestion. *Digestive Diseases and Sciences, 9*(3), 125–132

Van Caillie-Bertrand, M., Degenhart, H. J., & Fernandes, J. (1984). Selenium status of infants on nutritional support. *Acta Paediatrica Scandinavica, 73*(6), 816–819.

VandenBerg, K. A. (1990). Nippling management of the sick neonate in the NICU: The disorganized feeder. *Neonatal Network, 9*(1), 9–16.

Vandenplas, Y. (1993). Pathogenesis of food allergy in infants. *Current Opinions in Pediatrics, 5*(5), 567–572.

Vandenplas, Y., Belli, D. C., Benatar, A., Cadranel, S., Cucchiara, S., Dupont, C., Gottrand, F., Hassall, E., Heymans, H. S., Kearns, G., Kneepkens, C. M., Koletzko, S., Milla, P., Polanco, I., & Staiano, A. M. (1999). The role of cisapride in the treatment of pediatric gastroesophageal reflux. The European Society of Paediatric Gastroenterology, Hepatology and Nutrition. *Journal of Pediatric Gastroenterology and Nutrition, 28*(5), 518–528.

Vandenplas, Y., Derde, M. P., & Piepsz, A. (1992). Evaluation of reflux episodes during simultaneous esophageal pH monitoring and gastroesophageal reflux scintigraphy in children. *Journal of Pediatric Gastroenterology and Nutrition, 14*(3), 256–260.

Varela-Moreiras, G., Antoine, J. M., Ruiz-Roso, B., & Varela, G. (1992). Effects of yogurt and fermented-then-pasteurized milk on lactose absorption in an institutionalized elderly group. *Journal of the American College of Nutrition, 11*(2), 168–171.

Varney, K. (1988). *Metamusic with Hemi-Sync as an adjunct to intervention with developmentally delayed young children.* Unpublished doctoral dissertation, Virginia Commonwealth University, Richmond VA.

Vegter, F., Hage, J. J., & Mulder, J. W. (1999). Pierre Robin syndrome: Mandibular growth during the first year of life. *Annals of Plastic Surgery, 42*(2), 154–157.

Veit, F., Heine, R. G., & Catto-Smith, A. G. (1994). Dumping syndrome after Nissen fundoplication. *Journal of Paediatrics and Child Health, 30*(2), 182–185.

Velanovich, V. (1994). The transverse-vertical frenuloplasty for ankyloglossia. *Military Medicine, 159*(11), 714–715

Verny, T., & Kelly, J. (1981). *The secret life of the unborn child.* New York: Dell.

Vieth, A. Z., & Trull, T. J. (1999). Family patterns of perfectionism: An examination of college students and their parents. *Journal of Personality Assessment, 72*(1), 49–67.

Vu, M., Straathof, J., v. d. Schaar, P., Arndt, J., Ringers, J., Lamers, C., & Mascle, A. (1999). Motor and sensory function of the proximal stomach in reflux disease and after laparoscopic Nissen fundoplication. *American Journal of Gastroenterology, 94*(6), 1481–1489.

W

Wagner, C. L., Anderson, D. M., & Pittard, W. B. 3rd. (1996). Special properties of human milk. *Clinical Pediatrics, 35*(6), 283–293.

Wang, Y., Harvey, C. B., Hollox, E. J., Phillips, A. D., Poulter, M., Clay, P., Walker-Smith, J. A., & Swallow, D. M. (1998). The genetically programmed down-regulation of lactase in children. *Gastroenterology, 114*(6), 1230–1236.

Wasantwisut, E. (1997). Nutrition and development: Other micronutrients' effect on growth and cognition. *Southeast Asian Journal of Tropical Medicine and Public Health, 28*(Suppl. 2), 78–82.

Watson, L. R. (1998). Following the child's lead: Mothers' interactions with children with autism. *Journal of Autism and Developmental Disorders, 28*(1), 51–59.

Watson, R. L., Dowell, S. F., Jayaraman, M., Keyserling, H., Kolczak, M., & Schwartz, B. (1999). Antimicrobial use for pediatric upper respiratory infections: Reported practice, actual practice, and parent beliefs. *Pediatrics, 104*(6), 1251–1257.

Weber, F., Woolridge, M. W., & Baum, J. D. (1986). An ultrasonographic study of the organization of sucking and swallowing by newborn infants. *Developmental Medicine and Child Neurology, 28*(1), 19–24.

Weber, T. R., Sears, N., Davies, B., & Grosfeld, J. L. (1981). Clinical spectrum of zinc deficiency in pediatric patients receiving total parenteral nutrition (TPN). *Journal of Pediatric Surgery, 16*(3), 236–240.

Weiffenbach, J., & Thach, B. T. (1973). Elicited tongue movements: Touch and taste in the mouth of the neonate. In J. F. Bosma (Ed.), *Fourth Symposium on Oral Sensation and Perception.* Springfield, IL: Charles C. Thomas.

Weinberg, M. K., & Tronick, E. Z. (1998). The impact of maternal psychiatric illness on infant development. *Journal of Clinical Psychiatry, 59*(Suppl. 2), 53–61.

Welch, M. V., Logemann, J. A., Rademaker, A. W., & Kahrilas, P. J. (1993). Changes in pharyngeal dimensions effected by chin tuck. *Archives of Physical Medicine and Rehabilitation, 74*(2), 178–181.

Wesley, J. R., Coran, A. G., Sarahan, T. M., Klein, M. D., & White, S. J. (1981). The need for evaluation of gastroesophageal reflux in brain-damaged children referred for feeding gastrostomy. *Journal of Pediatric Surgery, 16*(6), 866–871.

Wharton, B. A., & Scott, P. H. (1996). Distinctive aspects of metabolism and nutrition in infancy. *Clinical Biochemistry, 29*(5), 419–428.

Whitelaw, A. (1990). Kangaroo baby care: Just a nice experience or an important advance for preterm infants? *Pediatrics, 85*(4), 604–605.

Wickwire, N. A., Gibbs, C. H., Jacobson, A. P., & Lundeen, H. C. (1981). Chewing patterns in normal children. *Angle Orthodontist, 51*(1), 48–60.

Widstrom, A. M., Marchini, G., Matthiesen, A. S., Werner, S., Winberg, J., & Uvnas-Moberg, K. (1988). Nonnutritive sucking in tube-fed preterm infants: Effects on gastric motility and gastric contents of somatostatin. *Journal of Pediatric Gastroenterology and Nutrition, 7*(4), 517–523.

Wilbarger, P., & Wilbarger, J. L. (1991). *Sensory defensiveness in children aged 2–12: An intervention guide for parents and other caretakers.* Santa Barbara, CA: Avanti Educational Programs.

Williams, L., Davis, J. A., & Lowenthal, D. T. (1993). The influence of food on the absorption and metabolism of drugs. *Medical Clinics of North America, 77*(4), 815–829.

Williams, P. D., Press, A., Williams, A. R., Piamjariyakul, U., Keeter, L. M., Schultz, J., & Hunter, K. (1999). Fatigue in mothers of infants discharged to the home on apnea monitors. *Applied Nursing Research, 12*(2), 69–77.

Wilson, P. G., Reid, D. H., Phillips, J. F., & Burgio, L. D. (1984). Normalization of institutional mealtimes for profoundly retarded persons: Effects and noneffects of teaching family-style dining. *Journal of Applied Behavior Analysis, 17*(2), 189–201.

Wo, J. M., Trus, T. L., Richardson, W. S., Hunter, J. G., Branum, G. D., Mauren, S. J., & Waring, J. P. (1996). Evaluation and management of postfundoplication dysphagia. *American Journal of Gastroenterology, 91*(11), 2318–2322.

Wodarski, L. A. (1990). An interdisciplinary nutrition assessment and intervention protocol for children with disabilities. *Journal of the American Dietetic Association, 90*(11), 1563–1568.

Wolf, L. S., & Glass, R. P. (1992). *Feeding and swallowing disorders in infancy: Assessment and management.* San Antonio, TX: Therapy Skill Builders.

Wolff, R. P., & Lierman, C. J. (1994). Management of behavioral feeding problems in young children. *Infants and Young Children, 7*(1), 14–23.

Wolfson B. J., Allen, J. L., Panitch, H.B., Karmazin, N. (1989). Lipid aspiration pneumonia due to gastroesophageal reflux: A complication of nasogastric lipid feedings. *Pediatric Radiology, 19*(8), 545?547.

Woods, N. S., Eyler, F. D., Conlon, M., Behnke, M., & Wobie, K. (1998). Pygmalion in the cradle: Observer bias against cocaine-exposed infants. *Journal of Developmental Behavioral Pediatrics, 19*(4), 283–285.

Woodson, R., & Hamilton, C. (1988). The effect of nonnutritive sucking on heart rate in preterm infants. *Developmental Psychobiology, 21*(3), 207–213.

Woolridge, M. W. (1986). The anatomy of infant sucking. *Midwifery, 2*(4), 164–171.

Wu, C. H., Hsiao, T. Y., Chen, J. C., Chang, Y. C., & Lee, S. Y. (1997). Evaluation of swallowing safety with fiberoptic endoscope: Comparison with videofluoroscopic technique. *Laryngoscope, 107*(3), 396–401.

Y

Yamreudeewong, W., Henann, N. E., Fazio, A., Lower, D. L., & Cassidy, T. G. (1995). Drug-food interactions in clinical practice. *The Journal of Family Practice, 40*(4), 376–384.

Yannicelli, S., Rohr, F., & Warman, M. L. (1994). Nutrition support for glutaric acidemia type I. *Journal of the American Dietetic Association, 94*(2), 183–188,191; quiz 189–190.

Yirmiya, N., Kasari, C., Sigman, M., & Mundy, P. (1989). Facial expressions of affect in autistic, mentally retarded and normal children. *Journal of Child Psychology and Psychiatry and Allied Disciplines, 30*(5), 725–735.

Yoder, P. J., Kaiser, A. P., Alpert, C., & Fischer, R. (1993). Following the child's lead when teaching nouns to preschoolers with mental retardation. *Journal of Speech and Hearing Research, 36*(1), 158–167.

Yokoyama, S., Fujimoto, T., & Mitomi, T. (1988). [Long-term TPN for short bowel syndrome]. *Nippon Geka Gakkai Zasshi, 89*(9), 1403–1405.

Yu, V. Y. H. (1975). Effect of body position on gastric emptying in the neonate. *Archives of Disease in Childhood, 50,* 500–504.

Z

Zand, J., Walton, R., & Roundtree, B. (1994). *Smart medicine for a healthier child: A practical A-to-Z reference to natural and conventional treatments for infants and children.* Garden City Park, NY: Avery Publishing.

Zeisel, S. H. (1986). Dietary influences on neurotransmission. *Advance Pediatrics, 33,* 23–47.

Ziegler, E. E., & Fomon, S. J. (1983). Lactose enhances mineral absorption in infancy. *Journal of Pediatric Gastroenterology and Nutrition, 2*(2), 288–294.

Zlotkin, S., Stallings, V., & Pencharz, P. B. (1985). Total parenteral nutrition in children. *Pediatric Clinics of North America, 32*(2), 381–400.

Zuckerman, B., Bauchner, H., Parker, S., & Cabral, H. (1990). Maternal depressive symptoms during pregnancy, and newborn irritability. *Journal of Developmental and Behavioral Pediatrics, 11*(4), 190–194.

Index

Oral feeding *(continued)*
188–193, 195–197, 199, 201, 203, 207,
209, 212, 219, 224, 226–227, 236, 238,
240, 245, 247, 249–250, 253, 256,
263–265, 267, 270, 297–299, 304, 313,
332–333, 341, 348, 351, 353, 359,
361–362, 365, 368–371, 373–374,
376–379, 381–382, 386, 388, 390,
392–394, 397, 399, 401, 403–404, 408,
415, 424, 429–430, 432, 435, 443, 453,
455, 459–461, 463, 465, 472, 476, 479,
490–491, 493, 503, 511, 522, 531, 542,
548, 556, 568, 571, 574, 576, 578, 580,
588, 590, 596, 629–630, 639, 641, 644,
657, 660, 663, 669, 683–686, 691, 694
  readiness factors, 61, 72–73, 89, 90,
    94–95, 173, 211, 323, 357–358, 360,
    364, 398–400, 507–508, 521–524, 538,
    540, 546–547, 549, 551, 597, 611–615,
    617, 625, 656
  transition to, 70, 72, 75, 165, 211, 274,
    275, 323, 336, 338, 355, 380, 385, 400,
    421, 454, 471, 497, 538, 540, 549–551,
    562–563, 585, 598, 601–602, 610–612,
    614–616, 620, 625, 636, 656, 679, 687
  in tube-fed children, 95, 145, 200, 239,
    295–296, 337, 346, 349, 532–534, 549,
    575, 585, 587, 589, 591–592, 595–601,
    606–612, 615, 617, 619

Oral hypersensitivity, 400, 488, 495, 542,
574, 664
  and biting pattern, 126, 134, 136, 364
  and jaw clenching and tooth grinding,
    126, 136, 384
  and jaw thrust, 134, 136
  and tongue retraction, 384, 456
  and tongue thrust, 369
  and tonic bite reflex, 126, 134, 364

Oral-motor treatment program, 596

Oral movements, 51, 62–64, 69, 74, 89, 97,
101, 121, 123, 129, 130, 133, 182, 189,
195, 197, 219, 239, 332, 340, 348–349,
354–355, 357, 361, 367, 380, 383, 391,
395–397, 407, 411, 417, 421, 440–441,
444–445, 451, 458, 460, 469, 473,
477–478, 481, 485, 487–489, 493–494,
533–534, 542, 589, 595, 607–608,
684–685, 687, 690
  during cup feeding, 65, 68, 80, 125, 135,
    247, 368–369, 371–372, 375, 385–387,
    432, 437, 449, 462–463, 466–467, 686
  during spoon feeding, 66, 94, 125,
    135–136, 226–227, 364, 368–369, 375,
    385–386, 419, 437, 449, 452–453,
    462–463, 467, 531, 599, 606

Oral pharyngeal structures,
  anatomy and physiology of, 43
  movement of, 44, 101, 146–147

Oral pharyngeal tubes, 599

Oral reflexes, 74–76, 89–90, 106, 125, 129,
134, 204, 354, 364, 371, 387, 395–396,
399, 437, 447, 449, 467, 484, 501, 508,
542

Oral sensory development, 64–66, 69, 71,
75, 94, 97, 105, 119, 135–136, 167, 192,
209, 239, 242, 256, 324, 349, 354, 357,
361, 364, 366, 369, 373–375, 377–378,
380, 388, 391, 395–397, 454, 460, 463,
466–467, 469, 473, 475, 477, 486, 489,
491, 496, 521, 533, 534, 542, 587, 595,
604, 608, 617, 683, 686, 689

Oral stability, 51, 62–63, 73, 89–90, 102,
125, 129, 136, 219, 243, 298–299,
362–363, 367, 375, 386–387, 391, 397,
411, 430–431, 438, 441, 452–453, 467,
473, 538, 542, 548

Oral stimulation, 3, 187, 239, 390, 415,
437, 440, 453, 493, 495, 501, 576, 587,
592, 600, 610
  and hyperreaction, 365, 380, 420
  response to, 69, 365–366, 372, 380–381,
    389, 420, 446–449, 467, 469, 542, 547,
    597, 599, 604–607

Orogastric tubes, 113, 115, 192, 538, 542,
549, 552, 586–588

Oropharynx, 44, 145, 147, 153, 490

Osmolality, 333

P

Pacifier, 70–72, 95, 464, 471, 495–496,
502–503, 540, 556, 569–570, 601, 605,
613, 673
  criteria for, 497
  guidelines for use of, 497–498
  modification of, 471, 498, 606
  Numi-Med, 461

Pain, 9, 12, 19, 24, 66, 98–99, 105–106,
109, 113–114, 125, 152, 190, 195–196,
202, 204, 210, 250, 255–256, 265, 276,
281, 318, 330, 340, 342, 356, 361, 363,
365, 555, 557, 559, 561–562, 564,
567–570, 574, 578–579, 589, 598, 610,
614, 626, 675

Palate, 19, 52, 54, 67, 69, 78, 93, 133–134,
146, 173, 190, 297, 389, 437, 470, 512,
545, 639, 651, 653–656
  hard, 43, 53, 82, 98, 101–102, 127–129,
    191, 366, 376–377, 420, 438, 471, 650,
    685
  high, 129, 376–377, 541
  movement of, 46, 97, 121, 128, 142,
    210, 388, 438
  narrow, 129, 376–377
  soft, 43–44, 46, 48–52, 98, 101, 128,
    142, 191, 210, 376, 438, 541, 649–650,
    652

Palatal Obturator, 654–655

Palmomental reflex, 76

Parent Mealtimes Questionnaire,
  Eating and Drinking Skills, *175–178*
    Spanish Translation, *729–732*
  Tube Feedings and Beginning Oral
    Feedings, *181–184*
    Spanish Translation, *733–737*

Participation Experience, 128, 130, 170

Patent ductus arteriosis, 105

Pediatric undernutrition, *see also* Failure
  to thrive, 623–625

Percutaneous endoscopic gastrostomy
  (PEG) tube, 152, 589–591

Peristalsis, 45, 106, 108, 112, 154, 326, 342,
564, 567–568

pH probe, 150–154, 156, 565, 634
  Also, intraesophageal pH probe
  Also, intraluminal pH monitoring

Pharyngeal constrictors, 44, 50

Pharyngeal-esophageal junction (P-E juncture), 44, 46

Pharyngeal wall, 46, 146, 376, 603

Pharynx, 45–49, 54, 77, 83, 106, 115, 121,
126, 134–135, 141–142, 145–146,
152–154, 189, 210, 347, 370, 376, 387,
389, 391, 438, 471, 482, 490, 540, 558,
576, 586–590, 602–603, 606, 608,
612–613, 616–617, 620, 641–642, 649,
655, 659, 670–671, 678–679, 684–685,
668
  in adult, 44, 50–52, 101
  constrictors of, and swallowing, 44, 50
  in newborn, 52, 101

Phasic bite reflex, 126, 135

Physical environment, 7, 28, 72, 171,
237–238, 253, 262, 276, 356, 358–362,
364–366, 368–369, 371–374, 375–376,
379–379, 394, 608
  in feeding assessment, 171

Physiological limitations, 119, 353
  gastrointestinal, 100, 103, 105–106,
    109–110, 191
  oral-pharyngeal, 106
  respiratory-cardiac, 199, 211, 250,
    259–260, 267, 297, 302, 331, 340–343,
    348, 356, 368, 383, 387, 390, 392–394,
    405, 452, 455–456, 462, 473–474, 533,
    537, 539, 541, 550, 553, 564, 568, 588,
    598, 605–606, 610–611, 616–617,
    619–620, 626, 628, 630–631, 636,
    639–640, 684–685

Pierre Robin syndrome, 173, 366, 616

Poor appetite, 109, 152, 319, 334, 560, 577,
579, 619–620, 631, 636, 640

Positional stability, 62, 65, 80, 548

Positioning, 45, 62, 65, 80, 85, 102, 108, 127, 134, 137, 150, 156, 170, 205, 210, 217, 225, 258, 353, 360–361, 363–365, 371–373, 375–376, 385, 388–389, 396–400, 409–410, 418–420, 431, 433, 439, 445–448, 453, 457, 464–465, 468, 477, 486, 502, 565–567, 569, 572–573, 658
  for breast- or bottle-feeding, 28, 34–35, 73, 89–90, 94, 98, 101, 130, 143–145, 155, 161–162, 166, 190, 208, 226, 237, 294–296, 302, 384, 386, 462, 474, 498, 502–503, 509–510, 546, 548, 551, 601, 603, 653–657, 660, 693
  gastrointestinal positioning needs, 566–568
  mealtime, 28, 36, 161, 163–164, 166, 216, 222, 249, 279, 281, 293–306, 350, 355, 368, 407–408, 430, 449, 460, 463, 466, 469, 473, 475, 503, 539, 546, 550, 555, 557, 586, 592–593, 600, 606, 657–658, 660
  neurological positioning needs, 125, 279, 294, 296–297, 301, 564, 568, 599
  oral-facial positioning needs, 296, 460, 462–463, 466–467, 473, 481
  and options for feeding, 73, 141, 295–298, 306
  respiratory positioning needs, 101, 130, 154, 260, 296, 297, 302, 356, 405, 474, 550
  and self-feeding, 202, 295, 297, 394, 522

Postprandial period, 151, 153, 156, 565

Postural alignment,
  capital flexion, 402–403
  of head, neck, and trunk, 402–404, 408, 446–453, 455–456, 475, 477, 550
  symmetry, 403

Postural stability; see also Internal stability, 48, 53, 62, 65, 122, 237, 243, 254, 279, 304, 306, 684
  of head, neck, and trunk, 125–126, 129–130, 207, 209, 216–217, 402, 404, 406–407, 444, 449, 475, 524, 534, 603, 684–685, 688–689
  and jaw clenching and tooth grinding, 129, 406, 685
  and jaw instability, 125

Postural tone, 216, 450
  and drooling, 684
  and movement, 110, 122, 128–129, 131, 173, 188, 197, 200, 237, 245, 262, 279–280, 293, 297, 301, 304, 332, 362, 379, 384, 395–396, 406–407, 417, 443–444, 448–449, 457–459, 475, 477, 481, 488–489, 539, 607, 627, 684–685, 688
  and sensory threshold, 131–132, 378, 379, 417

Pre-feeding, 5, 59–60, 164, 210
  and drooling, 581
  and prematurity, 539
  in tube-fed children, 181, 239

Preemie nipples, 497, 548

Premature infant, 24, 318, 502, 509, 622
  breast-feeding in, 53, 319, 538, 540–541, 543–546, 548
  compared with term infant, 319, 578
  guidelines for feeding, 72, 74, 103, 535, 537–553, 578, 586–588

Principles and perspectives of treatment of feeding disorders, 692

Principles of learning, see Learning

Primary patterns of movement, 54, 91, 122, 127, 129–130, 135, 188, 226, 297, 301, 304, 345, 356, 368, 379–380, 389–390, 392–393, 397, 436, 438, 534, 599, 671, 685

Problem solving, 103, 157, 188, 216, 256, 273, 348, 427, 448, 511, 591
  model of, 205, 208, 211, 241
  setting priorities and, 187, 189, 193, 199, 201, 205, 213

Proprioceptive sensory information, 613, 621, 643, 645–646, 653–654, 422–423, 524, 640, 689

Protein, and weight gain, 314, 316, 334

Protraction and protrusion, 77, 82–84, 91, 93, 123–124, 127, 136, 198, 226, 299, 367–368, 369, 391–392, 406, 436, 452–454, 462, 474, 518, 532, 552, 603, 607, 688

Proximal stability, 63, 65, 78, 125, 417, 443–444, 455, 512, 541, 684

Pulmonary atresia, 105

Pulmonary stenosis, 105

Punished by Rewards (Kohn), 272

Pyloroplasty, 55, 108, 154, 351, 568, 570

Pyloric stenosis, 102, 147, 149, 555, 559

R

Respiratory distress, 114, 135, 250, 260
  protrusion, 127, 452, 462

Respiratory dysfunction, 387, 392, 393

Retching, 19, 108, 114, 154, 200, 202–204, 264–265, 275, 347, 493, 555, 557, 559–560, 569–570, 578, 598, 602, 639

Reverse swallow, 124

Rhythm, 4, 53, 67, 81, 95, 254, 357, 394, 419–420, 429, 441, 444, 449, 456, 466, 474–476, 480–481, 600, 605–607, 609
  in sucking, see Sucking, rhythm in, also Suckle-swallow, rhythmical

Rooting reaction, 35, 75, 89, 539, 542, 545, 547, 652
  Also, rooting reflex; rooting response

S

Sandifer Syndrome, 564

Satiation, 33, 116–117, 209, 250, 264, 388, 579, 601, 614–615, 659

Scapulae, 45, 62, 299, 402, 460

Scapular adduction, 599
  and nasal reflux, 376
  and tongue retraction, 299, 366, 369

Scheduled feedings, 549, 615

Scoliosis, 110

Seating and Positioning Considerations for Mealtime Support, 166, 294–295, 301, 303, *307–308*

Seizure disorder, 23, 318, 341, 422, 626
  and positioning, 297

Self-feeding, 25, 38, 64, 85, 202, 239, 295–297, 394, 429–430, 495, 500, 507–529, 671, 688
  and autism, 671
  minimal involvement, 688
  readiness factors for, 521
  and visual impairment, 189, 662, 666

Sensation and movement, 60, 69, 190, 207–208, 222, 259, 323, 388, 409, 411, 417, 476, 488, 600, 657

Senses, 49, 111, 113, 117, 226, 253, 277, 281–284, 286–287, 347, 377–378, 382, 524, 593, 612, 662–663, 670, 680, 693
  and movement, 64–65, 69, 121
  and stability, 64–65

Sensory-based feeding problems, 189–193, 265, 349, 524

Sensory defensiveness, 19, 60, 114, 118, 131–133, 137, 187, 189, 199, 201–204, 218, 223, 246, 255, 257, 275, 328, 349, 367, 375, 380–381, 386, 395–398, 418, 422–423, 436, 457, 470, 484, 493, 494, 521, 524, 533, 625, 627, 629–630, 640

Sensory discrimination, 71, 132, 137, 190, 204, 209, 211, 362, 378, 380, 397, 409, 414, 417, 432, 435–436, 442, 445, 457–459, 472, 478, 534, 595–596, 608, 686–688, 690

Sensory environment, 11, 26, 28–29, 35, 65, 69, 94, 99, 119, 167, 171, 189, 205, 207, 227–228, 236, 238, 246, 249, 253, 262–263, 276–279, 285–288, 306, 345, 356–358, 360, 364–367, 369, 372–373, 378–379, 381–385, 387–389, 391–392, 394–400, 409–411, 414–415, 417–419,

and sensorimotor development, 62, 688–689

Stability bite, 136, 362, 406, 449

State of regulation, 32–33, 71, 541–542, 544, 546–548

Sternum, 45, 420

Stimulation, normalizing the response to, 448, 604, 607

Stomach, 24, 34, 45–48, 50, 54–55, 98, 100, 102–103, 106–108, 112, 114–115, 117, 140, 142, 147–156, 192, 198, 201, 210, 265–266, 275, 297, 315, 320, 326–328, 333, 337–338, 342, 347, 490, 555, 557, 559–570, 574, 579, 586, 588–590, 592–594, 601–603, 611–612, 614–615, 629, 634

Stomach emptying; also Gastric emptying, 148, 150–153, 155–156, 170, 200–201, 210, 326, 408, 560, 566–569, 593, 601
  delayed stomach emptying; also delayed gastric emptying, 98, 108, 110, 154, 328, 334, 347, 564, 568, 570, 579, 589

Stomach motility, 108

Straws, 39, 61, 68, 79–80, 91–92, 250, 287–288, 296, 358, 363, 371, 432–436, 458, 467–468, 473, 481, 500, 503, 519–520, 577, 605,
  adaptors for, 468, 473, 500
  criteria for, 500
  guidelines for use of, 500
  and the physically challenged child, 500

Stress, and allergy, 12, 19, 22–23, 109, 112, 114, 324, 327, 342, 344–345, 350, 558–559, 574, 598, 602

Structural Limitations, 101, 103, 105, 110, 190–192, 387, 389, 490–491, 575, 625
  gastrointestinal, 102
  oral-facial, 100

Subcortical areas of brain, 159

Suck; see also Sucking; Suckling, 25, 30, 33, 34, 54, 70, 72–75, 80–81, 89, 92–93, 101, 125, 134, 141, 186, 196, 226, 254, 261, 296, 393, 452–454, 460–462, 468, 471, 483, 497, 500, 508, 517–520, 541–542, 545–546, 556, 576, 588, 590, 601, 606–607, 613, 631, 691
  pattern of, 24, 71–79, 82, 95, 127, 206, 383, 385, 388, 463, 498, 540, 547
  and suckle, similarities and differences, 78

Suck-swallow-breathe, 35, 44–45, 47–48, 51, 53, 56, 65, 67, 84–85, 89, 100–101, 104, 106, 110–111, 114, 142, 188, 210–211, 226, 250, 267, 328, 347, 366, 383–384, 388, 392–394, 438, 473–474, 539, 541–542, 547–548, 551, 590, 598, 626, 691, 693

Suck-swallow reflex, 75

Sucking; see also Suck; Suckling, 24, 33–34, 43–45, 47–48, 51–54, 60, 66, 71, 73, 76–82, 84–85, 89–95, 98, 101, 104–105, 123, 125, 127–128, 133–136, 142, 160, 195–196, 208, 213, 219, 226, 245, 249–250, 262, 269, 287, 294, 296–297, 355, 357, 367–370, 372, 374–376, 378, 380–384, 388, 398, 434–437, 452–453, 458–464, 466–469, 471, 474–475, 483, 486, 497–498, 500–501, 508, 517, 519–520, 529, 531, 543–546, 548, 563, 569–571, 575–576, 587–588, 595, 601, 606, 656, 658–660, 664, 683, 693
  before birth, 70, 75
  from bottle or breast, 54, 76–79
  with cleft palate, 78, 98, 101, 438, 649, 651–654, 657
  from cup, 79–80
  difficulty with, and bottle or breast-feeding, 98, 101, 116, 128, 206, 372, 383, 393, 462, 545
  facilitating food transitions, 74–75, 385,
  facilitating normal pattern of, 383–384, 469, 485, 491
  and flexion, 89
  and hypotonia, 373, 541
  negative pressure, 54, 652
  non-nutritive, 54, 69, 71–72, 118, 134, 383, 461, 540, 601, 673
  nutritive, 54, 71–72, 76, 78, 134, 383, 461, 673
  positive pressure, 54, 652
  in premature infants, 53, 72, 540–542, 545–548
  problems with, 128, 134, 383–384, 393, 541, 571, 613, 626
  rhythm in, 53, 79, 143, 384, 474, 599, 673
  soft solids from spoon, 81–82, 90
  swallowing and breathing, coordination of, 53, 56, 84, 100–101, 106, 110–111, 114, 167, 188, 206, 210, 267, 328, 366, 383, 388, 392–394, 438, 473–474, 539, 541–542, 551, 598, 626–627
  and suckling, similarities and differences, 78
  and tongue touch, 384, 462, 599
  and up-down tongue movement, 82, 367, 384

Sucking pads, 51–53, 89–90, 531, 542, 548

Suckle-swallow, 65, 77, 82–84, 90–91, 124, 208, 391, 449, 463, 469, 606, 610, 613
  rhythmical, 82, 606–607

Suckling; see also Suck; Sucking, 66, 70, 75, 78, 81, 90, 238, 283, 384, 462, 477, 519, 617
  in drinking, 385

patterns of, 64, 77–79, 90, 127, 136, 368, 383–385, 391, 437, 452–453, 460–462, 464, 477, 532, 607
  transition to sucking, 79, 355, 384–385, 437, 462, 477

Suggestion, and learning, 253, 255–256, 354

Sulcus, anterior and posterior, 47

Supplemental nursing system, 613
  Lact-Aid, 462, 503, 654

Surgery, and cleft palate, 656

Swallow reflex, 44, 46–47, 49–50, 106, 135, 387–388, 488, 605–606

Swallowing, 3–4, 24–25, 29–30, 33–34, 47, 52, 54, 56, 61, 64, 66–67, 73, 75–77, 80–82, 84, 86, 89–93, 95, 98, 101–102 104–105, 108, 110, 114–115, 117, 121, 124, 128–129, 134, 139–140, 142, 147–148, 151, 154, 160–162, 167, 186, 188, 190, 192–193, 196, 204, 206, 208, 226–229, 250, 258–259, 263, 267, 283, 287, 294, 296–297, 312, 328, 337, 340, 350, 357–358, 361, 364, 366, 373–376, 378, 380–383, 387, 389–394, 396–397, 434, 437, 440, 463, 466, 474–475, 480, 482, 488, 491, 499, 502–503, 508, 510, 521, 531–532, 534, 539–542, 544–546, 548, 556, 559, 563–564, 567–571, 587, 590, 596, 598, 601, 605, 608, 610, 613, 626–627, 630, 645, 649, 652–653, 655–656, 664, 683–684, 687, 690–691
  and aspiration, see Aspiration
  with cleft palate, 128
  coordination of, and food transitions, 551
  disorders of, 135, 140, 246, 595, 599
  and drooling, 84–85, 266, 390, 470, 472–473, 540, 683, 684
  facilitating mature pattern of, 391
  facilitating normal pattern of, in aspiration, 387, 388
  of food bolus, see Bolus
  and gagging, 48, 71, 83, 102, 202, 389, 400, 438, 485, 490–491, 558, 574–576, 589, 686
  and nasal reflux, 376
  oral pharyngeal structures in, 43–44
  oral phase/oral preparatory phase, 49, 53, 57, 134
  pharyngeal phase, 49–50, 58, 388
  problems with, 142, 146, 489
  process of, 49, 139, 142, 368
  of semisolids, 83–85
  swallow mechanism, 46, 74, 106, 139, 142, 155, 170, 589, 612
  and tracheostomy, 111, 470–471
  valving mechanism in, 49, 51

Syndactive theory of development, 544

T